ANESTHESIA and UNCOMMON DISEASES

Pathophysiologic and Clinical Correlations

Second Edition

JORDAN KATZ, M.D.

Professor and Vice Chairman,
Department of Anesthesia,
University of California, San Diego;
Chief, Anesthesia Service
Veterans Administration Hospital
La Jolla, California

JONATHAN BENUMOF, M.D.

Associate Professor of Anesthesia
University of California, San Diego
La Jolla, California

LESLIE B. KADIS, M.D.

Co-Director, Project Family,
Aptos, California
Family and Child Psychiatric Medical Clinic,
Campbell, California

W. B. SAUNDERS COMPANY

Philadelphia   London   Toronto   Mexico City   Rio de Janeiro   Sydney   Tokyo

W. B. Saunders Company: West Washington Square
Philadelphia, PA   19105

Library of Congress Cataloging in Publication Data

Katz, Jordan.

Anesthesia and uncommon diseases.

1. Anesthesia — Complications and sequelae.   I. Benumof,
   Jonathan, joint author.   II. Kadis, Leslie B., joint author.
   III. Title. [DNLM: 1. Anesthesia.   2. Pathology.
   WO235 A579]

RD82.5.K37 1981   617'.96   80–51961

ISBN 0–7216–5302–2

Listed here is the latest translated edition of this book together
with the language of the translation and the publisher.

Spanish (*1st Edition*)—Salvat Editores, S.A., Barcelona, Spain

Spanish (*2nd Edition*)—Salvat Editores, S.A., Barcelona, Spain

Anesthesia and Uncommon Diseases: ISBN   0-7216-5302-2
Pathophysiologic and Clinical Correlations

Last digit is the print number: 9   8

To my wife Ruby
and our sons, Ross, Scott, Marc, and Miles
"Nobis erat somnium quod non omnino erat somnium"

JORDAN KATZ

To Sherry, Benjamin, Sarah, Mom, and Dad

JONATHAN BENUMOF

To Ruth, whose continued support makes all things possible.

LESLIE KADIS

Contributors

J. ANTONIO ALDRETE, M.D., M.S.
Professor, Department of Anesthesiology, University of Alabama, Birmingham, Alabama.
Hematologic Diseases.

DAVID D. ALFERY, M.D.
Staff Anesthesiologist, St. Thomas Hospital, Nashville, Tennessee.
Pulmonary Diseases.

LAWRENCE V. BASSO, M.D.
Clinical Associate Professor of Medicine, Stanford University School of Medicine; Staff Endocrinologist, Stanford University Hospital; Endocrinologist, Palo Alto Medical Clinic, Palo Alto Clinic, Palo Alto, California.
Diseases of the Endocrine System.

JONATHAN L. BENUMOF, M.D.
Associate Professor of Anesthesiology, Department of Anesthesia, University of California, San Diego, School of Medicine, San Diego, California.
Anesthesia in the Geriatric Patient. Pulmonary Diseases.

RICHARD E. BERRYHILL, M.D.
Clinical Instructor in Anesthesia, University of California Medical Center, San Diego; Staff Anesthesiologist, Naval Regional Medical Center, San Diego, California.
Skin and Bone Disorders.

NORMAN H. BLASS, M.D.
Associate Professor of Anesthesiology, Obstetrics and Gynecology, Wright State University School of Medicine; Group Director in Obstetrical Anesthesia, Miami Valley Hospital, Dayton, Ohio.
Morbid Obesity and Other Nutritional Disorders.

JAMES L. BROOKS, JR., M.D.
Fellow in Cardiac Anesthesia, Emory University School of Medicine, Atlanta, Georgia; Staff Anesthesiologist, Orlando Regional Medical Center, Orlando, Florida.
Cardiac Diseases.

THOMAS B. CALDWELL III, M.D.
Clinical Assistant Professor of Anesthesiology, Vanderbilt University School

of Medicine; Attending Anesthesiologist, St. Thomas Hospital, Nashville, Tennessee.
Infectious Diseases. Anesthesia for Patients with Behavioral and Environmental Disorders.

CLIFF CHADWICK, M.D.
Assistant Professor in Anesthesia, University of Washington School of Medicine, Seattle, Washington.
Gastrointestinal Disorders.

RICHARD CHERLIN, M.D.
Clinical Instructor in Medicine, Stanford University School of Medicine; Attending Endocrinologist, Santa Clara Valley Medical Center, San Jose, California.
Genetic and Metabolic Diseases.

MICHAEL J. COUSINS, M.D., F.F.A.R.A.C.S., F.F.A.R.C.S.
Professor and Chairman, Department of Anaesthesia and Intensive Care, The Flinders University of South Australia, Bedford Park, South Australia.
Renal Diseases.

JOHN H. EISELE, JR., M.D.
Professor of Anesthesiology, Department of Anesthesiology, University of California, Davis, School of Medicine; Attending Staff, University of California, Davis, Medical Center.
Connective Tissue Diseases

FRANK GUERRA, M.D.
Assistant Clinical Professor of Anesthesiology and Psychiatry, University of Colorado School of Medicine; Staff Anesthesiologist and Psychiatrist, Presbyterian Hospital, Denver, and University Hospital, Denver Colorado.
Hematologic Diseases.

STEPHEN H. JACKSON, M.D.
Chairman, Department of Anesthesia, Good Samaritan Hospital of Santa Clara Valley, San Jose, California.
Genetic and Metabolic Diseases.

LESLIE KADIS, M.D.
Assistant Clinical Professor of Psychiatry, Langley Porter Neuropsychiatric Institute; Assistant Clinical Professor of Psychiatry and Behavioral Sciences, Stanford University School of Medicine; Co-Director, Project Family, Aptos, Family and Child Psychiatric Medical Clinic, Campbell, California.
Neurological Disorders.

JOEL A. KAPLAN, M.D.
Professor of Anesthesiology, Emory University School of Medicine; Director, Division of Cardiac Anesthesia, Emory University Hospital, Atlanta, Georgia.
Cardiac Diseases.

JORDAN KATZ, M.D.
Professor and Vice Chairman, Department of Anesthesia, University of California, San Diego, School of Medicine; Chief, Anesthesia Service, Veterans Administration Medical Center, San Diego, California.
Other Hereditary Disorders. Gastrointestinal Disorders.

CHINGMUH LEE, M.D.
Professor of Anesthesiology, University of California, Los Angeles, School of Medicine; Professor and Chairman, Department of Anesthesiology, Harbor-UCLA Medical Center, Torrance, California.
Muscle Diseases.

RICHARD I. MAZZE, M.D.
Professor of Anesthesiology, Stanford University School of Medicine; Chief, Anesthesiology Service, Veterans Administration Medical Center, Palo Alto, California.
Renal Diseases.

WALTER MILLAR, M.D.
Assistant Clinical Professor, Department of Anesthesia, University of California, San Diego, School of Medicine, San Diego, California.
Other Hereditary Disorders.

JORDAN MILLER, M.D.
Associate Professor of Anesthesiology, University of California, Los Angeles, School of Medicine; Attending Staff, University of California, Los Angeles, Hospital, Los Angeles, California.
Muscle Diseases.

JOHN WILLIAM PENDER, M.D.
Emeritus Professor of Anesthesiology, Stanford University School of Medicine; Senior Staff, Department of Anesthesiology, Palo Alto Medical Clinic, Palo Alto, California.
Diseases of the Endocrine System.

LAURENCE S. REISNER, M.D.
Associate Clinical Professor of Anesthesiology and Reproductive Medicine, University of California, San Diego, School of Medicine; Co-Director, Obstetric Anesthesia Service, University of California, San Diego, Medical Center.
The Pregnant Patient and the Disorders of Pregnancy.

RICHARD P. SAIK, M.D.
Associate Professor of Surgery, University of California, San Diego; Attending Surgeon, University of California, San Diego, Medical Center; Acting Chief of Surgery, Veterans Administration Hospital, San Diego, California.
Gastrointestinal Disorders.

DONALD SILCOX, M.D.
Clinical Associate Professor of Medicine, Department of Medicine, Section of Rheumatology, Stanford University Medical School; Medical Staff, Santa Clara Valley Medical Center, San Jose, California.
Genetic and Metabolic Diseases.

C. F. WARD, M.D.
Assistant Professor of Anesthesiology, University of California, San Diego, School of Medicine.
Diseases of Infants.

BARRY ZAMOST, M.D.
Clinical Instructor, Department of Anesthesia, University of California, San Diego, School of Medicine; Staff Anesthesiologist, Anesthesia Service Medical Group, San Diego, California.
Anesthesia in the Geriatric Patient.

BARRY L. ZIMMERMAN, M.D.
Assistant Clinical Professor of Anesthesiology, University of California, San Diego, School of Medicine; Staff Anesthesiologist, University of California, San Diego, Medical Center, San Diego, California.
Uncommon Problems in Acute Trauma.

Preface

The rather remarkable acceptance of the first edition by the anesthesiology community was the prime motivating force for the updating and expansion of this text. Both editors and contributors of the first edition realized the deficiencies in the published work. Many of these revolved around the paucity of meaningful information in the anesthesia literature concerning the topics written about. The authors presented as informed a treatise as possible with the data available. To this they added their own expertise and experience to mold a contribution which obviously met the needs of practitioners. Since the original publication there has been a marked expansion in our knowledge of much of the subject matter covered in the text. Although the reader will note that there is still some element of informed speculation concerning certain disease entities, the majority of the recommendations for management can now be based on more secure scientific evidence and clinical experience.

One additional factor prompted the need for a second edition. As anesthesia practice has become more sophisticated, subspecialization within the field has become more prominent. Many physicians (new and old) now restrict their practice to specific subspecialty areas. Thus some types of cases have become uncommon anesthesia experiences for them. These concerns have prompted the editors, in several cases, to expand upon existing chapters and also to consider the addition of new topics. This latter endeavor led to the production of three new chapters which the editors thought would be appropriate in a book of this type.

The second edition, for the most part, is a total rewrite of the subject areas covered. We believe that the information represents the best amalgamation of basic science and clinical information available to date. It also represents a critical evaluation by a selected group of highly qualified contributors. In addition, and somewhat in contrast to the first edition, many of our contributors have had an extensive personal experience with the diseases discussed.

By no means has the text met its ultimate objective—a definitive presentation of materials in the specific areas covered. It is doubtful if this text, or any text, will ever accomplish these goals since knowledge in all areas is very rapidly expanding. However, we are satisfied that we have come as close to this objective as possible.

The editors would like to acknowledge the help of the publishers, The W. B. Saunders Company, and in particular Ms. Mary Cowell. In addition a special thanks must be paid to the clerical staff of the Department of Anesthesiology at the University of California, San Diego. Ms. LeAnn Srite and Mrs. Donna Barnum must be singled out for their efforts.

JORDAN KATZ
JONATHAN BENUMOF
LESLIE KADIS

Contents

Chapter 1

GENETIC AND METABOLIC DISEASE.. 1

INBORN ERRORS OF METABOLISM... 1
Stephen H. Jackson, M.D.

OTHER HEREDITARY DISORDERS.................................... 68
Walter Millar, M.D., and Jordan Katz, M.D.

Chapter 2

**THE PREGNANT PATIENT AND THE DISORDERS
OF PREGNANCY** 81
Laurence S. Reisner, M.D.

Chapter 3

ANESTHESIA IN THE GERIATRIC PATIENT 98
Barry Zamost, M.D., and Jonathan L. Benumof, M.D.

Chapter 4

DISEASES OF INFANTS 119
C. F. Ward, M.D.

Chapter 5

DISEASES OF THE ENDOCRINE SYSTEM................................ 155
John William Pender, M.D., and Lawrence V. Basso, M.D.

Chapter 6

PULMONARY DISEASES 221
David D. Alfery, M.D., and Jonathan L. Benumof, M.D.

Chapter 7

CARDIAC DISEASES... 268
James L. Brooks, Jr., M.D., and Joel A. Kaplan, M.D.

Chapter 8

HEMATOLOGIC DISEASES 313
J. Antonio Aldrete, M.D., M.S., and Frank Guerra, M.D.

Chapter 9
GASTROINTESTINAL DISORDERS 384
Richard P. Saik, M.D., Cliff Chadwick, M.D., and
Jordan Katz, M.D.

Chapter 10
MORBID OBESITY AND OTHER NUTRITIONAL
DISORDERS 450
Norman H. Blass, M.D.

Chapter 11
RENAL DISEASES 463
R. I. Mazze, M.D., and M. J. Cousins, M.D.

Chapter 12
NEUROLOGICAL DISORDERS 485
Leslie B. Kadis, M.D.

Chapter 13
CONNECTIVE TISSUE DISEASES 508
John H. Eisele, Jr., M.D.

Chapter 14
MUSCLE DISEASES 530
Jordan Miller, M.D., and Chingmuh Lee, M.D.

Chapter 15
SKIN AND BONE DISORDERS 562
Richard E. Berryhill, M.D.

Chapter 16
INFECTIOUS DISEASES 588
Thomas B. Caldwell III, M.D.

Chapter 17
UNCOMMON PROBLEMS IN ACUTE TRAUMA 635
Barry L. Zimmerman, M.D.

Chapter 18
ANESTHESIA FOR PATIENTS WITH BEHAVIORAL AND
ENVIRONMENTAL DISORDERS 672
Thomas B. Caldwell III, M.D.

INDEX 779

1

Genetic and Metabolic Disease

Inborn Errors of Metabolism

By STEPHEN H. JACKSON, M.D.

Inborn Errors of Carbohydrate Metabolism
Hypoglycemia
Inborn Errors of Fructose Metabolism
Inborn Errors of Galactose Metabolism
Inborn Errors of Glycogen Metabolism
Hereditary Hepatic Porphyrias
Inborn Errors of Amino Acid Metabolism
Cystinuria
Phenylketonuria

Wilson's Disease
Gout
Inborn Errors of Lipid Metabolism
Familial Hyperlipoproteinemias
Familial Hypolipoproteinemias

INTRODUCTION

The human *gene* is composed of *deoxyribonucleic acid* (DNA), and about 50,000 separate gene pairs (*loci*) compose the twenty-three pairs of human chromosomes. The information inherent to each gene is determined by the sequence of purine and pyrimidine bases of the nucleotides that compose the DNA. DNA serves as a template for its own replication, but the structure of each gene is subject to variation (*mutation*). The altered genes at a given locus are called *alleles*. Certain genes dictate the sequential arrangement of the nucleotide bases of *ribonucleic acids (RNA)*, which, in turn, determine cellular function and tissue growth and differentiation. A *structural gene* indirectly specifies the amino acid sequence of a protein (polypeptide) by initially transferring its genetic information to a *messenger* RNA that, in turn, directs the ribosomal synthesis of the protein. The form and content of messenger RNA information is that of a triplet code:

three sequential nucleotides specify a single amino acid. The incorporation of each amino acid into the polypeptide is facilitated by a specific *transfer RNA* (carrier) molecule. Other genes can regulate the rate of protein synthesis, control the function of other genes, or even code the structure of the RNA that regulates general processes. Thus, when a gene mutation occurs, there is a change in either the quality or quantity of a specific protein. This change may be deleterious — either structurally or functionally — and ultimately impair the viability of the intact human. Mutation of a structural gene alters the structure of a specific protein and possibly the quantity of several other proteins. Mutation of a control or *regulatory gene*, on the other hand, changes the functional activity of one or more structural genes — and, therefore, the quantity of one or more proteins — without altering the structure of the protein molecules.

When only one of a pair of genes at a given locus has mutated (*heterozygous state*) and this mutant allele causes a clini-

1

cal disorder, then a dominant mode of inheritance is established. In the *homozygous state* each parent chromosomal locus must contribute an identical mutant allele in order for the disease to be expressed. Inborn errors of metabolism are, nevertheless, not entirely genetically determined. It usually is necessary for an abnormal genotype to have a specific environmental (biochemical) milieu in which the disease may become clinically manifest (phenotypic expression). Ten to twenty per cent of the loci of a normal human chromosome may be heterozygous in character, and as many as five of these loci may contain genetic information that, with homozygous representation, would result in a pathological state.

The sequelae of genetically determined changes in the quality or quantity of a protein relates to the function normally performed by that protein. In the ensuing chapters four basic pathobiochemical alterations will be encountered: 1) defect in membrane transport, wherein a specific protein essential for the transportation of a compound across a membrane is absent. In cystinuria there exists a defective transport mechanism for certain amino acids in the intestinal mucosa and renal tubules; 2) deficiency of specialized cell membrane, cytoplasmic, or nuclear receptor protein that normally would serve to bind biologically active molecules as a prerequisite to executing their normal function. In Type 2 hyperlipoproteinemia there is a deficiency of cell receptors for a specific type of lipoprotein, and this results in a decreased blood clearance and cellular metabolism of the lipoprotein and an interrelated loss of regulation of cholesterol biosynthesis; 3) impaired regulation of the rate of a biosynthetic pathway from which there results an overproduction of a biologically active compound. In intermittent acute porphyria a deficiency of a single enzyme involved with the synthesis of heme leads to a loss of repression of the activity of the enzyme controlling the rate-limiting step of the entire synthetic pathway. In gout caused by purine overproduction, a structurally and functionally aberrant enzyme augments the generation of the critical substrate for the rate-limiting reaction of purine synthesis; and 4) decreased or absent enzyme activity effects a metabolic block in which the product — or a substance derived from the product — of the blocked reaction is present in reduced quantity or is totally absent. In addition, there is an accumulation of the immediate precursor compound and/or the metabolite(s) of the precursor. Phenylketonuria, transferase deficiency galactosemia, and Type 1 glycogen storage disease are but three examples of this common type of inherited metabolic disorder.

The following section will cover several of the hundreds of known inborn errors of metabolism, and for each there will be depicted the 1) normal biochemistry, 2) specific genetically determined biochemical lesion(s), and 3) pathobiochemical and pathophysiological sequelae. The anesthetic management usually will be a logical consequence of this information. Because the objective scientific literature concerning such anesthetic management is, essentially, nonexistent, it is anticipated that the ensuing pages will stimulate and guide anesthesiologists to properly investigate and report their clinical experiences with such patients.

INBORN ERRORS OF CARBOHYDRATE METABOLISM

Carbohydrates play a major role in providing energy for cellular metabolism. The catabolism of mono- or polysaccharide carbohydrates produces smaller molecules and the release of energy. Glucose is the most important of the biological hexoses. Depending upon its energy requirements and its ability to utilize energy substrates other than glucose, each tissue and organ differs in its requirement for glucose. Glucose is initially metabolized via the Embden-Meyerhof glycolytic pathway to triose phosphates and/or pyruvate and thereby liberates about one third of the available free energy. In the presence of an adequate oxygen supply, the resultant pyruvate is converted to acetyl coenzyme A, which then enters the Krebs tricarboxylic acid cycle, whose enzymatic machinery catalyzes its combustion to carbon dioxide and water. This process provides the remaining two thirds of the available free energy in the form of compounds with high energy phosphate bonds such as *adenosine triphosphate* (ATP). The citric acid cycle not only serves a catabolic, energy-producing function but also provides molecular products to be used as substrates of other biosynthetic (anabolic) pathways. Thus, the smaller molecular products of fat and protein metabolism form a common interconvertible pool with those of carbohydrate metabolism, thereby biochemically linking these three interdependent pathways. Glucose may be derived directly from the alimentary canal or from glycogen via *glycogenolysis* (glucose polymer degradation), but it is also synthesized by the liver from smaller molecules via the anabolic process *gluconeogenesis*. Another important source of energy is the free fatty acids, which are broken down to acetyl coenzyme A via beta-oxidation and then enter the citric acid cycle. During the fasting state, most tissues can utilize free fatty acids and ketone bodies for energy. The central nervous system and erythrocytes predominantly depend upon glucose as an energy source. The hexose monophosphate shunt is another important alternate pathway of glucose metabolism, particularly in the newborn and in certain tissues, such as the adrenal cortex, erythrocytes, autonomic nervous system, and cerebral white matter.

Metabolism is regulated by an exquisitely sensitive set of interrelated checks and balances, these being partly extrinsic (environmental, physiological) and partly genetic in nature. This metabolic regulation is, essentially, synonymous with control of the enzymatic machinery involved therein. Two general methods are available for regulating the enzymatic apparatus. The first involves control of the rate and extent of enzyme biosynthesis, this being a slow and insensitive method. The second and more dynamically important process involves control of the functional activity of enzymes and, consequently, the biochemical reactions that they catalyze. The activity of certain enzymes is particularly crucial if such an enzyme facilitates the rate-limiting step of a series of reactions.

The sympathetic nervous system (via catecholamine secretion), as well as several other hormonal systems, influences carbohydrate homeostasis. Norepinephrine, present at postganglionic nerve terminals, and epinephrine, secreted by the adrenal medulla into the circulatory system for delivery to target organs, effect hyperglycemia and hyperlactatemia. Epinephrine is the more important of the two. The increased blood glucose is secondary to the beta$_2$ receptor stimulation of hepatic (and other organ) glycogenolysis. Although the catecholamines inhibit the uptake of glucose by skeletal muscle, they accelerate the glycolytic metabolism (also beta$_2$ effect) of the newly generated intracellular glucose to lactate, which is itself released into the circulation. The liver extracts this increased blood lactate supply and converts it to glucose via catecholamine-stimulated gluconeogenesis. In addition, the catecholamine-induced increase in oxidation of skeletal muscle free fatty acid (blood levels are also increased by the beta$_1$ lipolytic effect) interferes with pyruvate utilization and thereby contributes to the increased lactic acid production.

Other hormones exert important regulatory influences on carbohydrate metabolism. The pancreatic beta cell hormone insulin is released into the circulation in response to elevation of blood glucose levels. Insulin acts to lower blood glucose via two mechanisms: 1) it facilitates the membrane transport of glucose into skeletal muscle and adipose cells (insulin is not necessary for glucose uptake by most other organs) and 2) it enhances utilization of glucose. This latter effect is achieved by 1) storage of glucose as glycogen by virtue of an insulin-induced increase in the activity of glycogen synthase, and 2) oxidation of glucose via insulin's stimulation of pyruvate dehydrogenase, which accelerates the conversion of pyruvate to acetyl coenzyme A, which, in turn, enters the tricarboxylic acid cycle. Insulin also favors the biosynthesis of triglycerides, polypeptides, and nucleic acids from their respective building blocks (free fatty acids, amino acids, and mononucleotides) over their gluconeogenic conversion. "Anti-insulin" hormones oppose the hypoglycemic action of insulin by 1) stimulating enzymes favoring glycogenolysis (glucagon, catecholamines) and gluconeogenesis (glucagon, catecholamines, and glucocorticoids) and 2) diminishing the number (growth hormone) or the activity (glucocorticoids) of insulin receptors. In addition, the secretion of insulin is inhibited by the catecholamines. The pancreatic alpha cell hormone glucagon affects hepatic carbohydrate metabolism in a manner similar to that of epinephrine but has no effect on muscle phosphorylase and glycogenolysis. The pituitary adrenocorticotrophic hormone (ACTH) stimulates the adrenal cortex to synthesize and secrete glucocorticoid steroids, which cause hyperglycemia both by increasing hepatic gluconeogenesis and by decreasing peripheral glucose utilization.

Table 1–1 outlines the factors that influence blood glucose levels in the anesthetized patient; they are numerous, complex, interdependent, and particularly difficult to study in vivo. This is in sharp contrast to the controllable and relatively simplistic in vitro systems which have provided important information toward an understanding of the intact organism. The complexity of the human condition is underscored by the fact that even though most inhalational anesthetics effect hyperglycemia, the functional supply of glucose at the cellular level is not necessarily augmented because anesthetics may also impair the uptake and/or utilization of glucose.

Table 1–1 *Factors Influencing Blood Glucose Levels During Anesthesia*

Nutritional status
  Pre-existent
    Genetic
    Acquired
  Perianesthetic management

Direct effects of anesthesia (possibly dose-related, organ[s]–specific, disease-modified)
  Enzymes of glucose metabolism
    Glucose synthesis
      Glycogenolysis
      Gluconeogenesis
    Glucose degradation and utilization
      Glycolysis
      Tricarboxylic acid cycle (oxidative)
      Hexose monophosphate shunt
    Glucose storage
      Glycogenesis
  Hormones affecting glucose metabolism (insulin, cortisol, glucagon, epinephrine, growth hormone)
    Release (secretion) from synthesizing organ
    Functional activity at metabolic receptor site (cell membrane, intracellular)
  Transport of glucose across cell membrane
    Passive diffusion
    Facilitated (active)

Indirect effects of anesthetics
  Sympathoadrenal axis activity
    Basal
    Surgically evoked
  Alternate energy sources
    Generation
    Functional availability
  Renal clearance of glucose

The pre-existent nutritional status of the patient influences the degree of nutrient energy reserves. Superimposition of the fasting state and the psychological and physiological stresses (normal and/or pathological) of the preoperative period further alter the biochemical machinery and profile. The genetically determined and acquired disorders of carbohydrate metabolism that are discussed in this and other sections of this book further influence the body's ability to adequately adapt to metabolic derangements. Anesthesia then even further contributes to this deviation from normal metabolism (see Table 1–1). Each anesthetic drug is probably somewhat biochemically unique in each of these respects, and the degree of its effect may be determined by the depth and duration of anesthetic exposure.

Because plasma insulin levels simply reflect the dynamic balance between pancreatic secretion and peripheral consumption, determination of the effects of anesthetics on insulin levels has been of limited informational value. Only diethyl ether elevates plasma insulin, whereas cyclopropane, subarachnoid block, methoxyflurane, enflurane, halothane, and barbiturate-nitrous oxide effected no change. Because of the effect that blood glucose concentration has on pancreatic release of insulin, it has been suggested that the ratio of plasma insulin to blood glucose concentration (I/G) is a more informative parameter. Prior to the commencement of surgery, a decreased I/G has been found in patients anesthetized with cyclopropane, methoxyflurane, and halothane. However, this decrease largely reflects an increased blood glucose in the face of virtually unchanged plasma insulin. It is probable that this reduction of I/G is caused by a relative or absolute decrease of the release of insulin from the pancreas in response to hyperglycemia. Indeed, halothane and methoxyflurane inhibit glucose-stimulated insulin release in humans, at least part of this inhibition being a direct effect of the anesthetics. Although it is well established that catecholamines inhibit pancreatic insulin secretion, diethyl ether (a potent augmenter of sympathoadrenal activity) paradoxically increases I/G: both glucose and insulin are increased, but the latter to a greater degree, even though diethyl ether directly depresses insulin secretion.

The fact that hyperglycemia persists in the face of hyperinsulinemia suggests that insulin's hypoglycemic activity is impaired. Both enflurane and subarachnoid block effect no change of I/G, and superimposed surgical stimulation fails to alter the I/G associated with any anesthetic. Unfortunately, the I/G has limitations also: it fails to 1) elucidate the pathobiochemical change(s) of glucose metabolism and 2) consider the possibility of an anesthetic-induced modification of the metabolic activity of insulin in facilitating glucose transmembrane transport. Thus, the decreased I/G noted above for several anesthetics might also reflect a decreased functional potency of insulin, a possibility already raised for ether.

There is rather convincing evidence that anesthetics affect glucose transport across cell membranes: 1) anesthetics affect membrane structure and physical properties and therein have the potential for altering membrane-related function, 2) inhalational anesthetics depress facilitated (carbon dioxide-stimulated) glucose transport across erythrocyte membranes and noninsulin-mediated glucose uptake by skeletal muscle, 3) facilitated transport may even be involved in the diffusion of halothane across cell membranes, and halothane directly competes with glucose for the active carrier site, and 4) the hyperinsulinemic hyperglycemia evoked by ether will occur in the glycogen-depleted animal, thereby ruling out catecholamine-mediated glycogenolysis and supporting the concept of an impairment of insulin activity in the periphery. Perhaps of even greater importance is the fact that halothane decreases carrier-mediated glucose transport across the blood-brain barrier, possibly by competing with the glucose carrier and/or by altering the affinity of the carrier for glucose. Pentobarbital had no such deleterious influence. Interestingly, this same study demonstrated an increase of the simple diffusion of glucose, although the magnitude of this effect probably assumes only minimal clinical significance. It must, however, be noted that neither this depression of blood-brain glucose transport nor the 50 per cent reduction of brain glucose consumption can fully account for the two- to threefold increase in the ratio of brain to plasma glucose (which is independent of blood glucose concentration) encountered during anesthesia.

The final possible location of anesthetic action on glucose metabolism is within the cell. In this respect, skeletal muscle has been closely studied because it comprises a large body store of utilizable glucose responsive to both insulin and epinephrine; as such, it necessarily assumes a major role in the regulation of blood glucose concentration. Although both diethyl ether and halothane have no significant effect on insulin-mediated glucose uptake by skeletal muscle, they both 1) decrease the intracellular synthesis of glycogen from glucose in a dose-dependent manner and 2) increase the percentage of intracellular glucose that is glycolytically converted to lactate. Similarly, in the liver, halothane increases glycogenolysis and glycolysis while decreasing gluconeogenesis. The classic cellular and subcellular experiments by Fink and Cohen have clearly demonstrated anesthetic inhibition of mitochondrial oxidative respiration (the blocked site of electron transport is between NADH dehydrogenase and coenzyme Q) and a compensatory stimulation of glycolytic metabolism wherein ATP is anaerobically generated by the conversion of pyruvate to lactate. It is to be noted that the effects of anesthetics on muscle metabolism may be organ specific. In cardiac muscle, halothane and other inhalational anesthetics actually blocked glycolysis at the phosphoglucose isomerase-mediated step of the glycolytic pathway.

HYPOGLYCEMIA*

Hypoglycemia is a diminished blood concentration of glucose; it is also an indication of a regulatory inadequacy in the metabolism of glucose. Table 1–2 lists the etiologic possibilities of hypoglycemia and distinguishes two broad categories, fasting and reactive. The fasting group of disorders is often diagnostically more complicated, is associated with a severe degree of hypoglycemia, and may necessitate hormonal and/or surgical treatment.

Fasting hypoglycemia is the result either of diminished production or supply of glucose (such as decreased glycogenolysis or gluconeogenesis) or of increased cellular uptake and utilization.

---

*In collaboration with Richard Cherlin, M.D.

Table 1-2   *Causes of Hypoglycemia*

Fasting
  Decreased supply of glucose
    Glycogen storage disease (Types I, III, VI)
    Endocrine hormone deficiency
      Adrenal cortical insufficiency
      Glucagon deficiency (pancreas)
      ? Epinephrine deficiency
      Growth hormone deficiency
      Hypopituitarism
      Hypothalamic dysfunction
    Liver disease
      Hepatitis
      Congestion from congestive heart failure
      Neoplasm
      Toxicity (chemicals, drugs)
      Cirrhosis
    Starvation or malabsorptive state
    Drugs
      Alcohol
      Propranolol
      Salicylates
      Other
    Ketotic hypoglycemia of childhood
    Neonatal
      Prematurity
      Small for gestational age
      Enzyme deficiency
      Endocrine deficiency
    Ackee fruit ingestion (in Jamaica)
  Increased utilization
    Insulinoma
    Factitious
    Iatrogenic
    Non-islet cell tumors (mesenchymal, hepatoma, etc.)
    Neonatal
      Infant of diabetic mother
      Erythroblastosis fetalis
      Islet cell hyperplasia or neoplasia
      Critical illness (sepsis, respiratory)
    Lactation
    Hyperthermic, hypermetabolic states

Reactive
  Glucose-induced
    Functional
    Alimentary
    Early diabetes mellitus
    Post-hyperalimentation
  Non-glucose induced
    Transferase deficiency galactosemia
    Hereditary fructose intolerance
    Hereditary fructose-1,6-diphosphatase deficiency
    Leucine-induced

The glycogen storage diseases characterized by fasting hypoglycemia are discussed in detail in another section.

Glucocorticoids facilitate hepatic gluconeogenesis and have anti-insulin effects in peripheral tissues, possibly by virtue of changes in insulin receptors. Thus, a deficiency of glucocorticoids would decrease the amount of newly synthesized glucose and exaggerate the metabolic consequences of a given amount of insulin. Cortisol (hydrocortisone) may be deficient because of failure of the adrenal gland (Addison's disease), adrenogenital syndromes, diminished pituitary secretion of ACTH, or deficiency of the hypothalamic hormone corticotrophin releasing factor. Glucocorticoid replacement is therapeutic.

Glucagon deficiency is rare and may be involved in some forms of neonatal hypoglycemia. An absolute absence of epinephrine does not necessarily predispose to hypoglycemia, as those patients who have had bilateral adrenalectomies and who are on cortisol replacement do not develop hypoglycemia. Nevertheless, some studies have implicated a relative lack of epinephrine in some children with hypoglycemia. Hypopituitarism indirectly effects lowered blood glucose by its diminished output of both ACTH (and, therefore, cortisol) and growth hormone (GH) which provides gluconeogenic substrates and possesses an anti-insulin activity.

Severe hepatic dysfunction secondary to fulminant hepatitis, congestive heart failure, toxins (carbon tetrachloride, phosphorus, chloroform, urethane, or other drugs), cirrhosis, or metastatic cancer removes the primary glucose synthesizer, and glucopenia is the outcome.

Starvation, debilitating disease, and ethanol ingestion are all associated with hepatic glycogen depletion and thereby predispose to hypoglycemia. Ethanol also interferes with gluconeogenesis by altering the hepatic redox status. Other drugs causing hypoglycemia include the salicylates, haloperidol, chlorpromazine, monoamine oxidase inhibitors, and beta-adrenergic blockers (such as propranolol). The latter may also mask the signs and symptoms evoked by the sympathoadrenal homeostatic response to hypoglycemia.

Ketotic hypoglycemia of childhood is seen mostly in male infants 18 months of age or older but usually is outgrown by the fifth year of life. The underlying biochemical disorder may involve a deficiency of gluconeogenic precursors.

Neonatal hypoglycemia is defined as a blood glucose level below 40 mg./100 ml. Neonatal hypoglycemia on the basis of inadequate glucose production is a frequent finding in the premature (birth weight less than 2500 grams) infant and the "small" (below the tenth percentile) for gestational age neonate. In both situations there is a relative or absolute deficiency of the enzyme and/or hormonal systems involved with the generation of glucose in the face of hypoglycemia. The administration of glucagon usually is ineffective because of the absence of any hepatic glycogen stores and/or the absence of a full complement of mature glycogenolytic enzymes. In addition, the tendency of these neonates toward rapid heat loss and development of hypothermia imposes a further unfulfillable demand on the immature metabolic machinery that is called upon to generate energy substrates (such as glucose) that fuel heat production. The anesthetic management of the premature and otherwise small neonate therefore must necessarily include an awareness of the potential for the development of hypoglycemia. Prophylactic intravenous glucose administration, close and frequent monitoring of blood glucose concentrations, and vigorous treatment when necessary keynote the approach.

Increased utilization of glucose is generally the result of increased insulin or insulin-like hormone secretion. Pancreatic islet cell tumors (insulinomas) are a surgically remediable cause of hyperinsulinemia. Although microadenomatosis or hyperplasia has been reported, the majority are macroadenomas, 10 per cent being carcinomas. This disorder is encountered most frequently in the 30- to 60-year-old population, and may be insidious and unsuspected for years. These individuals may even be obese because of the frequent feedings necessary to avoid hypoglycemia. Their blood insulin levels are inappropriately increased at the time of hypoglycemia. Tolbutamide and glucagon tests have been employed to provoke excessive insulin release in cases where diagnosis is equivocal. Glucose tolerance tests produce extremely variable results and are not of diagnostic value.

Factitious hypoglycemia secondary to surreptitious injection of insulin mimics insulinoma because high immunoreactive insulin levels accompany hypoglycemia. Nurses, hospital technicians, and those individuals with a diabetic family member are especially predisposed to incurring this af-

fliction. Factitious hypoglycemia secondary to oral hypoglycemic agents such as sulfonylureas are diagnosed by urinary detection of the drug. Iatrogenic hypoglycemia in the diabetic patient may be the result of a diminished food intake or overmedication with insulin. This is not uncommon in the hospitalized diabetic patient and would be of potential concern in a fasting preoperative patient who receives insulin on the morning of surgery. Prophylactic instillation of intravenous glucose must be initiated prior to the insulin injection, and the intravenous cannula and flow rate must be inspected frequently to insure its proper functioning. It is obvious that the diabetic patient who is to have surgery is best scheduled as the first case of the day so as to minimize the problems imposed by prolonged fasting.

Extrapancreatic neoplasms, such as hepatomas and mesenchymal tumors (for example, retroperitoneal fibrosarcoma), have occasionally been associated with hypoglycemia. Because these neoplasms may achieve a large volume, they may consume very large amounts of glucose. In addition, many such tumors secrete a peptide that acts like insulin and may be one of the somatomedins.

Infants born of mothers with diabetes mellitus — juvenile or gestational — may develop blood glucose concentrations lower than 20 mg./100 ml. within the first two days of life, but they are most likely to do so within the initial two hours following birth. It is thought that chronic maternal hyperglycemia and transplacental transfer of glucose according to concentration gradients induce fetal hyperglycemia, islet cell hyperplasia, and hyperinsulinemia. Withdrawal of the maternal glucose supply at the time of birth presents the neonate with a hyperinsulinemia that outlasts the hyperglycemia as the demands for glucose utilization markedly increase with the onset of extrauterine life. Consequently, neonatal hypoglycemia often occurs within the first hours of life. The typically large neonate has accumulations of glycogen throughout its body, but it is only the hepatic stores that are of potential therapeutic benefit. The intravenous administration of 0.3 mg./kg. body weight of glucagon within the initial 15 minutes following birth catalyzes the mobilization of these hepatic glycogen stores and the glycogenolytic production of glucose. However, if the maternal picture was one of preeclampsia or eclampsia, the neonate may not have an adequate reservoir of glycogen in the liver. Regardless of the use or effectiveness of glucagon, the immediate establishment of an intravenous infusion of 10 per cent glucose at a rate of 80 ml./kg. body weight/24 hours will usually supply enough glucose to achieve euglycemia. The umbilical vein is always a readily accessible and easily achievable cannulation site. The goal is a blood glucose concentration of 80 to 120 mg./100 ml. Frequent, even hourly, monitoring of glucose levels is imperative so as to avoid not only hypoglycemia but also the hyperglycemia of overtreatment. The hyperosmolar state associated with hyperglycemia (and also rapid sodium bicarbonate therapy) has been implicated as a possible etiologic factor in the catastrophic event of neonatal intracerebral hemorrhage. Note that optimal control of the pregnant diabetic may reduce the incidence and severity of neonatal hypoglycemia. The rapid instillation of large volumes of dextrose-containing intravenous fluids to such an individual in the immediate prepartum period, as, for instance, prior to cesarean delivery under regional anesthesia, might induce an acute iatrogenic maternal hyperglycemia with the potential for subsequent neonatal hypoglycemia.

Increased glucose utilization effecting neonatal hypoglycemia also may be encountered in the infant with erythroblastosis fetalis (which is associated with islet cell hyperplasia) and in the "stressed" or critically ill neonate such as those with sepsis or respiratory distress.

Reactive hypoglycemia is a decreased blood glucose evoked by food ingestion. It is more common than fasting hypoglycemia, but it is an overdiagnosed and excessively abused medical entity. The criteria for establishing a diagnosis of functional hypoglycemia include the typical symptoms evoked by the autonomic responses to hypoglycemia approximately three hours after a glucose ingestion and a concomitant low blood glucose concentration. Conversely, no symptoms should be present when the blood glucose is normal. A low blood glucose during a glucose tolerance test without symptoms fails to prove a diagnosis of functional hypoglycemia. A diet high in protein

and low in carbohydrates usually maintains euglycemia.

Alimentary hypoglycemia is present in as many as 10 per cent of patients who have undergone gastric surgery. Their blood glucose rises to supranormal levels after glucose ingestion and rapidly declines below normal by the second hour. Rapid gastric emptying and stimulation of hormones (possibly gastric inhibitory peptide) which directly stimulate insulin secretion and postprandial hyperinsulinemia are proposed explanations of this form of reactive hypoglycemia.

Early diabetes mellitus may present with "late" hypoglycemia approximately five hours after glucose ingestion.

Patients receiving intravenous dextrose (glucose) — particularly the hypertonic dextrose employed for hyperalimentation — will have physiologically elevated insulin levels to prevent development of hyperglycemia. Abrupt withdrawal of the infusion may lead to hypoglycemia.

Although glucose is usually responsible for reactive hypoglycemia, galactose (transferase deficiency galactosemia) and fructose (hereditary fructose intolerance and hereditary fructose-1,6-diphosphatase deficiency) may cause hypoglycemia. Leucine is an amino acid and, by virtue of its ability to increase the release of insulin, may precipitate a hypoglycemic event. As such, ingestion of high protein meals is to be avoided and replaced by frequent feedings of carbohydrate-dominated foods.

The clinical manifestations of hypoglycemia are a result of both the direct effect on the central nervous system and of the compensatory response of the adrenal medulla. The rate of fall as well as the absolute level of blood glucose influence both the degree of central nervous system depression and the autonomic responses. The central nervous system is the organ most susceptible to hypoglycemia because of its basically absolute energy dependence on glucose; not only is glucose the "only" energy precursor allowed to pass through the blood-brain barrier but the brain's metabolic machinery can utilize "only" glucose as an energy substrate. Initially the patient may experience lightheadedness and hunger. Further dysfunction of the hypoglycemic brain is similar to that of cerebral anoxia and is manifested by aberrant behavior, confusion, irritability, and hyperactivity that may progress to convulsions and coma. When not depressed by impaired autonomic nervous system function or antiadrenergic drugs, the adrenal medulla responds to hypoglycemia by releasing epinephrine, the clinically detectable sequelae being hypertension, tachycardia, sweating, pallor, and anxiety. Nausea may also be a symptom. In the neonate weakness, hypotonia, cyanosis, and apneic episodes may dominate the clinical picture. Note: in the brain ketone bodies may partially substitute for glucose as an energy source.

The concentration of glucose in the blood is the result of a dynamic equilibrium between the glucose *input* from dietary sources and that released from the liver and kidney and the glucose *uptake* by organs and tissues, the most dominant of which are the brain, adipose tissue, erythrocytes, and skeletal muscle. There is no absolute blood glucose level that defines hypoglycemia in the non-neonate. Nevertheless, we arbitrarily define *a blood glucose concentration of less than 65 mg./100 ml.* as being a potentially significant hypoglycemia in the anesthetized state. In the anesthetized, insulin-treated diabetic a value of less than 100 mg./100 ml. is cause for concern.

Because the definitive therapy for hypoglycemia is simple, namely the immediate administration of a sufficient amount of glucose, the diagnosis of hypoglycemia becomes paramount. All anesthetics can mask the clinical manifestations of hypoglycemia, and therefore, its diagnosis must not rely upon clinical findings in the anesthetized state. In this regard, the history becomes of utmost importance in alerting the anesthesiologist to the potential for hypoglycemia. When such a possibility is suspected, then, regardless of the total anesthetic regimen to be employed, direct measurement of the blood glucose concentration is the only manner to establish the actual end result of said management.

Blood glucose concentration may be rapidly and accurately accomplished in the operating room with the use of the reagent strips that utilize the enzyme glucose oxidase, a single drop of blood, and a reflectance colorimeter. The glucose oxidase technology necessarily eliminates the variable and potentially significant fraction of the routine "blood sugar" concentration that is

attributable to the presence of non-glucose reducing substances. Care must be exercised to use only properly stored and fresh reagent test sticks so as to avoid altered reagent reactivity. The glucose oxidase catalyzes the oxidative conversion of glucose to glucuronic acid and hydrogen peroxide. Another enzyme on the strip, peroxidase, then facilitates the reaction of the hydrogen peroxide and a chromagen system, therein producing a characteristic color that can be read in a colorimeter. Because the color development is a continuing reaction, the test strip must be washed and blotted at exactly one minute. This colorimetric system employs a two-point calibration curve and a synthetic standard solution. This rapid technique compares favorably (slight negative bias) with the hexokinase procedure advocated as the national standard method for measuring glucose in biological fluids. Thus, the anesthetist may easily measure blood glucose levels as frequently as deemed necessary — every 30 minutes is an adequate practical approach — without the assistance of the clinical laboratory, which often meets with significant delays between sampling and reporting results. Nonetheless, an occasional blood sample should be sent to the laboratory to verify the accuracy of the colorimetric methodology. Note that all blood sampling should be performed at a site distant from the glucose infusion.

Frequent glucose determinations measure both the absolute level of glucose and the degree and rate of change. Appropriate glucose monitoring facilitates the early detection and treatment of any trend toward hypoglycemia and simultaneously precludes the overvigorous administration of glucose and ensuing hyperglycemia, thus assuming a particularly important position in the neonate.

The anesthetic management of the hypoglycemic patient depends in part on a good understanding of the pathobiochemistry (Table 1–1). Thus, in appropriate cases, proper dietary therapy should be enforced until the period of fasting must commence. Ideally, those individuals falling under the broad categorization of "fasting hypoglycemics" should be the first cases on the elective operating list in order to minimize the period of oral fast. The establishment of a continuous intravenous infusion of glucose is mandatory when the fast begins, and its uninterrupted function must be vigilantly guaranteed. In appropriate cases, nondietary drug and/or hormonal therapy should be continued, when feasible, uninterrupted through the intra- and post-anesthetic periods.

During anesthesia it is imperative that one maintain a steady infusion of intravenous glucose. In the adult a solution of 5 per cent glucose is adequate, whereas in the hypoglycemia-prone neonate, infant and small child, a solution of *at least* 10 per cent glucose should be administered continuously. If, despite glucose administration, blood tests indicate hypoglycemia, then the immediate injection of a 50 per cent glucose solution is indicated. Fructose solutions are not indicated because, as discussed above, glucose is the only sugar effective in combating hypoglycemia of the central nervous system. In all such patients it is imperative to have two routes for intravenous administration such that the glucose infusion may proceed independently of other intravenous therapy.

If anesthetic-induced preservation of sympathetic nervous system (catecholamine) mediated hyperglycemia (and other) metabolic homeostatic effects are sought, the agents of choice would be cyclopropane, fluroxene, nitrous oxide, and diethyl ether. However, halothane also has been demonstrated to be associated with the development of hyperglycemia in surgical patients without metabolic abnormalities. Sympathetic blockade induced by subarachnoid or epidural anesthesia would abolish any homeostatic adrenergic response to hypoglycemia. All other anesthetic drugs or techniques would induce some degree of sympathoadrenal inhibition, but this does not necessarily preclude the development of hyperglycemia. Catecholamine-induced gluconeogenesis is impaired in patients with severe hepatic dysfunction, when hepatic glycogen stores have been depleted by prolonged preanesthetic fasting, or in those patients in whom hepatic glycogen is unavailable. Although patients who have received adrenergic-blocking or -depleting drugs are more prone to hypoglycemia, beta adrenergic blockade with propranolol failed to eliminate the hyperglycemia associated with diethyl ether and cyclopropane anesthesias.

Cortisol is indicated in those patients receiving steroid therapy preoperatively. Prophylactic glucocorticoids may also prevent the development of profound unexplained hyperthermia during resection of an insulinoma. Additionally, it has been suggested that hypoglycemia might, on occasion, contribute to the mortality associated with the unsuccessful treatment of malignant hyperpyrexia.

Because of the potential masking of hypoglycemic symptoms, premedication with depressant drugs should be minimized or even avoided. Similarly, postoperative analgesia and sedation must be administered in guarded doses, preferably titrated with small intravenous increments. Antiemetic drugs should exclude the phenothiazines. The same prophylaxis, monitoring, and treatment provided pre- and intra-anesthetically must be continued throughout the postoperative period.

INBORN ERRORS OF FRUCTOSE METABOLISM

Fructose is a ketohexose (Fig. 1–1) that composes as much as one-third of our dietary carbohydrate supply. It is absorbed in the small intestine via a carrier-mediated diffusion process. Fructose is present in fruits and vegetables in the form of either a monosaccharide or (with glucose) a disaccharide, sucrose. Sorbitol is a naturally occurring hexitol and an isomer of mannitol that is used as 1) a urological irrigating solution for transurethral bladder and prostate surgery, 2) an osmotic diuretic, and 3) an "artificial" sweetener in diabetic foods. Sorbitol is biotransformed to fructose by the hepatic enzyme sorbital dehydrogenase. Inulin is a polymer of fructose and has been employed

CHO	CHO	CH_2OH
HCOH	HCOH	C=O
HOCH	HOCH	HOCH
HCOH	HOCH	HCOH
HCOH	HCOH	HCOH
CH_2OH	CH_2OH	CH_2OH
D-Glucose	D-Galactose	D-Fructose

Figure 1–1. D-Glucose, D-galactose, D-fructose.

in the measurement of glomerular filtration rates.

The following is a summary of the major metabolic disposition of fructose:

1. Fructose + ATP ← fructokinase → fructose-1-phosphate. This reaction occurs mainly in the liver, kidney and small intestine.

2. Fructose-1-phosphate ← fructose-1-phosphate aldolase → dihydroxyacetone phosphate + D-glyceraldehyde. Although this aldolase is most highly active in facilitating Reaction 2, it also catalyzes a) the reversible splitting of fructose-1,6-diphosphate to dihydroxyacetone phosphate and D-glyceraldehyde-3-phosphate, and, b) the condensation of these trioses to fructose-1,6-diphosphate (Reaction 4). This aldolase is composed of four subunits that dynamically dissociate and recombine into various hybrid forms that possess enzymatic activities of different degrees for each of these reactions it catalyzes.

3. D-Glyceraldehyde + ATP ← triose kinase → D-glyceraldehyde-3-phosphate.

4. Dihydroxyacetone phosphate + D-glyceraldehyde-3-phosphate ← fructose-1,6-diphosphate aldolase → fructose-1,6-diphosphate. Thus, fructose may be metabolized to trioses that are further glycolytically catabolized to pyruvate (and therein capable of passing through the tricarboxylic acid energy-producing cycle) or it may be converted by the liver and small intestine to glucose and/or glycogen. This latter conversion from fructose-1,6-diphosphate proceeds as follows:

5. Fructose-1,6-diphosphate ← fructose-1,6-diphosphatase → fructose-6-phosphate.

6. Fructose-6-phosphate ← phosphoglucoisomerase → glucose-6-phosphate.

7a. Glucose-6-phosphate ← glucose-6-phosphatase → glucose.

7b. Glucose-6-phosphate ← phosphoglucomutase → glucose-1-phosphate.

8. Glucose-1-phosphate + uridine triphosphate (UTP) + glycogen primer — UDP glucose phosphorylase and glycogen synthase → glycogen. In brain, erythrocytes, leukocytes, and adipose tissue, fructose is directly phosphorylated by the enzyme hexokinase to fructose-6-phosphate, but this reaction is inhibited by glucose, which has a much greater affinity for hexokinase. The direct conversion of fructose-1-phosphate to fructose-1,6-diphosphate is of only minor significance.

The plasma half-life of fructose (20 minutes) is about one half that of glucose. There is a rapid phosphorylation of fructose to fructose-1-phosphate (much of which ultimately is converted to glucose), which results in a rapid reduction of the serum inorganic phosphorus concentration. When compared with equivalent infusions of glucose, fructose effects a more rapid and significantly higher elevation of blood pyruvate and lactate levels. As such, fructose is more likely to lead to the development of a metabolic acidosis in the patient with diabetes mellitus. Because fructose does not cross the blood-brain barrier, it is not effective therapy for hypoglycemia. Insulin has no direct effect on fructose metabolism (the diabetic assimilates fructose in a normal fashion), but it does influence the ultimate disposition of fructose by increasing the amount that is converted to glucose by the liver.

Essential fructosuria is a benign, autosomal recessively transmitted disorder characterized by a deficiency of the enzyme fructokinase and a resultant blockade of Reaction 1. Frucotosuria appears after the affected individual receives fructose. There is an accompanying fructosemia, but blood pyruvate and lactate concentrations remain unchanged. Glucose and galactose metabolisms are unaltered. Because there are alternate routes of fructose metabolism, most of the fructose ultimately is metabolized. There are no clinical manifestations or sequelae of this disorder, and therefore, patients with essential fructosuria offer no specific management problems to the anesthetist.

Hereditary fructose intolerance is an autosomal recessively inherited disorder in which there is a marked deficiency of fructose-1-phosphate aldolase and a resultant blockade of Reaction 2, and, to a lesser extent, also Reaction 4. Ingestion or administration of fructose causes a marked fructosemia, but most importantly there is a very severe hypoglycemia that is resistant to glucagon therapy. The hepatic intracellular concentration of fructose-1-phosphate becomes markedly elevated and inhibits the hepatic generation and release of glucose by blocking a) gluconeogenesis from triose precursors at Reaction 4 and b) glycogenolysis at the level of the phosphorylase enzyme (see section on glycogen storage disease). This hypoglycemia is associated with normal serum insulin levels. Infants and children experience hypoglycemia more quickly and readily than do adults. These patients have normal biochemical responses to both glucose and galactose infusions, and either of these hexoses will prevent hypoglycemia when administered concomitantly with fructose. Infusion of the gluconeogenic precursor substrates dihydroxyacetone and glycerol fail to evoke euglycemia because of the blockade at Reaction 4. Along with the hypoglycemia is a prominent drop in the serum inorganic phosphorus concentration, this being attributable to the sequestration of phosphate by the liver in the form of fructose-1-phosphate and a hypermagnesemia.

Clincally this disease is not manifested until the affected individual ingests fructose-containing foods. As such, infants first develop signs and symptoms when they are weaned from breast milk and/or fructose is added to their diet. Following the chronic ingestion of fructose-containing foods, these infants begin to have protracted vomiting, severe growth-curve deterioration with failure to thrive (and gradual progression to cachectic death), hypoglycemia and all its sequelae (central nervous system dysfunction ranging from irritability to seizures and/or coma — see section on hypoglycemia), hepatosplenomegaly with clinical jaundice, and renal dysfunction characterized by alkaline urine, albuminuria, and aminoaciduria. The "wisdom of the body" is clearly demonstrated by their rapid development of a clear aversion to all sweets and fruits, for this disorder is totally averted by the cessation of fructose intake. Hence, the absence of the disease syndrome in older children and adults.

The hepatomegaly is accompanied by acute and chronic hepatocyte injury, and serum levels of hepatic enzymes and bilirubin are increased in proportion to the amount of ingested fructose. When unrecognized and/or untreated, the liver injury will progress to a state of cirrhosis and, ultimately, to death due to liver failure. Two possible mechanisms have been proposed to explain the hepatocellular damage: 1) toxicity of fructose-1-phosphate when present in high intracellular concentrations and 2) interference with generation of high-energy compounds within hepatocytes.

The intracellular accumulation of fructose-1-phosphate also has been incriminated as the cause of renal tubular dysfunction and the resultant inability to acidify the urine. The albuminuria and aminoaciduria reflect altered glomerular function as well. When hepatic function is so impaired that the blood amino acid nitrogen concentration is increased, an additional reason — exceeding the renal threshold — for the aminoaciduria is present.

The diagnosis is confirmed by a cautiously administered intravenous fructose tolerance test. Treatment is synonymous with prevention, that is, the total omission of fructose from the diet. Hepatic and renal dysfunction is entirely reversible if the diagnosis is confirmed and treatment initiated relatively early in the affected individual's life. Similarly, and unexplainedly, as long as the hypoglycemic events are not associated with hypoxemia or other cerebral damage during the convulsive episodes, central nervous system function and intelligence are preserved.

The patient whose diet has been properly managed should present no metabolic problem to the anesthetist, who must only insure that the appropriate diet is continued in the hospital. In the recently diagnosed or partially treated infant, one must be concerned with the tendency to hypoglycemia and dehydration with both electrolyte and acid-base derangements (the latter due to both prolonged vomiting and renal loss of base). These individuals should receive intravenous glucose and salt-containing solutions as a therapeutic endeavor to achieve normoglycemia and normovolemia accompanied by acceptable serum electrolyte concentrations prior to the commencement of anesthesia. A complete discussion of the anesthetic management of the hypoglycemia-prone patient is presented in another section. Fructose-containing intravenous solutions are obviously absolutely contraindicated. It also is mandatory to avoid the use of any urological irrigating solution that contains sorbitol, which may be absorbed into the blood stream, be metabolized to fructose, and trigger all the pathobiochemical events encountered in hereditary fructose intolerance.

For those patients with hepatic dysfunction, the anesthetic considerations would be similar to those for any patient with a similar degree of hepatic impairment. It would be practical to avoid or minimize the use of any anesthetic drug that possesses the potential for hepatocellular damage. Prolongation of neuromuscular blockade produced by succinyldicholine will occur only in those patients with liver damage advanced enough to produce hypopseudocholinesterasemia, and this can be determined by laboratory measurement preanesthetically. Depression of drug metabolism is not clinically significant until hepatic functional impairment is severe. Those patients who have moderate hepatic dysfunction do not display an increased sensitivity to the depressant effects of sedatives, tranquilizers, or analgesics (the non-volatile anesthetics). Similar considerations would apply to both the amide and ester groups of local anesthetics. Nevertheless, because the distinction between moderate and severe hepatic dysfunction is not always absolute and clear-cut, it would seem wise to employ these drugs only when clearly indicated and in doses smaller than usual. The activity of the non-depolarizing muscle relaxants and decamethonium should be clinically unaffected by hepatocellular injury unaccompanied by advanced renal dysfunction, although there have been reports of alleged resistance to d-tubocurarine in patients with cirrhosis. The phenothiazines may of themselves effect cholestatic jaundice.

The inability of affected individuals to acidify the urine (obligatory loss of fixed base) might counteract a tendency toward metabolic alkalosis such as may be present in the child with prolonged vomiting. If a severe metabolic alkalosis is encountered, it might be necessary to initiate intravenous therapy with arginine hydrochloride or ammonium hydrochloride solutions. The latter is contraindicated in those patients who have a predisposition to hyperammonemia as might be encountered in severe liver disease.

Hereditary fructose-1,6-diphosphatase deficiency is an autosomal recessively inherited trait in which the enzyme responsible for the conversion of fructose-1,6-diphosphate to fructose-6-phosphate (Reaction 5) is absent. As such, there is an accumulation of fructose-1,6-diphosphate and a blockade of gluconeogenesis from various precursors such as trioses, amino acids, lactate, and pyruvate. Therefore, when hepatic glycogen sources are deplet-

ed with the institution of the fasting state — neither glucagon nor epinephrine can effect hepatic release of glucose — there occurs within 14 hours a severe hypoglycemia that is responsive only to glucose therapy. There is a concomitant lacticacidemia which is caused by the metabolic conversion of gluconeogenic substrates to lactate because their synthetic pathways to glucose are inhibited. Infections and other catabolic states further increase the hepatic uptake of lactate precursors and their conversion to lactate, and therein accentuate the lactic acidosis.

The critical location of the metabolic blockade effects clinical manifestations very early in life. The signs and symptoms of hypoglycemia predominate (see pages 7–10). These infants may also present with hyperventilation which represents an attempt at a compensatory hypocarbia for their metabolic (lactic) acidosis. Unexplained hepatomegaly with fatty infiltration and hypotonic muscular function have also been described.

The assimilation of fructose precipitates the pathobiochemistry and the resultant clinical sequelae. However, these infants do not react to fructose with as much pathologic intensity as do those with hereditary fructose intolerance; nor do they develop an aversion to sweet foods. Their physical and mental growth pattern tends toward the normal range and they may even be somewhat obese.

The hypoglycemia of this disorder is treatable only with glucose. Because hepatic glycogen depletion necessarily precedes the onset of the fasting hypoglycemia that characterizes this disease, glucagon is not effective in restoring euglycemia. Neither glycerol or dihydroxyacetone can generate glucose production, and to the further detriment of the patient, they will augment the predisposition to lactic acidosis.

Treatment is prevention, and this involves 1) exclusion of fructose-containing foods from the diet, 2) a dietary regimen that eliminates periods of fasting exceeding four hours in infants and 10 hours in adults, and 3) when febrile, infectious, or any generally stressful state becomes manifest, the administration of glucose must be initiated and adequate supply guaranteed in order to prevent the development of both lacticacidemia and hypoglycemia.

The anesthetic management of these individuals is that of the patient with fasting hypoglycemia (see pages 6–10). Strict adherence to proper dietary measures must be insured pre- and post-anesthetically. Initiation of the typical fasting period preanesthetically must immediately be covered with intravenous glucose in adequate dosage in order to preserve hepatic glycogen and euglycemia. It is of great advantage to have these patients first on the operative list in the morning so as to minimize the fasting period. There is no specific choice of anesthetic, although if liver glycogen stores remain adequate, those drugs that elicit a catecholamine release into the circulation offer more of a protection against the development of hypoglycemia. Blood glucose levels must be closely monitored. Also, it is essential to monitor the acid-base status of such patients with frequent blood gas determinations; arterial cannulation facilitates such measurements. When metabolic acidosis (increasing base deficit) occurs, it must be treated vigorously, not only with sodium bicarbonate (sodium lactate and sodium acetate infusions are contraindicated) but also by increasing the intravenous supply of glucose. It is obvious that fructose solutions are contraindicated, as are also any lactated solutions. Sorbitol should never be utilized for urological irrigative fluids because it is metabolized to fructose. Hypothermia and hyperthermia both predispose to lactic-acidemia and, as such, appropriate monitoring of the patient's temperature is mandatory, as well as is the preparedness to treat any deviation from normothermia, this being of particular concern in the neonate and infant. Significant blood transfusion therapy increases the tendency to lactic acid accumulation. Naturally, any hypoxemic state would also amplify the development of a lactic acidosis.

INBORN ERRORS OF GALACTOSE METABOLISM

Milk is the single most important constituent of the diet of most neonates. The predominant carbohydrate of milk is the disaccharide lactose, which is hydrolyzed by intestinal cells to the monosaccharides glucose and galactose (Fig. 1–1). The most important biochemical pathway of galactose utilization involves its conversion to glucose, which is summarized:

1. Galactose + ATP + Mg^{++} ← galactokinase → galactose-1-phosphate + ADP. Galactokinase possesses the property of both high concentration of substrate and product inhibitions, this being of significance in view of the possible toxicity of galactose-1-phosphate (see below). The gene controlling galactokinase is located on chromosome 17, band q 21–22.

2. Galactose-1-phosphate + UDP glucose ← galactose-1-phosphate uridyl transferase → UDP galactose + glucose-1-phosphate. This transferase also has the property of high concentration of substrate (UDP glucose) and product (glucose-1-phosphate) inhibition. The gene controlling the transferase is located on chromosome 3.

3. UDP galactose ← uridine diphosphate galactose-4-epimerase → UDP glucose. By facilitating the reversible inversion of the hydroxyl group at carbon 4, the epimerase allows for the interconversion of glucose with galactose. This minor alteration of the hexose moiety has far-reaching biological significance because galactose is a key constituent of many complex molecules, such as brain cerebrosides, and in certain biological milieu glucose may be its only source. NAD is necessary for the epimerase's activity, and the ratio of NAD to NADH must be high. As such, drugs (such as ethanol) or physiological situations favoring NADH accumulation will block galactose metabolism and impair its plasma clearance. The normal regulation of galactose metabolism involves control of epimerase activity.

4. UDP glucose + pyrophosphate ← UDP glucose phosphorylase → UTP + glucose-1-phosphate. Note that this reaction, because it affects the metabolic levels of UDP glucose, necessarily is intimately related with the synthesis of glycogen (see page 17).

Two other alternative pathways of galactose metabolism have been described and, although under normal metabolic circumstances they assume quantitative insignificance, they might achieve pathobiochemical predominance when galactose accumulates to high tissue concentrations as in blockade of Reactions 1 and/or 2.

1a. Galactose + NADPH — aldose reductase→ galactitol. The product of this reaction is ultimately excreted in the urine in an unchanged form. Galactitol has been shown to be of particular cytotoxological importance in the state of galactose toxicity, especially in the formation of cataracts (see below). This reductive reaction is in contradistinction to the following oxidative reaction.

1b. Galactose + NAD— galactose dehydrogenase → galactonic acid. This product is ultimately catabolized and decarboxylated to xylulose.

Galactose is so rapidly and efficiently converted to glucose by the liver that the clearance of intravenously administered galactose has been employed to 1) measure hepatic blood flow and 2) quantitate hepatic dysfunction.

Two autosomal recessively transmitted disorders of galactose metabolism have been clearly delineated and will occupy the remainder of this chapter. Their incidence is estimated to range from 1:20,000 to 1:175,000.

Transferase deficiency galactosemia is a disorder that results from the complete absence or deficiency of galactose-1-phosphate uridyl transferase and resultant block of Reaction 2. The consequent accumulation of galactose and its derivatives, such as galactose-1-phosphate and galactitol, effects a toxicity syndrome manifested clinically by failure to thrive with vomiting and/or diarrhea within a few days following the initiation of milk intake. During the ensuing days, hepatomegaly with hepatocellular disease and cataract formation are added to the pathological picture. A severe hemolytic anemia may develop and accentuate the already present jaundice. Mental and motor retardation is noted within several months, and death is usually preceded by the development of ascites and liver failure. Although it is reasonably well established that galactitol is mechanistically involved with the lens changes, the other organ pathology remains unexplained. Nevertheless, it is clear that the formation and accumulation of galactose-1-phosphate is in some manner biochemically related to organotoxicity.

The laboratory correlates include hypergalactosemia, galactosuria, aminoaciduria with albuminuria (glomerular and renal tubular dysfunction), liver function tests reflecting hepatocellular injury, and a hy-perchloremic acidosis (both renal-tubular and gastrointestinal in origin). Hypoglycemia may develop and is thought to be secondary to hepatic dysfunction with diminished capacity to produce glucose. The response to glucagon of this nutritionally deprived and injured liver is, as expected, ineffective in restoring a euglycemic state. The diagnosis is established by the demonstration of a deficiency or absence of erythrocyte transferase activity. Note that premature or even normal neonates may have galactosuria for one to two weeks.

The management of the neonate with clinical disease consists of elimination of galactose from the diet, and in the initially severe case, intravenous glucose administration for several days. Specific dietary preparations are available for these infants: soybean milk and casein hydrolysates are empirically devoid of galactose. There is no improvement in the capacity of these individuals to metabolize galactose as they grow and develop, and, therefore, eternal dietary vigilance is mandatory. The deprivation of galactose does not impair normal growth and development, this being the result of Reaction 3's epimerization of glucose to galactose. It is both remarkable and fortunate that the galactose-free diet will effect a relatively rapid regression of the clinical sequelae of the transferase deficiency; mental retardation is the only manifestation of this disorder that is not entirely reversible. However, the severe depression of intelligence quotients that is encountered in phenylketonuric infants is usually not encountered in these transferase patients, even when proper dietary management is not initiated promptly. Nevertheless, even when intelligence appears normal, these patients may have learning impairments and psychological abnormalities. Proper dietary adherence can be monitored by assaying for the concentration of erythrocyte glucose-1-phosphate.

It is currently held that heterozygous women who are pregnant should be placed on galactose-free diets in order to minimize fetal exposure to galactose, which might otherwise cause permanent intrauterine brain damage. Certainly, amniocentesis may reveal an intrauterine diagnosis of transferase deficiency and these neonates would then be treated from birth with a prophylactic diet.

Current theory is that a structural gene mutation effects replacement of a critically situated (near the catalytic site) amino acid of the transferase molecule and results in an inactive enzyme. Indeed, the classic transferase patient has no detectable enzymatic activity. However, there are galactosemic individuals — usually of Negro origin — who have about 10 per cent residual transferase activity in their liver and intestinal mucosa (they have no erythrocyte activity) and who have a greater tolerance to galactose, particularly when they have reached several years of age. Interestingly, there is a Duarte gene that is allelic with the normal transferase gene and associated with an erythrocyte transferase activity that is half of normal. These individuals are clinically normal and probably represent a modified enzyme that is similar to transferase, but possessive of only half-normal activity.

Galactokinase deficiency galactosemia is a much milder form of galactosemia that is characterized by the essentially isolated clinical manifestation of premature cataract formation. There is a generalized absence of galactokinase that is most easily confirmed by erythrocyte enzymatic assay, and there is a resultant block of Reaction 1. A large percentage of administered galactose is reduced to galactitol, which is thought to be etiologically involved with the development of cataracts.

A totally benign autosomal recessively inherited absence of uridine diphosphate galactose-4-epimerase has also been described.

The patient with transferase deficiency galactosemia whose diet has been properly managed should offer the anesthetist no management problems, as the patient should be free of any active sequelae of this disorder. Laboratory determination of the concentration of erythrocyte galactose-1-phosphate concentration will ascertain the actual degree of adherence to the galactose-free diet. Those individuals who have been consuming even relatively minor amounts of galactose will have an abnormal erythrocyte value and usually a concomitant smoldering organotoxicity. When such individuals present for elective surgery, they should be postponed until proper dietary management quiets the disease activity. In any event, the anesthetist must insure that a galactose free diet is provided for these patients in the hospital.

In the recently diagnosed or partially treated transferase infant who is to have urgent or emergency surgery, the anesthetist is presented with a situation of multiple organ toxicity and many potentially lethal physiological alterations. If the blood hemoglobin is significantly lower than predicted for the patient's age, a hemolytic anemia should be suspected, confirmed, and treated with erythrocyte infusions. The hemoglobin may even be spuriously normal (or high) when the patient is dehydrated. Dehydration with both electrolyte and acid-base derangements secondary to both gastrointestinal and renal losses must be vigorously treated with adequate volumes of appropriate intravenous sodium- and potassium-containing solutions. Sodium bicarbonate is to be employed as indicated, but acetate and lactate buffers may be ineffective in the severely hepatotoxic individual. It is to be noted that the inability to acidify the urine (obligatory renal tubular loss of fixed base) might counteract the propensity to developing a metabolic alkalosis, such as is seen with prolonged vomiting. Should a severe metabolic alkalosis be present, the intravenous administration of arginine hydrochloride is indicated. Ammonium hydrochloride therapy is contraindicated in those patients who have a predisposition to hyperammonemia such as may be encountered in severe liver disease. Blood glucose determinations should be made relatively frequently because those patients with advanced hepatic dysfunction are likely to develop hypoglycemia. In any event, dextrose should be routinely and liberally included in all the intravenous solutions.

In infants with hepatocellular injury, the anesthetic considerations are those of any patient with a similar amount of hepatic functional impairment. It would be prudent to avoid or minimize the use of any anesthetic drug that possesses the potential to induce hepatocellular injury. Prolongation of neuromuscular blockade produced by succinyldicholine will occur in those individuals whose liver damage is severe enough to cause a hypopseudocholinesterasemia, which can be measured preanesthetically. Drug metabolism is otherwise rarely impaired before hepatic dysfunction is far advanced. Patients with moderate degrees of hepatic functional depression do not display an increased sensitivity to sedative, tranquilizer, or analgesic drugs. Considerations similar to those heretofore mentioned apply to both the amide and ester groups of local anesthetics. However, because the categorization of moderate or severe hepatic dysfunction is not always easily established, it is advisable to employ these drugs only when clearly indicated and in doses that are both incremental and smaller than usual. In the absence of renal failure, the activity of non-depolarizing muscle relaxants and decamethonium should be clinically unaffected by hepatocellular damage.

The debilitated and severely affected transferase deficiency infant who presents with an emergency surgical situation is best managed anesthetically with an awake endotracheal intubation followed by a mixture of nitrous oxide–oxygen sufficient to produce adequate oxygenation. Minimal incremental doses of non-depolarizing muscle relaxants may be added in the unlikely event that muscle relaxation is needed. Prior to initiation of the anesthetic, these fragile infants must be prepared as well as is practical and feasible according to the considerations listed above.

The patient with galactokinase deficiency galactosemia provides the anesthetist essentially no management problems other than the ensuring of proper dietary care.

Inborn Errors of Glycogen Metabolism

Glycogen is a glucose polymer. It is the storage form of glucose, the glucose reservoir that is utilized when demands for glucose exceed that which is readily available in the blood. Glycogen is thus appropriately entitled the "energy buffer."

The synthesis of glycogen is summarized here:

1. Glucose + ATP ← glucokinase → glucose-6-phosphate. In the nutritionally sound liver a very specific glucokinase catalyzes most of the phosphorylation of glucose. The remainder is facilitated by the less specific hexokinases, which are the only kinases found in muscle.

2. Glucose-6-phosphate ← phosphoglucomutase → glucose-1-phosphate. This is the only step in the synthesis and catabolism of glycogen that is a reversible reaction, and glucose-1,6-diphosphate is an intermediary compound.

3. Glucose-1-phosphate + uridine triphosphate (UTP) ← uridine diphosphate-glucose phosphorylase → uridine diphosphoglucose (UDPG).

4. UDPG + glycogen primer (an oligo- or polysaccharide) ← glycogen synthase (UDPG:glycogen α-1,4-glucosyltransferase) → glycogen primer-α-1,4-glucose + UDP. Glycogen synthase may exist in two forms: active and inactive. Insulin converts this enzyme, which in the well-fed state is mainly in the inactive form, to the active form, whereas glycogen promotes the inactive state. Both glucose and vagal stimulation increase the activity of glycogen synthase. The conversion from active to inactive forms is enzymatically mediated by a phosphorylating kinase that is activated by cyclic AMP (which, therefore, inhibits glycogen biosynthesis).

5. α-1,4-glycogen ← branching enzyme (α-1,4-glucan:α-1,4-glucan-6-glycosyltransferase) → α-1,4-α-1,6-glycogen. In the normal human glycogen molecule less than 10 per cent of the glucose residues are in the 1,6-linkage.

The breakdown of glycogen to glucose is summarized as follows:

6. α-1,4-α-1,6-glycogen ← α-1,4-glucan phosphorylase → glucose-1-phosphate + α-1,4-α-1,6-glycogen. The α-1,4-glucan phosphorylase is present in both muscle and liver and may exist in either an active or inactive form. In the liver glucagon activates this enzyme, whereas in muscle epinephrine is the primary activator. The sequence of biochemical events involved with this activation process is:

6a. Adenosine triphosphate (ATP) ← adenyl cyclase that is activated by epinephrine or glucagon → adenosine-3′,5′-phosphate (cyclic AMP).

6b. Inactive phosphorylase kinase ← cyclic AMP → active phosphorylase kinase.

6c. Active phosphorylase kinase + ATP + Mg^{++} + inactive α-1,4-glucan phosphorylase → active α-1,4-glucan phosphorylase.

This glycogen phosphorylase catalyzes glycogenolysis by cleaving glucosyl residues from the nonreducing end of the α-1,4-glucosyl chain of glycogen. This process proceeds in a stepwise fashion until there is a α-1,4-trisaccharide residue attached to a α-1,6-glucosyl linkage.

7. α-1,4-α-1,6-glycogen (limit dextrin) +α-1,4-α-1,6-glycogen ← oligo-(1,4→1,4)-glucan transferase → α-1,6-glycogen +α-1,4-α-1,6-glycogen. Thus the trisac-

charide residue is enzymatically removed from the limit dextrin and transferred to another glycogen molecule and attached by a 1,4-linkage. This now leaves the next glucose to be cleaved in an exposed 1,6-linkage, thereby amenable to the cleaving activity of the debrancher enzyme as delineated in Reaction 8.

8. α-1,6-glycogen $\leftarrow$ amylo-1,6-α-1,4-glucosidase $\rightarrow$ glucose + α-1,4-glycogen. This free glucose (about 10 per cent of the glucose derived from glycogen) is converted to glucose-6-phosphate (Reaction 1), and the glucose-1-phosphate derived from Reaction 6 is converted to glucose-6-phosphate via Reaction 2.

9. Glucose-6-phosphate + H_2O $\leftarrow$ glucose-6-phosphatase $\rightarrow$ glucose + phosphate. Glucose-6-phosphatase is a hepatic, intestinal and renal microsomal enzyme that also is a nonspecific hydrolase, pyrophosphatase, and weak kinase. Its activity is increased by fasting, fructose loading, hydrocortisone (cortisol) administration, and ethanol ingestion, whereas insulin depresses its activity. This enzyme allows for the ultimate conversion of glycogen to free glucose, the only form of glucose that may be released into the circulation.

Type I glycogen storage disease (von Gierke's disease) is autosomal recessively inherited and characterized by a deficiency of glucose-6-phosphatase and a resultant block of Reaction 9 in the liver, kidney, intestinal mucosa, and platelets. This effects a hepatorenal accumulation of glycogen and a severe fasting hypoglycemia that is essentially unresponsive to glucagon or epinephrine. In some patients these hormones cause a slight increase in the blood glucose concentration which is secondary to free glucose released from the breakdown of glycogen at the 1,6-linkages.

Biochemically there also is found 1) hyperlactatemia caused by the high level of activity converting pyruvate — via the abundantly present reduced nucleotide cofactors, NADPH and NADH — to lactate; 2) elevated free fatty acids caused by the a) hypoglycemia-stimulated release of free fatty acids from adipose tissue and b) increased synthesis of fatty acids facilitated by the increased availability of reduced nucleotide cofactors (from the high level of activity of both the phosphogluconic acid and tricarboxylic acid oxidative pathways)

and acetyl coenzyme A (from pyruvate); 3) hypercholesterolemia probably also related to the increased availability of NADPH and acetyl coenzyme A; and 4) hypertriglyceridemia possibly due to reduced clearance and low post-heparin serum lipoprotein lipase activity. The glucose tolerance test is diabetic in pattern, probably in part due to an unexplained decreased insulin secretory response to the glucose load. Galactose and fructose infusions cause no elevations of blood glucose (Reaction 9 is necessary for the conversion), but will increase lactic acid levels. Hyperuricemia is uniformly present and is thought to be caused by a) decreased uric acid excretion caused by lactate's competitive inhibition of renal tubular urate secretion and b) increased uric acid synthesis possibly related to increased ribose — and ultimately phosphoribosylpyrophosphate — synthesis (see section on gout). Intravenous glucose unexplainedly increases uric acid clearance without altering serum lactate levels.

These individuals have an impaired growth rate, a very large and protuberant abdomen secondary to the massive hepatomegaly (and to a lesser extent to renomegaly), osteoporosis, poor muscular development (but otherwise normal neuromuscular function), and tendency to obesity. The liver and kidney are laden with glycogen, but the liver function tests are normal; however, there is a significant disposition toward the development of hepatic adenomas with malignant potential. A coagulopathy most probably related to platelet dysfunction is usually present. The hyperuricemia is present from birth; the gouty syndrome usually becomes manifest in the second decade and may lead to all the significant morbidity — and even mortality — associated with gouty nephropathy (see section on gout). The Fanconi syndrome may also be encountered.

Hypoglycemia is most severe in the fasting state and may lead to the development of seizures. However, some affected individuals unexplainedly fail to have epileptic activity even at extraordinarily low blood glucose concentrations. Mental retardation is not encountered as long as convulsions have not led to hypoxemic brain injury, especially during the first years of life.

The diagnosis is confirmed by an open liver biopsy, which is preferable to closed techniques, in order to a) provide ample tissue for biochemical and histological studies and b) allow for direct control of any hepatic bleeding.

Treatment of this enzymatic deficiency is the oral or parenteral administration of glucose. Frequent feedings of normal protein–high glucose diets are very effective in preventing hypoglycemia. During the usual sleeping-fasting period of the night, the patient must have glucose, and nocturnal intragastric feeding techniques may have to be employed during this time. Diazoxide has been utilized with some success, probably related to its repression of both insulin release and hepatic glucose uptake as well as increasing 1,6-linkage glycogenolysis. Portacaval shunts have been successfully employed to increase the distribution of glucose-rich blood to non-hepatic tissues. In addition, liver glycogen is dramatically reduced, physical growth accelerated, and coagulopathy eliminated, but fasting hypoglycemia is unaltered. Such operative procedures must be preceded by a preoperative hyperalimentation period, which effects a partial reversal of hepatomegaly, biochemical abnormalities, and coagulopathy.

The anesthetic management primarily involves concern with prevention of hypoglycemia, and this is discussed in the section on hypoglycemia. Because catecholamines are essentially ineffective in inducing hyperglycemia, diethyl ether, cyclopropane, fluroxene, or nitrous oxide offer little or no advantage over other anesthetics in this respect. An intravenous infusion of glucose must be initiated and maintained at the time that the preanesthetic fast commences. In addition to monitoring blood glucose, one must also follow the acid-base status (via arterial pH and carbon dioxide tension); these patients have a chronic metabolic (lactic) acidosis which must not be allowed to worsen. If such deterioration is concomitant with hypoglycemia, then this is a clear signal that glucose is being administered in insufficient amounts; however, if euglycemia prevails, then other etiologies must be considered (hypoxia, hypotension, etc.). If the acidosis is severe enough, then sodium bicarbonate or other organic buffer may have to be employed; sodium lactate is absolutely contraindicated. Naturally, lactated intravenous solutions must not be used. The hemostatic defect is a strong relative contraindication to regional anesthesia, and excessive hemorrhage may contribute to interference with airway mechanics, especially following intraoral, laryngeal, or neck surgery. If bleeding becomes problematic, appropriate laboratory studies must rule out etiologies other than that of the platelet dysfunction found with this disorder. Should the latter, indeed, be the cause, then treatment with heterologous platelets (devoid of glucose-6-phosphatase deficiency) is the appropriate choice. Additional clinical considerations for the management of the patient afflicted with gout are fully discussed in the section on gout, and include the use of appropriate medications and the establishment and maintenance of an adequate flow of urine.

These patients must also be carefully monitored from a metabolic point of view in the postoperative period until the therapeutic dietary regimens may be reinstituted. Because of their generally poor muscular development, there must be special care and awareness of respiratory muscle function, for these individuals are more likely to develop a postoperative pneumonitis, atelectasis, and other pulmonary complications. Complete reversal of any muscle relaxants must be insured.

Type 2 glycogen storage disease (Pompe's disease, generalized glycogenosis) is an autosomal recessively transmitted disease in which there is a deficiency of α-1,4-glucosidase. This is a normal lysosomal enzyme located throughout the body that hydrolyzes linear oligosaccharides and the 1,4-linkages at the periphery of the glycogen molecule. Note that α-1,4-glucosidase was not involved with Reactions 1 through 9, all of whose enzymes are normal in this disorder.

This enzyme deficiency results in the cytoplasmic, intralysosomal accumulation of glycogen which cannot be degraded either from within (no enzyme), or from without by the extralysosomal, cytoplasmic glycogenolytic enzymatic complement. However, because the body's remaining carbohydrate machinery is intact, euglycemia and eulipidemia prevail, and the responses to epinephrine and glucagon are normal.

The most critically affected organs are the heart, the skeletal muscle, and central nervous system. The respective clinical sequelae are cardiomegaly with progressive and refractory myocardial failure, generalized hypotonia, and various neurologic deficits, including mental retardation. Macroglossia may be prominent. The clinical picture is unexplainedly broadly variable and ranges from death due to acyanotic cardiac failure and/or neuromuscular respiratory failure during the first months of life (infantile) to a more slowly progressive form terminating with death prior to the third decade of life (childhood) to a normal life expectancy marred only by a generalized muscular weakness.

The diagnosis involves demonstration of increased tissue concentrations of normally structured glycogen and the absence of the 1,4-glucosidase. There is no currently successful treatment. As such, prevention in the form of early gestational diagnosis via amniocentesis for fetal fibroblast enzymatic content is an option for affected families.

The anesthetic management of affected infants may be complicated by the macroglossia; therefore, an awake intubation of these hypotonic infants following glycopyrrolate (free of central nervous system effects) premedication is indicated. Induction and maintenance would probably best be accomplished with a pure inhalational (rapidly retrievable) technique, but it must be borne in mind that myocardial decompensation is imminent in such patients. Muscle relaxants are unnecessary in these hypotonic patients, who would also be prone to postoperative respiratory complications because of pathological involvement of their respiratory muscles.

Type 3 glycogen storage disease (Cori's Disease, limit dextrinosis) is an autosomal recessively transmitted disorder distinguished by a deficiency of amylo-1,6-glucosidase, the glycogen debranching enzyme (Reaction 8 is blocked) and the consequent accumulation of polysaccharide with a structure similar to that of limit dextrin. Three of every four Israelis who have a glycogen storage disease have Type 3. The abnormally structured glycogen accumulates to a significant degree in the liver, skeletal muscle, and heart, and may be found in the spleen, but the kidneys are spared. Many of the clinical manifestations are noted in early childhood, particularly hepatomegaly and hypoglycemia. The he-

patic involvement usually is associated with a chronic, low-grade hepatitis (mild enzyme elevation), but often the liver unexplainedly returns to normal size with cessation of inflammatory activity at the onset of puberty. A mild degree of hypoglycemia is the rule; however, prolonged fasting will precipitate a severe hypoglycemia and, eventually, coma and convulsions. Epinephrine and glucagon cause variable increases of blood glucose and are most effective after a feeding or an intravenous infusion of glucose, presumably because of the availability for cleavage of recently added 1,4-glucosyl units on the glycogen molecule. Because of the normal capability of gluconeogenesis, protein and amino acid administration result in an increased blood glucose. Because their metabolism is unaffected, both galactose and fructose are effective euglycemic agents.

Skeletal muscle involvement may lead to a progressive myopathy with weakness in adults. Cardiomegaly may be seen, but cardiac function remains normal. Growth retardation may be significant, especially if the major treatment, which is frequent feedings of a high protein diet, is not adhered to in a compulsory fashion. Portacaval shunting has been reported to be a successful mode of therapy in a few cases.

Hypoglycemia — particularly in the fasting state — may be severe and must be prevented (this is discussed in the section on hypoglycemia). Therefore, intravenous glucose must be instituted at the time preanesthetic fasting is initiated. Because catecholamines are potentially effective in promoting euglycemia, it may be advantageous to choose an anesthetic technique utilizing nitrous oxide, fluroxene, cyclopropane, or diethyl ether. However, this effect on blood glucose is variable and unreliable, and therefore, vigilant antihypoglycemic prophylaxis is clearly the mainstay of glucose regulation regardless of the choice of anesthesia. Note that preanesthetic glucose administration during the routine "fasting" period will enhance any potentially beneficial effects of epinephrine or glucagon mediated glucose mobilization.

Because of the chronic but benign hepatocellular inflammatory process often seen in these patients, the choice of anesthesia would best be one with a low potential for being invoked as a cause for further or accelerated hepatocellular injury. When splenomegaly is present, intrasurgical inadvertent splenic damage and hemorrhage must be considered in the differential diagnosis of unexplained hypotension. When skeletal muscle disease is present, the requirement for muscle relaxants is minimal or nonexistent. These hypotonic individuals also are candidates for postoperative respiratory complications, and, as such, must be carefully guided through appropriate respiratory care procedures. Fortunately, these patients are not at risk for the development of myotonia or dystonia.

Type 4 glycogen storage disease (Andersen's disease, amylopectinosis) is a very rare, probably autosomal recessively inherited disorder in which there is a deficiency of α-1,4-glucan:α-1,4-glucan-6-glucosyl transferase, the branching enzyme of Reaction 5. The synthesized glycogen has no branching in terms of 1,6-glucose-linked chains, and, therefore, it has an abnormal structure distinguished by long, unbranched 1,4-glucosyl chains similar to that of amylopectin. This glycogen does not accumulate to any abnormal degree, so in the strictest sense this is not truly a glycogen storage disease. However, the abnormal glycogen is very insoluble, and it has been postulated that the body reacts to this glycogen in a "foreign-body" manner, one that unfortunately results in infantile morbidity and mortality.

The clinical picture is dominated by hepatomegaly that develops within the earliest months of life. An unrelenting hepatocellular inflammatory process (transaminase is always elevated) inevitably leads to hepatic cirrhosis with liver failure and death before the age of three. Blood glucose and glucose tolerance testing are normal. That epinephrine and glucagon are variably effective in achieving an elevation of the blood glucose levels is possibly related to the severe degree of hepatic dysfunction rather than to a defect in glycogen catabolism. Splenomegaly, muscular hypotonia, and severe growth retardation are concomitant findings. The medical management of such unfortunate children centers about managing their liver disease, as there has been no successful therapeutic regimen that will overcome the basic biochemical disturbance.

The anesthetic management is that of a "failure-to-thrive" child with hypotonia, a space-occupying abdominal lesion, and impending hepatic insufficiency. There will be minimal resistance to an awake intubation, which may then be followed by controlled ventilation with a mixture of nitrous oxide and oxygen sufficient to provide adequate arterial oxygenation. Muscle relaxants are unnecessary. The hepatic dysfunction is best managed (if possible) by the avoidance of any drug that might be incriminated as a potential threat to hepatocellular integrity. Otherwise, anesthetic considerations would be those of any patient with a similar degree of hepatic dysfunction. Depression of drug metabolism is not clinically significant until hepatic functional impairment is of a severe degree, at which point any non-inhalational (fixed) anesthetic drugs should be used only with extreme caution regarding dosage. Because these children are also very prone to loss of heat, special attention must be paid to the maintenance of body temperature.

Type 5 glycogen storage disease (McArdle's disease) is an autosomal recessively transmitted disorder in which there is an absence of skeletal muscle α-1,4-glucan phosphorylase in the presence of normal hepatic α-1,4-glucan phosphorylase and muscle phosphorylase kinase; therefore, there is a block of Reaction 6 only in muscle. This disease underlines the presence in the human of separate genetic control of distinct organ-specific phosphorylases. There is a resultant accumulation of normally structured glycogen in skeletal muscle, and a significant restriction of the intracellular mobilization and availability of glucose as a source of ATP. Glycogenolysis as a source of ATP for muscle is required only during prolonged heavy exercise; until that point is reached, non-glycogenolytic glucose, fructose, and even fatty acids are employed as primary sources of ATP generation. This ultimate limitation of potential energy substrate supply effects a similar limitation of the potential for total muscle contractile activity over a given amount of time and hence a clinically manifested diminished skeletal muscle functional capacity. Consequently, phosphorylase deficiency is of clinical relevance only during excessive heavy muscular activities (mild to moderate exercise is well tolerated). When the demand for glycogenolysis finally does occur, the muscle becomes ATP depleted and loses function. The normal glycolytic production of lactate during exercise (skeletal muscle is the major contributor of lactate to the blood in this situation) does not occur. However, if this abnormal muscle is provided with lactate — as with intravenous lactated solutions — it is fully equipped biochemically to utilize lactate as a source of energy via the normal aerobic machinery. Clinically, this is manifested by exercise-induced fatigue, painful muscle cramping, stiffness, and, often, the development of myoglobinuria. The myoglobinuria has the potential for renal tubular blockage and may necessitate the induction of urinary alkalinization and diuresis to avoid renal failure. The muscular pathobiochemistry results in low grade muscle injury and a subsequent elevation of blood lactic dehydrogenase, creatine phosphokinase, and aldolase. Euglycemia prevails, and there is a normal hepatic regulation of the blood glucose concentration and a normal liver response to glucagon.

Clinically, these patients unexplainedly do not become symptomatic until they become teenagers. Until their third decade, their only symptom may be easy fatigability. However, in the succeeding decades they develop the exercise-related cramping and myoglobinuria, and ultimately muscle-wasting with significant functional weakness. With advanced age these individuals may become so weak and have such diminished exercise tolerance that they are essentially functional myasthenics. Renal failure may intercede at any time and is a major determinant of morbidity and mortality. Should these patients continue to exercise during muscle cramping — a dangerous idea from a renal point of view — they may become symptom free. This has been attributed to increased muscle blood flow and increased utilization of blood borne free fatty acids as an alternate energy supply.

Treatment consists of the avoidance of strenuous exercise and oral ingestion of adequate amounts of glucose and fructose, both sugars being readily utilizable precursors for skeletal muscle ATP production. Although an impractical drug therapy, isoproterenol does increase skeletal muscle blood flow and serum-free acid concentrations, which thereby provide muscle with a supply of utilizable alternate enrgy precursors.

Anesthetic management depends on the severity of the disease. In younger patients with milder disease there is no anesthetic drug of choice, and general anesthesia without the use of muscle relaxants is preferred. Patients with advanced myopathy obviously require no relaxants. Because muscle activity ultimately predisposes to muscle weakness, these patients resemble myasthenia gravis patients: their functional muscle reserve is limited. If muscle relaxants are deemed necessary, the nondepolarizing relaxants, d-tubocurarine, gallamine, metocurine, and pancuronium would provide the least biochemical trespass in that muscle contractile activity would be decreased, thereby preserving the maximum biochemical capacity for the crucial postoperative period. The disadvantage of the nondepolarizing muscle relaxants is that it is difficult to fully reverse their effect, and residual paresis would further compromise the already pre-existing decrease in muscle reserve. The depolarization and contraction caused by the depolarizing relaxants succinylcholine and decamethonium not only unnecessarily utilize the limited muscle energy supply but also may induce myoglobinuria. Regardless of the anesthetic approach, the keynote to successful postoperative recovery is the provision of good postoperative respiratory care to these biochemically "myasthenic" individuals.

Although exercise-related muscle cramping and stiffness are common complaints, these patients are not predisposed to the development of myotonic or dystonic states. However, when such symptomatology becomes manifest in the postanesthetic period, this should be considered as unequivocal evidence of excessive muscular activity and/or inadequate muscular energy substrate supply, as may be seen in postanesthetic shivering. Theoretically, individuals with this Type 5 disorder would be unlikely to develop malignant hyperpyrexia, as they would have a limited ability to generate the extreme hypermetabolic state in their skeletal muscle. On the other hand, they might have a decreased capacity for rewarming from a hypothermic state and an increased potential for generating myoglobinuria in achieving euthermia.

In essence, the biochemical lesion in this disorder is that of inadequate availability of energy substrate for skeletal muscle; therefore, the major therapeutic endeavor should be to provide such substrate. Glucose, fructose, lactate, and acetate are all substrates utilizable by skeletal muscle and may be furnished intravenously. Glucose, in order to enter muscle cells, requires the facilitative action of insulin and obviously would be functionally less effective in a patient who also has diabetes mellitus. Fructose, lactate, and acetate are independent of insulin activity. Provision of energy substrates must be assured throughout the postoperative period when the demand for such will invariably increase.

Type 6 glycogen storage disease (Hers' disease) is characterized by a decreased (but not absent) hepatic α-1,4-glucan phosphorylase (Reaction 6) and normal phosphorylase activating systems (Reactions 6a,b,c). There is a consequent increase in the glycogen content of the liver and a predisposition to hypoglycemia, particularly in the fasting state. Because of the relative — rather than absolute — functional unavailability of hepatic glycogen, the clinical sequelae are generally benign. The response to glucagon and epinephrine is variable but generally ineffective in restoring euglycemia. The major anesthetic consideration, therefore, is that of avoiding hypoglycemia (see section on hypoglycemia).

Type 7 glycogen storage disease is an extremely rare disorder in which there is a deficiency of the skeletal muscle glycolytic (glucose breakdown) regulatory enzyme, phosphofructokinase (ATP:D-fructose-6-phosphate-1-phosphotransferase), which catalyzes one of the two primary reactions of glycolysis: fructose-6-phosphate + ATP → fructose-1,6-diphosphate. As a result there is a Type 5-like clinical and biochemical picture with limited exercise capacity, myoglobinuria, and absence of hyperlactatemia with attempted heavy muscular activity. This is a glycogen storage disease because there is a concomitant increased activity of two muscle glycogenogenic enzymes, UDP phosphorylase (Reaction 3) and glycogen synthase (Reaction 4), which leads to an inappropriate synthesis and accumulation of muscle glycogen. A major difference from Type 5 is that glucose and fructose are not efficiently employed energy substrates; however, acetate, lactate, and fatty acids are utilized in a normal fashion. As the phosphofructokinase deficiency is

not absolute, there is a very small capacity for glucose and fructose utilization as energy precursors. The anesthetic management is otherwise similar to that of Type 5.

Type 8 glycogen storage disease is an X-linked, genetically transmitted disease in which there is a deficiency of hepatic phosphorylase kinase. This effects a depressed activity of hepatic α-1,4-glucan phosphorylase (Reaction 6c) and a resultant blockade of the cleavage of glucose residues from glycogen (Reaction 6). As the enzyme deficiency is not absolute, there remains a limited capability for activation of hepatic phosphorylase and, therefore, there is a relatively normal response to glucagon. The clinical manifestations include only a benign hepatomegaly (the liver contains an increased concentration of glycogen) and a tendency to hypoglycemia. As such, the anesthetic management is directed toward maintenance of euglycemia.

HEREDITARY HEPATIC PORPHYRIAS

The porphyrins are molecular components of heme, which functions in aerobic systems as the prosthetic group of several hemoproteins, larger molecules that are concerned with the essential functions of oxidation, electron transport, and hydroperoxidation. These hemoproteins include hemoglobin, myoglobin, mitochondrial and microsomal cytochromes, catalase, and tryptophan pyrrolase. Their basic biochemical functions involve the transport of molecular oxygen, activation of oxygen, and transfer of electrons to oxygen as the final receiver in the electron transport system. Interestingly, there is no known physiological role for free porphyrins, which also are chemically related to the plant chlorophylls and the vitamin B_{12} corrin ring. The biosynthesis of heme is summarized stepwise in the following equations:

1. Succinyl coenzyme A + glycine ← δ-aminolevulinic acid synthetase → δ-aminolevulinic acid (δ-ALA) + CO_2. This is an intramitochondrial reaction and therefore is not present in mature erythrocytes. The Krebs tricarboxylic acid cycle supplies most of the succinyl coenzyme A. Pyridoxal phosphate (vitamin B_6) is an obligate cofac-

tor in this step of heme synthesis, which is the only reaction in the entire synthetic process requiring a vitamin cofactor and energy. All subsequent reactions are strongly favored thermodynamically and are therefore basically irreversible. The initial part of this reaction is between pyridoxal phosphate and a sulfhydral group of the active site of δ-ALA synthetase; then follows the formation of a Schiff base with glycine, and, finally, a condensation reaction with succinyl coenzyme A. Most importantly, this step is the rate-limiting one of the entire biosynthetic pathway, and it is regulated through the mechanisms of feedback repression and inhibition as well as substrate, hormonal and chemical induction.

2. δ-ALA ← δ-ALA dehydrase → porphobilinogen (PBG). This and the following two reactions are extramitochondrial. Zinc is required at this step. Although δ-ALA dehydrase has the property of being feedback inhibitable by coproporphyrin III, protoporphyrin IX and heme, under normal conditions this enzyme has no regulatory control on the rate of heme synthesis; its peak reactivity velocity grossly exceeds that of δ-ALA synthetase.

3. 4 PBG ← uroporphyrinogen I synthetase (PBG deaminase), uroporphyrinogen III cosynthetase → uroporphyrinogen III.

4. Uroporphyrinogen III ← decarboxylase → coproporphyrinogen III. Note that only porphyrin isomers of type III are intermediates in this biosynthetic pathway.

5. Coproporphyrinogen III ← coproporphyrinogen oxidase (oxidative decarboxylase) → protoporphyrinogen IX. This and all subsequent steps are intramitochondrial.

6. Protoporphyrinogen IX ← protoporphyrinogen oxidase (dehydrogenase) → protoporphyrin IX.

7. Protoporphyrin IX + iron ← ferrochetatase → heme. Note that the catabolism of heme produces bile pigments and not porphyrins.

Because the synthesis of heme is an absolutely essential process (a total blockade of heme biosynthesis is incompatible with life), there are numerous compensatory mechanisms for any genetic and/or acquired enzymatic deficiencies. Thus, the maintenance of steady state heme homeostasis is very closely regulated, and the key to this regulation concerns the quality and activity of δ-ALA synthetase, in both the liver and erythroid cells. Negative feedback inhibition by heme could be achieved through: 1) decreasing δ-ALA synthetase activity. This is not thought to be a significant mechanism; 2) decreasing the synthesis of δ-ALA synthetase. This is considered to be an important mode of control as the biologic half-life of the enzyme and its messenger RNA is rather brief; 3) reducing the transfer of synthesized enzyme from the polyribosomes to the mitochondria, a regulatory site that has much recent investigational support.

In the opposite direction, biosynthesis of δ-ALA synthetase is inducible (capable of having its activity increased) by numerous chemical compounds with diverse structures such as steroids and lipid-soluble drugs. The mechanism of such induction involves the cytochrome P-450 system, a group of hemoprotein isoenzymes which function as terminal oxidases in drug metabolism. The primary function of this enzyme complex is to convert lipid-soluble, nonpolar drugs —a physicochemical property of most central nervous system depressants — into water-soluble, polar compounds that are then eliminated from the body by the kidney, the predominant organ of drug excretion. As an example, the rapid-acting barbiturates are lipid compounds that are available in the form of the more water-soluble sodium salts for intravenous administration even though the active drug form is the lipid soluble free acid. The kidneys readily filter these barbiturates through the glomerular apparatus, but then the tubular collecting system reabsorbs the vast majority of the filtered lipoid drug which then reappears in the circulation. The cytochrome P-450 system functions to biotransform these drugs into a polar, water-soluble form that will be more readily excreted by the kidney. The liver is the predominant area of cytochrome P-450 activity which, in turn, resides in the endoplasmic reticulum, a series of convoluted lipid membranes which upon mechanical fragmentation coalesce into spheres called microsomes. In fact, the biosynthesis of the cytochrome P-450 system is the major consumer of the heme produced by the liver.

A unique aspect of this enzyme-drug interaction is the capacity for the isoenzymes to combine with a wide variety of structurally unrelated compounds. The cytochrome P-450 enzyme combines with the lipid drug, activates molecular oxygen with electrons obtained from NADP or NADPH, oxidizes the drug, and then detaches from the newly polar, water-soluble compound. This biotransformational process is dose related and slow in response, possibly requiring hours to days in order to achieve its function. However, the cytochrome P-450 system possesses the capacity to increase its activity in response to substrate (drug) exposure, a phenomenon known as *induction*. Because this system is relatively nonspecific in nature, one drug *may* induce the biotransformational fate of another; each inducing drug induces a specific profile subspecies of the cytochrome P-450 system. Despite the slow and dose-related nature of this machinery, a single small dose of drug can and does effect induction. The extremely lipid-soluble drugs, because of their prolonged storage in fat depots, may bring about a profound and prolonged induction of enzyme activity.

The barbiturates' — particularly phenobarbital — enzyme-inducing capacity has been utilized for the stimulation of premature, under- or undeveloped bilirubin conjugating enzymes in the prevention and/or treatment of kernicterus. Steroids have been employed late in gestation to accelerate the functional maturation of the enzyme systems involved with pulmonary surfactant production. Ethyl alcohol (ethanol) induces the cytochrome P-450 system such that chronic ethanolics often are resistant to the effects of central nervous system depressants. Patients with seizure disorders receiving phenobarbital and/or phenytoin have a vastly induced cytochrome P-450 system, and this biochemical environment might augment the biotransformation of anesthetic drugs, such as methoxyflurane or enflurane, and even lead to a clinically significant and toxic level of metabolites such as fluoride. Withdrawal of inducing drugs will result in a slow return of the enzymatic activity toward normal by virtue of the cessation of new synthesis and natural degradation of older enzymes.

The induction of δ-ALA synthetase is achieved by an initial increase of the synthesis of the apoprotein of cytochrome P-450 (apocytochrome P-450), the production of which normally precedes that of heme and is the rate-limiting reaction. This new apocytochrome P-450 necessarily depletes the pool of heme so that the end product, cytochrome P-450, may be formed. This, in turn, creates an obligatory requirement for new heme synthesis that is effected through a decreased negative feedback inhibition of δ-ALA synthetase by the depleted level of heme. This induction usually results in a mild to moderate increase of δ-ALA synthetase activity, but another group of structurally unrelated compounds (such as allylisopropylacelylcarbamide, dicarbethoxydihydrocollidine, griseofulvin, and chlorinated hydrocarbons, as, for example, hexachlorobenzene) do effect extremely large increments of δ-ALA synthetase activity. These compounds do so by 1) reducing the synthesis of heme, thereby producing a partial derepression of δ-ALA synthetase, 2) inducing microsomal cytochrome P-450, again releasing negative feedback inhibition by demanding more heme synthesis, and, 3) increasing heme catabolism, which necessitates new anabolism.

Finally, there are several important endogenous and exogenous factors that modify the induction of δ-ALA synthetase: 1) glucose and/or protein administration inhibits induction, the underlying mechanism yet to be determined; fasting augments induction; 2) chelated iron augments induction by stimulating the breakdown of heme and cytochrome P-450; 3) steroids and several hormones (and their metabolites) augment induction.

Approximately 100 mg. of heme are synthesized by the human liver daily and 300 mg. by the erythroid tissues, but only a small amount of heme precursors is excreted in the urine and/or bile. This indicates a high degree of biosynthetic efficiency. δ-ALA, PBG, and uroporphyrinogens are excreted mainly in urine (porphyrinogens are converted to porphyrins upon exposure to light and air), while coproporphyrin is eliminated mainly in the bile and protoporphyrin is eliminated exclusively in the bile. The liver is the major site in which inherited and/or acquired defects in heme biosynthesis are expressed. Erythroid tissue has no concomitant impairment of heme (hemoglobin) synthesis even though the basic enzymatic defect also is present in extrahepatic tissue. The metabolic and clinical manifestations of the hepatic porphyrias emanate solely from the hepatic pathobiochemistry.

The hepatic porphyrias are a collection of diseases in which there is an elevation of the biosynthesis of porphyrin precursors and/or porphyrins by the liver. Table 1–3 summarizes the demonstrated or suspected partial enzymatic defect and the resultant distinct pattern of accumulation and excretion of heme intermediate compounds for the three genetically transmitted porphyrias: intermittent acute porphyria (IAP), hereditary coproporphyria, and variegate porphyria.

These hepatic porphyrias share the following common properties: 1) δ-ALA synthetase activity is increased, and is responsible for the inappropriate hypersynthesis of porphyrin precursors and/or porphyrins but not the specifically distinctive patterns of their urinary and fecal excretion; 2) the specific enzymatic step at which partial blockade occurs can mechanistically explain the characteristic intermediary accumulative and excretory patterns as well as the release of feedback repression of δ-ALA synthetase; 3) the initial chemical and clinical manifestations are rarely encountered prior to puberty and once present are modified by nutritional (glucose) and hormonal (menstruation, pregnancy) factors; genetic carriers may be asymptomatic throughout life; 4) acute attacks are precipitated by therapeutic doses of certain drugs, the majority of which are lipid soluble and have the property of inducing cytochrome P-450 and δ-ALA synthetase; 5) the neuropsychiatric manifestations of acute attacks are always accompanied by the excess presence of ALA and PBG; 6) genetic transmission is of an autosomal dominant pattern.

The clinical manifestations of the hepatic porphyrias are the consequence of neurologic lesions in scattered regions of the central, peripheral, and autonomic nervous systems, and, although always accompanied by excesses of ALA and PBG, no direct pathogenic properties have been demonstrated for these porphyrin precursors. However, there is some evidence that the oxidized products of porphyrins may adversely affect various metabolic processes within neural tissues. This neuropathologic

state classically causes abdominal symptoms, peripheral neuropathy, and various types of mental disturbances. The abdominal pain is of moderate to severe intensity, is frequently colicky, and is non-specific in location. Physical examination characteristically reveals a soft, non-tender or mildly tender abdominal wall without signs of peritoneal inflammation. A history may also be obtained that is consistent with gastroduodenal spasm (distention, vomiting) or intestinal obstruction (absence of bowel movements), and roentgenographic evaluation may demonstrate regions of spastic constriction with proximal loop obstruction. Acute episodes may last for days to weeks and periods of "remission" (low grade disease activity) may occur. Therefore, the patient may present with dehydration and a significant hypovolemic state, electrolyte abnormalities (particularly hypokalemia, hypochloremia and hyponatremia, this latter finding due possibly to hypothalamic injury and subsequent inappropriate antidiuretic hormone secretion), hypoproteinemia, vitamin deficiency, acid-base abnormalities, and weight loss or even cachexia. In the extreme situation, hypovolemic hypotension with prerenal oliguria (or even anuria) may occur. Mortality, albeit unusual, is the consequence of respiratory neuronal disease and resultant functional insufficiency.

Neurological lesions may manifest anywhere within the central, peripheral or autonomic nervous systems, so the clinical spectrum is extremely broad and variable, ranging from pain syndromes to sensory deficits or alterations, para- or quadriplegia, bulbar paralysis, semicomatose or comatose states, and seizures. Various forms of mental dysfunction and psychiatric ailments are common.

Chronic hypertension and/or sinus tachycardia is encountered in many patients. In fact, the pulse rate is considered to be a coarse barometer of the activity of the porphyria. However, the increased pulse rate might also be the result of hypovolemia, pain, hypoxemia, hypercarbia, or hypokalemia.

Liver function testing fails to reveal any abnormality except for some mild retention of sulfobromophthalein during acute exacerbations. Renal function is dependent upon the degree of damage elicited by repeated episodes of prerenal oliguric states:

Table 1-3 *Heme Precursor and/or Converted Porphyrin in Urine and Feces*

	Urine		Feces	
	Latent Phase	Acute Attack	Latent Phase	Acute Attack
Intermittent acute porphyria				
Enzymatic deficiency:				
Uroporphyrinogen I synthetase				
δ-aminolevulinic acid, porphobilinogen	Normal or mildly increased	Markedly increased (20–500 mg/day)	–	–
Note: increased plasma and cerebrospinal fluid levels during acute attacks				
Coproporphyrin III, protoporphyrin III	–	Often increased	–	Usually slightly to moderately increased
Hydrophilic porphyrin-peptide conjugates	–	–	–	Occasionally present
Variegate porphyria				
Enzymatic deficiency:				
?Protoporphyrinogen oxidase				
?Ferrochetalase				
δ-aminolevulinic acid, porphobilinogen	Normal or slightly increased	Markedly increased	–	–
Coproporphyrin III, protoporphyrin III	Usually slightly increased	Markedly increased	Increased	Markedly increased
Hydrophilic porphyrin-peptide conjugates	Normal or slightly increased	Increased	Increased	Increased
Hereditary coproporphyria				
Enzymatic deficiency:				
Coproporphyrinogen oxidase				
δ-aminolevulinic acid, porphobilinogen	Normal or slightly increased	Markedly increased	–	–
Coproporphyrin III	Normal or slightly increased	Increased	Markedly increased (2000 mg/day)	Markedly increased
Protoporphyrin III	–	–	Usually normal	Usually normal
Hydrophilic porphyrin-peptide conjugates	–	–	–	–

Note: may be increased in infections and hepatic carcinoma

Note: may be increased in obstructive liver disease, lead poisoning and hemolytic anemia

Normal values
δ-aminolevulinic acid – urine: 2–4 mg/day
–bile: negligible
Porphobilinogen – urine: <1.5 mg/day
–feces: negligible
Uroporphyrin III – urine: <3 μg/day
Coproporphyrin III – urine: 50–300 μg/day
–feces: 400–1000 μg/day
Protoporphyrin III – urine: negligible
–feces: 800–2000 μg/day

serum creatinine provides this information.

The clinical pattern of *intermittent acute porphyria* (IAP) is that of acute attacks (relapses) usually precipitated by an inducing entity superimposed upon a latent (or remissive) phase which is characterized by absent, less intense, or resolving pathology. Recovery from the neurological insults is variable in extent and speed of achievement. IAP is an autosomal dominantly transmitted disease with a highly variable phenotypic (clinical) expression. Many genetic carriers may even be asymptomatic throughout adult life, this fact perhaps highlighting the importance of exposure to porphyrogenic triggering compounds. Clinical manifestations are usually seen initially in the early adult years and there is a moderate preference for females. Although the worldwide incidence is estimated at only 1 per 80,000 people, its regional incidence may be 100 times higher.

The primary biochemical lesion in IAP is a generalized deficiency (but not absence) of uroporphyrinogen I synthetase (PBG deaminase), and there is a secondary, regulatory increase of hepatic δ-ALA synthetase. This creates a situation primed for inducibility by environmental factors, the most important of which are exogenous lipid-soluble compounds that induce hepatic cytochrome P-450. This, in turn, increases demand for hepatic heme, and therefore δ-ALA synthetase activity necessarily must be augmented. Another important consideration is that an impaired adaptive response of the cytochrome P-450 drug metabolizing system necessarily prolongs the half-life of the porphyrinogenic compounds. Uroporphyrinogen I synthetase activity remains unchanged during exacerbations of the disease, and erythrocyte levels allow for the detection of asymptomatic carriers of the IAP gene. Consistent with this mechanistic explanation of IAP is the demonstrated therapeutic effectiveness of hematin infusions during acute episodes of IAP.

Variegate porphyria is an inducible hepatic porphyria that is clinically similar to IAP, but it is distinguishable 1) clinically by cutaneous pathology and 2) chemically by its pattern of porphyrin excretion (see Table 1–3). Skin involvement is chronic — the usual locations being the face and the back of the hands — and is elicited by minimal

mechanical trauma. Such lesions are prone to infection and scarring. Additionally, the skin is photosensitive and hyperpigmentation and hypertrichosis often result. These cutaneous manifestations bear no chronologic relationship to neuropsychiatric events. The presence of the photobiologically active porphyrins in the skin is the probable cause of the photosensitivity. The primary enzymatic partial deficiency has been localized to the steps involving the conversion of protoporphyrinogen IX to protoporphyrin IX and heme, but the specific hepatic intramitochondrial enzymatic deficit — be it

Table 1–4 *Anesthetic Drugs Reported Safe for Hereditary Hepatic Porphyrias*

Tranquilizer
  Chlorpromazine
  Promazine
  Promethazine

Analgesic
  Morphine
  Meperidine
  Mefenamic acid

Sedative-hypnotic-narcotic
  Paraldehyde
  Chloral hydrate
  Propanidid

Dissociative
  Ketamine*

Local anesthetic
  Procaine

General anesthetic
  Nitrous oxide
  Cyclopropane
  Diethyl ether
  Halothane*
  Enflurane*

Muscle relaxant
  Succinyldicholine
  Decamethonium
  d-Tubocurarine
  Gallamine

Anticholinergic
  Atropine

Anticholinesterase
  Neostigmine

Antihypertensive
  Tetraethylammonium
  Pentolinium
  Rauwolfia alkaloids
  Sodium nitroprusside
  Nitroglycerine

Antitachycardic
  Neostigmine
  Propranolol

*Limited clinical experience.

protoporphyrinogen oxidase or ferrochetalase — has not been determined. There is a secondary augmentation of hepatic δ-ALA synthetase activity.

Hereditary coproporphyria is a very rare clinical syndrome indistinguishable from IAP but for its distinct pattern of excretion of porphyrin and porphyrin precursors (see Table 1–3). The primary enzymatic partial deficiency is that of hepatic intramitochondrial coproporphyrinogen oxidase, which mediates the oxidative decarboxylation of coproporphyrinogen III to protoporphyrinogen IX. There is a secondary derepression of hepatic δ-ALA synthetase activity.

Several analgesics, tranquilizers, sedative-hypnotics, spasmolytics, and antihypertensive drugs have been administered successfully and without adverse porphyric reactions in the treatment of acute porphyric attacks. Table 1–4 lists those drugs that may safely be employed for pre-, intra-, and postanesthetic purposes. Table 1–5, on the other hand, lists the porphyrogenic drugs, which *must be avoided.* Overwhelming evidence in humans indicates that *all barbiturate drugs are absolutely contraindicated in the active phase of the hereditary hepatic porphyrias.* On the other hand, a recent survey in Finland indicated that during the latent (or remissive) stage, the induction of clinical porphyric activity by barbiturates or other porphyrogenic anesthetic drugs is rare. This report notwithstanding, it would seem prudent to avoid all anesthetic drugs with acknowledged porphyrogenic properties in any patient with a hereditary hepatic porphyria, regardless of the state of activity of the disease, because alternative anesthetic combinations — albeit limited — are, indeed, available.

The appropriate anesthetic technique for the management of a known hereditary hepatic porphyric patient has not been established for the following reasons:

1. The relative paucity of porphyric patients and the resultant limited clinical anesthetic experience with such patients has not allowed for a proper evaluation and delineation of the porphyrogenic properties of most anesthetic drugs. In some instances, as with ketamine, contradictory laboratory and clinical experiences have been encountered. Extrapolation from laboratory experiments in other species may not be applicable to the human condition, and comparable interspecific drug dosages have not been defined. The moral propriety of human evaluation of suspected porphyrogenic drugs must be considered as well.

2. Porphyrias are rather unpredictable in the presence, intensity, and duration of their clinical disease activity.

3. The precipitation (or exacerbation), if any, and extent of disease activity by porphyrogenic compounds is not clearly predictable.

The potent inhalational anesthetics are metabolically degraded by the hepatic microsomal cytochrome P-450 drug metabolizing enzyme system. Although there is conflicting evidence concerning halothane, the inhalational anesthetics are considered to be inducers of cytochrome P-450, and this

---

Table 1–5 *Currently Available Porphyria-Inducing Drugs*

Anesthesia premedicants, anesthetics, intra-anesthesia therapeutics:
  The barbiturates
  The nonbarbiturate sedative and hypnotic drugs, meprobamate, diazepam, chlordiazepoxide, apronalide, ethinamate, glutethimide, methyprylon, carbromal
  The steroid configuration drugs, such as hydroxydione, Althesin (alfaxalone and alfadolone), pancuronium
  Ethyl alcohol
  The hydantoin anticonvulsants, such as phenytoin (which is also an antiarrhythmic drug)
  Nikethamide (central nervous system-cardiorespiratory stimulant)
  Pentazocine (benzomorphan analgesic)

Drugs not usually associated with anesthesia:
  The sulfonamides
  Sex hormones
  The antipyretic, analgesic, anti-inflammatory drugs aminopyrine and antipyrine
  Griseofulvin (anti-fungal)
  The hypoglycemic sulfonylureas tolbutamide and chlorpropamide
  Metapyrone (inhibitor of adrenal steroid synthesis)
  Ergot preparations
  Methyldopa (antihypertensive)

property would make these drugs porphyrogenic candidates. However, the available laboratory and clinical information points to the safety of the halogenated hydrocarbons, particularly halothane, as anesthetics for both induction and maintenance in the patient with hereditary hepatic porphyria. Ketamine's safety in humans has not been unequivocally established. Although pancuronium has not been demonstrated to be an inducing compound, its steroidal configuration and capacity for biotransformation, and the availability of other safe muscle relaxants, would preclude its use in the porphyric patient. On purely theoretical grounds, neostigmine has been questioned as to safety because of the anticholinesterase property possessed by some porphyrogenic insecticides, but clinically it has proven to be safe in the anesthetic management of porphyrics.

Because of the scattered occurrence and unpredictable onset of central and peripheral neuropathological lesions in these disorders, intrathecal anesthesia, epidural anesthesia, nerve blocks, ganglion blocks, and plexus blocks are best avoided; new disorders attributable to the blocked part of the nervous system might unjustly incriminate the injected anesthetic.

As can be seen in Table 1–4, the choice of a proved, safe anesthetic technique (particularly in operating rooms where the employment of flammable anesthetics is prohibited) is somewhat limited; there is no preferred method listed. In those cases in which endotracheal intubation either is necessary or facilitates anesthetic management, the utilization of an awake intubation can circumvent the need for any induction anesthetic drugs. The fully informed, well-motivated, and humanistically managed patient will tolerate this nihilistic approach. Once the patient is intubated, a balanced anesthetic technique with narcotics, muscle relaxants, and nitrous oxide might be employed.

The anesthetic approach to a patient with a hereditary hepatic porphyria must commence with a detailed preanesthetic evaluation. Particular attention must be given to the neurological examination, blood pressure and pulse patterns, intravascular volume status, serum electrolytes, blood creatinine concentration, serum protein levels, and respiratory system function (arterial blood gases, pulmonary function screening, inspiratory force measurement). The neurological examination should be repeated prior to the anesthetic induction in order to detect any recent adverse changes that might otherwise be attributed to the anesthetics to be utilized. It is important to delineate any tendency to hypertension as well as its degree of lability, because induction of anesthesia in hypertensive porphyrics often results in the precipitous development of hypotension. Antithetically, a significant number of adequately anesthetized porphyric individuals maintain or develop clinically significant hypertension that requires appropriate drug therapy. Hypertension combined with the sinus tachycardia frequently found in such patients poses a potentially seriously high myocardial oxygen demand, which, in turn, might lead to myocardial ischemia. Propranolol might be therapeutically indicated in such a situation. Hypokalemia and/or hyponatremia—often extreme in extent—must be judiciously corrected preanesthetically, both to prevent extreme hemodynamic changes and arrhythmias and to avoid excessive effects of neuromuscular relaxants. Unexplained or unexpected residual paresis or paralysis after the routine use of muscle relaxants could be the result of an intensification or exacerbation of the porphyric process and must be diagnostically evaluated with a peripheral nerve stimulator. The respiratory muscles are of primary importance in this respect and in all cases appropriate respiratory assistance and care must be provided until normal function can be demonstrated. Blood creatinine concentrations help to detect and evaluate the possible presence of renal dysfunction and any reversible component thereof. A prerenal cause may be seen in the severely dehydrated patient who will usually respond to appropriate fluid therapy guided by careful monitoring of vital signs, urine output, and, when necessary, appropriate central venous lines.

Because fasting may in itself induce cytochrome P-450 activity, and because of the reported efficacy of glucose in modifying porphyric attacks, it would be wise to begin an intravenous infusion of glucose concomitant with initiation of the routine preanesthetic fast. Particular care must be exercised with respect to the skin of the patient who has dermatologic manifestations of his porphyria. This involves the proper use of bland tapes, avoidance of tapes wherever possible, elimination of excessive pressure from all equipment, and protection from excessive exposure to photosensitizing light. Blood pressure cuffs and tourniquets should be padded. Intravenous puncture sites should be treated with antibiotic ointment prophylactically. In addition, the dermatologically fragile facial skin must be protected from mask-induced trauma during an inhalation induction.

Through all of the above discussion, the anesthetist is dealing with a known disease entity. However, it is possible to anesthetize a previously undetected porphyric patient and precipitate a porphyric attack during the anesthetic. None or all of the above-mentioned sequelae of this disease may be encountered intra- or postanesthetically. Certainly, one must consider porphyria in the differential diagnosis of the postanesthetic patient who 1) remains unexplainedly paralyzed or comatose at the termination of anesthesia, 2) demonstrates a peripheral nerve lesion (motor or sensory) upon awakening, or 3) complains of severe unexplained abdominal pain. The anesthetist confronted with the differential diagnosis of an acute adverse reaction to an induction dose of an anesthetic such as barbiturate or diazepam should consider, in addition to anaphylaxis and direct cardiovascular depression, the possibility of a porphyric attack. Finally, when providing respiratory care for the porphyric with pulmonary insufficiency, it is obviously critical to insure that the patient receives no porphyrogenic drugs.

No conclusive specific and definitive drug or biochemical treatment has been successfully introduced. Although intravenous procaine had been used with therapeutic success almost 30 years ago and has been shown to decrease the activity of hepatic δ-ALA synthetase of rats, procaine is not currently being advocated for the treatment of acute attacks. The administration of very large amounts of glucose is reportedly effective in modifying the activity of a porphyric episode. Most importantly, there have been recent reports of the dramatic effectiveness of the intravenous infusion of hematin (a repressor of δ-ALA synthetase) in bringing about remission from extreme and life-threatening porphyric attacks. Further work will be necessary to establish conclusively this rational biochemical treatment.

INBORN ERRORS OF AMINO ACID METABOLISM

The term protein is derived from the Greek word meaning "primary," and indeed proteins are involved with the entire spectrum of biological functions. They are the catalysts (enzymes) involved in regulation of all biological reactions, the building units of all subcellular and cellular architecture, the transport carriers of essential compounds, the regulators (hormones) of physiological relationships, the essential molecules (antibodies) of immune reactions, and the crucial molecules of the contractile process and mitotic apparatus. Proteins are macromolecules, polymers of the monomeric units, amino acids. All but two of the amino acids are alpha-amino acids, which have a primary amino group, and a primary carboxyl group joined to the same carbon atom; their general structure is

$$NH_2 — CHR — COOH$$

The two exceptions are the alpha-imino acids proline and hydroxyproline.

Several biochemically important amino acids and amino acid derivatives are not constituents of protein. Because the absolute configuration of all the amino acids obtained from human protein has been related to that of L-glyceraldehyde, they all are of the L-configuration. Each amino and carboxyl group of an amino acid has a characteristic pKa value. In the pH range of 4 to 9 an amino acid exists as a dipolar ion, and therefore is readily soluble in water but insoluble in the lipoproteinaceous cell membrane. Consequently, the transport of amino acids across cell membranes requires energy.

Amino acids may be obtained from food, catabolism of body (primarily skeletal muscle) protein, or biosynthesis. The human body is unable to synthesize several of the amino acids, which therefore must be obtained by dietary means; these are called essential amino acids. A nonessential amino acid (such as tyrosine) may be synthesized from an essential one (phenylalanine), but if this biosynthetic pathway is blocked (as in phenylketonuria), it too becomes an essential amino acid.

Amino acids have four major metabolic fates: 1) biosynthesis of protein, 2) biosynthesis of nonprotein nitrogen-containing molecules, 3) catabolism to end products that are excreted, and 4) conversion to compounds that are utilized metabolically. Catabolism of amino acids in man commences with the removal of the amino group by either oxidative deamination or transamination, the major end product being urea. The carbon skeleton of amino acids may enter into or be derived from lipid and carbohydrate metabolic pathways.

If all amino acids are functionally available to the body, then abnormalities of protein synthesis are affected only by aberrations of the nucleic acids determining such synthesis. Certain genetically determined diseases have been discovered in which there is a defect in the metabolism or transportation of amino acids.

CYSTINURIA

Cystinuria is a genetically determined disease that is an example of a defect in the transportation of amino acids across cell membranes. Specifically, cystinuria is a disorder of the transportation of the amino acid cystine and the dibasic amino acids lysine, arginine, and ornithine affecting the epithelial cells of the renal tubule and gastrointestinal tract.

In the normal kidney, amino acids are filtered at the glomerulus and are almost entirely reabsorbed in the proximal portion of the nephron. This reabsorptive mechanism has a maximal capacity, and aminoaciduria will occur when the filtered load exceeds this capacity. This situation is most frequently encountered when an extrarenal metabolic defect brings about an accumulation of amino acids in the plasma. Therefore, most aminoacidurias are not disorders of renal tubular function. In cystinuria, however, there is an excessive loss of cystine, the dibasic amino acids, and the mixed disulfide of cysteine-homocysteine in the face of low or normal concentrations of these amino acids. Because aminoaciduria occurs in the presence of a normal or reduced filtered load of amino acids, the reabsorptive capacity of the renal tubule is abnormal. This selective increase in the renal clearance and urinary excretion of these

amino acids is transmitted as an autosomal recessive trait. It is thought that cystine and the dibasic amino acids are in competition for a single reabsorptive site in the luminal brush border and that this site is defective in cystinuria. Intracellularly, cystine occurs almost exclusively in the form of the free thiol cysteine, which competes with lysine, arginine, and ornithine for efflux from the nephron, and it may be that this interaction is a key determinant in the regulation of cystine transport into the renal tubular cells. Because the cystinuric's clearance of cystine exceeds the filtered load at the glomerulus, it is thought that these patients also secrete abnormal amounts of cystine. Renal clearance of all other amino acids is normal in cystinuric patients.

A similar, but not identical, transportation defect has been demonstrated in the small intestine of cystinuric patients. Oral administration of the involved amino acids results in an increased fecal excretion of the acids and their bacterial breakdown products. This intestinal defect has been utilized as a sensitive genetic marker and has identified three allelic types of cystinuric homozygotes.

Cystine is a nonessential amino acid and may be synthesized from the essential amino acid methionine. Of the amino acids affected in cystinuria, only lysine is an essential amino acid. However, there appears to be no growth or developmental sequelae of its decreased gastrointestinal absorption. This probably is related to the ability of cystinurics to absorb lysine from the small intestine as oligo- and dipeptides, these subsequently being enzymatically degraded to lysine and other amino acids.

Although cystinuria is a rare disease, massive screening programs of newborns indicate its incidence to be approximately 1 in 7000, which makes cystinuria one of the most common of the inherited disorders of metabolism. Although there is no sexual preference, males are more likely to be severely affected.

The only definite clinical sequela of these metabolic derangements is the formation of renal and urinary tract calculi composed of the amino acid cystine. Cystine's solubility in aqueous solutions is the lowest of the naturally occurring amino acids and decreases with increasing acidity of the urine. These urinary tract calculi predispose to urinary tract obstruction, subsequent infection, and, ultimately, progressive loss of renal function. Renal colic is the most common presenting symptom, and, although clinical expression of cystinuria may occur at any time during the patient's life, it most frequently is initially encountered in the second and third decades.

Both cystine and uric acid stones are most likely to be generated in acid urine, but only cystine stones are radiopaque, owing to the density of the sulfur molecules. Calcium stones may appear at a later time, but they are formed only as sequelae to secondary urinary tract infections. Cystine calculi often are staghorn in anatomy, but multiple recurrent calculi may also be found. Diagnosis is made by observing the classical hexagonal cystine crystals on microscopic examination of the urine, but final confirmation of cystinuria depends on a positive cyanide-nitroprusside test and, ultimately, one of the more sophisticated processes of chromatography or electrophoresis. It has been demonstrated that cystine stones are most likely to form when the cystine urinary excretion rate is greater than 300 mg. cystine per gram of creatinine.

Because excessive stone formation will result in progressive renal failure, therapy is directed toward preventing the formation of calculi and/or dissolving or removing those calculi that already have formed. This is achieved by reducing cystine excretion and increasing the solubility of cystine, and these are respectively accomplished by 1) dietary restriction of the essential amino acid precursor methionine, thereby minimizing cystine synthesis and ultimate excretion, 2) increasing cystine solubility by: a) increasing urine volume in order to decrease the concentration of cystine, this diuresis being achieved by a high fluid intake, particularly at night, when urine production normally is low; because many cystinurics excrete about 1000 mg. of cystine each day, in order to maintain a urinary concentration under 300 mg. per ml., fluid intake must be at least 4 liters per day. Hydration therapy has successfully prevented calculus formation in about two of every three patients adhering to this approach. b) Alkalinization of the urine with sodium bicarbonate (2–6 gm./day) or sodium citrate (Shohl's Solution, 20–60 ml./day) ingestion and the administration of carbonic anhy-drase inhibitors; however, cystine solubility doesn't increase significantly until urinary pH is greater than 7.5, which, unfortunately, is almost the maximum physiologic urinary pH that may be achieved. c) D-penicillamine ($\beta\beta$-dimethylcysteine) therapy, a drug which, through a disulfide exchange reaction, combines with cystine to form the mixed disulfide of cysteine-penicillamine, a compound that is much more soluble in aqueous solutions than in cystine. This drug also has other poorly understood mode(s) of action in effecting a decreased plasma and urine cystine concentration. The usual dose of 1 to 2 grams daily will reduce cystine urinary excretion to 200 mg. or less of cystine per gram of creatinine, thereby preventing the cystine from reaching the supersaturation levels required for stone formation. D-penicillamine also may dissolve preformed calculi.

Although D-penicillamine has been safely administered to children and pregnant women, it has many adverse side effects. Hypersensitivity reactions manifest as skin eruptions of an urticarial or morbilliform nature; lymphadenopathy, anorexia and temperature elvations are seen in about one fourth of patients on this drug. Aplastic anemia, granulocytopenia, thrombocytopenia (or any combination of these three) are less frequently encountered forms of hypersensitivity reaction. A membranous glomerulopathy that may progress to a nephrotic syndrome, a lupus erythematosus-like syndrome, bullous-type skin lesions, easily traumatized skin, myasthenic syndrome, intrahepatic cholestasis, toxic hepatitis, loss of taste, intraoral and vulval lesions, and even a fatal Goodpasture-like syndrome are other potential adverse reactions to this drug. It has been demonstrated that D-penicillamine may react with the vitamin pyridoxine, and this demands appropriate pyridoxine supplementation (25 mg./day). In addition, its chelating properties (see Wilson's disease) cause an increased urinary excretion — and potential body depletion — of metals such as zinc, copper, calcium, cadmium, mercury, and iron. It is therein obvious that D-penicillamine treatment is associated with significant morbidity — and even mortality — and, therefore, its therapeutic utilization is restricted to those cystinurics in whom the more conservative modes of therapy have failed. These patients include the habitual calculus formers, particularly those who 1) have required surgical treatment for stone extraction, 2) have already lost one kidney to the disease process, and 3) have renal functional impairment. Patients who do develop a hypersensitivity reaction to D-penicillamine will become quiescent within one week of cessation of the drug therapy. It may then be judiciously reinstituted in microgram doses that are progressively increased until previous dosages are re-established. The simultaneous deployment of glucocorticoids and even antihistamines may facilitate the reintroduction of D-penicillamine by suppressing allergic-type activity. Such patients, however, will present as glucocorticoid-dependent individuals who will require appropriate coverage during the perioperative period. Another consideration is that of a smoldering hypersensitivity state and the prudence of avoiding the use of a halogenated hydrocarbon. Indeed, a "toxic" hepatitis and intrahepatic cholestasis have both been noted during D-penicillamine therapy. N-acetyl-D-penicillamine may have fewer side effects and has been used as a therapeutic alternative to its parent compound.

In view of the pathophysiochemical events leading to cystine stone formation (the only pathological consequence of cystinuria), the major anesthetic considerations are the establishment and maintenance of a diuresis and urinary alkalinization. The surgical patient normally receives potent antidiuretic stimuli, these including the preanesthetic fast (dehydration), the normal decrease in urine flow encountered during preoperative sleep, and the stresses of the pre-, intra-, and postanesthetic (operative) periods. The kidney usually responds homeostatically to these antidiuretic stimuli by decreasing the excretion of water (antidiuresis) and salt. Several endocrinologic systems — including the sympathoadrenal and the hypophyseal–pituitary axis — mediate and regulate such renal function. Therefore, anesthetics may effect this renal activity directly and also indirectly by influencing these endocrine systems. Antidiuresis is achieved by the kidney by several mechanisms: 1) augmentation of renal vascular resistance, 2) altered autoregulation and/or distribution of renal blood flow, 3) increased influence of the antidiuretic

hormone (ADH, vasopressin), 4) stimulation of the renin-angiotensin system, and 5) modification of renal tubular transport and secretory function. The potent inhalational anesthetics, irrespective of their effect on the level of sympathoadrenal activity, all decrease renal blood flow and glomerular filtration rate and increase the filtration fraction, therein causing water and salt retention. It is now thought that the "balanced" anesthetic combinations (nitrous oxide with narcotics, barbiturates, and/or neuroleptics) have a similar effect. Because ADH decreases free water clearance by increasing water reabsorption in the collecting ducts, attention has been given to the level of ADH activity during anesthesia and surgery. Anesthetics per se appear to have no direct effect on ADH secretion, but surgical stimulation clearly produces a hyperADHemia that can account for the antidiuresis associated with surgery. Hypoxemia, hypercarbia, hypothermia, hyperthermia, hypotension, hypovolemia, hyperosmolaremia, and drugs with cholinergic or adrenergic properties are all potent stimuli for pituitary release of ADH. Deeper levels of anesthesia may nevertheless diminish the intensity of this antidiuretic state. In fact, light anesthesia coupled with potent surgical stimuli may lead to such high blood levels of vasopressin that the pharmacologic pressor activity of vasopressin in the splanchnic, renal, and coronary vasculatures may become clinically manifest.

Prophylactic and therapeutic diuresis is achieved by forced-fluid intake to greater than 4,000 ml./day (proportionately less in children) and administration of alkaline compounds. Hydration is preferably by the oral route until the compulsory preanesthetic fasting state commences, at which time one should initiate an intravenous infusion of a balanced salt solution with a pH in the range of 7. The rate of infusion initially should be approximately 200 ml./hour and should be further regulated to guarantee a generous hourly urine output. Once established, this diuresis must be maintained during and following the anesthesia and surgery by appropriate administration of intravenous solutions until the patient is able to resume oral intake sufficient to maintain the diuresis. The potent diuretic drugs (furosemide, ethacrynic acid), ethanol (an anti-ADH drug), or even mannitol may be employed to create and/or maintain the diuresis, but care must be exercised to provide adequate salt and water intake, both of which may become depleted by this pharmacologic intervention and therein counterproductively lead to an antidiuretic state several hours later. Alkalinization is achieved prior to the fasting period with ʌoral sodium bacarbonate or citrate as discussed earlier. Alkalinization of the urine by direct addition of these compounds to the blood is rarely necessary. Acetazolamide, the potent carbonic anhydrase inhibitor, will effect both urinary alkalinization (loss of bicarbonate) and promotion of diuresis, but its use should be of an acute nature and only when the more conservative measures have failed.

Because these patients are prone to develop urinary tract infections, unless clearly indicated, catheterization of the bladder for monitoring urinary output should be avoided unless the duration of the surgical procedure predisposes to bladder distention and/or the patient is unable to void spontaneously within a reasonable period of time following termination of the anesthetic. Therefore, the duration of regional anesthetics should closely approximate the anticipated duration of the operation, and general anesthetics should be managed so as to allow the patient to be able to spontaneously void within a relatively short time following the termination of the anesthetic. Whenever possible and appropriate, the surgeon should intraoperatively empty the bladder during the latter stages of the operation.

Cystinurics who are receiving penicillamine therapy must be screened preanesthetically for all the possible side and adverse effects of this drug that have been discussed above. This should include a complete blood count, liver function tests, complete urinalysis, and chest roentgenogram. In addition, the skin should be evaluated for likelihood of damage by mask (friability, skin lesions present), and the patient should be informed that a small white papule might form at the venous cannulation site. A test dose of a nondepolarizing muscle relaxant should be administered intravenously prior to induction of anesthesia to evaluate any tendency toward a myasthenic syndrome. The development of a significant temperature elevation following induction of anesthesia should be considered to represent malignant hyperpyrexia until proven otherwise, but in those patients receiving D-penicillamine, particularly in the second to third week following initiation of this drug, this hyperpyrexia might indeed represent a drug fever reaction.

The anesthetic considerations for the management of a cystinuric with advanced renal dysfunction or renal insufficiency are discussed elsewhere.

PHENYLKETONURIA

Phenylalanine is an essential amino acid and the precursor of the amino acid tyrosine and is therefore necessary for the normal synthesis of protein. Figure 1–2 depicts the normal and alternate pathways of phenylalanine metabolism. The conversion to tyrosine is irreversible and dependent upon the enzyme phenylalanine hydroxylase. This reaction occurs only in the liver, kidney, and pancreas. Phenylalanine hydroxylase is an iron-containing dimer with a molecular weight of 100,000, and several isoenzymes have been identified. The obligatory cofactor for its activity is tetrahydrobiopterin. Figure 1–3 summarizes the cofactor transformations necessary for aerobic phenylalanine hydroxylation. After the dihydrobiopteridine is enzymatically reduced to tetrahydrobiopterin, the latter shuttles to and from the quinonoid and tetrahydro forms via the NADH-dependent dihydropteridine reductase pathway. The product of phenylalanine hydroxylation is tyrosine, which is the precursor of the catecholamines, thyroid hormone, melanin, and various biogenic amines. The phenylalanine not hydroxylated to tyrosine is normally metabolized to phenyllactic, phenylacetic, and phenylypyruvic acid derivatives that are excreted in the urine.

Because of a genetically determined (autosomal recessive transmission) absence of phenylalanine hydroxylase, the classic phenylketonuric patient cannot convert phenylalanine to tyrosine (which, in essence, becomes an essential dietary amino acid), and consequently a hyperphenylalaninemia will occur. Hyperphenylalaninemia may be caused not only by the complete absence of the phenylalanine hydroxylase but also by 1) gradations of defective phenylalanine hydroxylase and 2) other enzyme

PHENYLALANINE METABOLISM

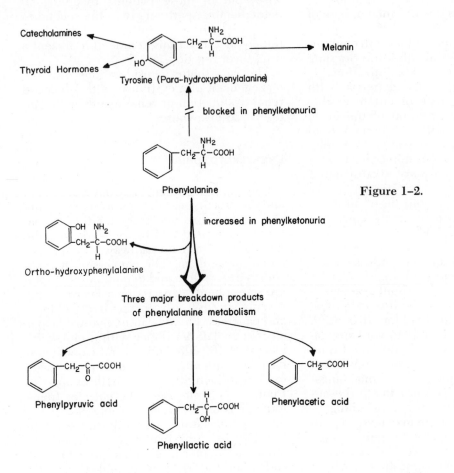

Figure 1–2.

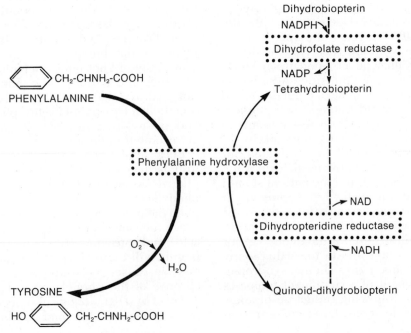

Figure 1–3. Conversion of phenylalanine to tyrosine and associated cofactor transformations.

defects that effect a secondary hyperphenylalaninemia (Table 1–6). Therefore, although classic phenylketonuria is only one of numerous hyperphenylalaninemias, it is clearly the most prevalent, its incidence ranging from 1:40 live births in certain gypsy populations to 1:7000 in West Germany and England to 1:15,000 in Japan and North America. This section will be limited to a discussion of classic or Type I phenylketonuria.

The phenylketonuric patient accumulates phenylalanine in the body, and the urinary excretion of this amino acid increases. The simultaneously increased utilization of the normal degradative metabolic pathways results in an elevated urinary excretion of these normal metabolites. The elevated tissue levels of phenylalanine and its metabolites have numerous biochemical sequelae, the underlying mechanisms involving the inhibition, to varying degrees, of a large number of enzymatic systems. For example, tyrosinase, an enzyme involved in melanin synthesis, is inhibited and probably explains the decreased pigmentation of affected individuals. Decreased blood catecholamine levels have been predicted and detected. In the central nervous system, tyrosine is a precursor of the key biogenic amines dopamine and norepinephrine. In addition, the transport and metabolism of the amino acid tryptophan is adversely affected, and there is a secondary alteration of the metabolism of the cerebral amine 5-hydroxytryptamine (serotonin), a tryptophan derivative.

Indeed, the major pathology in phenylketonuria is located in the brain; however, little is known about the mechanism by which brain development and function are disturbed. It is noteworthy that the brain of a fetus with phenylketonuria develops normally in intrauterine life even though there is a complete absence of fetal hepatic phenylalanine hydroxylase activity. Normal fetal liver has been demonstrated to have such activity as early as the seventh week of gestation. The most critical period of the growth and development of an infant's human brain occurs within the first six months of life. Because there is only a modicum of cerebral cell division beyond this time, the vast majority of further growth occurs by increments in the protein, DNA, and lipid content of these cells. Myelinization is not completed until the sixth year of life, and the major pathological finding in phenylketonurics is diffuse and/or focal demyelinization. It is unknown how phenylalanine excess impairs the complex process of myelinization, which involves stepwise elaboration of complex lipids and their lamination in lipoprotein layers about the nerves. Whereas the primary abnormality is defective myelinization, it has been suggested that the myelin so formed may be defective and prone to premature breakdown. In some fashion the immature brain, presented with an abnormal and deficient pattern of amino acids, cannot correctly construct its essential and permanent structural components as well as appropriate amounts of its pharmacodynamic amines. This abnormal biochemical environment effects an arrest of proper growth and differentiation of the central nervous system, and mental retardation results. However, once cerebral maturation has been completed (six years), hyperphenylalaninemia and its sequelae theoretically — and in practice (see dietary management) — have no adverse effect on

Table 1–6   *Hyperphenylalaninemias – Phenylketonuria and Its Variants*

Disorder	Enzymatic Disorder
Phenylketonuria	Absent phenylalanine hydroxylase
Transient neonatal hyperphenylalaninemia	Immature liver with delayed production of phenylalanine hydroxylase
Persistent hyperphenylalaninemia	Decreased phenylalanine hydroxylase
Dihydropteridine reductase deficiency	Decreased dihydropteridine reductase
Abnormal dihydropteridine reductase function	Abnormally functioning dihydropteridine reductase
Transient neonatal tyrosinemia	Immature liver with delayed maturation of para-hydroxyphenyl pyruvic acid oxidase
Hereditary tyrosinemia	Diminished para-hydroxyphenyl pyruvic acid oxidase
Transaminase deficiency	Decreased phenylalanine transaminase

further intellectual function or emotional development.

Phenylketonuric neonates are normal in appearance, but within the first four months of life they present vomiting, irritability, musty body odor, and/or eczema. The vomiting of early infancy has even led to surgery for suspected pyloric stenosis. The eczema occurs only in about 25 per cent of untreated infants. There is a progressive loss of hair and skin pigmentation, and the skin is easily traumatized. The musty body odor usually develops within the first three months and is caused by the phenylacetic acid in the sweat of those infants that tend toward hyperhidrosis. With increasing age, however, the key clinical manifestation, mental retardation, usually becomes obvious. Without appropriate therapy, the infant loses about 50 IQ points during the first year of life. Although about 25 per cent of such children have no detectable neurologic abnormalities, the remainder may have a wide range of findings, including hyperreflexia, muscular hypertonicity, unusual body motions, and behavioral abnormalities. One third to one half of the untreated phenylketonuria infants will develop seizures (grand and/or petit mal), but almost all will have an abnormal electroencephalogram. After the first year of life, other abnormalities noted include further delay of psychomotor development, microcephaly, prominent maxilla with widened interdental spaces, enamel hypoplasia, and decalcification of long bones.

Early detection and early initiation of a diet containing very low amounts of phenylalanine is mandatory for successful preventive therapy. The foundation upon which this low-phenylalanine diet rests is Lofenalac or PKVard formula, which is the primary source of protein. It is supplemented with fruits, vegetables and cereals. The diet is regulated to maintain blood phenylalanine levels between 3 and 10 mg./100 ml. Excessive restriction of phenylalanine may result in elevated blood phenylalanine levels due to tissue protein catabolism. Blood phenylalanine levels less than 3 mg./100 ml. have resulted in reduced growth and development, retarded bone age, frequent infections, hepatomegaly, hypoglycemia (possibly related to reduced catecholamine synthesis), and various neurologic sequelae. The upper phenylalanine blood level of 10 mg./100 ml. is open to question, as concentrations up to 20 mg./100 ml. have been associated with normal intellectual development. This dietary regimen is supplemented with a wider range and variety of foods as the child grows older, but these supplements ultimately are regulated by the blood phenylalanine levels. The current practice is to discontinue dietary regulation at the age of eight because hyperphenylalaninemia beyond this point of growth and development has no further detrimental effect on the brain, either intellectually or emotionally. However, because of the high percentage of congenital anomalies and intrauterine growth retardation and microcephaly detected in the fetuses of pregnant mothers with phenylketonuria and the apparent relationship of said abnormalities to maternal phenylalanine blood levels, there is concern that female patients should continue dietary treatment throughout their reproductive years. Dietary regulation is so effective that it will return a large percentage of abnormal electroencephalograms to normal. In addition, within several months of institution, seizure activity may even be controlled by diet alone.

The absence of specific signs of phenylketonuria in early infancy and its consequent devastating sequelae have prompted worldwide mass screening procedures for hyperphenlalanimeia or its metabolites in blood or urine. The older use of the ferric chloride reaction with urinary phenylpyruvic acid has gradually been replaced with the more sensitive determinations of blood phenylalanine levels within the first 72 hours of neonatal life in most states. Because 10 per cent of phenylketonuric individuals are missed at this time, repeat testing has been advised at the age of four to six weeks. Table 1–6 summarizes the variants of classic phenylketonuria that these mass screening procedures have uncovered and portrays the breadth of genetic metabolic heterogenicity for just one amino acid, phenylalanine. Infants without classic phenylketonuria may neither need nor benefit from the classic dietary therapy.

The early detection and proper dietary management of the phenylketonuric state have beneficially altered the clinical spectrum of central nervous system sequelae of this disease. In order to evaluate the adequacy of, and adherence to, dietary therapy, blood phenylalanine concentration may be determined within 72 hours of an electively scheduled operation for all phenylketonuric children until eight years of age. Excessive phenylalanine levels might predispose to epileptogenic activity and abnormal neurological and/or emotional behavior. Abnormally low levels might lead to hypoglycemia, hepatic dysfunction, and aberrant neurological and/or psychological activity. In an elective surgical setting, assessment and assurance of proper management and regulation of the phenylketonuric infant's or child's diet is of paramount importance for long-term normal functioning of the brain. Care should be taken not to create an excessive period of preoperative fasting, which would bring on a catabolic state characterized by tissue protein breakdown and consequent elevated blood concentration of phenylalanine. Therefore, these patients should be placed first on the elective surgical schedule.

The less fortunate phenylketonuric patients are, to varying degrees, mentally retarded. As such, preoperatively, the anesthesiologist may be unable to communicate with the patient and thereby fail to establish any significant humanistic relationship. The results of attempts to sedate such a retarded individual preanesthetically are quite unpredictable: the patient may be excessively depressed by normal or subnormal doses of tranquilizers, narcotics or hypnotics, or, on the other hand, may become excited and unmanageable. Large doses of premedicants have their obvious sequelae and may persist through the postanesthetic period. Therefore, premedication with only an anticholinergic drug is advised. Glycopyrrolate is a highly polar quaternary-ammonium anticholinergic compound that is more restricted in its passage across the blood-brain barrier than are the nonpolar tertiary amines atropine and scopolamine. Glycopyrrolate, therefore, is less likely to affect central nervous system function in these sensitive individuals who already possess abnormal central nervous system metabolism and altered neurotransmitter activity.

In infants and children it is probably most practical to proceed with an inhalational anesthetic utilizing nitrous oxide-oxygen-halothane for both induction and maintenance, thereby allowing for both a maximally controllable anesthetic and opportunity for rapid recovery and resumption of a therapeutic diet (when possible). An intravenous infusion of glucose should be initiated after induction to minimize the potential for the development of a fasting-induced catabolic state. Intravenous glucose administration must be continued postanesthetically until oral caloric intake is adequate. In older children and adults no longer requiring dietary management, it usually is more practical to induce aneshtesia via the intravenous route. There is no described abnormality of any organ other than the brain, and, as such, the choice of anesthetic drugs is to be influenced only by the aforementioned considerations. For those unfortunate individuals who already have developed central nervous system sequelae of phenylketonuria the major anesthetic management objectives remain: prevention of development of a catabolic state and rapid reinitiation of any therapeutic diet and medication.

General anesthesia is, of course, of therapeutic benefit for patients with seizure disorders. However, after emergence from anesthesia, these seizure-prone phenylketonurics would again be prone to developing a seizure, especially when the longer-acting barbiturates or diazepam have been omitted from the anesthetic technique. Therefore, if the patient has been receiving anticonvulsant therapy, the same or equivalent regimen should be continued throughout the day of the anesthetic. Frequently, this will involve substitution of parenteral for oral drug preparations during the pre- and postanesthetic periods in which the patient is to have nothing by mouth and/or is prone to emesis. Should the oral anticonvulsant be unavailable in parenteral form, an appropriate parenteral dose of phenobarbital (or other appropriate drug) may be substituted unless there is a history of hypersensitivity, excitement, and/or hyperactivity associated with barbiturate treatment. Anesthetic drugs with known epileptogenic properties, such as pentazocine, ketamine, enflurane, phencyclidine and gamma-hydroxybutyrate, should not be administered. Because it lowers the seizure threshhold, hypocarbia must be avoided and normocarbia confirmed by direct measurement or captographic analysis. Electroencephalographic monitoring for seizure activity, if available, would be an element of optimal management.

The phenylketonuric afflicted with epilepsy will have a prescribed schedule of anticonvulsant medication. A proper medical history should determine patient adherence to this schedule and its effectiveness in controlling the seizure activity. If the seizure activity has not been satisfactorily controlled, the drugs and/or their dosages should be adjusted and their efficacy evaluated, preferably prior to the realization of an elective operation. In the inadequately controlled individual, blood levels of the anticonvulsant drugs will determine whether the therapeutic range has been achieved. Even in the well-controlled patient, this information will be of value from the point of view of proximity to toxic concentrations. It is important to be aware of the toxic manifestations of the anticonvulsant drugs being administered to the phenylketonuric. For instance, phenytoin, perhaps the most commonly employed of these drugs, may produce nystagmus, ataxia, slurred speech, and even mental confusion in the lower toxic blood concentrations. Gross overdosage, as may be encountered during intravenous phenytoin administration, may involve significant central nervous and cardiovascular depression. Phenytoin also causes gingival hyperplasia, and these patients often have accompanying poor dentition. Phenytoin has the potential to cause bone marrow depression and hepatocellular injury. When the anesthetist changes phenytoin administration from the oral to the intramuscular route, there may be a decrease of the drug's blood level, because it is a highly insoluble compound that is much more slowly absorbed from intramuscular areas than from the gastrointestinal tract. Therefore, in the patient who is not expected to resume oral medications within 24 hours, it is recommended that the substitutive intramuscular phenytoin dose be increased by about 50 per cent over the previously established oral dose. Likewise, postoperative reinstitution of oral phenytoin must consider the continuing absorption from previous intramuscular injections.

Primidone is another frequently employed anticonvulsant which is metabolized to phenobarbital and phenylethylmalonamide, all three compounds possessing anticonvulsant activity. In the absence of a parenteral form of primidone and its known metabolic fate, any of the longer-acting barbiturates will be a satisfactory substitute.

It is to be noted that the major anticonvulsant drugs are enzyme-inducing agents and, as such, have considerable influence on the metabolism of anesthetic drugs from both the dose-effect and toxic biotransformational points of view.

Body temperature should be carefully monitored and precautions taken to prevent the development of hyperthermia, which, in conjunction with severe acidosis, has been implicated etiologically in seizures under anesthesia. Those phenylketonurics who are hypertonic preanesthetically are not more prone to malignant hyperpyrexia because the basic disorder is not of one of the neuromuscular mechanism but rather of the central nervous system.

Because of the tendency to develop hypoglycemia (which may enhance the epileptic state), the blood glucose level should be monitored (see section on hypoglycemia), and in infants the intravenous solution should contain at least 10 per cent glucose. For those phenylketonuric patients who require hyperalimentation, the commerically available amino acid containing intravenous solutions contain too high a concentration of phenylalanine. Therefore, they are to be employed only when clearly indicated and with frequent monitoring of the blood phenylalanine concentration.

The anesthetist must be aware of the sensitive skin of these patients, particularly when applying tape and using a face mask. Other specific anesthetic management considerations for these patients include brittle dentition and bones and the possible presence of anatomic airway abnormalities.

Although unrelated to the hyperphenylalaninemic disease states, it is worthwhile from a completeness viewpoint to mention the recent introduction of the use of D-phenylalanine as an analgesic-like drug. This dextrorotatory form of phenylalanine inhibits the enzymes that normally degrade the enkephalins which are endogenous morphine-like compounds.

WILSON'S DISEASE

Copper is an inorganic nutrient that is essential for human life; however, it is required in quantities that are minute when compared with calcium, phosphorus, and iron. The normal adult body contains only 75 mg. of copper. Only one third of the dietary requirement is absorbed from the intestine. In this energy-requiring process copper is attached to a metal-binding protein (metallothionein) originating from the intestinal mucosa, and then this complex is transported across the intestinal wall into the blood. Serum albumin strongly binds copper and is the major hematological transport molecule; copper also binds to various peptides and amino acids (particularly histidine and threonine). Although these latter relatively tightly bound copper complexes constitute only a very small percentage of the plasma copper, they assume major therapeutic importance because they are in exchange equilibrium with similarly bound copper and copper complexes residing in tissues. The liver is the main organ that takes up the transported copper, and hepatic copper may then undergo one or two metabolic fates: 1) it is incorporated into the globulin glycoprotein, ceruloplasmin, as this protein is synthesized, and ceruloplasmin is then released into the blood (normal concentration is 30 mg./100 ml.) wherein 90 per cent of plasma copper exists in this metalloprotein form, or 2) the liver may excrete copper into the bile, this being the normal body's predominant route for copper excretion. Unlike the copper complexes heretofore elaborated, the copper of ceruloplasmin is an integral constituent of the molecule, and, therefore, *not* in dissociative equilibrium with the remaining 10 per cent of the plasma copper; it is released only during the natural decay of the molecule. The exchangeable copper present in the body tissues and extracellular fluids is loosely complexed to amino acids or peptide-type molecules. Therefore, decoppering drugs may bind this dissociable copper (only 2 per cent of the total body copper) and upon urinary excretion increase the body's excretion of copper by as much as 20 times. The true tissue cuproteins in which copper is firmly integrated into the molecule both structurally and functionally include cytochrome C oxidase, superoxide dismutase, monoamine oxidase, and tyrosinase. Ceruloplasmin itself is also an oxidase that facilitates the transfer of electrons from various substrates to molecular oxygen and the conversion of ferrous iron to ferric iron. It is the former activity as it relates to various biogenic amines that has implicated ceruloplasmin as having a critical role in the normal biochemistry of the central nervous system. In this regard, it is of note that its oxidase activity is modified by the tricyclic antidepressants and phenothiazine-like drugs. The copper present in intracellular cytoplasm is largely bound to metallothionein.

Copper deficiency and excess (toxicity) states are rare. Copper deficiency occurs in Menkes' syndrome and may be encountered in long-term parenteral alimentation, malabsorption-like states, nephrotic syndrome, and malnutrition. Cuprotoxicity has been described in renal hemodialysis, the toxicity being related to inhibition of microsomal ATPase and several glycolytic pathway enzymes.

Wilson's disease is an autosomal recessively transmitted disorder of copper metabolism in which there is an accumulation within specific tissues, such as liver and brain, of toxic amounts of copper. There is no proven hypothesis as to the primary genetic defect. The rate of hepatic ceruloplasmin synthesis is diminished, and because the apoceruloplasmin is of normal composition and present in normal quantities, the blockade appears to be at the level of the incorporation of copper into the molecule. However, only 95 per cent of affected individuals have hypoceruloplasminemia, and some of the asymptomatic heterozygote carriers have hypoceruloplasminemia. In addition, there is no correlation between the degree of impairment of ceruloplasmin synthesis and the copper content of affected organs, and when appropriate drug therapy effects clinical improvement, even further depression of serum ceruloplasmin levels is noted. Estrogen administration may increase serum ceruloplasmin, but fails to alter the clinical state.

The gastrointestinal absorption of copper is entirely normal. There is, however, a severe inhibition of the biliary excretion of copper that is quantitatively sufficient to account for the positive copper balance in these patients. Biliary excretion is unrelated to serum ceruloplasmin concentrations. It is, indeed, possible that there is a primary genetic defect in the regulatory mechanism for biliary excretion of copper.

The clinical manifestations of Wilson's disease are variable with respect to 1) age of onset, 2) organ preference(s), 3) intensity of pathophysiologic activity, and, 4) chronologic course. The initial presentation is most commonly encountered in the second and third decades of life although the range is from the first to the fifth decades. With increased diagnostic acuity and index of suspicion an enlarging number of genetically affected individuals are being diagnosed at the early end of this spectrum.

Three organs are classically affected: 1) *Liver*—this may be the sole presenting pathology. An initial hepatosplenomegaly is associated with hepatocellular injury that may assume an acute, subacute, or chronic course. There is a progression to cirrhosis, esophageal varices, and/or ascites that may culminate with hepatic failure and death. The hepatic laboratory profile reflects the extent of liver damage, and, accordingly, during the initial stages of the disease there may be only minimal a) elevations of the hepatospecific enzymes such as the serum glutamic-pyruvic transaminase (SGPT) and gamma glutamyl transpeptidase (GGT), b) prolongation of the prothrombin time, or c) increased sulfobromophthalein retention. In some cases the clinical-pathologic picture assumes that of the alleged post-halothane hepatitic syndrome. The onset of hepatic encephalopathy has been confused with neuropsychiatric manifestations of Wilson's disease. 2) *Brain* —tremors of the upper extremities (pseudosclerosis) and a dystonic syndrome (lenticular degeneration) characterized by rigidity, painful spasticity, dysphagia, inability to control oral secretions, and dysarthria are the two most frequent neurological sequelae. Intellectural function is preserved, but psychological problems are often present and may even be the presenting symptom. Indeed, even schizophrenic behavior has been the harbinger of clinical symptomatology. Although uncommon, epilepsy may be a dramatic addition to the wide array of neuropathology. 3) *Cornea* — pathognomonic of this disorder is the development of green-brown, copper-containing Kayser-Fleischer rings at the margin of the cornea near the limbus. These consist of granular deposits in the inner surface of the cornea in Descemet's membrane that may be detectable only by slit-lamp examination. However, they may not be present in the very young patient with the pure hepatic presentation.

Patients with Wilson's disease may develop a hemolytic anemia. In the patient with advanced liver disease this anemia is chronic, of minor magnitude, and homeostatically compensated. However, severe acute episodes that are unrelated to — or even *precede* — any of the above triad may occur and be of life-threatening proportions. As in acute copper toxicity, this hemolysis is thought to be caused by a hypercupremic inhibition of erythrocyte glycolytic enzymatic systems. Another source of potential morbidity or even mortality is that of extreme fevers of unknown origin, as are often seen in the late stages of this disease.

Although not usually of clinical significance, generalized renal dysfunction is almost universally demonstrable at the laboratory level: decreased creatinine clearance, hematuria, aminoaciduria, defects in acidification and concentration, glycosuria, uricosuria, and proteinuria as well as the diagnostic hypercupriuria.

The clinical diagnosis of Wilson's disease incorporates any or all of the wide spectrum of clinical manifestations discussed heretofore. Because universally effective drug treatment modalities do exist, it behooves the physician to detect the presence of this disorder not only in the symptomatic person but also in the asymptomatic (pre-prodromal) individual. The pathognomonic corneal changes may not develop until the second or even third decade of life. In any event, laboratory confirmation is mandatory.

Normal neonates have physiologically low concentrations of both serum ceruloplasmin and copper, but these values increase to 40 mg. and 140 μg./100 ml. respectively during the first two years of life, after which they gradually decrease to the adult levels of 30 mg. and 110 μg./100 ml. respectively. Because hypoceruloplasminemia (30 mg./100 ml.) is 1) not present in 5 per cent of patients with Wilson's disease, 2) may be present in the asymptomatic heterozygote carrier, and, 3) may be encountered in malnutritive and malabsorptive states, hereditary tyrosinemia, protein-losing enteropathy, and nephrotic syndrome, the presence of hypoceruloplasminemia is *not, per se,* diagnostic. Similarly, hypocupremia is usually, but not inevitably, present. There is an increase in the serum concentration of nonceruloplasmin-bound copper, but as this represents only a modicum of the total serum content, when hypoceruloplasminemia is present the total serum content usually is reduced.

A hypercupriuria of 100 μg./day always is present (normal is 40 μg./day) and increases dramatically with initiation of decoppering drug therapy. Liver biopsy demonstrates a large increase in copper content, but similar values are obtained with chronic cholestatic conditions. It is of interest that copper deposition is widespread in the brain, but is most prominent in the basal ganglia. Although the neurons are histopathologically affected, copper is predominantly located in the glial cells.

Treatment involves 1) decreasing the amount of absorbable alimentary tract copper by eliminating those foods that have high copper content and by ingesting copper-binding sulfides, and 2) removal and excretion of excessive tissue copper. The first significant human decoppering drug was 2,3-dimercaptopropanol. Its drawbacks included painful intramuscular administration and frequent adverse drug reactions. A more effective oral medication with significantly fewer side effects is D-penicillamine ($\beta\beta$-dimethylcysteine). The usual dose is one to two grams daily for patients over 10 years of age (including pregnant women), proportionately smaller doses being prescribed for younger children. Clinical improvement may not be noticeable during the first weeks of therapy, albeit the urinary excretion of copper will markedly increase. Reversal of the disease syndrome is gradual and usually complete except for those cases in which treatment is initiated during an advanced stage of organopathology. D-penicillamine therapy may be monitored by measuring the increase in urinary copper excretion (1,000 μg./day). When the body's excess copper stores have been effectively diminished, the hypercupriuria will likewise diminish. Unfortunately, D-penicillamine is not without potentially significant adverse reactions. Within the first week of therapy, about one fourth of patients will develop a hypersensitivity reaction characterized by fever, lymphadenopathy, anorexia, and various dermatologic lesions of an urticarial or morbilliform nature, and there may even be pancytopenia, although granulocytopenia and thrombocytopenia are most commonly seen. Cessation of the drug usually effects quiescence of this hypersensitivity activity within a week, and the drug is then judiciously reinstituted in microgram dosages followed by progressive increments until previous doses are reestablished. The simultaneous deployment of glucocorticoid—and even antihistamine—drugs may facilitate the reintroduction of penicillamine. Therefore, such patients may present themselves to the anesthetist as adrenal-suppressed individuals requiring glucocorticoid coverage during the intra- and postanesthetic periods. The existence of a smoldering hypersensitivity state might be a consideration concerning the utilization of a halogenated hydrocarbon. In addition, a "toxic" hepatitis and intrahepatic cholestasis also have been encountered during D-penicillamine therapy. Because D-penicillamine does have some of the anti-pyridoxine activity that its L-isomer possesses, 25 mg./day pyridoxine should accompany D-penicillamine treatment. Pyridoxine is therapeutic should an optic neuritis occur.

Nonhypersensitivity-related dermatologic complications include desquamative processes, easy friability, and bullous-type lesions. Various intraoral and vulval lesions may also appear, and the sense of taste often is impaired. Occasionally more serious and potentially lethal adverse reactions to D-penicillamine may necessitate its cessation: a lupus erythematosus-like syndrome, membranous glomerulopathy that may progress to a nephrotic syndrome, and Goodpasture's syndrome. Finally, the chelating properties of D-penicillamine are not confined to copper, and include zinc, mercury, iron and cadmium, thereby providing for a potential deficiency of these metals.

A newer and possibly less toxic decoppering drug, triethylene tetramine dihydrochloride, awaits fuller clinical evaluation. Liver transplantation is to be considered only in those individuals unable to tolerate decoppering therapy.

Both the variable intensity and organ involvement of the disease and the response to drug therapy require that the anesthetic management be adapted to the specific individual to be anesthetized. If the patient is psychologically normal, routine premedications may be administered. This would be modified only in the patient with severe hepatic dysfunction wherein drug detoxification may be impaired. Many of these patients are, however, psychologically abnormal. In such cases, the preoperative visit may assume significant importance in the preanesthetic management and might even obviate the requirement for any premedication. On the other hand, the preanesthetic visit may be of limited success and the patient's supratentorial reaction to premedicant drugs could be unpredictable, with possible excessive depression or excitation from routine doses. The highly polar quaternary-ammonium anticholinergic drug glycopyrrolate is preferred to the nonpolar tertiary amines atropine and scopolamine because it does not cross the blood-brain barrier and, therefore, would be less likely to adversely affect an already aberrant central nervous system function.

In the choice of anesthesia one must recognize the potential for incrimination of halothane and other halogenated hydrocarbon anesthetics should hepatic function worsen postanesthetically. This consideration may be of even greater importance in the patient who displays hypersensitivity to D-penicillamine treatment. There should be clear delineation of liver function prior to the provision of anesthesia: SGPT and GGT are perhaps the most sensitive indicators. If possible, liver function testing should be performed once weekly for two to three weeks prior to the operation so as to establish the level and direction of any pathological liver function, which assumes an unpredictable course in Wilson's disease. Measurement of 24-hour urinary copper excretion on a proper diet in the hospital and under appropriate D-penicillamine therapy provides vital information regarding the probable level, if any, of the disease activity at a total body level.

An anesthetic technique that allows for early postanesthetic neurological evaluation without the residual influences of anesthetic drugs would be preferred in those individuals with significant neuropathology. General anesthesia is of therapeutic benefit for patients with seizure disorders. However, after emergence from anesthesia, these patients would again be prone to epileptic activity, especially if long-acting barbiturates or diazepam have been omitted from the anesthetic technique. Such patients must be carefully and preparedly monitored in the recovery room. Because the neurological pathology is largely confined to the brain, regional anesthesia is not contraindicated in the patient with Wilson's disease and, in fact, offers an appropriate

and acceptable alternative to general anesthesia.

It is of obvious importance to ensure proper dietary management in the hospital setting, but most of the patients are quite aware of those specific foods that have high copper content. The commonly used intravenous solutions do not contain copper and, as such, are of no concern. Proper handling of any steroid medications has been mentioned above. Optimal management aims at early resumption of preoperative medications, including any anticonvulsant drugs.

If the anemia associated with Wilson's disease is of a chronic, low-grade nature, then the patient suffers only from a decreased reserve of erythrocytes and is otherwise normovolemic and hemodynamically stable. The need for packed cell transfusion would be similar to that of any other basically normal individual. However, a recent hemolytic episode might result in a hemodynamically and/or hemopoietically unstable patient — possibly requiring erythrocyte therapy — and, additionally, could be an indicator of poor control of copper homeostasis. Acute hemolytic reactions during anesthesia — particularly during a blood transfusion — may present not only an acute medical emergency but also a problem in diagnosis and therapy, because general anesthesia masks the clinical presentation of such events. The first signs may include hypotension, fever, tachycardia, hemoglobinuria, or coagulopathy (abnormal bleeding). In those operative procedures wherein large blood loss is anticipated, the use of an erythrocyte-saving system and reautotransfusion would obviate the diagnostic problems that might be introduced by heterologous blood.

Those patients receiving D-penicillamine should be evaluated for, and advised of, the likelihood of injury to their skin by mask, intravenous cannula, blood pressure cuff, and even electrocardiogram electrodes. A subclinical test dose of a nondepolarizing muscle relaxant should be administered intravenously prior to anesthetic induction to ascertain any proclivity toward a myasthenic-like syndrome associated with D-penicillamine. The development of a significant temperature elevation during anesthesia must be considered to reflect a state of malignant hyperpyrexia until proven otherwise, but 1) those patients receiving D-pencillamine, especially in the second or third week of therapy, might be having a drug fever reaction, and 2) severe fevers of unknown origin are not uncommon, particularly in the advanced stages of Wilson's disease.

GOUT*

Uric acid (2,6,8-trioxypurine) is the major end product of purine (adenine and guanine) catabolism, the purines being essential components of nucleic acids and high-energy phosphorylated compounds. Uric acid possesses no physiologic function, but its low solubility in aqueous solutions is of pathophysiologic significance.

Gout is a metabolic disease that is manifested by 1) an increase in the concentration of serum uric acid (hyperuricemia), 2) recurrent attacks of arthritis in which crystals of monosodium urate are deposited in synovial tissue in and around joints, 3) renal disease in which hypertension is a common event, and 4) urate and uric acid urolithiasis.

The biochemical hallmark of gout is hyperuricemia. Because sodium is the most prevalent extracellular fluid cation, uric acid exists primarily as sodium urate. The binding of uric acid to plasma proteins is quantitatively small (0.3 mg./100 ml.) and devoid of physiological significance. A definition of hyperuricemia on a purely physiochemical basis is related to the limited solubility of sodium urate in extracellular fluid, which is about 6.4 mg. per 100 ml. It has been arbitrarily decided that hyperuricemia exists in males with a serum urate concentration of 7 mg. per 100 ml. or greater, and in females with a value of 6 mg./100 ml. or greater. There is, nevertheless, a significant overlap in the distribution of values in the 6.0 to 7.5 mg. per 100 ml. range for individuals with and without the diagnosis of gout. Automatic, multiphasic-screening laboratory determinations may produce values as much as 1 mg. per 100 ml. greater than standard, individual assays.

Hyperuricemia can arise on the basis of several mechanisms that can operate alone or in combination; increased uric acid production and decreased uric acid renal excre-

tion are the most important. Other mechanisms such as increased gastrointestinal purine absorption and increased serum binding of urate are of minor consequence in the pathogenesis of the hyperuricemia of gout.

Traditionally, hyperuricemia and gout have been classified as being either primary or secondary. The primary group includes 1) idiopathic gout in which the basic metabolic defect is essentially unknown and 2) gout associated with specific enzyme or metabolic defects. In secondary gout the hyperuricemia is part of some other acquired disorder. The difficulty with this classification is that the distinction between the two groups is often unclear. A more physiological classification is based on the 24-hour urinary uric acid excretion. On a diet essentially free of foods that contain purines, normal people excrete from 264 to 588 mg. (mean of $426 \pm$ two standard deviations) of uric acid per day. Patients who excrete more than 600 mg. of uric acid per day while on a purine-free diet are therefore classified as overproducers (or overexcretors) of uric acid. They make up approximately 10 to 15 per cent of all patients with gout. The remaining 85 to 90 per cent excrete less than 600 mg. of uric acid per day, and the overwhelming percentage are normoexcretors; that is, they excrete more than 264 mg. of urinary uric acid in 24 hours. Normoexcretors have a defect in tubular secretion of urate in which the renal proximal tubular cells require an elevated plasma uric acid concentration to achieve a secretory rate equivalent to that of normal people. This form of primary gout is labeled idiopathic because the mechanism underlying this tubular defect is unknown.

Two mechanisms are known to cause increased urinary excretion of uric acid: 1) de novo increase in the rate of purine biosynthesis and 2) excessive rate of purine nucleotide turnover.

The pathway of purine biosynthesis is shown in Figure 1–4. Attention is to be focused on the high energy compound 5-phosphoribosyl-l-pyrophosphate (PP-ribose-P or PRPP). PRPP is a substrate that combines with 1) glutamine in the presence of magnesium and amidophosphoribosyl transferase to form β-phosphoribosylamine, the first compound specific to the synthesis of purine ribonucleotides, and 2) purine

*In collaboration with Donald Silcox, M.D.

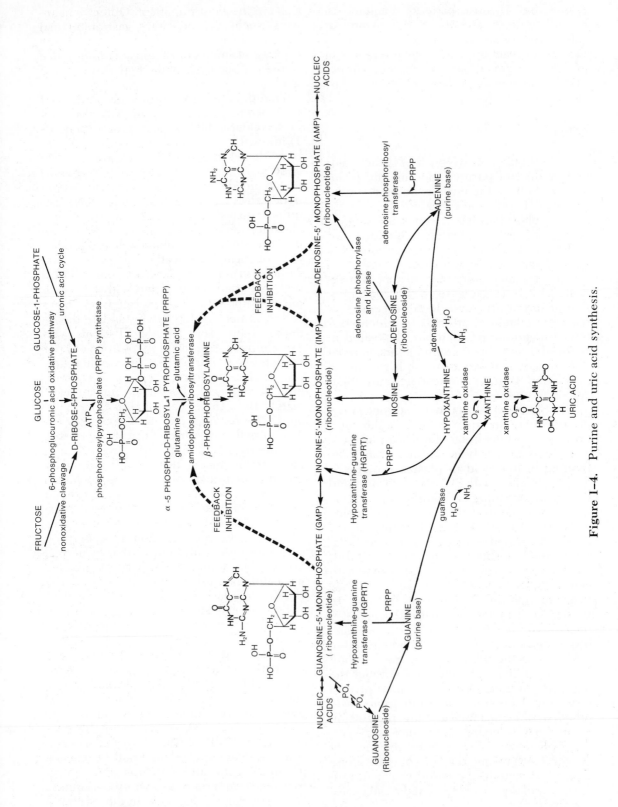

Figure 1-4. Purine and uric acid synthesis.

bases, such as guanine and adenine, to form purine-ribonucleotides as facilitated by specific phosphoribosyl transferase enzymes. The amidophosphoribosyl transferase reaction is the rate-determining reaction for purine biosynthesis, and the intracellular concentration of PRPP (substrate) is the most dominant factor in regulating the rate of this reaction. However, another key aspect to be noted is the feedback inhibition of the activity of amidophosphoribosyl transferase by the purine ribonucleotides guanosine-5-monophosphate (guanine monophosphate or GMP), adenosine-5-monophosphate (adenosine monophosphate or AMP), and inosine-5-monophosphate (inosine monophosphate or IMP). AMP and GMP are the purine nucleotide components of nucleic acids. Thus it is seen that the reaction catalyzed by amidophosphoribosyl transferase is a common step at which PRPP, glutamine and the purine ribonucleotides all may exert their role in the regulation of purine biosynthesis. The enzymes hypoxanthine-guanine phosphoribosyl transferase (HGPRT) and adenine phosphoribosyl transferase (APRT) are involved with an important salvaging mechanism for purine ribonucleotides. Only adenosine appears to have a nucleoside phosphorylase-kinase activity that is of physiological significance. Note that a deficiency of HGPRT or APRT would effect a marked increase in de novo purine biosynthesis because of the reduced amounts of "salvaged" feedback inhibitors.

To date, only three enzyme defects associated with purine metabolism are known to cause de novo increase in the rate of purine biosynthesis: 1) glucose-6-phosphatase deficiency as seen in glycogen storage disease, Type 1, 2) hypoxanthine-guanine phosphoribosyl transferase (HGPRT) deficiency, and 3) increased activity of PRPP synthetase.

In glucose-6-phosphate deficiency there is a hyperlacticacidemia and hyperbetahydroxybutyratemia, both compounds being potent depressants of renal excretion of uric acid. In addition, there is an augmented synthesis of uric acid, the underlying mechanism being an excess of intracellular carbohydrate intermediary compounds that, being unable to be released as free glucose, are converted to phosphorylated ribose compounds such as PRPP. The presence of supranormal levels of intracellular PRPP would then predispose to overproduction of purine-ribonucleotides. The hyperuricemia encountered in these individuals often is an extreme one. This disease is more comprehensively discussed in the section on glycogen storage diseases.

Virtual absence of hypoxanthine-guanine phosphoribosyl transferase (HGPRT) results in the Lesch-Nyhan syndrome, which is inherited in a sex-linked (X-chromosome) recessive manner and is characterized by early childhood uric acid uropathy, spasticity, self-mutilation, choreoathetosis and mental and growth retardation. The mechanism underlying the central nervous system dysfunction (no characteristic pathologic alterations have been detected) remains undetermined. HGPRT deficiency is also accompanied by an increased intracellular concentration of PRPP. Purine overproduction could result from the increased supply of substrate (PRPP) for the rate-limiting step in the synthetic pathway. As portrayed in Figure 1–4, HGPRT deficiency causes reduced levels of GMP and IMP, and both of these ribonucleotides are potent feedback inhibitors of purine biosynthesis. Less seriously affected patients may present in early adulthood with only spasticity, uncoordination, or even epilepsy. Heterozygote carriers are usually clinically normal, albeit mildly hyperuricemic.

Hyperactivity of PRPP synthetase is a very rare disorder that appears to be transmitted in an X-linked fashion with marked genetic heterogenicity. Increased PRPP synthetase activity may be a disordered regulatory phenomenon in which there is a resistance to feedback inhibition by purine nucleotides, or there may be a structurally modified synthetase with a supranormal biological activity. There are no distinguishing clinical features for this group of purine hyperproducers, but the gouty syndrome does appear at an early age.

The second mechanism leading to hyperexcretion of uric acid is that of excessive rate or purine nucleotide turnover. An increase in the rate of proliferation of cells of any type will increase purine (nucleic acid) synthesis and degradation, thus resulting in an increase in the urate pool that causes hyperuricemia and increased renal excretion of uric acid. This is common in myelo- and lymphoproliferative disorders, but may occur in widespread dissemination of solid cell tumors or during the chemo- or radiotherapeutic attack on any of these disorders. In acute leukemias the serum urate may be measured above 20 mg. per 100 ml. Precipitation of uric acid crystals in the renal tubules may occur and result in acute renal failure. Hyperuricemia is uncommon in chronic lymphocytic leukemia but may be present in one half the patients with chronic myelogenous leukemia.

Hyperproducers of urate usually have normal renal urate clearance, and their renal tubular secretory site responds normally to changes in their serum urate level.

Hypoexcretion of uric acid (< 264 mg./day) may be caused by plumbism and a wide variety of metabolic disturbances. Chronic lead intoxication leads to lead nephropathy characterized by granular, contracted kidneys. Creatinine clearance may only be slightly decreased in these patients, but uric acid clearance is markedly reduced, resulting in hyperuricemia and saturnine gout. Hyperuricemia occurs in uncontrolled diabetes, in starvation, and after exercise. This is due to accumulation in the serum of ketones (such as betahydroxybutyrate) and lactic acid, both causing inhibition of tubular secretion of uric acid. In fact, the serum level of uric acid correlates best with the concentration of betahydroxybutyrate. Hypothyroidism, hyperparathyroidism, and hypoparathyroidism have all been associated with hyperuricemia, probably because of reduced renal excretion of uric acid.

Drugs that may induce hyperuricemia and gout include diuretics, alcohol, aspirin in low doses, and pyrazinamide. The diuretics are the most common offenders, the ones most frequently implicated being the thiazides and ethacrynic acid. Indeed, the only diuretics that have not been implicated as a cause of hyperuricemia are spironolactone and ticrynafen (uricosuric). The mechanism of diuretic-induced hyperuricemia is at present unclear. It is probable that a prerequisite is sufficient salt and water loss to produce volume contraction. It is known that the administration of thiazide diuretics both increases the tubular reabsorption of filtered urate and inhibits the tubular secretion of urate. However, these effects do not represent a direct action on tubular transport of urate, because urate excretion remains near normal when volume depletion is prevented by replacement of urinary salt and water losses.

The relationship between overindulgence of ethanol and acute gout is well known. In addition, the daily ingestion of alcohol in significant but well-tolerated amounts (i.e., 100 mg./24 hours) may also be associated with hyperuricemia and increased urinary excretion of uric acid. It may take a number of days for the hyperuricemia and increased urinary uric acid secretion to return to normal. It is well known that hyperlacticacidemia results from the metabolism of ethanol, and the levels of lactic acid produced are adequate to suppress the renal excretion of uric acid and to induce hyperuricemia. Nevertheless, hyperuricemia and increased urinary excretion of uric acid with alcohol infusion or chronic ingestion of alcohol are not explained solely by the hyperlacticacidemia. A stimulatory effect upon purine synthesis may also be involved.

Aspirin in doses of less than 2 grams per day may increase the serum uric acid concentration. Doses in excess of 2 grams per day are generally uricosuric. This paradoxical effect is due to tubular inhibition of uric acid secretion in low doses of aspirin and inhibition of uric acid reabsorption in higher doses.

Pyrazinamide, an infrequently used antituberculous agent, is a potent inhibitor of renal tubular urate secretion. Also, its deaminated form, pyrazinoic acid, inhibits renal tubular urate secretion. Nicotinic acid (niacin), which is structurally similar to pyrazinoic acid, similarly decreases renal excretion of uric acid. Three to six grams of nicotinic acid per day will increase the serum urate concentration greater than 1 mg. per 100 ml. Nicotinic acid also stimulates purine biosynthesis. Ethambutol, levodopa, and methoxyflurane (see below) administration also have led to hyperuricemia. Fructose, by virtue of its rapid degradation to adenine nucleotides, also produces hyperuricemia.

Uric acid excretion is quantitatively determined by the amount of purine biosynthesis and is achieved mainly via the kidney. Normally about 98 per cent of the filtered urate load is reabsorbed, the nonabsorbed fraction accounting for approximately 20 per cent of the total renal excretion. The remaining 80 per cent is accomplished by distal tubular secretion of urate. The group of gout patients who are normoproducers usually have a decreased renal urate clearance because of an inability of their renal tubular secretory site to respond in a normal manner to a given serum urate level. Obviously, renal dysfunction or insufficiency due to any cause will interfere with renal urate clearance.

Renal disease is the most frequent extra-articular manifestation of gout and often antedates or is unaccompanied by arthritis. The only pathognomonic renal pathology in gout is the presence of monosodium urate crystals in the interstitium, medulla, or pyramids and an encirculating giant-cell reaction. An important factor predisposing to monosodium urate deposition in the renal medulla is a high sodium concentration: the sodium concentration is normally two to three times higher in the tip of the renal papilla than in the plasma, and with dehydration this concentration increases. Since higher sodium concentration lowers the solubility of monosodium urate, crystal deposition may occur. Because the highest concentration of urate is in the region of the loop of Henle, it is thought that the primary site of injury to the tubular epithelium is at this site. The crystals deposited in the collecting ducts are predominantly uric acid. The pK of uric acid is 5.75 and, therefore, at urinary pH of 4.5 to 5 the majority of sodium urate has been converted to uric acid, which, unfortunately, is only about 1/20 as soluble in water as is sodium urate. Uric acid crystals will spontaneously precipitate out of solution when supersaturation prevails, and supersaturation occurs when the urinary pH is less than 5.5. Thus, if urinary alkalinization is maintained at a pH above 6, most pure uric acid stone formation will be prevented. Liberal hydration with large quantities of fluids also counters the tendency to supersaturation by diluting the concentration of uric acid in the urine. There is a strong correlation between the clinical severity of gout and the extent of hyperuricemia with the amount and severity of histopathological changes in the kidney.

Acute uric acid nephropathy is not uncommon in the myeloproliferative and lymphoproliferative disorders and during the initial phases of chemotherapy. Acute uropathy on the basis of uric acid deposition in

patients over 10 years of age may be differentiated from other forms of acute renal failure by measurement of the ratio of urinary concentration of uric acid to creatinine: if greater than one, then uric acid nephropathy is the probable etiology. This ratio is greater than one in many normal children under the age of 10. These patients must be vigorously treated with hydration and urinary alkalinization. In severe cases wherein prompt and appropriate preventive or therapeutic efforts are unsuccessful, acute hemodialysis may be necessary.

Gouty nephropathy is most commonly a slowly progressive disorder that does not reduce life expectancy. However, the incidence of concomitant proteinuria and hypertension are each approximately 30 per cent. Renal insufficiency may ultimately develop in as many as 40 per cent of patients with gout. This correlates best with age, rather than with severity of the disease. There is no evidence that long-standing hyperuricemia per se predisposes to gouty nephropathy and chronic renal insufficiency. Allopurinol (see below) has not been shown to have any protective effect in the development of renal insufficiency in asymptomatic hyperuricemic subjects, but its use in patients who have renal deterioration has been shown to improve renal function in some cases.

There is a clear association of hyperuricemia with hypertension. The incidence of hyperuricemia in patients with hypertension ranges from approximately 25 per cent in those hypertensives without renal disease to 67 per cent in hypertensive patients on antihypertensive therapy with renal disease. In most hypertensive patients, hyperuricemia appears to be related to reduced renal clearance of uric acid. As a general rule, the hypertension found in gout patients is benign.

Patients with gout have two times the risk of coronary heart disease as those without gout. However, patients with asymptomatic hyperuricemia did not have an increased risk for coronary artery disease. Incubation of monosodium urate crystals with platelets results in rapid release of serotonin, ATP, and ADP, which indicates platelet activation and platelet aggregation. It is presently considered that platelet aggregation may be an important initiating event in atherosclerosis and thrombophlebitis.

Gout begins with asymptomatic hyperuricemia and progresses over many years, if untreated, to chronic tophaceous gout. In those patients with hyperuricemia due to a specific enzyme deficiency, asymptomatic hyperuricemia is present from birth. In the classic form of gout, affecting the patient with no known enzyme defect and with normal excretion of uric acid, the hyperuricemia begins at puberty in men but is delayed to menopause in women. This explains the rarity of clinical gout in premenopausal females. Asymptomatic hyperuricemia may last throughout the lifetime of an individual. Because the upper limit of normal for serum urate closely approximates the solubility of sodium urate in human plasma at physiologic pH, higher concentrations of urate result in supersaturation. Given the necessary pathophysiological circumstances, precipitation and tissue (cartilage, tendon, subchondral bone, and kidney) deposition will occur. The mechanism, or mechanisms, underlying the precipitation of urate crystals in a given tissue at a given time is poorly understood, but such factors as local decrease in pH, trauma, plasma urate-binding protein deficiency, cold, and relative affinity of chondroitin sulfate for urate have been implicated. Chances of an acute gouty arthritic attack increase as the serum uric acid concentration increases, but also are associated with the amount of urinary uric acid excretion. The most common initial clinical event is that of a spontaneous attack of acute gouty arthritis in a patient who has had hyperuricemia for a number of years. However, between 10 and 40 per cent of gouty subjects have nephrolithiasis before the onset of clinical gouty arthritis. The onset of clinical gout before the age of 30 is unusual and should raise the question of an underlying enzymatic defect leading to overproduction of purines.

In the first attack, involvement of a single joint is most commonly seen. The peripheral joints are more commonly affected than the proximal joints; the spine and the sacroiliac joints are rarely involved.

Acute attacks of gouty arthritis may be precipitated or brought on by a number of specific events. The most common are trauma, drug and alcohol ingestion, and surgery. Acute gout is known to occur from extended overwork of joints, as can occur when walking more than usual or that can occur with specific joints which are overused in certain occupations. The drugs that induce hyperuricemia have previously been described, but it is important to recognize that drugs which cause hypouricemia may also precipitate a gouty attack. Patients given allopurinol and probenecid without being "covered" with colchicine or a nonsteroidal anti-inflammatory drug may develop an acute attack of gout (see below). Other drugs that have been associated with precipitating attacks of gout include thiamine, insulin, and penicillin. ACTH withdrawal has also been implicated.

Patients who have hyperuricemia are at risk to develop gouty arthritis in the postoperative period; this usually occurs between the third and fifth postoperative day but may be as late as the tenth day. It is especially true in those patients with known gout who have not had perioperative colchicine or nonsteroidal anti-inflammatory drug therapy.

Chronic tophaceous gout occurs when the body is unable to dispose of urate as rapidly as it is produced. The total amount of urate in the body increases, and crystalline deposition occurs in the synovial membrane of the joints and cartilage as well as in the periarticular structures. The duration of time from the initial attack of gout to the beginning of chronic tophaceous gout averages about 11.6 years (3 to 42 years). Prior to the use of uricosuric agents and allopurinol, 70 per cent of patients developed tophi; currently this figure is only 17 per cent.

The goals of therapy of gouty arthritis are divided into two phases. First, the acute gouty attack is brought under control. Once this has been attained, appropriate antihyperuricemic therapy is instituted in order to prevent recurrences of acute gouty arthritis and the other complications described heretofore.

Colchicine remains the drug of choice in most cases of acute gouty arthritis. The drug is given orally in 0.5 mg. increments every hour until relief is obtained or side effects occur; often between seven and ten doses are required. Diarrhea frequently is produced. Intravenous colchicine may be necessary should the acute event occur in the postoperative period; 2 to 3 mg. are diluted in 20 ml. of normal saline and given slowly. With the oral colchicine, improvement is noted in 12 to 24 hours, with complete resolution by the second day. With intravenous colchicine, improvement is noted in 6 to 8 hours, and complete relief occurs within 24 hours.

Although numerous theories have been proposed to explain the therapeutic effectiveness of colchicine in gouty arthritis, ranging from depolymerization of microtubules to interference with leukocyte function, the mechanism underlying its anti-inflammatory property remains undetermined. Colchicine readily enters cells, forms reversible covalent complexes with subunit protein of microtubules, and inhibits the movement of intracellular granules and molecular complexes. Microtubules and microfilaments are present in all eukaryotic cells as essential components of the cytoskeleton and in organelles such as cilia, flagella, axopods, and mitotic spindle. As such, they are intimately involved with the molecular events underlying cytoplasmic translocation. They also are morphologically indistinguishable from the neurotubules and neurofilaments present in axons and dendrites of nerve cells, and they are probably responsible for both neuritic elongation and maintenance, albeit not for the propagation of nerve impulses. It has even been proposed that the reversible depolymerization of neuronal microtubules and/or microfilaments might be a basis for general anesthesia, but the experimental data with colchicine and halothane have failed to validate this theory. However, one logical consequence of this proposed mechanism of anesthesia is that the effects of colchicine and general anesthetics are additive, that is, patients receiving colchicine would have reduced anesthetic requirements. Indeed, colchicine is of itself a weak anesthetic and central nervous system depressant, and it potentiates the hypnotic effect of barbiturates, chloral hydrate, cyclopropane, and nitrous oxide.

The major side effect of colchicine is gastrointestinal toxicity (nausea, vomiting, diarrhea, painful abdomen), but aplastic anemia, granulocytopenia, thrombocytopenia, alopecia, respiratory depression, seizures, myopathies, neuropathies, and even ascending paralytic syndromes have been described. Importantly, hepatocellular damage has been reported and is more severe in those patients with pre-existent liver disease.

Indomethacin is another effective anti-inflammatory drug that is administered orally, beginning with 75 mg. and followed by 50 mg. every six hours, with a gradual reduction as the inflammation recedes. Phenylbutazone is also quite effective, as are the newer nonsteroidal anti-inflammatory drugs such as naproxen, ibuprofen, and fenoprofen. Unfortunately, all of these drugs possess potentially severe gastrointestinal side effects that include ulceration, acute and chronic hemorrhage, and perforation.

When monoarticular arthritis occurs, especially in a large joint, arthrocentesis is frequently effective in quickly reducing pain. Antihyperuricemic therapy should not be instituted until the acute attack of gouty arthritis is controlled because such therapy may prolong the duration of the acute attack. The anti-inflammatory drugs previously described should be utilized at a maintenance dosage at least during the initial phase of the use of hypouricemic drugs.

Despite the relative lack of importance of dietary limitation of purine ingestion, it would be wise to limit the intake of dietary nitrogenous precursors during the week prior to elective surgery.

Sustained lowering of the serum urate concentrations to levels below 6 mg. per 100 ml. prevents new urate deposition and may decrease the size of pre-existent urate deposits. The reduction of serum uric acid to appropriate levels of 5.5 mg. per 100 ml. or less can be achieved through drugs that 1) increase uric acid excretion, and, 2) decrease uric acid production. This pharmacologic intervention shifts the body's uric acid balance to a negative state. The uricosuric drugs that are widely used include probenecid, sulfinpyrazone, benzbromarone, and zoxazolamine. They block tubular reabsorption of uric acid and are indicated if the patient excretes less than 600 mg. of uric acid per 24 hours. It is important to realize that initiation of treatment with a uricosuric drug results in increased uric acid excretion and predisposes to renal calculus formation. Therefore, concomitant forced hydration and alkalization of the urine to a pH greater than 6 is necessary. Probenecid is begun in a dose of 250 mg. twice a day and increased to a maximum of 3 grams per day. The half-life of probenecid in plasma ranges from 6 to 12 hours, the duration depending on the dose, but if used in conjunction with allopurinol, its half-life is prolonged. Probenecid is rapidly metabolized by the liver. Its uricosuric effect is reduced by salicylates in low dosage; conversely, probenecid may delay the renal excretion of salicylic acid. A modest salt and water diuresis may occur and must be treated by replacement. Hepatic uptake of a number of drugs is reduced and, consequently, drugs such as indomethacin must be used in lowered dosage. The anticoagulant effect of heparin may be increased, and the activity of some antibiotics (ampicillin, nafcillin, and cephaloridine) may be reduced. Probenecid may also block the efflux of serotonin and dopamine from cerebrospinal fluid. Sulfinpyrazone, a derivative of phenylbutazone, has a high incidence of bone marrow changes.

Despite adequate trial with a uricosuric drug, one fourth of patients fail to achieve serum urate levels less than 7 mg. per 100 ml. In this group, and certainly in those individuals who excrete greater than 600 mg. per day, the addition of allopurinol is necessary. Allopurinol inhibits the activity of xanthine oxidase, the enzyme responsible for the conversion of hypoxanthine to xanthine and xanthine to uric acid (see Fig. 1–3). Xanthine oxidase is present in significant amounts only in the liver and small intestine and is capable of oxidizing purines, pteridines, and aldehydes. Allopurinol, an analogue of hypoxanthine, is the premier drug in the control of hyperuricemia accompanied by uric acid stone formation. It is metabolized to oxypurinol, which also inhibits xanthine oxidase. This blockade causes the hypoxanthine and xanthine to be reconverted to the nucleotide form, which, in turn, decreases de novo purine synthesis by 1) augmented feedback inhibition of the amidophosphoribosyltransferase reaction, and, 2) increased salvage reactions' competitive consumption of PRPP. The usual dose of allopurinol is 200 to 300 mg. per day, but may be twice as high in more severe gout. If renal function is normal, remarkable decreases in serum and urinary uric acid values occur within two days. Allopurinol itself has a half-life of only 2 to 3 hours; however, oxypurinol has a half-life of 28 hours. Clinical improvement and/or cessation of pathophysiological activity invariably occurs as the hyperuricemia is controlled to appropriate levels. When used in conjunction with uricosuric drugs, however, the urinary clearance of oxypurinol is increased, and the dose of allopurinol may have to be increased.

Allopurinol has several metabolic effects other than xanthine oxidase inhibition, but these are of little clinical consequence. However, allopurinol does interact with a number of drugs; it will prolong the half-life of drugs metabolized by hepatic microsomal cytochrome P-450 oxidizing system. Because 6-mercaptopurine and azathioprine are inactivated by xanthine oxidase, their effects are potentiated by allopurinol. Also, the effect of cyclophosphamide appears to be enhanced. Allopurinol has few side effects, the main ones being an increased incidence of acute attacks of gouty arthritis when therapy is initiated and the formation of xanthine nephrolithiasis (xanthine is also very insoluble in acid urine, the pK being 7.7), the latter situation mimicking the syndrome associated with the congenital absence of xanthine oxidase (hereditary xanthinuria).

Pseudogout also causes acute arthritis. The arthritis is due to deposition of calcium pyrophosphate dihydrate crystals in the synovial fluid. Unlike gout, there is no correlation between serum pyrophosphate and the development of an acute attack of pseudogout. Pseudogout may mimic gout, and, therefore, one may find a patient with pseudogout on a therapeutic regimen for gout. Acute attacks of pseudogout occur in the postoperative period, and colchicine is not nearly as effective in pseudogout as it is in gout. Arthrocentesis or institution of nonsteroidal antiinflammatory drugs are effective. Pseudogout is associated with several metabolic disorders, the most important being hyperparathyroidism. Approximately 10 per cent of patients with pseudogout will be found to have parathyroid adenomas. Therefore, it is imperative that a patient who has pseudogout be screened for hypercalcemia prior to surgery. Other metabolic disorders that have been associated with pseudogout include diabetes mellitus, hemochromatosis, Wilson's disease, and hypothyroidism. Differentiation between gout and pseudogout can readily be made by means of arthrocentesis and examination of the synovial fluid under polarized light microscopy.

Because both increased urinary acidity

and decreased excretion of free water increase the urinary concentration of undissociated uric acid, the critical determinant of supersaturation and stone formation, the anesthetist must guarantee an uninterrupted diuresis and urinary alkalization (avoidance of inordinate acidity). Unfortunately, the surgical patient normally receives potent antidiuretic stimuli, these including the preanesthetic fast (dehydration), the normal decrease in urine flow encountered during preoperative sleep, and the stresses of the pre-, intra-, and postanesthetic (operative) periods. The kidney usually responds homeostatically to these antidiuretic stimuli by decreasing the excretion of water (antidiuresis) and salt. Several endocrinologic systems — including the sympathoadrenal and the hypophyseal–pituitary axis — mediate and regulate such renal function. Therefore, anesthetics may affect this renal activity directly and also indirectly by influencing these endocrine systems. Antidiuresis is achieved by the kidney by several mechanisms: 1) augmentation of renal vascular resistance, 2) altered autoregulation and/or distribution of renal blood flow, 3) increased influence of the antidiuretic hormone (ADH, vasopressin), 4) stimulation of the renin-angiotensin system, and 5) modification of renal tubular transport and secretory function. The potent inhalational anesthetics, irrespective of their effect on the level of sympathoadrenal activity, all decrease renal blood flow and glomerular filtration rate and increase the filtration fraction, therein causing water and salt retention. It is now thought that the "balanced" anesthetic combinations (nitrous oxide with narcotics, barbiturates, and/or neuroleptics) have a similar effect. Because ADH decreases free water clearance by increasing water reabsorption in the collecting ducts, attention has been given to the level of ADH activity during anesthesia and surgery. Anesthetics per se appear to have no direct effect on ADH secretion, but surgical stimulation clearly produces a hyperADHemia that can account for the antidiuresis associated with surgery. Hypoxemia, hypercarbia, hypothermia, hyperthermia, hypotension, hypovolemia, hyperosmolaremia, and drugs with cholinergic or adrenergic properties are all other potent stimuli for pituitary release of ADH. Deeper levels of anesthesia may nevertheless diminish the intensity of this antidiuretic state. In fact, light anesthesia coupled with potent surgical stimuli may lead to such high blood levels of vasopressin that the pharmacologic pressor activity of vasopressin in the splanchnic, renal, and coronary vasculatures may become clinically manifest.

Prophylactic and therapeutic diuresis is achieved by forced-fluid intake to greater than 4000 ml. per day (proportionately less in children) and administration of alkaline compounds. Hydration is preferably by the oral route until the mandatory preanesthetic fasting state begins, at which time one should initiate an intravenous infusion of a glucose, nonlactate-containing solution with a pH of approximately 7 at a rate of at least 200 ml. per hour. The flow rate should be regulated to guarantee a generous hourly urine output. As discussed earlier, the presence of glucose in the intravenous solution prevents the generation of lactate and other tubular inhibitory organic acids associated with the fasting state, and the absence of lactate also avoids fostering any elevation of serum lactate levels, which at threshold concentration will inhibit renal tubular excretion of urate. Once established, this diuresis must be maintained during and following the anesthesia and surgery by appropriate intravenous therapy until the patient is able to resume an oral intake sufficient to sustain the diuresis. Intravenous ethanol, even though a potent anti-ADH drug, is contraindicated because it also leads to hyperlactatemia. For reasons discussed above, the use of the potent diuretic drugs (furosemide, ethacrynic acid) or even mannitol to create and/or maintain a diuresis in the gouty patient is counterproductive and ultimately may enhance the already pre-existent pathophysiology within the kidney.

Alkalization may be effected with oral sodium bicarbonate (2–6 gm./day) or sodium citrate (Shohl's solution, 20–60 ml./day) prior to the preanesthetic fast. Alkalization of the urine by directly alkalizing the blood is usually unnecessary. Acetazolamide, the potent carbonic anhydrase inhibitor, will bring about both urinary alkalization (loss of bicarbonate) and promotion of diuresis, but its use in gout has been infrequent.

The anesthetist should also insure continuation of gout-related drug therapy, when feasible, throughout the perioperative period. Oral medications, therefore, should be continued through the time of initiation of the fasting state, and surgical procedures are preferably scheduled at the start of the operative day (also a consideration for hydration and avoidance of prolonged fasting-starvation). It is generally accepted that the administration of colchicine to gouty patients prior to and following surgery (parenteral form is available) will minimize the high incidence of acute gouty arthritis associated with surgical procedures. Colchicine does potentiate the anesthetic effects of some central nervous system depressant drugs, but studies concerning the effect of colchicine on the minimal alveolar concentration of the halogenated hydrocarbon anesthetics remains to be determined. Finally, there should be a determined effort to resume oral medications at the earliest possible postoperative time.

The primary anesthetic considerations for gouty patients are usually dictated by factors other than their gout. The majority of such individuals are elderly and obese, and suffer from the usual cardiovascular dysfunction associated with their age and weight. Because emotional upset may precipitate an acute attack of gouty arthritis, a truly humanistic preanesthetic approach toward establishing a mutually beneficial doctor-patient relationship assumes major importance. The patient should be well-adjusted with respect to the total perioperative and hospitalization experience, and should arrive in the operating room in an appropriately relaxed state. There is no choice of anesthetic per se, but *methoxyflurane is an absolute contraindication.* Methoxyflurane is biodegraded to fluoride and oxalate, the former being a potent tubular nephrotoxin when toxic blood fluoride concentrations are achieved, and the latter offering the possibility of urinary oxalate stone formation. This biotransformation is augmented by previous exposure to inducing drugs (see section on porphyria). Hyperuricemia and reduced renal clearance of urate clearly are proven potential pathophysiologic sequelae of the administration of methoxyflurane. All of the other currently available potent halogenated hydrocarbon inhalational anesthetics are to be considered safe for use in the patient with gout, although enflurane possesses the theoretical potential for producing elevated blood

fluoride concentrations. The anesthetic considerations for those patients with renal disease are similar to those for any patient with a similar degree of renal functional impairment.

Gouty arthritic involvement of the temporomandibular joint may be present and evaluated preanesthetically because it is a potential source of difficulty in 1) achieving adequate exposure for direct laryngoscopy and endotracheal intubation, and 2) manipulating the temporomandibular joint for maintenance of an unobstructed airway.

INBORN ERRORS OF LIPID METABOLISM

The lipids present in the human represent a mixture of a variety of classes of substances and include the fatty acids, triglycerides (fatty acid esters of glycerol), phospholipids (derivatives of sphingosine phosphate and glycerol phosphate), and nonphosphorylated lipids (the steroids, the most abundant of which is cholesterol). Free fatty acids may be metabolized to provide energy, or they may be stored as a readily reconvertible energy reserve in the form of triglycerides. The phospholipids serve as essential structural components of cellular (plasma) and subcellular (mitochondrial, microsomal) membranes. These water-insoluble lipids concentrate at polar-apolar interfaces and stabilize lipoprotein structures in the basically aqueous milieu of the body. In addition to being a precursor of steroid hormones and bile acids, unesterified cholesterol is also an important component of cell membranes. The cholesterol esters are found mainly in the plasma, adrenals, and liver, but their function remains unclear.

A close interrelationship exists between fatty acid and carbohydrate metabolism. Energy is stored in the form of fatty acids when glucose is readily available to the cell (postprandial), and is derived from fatty acids when glucose availability diminishes. In fact, it has been estimated that in the basal state, free fatty acids provide as much as one-half of the caloric demands of the body.

Fatty acid metabolism is strongly influenced by hormones. Norepinephrine, released at the postganglionic adrenergic nerve endings, is more potent than epinephrine (blood-borne from the adrenal medulla) in affecting lipid metabolism in the human. These catecholamines mobilize adipose tissue triglycerides and cause release of the hydrolytic products into the circulation, thereby effecting an elevation of the levels of free fatty acid and glycerol in the blood.

The biochemical mechanism involved is as follows:

1. Norepinephrine increases the activity of the enzyme adenyl cyclase.

2. Adenyl cyclase catalyzes the conversion of adenosine triphosphate (ATP) to adenosine 3′,5′-phosphate (cyclic AMP, cyclic adenylic acid).

3. Adenosine 3′,5′-phosphate increases the activity of the intracellular enzyme lipase.

4. Lipase catalyzes the hydrolytic degradation of triglycerides to free fatty acids plus glycerol.

There is a concomitant increase in fatty acid uptake and utilization (for energy) by the vital organs and skeletal muscle. The liver may re-esterify the fatty acids and glycerol and release the triglyceride product into the blood, thereby causing a hypertriglyceridemia. Overnight fasting and/or preoperative apprehension will invariably effect such a lipid profile in an otherwise metabolically normal patient. Both alpha- and beta-adrenergic blocking drugs will partially inhibit fat mobilization from adipose tissue. Insulin, whose secretion by the pancreatic beta cells is stimulated by increased blood levels of free fatty acids (and inhibited by catecholamines), is a potent inhibitor of adipose tissue lipase and is thereby an antagonist of the fat-mobilizing properties of the catecholamines.

The actual blood levels of fatty acids may vary as much as 30-fold when the extremes of the normal postprandial state and diabetic ketoacidosis are considered, but they constitute an insignificant percentage of the total serum lipids. Free fatty acids are normally transported by albumin, but even in the analbuminemic patient, the free fatty acid serum level is only minimally diminished, their transport being handled by the lipoproteins. There is no proved disease entity that specifically involves a defect in fatty acid metabolism, although pathophysiologic effects of very high blood levels of unbound fatty acids have been suggested by several studies.

Without an interaction with specific plasma proteins only a small fraction of the water-insoluble lipids would be in true molecular solution and thereby available for blood transport. Although most plasma proteins bind little or no lipid, except for free fatty acids, apolipoproteins possess the unique property of binding from one to 12 times their weight of lipid. The apolipoprotein-lipid complex is called lipoprotein, and its structure is such that the protein and phospholipid surround other lipids in the core of the macromolecular complex. The plasma lipoproteins function to transport water-insoluble lipids in a stable colloidal form. Although both the lipid and protein compositions of the lipoproteins are in a dynamic state, there nevertheless is a characteristic composition for each of the major classes of lipoproteins: chylomicrons, very low density lipoproteins (VLDL), intermediate density lipoproteins (IDL), low density lipoproteins (LDL), and high density lipoproteins (HDL). These are characterized in Table 1–7. The lipid-free protein component of the plasma lipoproteins are called apolipoproteins, or apoproteins, and the apolipoprotein constituency of each of the major lipoprotein classes is heterogeneous. Table 1–8 summarizes the known structure and function of the major apolipoproteins.

Dietary fatty acids with an aliphatic chain length of 12 or more are rapidly reassembled into triglycerides after they enter the intestinal cells. These triglycerides and small amounts of cholesterol esters are then released into the intestinal capillary lymph as the core of chylomicrons, which are large-sized particles enclosed by a monolayer surface film composed of phospholipids, diglycerides, apolipoproteins and unesterified cholesterol. Chylomicrons function to transport dietary fats and sterols originating from the jejunum, and they are removed from the circulation within an hour. In adipose tissue and the mammary glands of lactating females, the chylomicrons are exposed to lipoprotein lipase, an enzyme that is attached to the lining of the capillary blood vessels. Most of the triglycerides are therein hydrolyzed to free fatty acids and glycerol, and there is a resultant increase in blood concentration of free fatty

Table 1-7   *Lipoprotein Properties and Composition*

	Chylomicrons	Very Low Density Lipoproteins (VLDL)	Intermediate Density Lipoproteins (IDL)	Low Density Lipoproteins (LDL)	High Density Lipoproteins (HDL)
Ultracentrifugal definition					
Density (gm/ml)	0.94	0.94–1.006	1.006–1.019	1.019–1.063	1.063–1.210
Corrected flotation rate (Svedberg units)					
at density = 1.063	400–100,000	20–400	12–20	0–12	–
at density = 1.20	–	–	–	–	0–9
Electrophoretic mobility	None	Pre-beta	Btwn beta & pre-beta	Beta	Alpha
Particle size (Angstrom units)	750–12,000	290–750	210–320	180–250	50–120
Lipoprotein constituents (% dry weight)					
Triglyceride	90	52	21	10	4
Unesterified cholesterol	2	6	8	8	4
Esterified cholesterol	3	18	37	39	16
Protein	1	8	15	22	50
Phospholipid	4	16	19	21	26
Major apoprotein constituents (in order of % dry weight)	C–I, II, III B A–I, II	C–I, II, III B E	B	B	A–I, II

Table 1-8   *Apolipoprotein Structure and Function*

Apolipoprotein	Structure	Function
A–I	Single chain polypeptide of 245 amino acids, but excluding the basic amino acid group; without glycosidic linkage	Activate lecithin: cholesterol acyltransferase (LCAT), which catalyzes the catabolism of triglyceride-rich lipoproteins after initial step of hydrolysis Regulate membrane lipid constitution Bind phospholipid Regulate membrane fluidity
A–II	Two identical polypeptide chains joined by disulfide bond	Unknown
B	Poorly characterized: molecular weight 30,000; beta structure with an alpha helix	Transport of triglycerides from liver and intestine into plasma
C–I	Single chain polypeptide of 57 amino acids	Bind phospholipid Activate LCAT
C–II	Polypeptide of 80 amino acids	Specifically activates lipoprotein lipase (which catalyzes triglyceride hydrolysis) of post heparin plasma and adipose tissue by enhancing the binding of the enzyme to a hydrophobic area of chlomicrons Note: does not activate hepatic lipoprotein lipase
C–III	Single chain polypeptide of 79 amino acids; has glycosidic linkage to a carbohydrate chain containing sialic acid	Not clearly established: possibly inhibits or inactivates lipoprotein lipase, and possibly bind phospholipid
E	Polypeptide with high concentration of arginine; molecular weight 33,000	Regulation of cholesterol transport

acids. In the fed state, most of these fatty acids enter the fat cells where re-esterification and triglyceride storage occur, but in the fasting state there is a rapid oxidation of the fatty acids. In either event, the remnants of the chylomicron metabolism now contain relatively more cholesterol esters and phospholipids, and they are removed from the circulation by the liver. The VLDL function to transport endogenous hepatic-synthesized triglycerides. The metabolic degradation of VLDL is similar to that of the chylomicrons in that the majority of triglycerides are hydrolyzed in extrahepatic peripheral tissues with the remnants ultimately extracted by the liver. The C-apolipoproteins associated with chylomicrons and VLDL are not biosynthesized by the intestinal mucosal cells; they are provided by the HDL in extra-intestinal tissues. When the chylomicrons and VLDL are catabolized, the C-apolipoproteins are retransferred to HDL. The A- and B-apolipoprotein constituents are synthesized by the intestinal cells. The B-apolipoprotein of degraded VLDL reappears in the plasma as a constituent of LDL.

The LDL are the product of the catabolism of triglyceride-rich lipoproteins and, in turn, ultimately are metabolized. The LDL function to transport hepatic cholesterol — which is derived from endogenous biosynthesis and remnant catabolism — to numerous tissues via an interaction with a specific cell surface receptor, the LDL receptor. LDL also receives cholesterol in the plasma through transfer facilitated by the enzyme lecithin-cholesterol acyltransferase (LCAT). The metabolic regulation of LDL is intimately related to the regulation of cholesterol synthesis in peripheral tissues. Cholesterol homeostasis ultimately is achieved by HDL-facilitated transport to the liver for bile excretion. HDL is synthesized both in the liver and intestine, and functions as a receptor vehicle for the transport of unesterified cholesterol derived from extrahepatic cell membranes to the liver, which is the predominant catabolizer of HDL. The cholesterol is, in turn, esterified via the LCAT enzyme system.

Hyperlipidemia is an increase in the plasma lipid concentration, and hyperlipoproteinemia is an increase in the plasma of specific lipoprotein particles. The general population displays a continuous distribution of plasma concentrations of both lipids and lipoproteins, which are measured after a twelve-hour fasting period. The uppermost five percent of these distributions have been arbitrarily designated as being abnormally elevated. The majority of these abnormal individuals have complex interactive etiologies that include multiple-gene determinations and numerous environmental (nongenetic) factors. Only 20 per cent of these hyperlipidemic or hyperlipoproteinemic individuals have a single-gene determined form of their disease. The definitive diagnosis of these individuals necessarily utilizes additional biochemical, clinical, and genetic analysis and information. In this section, we shall discuss six single-gene determined hyperlipoproteinemias. However, even among these six relatively well-defined entities there probably exists a significant degree of genetic heterogeneity, such that several types of single-gene mutations at one or more gene loci may each effect the same disorder. The normal upper limits for plasma concentrations of cholesterol and triglyceride are, respectively, 230 mg. per dl. and 140 mg. per dl. at the age of 10, and these increase to respective values of 330 mg. per dl. and 190 mg. per dl. at the age of 60. Cholesterol and triglyceride are distributed unevenly in the major lipoprotein groups: 50 to 75 per cent of plasma cholesterol is contained in LDL, 20 to 45 per cent in HDL, and 5 to 10 per cent in VLDL. In contrast, plasma triglycerides are mainly present in the chylomicrons and VLDL.

Lipoprotein lipase is a glyceryl-ester hydrolase that catalyzes the extrahepatic removal of triglyceride-rich lipoproteins from the blood. It possesses positional specificity for the primary ester bond of triglycerides and diglycerides: 2-monoglycerides must first be isomerized to 1- or 3-monoglycerides for lipoprotein lipase to be effective. This enzyme also facilitates the cleavage of the primary acyl ester bond of phosphatidylcholine. Lipoprotein lipase is most prevalent in the adipose tissue and mammary glands of lactating females (under control of the hormone prolactin), but it is also found in the heart, skeletal muscle, lung, and liver. Increase in lipoprotein lipase activity is induced by insulin and high-caloric and high-fat intake. Plasma lipoprotein lipase activity increases in response to the administration of intravenous heparin (10–100 international units/kg.) because heparin releases the enzyme from lipoprotein lipase-containing tissues. The enzyme is rapidly removed from blood by the liver. Heparin actually releases two distinct triglyceride hydrolases: 1) lipoprotein lipase, which is extrahepatically synthesized, requires C-II apolipoprotein as an activator, is inhibited by protamine and high salt concentrations, and has activity that is equipotent in chylomicrons, VLDL, and triglyceride emulsions, and 2) hepatic lipase, which is synthesized in the liver, does not require an activating apolipoprotein, is resistant to inhibitory effects of protamine and salt, and has its maximal activity in triglyceride emulsions. Lower doses of heparin effect an increase of both lipases that peak within 30 minutes and return to baseline within two hours, whereas higher doses of heparin produce an earlier peak of the hepatic lipase. Young men have higher lipoprotein lipase levels than do young women, but this sexual preference disappears with age.

FAMILIAL HYPERLIPOPROTEINEMIAS

Familial lipoprotein lipase deficiency—Type 1 hyperlipoproteinemia—is a rare, autosomal-recessive, genetically determined disease that requires two mutant alleles for phenotypic expression. It is biochemically characterized by a very low level of lipoprotein lipase activity in postheparin plasma, and this enzymatic deficiency results in severe impairment of the removal of lipoprotein particles containing dietary fat as well as a resultant massive hyperchylomicronemia and hypertriglyceridemia with concomitant decreased levels of other lipoproteins. It has not been determined whether the diminished lipoprotein lipase activity is the result of absence of the enzyme, of structurally altered enzyme with diminished or absent activity, or of deficient binding of the enzyme to the target cells. The Type 1 profile of severe hyperchylomicronemia and normal or subnormal concentrations of VLDL, LDL, and HDL may also be encountered in systemic lupus erythematosus, multiple myeloma and other dysglobulinemias, hypothyroidism, and oral contraceptive users. The serum triglyceride

concentration is very high (2,000–12,000 mg./dl.), and the plasma cholesterol may be increased when the triglycerides are > 3,000 mg. per dl.; however, the cholesterol to triglyceride ratio is approximately 1:10 and reflects the ratio of these substances in the chylomicrons. In a like fashion, the ratio of unesterified to esterified cholesterol is about 1:1 (as in the chylomicrons). Dietary elimination of fat for five days effects a disappearance of the chylomicrons, a reduction of the triglycerides to < 400 mg. per dl., and a decrease of the cholesterol to < 250 mg. per dl. On the other hand, the LDL and HDL remain unchanged at subnormal levels. Although these patients have no glucose intolerance, insulin-dependent diabetics bordering on ketoacidosis may display a Type 1 lipoprotein profile.

Both low and high dose heparin administration (10–100 IU/kg.) effect very low levels of plasma lipoprotein lipase. Assay of adipose tissue lipoprotein lipase activity similarly reveals extremely low levels of enzymatic activity. The vast majority of patients with hypertriglyceridemia and some degree of hyperchylomicronemia do not have familial lipoprotein lipase deficiency.

Clinically, the major presenting symptom is repeated episodes of unexplained abdominal pain. This pain may be variously located and of any degree of intensity, and it usually — but not invariably — is associated with excessive fat intake and hyperchylomicronemia. The abdominal pain may even be associated with fever, leukocytosis, anorexia, muscle spasm, rigidity, and rebound tenderness, and therein prompt a laparotomy, which simply reveals a milky intraperitoneal exudate. There often is an associated pancreatitis, which may explain some of the pain pattern such as radiation to the back. The pancreatitis is caused by an enzymatic autodigestion of the pancreas. Phospholipase A will, in the presence of bile salts, break down phospholipids such as lecithin in the cell membrane, and this causes the formation of cytodestructive chemicals. Serum lipase will be increased early in the attack and remain elevated for several days. The serum amylase may be spuriously normal, but urinary amylase excretion will always be elevated. Serum calcium concentration may be reduced secondary to the reaction of calcium with the fatty acids released from the retroperitoneal fat by the spilled lipase. However, in spite of repeated attacks of pancreatitis, pancreatic calcification is rare. The major sequelae of the pancreatitis include abscess and/or pseudocyst formation, fluid and electrolyte disturbances that may be of an extreme degree (due to the potential for a very large sequestration of inflammatory fluid in the retroperitoneal space), gastrointestinal and/or intraperitoneal bleeding, and disturbance of ventilation to perfusion ratios in the lung, which results in arterial hypoxemia. This latter clinical finding may be caused by a damaging of pulmonary surfactant by lipolytic enzymes released into the serum and/or by a frequently encountered hypercoagulable state and resultant diffuse pulmonary microemboli. The appropriate therapy for such patients includes: 1) correcting the hyperlipoproteinemic state (see later in this section), 2) intravenous replacement of lost fluids and colloids or blood, employing, whenever indicated, central venous lines and urine output, 3) correction of electrolyte abnormalities, 4) gastric suction and anticholinergic drugs to reduce secretory stimuli to the pancreas, 5) administration of analgesic drugs that do not cause spasm of the sphincter of Oddi, such as meperidine, 6) antibiotics as indicated, and, 7) supplemental oxygen to provide an acceptable arterial oxygen tension. Because of the often dramatic alterations in oxygen exchange that may occur over relatively short periods of time, it is important to closely monitor arterial oxygen tension.

Hepatosplenomegaly — unaccompanied by hepatic dysfunction or hypersplenism — may be detected in most patients and is caused by chylomicron accumulation in the cells of the reticuloendothelial system. About half of these patients develop eruptive xanthomas, which are acute, nontender, small yellow nodules with an erythematous base that may last for several weeks. There is no associated coronary arterial disease.

This disease has no sexual preference. The majority of affected individuals are diagnosed before the age of 10, although afflicted infants with colic and/or splenomegaly have been diagnosed in the early months of life; others have not been detected until their fourth decade. Treatment of this disorder involves dietary restriction of fats at a level of 40 to 60 gm. per day. The degree of fatty acid saturation or desaturation is not important. Medium-chain triglycerides are absorbed by the portal circulation and do not reaccumulate as chylomicrons in the circulation, and these substances are utilized as dietary supplements. The effectiveness of the diet is monitored by following the plasma triglycerides, which should decrease to the 1000 to 2000 mg. per dl. range.

Cholesterol is a major component of cell membrane. It is obtained either from intestinal absorption (entering the plasma as a constituent of chylomicrons) or from biosynthesis by tissues, primarily the liver and intestine. There is an inverse relationship between dietary and biosynthetic sources of cholesterol such that adequate dietary supplies inhibit cellular production and dietary deprivation stimulates the synthetic machinery. Dietary cholesterol is transported to the liver in the form of LDL. When received by hepatocytes, this cholesterol suppresses (feedback inhibition) the biosynthetic activity of the microsomal enzyme 3-hydroxy-3-methylglutaryl coenzyme A reductase (HMGCoA reductase), which normally facilitates the irreversible conversion of HMGCoA (derived from acetate) to mevalonate in the presence of NADPH. Mevalonate is subsequently converted to cholesterol.

Cholesterol is also manufactured in tissues other than liver and intestine, but this synthetic rate is normally very low owing to a suppression by LDL, which binds to specific *cell surface LDL receptors* and then is incorporated into the cell. The LDL apolipoprotein is hydrolyzed by lysosomal enzymes and the cholesterol ester is hydrolyzed by a lysosomal acid lipase. The resultant free intracellular cholesterol then 1) suppresses the activity of HMGCoA reductase and thereby stops cellular synthesis of cholesterol and 2) activates fatty acid CoA:cholesterol acyltransferase, which facilitates cholesterol esterification and intracellular storage. Cells saturated with cholesterol and cholesterol esters decrease their production of LDL receptor protein and therein regulate against excessive cholesterol accumulation. Thus it is clear that *the LDL cell surface receptor is the key factor in the body's cholesterol homeostasis* because it controls the degradation (clearance) of plasma LDL.

Hepatic cholesterol may be utilized in the following ways: 1) incorporation into LDL for secretion into plasma and transport to other tissues, 2) conversion to bile acids, 3) excretion into the biliary tract as neutral sterols, or, 4) esterification with long chain fatty acids into cholesterol esters and storage within the liver cells. The cholesterol transported to peripheral tissue is utilized mainly for cell membrane synthesis. Because these membranes have a high turnover rate, there is a significant excretion of cholesterol by the cells into the plasma where it is incorporated into HDL and ultimately esterified with fatty acids via the LCAT enzyme.

Familial hypercholesterolemia — Type 2a hyperlipoproteinemia — is the most common, simply inherited (mendelian autosomal-dominant, highly penetrant) genetic disorder affecting humans, with a heterozygote frequency in English-speaking countries of as much as 1 in 200 persons. These individuals have a genetically determined deficiency of the cell surface receptor that binds LDL, and this results in the absence of the normal regulatory mechanisms controlling the clearance and degradation of plasma cholesterol. Consequently, the plasma concentration of LDL cholesterol is elevated. However, familial hypercholesterolemia accounts for only a small percentage (5%) of those humans who have hypercholesterolemia caused by elevated LDL. The majority of such individuals have undefined complex interactive etiologies that are of polygenic and environmental origin.

Studies with fibroblast cell cultures from homozygotes have demonstrated that there may be two types of allelic mutations of the LDL cell receptor:molecule, functionless and defective. Either type effects decreased LDL catabolism (clearance) and transport of cholesterol into cells, with a consequent loss of suppression of HMGCoA reductase and the subsequent cholesterol biosynthesis. As a result, in spite of a plasma hypercholesterolemia, there is an inappropriate cellular overproduction of cholesterol that ceases only when the de novo intracellularly synthesized cholesterol suppresses its own synthesis.

Heterozygotes possess half the normal amount of normal LDL cell receptors. Their two- to threefold elevation of the concentration of plasma LDL results in a normal amount of LDL binding and, consequently, a normal rate of LDL catabolism and cellular cholesterol synthesis. Homozygotes have plasma cholesterol concentrations of 600 to 1200 mg per dl. and the heterozygotes average 350 mg. per dl., although there often is great variability amongst heterozygotes. This elevated cholesterol is only that within the LDL, which otherwise is of normal structure and composition. In both homo- and heterozygotes about 75 per cent of the cholesterol is in the form of cholesterol esters; phospholipids are only moderately increased, and triglyceride levels are essentially normal. Hypercholesterolemia is present at birth and, therefore, is the earliest manifestation of this disorder. The abnormal lipoprotein pattern of familial hypercholesterolemia may also be observed in hypothyroidism, hyperadrenalcorticism, acute intermittent porphyria, nephrotic syndrome, dysglobulinemias, hepatic tumors, and biliary cirrhosis, as well as in familial-combined hyperlipidemia (see below). The definitive diagnostic test is the measurement of LDL receptor functional activity in fibroblasts cultured from the affected individual.

The clinical sequelae of familial hypercholesterolemia are the result of cholesterol deposition as cytoplasmic droplets within histiocytic foam cells in various body tissues. Two of the three most prominent areas so affected are the tendons (xanthomas) and eyes (arcus cornea). In heterozygotes these lesions are initially detected in the latter part of the second decade, and they are present in half of these people by the end of the third decade. Note, however, that arcus cornea may be present in normal people, particularly in the black population. Homozygotes may have cutaneous xanthomas at birth and all will have these lesions by the fourth year. Homozygotes all develop tendon and eye pathology in childhood.

The third and only significant sequela is that of coronary arterial disease. Symptoms and signs of coronary artery disease include those of anginal syndrome, myocardial infarction, congestive heart failure, and arrhythmias; death due to myocardial disease ultimately will ensue. In homozygotes coronary artery disease is uniformly fatal within the first three decades, and generalized atherosclerotic vascular disease is commonly

‚encountered. Cholesterol accumulation in the aortic valve may even effect clinical aortic stenosis. Heterozygotes begin to demonstrate clinical evidence of coronary disease in their fourth (male) and fifth (female) decades. Fifty per cent of men will have had a myocardial infarction by the age of 50, whereas the same percentage of women will be so affected by the age of 60. The incidence of coronary problems is 25 times that of unaffected relatives.

As a result, when such a patient is to have an anesthetic, he or she is to be considered to have potentially-significant coronary arterial disease until proven otherwise. This means that even the asymptomatic individual (usually a heterozygote) must be fully investigated for the presence of any coronary disease before being brought to an elective operation. Documentation would include a thorough cardiac history, electrocardiogram, and, when indicated, a stress electrocardiogram test. Further radiographic and/or angiographic evaluation should be done when indicated, as for instance in the patient with severe ischemic changes at low work-load levels. Those patients who already possess a clinical coronary history obviously should be completely evaluated in order to specifically delineate the location and extent of coronary arterial disease and the degree, if any, of myocardial tissue damage. These individuals will often have been treated with drugs that are important considerations for the anesthetic management, as for example, beta blocking agents, vasodilators, anti-arrhythmic compounds and cardiotonic drugs (when failure is present).

Fortunately, heterozygotes do not display an increased incidence of hypertension, premature cerebrovascular disease, obesity, diabetes mellitus, or hyperuricemia, and peripheral vascular disease is much less prevalent than is coronary arterial disease.

Because there is no therapy that enhances entrance of plasma LDL into cells, the current therapeutic regimen aims at decreasing the plasma concentration of LDL-cholesterol. This therapeutic endeavor is based upon the hypothesis that a diminished plasma LDL-cholesterol either prevents or slows the process of atheroslcerosis. Dietary treatment effects a 15 per cent reduction of plasma cholesterol concentration in heterozygotes and includes a decreased dietary cholesterol intake to less than 300 mg. per day in adults (< 150 mg./day in children) and a decreased saturated-fat intake while increasing polyunsaturated-fat consumption. Note that the cholesterol esters of plasma LDL normally are rich in the polyunsaturated fatty acids (e.g., linoleate), in contradistinction to endogenously esterified cholesterol, which preferentially conjugates with monounsaturated fatty acids (e.g., oleate and palmitoleate).

Supplementation of this diet with the administration of bile acid sequestrants effects a 30 per cent reduction in plasma cholesterol, which brings the heterozygote values toward the upper limits of the normal range. Cholestyramine and colestipol (15-20 gm./day) are sequestrants, nonabsorbable anion-exchange resins that absorb bile salts in the intestinal lumen, thereby eliminating their absorption into the blood. Fecal excretion of bile salts is consequently increased, and there is a compensatory utilization of hepatic cholesterol for conversion to bile acids. Unfortunately, there normally also is a compensatory augmentation of hepatic cholesterol synthesis. Therefore, cholestyramine or colestipol increases the fractional catabolic rate of LDL without affecting the rate of LDL synthesis. Partial ileal-bypass surgery is a more drastic method for achieving the same results achieved by the sequestrating drugs.

The bile acid sequestrants also have a strong affinity for acidic drugs such as thyroid hormone, coumadin, phenobarbital, digoxin, digitalis, chlorthiazide, and phenylbutazone and, consequently, may diminish the anticipated effect of these drugs when administered orally. On the other hand, when sequestrant therapy is discontinued, there may be a sudden augmentation (even toxicity) of these drugs. These considerations are of particular importance to the anesthesiologist in that 1) digitalis toxicity or loss of digitalis effect may be encountered, 2) hypo- or hyperthyroidism may become manifest, and 3) decreased absorption of the fat-soluble vitamin K may lead to hypoprothrombinemia and the associated coagulopathy. Thus, in the patient with coronary artery disease receiving cholestyramine or colestipol, the critical balance of myocardial oxygen supply and demand may be disturbed, cardiac arrhythmias may become manifest, and regional anesthesia may be contraindicated. Therefore, preanesthetic measurement of digitalis and thyroid hormone levels as well as serum potassium and prothrombin time become imperative. Any detectable abnormalities are relatively easily corrected by adjusting drug doses, administration of supplemental potassium, and parenteral treatment with vitamin K. Folate deficiency anemia has also been reported.

Niacin (nicotinic acid) reduces both cholesterol and triglyceride concentrations in the serum. The underlying biochemical mechanism has not been determined even though niacin does possess several well-established biochemical properties. The routine dose of up to 3 to 6 gm. daily may produce cutaneous flushing, peptic ulcer, glucose intolerance, hyperuricemia, and even hepatocellular disease, all of which must be evaluated preanesthetically. Finally, because niacin may potentiate the hypotensive effects of ganglionic-blocking drugs, the anesthetist who wishes to regulate blood pressure with antihypertensive agents should avoid using ganglionic-blocking drugs, such as pentolinium and trimethaphan camsylate, or use them with extreme caution.

Because dextrothyroxine (the isomer of thyroid hormone) depresses serum cholesterol by increasing its catabolism in the liver, it has been used as a supplemental therapeutic modality. However, it also increases myocardial work and oxygen demand and, therefore, is contraindicated in those individuals who have any coronary artery disease, congestive heart failure, and/or cardiac arrhythmias. In addition, dextrothyroxine potentiates the action of digitalis-like drugs and anticoagulants.

Unfortunately, homozygotes have no change in plasma cholesterol with the above-mentioned therapeutic regimen, and several other approaches have been introduced: 1) intravenous hyperalimentation, the beneficial mechanism of which is as yet unexplained, 2) portacaval shunt, which decreases cholesterol and LDL biosynthesis and therein reduces plasma cholesterol even though there is a decreased fractional rate of LDL catabolism, and 3) plasma exchange therapy in which plasma cholesterol is physically removed from the blood. Following this latter technique, there is a gradual reaccumulation of cholesterol in the plasma, and therefore, this therapy must be repeated as needed.

Familial Type 3 hyperlipoproteinemia is a rare, genetically determined, autosomal-dominant transmitted disorder in which an abnormal lipoprotein called beta VLDL is detected in the plasma. It is differentiated from normal VLDL by its 1) higher proportion of cholesterol (mainly esters) relative to triglyceride and 2) deficiency of C- in relation to B-apolipoprotein content, as well as an absolute increase in E-apolipoprotein. Although the basic biochemical defect has not been determined, it has been postulated that it is involved with the catabolism of triglyceride-rich particles.

Plasma cholesterol and triglyceride concentrations are increased. The VLDL are increased, but the LDL and HDL are moderately decreased. However, the IDL are significantly elevated, and, uncharacteristically, the IDL contains C- and E-apolipoproteins. Half of these patients have hyperuricemia and a similar percentage will have glucose intolerance without progressing toward hyperglycemic ketoacidosis or insulin dependence.

Clinically, this disorder rarely manifests itself before the age of 20. Two thirds will have pathognomonic xanthomas in their palmar creases, although xanthomas also occur elsewhere. Obesity is common. By the fifth or sixth decade, over half of these individuals will have developed clinically significant atherosclerotic coronary and/or premature peripheral vascular (including the cerebral vessels) disease. As the atherosis is the main determinant of morbidity and mortality associated with this disorder, it behooves the anesthetist to have the patient fully evaluated and prepared from the point of view of coronary and cerebral arterial disease.

Treatment of familial Type 3 hyperlipoproteinemia can fully restore plasma cholesterol and triglyceride levels to normal, but the abnormal β-VLDL remain unchanged. The patient first must be dieted with reduced caloric intake down to ideal body weight. This weight is then maintained with a diet in which carbohydrates and fats each supply 40 per cent of the caloric intake, the fats consisting mainly of the polyunsaturated nature. Dietary cholesterol is not to exceed 300 mg. per day, and ethanol intake is prohibited.

After satisfying dietary requirements, the patient is given clofibrate (2 gm./day), a branched-chain fatty acid ester. Clofibrate effects a decreased synthesis of triglyceride and cholesterol, an increased secretion of sterols, a decreased free fatty acid release from peripheral tissue, and an increased clearance of VLDL and IDL. It is crucial to be aware of the side effects associated with clofibrate administration: 1) the potentiation of coumarin anticoagulants, such that careful evaluation of the patient's coagulation potential (particularly the prothrombin time) must be achieved prior to surgery, and, particularly, regional anesthesia, 2) increase of hepatic circulating enzymes, this necessitating preanesthetic baseline measurement and assuming particular importance for employment of a halogenated hydrocarbon, 3) cardiac dysrhythmias, and 4) inappropriate antidiuretic hormone secretion and the associated blood volume, electrolyte and renal functional consequences.

Nicotinic acid (niacin) is given as 0.5 gm. per day, gradually increasing to 3 to 6 gm. per day, and has effects equipotent to clofibrate. It is a component of the coenzymes NAD and NADP and suppresses free fatty acid release from peripheral adipose tissue stores with a consequent reduction of hepatic VLDL synthesis and secretion, and a resultant decreased concentration of plasma triglyceride. Ultimately there is a diminished plasma IDL and LDL and, therefore, cholesterol as well. Nicotinic acid, which has been employed by anesthetists for the treatment of post-spinal cephalalgia, may have significant side effects: glucose intolerance, hyperuricemia and/or hepatotoxicity will contraindicate its use in those patients with diabetes mellitus, gout, or liver disease. In addition, its cutaneous vasodilatory property may mimic an atropine flush. Patients with a peptic ulcer history cannot use nicotinic acid because of its propensity to induce gastritis and associated bleeding. Nicotinic acid's ability to augment the hypotensive effects of ganglionic-blocking drugs such as trimethaphan camsylate and pentolinium forces the anesthetist to use these agents in reduced doses and with extreme precaution.

D-Thyroxine, an analogue of L-thyroxine, is another alternative drug therapy, but is of pathophysiological potential when employed in the setting of coronary arterial disease, cardiac arrhythmias, or congestive heart failure. Of all the hyperlipoproteinemias, familial Type 3 displays the most gratifying therapeutic response in that xanthomas may disappear and peripheral vascular flow may even increase.

The final three monogenic familial hyperlipoproteinemias are less well delineated, poorly understood from a biochemical mechanistic point of view, and are rare in occurrence. These are briefly summarized:

Familial hypertriglyceridemia (Type 4 hyperlipoproteinemia) is characterized by an isolated increase of endogenously synthesized triglyceride as found in the VLDL. Thus, the plasma triglyceride is elevated, but the cholesterol concentration is normal. The affected individuals may display hyperglycemia, hyperuricemia, hyperinsulinemia, obesity, and a proclivity to develop premature coronary arterial disease.

Familial Type 5 hyperlipoproteinemia is a more exaggerated form of marked hypertriglyceridemia in which the VLDL are increased and postprandial hyperchylomicronemia occurs. Serum cholesterol is concomitantly elevated. Although the patients may have eruptive xanthomata, abdominal pain and pancreatitis, the postheparin plasma lipoprotein lipase activity is normal. Obesity and hyperglycemia are frequently encountered, but there is no increased frequency of premature cardiovascular disease.

Familial combined hyperlipoproteinemia is a disorder in which the affected individuals display a lipoprotein profile of Type 2 and/or Type 4 hyperlipoproteinemia. They are prone to premature coronary disease, obesity, and glucose intolerance.

The anesthetic management of the patient with coronary artery disease clearly depends on the sequelae of the deposition of coronary arterial atheromata, that is, the amount and location of myocardium that is in ischemic jeopardy and/or already has been permanently damaged. Basic information that is helpful includes: 1) left ventricular functional evaluation, such as left ventricular end-diastolic pressure (or pulmonary arterial wedge pressure), left ventricular ejection fraction and cineangiographic delineation of ventricular wall contractility, 2) presence, if any, of critically constrictive coronary arterial lesions and the amount of myocardium that is in ischemic jeopardy distal to these lesions, 3) propensity to cardiac arrhythmia, especially ventricular ectopy and atrioventricular block, 4) proclivity to hyperdynamic cardiovascular function, such as may be seen in hypertensive individuals, and 5) cardiovascular drug therapy, including antihypertensive drugs, beta adrenergic-blocking agents, cardiotonic compounds, vasodilator drugs, and antiarrhythmic agents.

The total anesthetic management of these unfortunate individuals extends from the appropriate preoperative evaluation and preparation through the initial postanesthetic days. Although a discussion of such management is beyond the scope of this section, the patient should be classified — and managed accordingly — into one of three categories: 1) hyperdynamic cardiovascular system, 2) failing myocardium, or 3) essentially normal cardiac and vascular function in the presence of ischemia. The hyperdynamic pattern requires an anesthetic that suppresses both the cardiovascular and the sympathoadrenal systems, whereas the patient with compromised myocardial function necessarily is managed with a technique that preserves homeostatic cardiovascular mechanisms. Excessive myocardial oxygen demands (tachycardia and hypertension) are to be avoided, while myocardial oxygen supply is to be optimally maintained. These same principles apply well into the postanesthetic phase, for only coronary artery bypass surgery can immediately improve the coronary flow situation.

The effect of anesthetic drugs on lipid metabolism has been only incompletely examined. Those anesthetics that are associated with elevated blood norepinephrine levels (fluoroxene, nitrous oxide, cyclopropane, and diethyl ether) would be expected to produce increased plasma free fatty acid (FFA) and triglyceride levels by virtue of the catecholamine effect on intracellular adipose tissue lipase. On the other hand, barbiturates, halothane, methoxyflurane, and enflurane would not be predicted to increase the FFA. However, investigators have been unable to demonstrate the expected FFA increases during diethyl ether anesthesia, and halothane unexpectedly effected a two- to threefold increase. Therefore, there are other undefined mechanisms that are critical determinants of plasma FFA and triglyceride concentrations during surgical anesthesia.

Fasting will effect an elevation of plasma FFA, but in humans significant lipolysis is not achieved until the fast has been at least of 24 hours' duration. Consistent with this temporal requirement is the fact that the FFA concentrations are relatively low in the typical "NPO after midnight" patient. However, when this partial fasting state is combined with the normal preanesthetic psychological and/or physical stresses (and accompanying heightened sympathoadrenal activity) the resulting metabolic milieu changes from that of a glycolytic biochemistry to one of predominant lipolysis and elevation of plasma FFA. Intravenous glucose, by preserving a euglycemic state as well as any available glycogen stores, would minimize the deployment of the body's homeostatic lipolytic mechanisms for maintaining an adequate supply of energy substrates. Hypercarbia, hypoxemia, and metabolic acidosis all have significant fat-mobilizing effects indirectly through sympathoadrenal stimulation.

Neurolept, balanced, and halothane anesthesias without superimposed surgical stress did not change plasma FFA levels. On the other hand, when combined with surgical stimulation, methoxyflurane, halothane, nitrous oxide, and cyclopropane (most pronounced) all increased plasma FFA concentrations. Thus, it is most probable that anesthetic drugs themselves assume only minimal etiologic importance in the overall hormonal and metabolic alterations affecting plasma FFA levels during and after surgery. Surprisingly, diethyl ether, an augmenter of sympathoadrenal activity, effected no change in plasma FFA levels, although this may be related to the ether-induced augmentation of hepatic clearance of FFA. Notwithstanding, the neurological impulses that are transmitted from the surgical site to the central and autonomic nervous systems are necessary components of the mechanisms that effect alterations in lipid metabolism. As such, a significant neurogenic blockade — sympathetic and somatic — effected by intrathecal or epidural anesthesia will inhibit the human response to surgical stress and does, indeed, prevent any increase in plasma FFA levels. Additionally, beta-adrenergic blocking drugs will prevent and/or reverse the elevation of plasma FFA normally induced by catecholamine-stimulating anesthetics such as cyclopropane.

Human adipose tissue lipolysis has been shown to be stimulated by low concentrations of halothane, and this has been attributed to the beta-adrenergic stimulating property of halothane. Higher clinical concentrations of halothane, however, inhibited this lipolysis by some as-yet-undetermined mechanism blocking the activation of intracellular lipase.

Elevated concentrations of plasma FFA might have profound effects on the management of an anesthetic. FFA are direct competitive inhibitors of barbiturates and other acidic drugs for albumin-binding sites and could therein result in increased plasma concentrations of the free (active) form of the barbiturates. This has been demonstrated for thiopental as FFA prolonged the duration of action of this barbiturate. Increased FFA levels detected in the post-myocardial infarction period have been etiologically incriminated for the high incidence of ventricular arrhythmias. Similarly, elevated plasma FFA has been associated with a lowering of the threshold for epinephrine-induced arrhythmias during halothane (but not barbiturate) anesthesia. The shift of glycolytic to lipolytic metabolism of the heart not only may affect the electrical stability of cardiac cell membranes but also may increase the sensitivity to the negative inotropic properties of anesthetics.

Cell membranes are complex structures containing phospholipids, neutral lipids (such as cholesterol), and protein. The phospholipids are arranged in the form of a bilayer, which may be the fundamental structure of the cell membrane. General anesthetics are simple chemical structures possessing relatively nonspecific binding properties, and they dissolve in the lipid bilayer. One of the membrane theories of anesthesia proposes that this physical dissolution causes an expansion of the lipid bilayer that affects the intramembranous protein or lipoprotein molecules that regulate electrical and/or chemical changes within the neuron. Hyperlipoproteinemic states might alter the ratios of the critical lipid compounds (cholesterol and phospholipids) that compose the lipid bilayer of the cell membrane, thereby creating a chemical membrane structure that is more or less receptive to — or affected by — an anesthetic molecule. Indeed, only those lipid bilayers with high cholesterol to phospholipid ratios are, in fact, disordered by anesthetic drugs. If patients with hyperlipoproteinemias have altered ratios of these key intramembranous lipids, then the nervous system (and other organs as well) might respond in an unusual manner when exposed to anesthetic drugs.

It has been demonstrated that local anesthetics inhibit the activity of phospholipase, an enzyme that catalyzes membrane-bound phospholipid breakdown. Halothane, chloroform, fluroxene, and ether stimulate (low dose) and inhibit (high dose) the turnover of synaptic phospholipids that are intimately involved with cellular depolarization. Halothane augments the synthesis of lipids in tissue culture preparations. However, whether these experimental findings would be altered in the hyperlipoproteinemic state and how this would ultimately affect the outcome of a clinical anesthetic remain to be determined. Thus, we see that there is only a smattering of information concerning the effect of anesthetics on aspects of lipid metabolism other than triglyceride lipolysis, and any statements concerning anesthesia and either normal or abnormal lipoprotein metabolism would be entirely conjectural.

The extent or degree of elevation of blood lipids in the lipid disorders already discussed varies from slight to massive, the latter being most spectacularly exemplified by a postprandial hyperchylomicronemic patient. It is interesting to speculate as to the effect that hyperlipemia would have on the blood-gas solubility coefficient of the volatile anesthetic drugs. Hyperlipemia would be expected to increase the partition coefficient and consequently alter the expected pattern of uptake and distribution of the anesthetic gas. For example, would a halothane anesthetic more closely simulate a methoxyflurane anesthetic? Or would a methoxyflurane or diethyl ether anesthesia be practically achieved? The hypolipoproteinemias might produce the opposite effects.

Another question of interest is whether the accumulation of lipid in the liver — as might be encountered in the fasting or nutritionally deprived state — might lead to the accrual of supranormal hepatic concentrations of lipid-soluble anesthetics. The role that this might play in the development of hepatocellular injury is even more speculative.

Fatty acids administered in the form of fat emulsions are an alternative source to glucose of nonprotein calories that are incorporated in the regimen of total parenteral administration. Fatty acids have a respiratory quotient (carbon dioxide produced divided by oxygen consumed) of 0.7, whereas that of glucose is 1.0. As such, calorie for calorie, the oxidative catabolism of fatty acids generates significantly less carbon dioxide than that of glucose. Thus, the substitution of fatty acids for glucose in supplying as much as one half of the caloric content of total parenteral solutions may assume particular importance in the patient with diminished or absent respiratory reserve. Manipulation of the caloric constituents may even prevent the development of respiratory insufficiency (alveolar hypoventilation and carbon dioxide retention) or facilitate the weaning of a patient from ventilatory support. The metabolism of fatty acids appears to be unaffected by anesthetic drugs. Fat emulsions (preferably soybean oil emulsions in which linoleic, linolenic, and oleic acids are the predominant fatty acids) have physicochemical characteristics and blood-clearance kinetics identical to those of chylomicrons.

Cholinesterase (previously referred to as pseudocholinesterase) is an enzyme that is synthesized by the liver and found in the serum, wherein it appears in two pools of activity: 1) the free form, the fraction that is routinely measured in the laboratory, and 2) bound to LDL. Cholinesterase may be involved in the biosynthesis, metabolism and structure of LDL. It facilitates the removal of the toxic choline esters formed as intermediary compounds during fatty acid metabolism. Serum and LDL cholinesterase levels are increased in several forms of the familial hyperlipoproteinemias, and this might accelerate the rate of enzymatic biodegradation—and recovery from—succinylcholine, procaine, cocaine, chloroprocaine and tetracaine. The relationship, if any, of absent, deficient or abnormal serum cholinesterase states to the metabolism of lipoproteins remains to be elucidated.

FAMILIAL HYPOLIPOPROTEINEMIAS

Three rare, genetically determined hypolipoproteinemias have been described: abetalipoproteinemia, hypobetalipoproteinemia, and Tangier disease (primary HDL deficiency). The most common of these is abetalipoproteinemia, which is chemically characterized by the absence of plasma apolipoprotein B, and consequently, a markedly reduced plasma cholesterol (absent LDL) and triglyceride (absent chylomicron and VLDL) concentrations. It is presumed that either the apolipoprotein is not synthesized or that it is synthesized but not assembled with its appropriate lipid. There is a concomitant decreased plasma phospholipid content and a reduction of the ratio of phosphatidylcholine to sphingomyelin. Clinically, this autosomal-recessively inherited disorder is manifested by the following:

1. Intestinal fat malabsorption that begins in the neonatal period and is accompanied by anorexia, vomiting, mild steatorrhea, and failure to grow. There is thought to be a variable deficiency of fat-soluble vitamins (A, D, E, K) and, in addition to the vitamin K-related hypoprothrombinemia and its associated bleeding tendencies, many of the clinical sequelae to be enumerated below may be, to some degree, attendant upon these vitamin deficiencies. Despite this malabsorptive syndrome, medium-chain triglycerides do not require chylomicron formation for transportation and absorption into the portal venous system and, as such, remain as an important utilizable source of caloric consumption.

2. Pigmentary degeneration of the retina and various other severe ocular disturbances.

3. Neuromuscular dysfunction, often detectable initially as neonatal psychomotor impairment but invariably culminating in severe ataxia within the first two decades of life. Spinocerebellar tract demyelination is the most prominent neuropathological finding. Kyphosis, scoliosis, and hyperlordosis are frequent sequelae.

4. Acanthocytosis, which is a geometric malformation of the erythrocyte (recall the role of phospholipids and cholesterol in determining cell membrane structure and function) that leads to premature hemolysis and accompanying low-grade, chronic anemia with reticulocytosis, hyperbilirubinemia and hypohaptoglobinemia. The anemia is most prevalent in younger children.

5. Cardiac and/or hepatic dysfunction of variable nature and extent may be encountered.

Treatment with pharmacologic doses of vitamin A has been utilized with moderate success for the ocular abnormalities, and pharmacologic doses of vitamin E have been employed with encouraging results for the neuromuscular and hemolytic sequelae. Vitamin K is definitive therapy for hypoprothrombinemia. The dietary restriction of triglycerides containing long-chain (C16-C24) fatty acids is mandatory for relieving the gastrointestinal syndrome, but caloric substitution must be achieved with either medium-chain (C8-C14) triglycerides or protein and carbohydrates.

The anesthetic management begins with attention to continued dietary adherence during the hospitalization. Because triglyceride-poor diets are problematic wth respect to achieving adequate caloric intake, carbohydrate calories in the form of glucose must be supplied in generous quantities both intra-anesthetically and in the postoperative period until the routine therapeutic diet is resumed. Fat emulsions contain large amounts of long-chain fatty acids, and therefore are relatively contraindicated as a source of calories. Hyperalimentation with protein hydrolysates and glucose is an acceptable alternate approach. Because most of these infants and children are very small on a weight for age basis, the anesthetist must be prepared to use pediatric equipment that is appropriate for the patient's size, rather than age.

Neuromuscular transmission and muscle tone and function are normal, but the dose of muscle relaxants, as calculated on a mg. per kg. basis, will be small. Dystonic states are not encountered. The ataxia requires provision of specific care and assistance for any locomotive activity, such as transferring to and from beds or operating table. Once the anesthetic premedications have been administered, the patient must remain in bed because any sedation of an ataxic individual will compromise any ability to achieve safe voluntary movement. Similar considerations apply postoperatively.

When such individuals have uncorrected kyphosis and/or scoliosis, pulmonary mechanics and functional capacity must be evaluated. Significant scoliosis in early childhood may cause alveolar hypodevelopment. Significant degrees of scoliosis will result in decreased vital capacity, total lung capacity, and maximal voluntary ventilation. Neither obstructive pulmonary impairment nor airway obstructive phenomena are encountered. Some degree of altered ventilation-perfusion relationships may exist and lead to impaired oxygen exchange. Diminished pulmonary functional reserve must be considered not only during anesthesia, wherein adequate ventilation and oxygenation should be confirmed by arterial blood gas determination, but also during the postanesthetic period when such patients are at increased risk to develop atelectasis, further aberration of ventilation-perfusion relationships, and pneumonitis. Appropriate aggressive respiratory care techniques must be employed, and arterial blood gas and vital capacity measurements must be done as indicated. The reversal of neuromuscular blocking drugs should be objectively determined with a peripheral nerve stimulator to prevent any further respiratory impediment. Inspiratory force measurements may be of additional informative value.

The pathological involvement of the spinocerebellar tract is not an absolute contraindication to regional anesthesia, but uncorrected hypoprothrombinemia is. Hyperlordosis may make any lumbar approach to regional anesthesia difficult to achieve. Because the acanthocytic anemia is of a chronic, low-grade nature and, therefore, usually well compensated, sympathetic blockage is well tolerated and erythrocyte transfusion is not indicated. Hepatic fatty infiltration is uncommon and usually not associated with enzymatic elevations, and, therefore, poses only a theoretical concern over the susceptibility to damage by halogenated hydrocarbon anesthetics.

Other Hereditary Disorders

By WALTER MILLAR, M.D., and JORDAN KATZ, M.D.

Marfan's Syndrome
Ehlers-Danlos
   Syndrome
Down's Syndrome (Trisomy 21)

Chediak-Higashi Syndrome
Weber-Christian Disease
Hemochromatosis

MARFAN'S SYNDROME

Marfan's syndrome is an autosomal dominant trait, characterized by a generalized defect of connective tissue. Although expression of the trait is variable, the most common diagnostic signs are disproportionate length of long bones (arachnodactyly), hypermobility of joints, prolapsed lens, and cardiac murmurs, most often the systolic click-murmur of mitral valve prolapse.

The underlying biochemical defect has not been identified but seems to be restricted to a deficiency of mechanical strength in connective tissue. When organ dysfunction or failure occurs, it is secondary to the absence of elasticity or tensile strength in the supporting matrix rather than to a parenchymal defect. The implications of this reduction in connective tissue strength in various organ systems help to define the surgical and anesthetic problems likely to be encountered in affected individuals.

Cardiovascular problems are the most common immediate cause of death. The mean age at death in published reports is early in the fourth decade; whether modern medical and surgical management will affect this early mortality remains to be proven. The click-murmur syndrome, produced by a "floppy" or prolapsing posterior mitral valve leaflet is characteristic of Marfan's but also occurs in a large percentage of the general population; its prognostic significance is still controversial.

Less obvious clinically, but more important prognostically, are lesions of the pulmonary artery, aorta, and distal arteries, involving degeneration of the elastic fibers of the media with replacement by collagen, which have collectively been labeled "cystic medial necrosis." The resulting weak-ness of the supporting media leads to the formation of saccular aneurysms, most commonly of the aortic root and ascending arch. Saccular expansion of the aortic root leads to dilatation of the aortic ring and eventually to aortic regurgitation and its sequelae of hypertrophy, dilatation, secondary mitral valve regurgitation, heart failure, and angina. Patients may present to surgery for repair of a leaking or dissecting arch aneurysm, coronary artery bypass grafts, valve replacement, repair of a distal aortic or arterial aneurysm or any combination of these. Medical therapy is directed at preventing these lesions by reducing aortic wall tension and controlling blood pressure changes as well as absolute level. Beta-adrenergic blockade by propranolol is a well tolerated and rational means to this end, but long-term results of such therapy have not been reported.

Pulmonary function is usually normal if scoliosis or pectus excavatum has not compromised chest wall mechanics. Vital capacity may be below that predicted by height owing to disproportionate leg length. Emphysema is not uncommon and is characterized by bronchogenic cysts and "honeycomb" appearance on chest x-ray.

Skeletal deformities vary in severity. Disproportionate growth of long bones is pathognomonic and leads to arachnodactyly, arm span greater than height, greater distance from sole to pubis than pubis to vertex, a high, arched palate, and an enlarged spinal canal. When this growth is asymmetrical, kyphoscoliosis or facial or chest wall deformities may occur. Pectus excavatum, when present, may be related to excessive rib growth.

Joint laxity is a constant feature; recurrent dislocations may require surgical repair.

The peripheral musculature is usually poorly developed, and defects in the abdominal wall lead to inguinal, femoral, umbilical, and diaphragmatic hernias.

Subluxation of the lens (ectopia lentis) is common and leads to visual impairment but is seldom repaired surgically.

In spite of the generalized nature of the connective tissue weakness, most surgical procedures are associated with good wound healing; vascular procedures are the exception to this rule if extensive tissue damage has ensued from aneurysm dissection.

The patient with Marfan's syndrome should be handled very gently, with minimal stress on the connective tissues. Preoperative evaluation should identify such complications of the syndrome as emphysema, aneurysms of the aorta, aortic regurgitation, heart failure, and arrhythmias. Beta-adrenergic blocking drugs should be continued through surgery unless a cogent reason exists to stop them. Antibiotic prophylaxis for bacterial endocarditis is indicated if significant valvular disease has developed.

Proper positioning and limb support of the patient prior to induction will help to avoid joint trauma or dislocation during anesthesia and surgery. Monitoring must be appropriate to the functional status of the patient and to the surgical procedure. An indwelling arterial line is a convenience, particularly when cardiac dysfunction has been identified preoperatively, but carries an increased risk of morbidity in a patient with already weakened arterial walls.

The anesthetic technique should be chosen to prevent any hypertension in response to intubation and surgery, because increased tension on the weakened arterial walls may lead to aneurysm dissection, and increased myocardial oxygen consumption may lead to ischemia or failure of hypertrophied myocardium.

The insertion of all tubes, probes, and monitors must be done with skill and patience to avoid perforation or damage to tissues. Laryngoscopy and intubation, if required, should avoid excessive traction on the temporomandibular joints. Positive-pressure ventilation may produce pneumothorax at inflation pressures considered safe for normal lungs.

The increased volume of the spinal canal may affect the required dose for spinal or epidural block, but no data have been reported to substantiate this notion.

EHLERS-DANLOS SYNDROME

Ehlers-Danlos syndrome (EDS) describes a group of inherited disorders of collagen synthesis. Eight types have been described by Beighton. All show hyperextensible, fragile skin that bruises easily and heals poorly, leaving wide, thin "cigarette-paper" scars. Other signs usually include hypermobile joints, easy or excessive bleeding after minor trauma, varicose veins, and premature birth because of early amniotic rupture. Collagen throughout the body is deficient in strength and may be reduced in amount.

Specific enzyme deficiencies have been identified for a few of the rare types. In the majority of affected individuals, the definiciency is unknown. The most common types are autosomal dominant, but an X-linked recessive and several autosomal recessive patterns have been identified, suggesting a polygenic etiology.

Cardiovascular manifestations range from no apparent lesion to arterial aneurysm, arterial rupture without aneurysm, varicose veins, aortic regurgitation, mitral valve prolapse, and conduction disturbances. In contrast to Marfan's syndrome, there does *not* seem to be a predictable succession of cardiovascular lesions.

A variety of connective tissue failures may bring the Ehlers-Danlos patient to surgery, including vascular disruption, spontaneous pneumothorax, rupture of viscus, recurrent joint dislocation, or hernia. Surgery may be complicated by excessive bleeding in spite of normal laboratory tests of coagulation, friable tissues in which sutures may tear, and poor wound healing. In type IV EDS (ecchymotic), a type III collagen deficiency, bleeding may be life-threatening after even minor surgery. Genetic consultation before elective surgery can identify this specific type.

Anesthetic considerations are generally similar to those for Marfan's syndrome (see above). Vascular fragility may make venous access difficult and makes hematoma a serious risk where needles are inserted for regional anesthesia, intramuscular premedication, or monitoring. A bleeding time determination will help to estimate the risk of regional anesthesia as well as that of surgical hemorrhage.

DOWN'S SYNDROME (TRISOMY 21)

Down's syndrome (DS) refers to a large but inconstant set of morphologic features characteristic of patients with extra chromosomal material from chromosome 21 in some or all cell lines. It is the only known autosomal aneuploidy consistent with prolonged survival into adulthood but is nevertheless associated with excess mortality at every stage from conception onward. The incidence is approximately 1.5 per 1000 live births, with minor, if any, differences between geographic or ethnic groups. Surgical correction of congenital defects and improved medical care have greatly reduced excess mortality in the postnatal period, so that survival past early adulthood is no longer uncommon. Approximately 100,000 afflicted individuals live in the United States at present; this number will likely increase as the population ages.

The extra chromosomal material responsible for the syndrome may arise by several mechanisms. By far the most common (>90%) is an extra chromosome 21, resulting in 47 chromosomes total, present in all cell lines. If both parents have normal karyotypes, the extra chromosome 21 occurs because the chromosome pair did not split, or disjoin, during meiosis. Nondisjunction of chromosome 21 results in a nonviable gamete lacking chromosome 21 and a gamete with two chromosomes 21. This dipoid gamete, when united with a normal gamete, produces a zygote with three chromosomes 21, which pattern is usually preserved in all subsequent mitotic divisions.

The incidence of trisomy 21 offspring, and presumably of meiotic nondisjunction, is related to maternal age and increases markedly after age 35, ranging from 0.6 per 100 live births at age 19 or less, to 1.3 at age 30 to 34, to 41.5 at age 45 or greater. An independent relationship to paternal age or other factors is more difficult to document, but recently developed techniques have demonstrated paternal origin of the extra chromosome in 20 to 30 per cent of cases.

The mechanism of translocation accounts for 3 to 5 per cent of Down's syndrome. Chromosomal breakage in a germ cell may result in a fragment of chromosome 21 becoming reattached to another chromosome. After meiosis, the resulting gamete will either have a deficiency, a normal total amount, or an excess (the translocated fragment) of chromosomal material from chromosome 21. Those with a deficiency are nonviable. Those with an excess produce offspring phenotypically indistinguishable from regular trisomy 21. Those with the normal amount of chromosomal material are phenotypically normal and have either a normal karyotype or a balanced translocation; the latter are "carriers" for DS. Spontaneous translocation is not related to parental age.

The remainder of DS is produced by trisomy 21 in some but not all cell lines, a condition known as mosaicism. The phenotypic expression varies from typical DS to clinically normal individuals identified only after they had parented several DS offspring. Hence, the true incidence of mosaicism is difficult to define.

The biochemical mechanism responsible for DS is as yet unknown. Gene mapping studies indicate that a specific portion of the chromosome, the distal portion of the long arm, is responsible for most of the clinical features. Nevertheless, few specific enzyme defects have been identified and these do not at present account for the generalized but inconstant failure of growth and development of organ systems.

The clinical features of DS vary from patient to patient, although it has been stated that DS patients resemble one another more than they do their own siblings. Most of the characteristic features are anatomic or physiological anomalies present from birth. DS babies are commonly both premature and small for gestational age. In contrast to other growth-retarded newborns, the placentas are of normal size and morphology. Growth remains depressed in infancy and throughout childhood.

Although the typical facies and features of DS are familiar, those anomalies relevant to anesthesia bear emphasis. Mental retardation ranges from moderate to profound. DS patients are reputed to be happy, docile, and obedient; however, the DS child or adult who presents for anesthesia in a strange environment may not fit this stereotype.

The CNS abnormality is not limited to

failure of growth and development. DS patients not uncommonly develop epilepsy in adulthood, and early senile dementia (Alzheimer's disease) has been reported in a number of DS patients.

Congenital heart disease is present in about 50 per cent of DS patients. Atrioventricularis communis, ventricular septal defect, atrial septal defect, tetralogy of Fallot, and persistent patent ductus arteriosus are the most common defects. Pulmonary artery hypertension develops more rapidly in DS than in normals with equivalent anatomic defects. In the absence of congenital heart disease, resting systemic blood pressure is lower in DS than in controls, with less tendency toward hypertension as age advances.

Immunologic deficiency is a particular problem. Infections, especially of the respiratory tract, are frequent and prolonged in DS and until recently often led to an early demise. Blood leukocyte counts are normal, although granulocytes are structurally and functionally abnormal. Antibody response to certain antigens is reduced, but serum gamma globulin levels are usually above normal. Cell mediated immunity defects have also been identified. Resting cortisol levels are normal, but adrenal response to ACTH is subnormal. This may account for a diminished general response to stress.

Abnormalities of both bone and soft tissue contribute to the facies characteristic of DS. The eyes appear to be set widely apart because of epicanthal folds and oblique palpebral fissures (which led to the archaic and offensive term mongolism). The skull is brachycephalic, and the facial bones are hypoplastic with a high, arched palate. The maxilla and mandible are small, resulting in a protruding tongue, which is usually furrowed. Dentition is frequently abnormal in number, location, and shape. The voice is usually low-pitched but the larynx may be small.

Formerly, the majority of surgical procedures in DS were for correction of congenital cardiac or gastrointestinal lesions in early childhood. Increasing survival into middle age makes other surgical interventions increasingly likely. General anesthesia is often necessary for relatively trivial procedures, for example, dental restorations.

The paucity of case reports or specific literature related to anesthetic problems in DS would indicate that anesthesia is usually well tolerated. Sedative premedication is indicated in the older child or adult who is likely to be frightened and uncooperative. Anticholinergics are routinely prescribed by many anesthetists on the assumption that hypersecretion is more common in DS.

The choice of anesthetic method or technique is dictated by the identified congenital anomalies (particularly cardiac) and the surgical procedure rather than by the diagnosis of DS. The propensity for respiratory infections requires stringent asepsis in equipment and technique and may present a difficult choice for the anesthetist, whether to proceed with or postpone necessary elective surgery in a patient who has an active respiratory infection which may never completely resolve.

Although a high, arched palate, small jaw, and protruding tongue might make intubation difficult, ligamentous laxity and muscular hypotonia seem to contribute to easy exposure of the larynx. The endotracheal tube required may be smaller than that predicted by age or height.

Whether DS patients have abnormal responses to sedative and anesthetic drugs, neuromuscular blockers, or autonomically active drugs has not been systematically studied; the persistent clinical impression that ordinary doses may produce exaggerated effects dictates caution.

CHEDIAK-HIGASHI SYNDROME

Chediak-Higashi syndrome is a rare disorder characterized by oculocutaneous albinism and impaired resistance to bacterial infection leading to early demise. It is probably an autosomal recessive trait and occurs in mice, mink, and cattle as well as man.

Research has been focused on the structural, biochemical, and functional abnormalities of the polymorphonuclear leukocyte (neutrophil). The cytoplasmic granules of these, as well as other granule-producing cells, are abnormally large. Although no deficiency in the granular enzyme content has been identified, impaired degranulation and bacterial killing by neutrophils has been related to impaired transfer of lysosomal contents into phagosomes, perhaps by disruption of the architecture or function of the cytoplasmic microtubules. Impaired neutrophil chemotactic migration also contributes to impaired response to bacterial invasion.

Function of the cytoplasmic microtubules, and hence chemotaxis and degranulation, is related to the intracellular balance of the cyclic nucleotides, cyclic AMP and cyclic GMP. Chediak-Higashi neutrophils have elevated levels of cAMP. Elevation of intracellular cGMP in vitro with cholinergic agonists, or reduction of cAMP in vivo or in vitro by administration of ascorbic acid, has been shown to enhance chemotaxis and bacterial killing.

Analogous defects in platelet structure and function have been described, which result in prolonged template bleeding times and presumably in hemostatic difficulties during surgery.

A poorly understood lymphoproliferative disorder, known as the accelerated phase of the syndrome, may supervene at any time. Anemia, neutropenia, lymphadenopathy, hepatosplenomegaly, and widespread mononuclear infiltration of tissues occurs. Splenectomy has been performed, but chemotherapy probably offers more hope for successful treatment.

The majority of patients identified have died in infancy or early childhood as a result of overwhelming sepsis or the accelerated phase. Improvements in prevention and therapy of infection will likely lead to improved survival and increasing numbers of patients presenting for anesthesia in the future. At this writing, the recommendations for anesthetic management are limited to meticulous supportive care of the patient, evaluation of platelet function by a template bleeding time preoperatively, and avoidance of iatrogenic infection by careful sterile technique.

WEBER-CHRISTIAN DISEASE

Weber-Christian disease, or nodular non-suppurative panniculitis, is a chronic recurring febrile disease characterized by tender painful nodules usually seen in the fat of the abdominal wall or thigh. They may occur with or without erythema, and generally all resolve into brown sunken atrophic areas. Pathologically, these are areas of inflammatory reaction within the fat that progress to phagocytosis of degenerative fat cells with giant cell formation, fibrosis and calcification, and occasionally with vascular involvement. The disease may occur in any fat deposit in the body. When it involves the mesenteric or retroperitoneal fat it may masquerade as an acute abdomen with pain, tenderness, and fever. If pericardial fat is involved, the clinical syndrome of elevated venous pressure and fixed cardiac output similar to restrictive pericarditis may occur. Fibrosis of the pericardial fat may be noted histologically. Seizures may occur when the disease involves the meninges. Involvement of the infrapatellar fat pad may resemble arthritis. Acute adrenal failure caused by adrenal infarction has been reported secondary to retroperitoneal panniculitis.

The etiology of Weber-Christian disease is unclear. Sensitivity to halogens such as iodides and bromides has been reported, but this is by no means a usual phenomenon in the disease. Local panniculitis without systemic involvement can be due to local exposure to cold, especially in infants. It has been reported secondary to ice packs applied to febrile infants as well as to popsicles resting on the corner of the mouth. Presumably this is due to the more easily congealed subcutaneous fat in infants.

The anesthetic management for patients with Weber-Christian disease should begin by avoiding any trauma to the subcutaneous fat whether by the application of heat, cold, or pressure. Since these patients are usually febrile in an acute exacerbation of the disease, pharmacologic attempts, rather than the use of ice, should be made to lower the temperature prior to surgery. The possible halogen sensitivity might contraindicate the use of some agents. Metabolism of the agent may release enough fluoride or bromide to trigger a relapse. There is no available literature to support or refute this speculation.

Patients with Weber-Christian disease may have a decreased cardiac reserve as a result of involvement of the pericardial fat, or adrenal insufficiency secondary to periadrenal fibrosis and adrenal infarct, or adrenal atrophy when steroids were used to treat the disease. In the patient with restricted pericarditis, any decrease in the venous return might be catastrophic in reducing cardiac output. The preanesthetic central venous pressure, usually higher than normal, should be maintained by judicious volume replacement. The pooling of intravascular volume in the peripheral vascular systems owing to rapid changes in position, ganglioplegics, alpha blocking agents, or regional anesthesia must be carefully assessed.

HEMOCHROMATOSIS

Hemochromatosis is a rare disorder in the regulation of iron absorption that is probably inherited as an autosomal dominant trait. Twenty-five to fifty per cent of first degree relatives show increased iron absorption, with no sex predominance, and the syndrome is highly correlated with certain histocompatability antigens. Nevertheless, the exact mode of inheritance is uncertain, because no reliable test will identify the abnormal gene.

The clinical expression of the disorder is secondary to the chronic toxic effects of excessive storage iron in the involved tissues, and thus it requires both the genetic predisposition to absorb excessive dietary iron and a positive overall iron balance for many years. In women, the iron loss obligated by menstrual blood loss may delay or prevent the accumulation of excessive tissue iron stores.

There is no known metabolic control mechanism for the excretion of iron; balance depends on small obligate daily losses in the sloughed epithelium of skin and intestine, the inconstant losses of bleeding, and the variable absorption of dietary iron, which is normally under precise metabolic control.

A typical Western diet contains 10 to 15 mg. of elemental iron per day. The adult in iron balance absorbs about 1 mg. from this diet to compensate for obligate losses. Growth, pregnancy, and erythropoiesis increase absorption of iron by the intestinal mucosa, while a high tissue level of storage iron (predominantly in the liver) is inhibitory. Biochemical details of the control mechanism are unknown.

In hemochromatosis, a relative lack of inhibition of gastrointestinal absorption causes much higher tissue levels than normal. At some tissue level — which may or may not be a toxic level — inhibition occurs; at this point, measured absorption will be normal and tissue iron level will be elevated but constant. The affected patient who has an altered inhibitory "set point" still below the toxic level, or who has remained in iron balance because of blood loss in spite of increased absorption, will likely escape detection. Conversely, the patient with elevated iron stores due to excessive iron intake may carry a false diagnosis of hemochromatosis.

Not every patient presents with the classic diagnostic triad of diabetes, cirrhosis, and skin pigmentation. The toxic effects of iron are manifest in pituitary, pancreas, liver, skin, heart, and joints. Cell necrosis and fibrosis lead to organ dysfunction which may or may not resolve with reduction of tissue iron levels. Gonadotrophic hormone secretion is most sensitive to pituitary injury, so that sexual or menstrual dysfunction may occur. Both pituitary and pancreatic islet cell injury have been implicated in the insulin deficiency that is the hallmark of hemochromatosis. A genetic association with diabetes mellitus has also been identified.

The liver, as the primary site for iron storage, is particularly susceptible to injury from iron overload. Diffuse hepatocellular fibrosis leads to cirrhosis but seldom to portal hypertension or ascites in the absence of other toxins. Ethanol may both enhance iron absorption and aggravate the liver injury. The skin is darkened ("bronze diabetes") by increased melanin and perhaps by iron itself. The heart is affected by a diffuse cardiomyopathy and, less often, by conduction defects. Polyarthralgia may develop early or late in the course and may mimic pseudogout or rheumatoid arthritis.

The syndrome is manifest only when organ dysfunction has occurred, after the accumulation of 15 to 20 grams excess storage iron. Onset of symptoms is usually in the fifth decade in males and later, if at all, in females. Regular phlebotomy is effective in reducing iron stores and prolonging life. Some reversal of organ dysfunction occurs with therapy, but hepatomas occur frequently in cirrhotic livers despite normalization of tissue iron.

Anesthetic management depends on the location and severity of organ dysfunction. Glucose intolerance is managed as it would be for diabetes mellitus of equivalent severity. Cirrhosis becomes a significant problem only when portal hypertension occurs or with incipient liver failure.

Cardiomyopathy yields a progressively diminished cardiac reserve and requires meticulous attention to fluid balance, anesthetic effects on the myocardium, and the need for inotropic support or antiarrhythmics. Blood replacement during surgery sufficient to maintain optimum oxygen delivery is indicated, even in the patient on a phlebotomy schedule.

REFERENCES

Lipid

Allison, S., Tomlin, P., and Chamberlain, M.: Some effects of anesthesia and surgery on carbohydrate and fat metabolism. Brit. J. Anaesth. *41*:588, 1969.

Bennis, J., and Smith, U.: Effects of halothane on lipolysis and lipogenesis in human adipose tissue. Acta Anaesthesiol. Scand. *17*:76, 1973.

Bennis, J., and Smith, U.: Studies of the dual effects of halothane on the lipolysis of human fat cells. Anesthesiology *45*:379, 1976.

Biebuyck, J.: Nutrition and metabolism in the surgical patient. American Society Anesthesiol. Refresher Courses 7:13, 1979.

Bosomworth, P., and Morrow, D.: Metabolic significance of catecholamines released during anesthesia. Internat. Anesth. Clin. 5:481, 1967.

Brown, M., and Goldstein, J.: Receptor-mediated control of cholesterol metabolism. Science *191*:150, 1976.

Bruce, D.: Anesthetic implications of fasting. Anesth. Analg. 50:612, 1971.

Cameron, J., Capuzzi, D., Zuidema, G., et al.: Acute pancreatitis with hyperlipemia: The incidence of lipid abnormalities in acute pancreatitis. Ann. Surg. *177*:483, 1973.

Cameron, J., Capuzzi, D., Zuidema, G., et al.: Acute pancreatitis with hyperlipemia. Amer. J. Med. 56:482, 1974.

Chu, M., Fontaine, P., Kutty, K., et al.: Cholinesterase in serum and low density lipoprotein of hyperlipidemic patients. Clin. Chim. Acta 85:55, 1978.

Cooperman, L.: Plasma free fatty acid levels during general anesthesia and operation in man. Brit. J. Anesth. 42:131, 1970.

Fredrickson, D., Goldstein, J., and Brown, M.: The familial hyperlipoproteinemias. *In* Stanbury, J. B., Wyngaarden, J. B., and Fredrickson, D. S. (eds.): The Metabolic Basis of Inherited Disease. New York, McGraw-Hill, 1978, pp. 604–655.

Ghoneim, M.: Fasting and metabolism. Anesthesiology 47:235, 1977.

Glueck, C.: Postheparin lipoprotein lipase. New Engl. J. Med. 292:1347, 1975.

Grundy, S.: Cholesterol metabolism in man. West. J. Med. *128*:13, 1978.

Hallberg, D., and Oro, L.: Free fatty acids of plasma during spinal anesthesia in man. Acta. Med. Scand. *178*:281, 1965.

Havel, R.: The autonomic nervous system and intermediary carbohydrate and fat metabolism. Anesthesiology 29:702, 1968.

Havel, R.: Lipoproteins and lipid transport. Adv. Exper. Med. Biol. *63*:78, 1975.

Herbert, P., Gotto, A., and Fredrickson, D.: Familial lipoprotein deficiency. *In* Stanbury, J. B., Wyngaarden, J. B., and Fredrickson, D. S. (eds.): The Metabolic Basis of Inherited Disease, New York, McGraw-Hill, 1978, pp. 544–588.

Jackson, R., Morrisett, J., and Gotto, A.: Lipoprotein structure and metabolism. Physiol. Rev. 56:259, 1976.

Jackson, S.: Inborn errors of lipid metabolism. *In* Katz, J., and Kadis, L. B. (eds.): Anesthesia and Uncommon Diseases. Philadelphia, W. B. Saunders, 1973, pp. 1–6.

Jaques, L.: Heparin: An old drug with a new paradigm. Science 206:528, 1979.

Kutty, K., Redheendran, R., and Murphy, D.: Serum cholinesterase: Function in lipoprotein metabolism. Experientia 33:420, 1977.

Mäkeläinen, A., Nikki, P., and Vapaatalo, H.: Halothane-induced lipolysis in rats. Acta Anaesthesiol. Scand. *17*:179, 1973.

Margolis, S.: Treatment of hyperlipemia. J.A.M.A. 239:2696, 1978.

Merin, R., Samuelson, P., and Schalch, D.: Major inhalation anesthetics and carbohydrate metabolism. Anesth. Analg. 50:625, 1971.

Merin, R.: Inhalation anesthetics and myocardial metabolism: Possible complications for functional effects. Anesthesiology 39:216, 1973.

Merin, R.: New implications of fasting. Anesthesiology 48:236, 1978.

Miletich, D.: Fasting and metabolism. Anesthesiology 47:235, 1977.

Miletich, D., Albrecht, R., and Seals, C.: Responses to fasting and lipid infusion of epinephrine-induced arrhythmias during halothane anesthesia. Anesthesiology 48:245, 1978.

Miller, J.: Anesthetics and phospholipid metabolism. *In* Fink, B. R. (ed.): Molecular Mechanisms of Anesthesia. New York, Raven Press, 1975, pp. 439–447.

Neely, J., and Morgan, M.: Relationship between carbohydrate and lipid metabolism and the energy balance of the heart muscle. Ann. Rev. Physiol. 36:413, 1974.

Oyama, T., and Takazawa, T.: Effect of methoxyflurance anaesthesia and surgery on human growth hormone and insulin levels in plasma. Canad. Anaesth. Soc. J. *17*:347, 1970.

Rudman, D., Bixler, T., and Del Rio, A.: Effects of free fatty acids on binding of drugs by bovine serum albumin, by human serum albumin and by rabbit serum. J. Pharmacol. Exp. Ther. 176:261, 1971.

Scherphof, G., Scarpa, A., and van Toorenbergen, A.: The effect of local anesthetics on the hydrolysis of free and membrane-bound phospholipids catalyzed by various phospholipases. Biochim. Biophys. Acta 270:226, 1972.

Singer, S., and Nicolson, G.: The fluid mosaic model of the structure of cell membranes. Science *173*:720, 1972.

Strong, L., Hartzell, C., and McCarl, R.: Halothane and the beating response and ATP turnover rate of heart cells in tissue culture. Anesthesiology 42:123, 1975.

Triner, L.: Lopilysis by halothane questioned. Anesthesiology 46:310, 1977.

Woodbury, J., D'Arrigo, J., and Eyring, H.: Molecular mechanism of general anesthesia: Lipoprotein conformation change theory. *In* Fink, B. R. (ed.): Molecular Mechanisms of Anesthesia. New York, Raven Press, 1975, pp. 439–447.

Wilson's Disease

Barzilia, D., Dickstein, G., Enat, R., et al.: Cholestatic jaundice caused by D-penicillamine. Ann. Rheum. Dis. 33:88, 1978.

Beart, R., Putnam, C., Porter, K., et al.: Liver transplantation for Wilson's disease. Lancet 2:176, 1975.

Brown, B., Jr., and Sipes, I.: Biotransformation and hepatotoxicity of halothane. Biochem. Pharmacol. 26:209, 1977.

Bunker, J., Forrest, W., Mosteller, F., and Vandam, L. (eds.): The National Halothane Study. A Study of the Possible Association Between Halothane Anesthesia and Postoperative Hepatic Necrosis. Washington, D.C., United States Government Printing Office, 1969.

Cooperman, L., Wollman, H., and Marsh, S.: Anesthesia and the liver. Surg. Clin. N. Amer. 57:421, 1977.

Dykes, M.: Hepatotoxicity of anesthetic agents. Internat. Anesth. Clin. 8:241, 1970.

Dykes, M.: Is halothane hepatitis chronic active hepatitis? Anesthesiology 46:233, 1977.

Evans, G.: Copper homeostasis in the mammalian system. Physiol. Rev. 53:535, 1973.

Friedman, M.: Chemical basis for pharmacological and therapeutic actions of penicillamine. Adv. Exp. Med. Biol. 86B:649, 1977.

Frommer, D.: Defective biliary excretion of copper in Wilson's disease. Gut 15:125, 1974.

Jackson, S.: Wilson's disease and anesthesia. In Katz, J., and Kadis, L. B., (eds.): Anesthesia and Uncommon Diseases. Philadelphia, W. B. Saunders, 1973, pp. 15–17.

Masters, C., Dawkins, R., Zilko, P., et al.: Penicillamine-associated myasthenia gravis, antiacetylcholine receptors and antistriational antibodies. Amer. J. Med. 63:689, 1977.

Meyer, R., and Zalusky, R.: The mechanisms of hemolysis in Wilson's disease: Study of a case and review of the literature. Mt. Sinai J. Med. N.Y. 44:530, 1977.

Moult, P., and Sherlock, S.: Halothane-related hepatitis. Quart. J. Med. 44:99, 1975.

Sass-Kortsak, A., and Bearn, A.: Hereditary disorders of copper metabolism. In Stanbury, J. B., Wyngaarden, J. B., and Fredrickson, D. S. (eds.): The Metabolic Basis of Inherited Diseases. New York, McGraw-Hill, 1978, pp. 1098–1126.

Sternlieb, I., and Scheinberg, I: Chronic hepatitis as a first manifestation of Wilson's disease. Ann. Intern. Med. 76:59, 1972.

Sternlieb, I.: Diagnosis of Wilson's disease. Gastroenterology 74:787, 1978.

Stoelting, R.: Estimation of hepatic function — effects of the anesthetic experience. Amer. Soc. Anesthesiol. Refresher Courses 4:139, 1976.

Strickland, G.: Febrile penicillamine eruption. Arch. Neurol. 26:474, 1972.

Trachtenberg, H.: Anesthesia for the patient with hepatic disease. Internat. Anesth. Clin. 8:437, 1970.

Vaughan, R., Sipes, I., and Brown, B., Jr.: Role of biotransformation in the toxicity of inhalation anesthetics. Life Sci. 23:2447, 1978.

Wright, R., Eade, O., Chisholm, M., et al.: Controlled prospective study of the effect on liver function of multiple exposures to halothane. Lancet 1:817, 1975.

Porphyria

Adler, A. (ed): The biological role of porphyrins and related structures. Ann. N.Y. Acad. Sci. 244:1, 1975.

Brown, B., Jr.: Hepatic microsomal enzyme induction. Anesthesiology 39:178, 1973.

Brown, B., Jr.: Enzymatic activity and biotransformation of anesthetics. Internat. Anesth. Clin. 12:25, 1974.

Brown, B., Jr., and Sagalyn, A.: Hepatic microsomal enzyme induction by inhalation anesthetics. Anesthesiology 40:152, 1974.

Brown, B., Jr.: Enzyme induction and anesthesia. Weekly Anesthesiology Update 2:No. 35, 1980.

Chang, T., and Glazko, A.: Biotransformation and disposition of ketamine. Internat. Anesth. Clin. 12:159, 1974.

Chapados, R., and Paiement, B.: A case of acute intermittent porphyria. Canad. Anaesth. Soc. J. 13:616, 1966.

Dean, G.: Mefenamic acid and chlorpromazine in porphyria variegata. S. Afr. Med. J. 41:925, 1967.

Dean, G.: A report on propranidid, an intravenous anesthetic, in porphyria variegata. S. Afr. Med. J. 43:227, 1969.

Dean, G.: The Porphyrias. A Story of Inheritance and Environment. London, Pitman, 1971.

DeMatteis, F.: Disturbances of liver porphyrin metabolism caused by drugs. Pharmaco.. Rev. 19:523, 1967.

DeMatteis, F.: Drugs and porphyria. S. Afr. J. Lab. Clin. Med. 17:126, 1971.

Doss, M. (ed.): Porphyrins in Human Disease. Basel, Karger, 1976.

Douer, D., Weinberger, A., Pinkhas, J., et al.: Treatment of acute intermittent porphyria with large doses of propranolol. J.A.M.A. 240:766, 1978.

Dundee, J., McCleery, W., and McLoughlin, G.: The hazard of thiopental anesthesia in porphyria. Anesth. Analg. 41:567, 1962.

Eales, L.: Porphyria and thiopentone. Anesthesiology 27:703, 1966.

Eales, L.: Drugs and the porphyrias: Acute porphyria. S. Afr. Med. J. 41:566, 1967.

Eales, L.: The acute prophyric attack. III. Acute porphyria: The precipitating and aggravating factors. South African J. Lab. Clin. Med. 17:120, 1971.

Elder, G., Gray, C., and Nicholson, D.: The porphyrias: A review. J. Clin. Path. 25:1013, 1972.

Fischer, P., Ferizovic, A., Neelson, I., et al.: Porphyria-inducing activity of alfaxolone and alfadolone acetate in chick embryo liver cells. Anesthesiology 50:350, 1979.

Fox, O., Wilkinson, R., and Ralsow, F.: Thiopental anaphylaxis: A case and a method for diagnosis. Anesthesiology 35:655, 1971.

Fromke, V., Bassenmaier, I., Cardinal, R., et al.: Porphyria variegata: study of a large kindred in the United States. Am. J. Med. 65:80, 1978.

Grabschmidt, H.: A case of acute porphyria: Remissions induced with procaine intravenously. Calif. Med. 72:243, 1950.

Jackson, S.: Hereditary hepatic porphyrias. In: Katz, J., and Kadis, L. B. (eds.): Anesthesia and Uncommon Diseases. Philadelphia, W. B. Saunders, 1973, pp. 10–15.

Kosekelo, P., and Tenhunen, R. (eds.): International Conference on Porphyrin Metabolism. Ann. Clin. Res. 8(Suppl. 17); 1976.

Kostrezewska, E., and Greger, A.: Ketamine in acute intermittent porphyria—dangerous or safe? Anesthesiology 49:376, 1978.

Lepinskie, F.: Porphyria as a problem in anesthesia. Canad. Anaesth. Soc. J. 10:286, 1963.

Linde, H., and Berman, M.: Nonspecific stimulation of drug-metabolizing enzymes by inhalational anesthetics. Anesth. Analg. 50:656, 1971.

Mazze, R., Hitt, B., and Cousins, M.: Effect of enzyme induction with phenobarbital on the in vivo and in vitro defluorination of isoflurane and methoxyflurane. J. Pharmacol. Exp. Ther. 190:523, 1974.

McEwin, R.: Acute intermittent porphyria Aust. N.Z.J. Surg. 42:327, 1973.

Mees, D., Jr., and Frederickson, E.: Anesthesia and the porphyrias. Southern Med. J. 68:29, 1975.

Meyer, U., and Schmid, R.: The porphyrias. In: Stanbury, J. B., Wyngaarden, J. B., and Fredrickson, D. S. (eds.): The Metabolic Basis of Inherited Disease. New York, McGraw-Hill, 1976, pp. 1166–1220.

Murphy, P.: Acute intermittent porphyria. Brit. J. Anaesth. 36:801, 1964.

Mustajoki, P., and Heinonen, H.: General anesthesia in "inducible porphyrias." Anesthesiology 53:15, 1980.

Norris, W.: Anesthesia in porphyria. Brit. J. Anaesth. 32:505, 1960.

Parikh, R., and Moore, M.: Anesthetics in porphyria: Intravenous induction agents. Brit. J. Anaesth. 47:907, 1975.

Parikh, R., and Moore, M.: Effects of certain anaesthetic agents on the activity of rat hepatic δ aminolaevulinate synthase. Brit. J. Anaesth. 50:1099, 1978.

Parikh, R., and Moore, M.: Anaesthetics and porphyria. Brit. J. Anaesth. 51:809, 1979.

Peterson, A., Bossenmaier, I., Cardinal, R., and Watson, C.: Hematin treatment of acute porphyria. J.A.M.A. 235:520, 1976.

Rizk, S., Jacobson, J., and Silvay, G.: Ketamine as an induction agent for acute intermittent porphyria. Anesthesiology 46:305, 1977.

Rizk, S.: Ketamine is safe in acute intermittent porphyria. Anesthesiology 51:184, 1979.

Silvay, G., and Miller, R.: Porphyrias. Anesthesiology Rev. 6:51, 1979.

Slavin, S., and Christoforides, C.: Thiopental administration in acute intermittent porphyria without adverse effect. Anesthesiology 44:77, 1976.

Stein, J., and Tschudy, D.: Acute intermittent porphyria: A clinical and biochemical study of 46 patients. Medicine 49:1, 1970.

Stone, D., and Munson, E.: Anaesthetics and porphyria. Brit. J. Anaesth. 51:809, 1979.

Sumner, E.: Porphyria in relation to surgery and anaesthesia. Ann. R. Coll. Surg. Engl. 58:81, 1975.

Tschudy, D., Valsamis, M., and Magnussen, C.: Acute intermittent porphyria: Clinical and selected research aspects. Ann. Intern. Med. 83:851, 1975.

Ward, R.: Porphyria and its relation to anesthesia. Anesthesiology 26:212, 1965.

Watkins, J., and Clarke, R.: Report of a symposium: Adverse responses to intravenous agents. Brit. J. Anaesth. 50:1159, 1978.

Watson, C.: The problem of porphyria. New Engl. J. Med. 263:1205, 1976.

Amino Acid

Barzilia, D., Dickstein, G., Enat, R., et al.: Cholestatic jaundice caused by D-penicillamine. Ann. Rheum. Dis. 37:88, 1978.

Bastron, R., and Deutsch, S.: Anesthesia and the kidney. New York, Grune and Stratton, 1976.

Bender, D.: Amino Acid Metabolism. New York, John Wiley, 1975.

Berry, H.: Hyperphenylalaninemias and tyrosinemias. Clin. Perinatol. 3:15, 1976.

Biebuyck, J., Dedrick, D., and Scherer, Y.: Brain cyclic AMP and putative transmitter amino acids during anesthesia. In: Fink, B. R., (ed.): Molecular Mechanisms of Anesthesia. New York, Raven Press, 1975, pp. 451–470.

Biebuyck, J.: Nutrition and metabolism in the surgical patient. Amer. Soc. Anesthesiol. Refresher Courses 7:13, 1979.

Burchiel, K., Stockard, J., Calverly, R., et al.: Electroencephalographic abnormalities following halothane anesthesia. Anesth. Analg. 57:244, 1978.

Cassels, W., Becker, T., and Seevers, M.: Convulsions during anesthesia. Anesthesiology 1:56, 1940.

Cohen, D., and Young, J.: Neurochemistry and child psychiatry. J. Amer. Acad. Child Psychiatry 16:353, 1977.

Cranford, R., Leppik, I., Patrick, B., et al.: Intravenous phenytoin in acute treatment of seizures. Neurology 29:1474, 1979.

Crooke, J., Towers, J., and Taylor, W.: Management of patients with homocystinuria requiring surgery under general anesthesia. Brit. J. Anaesth. 43:96, 1971.

Delaney, A., and Gal, T.: Hazards of anesthesia and operation in maple-syrup urine disease. Anesthesiology 44:83, 1976.

Greer, M.: Anesthesia and seizures. Internat. Anesth. Clin. 6:351, 1968.

Hoover, H. Jr., Grant, J., Gorschbath, M., et al.: Nitrogen-sparing intravenous fluids in postoperative patients. New Engl. J. Med. 293:172, 1975.

Jackson, S.: Inborn errors of amino acid metabolism. In Katz, J., and Kadis, L. B. (eds.): Anesthesia and Uncommon Diseases, Philadelphia, W. B. Saunders, 1973, pp. 6–10.

Jackson, S., Dueker, C., Grace, L.: Seizures induced by pentazocine. Anesthesiology 35:92, 1971.

Knox, W.: Phenylketonuria. In Stanbury, J. B., Wyngaarden, J. B., and Fredrickson, D. S. (eds.): The Metabolic Basis of Inherited Disease, New York, McGraw-Hill, 1972, pp. 265–295.

Kramer, M., and Poort, C.: Influence of anesthetic drugs on amino acid incorporation in the rat pancreas. Biochem. Pharmacol. 21:441, 1972.

Lockman, L., Kriel, R., Zaske, D., et al.: Phenobarbital dosage for control of neonatal seizures. Neurology 29:1445, 1979.

Manku, R.: Effect of anesthesia on protein metabolism in patients undergoing hernioplasty. Anesth. Analg. 49:446, 1970.

Mullen, P.: Optimal phenytoin therapy: A new technique for individualizing dosage. Clin. Pharmacol. Ther. 23:228, 1978.

Neigh, J., Garmen, J., and Harp, J.: The electroencephalographic pattern during anesthesia with ethrane. Anesthesiology 35:482, 1971.

Neundoerfer, B., and Klose, R.: Changes in the child's

EEG during enflurane inhalation anesthesia. Electroencephalogr. Clin. Neurophysiol. 40:197, 1976.

Nyhan, W.: Heritable Disorders of Amino Acid Metabolism. New York, John Wiley, 1974.

Opitz, A., Brecht, S., and Stenzel, E.: Enflurane anesthesia for epileptic patients. Anesthetist 26:329, 1977.

Parker, C.: Diseases of phenylalanine metabolism. West. J. Med. 131:285, 1979.

Philbin, D., and Coggins, C.: Plasma antidiuretic hormone levels in cardiac surgical patients during morphine and halothane anesthesia. Anesthesiology 49:95, 1978.

Philbin, D.: Anesthesia and antidiuresis. Weekly Anesthesiology Update 2:No. 39, 1980.

Scriver, C., and Rosenberg, L.: Amino Acid Metabolism and Its Disorders, Philadelphia, W. B. Saunders, 1973.

Thier, S., and Segal, S.: Cystinuria. In Stanbury, J. B., Wyngaarden, J. B., and Frederickson, D. S. (eds.): The Metabolic Basis of Inherited Disease. New York, McGraw-Hill, 1978, pp. 1578–1592.

Tourian, A., and Sidbury, J.: Phenylketonuria. In Stanbury, J. B., Wyngaarden, J. B., and Fredrickson, D. S. (eds.): The Metabolic Basis of Inherited Disease. New York, McGraw-Hill, 1978, pp. 240–255.

Van Duyteren, G., and Wiggelinkhuizen, J.: Dissolution of bilateral staghorn cystine renal calculi. Arch. Dis. Child. 54:795, 1979.

Volep, J.: Management of neonatal seizures. Crit. Care Med. 5:43, 1977.

Weitzman, R., and Kleeman, C.: The clinical physiology of water metabolism: I. The physiologic regulation of arginine vasopressin secretion and thirst. West. J. Med. 131:373, 1979.

Winters, W.: Epilepsy or anesthesia with ketamine. Anesthesiology 36:309, 1972.

Gout

Allison, A., and Nunn, J.: Effects of general anesthetics on microtubules. Lancet 2:1326, 1968.

Balek, R., Kocsis, J., and Geiling, E.: Potentiating of several hypnotic and anesthetic agents by colchicine. Arch. Internat. Pharmacodynamie Thérapie 111:182, 1957.

Bastron, R., and Deutsch, S.: Anesthesia and the Kidney. New York, Grune and Stratton, 1976.

Coe, F.: Hyperuricosuric calcium oxalate nephrolithiasis. Kid. Intern. 13:418, 1978.

Fox, I., and Kelley, W.: Management of gout. J.A.M.A. 242:361, 1979.

Gomez, G., Stutzman, L., and Chu, T.: Xanthine nephropathy during chemotherapy in deficiency of hypoxanthine-guanine phosphoribosyltransferase. Arch. Intern. Med. 138:1017, 1978.

Hinkley, R., Jr., and Telser, A.: The effects of halothane on microfilamentous systems in cultured neuroblastoma cells. In Fink, B. R. (ed.): Molecular Mechanisms of Anesthesia. New York, Raven Press, 1975, pp. 103–118.

Jackson, S.: Gout and anesthesia. In Katz, J., and Kadis, L. B. (eds.): Anesthesia and uncommon diseases. Philadelphia, W. B. Saunders, 1973, pp. 17–20.

Kelley, W.: Pharmacologic approach to the maintenance of urate homeostasis. Nephron 14:99, 1975.

Kelton, J., Kelley, W., and Holmes, E.: A rapid method for the diagnosis of acute uric acid nephropathy. Arch. Intern. Med. 138:612, 1978.

Kleinman, H., and Ewbank, R.: Gout of the temporomandibular joint. Oral Surg. Oral Med. Oral Pathol. 27:281, 1969.

Liang, M., and Fries, J.: Asymptomatic hyperuricemia: The case for conservative management. Ann. Intern. Med. 88:666, 1978.

Mazze, R., Shue, G., and Jackson, S.: Renal dysfunction associated with methoxyflurane anesthesia. J.A.M.A. 216:278, 1971.

Okun, R., and Beg, M.: Ticrynafen and hydrochlorothiazine in hypertension. Clin. Pharm. Ther. 23:707, 1978.

Philbin, D., and Coggins, C.: Plasma antidiuretic hormone levels in cardiac surgical patients during morphine and halothane anesthesia. Anesthesiology 49:95, 1978.

Philbin, D., Coggins, C., Emerson, C., et al.: Plasma vasopressin levels and urinary sodium excretion during cardiopulmonary bypass: A comparison of halothane and morphine anesthesia. J. Thorac. Cardiovasc. Surg. 77:582, 1979.

Philbin, D.: Anesthesia and antidiuresis. Weekly Anesthesiology Update 2:No. 39, 1980.

Rieselbach, R., Sorenson, L., Shelp, W., et al.: Diminished renal urate secretion per nephron as a basis of primary gout. Ann. Intern. Med. 73:359, 1970.

Sauberman, A., and Gallagher, M.: Mechanisms of general anesthesia: failure of pentobarbital and halothane to depolymerize microtubules in mouse optic nerve. Anesthesiology 38:25, 1973.

Steele, T., and Rieselbach, R.: The renal handling of urate and other organic ions. In Brenner, B. M., and Rector. F. C., Jr. (eds.): The Kidney. Philadelphia, W. B. Saunders, 1976, Vol. I, pp. 442–476.

Weinman, E., and Knight, T.: Renal tubular tramsport of urate. Min. Elect. Metab. 1:121, 1978.

Weitzman, R., and Kleeman, C.: The clinical physiology of water metabolism: 1. The physiologic regulation of arginine vasopressin secretion and thirst. West. J. Med. 131:373, 1979.

Wyngaarden, J., and Kelley, W.: Gout and Hyperuricemia. New York, Grune and Stratton, 1976.

Wyngaarden, J., and Kelley, W.: Gout. In Stanbury, J. B., Wyngaarden, J. B., and Fredrickson, D. S. (eds.): The Metabolic Basis of Inherited Disease. New York, McGraw-Hill, 1978, pp. 916–1010.

Carbohydrate

Alexander, S., Colton, E., Smith, A., and Wollman, H.: The effects of cyclopropane on cerebral and systemic carbohydrate metabolism. Anesthesiology 32:236, 1970.

Alexander, S., Colton, E., and Taylor, J.: Some effects of α and β adrenergic blockade on the metabolic response to ether anesthesia in man. In Fink, B. R. (ed.): Cellular Toxicity of Anesthetics, Baltimore, Williams & Wilkins, 1972, pp. 312–320.

Allison, S., Tomlin, P., and Chamberlain, M.: Some effects of anesthesia and surgery on carbohydrate and fat metabolism. Brit. J. Anaesth. 41:588, 1969.

Berdanier, C. (ed.): Carbohydrate Metabolism: Regulation and Physiological Role. New York, Halsted-Wiley, 1976.

Bevan, J., and Burn, M.: Acid base and blood glucose levels of pediatric cases at induction of anaesthesia: The effect of preoperative starving and feeding. Brit. J. Anaesth. 45:115, 1973.

Biebuyck, J.: Effects of anesthetic agents on metabolic pathways: Fuel utilization and supply during anaesthesia. Brit. J. Anaesth. 45:263, 1973.

Biebuyck, J.: Nutrition and metabolism in the surgical patient. Amer. Soc. Anesthesiologists Refresher Courses 7:113, 1979.

Biebuyck, J., Lund, P., and Krebs, H.: The effect of halothane on glycolysis and biosynthetic processes of the isolated perfused rat liver. Biochem. J. 128:711, 1972.

Blackburn, G., Maini, B., and Pierce, E., Jr.: Nutrition in the critically ill patient. Anesthesiology 47:181, 1977.

Bosomworth, P., and Morrow, D.: Metabolic significance of catecholamines released during anesthesia. Internat. Anesth. Clin. 5:481, 1967.

Britt, B., Kalow, W., and Endrenyi, L.: Effects of halothane and methoxyflurane on rat skeletal muscle mitochondria. Biochem. Pharmacol. 21:1159, 1972.

Bromage, P., Shibata, H., and Willoughby, H.: Influence of prolonged epidural blockadge on blood sugar and cortisol responses to operations upon the upper part of the abdomen and thorax. Surg. Gynecol. Obstet. 132:1051, 1971.

Brown, B., Jr., and Sipes, I.: Biotransformation and hepatotoxicity of halothane. Biochem. Pharmacol. 26:209, 1977.

Bruce, D.: Anesthetic implications of fasting. Anesth. Analg. 50:612, 1971.

Brunner, E.: Normal nutrition in man: Anesthesiologic implications. Anesth. Analg. 50:620, 1971.

Brunner, E.: The effects of diethyl ether on carbohydrate metabolism in skeletal muscle. Anesthesiology 30:24, 1969.

Brunner, E., Cheng, S., and Berman, M.: Effects of anesthesia on intermediary metabolism. Ann. Rev. Med. 26:391, 1975.

Cataland, S.: Hypoglycemia: A spectrum of problems. Heart Lung 7:455, 1978.

Cervenko, F., and Greene, N.: Effects of cyclopropane anesthesia on glucose assimilation coefficient of man. Anesthesiology 28:914, 1967.

Clarke, R.: The hyperglycemic response to different types of surgery and anaesthesia. Brit. J. Anaesth. 42:45, 1970.

Cohen, P., and McIntyre, R.: The effect of general anesthesia on oxygen uptake and respiratory control of rat liver mitochondria. In Fink, B. R. (ed.): Cellular Toxicity of Anesthetics. Baltimore, Williams & Wilkins, 1972, pp. 109–116.

Cohen, R., and Simpson, R.: Lactate metabolism. Anesthesiology 43:661, 1975.

Cohn, R., and Segal, S.: Galactose metabolism and its regulation. Metabolism 22:627, 1973.

Comeaux, G., Shutts, P., and Rigor, B.: Anesthetic management of the patient with hypoglycemia. Anesth. Rev. 5:36, 1978.

Cooperman, L.: Plasma free fatty acid levels during general anaesthesia and operation in man. Brit. J. Anaesth. 42:131, 1970.

Cooperman, L., Wollman, H., and Marsh, M.: Anesthesia and the liver. Surg. Clin. N. Amer. 57:421, 1977.

Cornblath, M., and Schwartz, R.: Disorders of Carbohydrate Metabolism In Infancy. Philadelphia, W. B. Saunders, 1976.

Cox, J.: Anesthesia and glycogen-storage disease. Anesthesiology 29:1221, 1968.

Crawley, B., and Seager, R.: Monitoring of blood sugar during surgery. Anesthesia 25:73, 1970.

Dykes, M.: Is halothane hepatitis chronic active hepatitis? Anesthesiology 46:233, 1977.

Edelstein, G., and Hirshman, C.: Hyperthermia and ketoacidosis during anesthesia in a child with glycogen-storage disease. Anesthesiology 52:90, 1980.

Engquist, A., Brandt, M., Kehlet, H., et al.: Anesthesia does not cause metabolic stress. Anesthesiology 49:54, 1978.

Fajans, S., and Floyd, J. Jr.: Fasting hypoglycemia in adults. New Engl. J. Med. 294:766, 1976.

Fink, B., and Kenny, G.: Metabolic effects of volatile anesthetics in cell culture. Anesthesiology 29:505, 1968.

Fink, B., Kenny, G., and Simpson, W. III: Depression of oxygen uptake in cell culture by volatile, barbiturate and local anesthetics. Anesthesiology 30:150, 1969.

Folkman, J., Philippart, A., Tze, W., et al: Portacaval shunt for glycogen-storage disease: Value of prolonged intravenous hyperalimentation before surgery. Surgery 72:306, 1972.

Froesch, E.: Essential fructosuria, hereditary fructose intolerance and fructose-1,6-diphosphatase deficiency. In Stanbury, J. B., Wyngaarden, J. B., and Fredrickson, D. S. (eds.): The Metabolic Basis of Inherited Disease. New York, McGraw-Hill, 1978, pp. 121–136.

Gingerich, R., Paradise, R., and Wright, P.: Inhibition by ether of glucose-stimulated insulin secretion in isolated pieces of rat pancreas. Anesthesiology 51:34, 1979.

Gingerich, R., Wright, P., and Paradise, R.: Inhibition by halothane of glucose-stimulated insulin secretion in isolated pieces of rat pancreas. Anesthesiology 40:449, 1974.

Greene, N.: Carbohydrate metabolism and anesthesia. Internat. Anesth. Clin. 5:411, 1967.

Greene, N.: Halothane and metabolism. Clin. Anesth. 1:182, 1968.

Greene, N.: Insulin and anesthesia. Anesthesiology 41:75, 1974.

Greene, N., and Cervenko, F.: Inhalation anesthetics, carbon dioxide and glucose transport across red cell membrane. Acta Anesth. Scand. (suppl. 28):3, 1967.

Greene, N., and Webb, S.: Facilitated transfer of halothane in human erythrocytes. Anesthesiology 31:548, 1969.

Hashimoto, Y., Watanabe, H., and Satou, M.: Anesthetic management of a patient with hereditary fructose-1,6-diphosphatase deficiency. Anesth. Analg. 57:503, 1978.

Havel, R.: The autonomic nervous system and intermediary carbohydrate and fat metabolism. Anesthesiology 29:702, 1968.

Howell, R.: The glycogen-storage diseases. In Stanbury, J. B., Wyngaarden, J. B., and Fredrickson, D. S. (eds.): The Metabolic Basis of Inherited Disease. New York, McGraw-Hill, 1978, pp. 137–159.

Jackson, S.: Inborn errors of carbohydrate metabolism. In Katz, J., and Kadis, L. B. (eds.): Anesthesia and Uncommon Diseases. Philadelphia, W. B. Saunders, 1973, pp. 20–31.

Kekomäki, M., Suutarinen, T., and Mattila, M.: Redox state of the liver during anaesthesia as studied by parenteral galactose loads in children. Brit. J. Anaesth. 42:865, 1970.

Ko, K., and Paradise, R.: Contractile depression of rat atria by halothane in absence of glucose. Anesthesiology 34:152, 1971.

Ko, K., and Paradise, R.: The mechanism of negative inotropic effect of methoxyflurane on isolated rat atria. Anesthesiology 36:64, 1972.

Madsen, S., Brandt, M., Engquist, A., et al.: Inhibition of plasma cyclic AMP, glucose and cortisol response to surgery by epidural analgesia. Brit. J. Surg. 64:669, 1977.

Mahler, R.: Disorders of glycogen metabolism. Clin. Endocrin. Metab. 5:579, 1976.

Maze, A., and Samuels, S.: Hypoglycemia-induced seizures in an infant during anesthesia. Anesthesiology 52:77, 1980.

Merin, R.: New implications of fasting. Anesthesiology 48:236, 1978.

Merin, R.: The relationship between myocardial function and glucose metabolism in the halothane-depressed heart. II. The effects of insulin. Anesthesiology 33:396, 1970.

Merin, R., Samuelson, P., and Schulch, D.: Major inhalation anesthetics and carbohydrate metabolism. Anesth. Analg. 50:625, 1971.

Miranda, L., and Dweck, H.: Perinatal glucose homeostasis: The unique character of hyperglycemia and hypoglycemia in infants of very low birth weight. Clin. Perinat. 4:351, 1977.

Moult, P., and Sherlock, S.: Halothane-related hepatitis. Quart. J. Med. 44:99, 1975.

Nemoto, E., Stezoski, S., and MacMurdo, D.: Glucose transport across the rat blood-brain barrier during anesthesia. Anesthesiology 49:170, 1978.

Nikkilä, E., and Huttunen, J.: Clinical and metabolic aspects of fructose. Acta Med. Scand. 193(suppl.):542, 1972.

Oyama, T., and Takazawa, T.: Effects of diethyl ether anesthesia and surgery on carbohydrate and fat metabolism in man. Canad. Anaesth. Soc. J. 18:51, 1971.

Oyama, T., and Takazawa, T.: Effects of methoxyflurane anesthesia and surgery on human growth hormone and insulin levels in plasma. Canad. Anaesth. Soc. J. 17:347, 1970.

Oyama, T., and Takiguchi, M.: Plasma levels of ACTH and cortisol in man during halothane anesthesia and surgery. Anesth. Analg. 49:363, 1970.

Paradise, R., and Ko, K.: The effect of fructose on halothane-depressed rat atria. Anesthesiology 32:124, 1970.

Permutt, M.: Postprandial hypoglycemia. Diabetes 25:719, 1976.

Rosenberg, H., Haugaard, N., and Haugaard, E.: Alteration by halothane of glucose and glycogen metabolism in rat skeletal muscle. Anesthesiology 46:313, 1977.

Segal, S.: Disorders of galactose metabolism. In Stanbury, J. B., Wyngaarden, J. B., and Fredrickson, D. S. (eds.): The Metabolic Basis of Inherited Disease. New York, McGraw-Hill, 1978, pp. 160–181.

Starzl, T., Putnam, C., Porter, K., et al : Portal diversion for the treatment of glycogen-storage disease in humans. Ann. Surg. 178:525, 1973.

Stewart, T.: Evaluation of a reagent-strip method for glucose in whole blood, as compared with a hexokinase method. Clin. Chem. 22:74, 1976.

Stoelting, R.: Estimation of hepatic function — effects of the anesthetic experience. Amer. Soc. Anesthesiologists Refresher Courses 4:139, 1976.

Tarhan, S., Fulton, R., and Moffitt, E.: Body metabolism during general anesthesia without superimposed surgical stress. Anesth. Analg. 50:915, 1971.

Vaughan, R., Sipes, I., and Brown, B. Jr.: Role of biotransformation in the toxicity of inhalation anesthetics. Life Sci. 23:2447, 1978.

Watson, B.: Blood glucose levels in children during surgery. Brit. J. Anaesth. 44:712, 1972.

Wright, R., Eade, O., Chisholm, M., et al.: Controlled prospective study of the effect on liver function of multiple exposures to halothane. Lancet 1:817, 1975.

Yoshimura, N., Kodama, K., and Yoshitake, J.: Carbohydrate metabolism and insulin release during ether and halothane anesthesia. Brit. J. Anaesth. 43:1022, 1971.

Marfan's Syndrome

Brown, O. R., Demots, H., Kloster, F. E., Roberts, A., Menashe, V. D., and Beals, R. K.: Aortic root dilatation and mitral valve prolapse in Marfan's syndrome: An echocardiographic study. Circulation 52:651–657, 1975.

McKusick, V. A.: Heritable Disorders of Connective Tissue. 4th ed., St. Louis, C. V. Mosby, 1972.

Roberts, W. C.: Congenital cardiovascular abnormalities usually "silent" until adulthood: morphologic features of the floppy mitral valve, valvular aortic stenosis, discrete subvalvular aortic stenosis, hypertrophic cardiomyopathy, sinus of Valsalva aneurysm, and the Marfan syndrome. Cardiovasc. Clin. 10:407–453, 1979.

Ehlers-Danlos Syndrome

Beighton, P.: Cardiac abnormalities in the Ehlers-Danlos syndrome. Br. Heart. J. 31:227–232, 1969.

Beighton, P., Price, A., Lord, J., et al.: Variants of the Ehlers-Danlos syndrome. Ann. Rheum. Dis. 28:228–245, 1969.

Dolan, P., Sisko, F., and Riley, E.: Anesthetic considerations for Ehlers-Danlos syndrome. Anesthesiology 52:266–269, 1980.

Hollister, D. W.: Heritable disorders of connective tissue: Ehlers-Danlos syndrome. Pediatr. Clin. North Am. 25:575–591, 1978.

Wooley, M. M., Morgans, S., Hays, D. M.: Heritable disorders of connective tissue. Surgical and anesthetic problems. J. Pediat. Surg. 2:325–331, 1967.

Down's Syndrome

Breg, W. R.: Down's syndrome: A review of recent progress in research. Pathobiol. Ann. 7:257–303, 1977.

Federman, D. D.: Down's syndrome. Clin. Pediat. 4:331, 1965.

Millini, R., and Zanvio, L.: Problemi anesthesiologici nel mongolismo. Attual. Ostet. Ginecol. 14:511–518, 1968.

Richards, B. W., and Enver, F.: Blood pressure in Down's syndrome. J. Ment. Defic. Res. 23:123–135, 1979.

Chediak-Higashi Syndrome

Boxer, L. A., Watanabe, A. M., Rister, M., Besch, H. R., Allen, J., and Baehner, R. L.: Correction of leukocytic function in Chediak-Higashi syndrome by ascorbate. New Engl. J. Med. 295:1041–1045, 1976.

Leader, R. W.: The Chediak-Higashi anomaly — an evolutionary concept of disease. National Cancer Institute Monograph 32:337, 1969.

Oliver, J. M.: Impaired microtubule function correctable by cyclic GMP and cholinergic agonists in the Chediak-Higashi syndrome. Am. J. Pathol. 85:395–418, 1976.

Wintrobe, M.: Clinical Hematology, Philadelphia, Lea and Febiger, 1974, pp. 1323–1325.

Weber-Christian Disease

Epstein, E. J., Jr., and Oren, M. E.: Popsickle panniculitis. New Engl. J. Med. 282:966, 1970.

Hutt, M. S. R., and Pinninger, J. L.: Adrenal failure due to bilateral suprerenal infarction associated with systemic nodular panniculitis and endarteritis. J. Clin. Path. 9:316, 1956.

March, E. R., Jr., Turk, R. E., Scott, C. W.: Medical grand rounds from University of Alabama Medical Center. South. Med. J. 63:517, 1970.

Niedermayer, A. J., and Moran, T. J.: Relapsing febrile nodular nonsuppurative panniculitis: Report of a case treated with penicillin. Ann. Intern. Med. 29:958, 1948.

Spivak, J. L., Lindo, S., Coleman, M.: Weber-Christian disease complicated by consumption coagulopathy and microangiopathic hemolytic anemia. Johns Hopkins Med. J. 126:344, 1970.

Hemochromatosis

Hemochromatosis — Medical Staff Conference, University of California, San Francisco. West. J. Med. 128:133–141, 1978.

Pollycove, M.: Hemochromatosis. *In* Stanbury, J. B., Wyngaarden, J. B., and Fredrickson, D. S. (eds.): The Metabolic Basis of Inherited Disease. 4th ed., New York, McGraw-Hill, 1978, pp. 1127–1164.

2

The Pregnant Patient and the Disorders of Pregnancy

By LAURENCE S. REISNER, M.D.

Physiologic Alterations of Concern to the Anesthesiologist
Cardiovascular Changes
Respiratory System Changes
Clinical Application of the Physiologic Alterations in Pregnancy
Uteroplacental Perfusion

Drugs, the Developing Fetus and Newborn
Disorders of Pregnancy
Toxemia of Pregnancy
Hydatidiform Mole
Ectopic Pregnancy
Incompetent Cervix

The pregnant patient who requires an anesthetic for a surgical or obstetrical procedure presents a unique and challenging situation for the anesthesiologist. One must consider the physiologic alterations of pregnancy and their interaction with anesthetic agents. A knowledge of the principles of the placental transfer of drugs and their potential effects on the developing fetus is essential. The hemodynamics of uteroplacental perfusion and those trespasses that alter it need to be understood, and the potential for inducing premature labor or abortion needs to be considered. In addition to this basic knowledge, the relative importance of each of these factors during the three trimesters of pregnancy plus the puerperium should be known.

PHYSIOLOGIC ALTERATIONS OF CONCERN TO THE ANESTHESIOLOGIST

CARDIOVASCULAR CHANGES

Blood Volume. Blood volume increases gradually reaching a peak at 24 to 34 weeks of gestation. The magnitude of this increase is quite variable, 20 to 100 per cent, but, with a singleton fetus, seems to average out at 35 to 44 per cent over non-pregnant levels.[1, 2, 3] This tends to remain stable until term; it then declines gradually after delivery and returns to non-pregnant levels by six weeks post-delivery. Although a rise in blood volume has been suggested to occur in the early puerperium,[4] more recent work indicates that there is a steady decline from the time of delivery.[3] The degree of decline during the first three postpartum days appears to reflect the amount of intrapartum blood loss.

The increase in blood volume is due to an increase in both plasma volume and red cell mass. However, the increase in plasma volume is somewhat greater; therefore, the hematocrit and hemoglobin levels fall slightly below prepregnant values.[2] The increase in blood volume appears to adequately compensate for maternal blood loss at vaginal delivery, as there is little change in hematocrit. Patients who undergo cesarean section experience a greater blood loss than those having vaginal delivery (1000 cc vs. 500 cc) and have a slight decline in their hematocrit during the postpartum period.[3]

Cardiac Output. Traditional teaching of maternal cardiovascular physiology includes the statement that cardiac output begins to increase at the end of the first trimester and then rises gradually to peak at 30 to 50 per cent above prepregnant levels at 28 to 32 weeks of gestation. It was then reported to decrease toward non-pregnant levels by the end of pregnancy.[2, 5] Some early investigators did have findings obtained by direct cardiac catheterization suggesting that the peak increase in cardiac output is reached at an earlier time in pregnancy[6] and that cardiac output does not decline but remains elevated until term.[7] The reasons for these differences lie probably with differences in techniques and whether or not the patient was supine during the study in later pregnancy. Supine positioning results in vena caval and aortic compression and would alter the results. Rubler et al. have recently studied 40 pregnant patients using the noninvasive technique of echocardiography.[8] They found an increase in cardiac output of 54 per cent in the earliest group of patients studied (13–23 weeks), with essentially no change until delivery if the patients were evaluated in the lateral position. When placed supine, cardiac output was only 18 per cent above non-pregnant levels, the primary reduction being a decrease in stroke volume. They confirm that the observed increase in cardiac output was due to increases in stroke volume and heart rate. The magnitude of the heart rate change is 10 to 12 beats per minute.

Changes in cardiac output during labor are quite variable and depend upon patient position and the analgesic techniques employed. Elevations of cardiac output to 80 per cent over baseline have been recorded in patients with unmedicated labors who delivered under local anesthesia.[9]

Peripheral Resistance. Systemic vascular resistance has been shown by many investigators to decrease during pregnancy, reaching a maximum decline of 15 to 20 per cent at 20 to 24 weeks.[5, 6, 10] This is felt to be a hormonal effect of estrogen and progesterone resulting in vascular smooth muscle relaxation.[10] A slight decrease in blood pressure is commonly observed during the second trimester when resistance is at its lowest. These same hormones probably contribute to the increase in cardiac output as well.[11, 12]

RESPIRATORY SYSTEM CHANGES

Mechanics of Ventilation. The changes that take place in the mechanics of ventilation are due to the enlarging uterus causing diaphragmatic elevation. This leads to a reduction in residual volume as well as a decrease in expiratory reserve volume. The net change is a 15 to 25 per cent decrease in functional residual capacity at term.[5, 13] The change is gradual and does not become evident until the fifth or sixth month of gestation. As there is an increase in inspiratory capacity, there is essentially no change in vital capacity. A current wave of interest has focused on the closing volume or closing capacity (residual volume + closing volume) and their relationship to functional residual capacity as an indicator of small airway disease or impairment.[14] If the closing capacity approaches or exceeds the functional residual capacity, an abnormal state exists and oxygenation may be impaired. While there has been some variation in findings from investigator to investigator, it appears that there is little change in closing capacity during pregnancy. The reduction in the difference between functional residual capacity and closing volume is due to the reduction in functional residual capacity.[15]

Lung compliance appears to undergo little or no change in pregnancy but total compliance is decreased, probably due to elevation of the diaphragm and the weight of the parturient's engorged breasts.[16] Airway resistance is decreased during pregnancy.[13, 16, 17] The mechanism is felt to be either a progesterone effect or the result of increased corticosteroid production.[16, 17]

Ventilation. Minute ventilation is increased above non-pregnant levels by 50 per cent. This peak increase is effected by the twelfth to sixteenth week of gestation and is due primarily to an increase in tidal volume, although there is some increase in respiratory rate as well.[16] Dead space is unchanged; therefore, alveolar ventilation is also significantly increased. This leads to a slight increase in arterial oxygenation and mild hypocarbia. The increase in ventilation is brought about by the action of progesterone, which appears to increase the sensitivity of the respiratory center to carbon dioxide.[5, 16]

Respiration. Oxygen consumption is increased over non-pregnant levels as a result of the demand of the growing uterus and its products of conception. Increased oxygen requirements are also generated by the alterations in maternal metabolism as well as by increased cardiovascular performance. This increase in oxygen consumption approximates 15 to 20 per cent at term.[18] Carbon dioxide production is increased significantly from 19 weeks of gestation on, but there is no change in the respiratory quotient at rest. It is increased during exercise.[19]

Gastrointestinal Tract. The gastrointestinal tract is influenced by both the anatomic and hormonal changes of pregnancy. The gastroesophageal junction is rendered less competent and the normal anatomic relationship of the pyloric valve is altered by the enlarging uterus. This slows gastric emptying and increases the probability of reflux, regurgitation, and pulmonary aspiration. The gestational hormones (e.g., estrogen and progesterone) have been suspected of relaxing intestinal smooth muscle and thus delaying gastric emptying. Intraabdominal pressure is increased by the enlarged uterus, and manipulations of the uterus during labor, delivery, or cesarean section tend to raise this pressure further. There is an increase in gastric secretions and acid concentration in the second half of pregnancy, possibly stimulated by an increase in gastrin production.[20]

The patient in labor has, in addition to the above, a further delay in gastric emptying due to anxiety, pain, narcotic analgesics,[21] or belladona drugs. There may also be an increase in gastric acid secretion due to starvation ketosis.

Gastric emptying seems to regain some semblance of normality during the first eight hours postpartum. In one study, a group of postpartum patients undergoing tubal ligation were compared to elective surgical patients. The postpartum patients were all more than eight hours post-delivery, and there was no difference in gastric volume or pH when compared to controls. Significant numbers of patients in both groups, however, had volumes in the at-risk range (>25 ml) and a pH in the at-risk range (<2.5) for the pulmonary acid aspiration syndrome.[22]

The reduction of the risk of acid aspiration has become a key issue in obstetric anesthesia, and several authors recommend the routine use of antacids.[23-25] However, the safety of administering large volumes of antacids to pregnant patients with decreased gastric emptying has come under question. Case reports of significant pulmonary problems after antacid aspiration have appeared in the literature.[26, 27] Moreover, a carefully conducted study in dogs has revealed that the aspiration of emulsion type antacids produced a hypoxic syndrome that was as severe and as long in duration as hydrochloric acid aspiration. However, one month later, the animals that had hydrochloric acid instillation had normal lung pathology examinations, while those that received antacid solutions still showed chronic inflammatory changes.[28] Alternatives to emulsion antacids are being sought in compounds such as cimetidine, but their safety for obstetric practice has yet to be evaluated.[29] It is this author's practice to not prescribe oral antacids for laboring patients, but to have a 15 milliliter dose given at least 30 minutes prior to anesthesia for operative or potentially operative deliveries.

CLINICAL APPLICATION OF THE PHYSIOLOGIC ALTERATIONS IN PREGNANCY

The cardiovascular changes that take place during pregnancy have no substantial effect on normal patients. However, the patient with pre-existing cardiac disease may be severely stressed at each of four critical periods involving pregnancy. The first critical period is when maximum cardiac output during gestation is reached, and the second is when maximum blood volume is attained. These may occur at approximately the same time, and place a tremendous burden upon the patient's cardiovascular system. The third critical time is during labor. The increases in cardiac output during uterine contractions may exhaust the myocardial reserve of these patients. The Valsalva maneuver and raising of the legs in stirrups are to be avoided. The fourth major risk period is the immediate puerperium, when major shifts in circulation and resistance take place and the effects of any administered anesthetic dissipate.

The pulmonary changes observed have

major significance to the anesthetist. First, the reduction in *functional residual capacity* means that an inhalation agent will equilibrate more quickly between the alveoli and the blood stream during induction. Second, this reduction means that there is less reserve oxygen available during apnea, and this coupled with the increased cardiac output and increased oxygen consumption leads to a more rapid onset of hypoxemia. This can be minimized by adequate preoxygenation, a feat more easily accomplished because of the reduced functional residual capacity. In addition, it is easier for the anesthetist to overventilate the patient. This might result in a decrease in fetal oxygen saturation because maternal hypocapnia and alkalosis lead to a decrease in umbilical blood flow and a shift of the maternal oxygen-hemoglobin dissociation curve to the left in the pregnant ewe.[30] Although these changes are probably not significant to a normal fetus, they may represent a significant compromise to one already stressed. The third implication is that because of the increase in alveolar ventilation, equilibration during induction of anesthesia will take place more quickly and with a lower concentration of inhalation anesthetic drug. It is important to remember that while the changes in minute ventilation take place early in pregnancy, the alterations in lung volumes are not evident until after the fifth month.

The physiologic and anatomic alterations to the gastrointestinal system require that we consider each pregnant patient to be a full-stomach patient after 20 weeks of gestation. This is critical regardless of when the last oral intake actually took place. If a general anesthetic technique is employed, an attempt at gastric drainage and/or neutralization of the acid gastric contents should be utilized. A rapid induction with rapid intubation during the maintenance of cricoid pressure should be used. Awake intubation must always be considered for those patients who would appear to have a difficult airway on physical examination.

UTEROPLACENTAL PERFUSION

Uteroplacental perfusion is of interest to the anesthetist because it not only involves maintenance of adequate nutritional, respiratory and acid-base status in the fetus but also is the means by which drugs that have been administered will reach the conceptus. Uterine blood flow increases gradually throughout pregnancy from approximately 52 ml at 10 weeks' gestation to about 700 ml at term.[2, 5] The uteroplacental circulation is felt to be maximally dilated and to possess little or no autoregulatory capabilties.[31] This means that the uteroplacental circulation is a pressure dependent system. The net perfusion pressure will be the mean arterial pressure minus uterine venous pressure. The latter will be influenced by uterine muscle tone. It is generally felt that a mean arterial pressure of 70 torr or greater provides the optimum in uteroplacental perfusion.

Anesthetic techniques may affect uteroplacental perfusion by one or more of the following mechanisms.

1. *Hypotension.* Hypotension from any cause, such as spinal or epidural anesthesia or deep general anesthesia, will decrease the perfusion pressure to the uterus. A decrease in maternal systolic blood pressure of 25 per cent or more, or any systolic blood pressure below 100 torr, is considered significant hypotension and therapy is warranted. The effects of sustained hypotension on the fetus in early pregnancy are unknown but might include spontaneous abortion or congenital malformation if flow was inadequate during a critical period in development. Although there is theoretical risk to the fetus, this author and others have utilized induced hypotension in pregnant patients during the second trimester for essential neurosurgical procedures.[32] Systolic pressures were maintained at 50 torr for cerebral aneurysm clipping without ill effect on the fetus. We employed continuous Doppler monitoring of fetal heart rate and observed no significant changes. Donchin observed transient fetal bradycardia.[32] If unscheduled hypotension should occur during the course of a regional anesthetic, the appropriate measures would include left uterine displacement, for the reasons discussed below, leg raising, volume infusion, maternal supplemental oxygen, and the administration of an appropriate vasopressor. While a healthy lamb fetus can withstand reductions in uterine blood flow of 50 to 60 per cent for five minutes with no significant acid-base changes, this may not apply to a compromised or even a healthy human fetus.[33]

2. *Aortocaval Compression.* Aortocaval compression and its physiologic consequences is one of the simplest problems we deal with, yet it is often ignored. Few pregnant women after the middle of the second trimester choose to assume the supine position, yet medical personnel frequently ask them to do so. The difficulty lies in the fact that the heavy and enlarged uterus, which tends to dextrorotate in most pregnancies, compresses the aorta against the lumbar spine at the third lumbar vetebral body and occludes the inferior vena cava as well.[34, 35] Vena caval occlusion occurs in virtually all patients to some degree. This can affect the fetus in utero adversely by two mechanisms. The first is hypotension. Occlusion of the inferior vena cava for five to 15 minutes results in a decrease in cardiac return. Initially pulse rate increases and pulse pressure decreases as compensatory mechanisms are invoked. But in 10 to 20 per cent of patients obvious symptoms of hypotension ensue. This problem was appropriately recognized nearly 30 years ago and named the "supine hypotensive syndrome."[36] While this is occasionally an obvious means by which a decrease in uteroplacental perfusion may be brought about, the second mechanism, that of aortic compression, is equally important. The compression of the aorta takes place above the bifurcation, and since the hypogastric arteries (the vessels from which the uterine arteries originate) lie below this level, they may be effectively deprived of their blood flow, even though the maternal brachial artery pressure remains normal. This effect may be easily assessed by palpating the right femoral pulse in a supine patient, and then manually displacing the uterus upward and to the left. A significant change in the tactile pulse contour reveals that aortic compression has taken place.

Aortocaval compression is a problem most often observed during labor, especially when regional analgesia is used. Left uterine displacement by a wedge under the right buttock, assuming the left lateral decubitus position, or use of a mechanical device is an easily applied modality that will minimize the problem.

3. *Direct Anesthetic Effect.* Some anesthetics have an effect on uterine muscle tone. Of the volatile agents in common use today, halothane, enflurane, and isoflurane all relax the myometrium in a dose related fashion.[37] If this accompanies hypotension, uteroplacental flow will be decreased; however, if normotension and uterine displacement are maintained, there should be no ill effect. There may be maternal considerations, however, if uterine hypotonus is induced by these agents post-delivery. Increased bleeding will occur from both decreased myometrial tone and decreased sensitivity to oxytocin. Ketamine has an opposite effect of the inhalation anesthetics. It tends to increase uterine tonus in a dose-related fashion. Doses of 1.1 mg per kg or less have only a small effect on uterine tone, but doses above this result in substantial increases.[38] This may well reduce uteroplacental perfusion. Another anesthetic event that may compromise uteroplacental perfusion is light anesthesia, particularly during laryngoscopy and intubation. This results in a substantial elevation in plasma catecholamine levels, often enough to cause significant maternal hypertension. The presence of high catecholamine levels produced by maternal stress in the ewe have been shown to be associated with significant falls in uterine blood flow.[39] Although similar events in humans have yet to be documented, some investigators have observed a parallel response in monkeys.[40] The currently available muscle relaxant drugs have no direct effect on uterine tone or uteroplacental perfusion.

The use of any of the agents or techniques just discussed is not specifically contraindicated. However, the anesthetist should be aware of their potential adverse effects and suitably apply them when circumstances are appropriate. For example, a high-dose ketamine induction would be inappropriate for cesarean section for abruptio placentae, a situation already involving elevated uterine tone, whereas low-dose ketamine would be suitable for a cesarean section being performed for a bleeding placenta previa with maternal hypovolemia. Careful consideration of all of the factors involving the fetus and the mother is essential.

4. *Vasopressors.* When maternal hypotension occurs as the result of regional anesthesia, prompt and appropriate management is called for. Blood pressure declines with regional anesthesia because of venous pooling induced by sympathetic blockade. This leads to a decrease in cardiac return and a subsequent fall in cardiac output and blood pressure. To re-establish satisfactory cardiac return, left uterine displacement, leg raising, and an intravenous volume load often suffice. However, if the pressure cannot be adequately restored by the use of these maneuvers, the administration of a vasopressor is indicated. Although there are several in our armamentarium, only a few are satisfactory for use in the pregnant patient. Those agents that work primarily by causing peripheral arteriolar constriction, such as methoxamine, phenylephrine, and norepinephrine, cause uterine artery constriction and subsequently do not allow uteroplacental perfusion to return to pre-hypotensive levels, in spite of the fact that maternal blood pressure is restored.[41] If these agents are administered to a normotensive patient, one sees a fall in uterine blood flow as maternal arterial pressure is elevated.[33, 42]

These same investigators have found, however, that drugs that elevate blood pressure by causing an increase in cardiac output as the result of enhanced inotropy and chronotropy and venous tone, improve uterine blood flow. These drugs, ephedrine and mephentermine, are indirect acting with primarily beta adrenergic activity. Uterine blood flow is restored to 85 to 90 per cent of the pre-hypotensive level with these drugs.[41]

The more potent catecholamine-type pressors are rarely indicated in common clinical practice. Epinephrine administration, although it decreases uterine tone, is associated with an increase in uterine artery resistance and a decrease in uteroplacental perfusion.[43] Isoproterenol infusion results in vasodilatation and a net fall in mean arterial pressure and uterine blood flow.[44] Dopamine when administered in dosages that do not elevate maternal peripheral resistance may transiently increase uterine blood flow but when given in dosages that elevate maternal blood pressure causes a fall in uterine perfusion.[44] When dopamine is used as a vasopressor to correct the hypotension of spinal anesthesia, uterine blood flow is not restored in the pregnant ewe.[45]

The treatment of significant maternal hypotension that requires vasopressor use is best undertaken with ephedrine or mephentermine. The exception to this general practice would be for some patients with significant cardiac disease who cannot tolerate the increased demands of beta adrenergic stimulation. Under these circumstances,

a dilute infusion of metaraminol or phenylephrine would be appropriate.

The adequacy of maintenance of uteroplacental perfusion may be indirectly monitored by using the continuous fetal heart rate monitor during anesthesia. The presence of a normal fetal heart rate of 120 to 160 bpm is reassuring, and the occurrence of a significant tachycardia or bradycardia is an indication of fetal distress.

DRUGS, THE DEVELOPING FETUS AND NEWBORN

One of the major concerns of anesthetists and surgeons alike when faced with the possibility of operating on a pregnant patient is what effect the anesthetic drugs and adjuvants will have on the developing fetus. Numerous individual studies and reviews fill the literature with information on this subject.[46-51] When considering such information, the following principles of teratology need to be kept in mind:

1. The *specificity* of the substance could be quite broad or limited to a single species.

2. The *dosage* of the agent reaching the conceptus will determine the degree of teratogenic effect. This is also dependent on those factors governing placental transfer; e.g., some of the muscle relaxants are teratogenic to the chick embryo when directly injected, but cross the placenta in such minuscule quantities as to not be a hazard in clinical practice.[52]

3. The *time* during *embryogenesis* at which exposure takes place is critical. The effects of a given drug will vary at different times during development. For instance, a specific drug may either kill the blastocyst or allow it to develop entirely normally if exposure occurs during the first two weeks, as the cells are totipotential. If given after twelve weeks, organogenesis is complete and only organ size or brain development may be affected.

The mechanisms of teratogenicity are mutation, chromosal dysjunction, interference with substrate precursors, depletion of energy sources, enzyme inhibition, altered membrane characteristics, or osmolar imbalance. These may result in excess cell death, reduced proliferation, decreased cellular interactions, impeded morphogenic movements, reduced biosynthesis, or mechanical disruption. The ultimate change is a lack of cells.[53]

To establish proof of teratogenicity one must look at both retrospective and prospective evidence. Retrospectively there should be a sudden increase in an anomaly beginning at the time of the drug's introduction. The exposure should have occurred at the appropriate time during development, and a reasonable dose-response curve might be evident. Prospectively, confirmatory animal studies need to be undertaken.

The potential for the teratogenicity of anesthetic agents and the adjunctive drugs used as premedicants, etc., has been thoroughly reviewed in two recent writings.[54, 55] It is clear that virtually every drug and every inhalation anesthetic including nitrous oxide is teratogenic to some species under some conditions. However, in the words of Shnider and Levinson: "At present, *no* anesthetic drug, premedicant, intravenous induction agent, inhalation agent or local anesthetic ... has been *proved* to be teratogenic in humans." In fact, the studies that have attempted to identify the relationship between anesthesia for surgery and congenital malformations were unable to do so.[56, 57] Although this scanty evidence is encouraging, we cannot assume that some potential for teratogenicity does not exist. The wisest course would be to postpone elective surgery until after pregnancy if possible. If surgery must be performed during gestation, the period of organogenesis, that is the first twelve eeks, should be avoided. When administering an anesthetic to a patient during pregnancy, only those agents and techniques that have had wide usage and evaluation should be employed, such as barbiturates, narcotics, halothane, muscle relaxants, and nitrous oxide if general anesthesia is used. If circumstances are appropriate for regional anesthesia, spinal anesthesia may be preferred over epidural anesthesia. This is for two reasons. First, there is no drug transfer to the infant, so the teratogenic risk, if any, is reduced, and second, if premature labor and delivery follow the operation, the neonate will not have to deal with the distribution and metabolism of the drug.

A final consideration for drug transfer to the infant is in the postpartum period. Nearly all substances given to the mother will be excreted in the breast milk. This consideration should be given to the lactating mother, particularly if she chooses not to have her infant exposed, and regional (spinal) anesthesia used when applicable. There is no evidence, however, that a single maternal exposure to routine anesthetic drugs in commonly employed doses has any effect on the breast-fed neonate.[58] The major difficulties arise with chronic drug use.

The major considerations, then, for providing appropriate anesthetic care for the pregnant patient are as follows:

1. Attention to the maternal physiologic adjustments and their influence on anesthetic techniques to provide maximum maternal and fetal safety.

2. Maintenance of adequate uteroplacental perfusion by avoiding and/or treating hypotension and aortocaval compression.

3. Selection of drugs and techniques that have a good record for fetal safety.

4. Provide surveillance of fetal well being by observing fetal heart rate and uterine activity whenever possible by the use of the fetal monitor.

The significance of the physiologic changes of pregnancy and the potential effects of anesthetic drugs and techniques have been reviewed. These principles will now be applied to some specific disorders of pregnancy that the anesthetist may become involved with.

DISORDERS OF PREGNANCY

TOXEMIA OF PREGNANCY

The Disease

The toxemias of pregnancy, e.g., preeclampsia and eclampsia (preeclampsia plus convulsions), are distinguished by being among those disorders for which we have no known etiology or specific pharmacologic therapy; yet, we symptomatically treat them with regularity in our labor and delivery suites. The overall incidence is seven percent of all pregnancies in the United States.[59] Preeclampsia most commonly presents during the third trimester of pregnancy, although it is not infrequently found in association with molar pregnancy during the first or early second trimesters. It is characterized by the classical triad of hypertension, edema of the face and upper extremities, and proteinuria.

Hypertension is the most significant diagnostic criterion and is defined as 1) a 30 torr increase in systolic blood pressure, 2) a 15 torr increase in diastolic pressure, or 3) any blood pressure increase to 140/90 torr or greater. The presence of proteinuria signifies renal involvement and is of prognostic significance. The edema of preeclampsia is not the lower extremity swelling commonly observed in pregnancy due to vena caval obstruction but is generalized and anasarca-like in quality.

Preeclampsia is classified as either mild or severe. The severe preeclamptic is a far more difficult management problem and is identified by the presence of 1) a blood pressure of 160/110 torr or greater, 2) proteinuria of 5 grams per day or greater, 3) oliguria (400 cc or less per day), 4) cerebral or visual symptoms, and 5) pulmonary edema or cyanosis. Any one of the preceding classifies the patient as a severe preeclamptic.

While the specific etiology of the disease remains unknown, much of the available evidence suggests that a reduction in uteroplacental bed perfusion initiates the many pathophysiologic changes seen. The disease is somehow related to the existence of a placenta, as the termination of pregnancy results in an amelioration of symptoms. Some investigators have proposed that a placental vasculitis occurs during the first trimester of pregnancy, which sets the stage for uteroplacental bed ischemia.[60, 61] This then leads to increased sodium and water reabsorption due to activation of the renin-angiotensin-aldosterone system and the subsequent stigmata of the disorder.

Pathophysiologic Alterations

The commonly noted pathophysiologic alterations are 1) a decrease in circulating blood volume, primarily plasma volume, in spite of an excess of total body sodium and water, resulting in hemoconcentration;[62] 2) a coagulopathy characterized initially by a reduction in platelet count[63] and later by a rise in fibrin degradation products, a fall in fibrinogen level and prolongation of partial thromboplastin time and prothrombin time; 3) a decrease in renal blood flow and an elevation of serum uric acid (6.6 mg/100 ml) over normal pregnant levels (3.0 ± 0.17 mg/100 ml)[63] secondary to an increased tubular reabsorption of sodium; 4) increased

vascular sensitivity to vasoactive substances such as catecholamines due to swelling of the arteriolar walls as a result of an increased sodium content within them;[64] 5) elevated catecholamine levels;[64] 6) retinal arteriolar spasm;[65] and 7) hepatic dysfunction in the more advanced case.[66] It is not clear if the hyperreflexia often seen with preeclampsia is a central nervous system or a peripheral nervous system manifestation.

Therapy

The therapeutic goals are to control blood pressure so as to prevent cardiac and vascular accidents, prevent seizures, maintain renal function, and provide optimum conditions for the fetus. While this may be achieved by bedrest and sedation for the mild preeclamptic, the patient with more severe disease requires pharmacologic intervention. If this fails, then early delivery is the only cure.

The conventional therapy for prevention of convulsions in the United States is magnesium sulfate. It is administered intramuscularly, as an intravenous bolus or as a continuous intravenous infusion, and tends to relax uterine muscle tone, therefore improving uterine blood flow. The therapeutic range is between 6 and 8 meq/L of magnesium. Patients receiving magnesium sulfate must have respiration, deep tendon reflexes, and urine output carefully observed. The drug is eliminated from the body only by renal excretion, and when toxic levels are approached deep tendon reflexes disappear before respirations are lost. Magnesium acts at the motor end-plate by inhibiting the release of acetylcholine, decreasing motor end-plate sensitivity and decreasing muscle membrane excitability. Magnesium also is a mild direct vasodilator, depresses myocardial conduction in larger doses, and decreases myocardial contractility at levels of 12 to 15 meq/L. It may also be a central nervous system depressant. The antidote for magnesium overdose is calcium, either as the chloride or gluconate. Another effect of magnesium of interest to the anesthetist is that it potentiates both depolarizing and non-depolarizing muscle relaxants because of its actions at the moter end plate.[67, 68] DeVore has demonstrated that defasciculation prior to a dose of succinylcholine is not necessary if the patient has received magnesium sulfate.[69]

The threshold for pharmacologic intervention in the management of hypertension is 170/110 torr. Blood pressures above this level are considered dangerous, as cerebral vascular accidents may occur, and therapy is directed at reducing diastolic pressure to 100 torr or only slightly below. This is because of the concern for maintaining a perfusion pressure sufficient to maintain uteroplacental blood flow. This concept has been recently challenged as a result of newer studies, in normal animals, of uteroplacental perfusion which suggest that lower mean arterial pressures might suffice.[70] Hydralazine has proven most popular, as it is a direct acting vasodilator that appears to maintain or increase renal and uterine blood flows.[71] It may be administered orally, intramuscularly, or intravenously. Tachycardia and an increase in cardiac output without a decrease in blood pressure occasionally occurs, and this may be corrected with propranolol. Other potent antihypertensives may be utilized to treat the maternal emergency but with caution. Diazoxide has been associated with precipitous decreases in blood pressure and fetal demise. Sodium nitropresside has been found to induce fetal cyanide toxicity.[72] Trimethaphan has been useful in some cases, and nitroglycerin, while it has promise, has not yet been adequately evaluated.[73] Regardless of the agent chosen, careful attention to blood volume restitution before or during antihypertensive therapy should avert precipitous changes in blood pressure. This often requires the insertion of a central venous pressure line, arterial line, and/or a Swan-Ganz catheter.

Diuretics have essentially no role in the modern care of the preeclamptic patient. They simply further aggravate the state of volume depletion.

Anesthetic Considerations

The anesthetic implications for the care of a patient with severe preeclampsia are as follows.

1. *Blood Volume.* There is a reduction in circulating blood volume with *hemoconcentration.* This may mask the presence of an anemia. The volume depletion may lead to an exaggeration of the response to aortocaval compression; therefore, left uterine displacement must be employed for all patients who have passed the middle of the second trimester to avoid the subsequent hypotension and decreased uteroplacental perfusion. Intravenous fluid loading may be necessary for the safe conduct of regional or general anesthesia. This may be accomplished with colloids such as plasma protein fraction or albumin, as there is often a significant decrease in colloid osmotic pressure. It is essential to remember that volume loading is a short-term therapy so that the patient will tolerate the trespasses of anesthesia. It is not a treatment for the disease. This should be undertaken only with careful monitoring of the cardiovascular system so as to avoid administering a volume excess, which could lead to ascites, anasarca, pleural effusion, or pulmonary edema.

2. *Vascular Reactivity.* The increase in vascular reactivity results in an intensified response to circulating catecholamines. This is a particular problem with light general anesthesia and endotracheal intubation.[74] This may be prevented by the administration of an intravenous bolus of lidocaine (1.5 mg/kg) or sodium nitroprusside (1 μg/kg) just prior to induction.[75] There will also be a more potent response from the administration of vasopressor agents. If they are required, the initial dose should be reduced by from 30 to 50 percent.

3. *Laryngeal edema* is more common in pregnancy and particularly in edematous preeclamptic patients. It may make intubation more difficult or result in postoperative airway problems.[76]

4. *Drug interactions* between therapeutic drugs and anesthetic agents may take place and compromise the patient. The interaction between the muscle relaxants and magnesium sulfate was mentioned above. This may best be avoided by utilizing lower doses of relaxants and employing a peripheral nerve stimulator to assess the degree of blockade.

Cardiovascular depression may occur from the addition of anesthetic adjuvants to pre-existing antihypertensives such as propranolol. If plasma proteins are low, some anesthetic drugs that are highly protein bound will need to be given in reduced dosage.

5. The *coagulopathy* of preeclampsia should be carefully assessed by a platelet count, fibrinogen level, fibrin degradation products, prothrombin time, and partial

thromboplastin time. Any significant abnormality represents a contraindication to regional anesthesia because continued bleeding in the epidural space and an epidural hematoma may result. Invasive monitoring techniques should be performed with consideration for potential bleeding subsequent to vascular puncture.

6. *Monitoring aids* are indispensable when caring for the preeclamptic patient. The minimum requirements for the severe preeclamptic undergoing anesthesia and surgery are a blood pressure cuff, stethoscope, cardioscope, and a Foley catheter. A central venous line or a Swan-Ganz catheter is extremely useful, and an arterial line provides second to second information on blood pressure responses. An external fetal heart rate monitor should be applied whenever feasible to ensure satisfactory fetal status. With full cardiovascular monitoring, one can determine cardiac output and resistance values for more precise guides to fluid and drug therapy.

The actual choice of anesthetic will depend on the surgical procedure itself, the status of the patient, and the condition of the fetus if still in utero. General anesthesia is favored by many and can be successfully utilized providing the appropriate precautions are taken. Regional anesthesia, for example, spinal or epidural, would be acceptable for procedures of the lower extremities and some intra-abdominal surgery. While considerable controversy has raged over the application of epidural anesthesia for cesarean section in the preeclamptic patient, most agree that with careful monitoring and fluid balance it can be administered safely. Epidural anesthesia usually results in a slower onset of sympathetic blockade and hypotension, thus avoiding the precipitous changes often seen with spinal anesthesia. Spinal anesthesia would prove more useful for those procedures requiring a level no higher than the tenth thoracic dermatome. When epidural or axillary block anesthesia is performed, the same considerations about drug transfer and fetal disposition that are used in routine obstetric practice must be invoked.[77] The addition of epinephrine, while reducing the blood level of local anesthetics, may have significant detrimental effects on maternal cardiovascular performance and uteroplacental perfusion, particularly in the hypertensive patient.

This unique and complex disease continues to be an enigma. The application of the above-mentioned principles will assist in providing a safer course of anesthesia and surgery for both mother and infant.

HYDATIDIFORM MOLE

The Disease

Hydatidiform mole and choriocarcinoma compose the disease entity known as gestational trophoblastic disease. Choriocarcinoma is a rare tumor, occurring either de novo, from germinal epithelium in the ovary or embryonic rests, or more commonly following either a normal or molar pregnancy.[78] Hydatidiform mole is a benign neoplasm in which part or all of the chorionic villi are converted into a mass of clear grapelike vesicles. Usually there is no fetus or embryo present, but there have been occasional reports of a mole with a coexistent fetus.[79] Varying degrees of trophoblastic proliferation take place. The incidence of molar pregnancy ranges from 1:2500 in the United States to 1:173 live births in the Philippines.[80] The diagnosis is suspected when fetal heart tones are not detectible by Doppler device or auscultation at the end of the first or beginning of the second trimester of pregnancy. A presumptive diagnosis may be rendered if serum or urine human chorionic gonadotropin levels are found to be quite high. This assay might be obtained for a patient who has no fetal heart tones or some of the other clinical stigmata of molar pregnancy. Confirmation of the diagnosis would be made by amniography or ultrasound study.[79, 81] Complicated moles are classified into three groups. Retained mole refers to the presence of molar tissue in the uterine cavity after prior evacuation. An invasive mole is one in which the villi have penetrated into the uterine wall. A metastatic mole is one that has spread via the venous system to extrauterine sites and is a far more serious disease. Eighty per cent of molar pregnancies are discovered between 12 and 18 weeks of gestation and are uncomplicated.

Pathophysiology

The patient with molar pregnancy may have no symptoms at all and will be discovered only because her physician has a high index of suspicion. More commonly, though, the patient will present with significant vaginal bleeding and a uterus that is larger than appropriate for the stage of gestation.[82] This is usually during the latter portion of the first, or during the second trimester of pregnancy. Approximately one fourth of the patients will have the signs and symptoms of toxemia, for example, hypertension, edema, and proteinuria. Some will have excessive nausea and vomiting. While thyroid function tests will be elevated in a large proportion of patients, only a few will demonstrate clinical signs of thyrotoxicosis.[83, 84] Trophoblastic embolization occurs in 2 per cent or less of the cases, and while often fatal, has responded favorably to chemotherapeutic agents and more current pulmonary therapeutic modalities such as mechanical ventilation with positive-end-expiratory pressure.[85, 86]

Therapy

The initial treatment of molar pregnancy is evacuation of the uterine contents. This may be accomplished by dilatation of the cervix followed by sharp curettage for patients with small uteri. The most common method of emptying the uterus today, however, is by suction curettage.[80] Under some circumstances hysterotomy with uterine evacuation or hysterectomy may be performed. Non-surgical evacuation of the uterus has been recommended by some authors by the use of oxytoxic agents or prostaglandins.[87] Regardless of the mode of uterine evacuation, the patient is then carefully followed for persistence of trophoblastic tissue by sensitive human chorionic gondotropin assays. Persistent trophoblastic disease is usually treated by chemotherapy with methotrexate and/or actinomycin D.

Anesthetic Considerations

The patient presenting for evacuation of a molar pregnancy requires assessment and consideration of the following:
1. *Blood volume* may be depleted as a result of vaginal bleeding. Anemia may be masked by hemoconcentration secondary to toxemia or dehydration. Since blood loss may be substantial at surgery, deficits should be corrected and additional blood

and blood products be available. Hemorrhage may occur at the time of dilatation or during the evacuation. Post-evacuation bleeding may occur as the result of uterine perforation, cervical laceration, or uterine atony. Intravenous lines of adequate caliber and number should be placed. Central venous pressure monitoring may well be indicated.
2. *Fluid and electrolyte* status should be assessed, as hyperemesis may lead to derangement of both.
3. If *toxemia* is present, blood pressure and volume should be under control prior to surgery. Appropriate monitoring (e.g., central venous pressure and/or arterial line) and pharmacologic therapy should be instituted as for other preeclamptic patients.
4. The potential for *thyroid storm* needs to be evaluated by performing thyroid function tests, and specific therapeutic modalities, such as iodine, steroids, adrenegic blocking agents, and antithyroid drugs must be ready at hand.[88]
5. *Uterine relaxation* will further increase blood loss; therefore, inhalation anesthetics with known tocolytic qualities, such as halothane, enflurane, and isoflurane, should be used in low concentrations, if at all.[37]
6. *Oxytocin*, usually as an infusion, will be required before, during, and after curettage. It should be remembered that an intravenous bolus of 5 units or more, or rapid infusion of a highly concentrated solution, will result in hypotension lasting from three to five minutes.[89] On occasion the surgeon will request ergotrate for increased uterine contractility. A pressor effect may be seen in from 22 to 48 per cent of patients after ergotrate administration.[90] Dangerous levels of hypertension have been observed after intravenous administration, and it is therefore recommended primarily for intramuscular use. It should not be used in combination with a vasopressor or in patients with signs and symptoms of preeclampsia.

The anesthetic management of the patient for evacuation of a molar pregnancy is based on the degree of symptoms and physiologic alterations present. On some occasions regional anesthesia is acceptable if the uterus is small and hypovolemia is not present. Appropriate monitoring and preparation for blood loss, extended surgical procedures, metabolic derangements, and hypertensive crises are among the requisite considerations for a safe intraoperative course.

ECTOPIC PREGNANCY

The Disease

Ectopic pregnancy occurs in the United States with a frequency of 1:100 to 1:200 live births.[91] It is currently responsible for 10 per cent of the maternal deaths in this country.[92] The most common location of an ectopic pregnancy is in the isthmus of the fallopian tube, although implantation on other abdominal organs or in the cornua of the uterus may take place. The usual cause of tubal pregnancy is prior salpingitis with subsequent narrowing of the tube. Other, less frequent, mechanisms include endometriosis, adhesions from prior abdominal or pelvic surgery, tuberculosis, or adhesions from other intra-abdominal infection. The surgeon may encounter an intact tubal pregnancy, a ruptured tubal pregnancy, a tubal abortion where in the conceptus has been expelled from the fimbriated end of the tube, or a chronic ectopic pregnancy. The diagnosis of ruptured ectopic pregnancy or tubal abortion requires immediate laparotomy, while intact and chronic ectopic pregnancies may require diagnostic operative procedures such as laparoscopy or culdoscopy.

The diagnosis is suspected when a female of child-bearing age presents with lower abdominal pain. If rupture has occurred, shoulder pain due to diaphragmatic irritation by the blood in the peritoneal cavity may be present. Signs and symptoms of neurogenic or hypovolemic shock may be manifested. Often, however, the patient will complain of vague symptoms, vaginal bleeding, or other nonspecific pelvic complaints, and the diagnosis will be delayed.[92] The usual signs and symptoms of pregnancy may be present and a pregnancy test may be positive.

Pathophysiology and Therapy

The pathophysiology of this problem is straightforward. The patient with a ruptured ectopic pregnancy or tubal abortion continues to bleed intra-abdominally. Initially, fainting from neurogenically induced causes occurs but the situation will soon progress to the familiar one of hemorrhagic shock. The unruptured ectopic pregnancy presents no immediate threat, and the chronic ectopic gestation tends to bleed slowly or intermittently, leading to anemia but not acute hypovolemia, unless rupture occurs. When a tubal pregnancy is suspected, a culdocentesis is performed. The finding of nonclotting blood within the peritoneal cavity identifies hemoperitoneum, and laparotomy is indicated. The surgical procedure begins by obtaining hemostasis, and then either salpingectomy, salpingo-oophorectomy, or hysterectomy will be performed. Salpingectomy is the most common operation.[91]

If culdocentesis is negative but an ectopic pregnancy is still suspected, diagnostic procedures such as ultrasound[93] or laparoscopy[94] will aid in the diagnosis. Once an ectopic pregnancy is identified, surgical removal is appropriate as soon as feasible to avoid the possibility of rupture.

Anesthetic Considerations

The anesthetist will be faced either with a patient who has an acute ruptured ectopic pregnancy about to undergo emergency surgery or with one who is to undergo a diagnostic operative procedure, possibly followed by definitive surgery.

The ruptured ectopic pregnancy patient usually has postural signs of *hypovolemia* and will need intravenous volume restoration and maintenance; therefore, additional intravenous access is advisable. Although these patients are usually young and have a healthy cardiovascular system, a central venous pressure monitor and a Foley catheter are very useful in guiding volume therapy. Since these patients have only recently had hemodynamic stability restored, it is often wise to delay induction until the abdomen is prepared and draped and the surgeon is ready to proceed. An interesting device to help control abdominal bleeding and support the cardiovascular system until surgery can begin is the G-suit or medical antishock trousers. The ability of this apparatus to arrest life-threatening intra-abdominal bleeding has been documented in animals and humans.[95] The suit is an inflatable device that covers the abdomen and both legs. Optimal inflation pressures are 20 to 25 mm Hg, as this is sufficient to compress the capacitance vessels in the legs and splanchnic bed and to decrease the transarterial pressure gradient intra-abdominally. This increases circulating blood volume while controlling the hemorrhage by compression. Once inflated, the pressure should not be released until the patient has had adequate fluid resuscitation and surgery is ready to begin, as a pressure drop of 40 to 60 torr may suddenly occur on deflation.[96] If possible, the legs should be deflated first and further volume given, if needed, prior to decompressing the abdominal bladder. Regardless, when the abdomen is surgically opened the patient will most likely experience a sudden drop in blood pressure; therefore, anesthetic maintenance needs to be light until hemostasis is gained.

These patients should be considered full-stomach patients. Since regional anesthesia is precluded by the hypovolemia, a rapid induction with prompt endotracheal intubation with cricoid pressure application should be employed to reduce the possibility of regurgitation and aspiration of gastric contents.

The patient who is to have diagnostic laparoscopy and removal of an intact ectopic pregnancy, if present, is not a major anesthetic problem. However, there are some specific considerations for anesthesia for laparoscopy. Although local[97] and regional anesthesia have been used, most anesthetists prefer to use general anesthesia.

1. *Endotracheal intubation* is necessary because when the abdomen is inflated with gas, usually CO_2, there is elevation of the diaphragm and increased work of breathing. Assisted or controlled ventilation is required to maintain adequate arterial blood gases.[98] The increased intra-abdominal pressure predisposes to regurgitation; therefore, the airway should be protected by a cuffed endotracheal tube.

2. The effects of Trendelenburg's position must be taken into account. They include the cardiovascular effects of increased venous return, impairment of ventilation, regurgitation of gastric contents, a shift in the tracheobronchial tree and subsequent endobronchial intubation, and brachial plexus palsy from misplaced shoulder braces.[99]

3. The hemodynamic effects of pneumoperitoneum, particularly if pressures exceed 25 torr, result in hypotension secondary to vena caval obstruction, vagal reflexes, and cardiac arrhythmia if CO_2 retention oc-

curs.[100, 101] Release of the pressure should correct the situation.

4. Complications that may occur during laparoscopy include CO_2 embolization,[102] hemorrhage secondary to laceration of mesenteric vessels,[103] subcutaneous emphysema, pneumomediastinum, and pneumothorax.[45] In addition, gastric or intestinal perforation may occur; on occasion, this may be due to distention from bag and mask ventilation or esophageal intubation.[50]

5. Laparoscopy would be contraindicated for patients in shock or for those with significant cardiovascular disease, significant pulmonary disease, or extreme obesity.

The care of the patient with an ectopic pregnancy is best facilitated by advance preparation and anticipation of the probable intraoperative events.

INCOMPETENT CERVIX

The patient with an incompetent cervix usually has a history of late first or second trimester pregnancy loss with painless dilatation of the cervix, prolapse followed by rupture of the membranes, and subsequent expulsion of the conceptus. Many women with this history have had prior surgical manipulation of the cervix for diagnostic reasons or therapeutic abortion.[105] The diagnosis is made either by history or by finding the cervix dilated at an early stage of pregnancy. The problem is treated by placing a suture or a band around the cervix (i.e., a cerclage procedure) to prevent loss of the uterine contents. This is usually performed between 12 weeks and 28 weeks of gestation, provided the patient has intact membranes and is not in premature labor. The commonly used operation early in pregnancy is one described by Shirodkar and modified by Barter wherein a Mersilene band is placed submucosally. The MacDonald procedure is useful at later stages of pregnancy, as it merely involves placing a pursestring suture around the cervix. The Wurm procedure (i.e., the placement of mattress sutures at right angles to close the cervical os) is less frequently used, and the Lash procedure, a resection of part of the cervix, is performed in the non-pregnant state only.[106] When the patient is to be delivered, either the cerclage is removed or cesarean section is performed.

The anesthetic care and its implications

will depend to some degree on the stage of pregnancy at the time of surgery. The author prefers to use low spinal anesthesia (T-10), as it provides adequate surgical conditions and is not associated with significant hypotension or nausea. Hypotension will reduce uteroplacental blood flow, and the retching associated with nausea will bulge the membranes and stress the suture, possibly leading to rupture of the membranes. Another advantage is that virtually no drug is transferred to the fetus. Others prefer general anesthesia with halothane, as it relaxes the uterus and may decrease the spontaneous onset of labor in response to cervical manipulation.[54]

The following points need to be considered when administering anesthesia for this operation.

1. There is an increased risk of the *acid aspiration* syndrome in pregnancy. An antacid should be administered at least one half hour prior to the procedure. If general anesthesia is used, a rapid induction, rapid intubation sequence with cricoid pressure is indicated.

2. *Uteroplacental perfusion* must be maintained. Aortocaval compression becomes significant in the second trimester; therefore, left uterine displacement must be accomplished with a wedge or table tilt.[107] If regional anesthesia is selected, an intravenous volume load prior to the block is advised to prevent hypotension. If a vasopressor is required, one such as ephedrine should be used, as it restores circulatory balance by improving cardiac output, not by vasoconstriction.[33] Should an epidural or caudal anesthetic be selected, epinephrine should be omitted from the anesthetic solution, as it may reduce uterine blood flow.[43]

3. *Local anesthetic drugs* should be selected with thought given to their fetal disposition.[77] Caudal and epidural anesthesia would best be performed with chloroprocaine or bupivacaine, since premature labor frequently follows this operative procedure. These local anesthetics appear to be better tolerated and more quickly eliminated by the fetus than other drugs.

4. While adequate evidence is still lacking in humans, all of the volatile anesthetics have some teratogenic action in some animal species.[54] Their avoidance except when specifically indicated is advisable.

5. Ketamine significantly increases uterine tone in doses greater than 1.0 mg

per kg and should be avoided for this procedure.[108]

6. Fetal heart rate and uterine activity can be easily monitored with external devices today, and these should be employed throughout the perioperative period.[109]

7. Because many obstetricians use uterine suppressants such as ethanol, isoxsuprine, or terbutaline in the immediate postoperative period, it is wise to be aware of their side effects, as the anesthetist may be called upon to deal with them.[110]

It must be stressed that the anesthetic care of the pregnant patient, whether in the labor and delivery suite, the cesarean section room, or the operating room, depends upon a thorough knowledge of the normal physiologic alterations of pregnancy and the pathophysiologic changes of the situation requiring intervention. This must be coupled with a knowledge of the pharmacology of the drugs we use, in order to provide the safest possible anesthetic plan. Monitoring devices, both invasive and non-invasive, can provide invaluable information and permit the most precise management of difficult situations. Indeed, the uncomplicated pregnant patient who comes to the operating room is an interesting enough entity, while the parturient with a disorder of pregnancy presents a formidable challenge.

REFERENCES

1. Pritchard, J. A.: Changes in the blood volume during pregnancy and delivery. Anesthesiology 26:393, 1965.
2. Hytten, F. E., and Leitch, I.: The Physiology of Human Pregnancy. 2nd ed., Oxford, Blackwell Scientific Publications, 1971.
3. Ueland, K.: Maternal cardiovascular dynamics VII. Intrapartum blood volume changes. Am. J. Obstet. Gynecol. 126:671, 1976.
4. Landesman, R., and Miller, M. M.: Blood volume changes during the immediate postpartum period. Obstet. Gynecol. 21:40, 1963.
5. Bonica, J. J.: Principles and Practice of Obstetric Analgesia and Anesthesia. Philadelphia, F. A. Davis Co., 1972, pp. 11–39.
6. Bader, R. A., Bader, M. E., Rose, D. J., et al.: Hemodynamics at rest and during exercise in normal pregnancy as studied by cardiac catheterization. J. Clin. Invest. 34:1524, 1955.
7. Lees, M. M., Taylor, S. H., and Scott, D. B.: A study of cardiac output at rest and throughout pregnancy. J. Obstet. Gynecol. Brit. Comm. 74:319, 1967.
8. Rubler, S., Prabodhkumar, M. D., and Pinto, E. R.: Cardiac size and performance during pregnancy estimated with echocardiography. Amer. J. Cardiol. 40:534, 1977.

9. Ueland, K., and Hansen, J.: Maternal cardiovascular dynamics III. Labor and delivery under local and caudal analgesia. Am. J. Obstet. Gynecol. 103:8, 1968.

10. Hansen, J. M., and Ueland, K.: Maternal cardiovascular dynamics during pregnancy and parturition. In Marx, G. (ed.): Clinical Anesthesia 10/2. Parturition and Perinatology. 1973, pp. 21–36.

11. Ueland, K., and Parer, J. T.: Cardiovascular changes during pregnancy in ewes. Am. J. Obstet. Gynecol. 96:400, 1966.

12. Walters, W. A., Lim, Y.L.: Cardiovascular dynamics in women receiving oral contraceptive therapy. Lancet 2:879, 1969.

13. Gee, J. B. L., et al.: Pulmonary mechanics during pregnancy. J. Clin. Invest. 46:945, 1967.

14. Juno, P., et al.: Closing capacity in awake and anesthetized-paralyzed man. J. Appl. Physiol. 44:238, 1978.

15. Craig, D. B., and Toole, M. A.: Airway closure in pregnancy. Canad. Anaesth. Soc. J. 22:665, 1975.

16. Bonica, J. J.: Maternal respiratory changes during pregnancy and parturition. In Marx, G. (ed.): Clinical Anesthesia 10/2. 1973, pp. 1–19.

17. Rubin, A., Russo, N., and Goucher, D.: The effect of pregnancy upon pulmonary function in normal women. Am. J. Obstet. Gynecol. 72:963, 1956.

18. Pernoll, M. L., Metcalfe, J., Schenkler, T. L., et al.: Oxygen consumption at rest and during exercise in pregnancy. Resp. Physiol. 25:285, 1975.

19. Pernoll, M. L., Metcalfe, J., Kovach, P. A., et al.: Ventilation during rest and exercise in pregnancy and postpartum. Resp. Physiol. 25:295, 1975.

20. Attia, R. R., Ebeid, A. M., and Fischer, J. E.: Gastrin: Placental, maternal and plasma cord levels. Its possible role in maternal residual gastric acidity. In Abstracts of Scientific Papers, Annual Meeting, American Society of Anesthesiologists, San Francisco, 1976, pp. 547–548.

21. Holdsworth, J. D.: Relationship between stomach contents and analgesia in labour. Br. J. Anaesth. 50:1145, 1978.

22. Blouw, T. B., Scatliff, J., Craig, D. B., et al.: Gastric volume and pH in postpartum patients. Anesthesiology 45:456, 1976.

23. Taylor, G., and Pryse-Davies, J.: The prophylactic use of antacids in the prevention of the acid-pulmonary aspiration syndrome (Mendelson's syndrome). Lancet 1:288, 1966.

24. Roberts, R. B., and Shirley, M. A.: Reducing the risk of acid aspiration during cesarean section. Anesth. Analg. (Cleve.) 53:859, 1974.

25. Wheatley, R. G., Kallus, F. T., Reynolds, R. C., et al.: Milk of magnesia is an effective pre-induction antacid in obstetric anesthesia. Anesthesiology 50:514, 1979.

26. Taylor, G.: Acid pulmonary aspiration after antacids. Br. J. Anaesth. 47:615, 1975.

27. Bond; V. K., Stoelting, R. K., Gupta, M. B.: Pulmonary aspiration syndrome after inhalation of gastric fluid containing antacids. Anesthesiology 51:452, 1979.

28. Gibbs, C. P., Schwartz, D. J., Wynne, J. W., et al.: Antacid pulmonary aspiration in the dog. Anesthesiology 51:380, 1979.

29. Stoelting RK: Gastric fluid pH in patients receiving cimetidine. Anesth. Analg. (Cleve.) 57:675, 1978.

30. Levinson, G., Shnider, S. M., deLorimer, A. A., et al.: Effects of maternal hyperventilation on uterine blood flow and fetal oxygenation and acid-base status. Anesthesiology 40:340, 1974.

31. Parer, J. T.: Uteroplacental circulation and respiratory gas exchange. In Shnider, S. M., and Levinson, G. (eds.): Anesthesia for Obstetrics. Baltimore, William and Wilkins, 1979, pp. 12–22.

32. Donchin, Y., Amirav, B., Sahar, A., et al.: Sodium nitroprusside for aneurysm surgery in pregnancy. Br. J. Anaesth. 50:849–851, 1978.

33. Ralston, D. H., Shnider, S. M., and deLorimer, A. A.: Effects of equipotent ephedrine, metaraminol, mephentermine, and methoxamine on uterine blood flow in the pregnant ewe. Anesthesiology 40:354, 1974.

34. Bieniarz, J., Crottogini, J. J., Curuchet, E., et al.: Aortocaval compression by the uterus in late human pregnancy. II. An angiographic study. Am. J. Obstet. Gynecol. 100:203, 1968.

35. Kerr, M. G., Scott, D. B., and Samuel, E.: Studies of the inferior vena cava in late pregnancy. Br. Med. J. 1:532, 1964.

36. Howard, B. K., Goodson, J. H., and Mengert, W. F.: Supine hypotensive syndrome of late pregnancy. Obstet. Gynecol. 1:371, 1953.

37. Munson, E. S., and Embro, W. J.: Enflurane, isoflurane, and halothane and isolated uterine muscle. Anesthesiology 46:11, 1977.

38. Galloon, S: Ketamine for obstetric delivery. Anesthesiology 44:522, 1976.

39. Shnider, S. M., Wright, R. G., Levinson, G., et al.: Uterine blood flow and plasma norepinephrine changes during maternal stress in the pregnant ewe. Anesthesiology 50:524, 1979.

40. Adamson, K., Mueller-Heuback, E., and Myers, R. E.: Production of fetal asphyxia in the rhesus monkey by administration of catecholamines to the mother. Am. J. Obstet. Gynecol. 109:248, 1971.

41. James, F. M., Greiss, F. C., Jr., and Kemp, R. A.: An evaluation of vasopressor therapy for maternal hypotension during spinal anesthesia. Anesthesiology 33:25, 1970.

42. Eng, M., Berges, P. V., Ueland, K., et al.: The effects of methoxamine and ephedrine in normotensive pregnant primates. Anesthesiology 35:354, 1971.

43. Rosenfeld, C. R., Barton, M. D., and Meschia, G.: Effects of epinephrine on distribution of blood flow in the pregnant ewe. Am. J. Obstet. Gynecol. 124:156, 1976.

44. Smith, B. E., and Hess, D. G.: The effects of dopamine and other catecholamines on uterine blood flow in pregnant ewes. In Abstracts of Scientific Papers, Annual Meeting, American Society of Anesthesiologists, New Orleans, 1977, pp. 439–440.

45. Rolbin, S. H., Levinson, G., Shnider, S. M., er al.: Dopamine treatment of spinal hypotension decreases uterine blood flow in the pregnant ewe. Anesthesiology 51:36, 1979.

46. Adamsons, K., and Joelsson, I.: The effects of pharmacologic agents upon the fetus and newborn. Am. J. Obstet. Gynecol. 96:437–459, 1966.

47. Sutherland, J. M., and Light, I. J.: The effects of drugs upon the developing fetus. Pediatr. Clin. North Am. 12:781, 1965.
48. Bussard, D. A., Stoelting, R. K., Peterson, C., et al.: Fetal changes in hamsters anesthetized with nitrous oxide and halothane. Anesthesiology 41:275, 1974.
49. Pope, W. D. B., Halsey, M. J., Lansdown, A. B. G., et al.: Fetotoxicity in rats following chronic exposure to halothane, nitrous oxide, or methoxyflurane. Anesthesiology 48:11, 1978.
50. Smith, R. F., Bowman, R. E., and Katz, J.: Behavioral effects of exposure to halothane during early development in the rat. Anesthesiology 49:319, 1978.
51. Smith, B. E., Gaub, M. L., and Moya, F.: Investigations into the teratogenic effects of anesthetic agents: The fluorinated agents. Anesthesiology 26:260, 1965.
52. Drachman, D. B., and Coulombre, A. J.: Experimental clubfoot and arthrogryposis multiplex congenita. Lancet 2:523, 1962.
53. Simpson, J. L.: Personal communication.
54. Pedersen, H., and Finster, M.: Anesthetic risk in the pregnant surgical patient. Anesthesiology 51:439, 1979.
55. Levinson, G., and Shnider, S. M.: Anesthesia for operations during pregnancy. In Shnider, S. M., and Levinson, G. (eds.): Anesthesia for Obstetrics. Baltimore, Williams & Wilkins, 1979, pp. 312–330.
56. Shnider, S. M., and Webster, G. M.: Maternal and fetal hazards of surgery during pregnancy. Am. J. Obstet. Gynecol. 92:891, 1965.
57. Smith, B. E.: Fetal prognosis after anesthesia during gestation. Anesth. Analg. (Cleve.) 42:521, 1963.
58. Knowles, J. A.: Excretion of drugs in milk — a review. Ped. Pharm. Ther. 66:1068, 1965.
59. Ferris, T. F.: Toxemia and hypertension. In Burrow, G. N., and Ferris, T. F. (eds.): Medical Complications During Pregnancy. Philadelphia, W. B. Saunders Co., 1975, pp. 53–104.
60. Nadji, P., and Sommers, S. C.: Lesions of toxemia in first trimester pregnancies. Am. J. Clin. Pathol. 59:344, 1973.
61. Speroff, L.: Toxemia of pregnancy: Mechanism and therapeutic management. Am. J. Cardiol. 32:582, 1973.
62. Soffronoff, E. C., Kaufman, B. M., and Connaughton, J. R.: Intravascular volume determinations and fetal outcome in hypertensive diseases of pregnancy. Am. J. Obstet. Gynecol. 127:4, 1977.
63. Redman, C. W. G., Bonnar, J., and Beilin, L: Early platelet consumption in preeclampsia. Br. Med. J. 1:467, 1978.
64. Zuspan, F. P.: Pregnancy induced hypertension. I. Role of sympathetic nervous system and adrenal gland. Acta Obstet. Gynecol. Scand. 56:283, 1977.
65. Finnerty, F. A., Jr: Hypertension in pregnancy. Clin. Obstet. Gynecol. 18(3):145, 1975.
66. Sheehan, H. L., and Lynch, J. B.: Pathology of toxemia of pregnancy. Baltimore, Williams & Wilkins, 1973.
67. Giesecke, A. H., Morris, R. E., Dolton, M. D., et al.: Of magnesium, muscle relaxants, toxemic

parturients, and cats. Anesth. Analg. (Cleve.) 47:689, 1968.
68. Ghoneim, M. M., and Long, I. P.: Interaction between magnesium and other neuromuscular blocking agents. Anesthesiology 32:23, 1970.
69. DeVore J: Personal communication.
70. Venuto, R., Cox, J. W., Stein, J. H., et al.: The effect of changes in perfusion pressure on uteroplacental blood flow in the pregnant rabbit. J. Clin. Invest. 57:938, 1976.
71. Hibbard, B. M., and Rosen, M: The management of severe preeclampsia and eclampsia. Br. J. Anaesth. 49:3, 1977.
72. Naulty, J. S., Cefalo, R., and Rodkey, F. L.: Placental transfer and fetal toxicity of sodium nitroprusside. In Abstracts of Scientific Papers, Annual Meeting, American Society of Anesthesiologists, San Francisco, CA, 1976, pp. 543–544.
73. Snyder, S. W., Wheeler, A. S., and James, F. M.: The use of nitroglycerin to control severe hypertension of pregnancy during cesarean section. Anesthesiology 51:563, 1979.
74. Fox, E. J., Sklar, G. S., Hiu, C. H., et al.: Complications related to the pressor response to endotracheal intubation. Anesthesiology 47:524, 1977.
75. Stoelting, R. K.: Attenuation of blood pressure response to laryngoscopy and tracheal intubation with sodium nitroprusside. Anesth. Analg. (Cleve.) 58:116, 1979.
76. MacKenzie, A. I.: Laryngeal oedema complicating obstetric anesthesia. Anaesthesia 33:271, 1978.
77. Ralston, D. H., and Shnider, S. M.: The fetal and neonatal effects of regional anesthesia in obstetrics. Anesthesiology 48:34, 1978.
78. Hertig, A. T., and Mansell, H.: Atlas of Tumor Pathology. Tumors of the Female Sex Organs. Part I. Hydatidiform Mole and Choriocarcinoma. Washington, D.C., Armed Forces Institute of Pathology, 1956, Sect LX, Fasc. 33.
79. Rubino, S. M.: Diagnosis of an intact hydatidiform mole with co-existent fetus by amniography. Obstet. Gynecol. 46:364, 1975.
80. Goldstein, D. P.: Surgery of moles and choriocarcinoma. In Barber, H. R. K., and Graber, E. A. (eds.): Surgical Disease in Pregnancy. Philadelphia, W. B. Saunders Co., 1974, pp. 494–513.
81. Baird, A. M.: The ultrasound diagnosis of hydatidiform mole. Clin. Radiol. 28(6):637, 1977.
82. Goldstein, D. P.: Five years' experience with the prevention of trophoblastic tumors by the prophylactic use of chemotherapy in patients with molar pregnancy. Clin. Obstet. Gynec. 13:945, 1970.
83. Bruun, T., and Kristoffersen, K.: Thyroid function during pregnancy with reference to hydatidiform mole and hyperemesis. Acta Endocrinol. 88:383, 1978.
84. Nagalaki, S., Mizuno, M., Sakamoto, S., et al.: Thyroid function in molar pregnancy. J. Clin. Endocrinol. Metab. 44:254, 1977.
85. Lipp, R. G., Kendschi, J. D., and Shmitz, R.: Death from pulmonary embolism associated with hydatidiform mole. Am. J. Obstet. Gynecol. 83:1644, 1962.
86. Natonson, R., Shapiro, B. A., Harrison, R. A., et

al.: Massive trophoblastic embolization and PEEP therapy. Anesthesiology 51:469, 1979.

87. Southern, E. M., et al.: Evacuation of the uterus in benign gestational trophoblastic disease with prostaglandins. In Karim, S. M. (ed.): Obstetric and Gynaecologic Use of Prostaglandins. MTP Press, 1976, pp. 247–251.

88. Stehling, L. C.: Anesthetic management of the patient with hyperthyroidism. Anesthesiology 41:585, 1974.

89. Weis, F. R., and Peak, I.: Effects of oxytocin on blood pressure during anesthesia. Anesthesiology 40:189, 1974.

90. Abouleish, E.: Postpartum hypertension and convulsion after oxytocic drugs. Anesth. Analg. (Cleve.) 55:813, 1976.

91. Sedlis, A.: Surgery of the fallopian tubes in pregnancy. In Barber, H. R. K., and Graber, E. A. (eds.): Surgical Disease in Pregnancy. Philadelphia, W. B. Saunders Co., 1974, pp. 339–407.

92. Schneider, J., Berger, C. J., and Cattell, C.: Maternal mortality due to ectopic pregnancy. A review of 102 deaths. Obstet. Gynecol. 49:557, 1977.

93. Cadkin, A. V., and Sabbagha, R. E.: Ultrasonic diagnosis of abnormal pregnancy. Clin. Obstet. Gynecol. 20(2):265, 1977.

94. King, R.: Diagnosis of unruptured ectopic pregnancy by the use of laparoscope. J. Tenn. Med. Assoc. 71:19, 1978.

95. Pelligra, R., and Sandberg, E. C.: Control of intractable abdominal bleeding by external counter-pressure. J.A.M.A. 241:708, 1979.

96. Cutler, B. S., Daggett, W.: Application of the g-suit to the control of hemorrhage in massive trauma. Ann. Surg. 173:511, 1971.

97. Diamant, M., Benumof, J., Saidman, L. J., et al.: Laparoscopic sterilization with local anesthesia: Complications and blood-gas changes. Anesth. Analg. (Cleve.) 56:335, 1977.

98. Baratz, B. A., and Karis, J. H.: Blood gas studies during laparoscopy under general anesthesia. Anesthesiology 30:463, 1969.

99. Calverley, R. K., and Jenkins, L. C.: The anesthetic management of pelvic laparoscopy. Canad. Anaesth. Soc. J. 20:679, 1973.

100. Diamant, M., Benumof, J., and Saidman, L. J.: Hemodynamics of increased intra-abdominal pressure. Anesthesiology 48:23, 1978.

101. Lee, C. M.: Acute hypotension during laparoscopy: A case report. Anesth. Analg. (Cleve.) 54:142, 1975.

102. Clark, C. C., Weeks, D. B., and Gusdon, J. P.: Venous carbon dioxide embolism during laparoscopy. Anesth. Analg. (Cleve.) 56:650, 1977.

103. Loveday, R.: Laparoscopy hazard. Brit. Med. J. 1:348, 1971.

104. Reynolds, R. C., and Pauca, A. L.: Gastric perforation, an anesthesia-induced hazard in laparoscopy. Anesthesiology 38:84, 1973.

105. Forster, F. M.: The incompetent cervix — the challenge. Med. J. Austral. 17(2):568, 1977.

106. Robboy, M.: The management of cervical incompetence. Obstet. Gynecol. 41(1):108, 1973.

107. Ekstein, K. L., and Marx, G. F.: Aortocaval compression and uterine displacement. Anesthesiology 40:92, 1974.

108. Marx, G. F., Hwang, H. S., and Chandra, P.: Postpartum uterine pressures with different doses of ketamine. Anesthesiology 50:163, 1979.

109. Katz, J. D., Hook, R., and Barash, P. G.: Fetal heart rate monitoring in pregnant patients undergoing surgery. Am. J. Obstet. Gynecol. 125:267, 1976.

110. Caritis, S. N., Edelstone, D. I., and Mueller-Heubach, E.: Pharmacologic inhibition of preterm labor. Am. J. Obstet. Gynecol. 133:557, 1979.

3

Anesthesia in the Geriatric Patient

By BARRY ZAMOST, M.D.,
and JONATHAN L. BENUMOF, M.D.

General Considerations
  Body Mass
  Composition of Body Fluids
  Temperature Regulation
  Progeria
Structural Characteristics:
  Musculoskeletal System, Skin, Dentition
  Total Hip Replacement
Cardiovascular System
  Pacemakers
Pulmonary System
Nervous System
Excretory System
  Transurethral Resection of the Prostate
Gastrointestinal System

Endocrine System
  Pituitary
  Adrenal
  Thyroid
  Parathyroid
  Ovary
  Testis
  Endocrine Pancreas
Pharmacology
Anesthetic Management
  Preanesthetic Medication
  Monitoring
  General Anesthesia
  Regional Anesthesia
  Recovery Period

The elderly patient is a high risk patient for anesthesia and surgery. Early studies demonstrated an operative mortality in patients over age 70 ranging from 15 to 45 per cent. The higher mortality rates occurred with abdominal, thoracic, and major vascular procedures. The highest mortality rate occurred with emergency operations. More recent studies indicate a reduction in overall mortality to under 5 per cent for elective procedures and under 10 per cent for emergencies. However, these mortality rates are still very high when compared with those of other ages. Abdominal, vascular, and thoracic operations and the development of postoperative complications still determine and dominate the mortality statistics.

The reason for these high mortality rates for the elderly surgical patient is that the elderly face surgery with an increased amount of pre-existing disease, the amount of which is increased for several reasons. First, specific diseases such as neoplasia, artherosclerosis, and degenerative diseases occur with aging. Second, the elderly are more likely to have suffered organ damage as a result of previous exposure or involvement with disease. Third, the aging process directly and adversely affects specific organ function.

At present, 10 per cent of the population of the United States is over the age of 65. The population size over 65 years of age diminishes exponentially, so that less than 1 per cent of the population is older than 75 years of age (the very aged). Since only a small fraction of these patients undergo surgery, the very aged patient not only is at high risk but also is a relatively uncommon candidate for anesthesia. Consequently, special emphasis must be directed toward the evaluation and preparation of these patients for anesthesia and surgery, and every effort must be made to identify and treat conditions that might cause complications postoperatively.

The following chapter describes the alterations in the structure and function of organ systems brought about by aging. The specific anesthetic implications of these age related organ changes will be discussed as they naturally arise in the text. Similarly, specific surgical procedures that are almost exclusively confined to the aged, such as total hip replacement, transurethral prostate resection, and cardiac pacemaker implantation, will be discussed as they arise in the text. In the final section of this chapter, a general overview of the anesthetic approach to the geriatric patient will be provided.

GENERAL CONSIDERATIONS

BODY MASS

Aging tissues show a decrease in the number of functioning parenchymal cells, together with an increased amount of interstitial substances. This loss of active metabolizing protoplasm causes a decrease in lean body mass and explains the 15 to 20 per cent decrease in basal metabolic rate observed in the elderly. Since fat tissue increases 10 to 20 per cent with aging, there is no consistent change in total body weight.

COMPOSITION OF BODY FLUIDS

Total body water content diminishes 10 to 15 per cent with age, from 60 per cent of the body weight in young individuals to 48 per cent of the body weight in the elderly. Extracellular fluid volume remains constant with normal aging; thus, the reduction in total body water is a reflection of decreased intracellular fluid, presumably due to cell loss with age. Blood, plasma, and red cell volume remain essentially unchanged with age. Total plasma proteins also remain unaltered with age. Serum albumin levels decrease slightly with age, while serum globulin levels increase slightly. Sodium, potassium, chloride, bicarbonate, and pH levels are not significantly altered with age under basal conditions.

TEMPERATURE REGULATION

Adaptive responses to heat and cold are less effective in the aged owing to a loss of integumentary function. Decreased numbers of skin capillaries cause a reduced capacity for vasoconstriction and vasodilation, while atrophy of the sweat glands causes a reduced capacity for sweating. The diminished ability to adapt to ambient temperature changes makes the elderly patient more susceptible to hyperthermia in overly heated operating rooms or when excessive surgical draping occurs and to hypothermia in cold operating rooms or with the use of cold intravenous fluids and drugs. The adverse effects of extremes of body temperature may be more pronounced in the elderly patient whose metabolic and organ functions are already compromised. Thus, efforts to preserve normothermia during anesthesia should be undertaken, and include continuous monitoring of body temperature, maintenance of an appropriate room temperature, proper draping of the patient, use of the temperature regulated surface blankets, and proper warming of intravenous solutions and blood.

PROGERIA

The syndrome of premature aging, or progeria, is a rare disorder characterized by early development (first or second decade) of cardiovascular disease, cerebral vascular disease, hypertension, diabetes, arthritis, and other stigmata of advanced aging. These patients are typically thin skinned and malnourished. Mandibular hypoplasia and micrognathia may lead to problems in airway management and endotracheal intubation. A narrowed glottic opening may require a smaller than normal endotracheal tube, and even minimal swelling of the glottis may greatly compromise the integrity of the airway. Most of the anesthetic management guidelines discussed in the last section of this chapter apply to the management of these patients.

STRUCTURAL CHARACTERISTICS: MUSCULOSKELETAL SYSTEM, SKIN, DENTITION

Evaluation of the physical characteristics of the aged is easily accomplished because most of the elements are readily visible. The important elements include bone, joints, muscle, skin, and teeth, and all show changes with aging that, when carefully considered, can influence the choice of anesthesia.

Posture in the elderly is one of general flexion, with the head and neck carried slightly forward and the dorsal spine becoming gently kyphotic. The flexed posture of old age is due to degenerative changes in the vertebral column, intervertebral discs, paraspinal tendons and muscles, and the extrapyramidal nervous system. The spine becomes fixed and rigid and offers a great deal of resistance to passive movement.

Osteoporosis, which is a progressive, age related decrease in total bone mass, is frequently encountered in women over 45 years of age and in men over 55 years of age. Osteoporotic bone is qualitatively normal, but there is a decreased amount of bone and the bone that is present is less dense. This predisposes the aged patient to fractures, especially of the hip and femur, which can follow seemingly negligible amounts of trauma. Vertebral bodies are also severely affected, making them susceptible to collapse, with development of the picture of kyphosis mentioned above. It is not known whether osteoporosis is a manifestation of the normal process of aging or a distinct disease entity.

Joint changes secondary to osteoarthritis are present universally with advancing age. Pathological changes include thinning of the joint cartilage, loss of joint fluid, hardening of the joint capsule and synovium, and proliferation of adjacent bone, all of which contribute to fixation and reduction in mobility of joints. Osteoarthritis commonly affects the weight bearing joints (knees, hips, lumbar spine), shoulders, cervical spine, and terminal interphalangeal joints of the fingers, and often involves the temporomandibular joints as well. The spine is the most common site of radiologic change due to osteoarthritis. In this location the pathologic process is degeneration of the intervertebral disc, with subsequent reduction in the size of the intervertebral space, and osteophyte formation leading to narrowing of the intervertebral foramina. Compression of nerve roots or spinal cord can result, especially in the cervical and lumbar areas, and can cause neurologic symptoms and signs to appear in those distributions. As in osteoporosis, it is not clear whether osteoarthritis is the result of senescent changes in cartilage or of cumulative injury to joints.

Skeletal muscle wasting and a general decrease in muscular strength, endurance, and agility are common in the aged, owing in part to a decrease in both the number and size of individual muscle fibers and degeneration of some motor end plates. Impairment of the extrapyramidal nervous system pathways leads to a general decrease in movement in the aged person, and is also responsible for the presence of tremors.

Aging produces readily visible changes in the skin, such as a general wasting with loss of elasticity, vascularity, and tensile strength. Degeneration of sebaceous gland activity results in dehydration of the skin. Subcutaneous fat decreases with age, which exaggerates the above described changes in the skin and additionally makes the skin more vulnerable to trauma.

Orofacial structures undergo changes related to the aging process. Loss of elasticity and tone in the muscles about the mouth leads to a collapsed appearance of the lower face and cheeks. Resorption of alveolar bone and weakening of the support results in lost or loose teeth. Absent dentition further contributes to the concavity of the cheeks.

Anesthetic considerations based on the physical characteristics of the aged individual are numerous and important. First there is the problem of airway management. Loss of orofacial supportive tissues in conjunction with loss of teeth makes a tight mask fit difficult to maintain. In many instances dentures can be electively left in place, or gauze can be inserted along the buccal surface of the mouth to help achieve a sealed mask fit. Loose teeth or dentures impose the possibility of dislodgement and aspiration of these structures should endotracheal intubation be undertaken. Neck and jaw mobility should be evaluated prior to intubation, since osteoarthritic involvement of the cervical spine and temporomandibular joints can reduce the ability of the anesthetist to position the head, neck, and jaws so that the larynx can be properly visualized. Cervical osteoarthritis can impair blood flow through the vertebral arteries by reducing the size of the transverse process vascular canal. Vigorous manipulation of the head should, therefore, be avoided since further compromise of blood flow could result in vertebral-basilar vascular insufficiency or cerebral ischemia, or both.

The rigid posture and intervertebral narrowing and calcification make it difficult to perform a subarachnoid or peridural block. The presence of spinal cord or nerve root symptoms may deter the anesthesiologist from administering regional anesthesia. The skeletal and arthritic changes discussed above make it difficult and uncomfortable for affected individuals to assume awkward positions such as the lithotomy position. Fusion of the costosternal joints results in a rigid thorax, which can interfere with ventilation.

During surgery, fragile bones, joints, and skin of elderly individuals are susceptible to trauma caused by tape, monitoring electrodes, stirrups, restraining straps, intravenous catheters, and constricting tourniquets. Close attention to pressure points and superficial nerves when the patient is placed on the operating table can reduce the chances of postoperative neuropathy and tissue necrosis.

Skin and mucosal atrophy lead to numerous problems in the elderly. Intravenous cannulation can be more difficult because skin and veins are more fragile and mobile. Pressure infusions are more likely to cause infiltration, and extravasation can be extensive. Consequently, if possible, cannulation sites should be visible in order to detect these complications. Nasal mucosa is also more atrophic and more likely to bleed from improperly placed tubes or airways.

As a consequence of senile muscle atrophy, the dose of muscle relaxant necessary to produce satisfactory operating conditions is reduced in the elderly. Any residual postoperative neuromuscular block is more significant, since the capacity of the remaining unblocked end plates to increase function is limited.

TOTAL HIP REPLACEMENT

Hip operations are one of the five most common procedures performed in patients 65 years of age or older. The use of methylmethacrylate bone cement in certain types of hip surgery is well established and is of interest to the anesthesiologist because of its association with various adverse effects. Cardiac arrests have been reported subsequent to insertion of the cement. Transient hypotension is a more common occurrence, probably as a result of vasodilatation. Embolization of methyl methacrylate, fat, air, and bone has been observed following application of the cement, with concomitant decreases in Pa_{O_2}.

These observations are of special interest in regard to the aged for two reasons. First, there is a direct correlation between advancing age and the degree of hypotension observed following methyl methacrylate cementing. This may be related to the fact that, in general, patients with preoperative hypertension or inadequate volume replacement become hypotensive more frequently and to a greater degree following the use of methylmethacrylate. Second, patients with rheumatoid arthritis have excessive and liquid marrow fat and may be more likely to develop fat embolism during pressurization of long bone shafts.

Anesthetic management of hip operations should be directed toward preventing and detecting complications. In addition to the routine monitoring (ECG, temperature, pulse, blood pressure, heart and breath sounds), direct intra-arterial catheterization may be indicated. Serial arterial blood gas determinations can insure that the arterial PO_2 is adequate before and after cement insertion. Volume replacement should be carefully maintained because hypovolemia is associated with greater incidence and degree of hypotension. Precise volume replacement, however, may be difficult because of unmeasured blood loss into large muscles around the hip and rapid blood loss from bone reaming. In addition, CVP measurement in the lateral position and in patients with heart disease may be inaccurate. Thus, in selected patients pulmonary artery wedge pressure measurement may be indicated. Finally, since the lung is the primary route for elimination of volatile methyl methacrylate monomer, high flow or nonrebreathing anesthesia breathing systems should be used to hasten the elimination of absorbed monomer during cementing.

CARDIOVASCULAR SYSTEM

Age and cardiovascular disease disability and mortality have a strong positive correlation. Awareness of the cardiovascular problems of the aged is prerequisite for the appropriate anesthetic management of the geriatric patient.

The aging cardiovascular system undergoes several anatomical and physiological changes that cause multiple clinical manifestations of heart disease and altered responsiveness to therapy. Some of these changes are attributable to a cardiopathy of aging, which may result from recurrent hemodynamic stress, and some of the changes are the result of pathologic conditions such as coronary artery disease, systemic and pulmonary hypertension, and valvular disease.

On gross inspection, the aged heart has an increased amount of subpericardial fat, and fat tissue appears at the entry of the pulmonary veins, the superior vena cava, and the base of the aorta. Thickened whitish adipose-fibrotic patches are noted in the endocardium and papillary muscles, along with fibrosis, thickening, and rigidity of the valves. Other age induced gross changes include alterations in heart size and geometry which consist mainly of an increase in left ventricular wall thickness and mass and corresponding decrease in the size of the left ventricular cavity. In addition, the left atrium enlarges and the aorta becomes wider and shifts to the right.

Histologically, the aged myocardium has a decrease in both the size and number of individual muscle fibers as well as focal (compensatory) hypertrophy of other fibers. There is an increase in pericardial elastic fiber tissue. The sinoatrial node and internodal tracts of elderly patients show a decrease in the amount of muscle and an increase in the amount of fibrosis and adipose tissue. The ventricular conduction system may become involved in the fibrosis and calcification of endocardial skeleton. These changes may account for the increased incidence of arrhythmias seen in older patients.

There are major changes in the composition of vessel walls as a function of age. The intima and muscle layers undergo a progressive structural deterioration, and the elastic media demonstrate fragmentation and loss of lamination. Thus, vessel walls become less resilient and are therefore less able to accommodate wide changes in arterial pressure. As a consequence, major vessels that are exposed to an increased blood pressure tend to dilate and become tortuous. Superimposed on these age related vascular changes is the development of atherosclerosis, a process that might also be considered a normal aspect of aging. Atherosclerosis includes three major morphologic lesions: fatty streaks, fibrous plaques, and atheromatous plaques.

Physiological changes accompany the anatomic changes of the aged cardiovascular system. Cardiac output diminishes from an average of 6.5 L/min at age 25 to 3.8 L/min at age 80. The decrease in cardiac output is the result of both a decreased stroke volume and a decreased heart rate. Circulation time is prolonged by 33 per cent at age 80 compared with that at age 30. Arteriosclerotic vessel lumen narrowing causes vascular resistance to increase in all tissues and reduces tissue perfusion.

Systemic blood pressure changes in the aging person are caused by the loss of compliance in the walls of the larger arteries. Systolic blood pressure usually increases with advancing years, while the diastolic pressure may increase slightly or remain unaffected. A practical upper limit of normal blood pressure in the elderly patient is 160 torr systolic and 100 torr diastolic.

With aging, arteriosclerotic lesions, subsequent tissue ischemia, and deterioration of specific neuron groups cause medullary cardiovascular control center changes that produce alterations in autonomic responses and adaptive ability of the cardiovascular system. Thus, normal resting autonomic tone is altered, resulting in increased vagal tone (slow heart rate, diminished response to atropine) and increased sensitivity to carotid sinus stimulation. Decreased sympathetic nervous system activity results in decreased compensatory or adaptive responses. The loss of autonomic reactivity together with the decreased myocardial contractility and heart rate results in a diminished cardiac reserve, which may not be apparent during routine activities but which could precipitate cardiac decompensation during periods of stress.

Cardiovascular changes in the elderly are caused not only by the normal aging process but also by superimposed pathologic processes of heart disease such as ischemic heart disease, hypertension, cardiac arrhythmias, and congestive heart failure. All of these diseases are age related disorders, and the presence of such organic heart disease or its complications will aggravate the normal deterioration of aging described above and will further limit the ability to respond to stress.

For the anesthesiologist the practical implications of the changes in the cardiovascular system with aging are much the same as in any patient with heart disease who requires surgery. The stress of anesthesia and surgery may overwhelm the limited cardiovascular reserve. Maintenance of vital signs near baseline, adequate oxygenation and ventilation, and favorable ratio of myocardial oxygen supply to demand and blood flow to peripheral organs and tissues are essential. Prolonged circulation time and advancing age slow the onset of action of drugs given intravenously and may lead to drug overdose unless injection rates or amounts are reduced. Myocardial depressant effects of intravenous barbiturates and volatile anesthetic agents will be exaggerated in the presence of an already reduced cardiac output. Diminished autonomic control reduces the ability to compensate appropriately for changes in vascular volume, position, and surgical stimulation.

PACEMAKERS

Elderly patients with pacemakers require surgery for battery change and also for reasons unrelated to their pacemakers. More than half of these patients are 70 years of age or older. The safe management of a patient who has a pacemaker requires that the anesthesiologist be familiar with the problems presented by pacemakers so that perioperative complications can be anticipated and avoided.

A permanent artificial cardiac pacemaker is indicated when the patient has complete heart block, sick sinus syndrome, or bradycardia with symptoms. In these conditions there is a defect in impulse formation or impulse conduction resulting in a heart rate and cardiac output that do not provide adequate cerebral and coronary perfusion; thus syncope, heart failure, angina, or dysrhythmias result. Heart block occurs most commonly in the sixth and seventh decades of life and is most commonly caused by Lev's and Lenegre's degenerative conduction system diseases. The former disease consists of fibrosis and calcification of the endocardial skeleton of the heart with impingement on the atrioventricular conduction system, and the latter disease is an idiopathic fibrosis of the conduction system. Degeneration of the sinus node together with fibrosis and scarring of the intra-atrial conducting system also occur with aging. The next most common cause of heart block is coronary artery disease, in which the interruption of conduction may be due to a myocardial infarction or ischemia. The type and severity of the heart block will depend upon the vessel affected. Heart block is also encountered in rheumatic heart disease and cardiomyopathies, and in association with surgical correction of congenital heart disease. Certain drug intoxications cause heart block, including digitalis, quinidine, procainamide, propranolol, and potassium.

A thorough preoperative evaluation of the patient with a pacemaker is important. The reason for the implantation of the pacemaker should be known. Since many of these patients have significant underlying cardiovascular disease, they should be evaluated for any progression of symptoms and for adequacy of medical therapy, as well as for electrolyte imbalances prior to any elective procedure. Once the status of the heart and the nature of the dysrhythmia are known, endocarditis prophylaxis should be considered. The type and specifications of the pacemaker should be known, and it should be established that the pacemaker is functioning properly in its ability to pace the heart. Failure of pacing may be due to a battery failure, wire disruption, or failure to capture the conducting tissue at the myocardial level.

Careful attention and special precautions must continue in the operating room in the management of the patient with a pacemaker. Care must be taken to avoid trauma to the battery or damage to the leads. Patients with temporary pacemakers must be transported and positioned carefully so that electrodes do not become dislodged or perforate the ventricle. For example, when the temporary electrode is in an arm vein, that arm must be stabilized and not placed in hyperextension; if the temporary electrode is in the femoral vein, the trunk should not be flexed or hyperextended. The controls of the external pulse generator of a temporary pacemaker should be accessible to the anesthesiologist, and continuous EKG monitoring is necessary to confirm proper pacemaker functioning and to detect arrhythmias.

Inhalation anesthesia, balanced technique, neuroleptanesthesia and regional techniques have all been used successfully in patients with pacemakers. Since patients with pacemakers have underlying cardiac pathology, maintenance of stable vital signs, adequate oxygenation, and normocapnia are of paramount importance during any form of anesthesia. Untoward physiologic changes during anesthesia may adversely affect the performance of the pacing system by altering the cardiac pacing threshold. A decrease in the cardiac conduction threshold may induce ventricular fibrillation. Causes of a decreased cardiac conduction threshold include myocardial ischemia (due to decreased cardiac output from hemorrhage, position changes, high positive airway pressures, and drug overdose), increased release of sympathomimetic amines, and hypoxia. An increase in pacing threshold may lead to intermittent or permanent failure of pacing. Succinylcholine, hyperkalemia, and acid-base disturbances can all increase the cardiac conduction threshold.

Perhaps the most important intraoperative concern in the patient with a cardiac pacemaker is the potentially dangerous effect of electromagnetic fields. Fixed rate (asynchronous) pacemakers are relatively insensitive to electrical interference and do not present a large problem in this regard. However, a pacemaker in the fixed rate mode still creates the danger of interaction between paced and spontaneous beats, wherein a pacemaker impulse that occurs during the vulnerable period (T wave) of a sinus beat may precipitate ventricular fibrillation. Demand pacemakers (synchronous) have their pulse generators suppressed when a spontaneous P or R wave occurs. The risk with a demand pacemaker is that the electronic sensing circuit may detect electrical activity from sources other than the heart. Therefore, if the pulse generator is suppressed, the patient will revert to the rhythm for which the pacemaker therapy was instituted, and cardiac standstill may ensue. Electromagnetic interference with the pacemaker may be transmitted from the environment by radar, orthopedic saws, and monitoring and telemetry devices. Spontaneous skeletal muscle contractions are common in the perioperative period, and may be capable of generating sufficiently large potentials to interfere with demand pacemakers.

The most common source of electromagnetic interference in the operating room is current from the electrocautery device. This stray current may be detected by the demand pacemaker and interpreted as spontaneous cardiac activity, with subsequent pacemaker suppression and periods of asystole. To reduce the possibility of this occurrence, the indifferent plate of the electrocautery unit should be placed as far away from the pulse generator as possible. Although the patient should be electrocardiographically monitored for arrhythmias and proper pacemaker function, palpation of the pulse or auscultation of the heart with a stethoscope is necessary to detect inhibition of the pacemaker during electrocautery, since these electrical surges will render the ECG useless. Demand pacemakers will ordinarily resume normal function as soon as the offending electromagnetic field is turned off. Therefore, the frequency and duration of electrocautery should be kept to a minimum in order to avoid repetitive and prolonged asystolic periods. In addition, many synchronous units will convert to asynchronous mode in the presence of electromagnetic interference. If it is disadvantageous to limit electrocautery, or if reversion to fixed rate mode does not occur spontaneously, a high power external magnet should be applied directly over the pacemaker to manually convert to asynchronous mode. The risk of inducing ventricular fibrillation by competing rhythms is small as long as there is low output from the generator, hypoxia is avoided, and electrolyte and acid-base balance is maintained.

Electrocautery presents an additional hazard in the presence of improperly insulated pacemaker electrodes. Since the electrodes are a direct electrical pathway to the heart, electrostatic energy may be transmitted directly to the myocardium and cause ventricular fibrillation or cauterize the myocardium, rendering it insensitive to pacing impulses.

Anesthesiologists are frequently involved in the intraoperative care of a patient for permanent pacemaker implantation or battery change. Monitoring considerations are the same as described for the patient with a temporary pacemaker, and a DC cardiac defibrillator and drugs necessary for cardiac resuscitation should be on hand as well. Patients who have heart block with symptoms may develop cardiac standstill, ventricular tachycardia, or ventricular fibrillation if they are submitted to general anesthesia. Therefore, it is recommended that the electrodes and battery be inserted under local anesthesia with light sedation. Epicardial leads require a thoracotomy, and such patients should have a temporary transvenous pacemaker inserted beforehand under local anesthesia. With a method of cardiac pacing first secured in this way, the epicardial leads may then be implanted more safely under general anesthesia. It should be recognized that there is a critical point during battery changes when the functioning battery is removed and the new battery is not yet secured to the leads; at this time cardiac standstill may occur.

When a patient with heart block presents for surgery, the question arises as to whether to insert a temporary pacemaker specifically for the purpose of making the conduct of anesthesia safer. If the patient must undergo emergency surgery and the heart block is due to either a myocardial infarction or digitalis toxicity, then a temporary pacemaker is indicated. Likewise, a patient with a complete heart block who must have a permanent pacemaker implanted should have a temporary pacemaker inserted first. The indications for temporary pacing of patients with bifascicular block who must undergo surgery include patients with a history of syncopy and those patients who have a reasonable chance to develop hypotension, major fluid shifts, or acid base and electrolyte disturbances intraoperatively.

PULMONARY SYSTEM

The effects of aging on lung structure and function are important to the anesthesiologist because of the increased need for homeostasis in gas exchange and the central role of the lungs in the uptake and elimination of anesthetic gases. Progressive structural changes occur in the senescent lung which involve airways, blood vessels, and the non-parenchymal support elements. Alveolar septal membranes are weakened and disrupted, causing a coalescence of alveoli, which become enlarged in size but reduced in number. These changes result in a linear decrease in alveolar surface area between the ages of 20 and 80 years, so that by 80 years the area available for gas exchange is reduced by 30 per cent. Pulmonary vascular resistance increases with age because of intimal and medial layer proliferation and fibrosis. The amount and density of elastic and fibrous connective tissue of the lung, airways, and pleura increase with age. Calcific and arthritic changes occur in the cartilages and joints of the thorax and bronchi, and the ventilatory muscles become weaker.

The degenerative pulmonary changes with advancing age noted above result in generalized rigidity and stiffness of the lung parenchyma, tracheobronchial tree, and thorax and affect the mechanical properties of the lung. Inspiration becomes more energy inefficient because of diminished chest wall mobility and muscular strength. Expiration also becomes more energy inefficient because elastic recoil is decreased. These changes in the mechanical forces of the lung lead to an increase in the total work of breathing in the elderly.

The aging lung also undergoes considerable alterations in lung volumes. Total lung capacity does not change significantly with age, but the residual volume and functional residual capacity increase at the expense of the vital and inspiratory capacities. The vital capacity progressively decreases, so that by age 70 it is approximately 70 per cent of the value at age 17, while the residual volume increases nearly 50 per cent during the same period of time. The volume of lung at which some airways collapse (closing volume) increases with age. The volume of anatomic dead space increases with age, so the per cent of the tidal volume that ventilates dead space increases from 20 per cent at age 20 to 40 per cent at age 60. Tidal volume and minute ventilation decrease slightly with age, and the maximum breathing capacity is diminished, as the result of decreased muscle strength and an inability to increase respiratory rate. Flow resistance increases with age, especially during forced exhalation, resulting in reduced maximal flow rates and forced expiratory volumes. Regulation of ventilation is altered in the elderly, as manifested by a reduced ability to respond to challenges of hypoxia or hypercarbia with a compensatory increase in ventilation. The increase in closing volume is the most important change, for it results in ventilation-perfusion imbalance.

The volume at which small airways collapse during exhalation increases with age because of the changes in elastic recoil and small airway morphology noted earlier. When closing volume exceeds functional residual capacity (the volume of lung that exists at the end of a normal exhalation), the closing volume will be within the tidal volume, and some airways will collapse during normal tidal breathing. The airways in question will remain closed until inspiration increases lung volume enough to open them once again. Since these airways are closed during part of the ventilatory cycle, they have less time to participate in fresh gas exchange, and they must therefore function as low ventilation to perfusion units, with consequent derangement of gas exchange. With a normal patient in the supine position, closing volume starts to exceed functional residual capacity at 36 years of age. At 65 years of age, the closing volume exceeds functional residual capacity even in the sitting position. Thus, in the elderly some airways will be closed in all positions at normal tidal breathing, leading to development of low ventilation to perfusion units and reduced arterial oxygen tension.

The age related changes in lung mechanics, volumes, and ventilation-perfusion imbalance result in reduced gas exchange efficiency in the elderly. The normal reduction of arterial oxygen tension that is progressive with age is well established, and can be reliably predicted by the equation: $Pa_{O_2} = 109$ mm Hg $- 0.43 \times$ age (in years). Since alveolar PO_2 remains relatively constant throughout life, the linear decrease in arterial PO_2 with age is accompanied by a linear increase in the alveolar-arterial PO_2 difference, from approximately 8 torr at age 20 to nearly 30 torr at age 70.

The elderly individual is subjected not only to the pulmonary problems related to the biologic process of aging but also to a lifetime of specific pulmonary disease entities and the cumulative effects of prolonged exposure to a polluted urban or occupational environment. The incidence of chronic obstructive pulmonary disease increases with age and adds to the physiologic consequences of aging mentioned above. Pneumonia also occurs frequently in the geriatric population, either sporadically or as a complication of another disease process or surgery. Tuberculosis is relatively frequent in the elderly. Carcinoma of the lung mainly occurs in middle years but is often seen in the aged. The decision to attempt curative resection in the elderly must be carefully considered because the mortality rates of pneumonectomy and lobectomy in those over age 70 are 30 per cent and 15 per cent, respectively. The postoperative elderly individual is more likely to develop life threatening pulmonary embolism because of pre-existing chronic venous disease and tissue blood flow stasis and longer periods of postoperative immobility. The adult respiratory distress syndrome can be observed following a variety of conditions in the elderly, including prolonged or severe hypotension, prolonged inhalation of high oxygen concentrations, pulmonary infections, and sepsis, or as a consequence of massive surgery, trauma, or prolonged anesthesia.

The progressive impairment of pulmonary function and narrowed margin of reserve with age are clear indications that the elderly will not tolerate the stress of anesthesia and surgery as well as younger people, and are at increased risk for the development of postoperative respiratory failure. The pre-existing pulmonary changes associated with aging and the superimposed problems produced by specific pulmonary disease may become exacerbated during anesthesia and surgery. Vital capacity, for example, has been observed to decrease as much as 50 to 70 per cent after upper abdominal and thoracic procedures and 25 to 35 per cent after lower abdominal procedures. Induction of anesthesia can lead to a reduction in lung volume, especially in older patients, resulting in further airway closure and uneven distribution of inspired gas. The effects of positive pressure mechanical ventilation, endotracheal intubation, decreased mucociliary transport, central depression from anesthetic agents, and residual neuromuscular block are additional threats to the aged respiratory system. The deleterious effects of aging, prior pulmonary disease, and perioperative impairment of pulmonary function can be synergistic in promoting the development of atelectasis, increased ventilation to perfusion imbalance, and hypoxemia. Anesthetic management should include preoperative evaluation. the goal being to quantify pulmonary function and to minimize or correct risk factors such as smoking, infection, and bronchospasm. Attention to adequate tracheobronchial toilet is an important intraoperative consideration. Elderly patients who are not fully responsive postoperatively should be left intubated and placed on a progressively decreasing intermittent mandatory ventilation (IMV) rate. When the IMV rate is less than two per minute and the patient demonstrates an adequate vital capacity (>15 ml/kg) and peak inspiratory force (>−30 cm H_2O) and has satisfactory arterial blood gases, extubation can be considered. If this kind of postoperative ventilatory support is necessary, hypoxemia secondary to airway collapse can be minimized by the use of positive end-expiratory pressure. Post extubation supplemental oxygen should be administered (nasal prongs, face mask) and a vigorous respiratory care regime instituted (turning, suctioning, chest physiotherapy, ambulation as soon as possible, and incentive spirometry).

NERVOUS SYSTEM

It is axiomatic that age-related changes in the structure or chemistry of the central nervous system will greatly influence the anesthetic state. Consequently, it is important to be aware of the changes that occur in the nervous systems of aging humans. It must be remembered, however, that it is difficult to distinguish between natural changes as a direct result of the aging process and pathologic alterations that occur as the result of disease.

Grossly, the weight of the brain decreases linearly with age to about 80 to 90 per cent of its peak value. The loss of brain substance is due to nerve cell loss in the cerebral and cerebellar cortexes and the thalamus. Degenerative changes in nerve axons include loss of myelin, reduction of synapses, and reduction in number of fibers in tracts. As the brain atrophies during aging, the cerebral cortical gyri shrink, the cranial cavity dead space increases, the sulci become wider and deeper, and the membranes covering the central nervous system become thickened. The arachnoid villi become fibrotic and the ventricles may become engorged with cerebrospinal fluid. There is glial cell proliferation.

Numerous chemical processes of neurotransmission are altered during aging. Brain activity levels of the enzymes tyrosine hydroxylase and aromatic L-amino acid decarboxylase are reduced in senescent humans. Thus the rates of conversion of tyrosine or dopa to catecholamine neurotransmitters decline. The activities of the two major enzymes involved in brain catecholamine catabolism, monoamine oxidase and catecho-o-methyl transferase, increase with age. Hence, catecholamine biosynthesis declines while catabolism increases, and the concentration of dopamine and norepinephrine is correspondingly lower in the elderly. The decrease in the presynaptic nerve terminal catecholamine concentration can cause corresponding changes in the postsynaptic effector cell function or sensitivity. The sum total of these changes suggests that brain catecholamine neurotransmission might be impaired in elderly individuals.

Similar age dependent alterations occur in other neurotransmitter compounds. The rate of synthesis of serotonin declines, while its rate of catabolism increases. Thus brain levels of serotonin are reduced. The activity of choline acetylase, the enzyme involved in the synthesis of acetylcholine, and acetylcholinesterase, the enzyme involved in its degradation, both decline late in life.

Physiologic and behaviorial responses in the elderly reflect the physical and chemical alterations of the central nervous system described above. Thus, organic dementia is common and is manifested by varying degrees of confusion, memory deficit, and emotional lability, and makes communication difficult and frustrating. Loss of hearing and poor eyesight are common and add to the communication difficulties. Pain perception is diminished. Motor changes of late life include weakness, tremors, and impaired coordination. Reflexes and compensatory mechanisms in general become depressed, and laryngeal and pharyngeal reflexes specifically become less reactive with age. The pupils tend to become miotic and sluggish in their reflex response to light and accommodation.

Against the background of age induced physical and chemical degenerative change in nervous tissue there may occur a number of diseases. The incidence of cerebrovascular disease increases with age, and the mortality of a cerebrovascular accident is directly related to the age of the patient. Other neurological disorders common in the geriatric population include cerebral neoplasms, metastatic tumors, nutritional deprivation states, toxic disorders, and meningeal and central nervous system infections.

There are several anesthetic implications of the central nervous system changes described. Since there is an overall reduction in the level of nervous system activity that anesthetic drugs have to depress, there is a corresponding decrease in analgesic and anesthetic drug requirement. Hence, aged patients obtain more pain relief from a standard dose of narcotic and will tolerate a less than perfect local or regional anesthetic better than younger individuals. The loss of protective airway reflexes with aging makes the elderly patient more prone to airway obstruction and aspiration, especially after a dose of narcotic or other CNS depressant. The presence of abnormal CNS function (weakness, tremors) requires chart documentation and consideration before inducing regional blockade. Ability to communicate adequately should be another factor involved in the choice of regional anesthesia. Confusion is common preoperatively and, if present, should be communicated to the recovery personnel. Confusion can progress to disorientation and hallucinations (the "sundowner syndrome") when aged patients are left in poorly lighted areas. Elderly patients with Parkinson's disease taking levodopa may develop arrhythmias, hypotension, or chest wall rigidity in the perianesthetic period. Phenothiazines, droperidol, and Innovar may cause extrapyramidal signs and should be avoided. Levodopa should be discontinued the evening before surgery and resumed as early as possible.

EXCRETORY SYSTEM

The kidney undergoes well documented age related changes in structure and function. As in other organ systems, it is difficult to distinguish between the involutional, time-related phenomena and the effects of specific renal disease. After the fourth decade of life there is a steady decline in renal mass with a greater loss of cortex relative to medulla. Distinctive intrarenal vascular changes also occur. In the cortex, obliteration of the lumina of the preglomerular arterioles causes a reduction in cortical blood flow; while in the medulla glomerular sclerosis causes shunting of blood flow from afferent to efferent arterioles, thus maintaining a relatively nonfunctional perfusion of the medulla.

These morphologic changes are accompanied by a progressive deterioration in renal function. After age 40 there is a decrease in total renal blood flow, which causes a 10 per cent per decade reduction in effective renal plasma flow. Glomerular function declines with age so that the glomerular filtration rate at age 90 is about 50 per cent below that at age 20. The BUN at age 20 averages 10 mg per 100 ml; at age 40, 13 mg per 100 ml; and at age 70, 20 mg per 100 ml. Starting at age 35 there is a reduction in creatinine clearance to about one half normal after age 65. Since the decrease in creatinine excretion is matched by a decrease in creatinine production from the reduced body muscle mass, the net effect is a constancy of the serum creatinine concentration. Thus, even a mild elevation of serum creatinine in an elderly individual usually indicates renal disease, and its use as an estimate of renal function is less sensitive than the creatinine clearance. Blood urea nitrogen may be even a less sensitive indicator of renal function, since it can be influenced by such non-renal factors as dietary protein intake, hepatic disease, state of hydration, and gastrointestinal bleeding. Renal tubular function is compromised by aging, as demonstrated by a reduced concentrating ability. The excretory and resorptive function of the renal tubules also declines, especially the ability to conserve sodium and excrete acid. Finally, renin-aldosterone responsiveness to acute stimuli becomes sluggish with advancing age.

Specific organic diseases may be superimposed on these age related changes in renal structure and function. Some degree of prostatism with outlet symptoms is present in three fourths of males over age 65, increasing the likelihood of developing obstruction of the lower urinary tract with consequent infection and deterioration of renal function. Co-existing renal disease, including the immunologic reactions (glomerulonephritis, nephrotic syndrome), the degenerative diseases (arteriosclerosis, diabetes, hypertension), and tubular and calculous diseases, may cause further renal impairment. Finally, extrarenal problems such as cardiac failure, injudicious use of diuretics, and intravascular volume deficit secondary to inadequate intake or abnormal losses are common in the elderly and can result in a further deterioration of renal function.

The decline in renal function with age has important implications for the anesthetic management of older patients. Renal excretion of drugs is impaired, which is another reason why the dosage of drugs eliminated primarily by renal mechanisms should be reduced. Since the ability to excrete acid is diminished, the aged patient has difficulty compensating for a metabolic or respiratory acidosis. Furthermore, since cardiac disease may coexist with renal disease, extremely careful titration of volume and fluid replacement in the geriatric patient is mandatory.

The induction of general anesthesia may aggravate deleterious effects of aging on renal function. Ordinarily anesthesia and surgery cause a reduced renal blood flow and glomerular filtration rate. Inhalation drugs cause the most depression, nitrous-narcotic techniques cause moderate depression, and regional techniques have the least impact. Thus, the elderly patient with borderline renal function needs careful attention to maintenance of urine output during the perianesthetic period. In addition, consideration should be given to the avoidance of drugs that are metabolized to inorganic fluoride and thus may be nephrotoxic.

The decline in renal function with age can interact adversely with other factors in the perianesthetic period. The decline in water conserving capacity in the geriatric patient may become important if fluid intake has been limited preoperatively, or if pituitary diabetes insipidus develops as a postoperative complication. Under these circumstances the serum sodium concentration may increase to levels that may impair central nervous system function and result in obtundation. Conversely, surgery and anesthesia in the elderly may result in water intoxication due to excess ADH secretion. Thus, the effects of aging on the kidney in conjunction with an anesthetic challenge may predispose the elderly patient to two life threatening, but opposite, complications. Anesthesiologists should have a high degree of suspicion of these two complications when faced with lethargic, confused, or obtunded older patients in the perioperative period.

Transurethral Resection of the Prostate

There is a high incidence of benign prostatic hypertrophy in elderly males, which is usually treated surgically. A transurethral resection is usually the preferred operative procedure because it has a lower morbidity and mortality when compared with open procedures. The major anesthetic considerations for this procedure include blood loss, bladder perforation, sepsis, and venous absorption of irrigating fluid.

Blood loss from the prostatic venous plexus can be substantial but very difficult to quantify, since the shed blood is diluted by the irrigating fluid. Hemolysis, once a problem with hypotonic irrigating solutions, is prevented by use of isotonic fluids containing amino acids or large-molecule sugars. During prostatic resection, activators are released that convert plasminogen to plasmin and may cause fibrinolysis with consumption of platelets and clotting factors.

Bladder perforation may occur during urethral instrumentation. This catastrophe may be experienced by an awake patient as abdominal discomfort or pain in the shoulder but will be masked by general anesthesia. Instrumentation of an infected urinary tract can cause a bacteremia and possibly septic shock.

Large amounts of irrigating fluid may be absorbed through open venous sinuses during resection. A sudden large infusion of electrolyte-free fluid can cause an acute increase in the intravascular volume and acute dilutional decrease in serum sodium concentration. Signs of acute fluid absorption include hypertension, tachycardia, congestive heart failure (dyspnea, rales, increased central venous pressure), and the sequelae of hyponatremia — disorientation, convulsions, and coma. When irrigating fluid absorption is suspected, resection should be stopped and the hyponatremia corrected with diuretics, fluid restriction and, rarely, intravenous infusion of 3 per cent saline. Limiting the time of resection to one hour helps to minimize the risk of fluid absorption. In general, regional anesthesia is preferred for transurethral resection because it permits early detection of a change in the patient's mental status (hyponatremia), breathing status (congestive heart failure), or occurrence of abdominal pain (bladder perforation).

GASTROINTESTINAL SYSTEM

The gastrointestinal tract shows evidence of degenerative changes with age. The mucosa of the stomach atrophies, and diminished gastric secretions and achlorhydria result. Since the aged patient's stomach has a limited capacity to produce acid, he or she is more prone to develop an alkalosis as a result of vomiting. In addition, oral administration of medications that are weak acids will produce variable and generally weaker effects because such compounds are rapidly absorbed only in the non-ionized form, and are thus dependent upon the presence of strong gastric acidity. The strength and rate of gastric contractions are decreased in older persons, resulting in delayed gastric emptying. These considerations are important in the assessment of whether or not an elderly patient has a full stomach prior to surgery.

Structural and physiological information about the aging process in other gastrointestinal organs is not as well documented. In the small and large intestines there is atrophy of the mucosal and muscular layers leading to loss of tone of the bowel wall, diminished peristalsis, and probably decreased secretory and absorption activity as well. Pancreatic structure in the aged person shows evidence of fibrous or fatty change and cavity formation, and pancreatic enzyme secretion is diminished. Atrophy of the salivary glands leads to xerostomia, a condition of diminished salivary secretions, and a change in secretion composition from serous to mucinous. Thus, premedication with anticholinergics for their antisalivary effect is less indicated in the elderly.

The liver shows no evidence of structural or functional deterioration that is attributable exclusively to advancing years. Liver blood flow declines in proportion to the cardiac output in the aging person. Serum levels of alkaline phosphatase, bilirubin, and SGOT do not show an age dependency. Although the total serum protein concentration remains constant in old age, albumin is reduced and globulin is increased by 20 per cent. When superimposed liver disease is present, the anesthetic considerations, such as impaired carbohydrate and protein metabolism, reduced detoxification of drugs, coagulation abnormalities, and avoidance of potentially hepatotoxic agents, are the same as for the younger individual.

In spite of the age related changes in the gastrointestinal system, there is no disease of older people that is attributable solely to the gastrointestinal system aging process.

Although the incidence of gallbladder calculi, peptic ulcer disease, intestinal obstruction, mesenteric vascular occlusion, and gastrointestinal malignancies increases with advancing age, these maladies are generally due to secondary factors. In patients over 60 years of age the incidence of hiatus hernia has been reported to be as high as 67 per cent, and although the majority of these hernias are asymptomatic, affected individuals are more prone to silent regurgitation and aspiration.

The elderly are especially prone to the possible effects of nutritional insufficiency, but this is not always a result of gastrointestinal disease. The diets of individuals in this age group are often nutritionally inadequate because of socioeconomic factors such as poverty, isolation, and ignorance, but more importantly motivation is often lacking.

ENDOCRINE SYSTEM

Although it has been proposed that endocrine factors function as pacemakers for many cellular and physiologic aspects of aging, the evidence for this is sparse and conflicting. As opposed to the idea of causing senescence, the endocrine glands more likely undergo the same aging process that involves the rest of the body.

PITUITARY

Age induced changes in the anatomy and histology of the pituitary gland include a 25 per cent decrease in weight by age 80, a reduction in blood supply, and a relative increase in the number of chromophobe and basophilic cells, with a relative decrease in the number of acidophilic cells. Failure of the aged patient to withstand stresses has been postulated to be caused by a deficient pituitary response, but no significant alteration in the secretory function of the pituitary gland with age has been shown to occur. ACTH release during stress is not altered by age.

ADRENAL

Fibrosis, hyperplasia, and nonfunctional tumor growth are the most important age related changes observed in the adrenal glands. Although adrenal hypofunction due to a decrease in adrenal reserves has long been suggested on a clinical basis, there is no evidence that this happens as the result of age alone.

The ability of the adrenals to secrete cortisol as a result of ACTH stimulation is maintained in the aged, as are the circadian rhythm pattern of activity and the system of negative feedback between pituitary and adrenal glands. Secretion of aldosterone, however, is significantly decreased in the elderly to more than one half that of young subjects.

THYROID

Age related thyroid gland changes include fibrosis, a progressive increase in weight and nodularity, and a decrease in blood supply. Circulating levels of T_3 and T_4 decrease during aging, but these changes are gradual and do not indicate hypothyroidism, nor do they require treatment. Myxedema is the most common thyroid disorder of old age, but it is often unrecognized because the symptoms are often confused with those of other diseases that are common to later life. Hyperthyroidism is uncommon in patients over 60 years of age, but it is not rare, accounting for 10 to 17 per cent of the thyrotoxic population.

PARATHYROID

The most striking change in aging parathyroids is an increase in the number of oxyphilic cells. However, the significance of this change is unknown, since parathormone secretion and parathyroid gland function remain normal throughout life. The fact that bone metabolism is severely altered while parathyroid function remains normal in the aged is compatible with the observation that thyrocalcitonin levels decrease with advancing age.

Forty per cent of parathyroid tumors are in patients over 50 years of age. Two thirds of primary hyperparathyroidism patients are over 50 years of age. Hypoparathyroidism in the elderly is rare, and is most always secondary to surgical excision.

OVARY

Perhaps the most significant endocrine changes in aging females are those associated with menopause. On gross examination, the senescent ovary is smaller and more fibrotic than in younger women. There is a decrease in the number of primary follicles, but the stroma, the source of steroid synthesis, does not appear to undergo atrophic changes. Estrogen concentration in postmenopausal women is one third to one half of that observed in younger women. The cause of the onset of menopause is unknown, but may be related to an alteration of ovarian sensitivity to gonadotropins.

TESTIS

The alterations in the histology of the testis with age include tubular fibrosis and atrophy, scarcity of Leydig cells, and reduction of spermatogenic activity. Testosterone levels fall with age, possibly as a result of reduced responsiveness of the testicular parenchyma to endogenous gonadotropins.

ENDOCRINE PANCREAS

Pancreatic structure in the aged shows evidence of fibrosis and cavity formation, but it is not known whether these changes impair the function of the gland.

Diabetes mellitus has become one of the most common diseases among older people, with a prevalence approaching 20 per cent of the population over the age of 65 years. Older people in general have a reduced insulin response to intravenous glucose. This decline in glucose tolerance is explained on the basis of a decreased sensitivity of the beta cells of the pancreas to blood sugar levels, leading to a diminished rate of insulin release. This change presents a problem in deciding what level of plasma glucose should be considered acceptable for an aged individual. Even when unequivocally present, diabetes in older people may be entirely asymptomatic. Urine glucose determinations may be misleading, since the threshold for urinary glucose secretion increases with age. When the onset of diabetes is particularly insidious, the aged individual may slip into severe hyperglycemia, dehydration, and ketoacidosis before the diagnosis is made.

The complications of diabetes in the elderly are the same as they are in the younger diabetic, although the presence of other problems, such as cardiovascular disease, introduces increased risks for the elderly. The practical aspects of the perioperative management of diabetes are the same in older persons as in younger persons.

PHARMACOLOGY

Geriatric anesthetic pharmacology is often complex because anesthetic drugs are often superimposed on multiple chronically administered medications. In addition, the physiological changes that occur with aging alter pharmacokinetics and pharmacodynamics, which in turn alter drug responsiveness. In the presence of multisystem disease and multiple drug exposure, altered drug responsiveness predisposes the elderly to complex drug interactions, diagnostic and therapeutic enigmas, and bizarre overdose and toxicity problems. Since anesthesiologists are often confronted with and may contribute to this confusing clinical situation, it is important to review the effects of aging on drug disposition and the implications that these changes have on the rational use of drugs in the elderly.

The pharmacokinetic processes of absorption, distribution, metabolism, and excretion govern the time course of a drug in the plasma, and each of these processes is influenced by aging. Alterations in gastrointestinal physiology of the aged affect the rate and extent of systemic absorption of orally administered drugs. Hypochlorhydria (increased gastric pH) in the elderly can alter the ionization and solubility of some drugs. Delayed gastric emptying can cause the breakdown of drugs that are acid labile or are extensively metabolized by the gastric mucosa or have a short half-life. Since the small bowel is the site of maximum drug absorption (large surface area), a decrease in intestinal mobility may provide a long mucosal contact time and excessive uptake. On the other hand, a reduced intestinal absorption capacity caused either by a reduction in the number of absorbing cells or by impairment of cell membrane transport enzyme systems could decrease drug absorption. Age related reduction in intestinal blood flow might also influence rates of absorption.

Distribution is the process of transferring drug molecules in the plasma to other parts of the body, and is influenced by a number of age dependent physiologic factors. Body composition is one important determinant of drug distribution. Since aging causes a decrease in total body water and skeletal muscle (decreased lean body mass), dosage schedules that are based on the usual estimates of body size, such as total body weight or surface area, result in higher blood or tissue levels of drugs whose distribution is limited to the lean body mass. This alteration in the apparent volume in distribution may account for the prolonged half-life of diazepam in aged subjects, which increases from 20 hours at 20 years to 90 hours at 80 years, and may also explain the increased depressant effect of diazepam on the central nervous system. The relative increase in total body fat might result in accumulation and prolongation of drugs that preferentially partition into lipoid tissue, such as thiopental and the lipid soluble volatile anesthetic agents. The decreased plasma albumin concentration in the elderly results in reduced protein binding, which can result in increased free drug concentration and enhanced pharmacological response. Meperidine and thiopental are two drugs that have marked increase in free drug concentration in the plasma with increasing age as a result of decreased protein binding of the drug. The decline in cardiac output associated with aging could decrease the rate of delivery of the drug to the target tissue. Alternatively, if the depressed cardiac output is redistributed preferentially to the cerebral and coronary circulations, then drugs known to depress these organs may accumulate in dangerously high levels if dosages are not reduced. Increase of permeability of the blood-brain barrier has been thought to influence drug availability and distribution in the elderly, which may explain why the elderly are more sensitive to central nervous system depressants.

The activity of many drugs is influenced by biotransformation. Many drugs that are initially lipid soluble must be made water soluble by the liver before they can be excreted by the kidney. Both liver mass and liver blood flow diminish with age, and this may decrease the rate of removal from plasma of some drugs. Alternatively, an impaired ability to metabolize some drugs can be due to reduced levels or decreased activity of hepatic microsomal enzymes. Drugs metabolized extrahepatically may also be affected by age related changes. For example, cholinesterase activity in the plasma is 24 per cent lower in older subjects; thus the potential exists for a longer duration of action of succinylcholine and ester-type local anesthetics.

The ultimate elimination of a drug or its metabolites from the body is predominantly through the kidneys, and renal changes can produce significantly altered drug levels in the elderly. The age related decline in renal hemodynamics, nephron mass, and glomerular and tubular function reduce the efficiency of drug excretion by the kidney. As previously mentioned, the creatinine clearance rather than BUN or serum creatinine should be used to estimate renal function and should be preferred as a guide for determining appropriate drug doses.

Age related changes in organs may mechanically limit the response of an organ to a drug's action. For example, changes in the number or state of receptor sites may explain altered drug responsiveness in the elderly. The reduced chronotropic activity of atropine has been explained on the basis of fewer cholinergic receptors. In some elderly patients barbiturates cause a paradoxical effect in that stimulation results rather than depression. The paradoxical result can be explained by the fact that the receptors stimulated by barbiturates deteriorate less with age than the receptors that are depressed by barbiturates. Disease states may influence the response to a drug. Impairment of hepatic, renal, or cardiac function may allow drugs to accumulate at high levels when standard doses are given. Specific diseases of organs may influence the response of the organ to a particular drug. For example, elderly patients with atrophic limbs resulting from cerebral vascular accidents may have a hyperkalemic response to succinylcholine. The presence of other factors such as myocardial and cerebral vascular disease, electrolyte and acid base disturbances, and endocrine imbalances is not uncommon in the elderly and can alter drug sensitivity. Finally, drug-drug interactions can result in the development of exaggerated or reduced pharmacologic responses.

ANESTHETIC MANAGEMENT

Careful preoperative evaluation and preparation are important in the management of the geriatric patient. Preoperative baseline evaluation of cardiac, pulmonary, renal, and neurologic status should be undertaken to detect the presence and severity of age related alterations in organ function and the presence of specific pre-existing systemic diseases. In addition, an accurate medication history is important.

Hypertension is an expected malady of old age. Antihypertensive medication should be continued up to the time of surgery. Patients receiving diuretics for blood pressure control often have significant depletion of total body potassium, and potassium replacement may be necessary, especially if the patient is also receiving digitalis.

Coronary artery disease, with its complications, is another ailment common to the elderly. Digitalis therapy for congestive heart failure or arrhythmias is commonly seen in the elderly and is often combined with propranolol if angina and/or hypertension is also present. Nitroglycerin, orally or as skin paste, is also a commonly administered preoperative drug, and is being used in the operating room to treat signs of myocardial ischemia and increases in pre-load. These drugs are being maintained up to the time of surgery now that their compatibility with general anesthesia and their protective action against undesirable increases in myocardial oxygen demand are known.

There are several other important preoperative cardiac concerns. The risk of reinfarction is increased if anesthesia and surgery are performed within six months of a myocardial infarction. Arrhythmias are also common in the elderly; they should be precisely identified and treated, when possible, preoperatively. A patient with a history of heart failure who is to undergo a procedure that can cause sudden intravascular volume changes is a candidate for intraoperative pulmonary artery occlusion pressure measurement.

Non-cardiac drug medication history is important. When diabetes is present in the aged, insulin requirements and maintenance of adequate serum glucose levels are important perioperative concerns. Elderly patients often receive psychotropic medications that can interact adversely with other drugs. Tricyclic antidepressants may cause arrhythmias or they can interact with vasopressors to cause paroxysmal hypertension. MAO inhibitors may cause severe hypertension when combined with vasopressors or meperidine. Lithium can cause atrial arrhythmias and may potentiate muscle relaxants. Elderly patients may be receiving steroids for arthritis, and since adrenal suppression is possible, preoperative steroid coverage is usually prudent. Aspirin therapy for arthritis may warrant tests of clotting and platelet function. Echothiophate eye drops may lead to prolonged action of succinylcholine because of pseudocholinesterase inhibition. Patients on L-dopa for parkinsonism may be prone to hypotensive episodes and chest wall rigidity and can develop extrapyramidal signs if phenothiazines or butyrophenones are administered. Finally, many antibiotics often used in elderly patients are known to potentiate the action of muscle relaxants.

Chronic lung disease is frequently present in the elderly. Pulmonary function tests can quantitate the degree of impairment and indicate whether therapy should be instituted preoperatively. Incentive spirometry, chest physical therapy, breathing and coughing instructions, and the use of medications where appropriate can help reduce the incidence of postoperative respiratory complications. Preoperative participation by the family in these matters can aid postoperative care immeasurably.

After assessment of the patient for any chronic illnesses, current medications, and major organ system function, the preoperative physical examination should emphasize the presence of pressure sores, the ability of the patient to tolerate the intended surgical position, airway anatomy and accessibility, vascular access, and vertebral anatomy. The patient's head should be placed in various positions to see if any position produces symptoms of cerebral ischemia. The results of the hemogram, serum electrolytes, ECG, and chest x-ray should be reviewed. Liver and renal function studies and arterial blood gases should be obtained in most instances.

The elderly patient is often dehydrated and has an inadequate intravascular volume for the induction of either a general or a regional anesthetic. Both of these anesthetic techniques can be accompanied by significant vasodilation, and consequently the effects of any pre-existing hypovolemia will be accentuated. On admission, dehydrated elderly patients may have a normal hematocrit, and upon rehydration the patient may become anemic. The tilt test is useful in the evaluation of volume status; if more than a 10 per cent increase in pulse rate or decrease in systolic blood pressure occurs when the patient sits upright for one minute, a volume deficit is most likely present. Dry mucosal surfaces, loss of tissue turgor, and oliguria are late signs of dehydration and hypovolemia. If time allows, correction of hypovolemia should be done slowly to permit adequate interstitial and intracellular volume adjustments as well. In selected patients, central venous pressure and pulmonary artery occlusion pressure measurements may serve as useful guidelines to preoperative volume replacement.

PREANESTHETIC MEDICATION

A variety of medications can be given preoperatively to decrease pain, relieve anxiety, and provide a smoother induction, maintenance, and emergence from anesthesia. In general, the more elderly and ill the patient is, the less amount of sedative and analgesic drug is required. In particular, an already clouded mental status or compromised cardiovascular or respiratory status should not be further jeopardized by depressant premedication. Elderly patients have a high incidence of hiatus hernia and regurgitation. Oral cimetidine can help to reduce gastric acidity and minimize the complications of aspiration. The decrease of oropharyngeal secretions with age obviates the need for routine preoperative administration of antisialogogues.

MONITORING

Elderly patients have diminished ability to withstand stress. Thus it is especially important to monitor vital functions in order to avoid wide deviations and to provide early warning of adverse trends. The electrocardiogram, blood pressure, minute ventilation, temperature, and urine output should be routinely monitored. Arterial, central venous, and pulmonary artery catheters are frequently indicated in geriatric patients to provide hemodynamic measurements as well as sites for fluid and drug administration and serial blood sampling. Since the aged have a high incidence of peripheral vascular disease, the adequacy of collateral flow should be tested before radial artery cannulation. Similarly, internal jugular vein cannulation should be performed with caution, since carotid artery puncture or plaque dislodgement could severely compromise the cerebral circulation. Non-tapered Teflon catheters are thought to provide the lowest incidence of thrombosis. During regional anesthesia, maintenance of verbal contact with the patient provides a monitor of the sensorium, and observation for agitation, restlessness, confusion, or pain may allow detection of hypoglycemia, coronary or cerebral ischemia, and hypoxia.

GENERAL ANESTHESIA

Advanced age is not a contraindication to general anesthesia, and it is not less safe than regional anesthesia for the elderly as once believed. In fact, general anesthesia is frequently more indicated than regional anesthesia when airway control, mechanical ventilation, and tracheobronchial toilet are of primary importance.

The prolonged circulation time of the elderly requires that intravenous induction drugs be administered in small incremental doses so that time is allowed for the full development of drug effect and observation of physiologic changes. The presence of hypovolemia and a diminished ability of the circulatory system to compensate for vasodilation can result in marked hypotension following a bolus of intravenous barbiturate. Unfortunately, subsequent laryngoscopy and endotracheal intubation may cause marked hypertension. The sequence of myocardial depression and hypotension after thiopental followed by hypertension and tachycardia associated with laryngoscopy and tracheal intubation must be avoided, since it may cause myocardial ischemia. A smooth, well controlled induction can be accomplished with small, incremental doses of narcotics combined with small doses of diazepam or barbiturates and/or by inhalation of volatile anesthetic by mask. Circulatory responses to airway stimulation can be attenuated with intratracheal or intravenous lidocaine. A reduction in systemic vascular resistance by intravascular infusion of nitroprusside or nitroglycerin is another alternative.

Anesthesia can be maintained by inhalation of volatile anesthetic or by a balanced technique (N_2O-narcotic). However, it should be remembered that the volatile drugs and N_2O can cause direct and reflex depression of myocardial activity and peripheral vascular tone. Ketamine has sympathomimetic effects in small doses, and has been used with good results in properly selected geriatric patients. It should always be remembered that age and anesthetic requirements have an inverse relationship. Thus, MAC for halothane in the newborn and for the octogenarian are 1.08 and 0.64 per cent, respectively. Similar MAC for isoflurane in the young adult and for the 80 year old patient are 1.30 and 9.95 percent, respectively.

The use of neuromuscular blocking agents in the elderly warrants certain precautions. Curare can cause hypotension and bronchospasm due to ganglionic blocking and histamine releasing properties. Pancuronium is vagolytic and can cause a tachycardia. Although a succinylcholine drip is ordinarily benign, elderly patients may have a hyperkalemic and/or phase-two block response. Dimethylcurare (metocurine) may be the relaxant of choice in the elderly since this drug has minimal vagolytic action, histamine release, and ganglionic blockade. Pyridostigmine may be preferred to neostigmine for reversal of neuromuscular block in geriatric patients because there is a lower incidence of arrhythmia and bradycardia, particularly in patients with hypertension, coronary artery disease, and conduction defects. In this regard, glycopyrrolate may be a better choice than atropine to antagonize the unwanted cholinergic side effects of these anticholinesterase drugs, since glycopyrrolate produces less tachycardia and has minimal CNS effects.

Deliberate hypotensive anesthesia can be used safely and without detrimental effect on mental function in the elderly. However, the safe use of deliberate hypotension in elderly patients requires that all selected patients be suitable in all the other important respects, such as being normovolemic and without cardiovascular disease.

REGIONAL ANESTHESIA

Regional anesthesia is often very useful for many procedures in the elderly. With most blocks analgesia and muscle relaxation are profound and there is no loss in consciousness. While wakefulness is ordinarily an advantage in monitoring related diseases (diabetes, angina, cerebral insufficiency) intraoperatively, it is a disadvantage with an uncooperative or uncomfortable patient who attempts to move his body. Injudicious intravenous sedation may progress to the point of administering an uncontrolled general anesthetic without benefit of airway or ventilatory control.

Single dose administration of spinal anesthesia is a common technique. Calcification of ligaments and decreased ability to flex the vertebral column may make lumbar puncture difficult via the midline approach. A paramedian approach, with entry through the skin 1 centimeter lateral to the vertebral spine, will bypass these ligaments and allow entry into the interspinous space. Larger gauge needles may be used for lumbar puncture, since the incidence of postspinal headache is low in the elderly. Efforts should be made to retain as much sympathetic response as possible to help minimize the cardiovascular depression. In this regard, hypobaric or hyperbaric solutions may be employed, depending on the patient's position, to achieve a low level or unilateral block, thus permitting maximal sympathetic compensation. Clinical impression holds that for a given dose the duration of spinal anesthesia is proportional to age.

Epidural anesthesia provides a slower onset of sympathectomy than spinal anesthesia, which allows more time for hemodynamic stabilization. Local anesthesia requirement per epidural segment decreases with age. However, epidural anesthesia may be technically difficult to perform in the elderly.

RECOVERY PERIOD

The same level of intensity in monitoring the vital signs, electrocardiogram, and temperature should continue into the recovery period. Early mobilization will help prevent thromboembolic phenomena.

The possible prolonged effects of anesthetic agents or adjuncts cause a particular problem in the elderly. In particular, narcotic and volatile drug ventilatory depression may require continued endotracheal intubation. Intravenous Narcan should be titrated to effect, for an excessive dose can result in agitation, hypertension, and arrhythmias. It should be remembered that Narcan has a shorter duration of action than narcotics and that a second peak of ventilatory depression may occur. Small doses of physostigmine may reverse some confusion or somnolence when diazepam or droperidol has been used. Adequacy of muscle relaxant reversal should always be assessed.

The waning of a regional anesthetic is sometimes difficult to assess in the elderly patient. Motor and sensory function may return while a sympathetic block persists; thus blood pressure stability should be ensured before moving the patient from the recovery area.

Postoperative hypertension, anemia, oliguria, and other medical problems should be evaluated and treated. The appearance of arrhythmias, wheezing, or confusion may signal a dire change in the patient's condition such as infarction, congestive heart failure, pulmonary embolus, or CVA. If there is any doubt about the stability of an elderly patient, he or she should go to an intensive care unit from the recovery room.

REFERENCES

General

1. Butler, R. N.: The doctor and the aged patient. Hosp. Pract. *13*:99, 1978.
2. Chadwick, D. A.: Reducing anesthetic risks for the geriatric surgical patient. Geriatrics 28:108, 1973.
3. Cogbill, C.: Operation in the aged. Arch. Surg. *94*:202, 1967.
4. Cole, W. H.: Medical differences between the young and the aged. J. Amer. Geriatr. Soc. *19*:589, 1970.
5. Djokovic, J. L., et al.: Prediction of outcome of surgery and anesthesia in patients over 80. J.A.M.A. *242*:2301, 1979.
6. Ellison, N.: Problems in geriatric anesthesia. Surg. Clin. North Am. 55:929, 1975.
7. Evans, T. I.: The physiologic basis of geriatric general anesthesia. Anaesth. Intensive Care *1*:319, 1973.
8. Levin, I., et al.: Physical class and physiologic status in prediction of operative mortality in aged sick. Ann. Surg. *174*:217, 1971.
9. Lorhan, P. H.: Emergency anesthesia for the aged. Int. Anesth. Clin. 9:29, 1971.

10. Lorhan, P. H.: Anesthesia for the aged. C. C Thomas, Springfield, Ill. 1971.

11. Martin, G.: Genetic and evolutionary aspects of aging. Fed. Proc. 39:1962, 1979.

12. Masoro, E. J., et al.: Analysis and exploration of age related changes in mammalian structure and function. Fed. Proc. 38:1956, 1979.

13. Miller, R., et al.: Anesthesia for patients over ninety years. N. Y. State J. Med.: August, 1977, pp 1421.

14. Reichel, W.: The geriatric patient. Hosp. Prac. 11:15, 1976.

15. Reichel W: Clinical Aspects of Aging. Baltimore, Williams & Wilkins, 1978.

16. Shock, N. W.: Systems physiology and aging. Fed. Proc. 38:161, 1979.

17. Siegel, J., and Chodoff, P.: The Aged and High-Risk Surgical Patient. New York, Grune and Stratton, 1976.

18. Wallace, D. J.: The biology of aging. J. Am. Geriatr. Soc. 25:104, 1977.

19. Ziffren, S. E., and Hartford, C. E.: Comparative mortality for various surgical operations in older versus younger age groups. J. Am. Geriatr. Soc. 20:485, 1972.

Cardiovascular System

1. Adelman, R.: Loss of adaptive mechanisms during aging. Fed. Proc. 38:1968, 1979.

2. Berg, G., et al.: Significance of bilateral bundle branch block in the preoperative patient. Chest 59:62, 1971.

3. Bierman, F.: Atherosclerosis and aging. Fed. Proc. 37:2832, 1978.

4. Duke, P.: The effects of age on baroreceptor reflex function in man. Canad. Anaesth. Soc. J. 23:111, 1976.

5. Harris, R.: Cardiac changes with age. *In* Goldman, R., and Rockstein, M. (eds.): Physiology and Pathology of Human Aging. New York, Academic Press, 1975.

6. Lakatta, E.: Alterations that occur in the cardiovascular system with advanced age. Fed. Proc. 38:163, 1979.

7. Lerner, S.: Suppression of a demand pacemaker by transurethral electrosurgery. Anesth. Analg. 52:703, 1973.

8. Roberts, J., et al.: Changes in responsiveness of the heart to drugs during aging. Fed. Proc. 38:1927, 1979.

9. Rooney, S., et al.: Relationship of RBBB and marked LAD to complete heart block during general anesthesia. Anesthesiology 44:64, 1976.

10. Simon, A. B.: Perioperative management of the pacemaker patient. Anesthesiology 46:127, 1977.

11. Wynands, J. E.: Anesthesia for patients with heart block and artificial pacemakers. Anesth. Analg. 55:626, 1976.

Pulmonary System

1. Dahr, S., et al.: Aging and the respiratory system. Med. Clin. North Am. 60:1121, 1976.

2. Don, H.: Measurement of gas trapped in the lungs at FRC and effects of posture. Anesthesiology 35:582, 1971.

3. Gredinsky, C.: Postoperative pulmonary compli-cations in the geriatric age group. J. Am. Geriatr. Soc. 22:405, 1974.

4. Kitamura, H.: Postoperative hypoxemia: Contribution of age to V/Q. Anesthesiology 36:244, 1972.

5. Manderly, J.: Effect of age on pulmonary structure and function of immature and adult animals and man. Fed. Proc. 38:(2):173, 1979.

6. Pontoppidan, H., and Beecher, H. K.: Progressive loss of protective reflexes in the airway with the advance of age. J.A.M.A. 174:2209, 1960.

7. Pump, K. K.: Emphysema and its relation to age. Am. Rev. Resp. Dis. 114:5, 1976.

8. Wahba, W.: Body build (age) and preoperative arterial oxygen tension. Canad. Anaesth. Soc. J. 22:653, 1975.

9. West, J. B.: Blood flow to the lung and gas exchange. Anesthesiology 41:124, 1974.

Nervous System

1. Bellville, J. W., et al.: Age and pain relief. J.A.M.A. 217:1841, 1971.

2. Lytle, L. D., et al.: Diet, central nervous system and aging. Fed. Proc. 38:2017, 1979.

Excretory System

1. Epstein, M.: Effects of aging on the kidney: Fed. Proc. 38:1969, 1973.

Pharmacology

1. Bender, A. D.: Pharmacodynamic principles of drug therapy in the aged. J. Am. Geriatr. Soc. 22:290, 1974.

2 Gillette, J.: Biotransformation of drugs during aging. Fed. Proc. 38:1900, 1979.

3. Klotz, U., et al.: Effects of age and liver disease on the disposition and elimination of diazepam. J. Clin. Invest. 55:347, 1975.

4. Mather, L. E., et al.: Meperidine kinetics in man. Clin. Pharmacol. Ther. 17:21, 1975.

5. Medical Letter 21(10):43, 1979.

6. Pearce, C.: The respiratory effects of diazepam supplementation of spinal anesthesia in elderly males. Br. J. Anaesth. 46:439, 1974.

7. Richey, D. P., and Bender, A. D.: Pharmacokinetic consequences of aging. Ann. Rev. Toxicol. 17:49, 1977.

8. Vestal, R.: Aging and pharmacokinetics: Impact of altered physiology in the elderly. *In* Cherkin et al. (eds.): Physiology and Cell Biology of Aging. (Aging, Vol 8), New York, Raven Press, 1979.

Anesthetic Management

1. Bourke, D. L., et al.: Methylmethacrylate and the cardiovascular system. Anesthesiol. Rev. 4(3):27, 1977.

2. Bromage, P. R.: Aging and epidural dose requirements. Br. J. Anaesth. 41:1016, 1969.

3. Chapin, J. W., et al.: Progeria and anesthesia. Anesth. Analg. 58:424, 1979.

4. Dohi, S., et al.: Age related changes in blood pressure and duration of motor block in spinal anesthesia. Anesthesiology 50:319, 1979.

5. Gordon, J. L.: Planning a safe anesthesia for the elderly patient. Geriatrics 32:69, 1977.

6. Gregory, G.: The relationship between age and halothane requirements in man. Anesthesiology 30:488, 1969.

7. Jedeikin, R. J., and Hoffman, S.: The oculocardiac reflex in eye surgery anesthesia. Anesth. Analg. 56:333, 1977.

8. Lorhan, P. H.: Clinical appraisal of the use of ketamine hydrochloride in the aged. Anesth. Analg. 50:488, 1971.

9. Milliken, R. A.: Geriatric spinal anesthesia in 102 year old man. Anesth. Analg. 51:400, 1977.

10. Owens, W. D., Waldbaum, L. S., and Stephen, C. R.: Cardiac dysrhythmia following reversal of neuromuscular blocking agents in geriatric patients. Anesth. Analg. 50:186, 1978.

11. Rollason, W., et al.: Comparison of mental function in relation to hypotensive and normotensive anesthesia in the elderly. Br. J. Anaesth. 45:561, 1971.

12. Sharrock, N.: Epidural anesthetic dose responses in patients 20 to 80 years old. Anesthesiology 49:425, 1978.

13. Steen, P., et al.: Myocardial reinfarction after anesthesia and surgery. J.A.M.A. 239:2566, 1972.

14. Stevens, K., et al.: Anesthetic factors affecting surgical morbidity and mortality in the elderly male. J. Am. Geriatr. Soc. 17:659, 1975.

15. Stevens W. C., et al.: MAC concentrations of isoflurane with and without nitrous oxide in patients of various ages. Anesthesiology 42:197, 1975.

16. Tarhan, S., et al.: Myocardial infarction after general anesthesia. J.A.M.A. 220:1451, 1972.

4

Diseases of Infants*

By C. F. WARD, M.D.

Anesthetic Considerations in the Newborn
  Anatomy
  Physiology
  Pharmacology
  Fluid metabolism
  Temperature regulation
  Anesthetic management
Choanal Atresia

Pierre Robin Syndrome
Laryngeal Papillomas
Tracheal Esophageal Fistula
Neonatal Respiratory Distress Syndrome
Congenital Lobar Emphysema
Biliary Disease
Congenital Diaphragmatic Hernia
Abdominal Wall Defects

ANESTHETIC CONSIDERATIONS IN THE NEWBORN

The principles governing anesthesia for the newborn are essentially the same as those for adults; however, there are certain anatomical, physiological, and environmental concerns unique to the neonate. The limited ability of the newborn to withstand physiological and environmental stress implies that only those infants who absolutely demand surgical intervention should come to operation. The lack of organ maturation and function in the normal infant, when compared with the normal adult, may seem to those unfamiliar with the care of the newborn to create an unusual disease process. As the requirements for meticulous supportive care are especially great, a brief general review of pertinent anatomy, physiology, and pharmacology is necessary prior to addressing the specific details of each disease entity.

ANATOMY

A typical newborn weighs 3.5 Kg, and, since cardiac output is proportional to weight[3,4], the newborn infant has a much greater cardiac output per unit weight than its parent. Not only does the infant weigh approximately 20 times less than its parent but its body proportions are also much different. The child is one third the length of the adult. This has significance, for many pulmonary functions are related to body length rather than weight.

The relative surface area of the newborn is one ninth that of the adult. Since surface area is related to caloric and fluid requirements, and therefore to O_2 consumption (and CO_2 excretion), an increased surface area-to-weight ratio in infants, when compared with adults, means that infants have relatively greater ventilation and fluid requirements. Similarly, since heat loss from radiation, evaporation, and convection is also directly related to surface area, a baby loses heat much more rapidly than an adult. Additionally, because the limbs of a newborn constitute a higher percentage of surface area than those of an adult, and convection constants are related to the radius of curvature of the surface, there is an in-

*Supported by NIHGMS 24674A.

The author wishes to acknowledge with appreciation R. Johnson, M.D., and T. Canty, M.D., for reviewing the manuscript, and D. J. Barnum and J. A. Johnson for editorial assistance.

creased heat loss from an infant's limbs. The distribution of the relatively large surface area of the newborn is different in other important respects as well. The infant's head is relatively large and bulky with a prominent occiput, while the neck is so short as to appear nonexistent. The trunk and upper body form a larger percentage of the body length than later in life, and the baby's prominent abdomen constitutes a larger percentage of the trunk.

The anatomical differences between the adult and the newborn infant impact directly on anesthetic management. The infant's bulky head and short neck, and its inadequate musculature, force it to adopt characteristic postures to maintain an adequate airway. These postures generally involve turning the head to the side, frequently in the prone position. If the infant is placed in the supine position under anesthesia, the large occiput forces cervical flexion if the head is in the sagittal plane, unless this is opposed by supporting the chin. The relatively large tongue and absence of teeth allow apposition of the palate and tongue, making the child a nasal breather. Nasal obstruction, from any cause, may therefore require the insertion of an oral airway. Similarly, an oral airway may be necessary in anesthesia because of posterior tongue displacement.

The structure of the remainder of the upper airway also varies significantly from that of the adult. The epiglottis is longer, stiffer, "Ω" in shape, and protrudes posteriorly from the tongue, tending to cover or obscure the laryngeal aperture. The posterior angulation, along with the natural "sniffing" position of the head when held neutral, indicates the use of a straight laryngoscope blade in order to pick up the epiglottis and visualize the glottis. The more cephalad location of the vocal cords, namely opposite C3-C4, makes it easy to overshoot the airway completely and enter the esophagus when using a straight laryngoscope blade. Therefore, a short blade with the bulb close to the tip is recommended. The anterior attachment of the vocal cords is more caudad in the newborn and may potentially cause difficulty with the endotracheal tube passage at the anterior commissure owing to inadvertent but excessive anterior angulation of the tube. Finally, the narrowest portion of the infant's airway is normally the complete ring of cartilage located at the cricoid, permitting a tube that is actually too large for the patient to pass the cords but go no further.

The lower airway also differs from that of the adult in a fairly predictable way. The trachea is relatively short (4 cm), and to prevent endobronchial intubation, the tip of the endotracheal tube should pass only 1 cm beyond the vocal cords before fixation. Even so, auscultation and observation of the chest over both lung apices is always necessary to insure correct positioning. Poiseuille's law states that the resistance of the infant's smaller lower airway must be much higher than that of the adult. However, since the infant's lung moves much less gas at a much slower velocity during each breath, the l/resistance or conductance values encountered in life for the newborn and adult are comparable. This allows the infant to generate essentially the same pressures as the adult during breathing. However, it is important to recognize that the smaller airway of the newborn can be much more easily mechanically obstructed by edema or secretions.

PHYSIOLOGY

Respiration

During a normal vaginal delivery, the birth canal exerts a positive pressure of 60 cm of H_2O or more on the highly compliant neonatal thorax, causing extrusion of 5 ml of tracheal fluid from the oropharynx. Immediately after the thorax is delivered, the chest wall expands to its previous dimensions, generating a negative thoracic pressure that assists in establishing passive aeration of the lungs. Thermal, tactile, auditory, and proprioceptive stimuli probably all participate in initiating the first active breath, but the key factor appears to be an interaction between hypercapnia and hypoxia. The first series of breaths establishes a negative interstitial pressure that may possibly aide in mechanically "unkinking" pulmonary vessels. These first breaths also greatly increase PA_{O_2} and Pa_{O_2}, contributing to the profound fall in pulmonary vascular resistance and rise in pulmonary blood volume that occurs in the first 24 hours of life. The liquid contained in the lung is rapidly mobilized via the circulation and lymphatics, the majority being cleared within the first 24 hours. Over the next several weeks, there is a decrease in the muscular thickness of the pulmonary arteries which is accompanied by further gradual decline in pulmonary vascular resistance. Therefore, a considerable period of time is required before the pulmonary circulation fully resembles that of the adult.

Since the newborn has a relatively increased body surface area and metabolic requirement, alveolar ventilation per kg in the newborn is roughly twice that of the adult (Table 4–1). The control mechanism responsible for the increased respiration is clinically relevant. For the first week of life, the human infant behaves as though he were acclimated to high altitude and hypoxemia (as indeed he was) and demonstrates an unsustained response to hypoxia. This reverts to sustained hyperventilation during exposure to hypoxia after the first week of life. The typical newborn CO_2 response curve is well to the left of the adult curve, resulting in a resting Pa_{CO_2} of $\cong 34$ torr. This further hyperventilation during the first week of life may be a result of a residual progesterone effect from the mother. The increased ventilation is accomplished by an increased respiratory frequency rather than tidal volume, which minimizes respiratory work.

Periodic respiration occurs often in the neonate. Apnea of more than five seconds' duration occurs approximately six times per hour in term infants and considerably more often in prematures. Normally, the infant spontaneously recovers, but such pauses may extend for 30 seconds or longer in some patients, resulting in bradycardia and cyanosis that require intervention. The cause of the prolonged apnea is currently unclear but may be related to the immaturity of respiratory control feedback mechanisms. The bradycardia is vagally mediated and can be abolished with atropine.

The chest wall of the infant is substantially more compliant than that of the adult, as might be expected for a thorax required to transit the birth canal. Although the pressure-volume curve of the lung is similar to that of the adult, a striking increase in compliance of the thorax reflects a lack of skeletal and muscular rigidity and explains the presence of both diaphragmatic respiration and chest retraction during inspiration. The lack of skeletal and muscular rigidity also greatly decreases chest wall recoil, which in turn causes the lung-chest wall combination to balance at end expiration at a reduced functional residual capacity (FRC). The decreased FRC falls within the range of closing volume during quiet respiration so that substantial "gas trapping" occurs during the first 10 days of life. After this time, the chest wall generally becomes more stable (by an as yet unknown mechanism) and the "gas trapping" decreases.

The distribution of ventilation and pulmonary perfusion differs somewhat in the newborn as compared with the adult. The chest of the supine infant is not subjected to the profound effects of gravity as is the upright adult chest. Thus, the infant lung has a remarkably good distribution of ventilation, often approaching the ideal of a uniform pattern. However, the infant lung has a propensity to trap gas behind closed airways. In addition, the infant has a venous admixture approaching three times that of the adult. Whether this represents fetal venoarterial circulation, atelectasis, or bronchial circulation is as yet unknown. The increased shunt persists for approximately 3 weeks, by which time Pa_{O_2} (and Pa_{CO_2}) have risen to adult levels.

The neonatal lung is disposed to intraoperative atelectasis and hypoxemia. Normally, ventilatory requirements are high while the chest bellows is only marginally effective and resembles a "flail" chest in function. Since FRC is reduced, significant

Table 4–1 Measurement of the Infant and Adult Human Lung

	Newborn	Adult
Body weight (kg)	3.5	70
Surface area (m²)	0.21	1.90
Tracheal diameter (mm)	8	18
Vital capacity (ml/kg)	33	52
Functional residual capacity (ml/kg)	30	34
Dead space (ml/kg)	2.2	2.2
Tidal volume (ml/kg)	6–8	7
Closing volume (ml/kg)	12	7
Respiratory rate at rest	40	20
Alveolar ventilation (ml/kg/min)	150–200	90
Oxygen consumption at rest (ml/kg/min)	6	3

gas trapping occurs during normal tidal ventilation and shunt is increased. The airways are small and easily obstructed, causing miliary atelectasis that is not easily detected without arterial blood gas tension measurement. If atelectasis occurs, the absence of pores of Kohn and therefore collateral ventilation (as in adults), coupled with the very small diameter of the alveoli, tend to promote persistence of atelectasis rather than reopening of areas to gas exchange. If respiratory depressants and surgery (often with restricted airway access) are added to the limited neonatal respiratory reserve, respiratory failure may ensue. For all of these reasons, it seems logical to intubate the newborn trachea and control ventilation, using positive end-expiratory pressure.

Cardiovascular Physiology

The circulatory transition following delivery is not as dramatic as the respiratory transition following the first breath, but it is equally complex. The precipitous fall in pulmonary vascular resistance (PVR) that occurs with the first breath is interlocked with an equally abrupt increase in systemic vascular resistance (SVR), well symbolized by the closure of a hemostat across the umbilical cord. However, prior to cord clamping the newborn normally receives a placental transfusion of up to 20 per cent of the "final" blood volume, with one third of the placental transfusion remaining intrathoracic. Obviously, the effects of gravity and the timing of cord clamping can significantly influence the volume of blood transfused, and this may in part account for the variation in blood volume reported for the newborn (82–107 ml/kg, average 93 ml/kg). The interruption of placental flow by clamping also transiently decreases venous return to the right heart until blood begins to return from the increased systemic circulation. Right atrial pressure therefore falls and left atrial pressure rises (as a result of increased pulmonary flow), thus functionally closing the foramen ovale. The fall in PVR and rise in SVR quickly reverse the unidirectional right-to-left flow in the ductus arteriosus to a bidirectional flow, and then finally to a unidirectional left-to-right pattern. Left ventricular output abruptly increases (from increased input), with a significant proportion of the output providing a functionally redundant flow to the lungs via the ductus. The ductus responds to the rise in blood oxygen tension in minutes to hours with muscular constriction, although this is readily reversible should hypoxia occur. After the first day of constriction, a period of obliterative degeneration takes place over a period of about two weeks, and finally, by about two months of age, 98 per cent of infants have a completely closed ductus. Interestingly, the ductus may close "on schedule" in cyanotic children, implying an unknown factor in the control of constriction.

Two points concerning the circulatory transition are worthy of additional reflection. First, the output of the left ventricle after birth is quite high, yet at birth it has less muscle mass than the right ventricle. Thus, the left ventricle must operate at nearly continuous full power to provide the required output. Consequently, depression of this ventricle by anesthetics may be poorly tolerated in the newborn. Second, the rapid placental transfusion suggests that the neonatal circulation may be transiently overdistended after birth, apparently without distress. This situation may not occur if the cord is quickly clamped or during cesarean section. The absence of significant neonatal responsiveness to volume overload gives some insight into neonatal vascular reactivity to vascular volume loss. If a neonate is subjected to a 10 per cent hemorrhage, baroceptor function causes a 10 to 15 per cent increase in heart rate, and an attempt is made to defend systemic blood pressure by a rise in systemic vascular resistance (to twice the adult value). However, very little venoconstriction occurs and, therefore, cardiac output, stroke volume, and ultimately blood pressure decrease substantially. Although it is teleologically attractive to relate minimal vascular responsiveness to a system that may receive an initial rapid volume augmentation, the lack of responsiveness provides the newborn with little in the way of defense against substantial blood loss.

Following the functional closure of the ductus, the neonatal circulatory pattern resembles that of the adult, and the ventricles pump in series. Data concerning the output of these chambers are not plentiful. Table 4–2 shows average values of normal human infant circulatory function; obviously, the

Table 4-2 *Average Values (± SD) on Normal Infants**

Age (hours)	10	±	5
	(range 2–28 hours)		
Weight (kg)	3.2	±	0.4
pH	7.39	±	0.02
PCO₂ (mm Hg)	33	±	2
Hematocrit (%)	54	±	6
O₂ Saturation (%) left atrium	97	±	1.6
Systemic atrial pressure (mm Hg)	56	±	8
Left atrial pressure (mm Hg)	2.0	±	1.5
Right atrial pressure (mm Hg)	0.0	±	1.4
O₂ Consumption (ml/kg/min)	6.9	±	11.0
Left ventricular (LV) output (ml/kg/min)	348		± 42
Right ventricular (RV) output (ml/kg/min)	233		± 44
Pulmonary blood flow (ml/kg/min)	305		± 41
L to R shunt (% of LV output)	38		± 11
R to L shunt (% of RV output)	20		± 3

From Burnard, E. D.: Influence of Delivery on the Circulation of the Newborn Infant. New York, Grune & Stratton, 1966, p. 52.

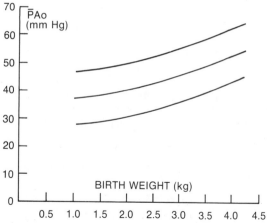

Figure 4–1. Parabolic regression (middle line) and 95% confidence limits (top and bottom lines) of mean aortic blood pressure on birth weight in normal newborn infants during hours 2 to 12 of life.

ductus is still open, since LV output is greater than RV output. However, even considering this, the value for RV output is substantially higher than the adult value of ≅70 ml per kg per minute. This high output state slowly subsides over the first year of life, in part perhaps due to improved O_2 delivery from adult hemoglobin.

The distribution of the neonatal cardiac output is not well defined. The pulmonary circulation has been discussed previously. Cerebral circulatory studies demonstrate flow values approximately equal to the adult values in ml per 100 grams of tissue per minute and intact autoregulation, although perinatal stress (i.e., hypoxia) may disrupt homeostasis quickly. Renal blood flow is impeded by high intrarenal vascular resistance, which decreases by about 30 per cent in a week and slowly thereafter for the next three to five months until adult levels are reached. Virtually nothing is known of the neonatal coronary circulation.

The systemic pressure is a function of the gestational age and the body weight; normal values for the first 12 hours of life are displayed in Figure 4–1. For infants weighing greater than 2 kg at term, this equates to a minimum blood pressure of 60/35 torr.

Values below this level suggest a possible need for vascular volume augmentation. The determinants of the neonatal blood pressure are probably largely passive and are related to considerations such as highly viscous blood flow through small vessels. How much active vascular control exists can be deduced from the response to hemorrhage, while the teleological reason for low blood pressure might be the lack of requirement to resist gravity over a large vertical distance, as in the upright adult.

PHARMACOLOGY

The technical and ethical problems encountered in drug research in infants have created a therapeutic orphan. Therefore, discussion of general neonatal pharmacologic principles is unfortunately vague.

Oral absorption of drugs in infants may be delayed during the first 48 hours of life by a relative gastrointestinal dysfunction and gut immaturity, and thereafter by gut immaturity alone. Intramuscular and subcutaneous injections may be ineffective in the newborn because of vasomotor instability, while pulmonary uptake of inhalational drugs often appears accelerated as a result of an increased minute ventilation.

An understanding of the distribution of drugs is aided by considering the concept of the Apparent Volume of Distribution

(AVD), the volume that must be filled to achieve a given plasma level. Minimal real data are available for children, but what data exist support the concept of an increased AVD in infants requiring an increased dose of most drugs in mg per kg. A better approximation of drug dose is mg per m² (BSA). AVD may be influenced by several factors, as shown in Table 4–3.

Metabolism is generally decreased in the infant as a result of enzyme immaturity, while excretion may be decreased (renal) or possibly increased (pulmonary).

Inhalation agents are frequently used in infants, and, in general, the pharmacology of the drugs is the same as in the adult. Uptake is accelerated by a high minute ventilation and high cardiac output, so that the infant can be thought of as entirely "vessel-rich." MAC for halothane is high in infants (1.1%) and unacceptable cardiovascular depression may be concomitantly present with equally unacceptable light planes of anesthesia in these patients. Presumably, the same situation holds true for enflurane.

Information regarding the intravenous agents is also sketchy. Extrapolation from the high MAC of halothane would result in the conclusion that an increased intravenous drug dosage is required for adequate anesthesia, but the variables in Table 2–3 may alter this conclusion. Whatever the dose, elimination will probably be relatively slow. Morphine appears to cause greater respiratory depression for equipotent doses than meperidine; there are no data regarding the relative effects of other narcotics. Ketamine in usual dose, as well as in low dose (0.1 - 0.2 mg/kg), has been used without unusual effect, while the pharmacology of the barbiturates in infants is almost unknown.

There is, however, reasonable experimental data on the use of relaxants. Succinylcholine kinetics have been examined in detail in children and, if the drug is given according to BSA, adult and infant effects are similar; however, the dose in mg/kg for infants will be higher. Recovery in infants, despite a low pseudocholinesterase level, is rapid, probably because of the increased AVD. Although early reports suggested that infants require only minimal doses of nondepolarizing drugs, recent studies state that if these drugs are administered according to clinical signs, infants may *seem* to need less drug. If administration is guided by peripheral nerve stimulation, the dose requirements (in mg/kg) in infants are essentially the same as in adults. However, there is considerable dose variation of nondepolarizing agents in infants. Reversal with anticholinesterase drugs is usually uneventful. The dose recommendations of these drugs are listed in Table 4–4. It is interesting to speculate that the active metabolites of pancuronium might significantly prolong a block using this drug. Thus far, this has not been reported.

Although oxygen therapy in infants has been the subject of intense investigation for decades, no firm safe guidelines have been established. The term infant (>44 weeks gestational age) is at no risk from elevated oxygen tension (Pa_{O_2}>80 torr) in the cerebral circulation, while a less mature newborn may develop retrolental fibroplasia (RLF) in similar circumstances. Indeed, RLF has been reported in an infant never exposed to supplemental oxygen, and for this reason it has been futile to recommend absolute rules. However, current guidelines for prematures support an FI_{O_2} to maintain Pa_{O_2} between 60 and 80 torr in the cerebral circulation. Changes in ventilation or the

---

Table 4–3 *Factors Affecting AVD in Infants*

Increased total body water
Increased blood volume
Decreased body lipid
  Higher fraction of lipid in CNS
Potentially "leaky" blood brain barrier
Decreased serum protein binding
  Lower serum albumin
  Decreased serum albumin binding affinity for some
    drugs
  Competition for binding sites from bilirubin

Table 4–4 *Dose Schedule for Relaxants and Reversal*

Succinylcholine	1.5 mg/kg IV
	2.0–4.0 mg/kg IM
Curare	0.3 mg/kg IV
Pancuronium	.06 mg/kg IV
Metocurine	0.2 mg/kg IV
Neostigmine	0.08 ⎫
+	+ ⎬ mg/kg IV
atropine	0.02 ⎭

addition of positive end expiratory pressure that might increase Pa_{O_2} without a change in FI_{O_2} also demand serious consideration. In some intraoperative circumstances the consequences of hypoxia are much more immediate and catastrophic, and it is not suggested that hypoxia is a tolerable state of affairs. Transcutaneous O_2 tension measurement may eliminate much of the current guess-work, but until that time, the recommendation to provide the lowest FI_{O_2} consistent with adequate Pa_{O_2} in prematures strongly, though inexactly, dictates management. A departure above or below this narrow range should be as strictly time-limited as possible.

FLUID METABOLISM

The term infant consists largely of water (80% of body weight), which is almost equally distributed between intracellular and extracellular compartments. Following a placental transfusion, approximately 12 per cent of the extracellular fluid is plasma, and the remainder is interstitial fluid. Fluid loss in the infant occurs as insensible loss (from lungs and skin) and urine. Insensible loss is a function of exposed surface area, relative humidity, ambient temperature, and respiratory minute volume, while urine production is a complex interaction between hormonal secretion, glomerular filtration, and tubular function. The sum of these two sources of loss is approximately 200 to 250 ml H_2O per 24 hours, with a large proportion of the loss being obligatory insensible loss.

The neonatal kidney is immature in several respects. The glomerular filtration rate (GFR) is initially low but increases five-fold in the first year of life. The initial low GFR restricts the infant's ability to withstand volume loading and indeed for the first three days of life there is no diuretic response to a water load. Tubular function also appears equally initially depressed (for most substances), although morphologically there appears to be a glomerulotubular imbalance. The concentrating power of the neonatal kidney is reduced (700 mOsm/L vs. 1200 mOsm/L in adults), but much of this limitation is due to low urea excretion in a highly anabolic newborn. The ability to control sodium excretion is also diminished.

The role of the kidney in acid-base regulation is limited, and is reflected by a decreased ability to excrete hydrogen ion and a lowered excretion threshold for bicarbonate. The latter limitation is unexplained and requires nearly a year to rise to adult values. Hydrogen ion excretion undergoes an initial rapid increase, but the kidney maintains a limited ability to increase excretion during stress for many months. The consequences of depressed renal function are rapidly apparent during any departure from health; the infant kidney, like the lung, is near the margins of compensation and can be easily overwhelmed.

TEMPERATURE REGULATION

The newborn has the ability to defend itself against a cold environment, but the mechanism, or mechanisms, responsible for this ability is not obvious. Shivering is possible at birth, but is not a prominent response to cold. Animal studies using relaxants have eliminated prolonged changes in muscle tone as a major cold adaptive response as well. Instead, non-shivering thermogenesis is largely responsible for heat production. This process takes place in brown fat stores in the neck, axillae, and mediastinum, and in the vicinity of the kidneys. Involved is a striking increase in O_2 consumption and norepinephrine secretion, with a subsequent thermal calorie addition to blood perfusing the brown fat. This mechanism may begin to operate whether an infant leaves thermal neutrality (defined as whatever environmental situation causes an abdominal skin temperature of 36° to 37° C.) and probably continues to aggressively defend body temperature down to an environmental temperature of 30° C. Control of the non-shivering thermogenesis mechanism is centrally mediated by the hypothalamus and may be disrupted by general anesthesia. Thus, in an era of air conditioned operating rooms, with significant airflow velocity (and wind-chill factor), the newborn may lose considerable body heat during anesthesia. The effects of this heat loss may be profound; during emergence from anesthesia the return to normal behavior, activity, and cardiorespiratory function may be very prolonged and a syndrome of cold injury may appear.

ANESTHETIC MANAGEMENT

Preanesthetic Evaluation. Post-delivery, there is generally a delay in a stable environment prior to operation. The duration of this delay may vary from hours to days, and valuable preoperative information can be obtained from the neonate's response to therapy during this period.

Fluid balance may have been established prior to surgery. If so, the route, volume, and composition of the infused fluid should be determined. The latter not only suggests the magnitude of electrolyte and/or glucose imbalance in the infant but also may dictate a need to change fluids because of drug–fluid incompatibility or concern for hyperosmolarity if the infusion rate is increased. The preoperative hematocrit should be between 40 and 50 per cent to insure adequate oxygen delivery and microcirculatory flow. A hematocrit above 50 may cause a hyperviscosity syndrome with perfusion impairment and should be reduced prior to surgery. Newborns should receive 1.0 mg of Vitamin K_1 oxide IM after birth to prevent hemorrhagic disease of the newborn, and following this injection clotting studies should be obtained. These infants may require supplemental fresh frozen plasma, especially if they have been transfused with packed cells and/or have undergone replacement transfusions. The latter maneuvers may also decrease the platelet count, which normally is the same in the newborn as in the adult.

Knowledge of the infant's present and past respiratory status is critical. A history of intubation minimizes the chance of the disquieting discovery of a major airway anomaly following induction of anesthesia. As in any other anesthetic procedure, a knowledge of the size of any previously used endotracheal tube is essential. The preoperative data should include the presence or absence of stridor, any history of apneic spells with or without bradycardia and, if the patient is intubated, the Fi_{O_2}, mechanical/spontaneous respiratory rate, and ventilator (or CPAP) settings. The current chest x-ray should be reviewed and arterial (or capillary) blood gas measurements should be obtained if appropriate. Reasonable efforts should be made preoperatively to obtain a pH of between 7.30 and 7.40.

Information regarding the cardiovascular system should specifically address the question of the presence of a patent ductus arteriosus and, if present, the apparent direction of the predominant shunt. The systemic blood pressure should be measured and the method (cuff with Doppler, arterial catheter) should be noted. Obviously, the physiologic impact of any other significant cardiovascular anomalies should be assessed as well.

The presence of sepsis should always be a major concern in the newborn, for the usually reliable indicator, fever, is of little use in many of these patients. The normally large surface area to weight ratio may prevent the development of hyperthermia in response to pyrogens and instead present a baby with cool extremities and vasoconstriction in a thermally neutral environment. Consequently, only positive cultures and/or a history of administration of potent antibiotics may hint of the presence of sepsis.

Transportation of an infant should always be regarded as stressful, and it is during movement that recently obtained baselines may shift. Significant efforts should be expended to maintain normal body temperature using either a heated incubator or wrapping the patient's body and limbs carefully. If the child is intubated, an incubator that includes provisions for artificial ventilation utilizing any required Fi_{O_2} from 0.21 to 1.0 should be used. It is desirable that someone who has the skills and equipment to reintubate the trachea accompany the infant in transit. Transport time should be limited and the infant moved only when operation is imminent.

Premedication should consist only of atropine, 0.02 mg/kg, optimally given IV in the operating room or subcutaneously 15 minutes prior to airway manipulation. This dose will decrease secretions and obtund vagal reactivity but does not eliminate the bradycardia associated with hypoxia.

Intraoperative Management. The operating room should be viewed as a giant incubator for the newborn. Room temperature should be raised to 28° to 32°C, rendered draft free (i.e., doors closed), and a heated water mattress placed on the OR table (maximum temperature 39° C). An overhead radiant warmer (output optimally 3 microns) is a desirable therapeutic addition. The "ideal" anesthesia machine should be capable of delivering air, with accurate gas flow meters calibrated in 100 ml increments below a 1 liter per minute flow rate. An in-line inspired O_2 analyzer and flow independent, temperature compensated vaporizers (to prevent failure to correct for elevated room temperature on vapor pressure) are logical additions. The ability to heat and humidify anesthesia gas will markedly aid temperature control and allow moderate room cooling after prepping and draping are completed.

The infant should be monitored with a precordial stethoscope, ECG, and rectal temperature. Unexpected but confirmed preoperative hypothermia may indicate sepsis and should be investigated. If infant activity prevents final placement of a Doppler transducer or photoplethysmograph until after the induction of general anesthesia, blood pressure should be determined preoperatively by palpation or with an oscillotonometer. If considered necessary for perioperative management, an arterial catheter may be inserted prior to the induction of anesthesia. Future preparation for surgery may proceed in either of two ways. If the child is intubated and has an intravenous catheter in situ, he may be paralyzed with a non-depolarizing agent, ventilated with an appropriate air/O_2 mixture while further monitors are applied, and positioned, prepped, and draped for surgery. Just prior to incision, anesthesia is induced. This method permits the assessment of the impact of controlled ventilation on cardiac output and blood pressure, and decreases the dose of anesthetic agent. Alternatively, a N_2O/O_2/potent inhalation agent mixture may be used to produce immobility, followed by the establishment of adequate intravenous access and monitoring. Endotracheal intubation is usually required in the newborn and can be performed either awake, following mask pre-oxygenation and paralysis with succinylcholine, or after the induction of general anesthesia. During an awake intubation, O_2 supplementation can be provided via an 8 French nasopharyngeal catheter. Finally, unless contraindicated by anatomy or surgery, gastric decompression with a 10 French catheter is recommended following intubation.

Two monitoring considerations deserve comment. First, determination of end-tidal CO_2 with an infra-red analyzer is a useful noninvasive way to assess minute ventilation. However, the technique is expensive and in neonates requires careful attention to sampling flow rates in order not to cause atelectasis and alveolar hypoxia. Second, transcutaneous O_2 and CO_2 measurement provides real-time assessment of tissue perfusion and oxygenation, with minimal risk of cutaneous thermal injury. However, this device requires single patient use of the applied probe and analyzer, is without pH capability, and has a price equal to two blood gas machines. Because of these limitations, the device presently remains largely a neonatal research instrument.

The choice of an anesthetic administration system depends on whether respiration is to be spontaneous or controlled. If ventilation is to be controlled, then any manageable low external dead space system will suffice. The advantages of a non-rebreathing system include control of Pa_{CO_2} with fresh gas flow during controlled ventilation and absence of valves, which may fail or stick and cause an increased amount of respiratory work during spontaneous ventilation. However, optimal use of a non-rebreathing system requires accurate flowmeters, humidification and warming of the inspired gas, and some method of exhausting waste anesthetic gas. The use of a circle system with CO_2 absorber eliminates some of these concerns, but makes it difficult to control Pa_{CO_2} during controlled ventilation, as minute ventilation cannot usually be measured with accuracy.

Accurate intraoperative fluid therapy is an extremely important component in successful anesthetic management. Since fluid and caloric requirements are closely related to body surface area, use of body weight (as is common) for fluid therapy requires some adjustment for the ratio of surface area to body weight. Using a solution of 5 per cent dextrose and 0.2 per cent saline with 20 mg of KCL added per liter, maintenance fluids can be approximated by administration of 4 ml/kg/hr for the first 10 kg of body weight and an additional 2 ml/kg/hr for the second 10 kg of body weight. The following adjustments may be required:

1. Use of 10 per cent dextrose to maintain adequate blood glucose (infrequent)
2. Reduction of fluid infusion by 20 per cent for mechanical ventilation with greater than 90 per cent humidified gas
3. Reduction of fluid infusion by 25 per cent in the first 24 to 36 hours after birth

4. Increased fluid infusion by a variable amount because of increased insensible loss (phototherapy, exceptionally low humidity)

If maintenance fluids are all that are required in a specific patient, it is advisable to calculate the preoperative fluid deficit and correct half of this deficit in the first hour, with further administration of fluid at 110 to 120 per cent of the baseline maintenance rate until the entire deficit is corrected. Generally, this simple approach is complicated by the trauma of surgery, requiring the intraoperative administration of substantially more fluid. The increased requirement may vary from 2 ml/kg/hr to 6 ml/kg/hr above the maintenance level and should consist of either lactated Ringer's solution or saline. It should be noted that doubling fluid requirements does not automatically double glucose requirements. Estimated blood volume (EBV) should be calculated, and in the newborn it is especially helpful to know the starting hematocrit, since there is a good correlation between a high hematocrit and placental transfusion. For the first few days after birth, a value of >55 per cent suggests a blood volume of approximately 90 ml/kg, while a value of <50 per cent suggests a blood volume value nearer 80 ml/kg. After the first two weeks, a blood volume value of approximately 80 ml/kg is reliable. If dehydration is present, then the hematocrit will grossly overestimate the initial blood volume. In the first week of life, in a patient with limited renal function, it seems reasonable to begin blood replacement early (i.e., loss equal to 5–8% EBV). After this age, replacement of a portion of blood loss by lactated Ringer's, with optional albumin, is acceptable. In general, blood should be transfused to maintain a hematocrit of approximately 40.

Fluids should be warmed prior to administration; room temperature is probably adequate for crystalloid, while blood should be passed through a warmer. This is especially true if the infusion catheter tip is located in the vicinity of the heart. Blood replacement will always be with adult hemoglobin, which unloads oxygen substantially more easily than fetal hemoglobin.

Emergence from Anesthesia. The desire to have an awake infant at the termination of the skin closure may prompt a premature reduction in depth of anesthesia, or an early reversal of paralysis. Such maneuvers are encouraged only if access to the child is unimpeded by drapes, for an unpremedicated, functionally vessel rich, high MAC requirement neonate may awaken rapidly and in an uncontrollable fashion. Thus it is generally desirable to make minimal reduction in inspired anesthetic concentrations until the wound is covered. Then, all inhaled agents are discontinued and ventilation with an FI_{O_2} of 1.0 is begun for 3 to 5 minutes (obviously an unnecessary step if N_2O was not used). Following this, the FI_{O_2} is reduced to a value of 0.1 to 0.2 higher than the preoperative FI_{O_2} value until the patient has recovered and/or gas tensions are measured. If mechanical ventilation was employed intraoperatively, a 30 per cent reduction in respiratory rate at the time of discontinuance of inhalational anesthesia will safely allow Pa_{CO_2} to increase gradually above the apneic threshold. Neuromuscular blockade is reversed by ensuring that the small volume of antagonist actually enters the circulation rather than remaining in the external IV system. If the child remains apneic after these measures, ventilation should be continued and gas tensions measured in 15 to 20 min. Extubation should ideally be performed on normothermic, vigorous infants who demonstrate adequate regular spontaneous ventilation over a period of several minutes.

Graduates of newborn intensive care nurseries who have had periods of apnea tend to become apneic following any general anesthetic for some months after leaving the ICU. Such infants should be given more than a few minutes of stability before extubation.

Whenever there is doubt, maintain ventilation until the doubt is removed. This is doubly true if the infant has been allowed to cool, although a sizable reduction in minute ventilation may be necessary to offset decreased CO_2 production.

After the expenditure of the effort to provide excellent pre- and intraoperative care, the anesthetist's job is finished only when the infant returns to the appropriate environment and there has been a thorough transfer of new data to the following physician. Fluid shifts, transfusion therapy, and drug effects require specific mention. Any complications should be explained in detail, and plans should be established concerning future fluid therapy and respiratory support. If the endotracheal tube was placed in the operating room and is to be left in situ, then a chest x-ray should be taken and reviewed, with optimal tube position confirmed or obtained by the anesthetist. The requirement for further participation in the patient's care is largely a function of the expertise of those following the infant; the details of postoperative care are beyond the scope of this text.

CHOANAL ATRESIA

This is a relatively rare (1 in 8000 births) defect of uncertain cause. The nasal airway may be obstructed unilaterally or bilaterally by a membranous or bony septum. Unilateral obstruction usually presents later in childhood as an excessive nasal discharge on the affected side; surprisingly, some cases of bilateral obstruction may also present in the same fashion. As a rule, however, infants with bilateral nasal obstruction present at birth or shortly thereafter with dyspnea. The term "cyclic" is often added to describe the sequence of hypoxia, followed by crying with mouth breathing and then a return to airway obstruction. Alternatively, the infant may become dyspneic only during feedings.

Diagnosis of bilateral choanal atresia can be made on the basis of respiratory distress relieved by an oral airway coupled with an inability to pass a catheter through either nostril. Confirmation can be obtained by instilling methylene blue and/or radiopaque dye into the nostril while the patient is supine. In those infants with bilateral obstruction, the immediate clinical necessity is to maintain an airway. This can be accomplished by inserting an oral airway or perforated rubber nipple into the mouth and keeping it taped firmly into place until the child develops the capacity to mouth breathe (about 3-4 weeks). Feeding remains a problem and may require the passage of an orogastric tube. Membranous obstructions have been repaired transnasally in the first day of life, while bony obstructions are usually approached transpalatally somewhat later. Transnasal correction using a laser has been reported; if this method is chosen, precautions against eye damage to the patient and operating room personnel should be taken (see section on laryngeal papillomatosis for further details). Although the procedure is somewhat controversial, the nasal passage is usually stented postoperatively in order to improve airway patency.

ANESTHETIC MANAGEMENT

Preoperatively, the final feeding should be of dextrose and water, and if an orogastric tube is in place, it should be aspirated (and probably removed) prior to induction of anesthesia to improve mask fit. The repair of choanal atresia poses the problem of maintaining an infant's airway within an operative field. A precurved endotracheal tube facilitates surgical exposure and is recommended. Induction and maintenance of anesthesia should be unremarkable, except for extra vigilance concerning blood loss into the oropharynx.

Emergence requires consideration of the repair and presence or absence of nasal stents. In general, both the patient's age and the nature of the procedure favor an awake extubation. The necessity for reintroduction of an oral airway will depend on the adequacy of the nasal passage and must be carefully considered before the infant is left unattended.

PIERRE ROBIN SYNDROME

The Pierre Robin syndrome, of unknown cause, consists of mandibular hypoplasia, glossoptosis, and often a cleft palate. The anomalad may occur by itself (incidence of 1:30,000 live births) or as part of a more complex syndrome. These infants commonly present with inspiratory airway obstruction, feeding difficulties leading to aspiration, and failure to thrive. Airway obstruction is usually ascribed to the unfavorable interaction between mandible length and tongue size. Recently, however, intrinsic tongue muscle maldevelopment has been proposed as the primary cause of obstruction, since the airway may improve prior to significant mandible growth. Placing the infant in a prone position or in cervical hyperextension may be required to maintain the airway. Feeding while upright and skin traction to the skull may also ameliorate moderate degrees of obstruction. Infants with severe feeding difficulties often benefit from gastrostomy performed under local anesthesia; they also may benefit from suturing the tongue to the alveolar ridge to maintain forward displacement. Alternatively, the tongue may be surgically repositioned anteriorly on the floor of the mouth. Acute and chronic upper airway obstruction has been associated with congestive heart failure in a few of these patients. Generally, the respiratory and feeding problems resolve with growth in two to four months. Surgery will be required for cleft palate repair and may be performed relatively early in life to improve feeding.

ANESTHETIC MANAGEMENT

For patients with an isolated Pierre Robin syndrome, the airway is the primary concern. Satisfactorily fitting a mask to a markedly recessed mandible may prove difficult, and placing the patient in the supine position may totally occlude the airway.

A nasal airway (available as small as 20 F) or an endotracheal tube used as a nasal airway may overcome inspiratory obstruction, but these do not necessarily allow for the application of positive airway pressure. Awake intubation provides the most safely established and secure airway, but is often difficult to accomplish. Although a precurved tube is helpful in maintaining the airway during palate surgery, technical difficulties in intubation may favor the use of a straight endotracheal tube in these patients. During laryngoscopy, oxygen should be continuously provided by nasopharyngeal catheter.

If visualization is inadequate to accomplish intubation with direct laryngoscopy, a fiberoptic device may prove useful. The fiberoptic laryngoscope (no suction available) or bronchoscope (suction available) can be passed orally or nasally and can function as a stylet over which an endotracheal tube (minus 15 mm connector) can be passed. Alternatively, if the small size of the endotracheal tube precludes this, the larynx can be visualized transnasally while the endotracheal tube is passed parallel to the fiberoptic bronchoscope via the other nostril. If either of these techniques is selected, supplemental oxygen, via catheter or endotracheal tube, should be provided during attempted intubation. Ketamine, in increments of 0.1 to 0.2 mg/kg intravenously,

may facilitate these maneuvers. Finally, intubation may be accomplished using a Hopkins rod-lens telescope as a stylet, again supplying supplemental oxygen during endoscopy. Tracheostomy should be reserved as a last resort except for patients with cor pulmonale secondary to obstruction. Following establishment of an airway, anesthetic management can be conventional. Postoperatively the patient should be extubated awake. While cleft palate repair improves the nasal airway, the preoperative mandible-tongue relationship remains unchanged. Consequently, airway maintenance measures should be continued postoperatively until proven unnecessary.

LARYNGEAL PAPILLOMAS

Laryngeal papillomas are the most common benign tumors of the upper respiratory tract in children. These exophytic lesions were first recognized as "warts in the throat" in the seventeenth century, and although there have been other histopathologic descriptions since that time, current thinking supports this initial label as probably correct. Several authors have reported an increased incidence of skin warts among family members of children with laryngeal papillomas, as well as an increased incidence of genital warts noted during pregnancies in mothers of children who develop laryngeal papillomas. These data, along with microscopic evidence, have generated significant interest in development of a vaccine against laryngeal papillomas. Until such a vaccine has been proven efficacious, primary therapy will be surgical removal.

The difficulty presented by laryngeal papillomas lies not in their size, but in their location and stubborn insistence on returning despite repeated surgical discouragement with chemicals, cautery, cryotherapy, or knife. Generally, laryngeal papillomas grow on the true vocal cords and extend into the ventricles. The disease may spread to the trachea and bronchi, and because of tissue friability and secondary infection may result in asphyxiation. The initial presentation of the disease is usually hoarseness, followed by dyspnea, cough, dysphagia, and eventually stridor.

The age at onset of symptoms may be

anytime after birth, although 12 months of age is most common. The duration of the disease is variably reported as 8 months to 40 years, with a recognized incidence of spontaneous regression, frequently at puberty, that makes evaluation of therapy difficult.

Surgical removal of these lesions has been accomplished with electrocautery, but a significant incidence of resultant airway stenosis has proven a major drawback. Various hormones, steroids, and podophyllin have been injected near, or applied to, the papilloma with variable results. Cryotherapy has been advocated, as has ultrasound, without clear-cut benefit being firmly established. The most thoroughly tested method is surgical removal under direct vision, via a laryngeal microscope. Recently, use of the laser has been tried as a unique method of removing these lesions. This device is unusual enough to require discussion of its anesthetic implications.

Lasers are devices that emit intense beams of monochromatic, tightly collimated, coherent light. The collimation and initial high energy level of the beam distinguish the laser from other light sources, as well as providing it with its biological effectiveness. The initial laser appeared in 1960, and since then a tremendous rate of development has produced lasers in the ultraviolet, infrared, and visible spectrum.

In the early 1970's, the CO_2 laser was introduced into medicine. This laser operates at a wavelength of 10.6 μ in the infrared spectrum and provides almost pure heat energy. The high water content of cells insures that more than 90 per cent of laser energy is absorbed within 0.5 mm of the irradiated surface, leading to a rapid vaporization of water as steam and to subsequent cell destruction. Since energy is delivered in short pulses, little heat is conducted away from the center of the field, although there is a thin layer of coagulation around the area. These features provide a unique surgical tool. The lesion is destroyed without bleeding and with minimal surrounding edema. Laser wounds heal rapidly, and scarring, with resultant contracture, is minimal.

Coupling this device with a microscope leads to extraordinarily precise control of surgery, requiring only a clear visualization of the lesion without concern for "working room." Seemingly the only disadvantage is the lack of pathologic specimens. However, the laser does have some drawbacks. Although the laser is firmly attached to the microscope and aimed in a straight line at the target tissue, there is a small potential for eye damage to the patient and operating room personnel. To avoid this, the patient's eyes should be taped shut following induction, and personnel in the room should wear glasses. A notice should be posted outside the room informing visitors (who always appear in response to the presence of unusual pieces of equipment) of the hazard to vision.

In addition, delivery of laser energy to the endotracheal tube can cause tube penetration, cuff failure, and intratracheal fires. Four different solutions have been developed for these endotracheal tube problems First, the tubes have been spirally wrapped in metallic foil in order to reflect the energy and disrupt the collimation. However, longitudinal foil application results in unacceptable tube bulk. Second (an extension of the metallic foil solution) is the use of a flexible metal endotracheal tube, which has been recently manufactured for this purpose. Third, the exposed endotracheal tube surface can be covered with continuously moistened sponges to dissipate the heat. This is especially useful to protect an in-situ tracheostomy tube. A fourth possible answer to this problem is to eliminate the endotracheal tube altogether and rely on high pressure Venturi ventilation from above the cords, utilizing intravenous agents for anesthesia. This is discussed more fully under anesthetic techniques.

A specific requirement when using laser systems is absolute target immobility. The operator generally has an aiming light, and when the laser is activated, what the aiming light touches is vaporized. There can therefore be no vocal cord motion, and this strongly suggests the use of muscle relaxants, thus eliminating insufflation techniques.

The question of a fire in the presence of N_2O and O_2, both of which support combustion, remains. Although the theoretical risk of a fire does exist, there is no risk of spontaneous combustion unless the unprotected endotracheal tube is struck often enough to actually burn. Wrapping the tube in metallic foil provides sufficient protection, and most experts continue to use N_2O and O_2 in the usual fashion.

ANESTHETIC TECHNIQUE

The patient may present for surgery with symptoms varying from minimal hoarseness to near-total airway obstruction. Premedication is important, not only for the current procedure but also for the "inevitable" repeat anesthetic next week/month/year. Although belladona alkaloids are useful to dry the airway, many of these patients will develop a hatred for (repeated) injections. Atropine, administered IV immediately after induction, will suffice in these situations. For the older child, diazepam by mouth, in a maximum dose of 0.4 mg/kg 120 minutes prior to surgery is useful, although results are somewhat difficult to predict. Other premedication schedules have been used, but care must be exercised to avoid any preoperative airway obstruction.

Mask induction using N_2O, O_2, and a potent volatile agent establishes a controlled plane of anesthesia prior to airway instrumentation. By far, the greatest experience is with halothane, although specific mention has been made of cardiac electrical stability with enflurane. Prior to surgical endoscopy, an intravenous infusion should be established and the vocal cords should be sprayed with local anesthetic. Anesthetizing the larynx has the added advantage of testing the depth of anesthesia prior to suspension laryngoscopy. Breath holding, coughing, or dysrhythmias suggest inadequate depth. Monitoring should include precordial stethoscope, blood pressure cuff, temperature, and electrocardiogram. The eyes should be taped closed and the globes padded to prevent damage. Thus far, there is general agreement in techniques.

Intubation would ordinarily be the next logical step; however, a few authorities feel this procedure carries a risk of spreading the disease and should not be performed. If a tracheostomy (highly undesirable for fear of disease spread) is not in place and intubation is eliminated, insufflation or Venturi ventilation remains as the only alternative to maintain gas exchange. For conventional (non-laser) surgery, insufflation leaves the airway unprotected from debris and also allows vocal cord motion with spontaneous respiration. In addition, the environment is grossly contaminated with anesthetic gas. Venturi ventilation, via a 16 gauge needle, can be accomplished in children but de-

mands axial alignment of the trachea and injector, close apposition of laryngoscope tip and larynx, mandatory gastric decompression, and an intravenous anesthetic technique. A useful compromise, outlined by Snow et al. for laser surgery, is to intubate the trachea with a small foil-wrapped tube, establish neuromuscular blockade with a succinylcholine infusion (monitored with a peripheral nerve stimulator), and then allow the surgeon to clear the lesions from the anterior one half to two thirds of the cords. This allows for a slow, careful laryngoscopy, with the endotracheal tube well out of the way (posterior) and eliminates concern for a ball-valve tracheal obstruction from a pedunculated lesion. Following this, the tube is removed and the posterior one half to one third of the cords is cleared, while ventilation is maintained using a Venturi injector with intravenous anesthetic supplementation. Placing the Venturi late in a stable anesthetic makes management easier and allows the anesthetist greater capability to coordinate injection to laser activation (if used). The coordination between Venturi injection and laser activation is necessary to prevent cord vibration from air movement as the burn is made. Alternatively, if the cords are cleared by blunt dissection, the coordination minimizes the possibility of blasting debris and blood into the trachea. Following either method, the surgeon can reanesthetize the vocal cords, using a long-acting topical spray supplied from a 22 gauge spinal needle attached to an extension tube and syringe. The suspension device is then removed, an oral airway is inserted, and the patient's ventilation is supported as required.

Intravenous steroids are advocated intraoperatively (even in laser surgery) by some; postoperative inspired gas humidification is recommended by all. This is especially crucial if bilateral anterior commissure lesions have been removed. The majority of reports dealing with laser use comment on the striking lack of difficulty encountered postoperatively by patients on whom it is used. Those patients who have laryngeal papillomas removed in a more traditional fashion are subject to the hazards of postoperative bleeding and edema in a small airway and should be managed accordingly.

Surgery is frequently repetitive in this

disease, and if these tiny lesions were located anywhere but the airway, outpatient procedures would clearly be preferable. In general however, the edema and bleeding associated with excision, coupled with intubation, suggest that a short (24-48 hour) inpatient stay is safest. An exception to this recommendation is the patient with a tracheostomy in situ whose lesions are localized above the stoma. Initial reports of laser surgery comment on the lack of postoperative difficulties, yet, even using this method, the fact that a very small airway is involved probably outweighs the convenience of outpatient surgery, and a short inpatient stay is recommended.

TRACHEAL ESOPHAGEAL FISTULA (TEF)

Esophageal atresia without TEF was initially described in 1670, followed in 1697 by the first case of atresia with TEF. In 1939 a patient survived a multiple-stage repair of atresia with TEF, and in 1941 the first successful single-stage repair was performed. Although many classification systems, using letters and numbers, are established in the literature, they do nothing to clarify the pathologic anatomy and will not be used here. Since esophageal atresia without tracheal fistula composes less than 10 per cent of the cases, and because the presence of a gastrointestinal-respiratory tract communication markedly influences anesthetic management, the emphasis of this discussion will be on TEF rather than esophageal atresia.

Development of the respiratory system begins at three weeks gestational age with the appearance of a diverticulum from the ventral wall of the foregut. Initially, the respiratory diverticulum remains in communication with the foregut, but it is soon separated from it by the esophagotracheal septum. Shortly thereafter, the primitive trachea and lung buds develop caudad while the larynx matures cephalad. If development proceeds normally, the gut and respiratory tract remain in communication only at the level of the laryngeal aditus. The intimate relationship between the developing airway and gut makes the possibility of a persistent communication easy to accept,

but it does not offer an explanation as to why it should occur. Mechanical impediments to esophageal development, such as anomalous vessels, have been suggested as causal but remain unsubstantiated.

The association of TEF with other anomalies is well established. One of the most interesting of these is the VATER association, first presented in 1973 by Quan and Smith. This consists of Vertebral defect, Anal defects, Trachea–esophageal fistula with Esophageal atresia and Renal dysplasia. Since the original paper, the V has become V^2 to include Ventricular septal defect while the R has become R^2 to include Radial dysplasia. Despite a remarkable amount of investigation, no common environmental or genetic cause for TEF, alone or as part of other anomalies, has been uncovered.

The number of possible pathologic anatomic variations is very large. The gastrointestinal tract connection with the airway can be anywhere between the larynx and the bronchi. The most cephalad connection is the laryngotracheoesophageal cleft. This exceedingly rare defect (approximately 50 reported since the first successful correction in 1955) may be smaller in length than the arytenoid cartilages or it may run the entire posterior aspect of the trachea. The most caudad connection is the bronchoesophageal fistula, a somewhat less rare but more easily repaired connection between the esophagus and a mainstem bronchus, usually close to the carina. In a few cases, the bronchoesophageal fistula has proved life sustaining, as a result of distal tracheal agenesis. Therapy in these cases has been extremely difficult.

Between these two extremes fall the majority of TEF, divided roughly into distal and proximal fistulas, depending on whether the trachea connects with the upper esophageal pouch (proximal and rare) or the lower segment (distal and common). Obviously, if two categories have been identified, a third can be created by combining them. Finally, esophageal atresia without TEF, and TEF without atresia (H type) are necessary to cover the remaining possible variants. Intermingled with these seven categories of fistula and/or atresia are over 90 anatomic variants involving multiple fistulas and segmental atresia of the esophagus, well described by Kluth in 1976. The statistics for all these anomalies have remained relatively constant throughout most series, and presented from the view of the anesthetist can be summarized as follows: 85 to 90 per cent of TEF will be between the distal trachea and lower esophageal segment, while only 7 to 9 per cent of cases have esophageal atresia without TEF. The incidence of TEF is between 1:3000 to 1:4500 live births.

The disease presents as difficulty in swallowing, recurrent pulmonary infection and/or aspiration, and abdominal distention. The urgency in making the diagnosis is in suspecting and preventing recurrent aspiration, not in performing definitive surgery. There will frequently be a history of polyhydramnios, and the baby is often noted to have excessive "foamy" oral secretions. Ideally, the diagnosis will be suspected at this point and NPO orders written. The infant may be intermittently cyanotic, especially if feeding is attempted, whereupon immediate regurgitation is common. Abdominal distention often develops, and if there is a delay in therapy, respiratory distress may occur from aspiration (gastric acidity is established within 24 hours after delivery). A chest x-ray frequently shows an air-filled upper pouch, and this can be confirmed by passing a radiopaque catheter down the esophagus as far as possible (usually 10-12 cm), followed by a repeat x-ray to rule out coiling of the tube if it seems to pass into the abdomen. The tip of the catheter should be placed underwater briefly before suction is applied; bubbles escaping with each breath suggest a proximal fistula. Analysis of the pH of the upper pouch contents is not useful, for an acid indication does not rule out the diagnosis. Esophageal atresia is established by the air esophagogram and the inability to pass the esophageal catheter, while a distal TEF is proved by air in the remainder of the gut. Confirmation of the diagnosis can be obtained by instilling a minimal amount of contrast medium into the esophagus and observing the total obstruction, although this is usually unnecessary.

The remainder of the x-ray should then be examined for infiltrates, cardiac abnormalities, bony defects, and the bowel air pattern. Obviously, in the case of an isolated proximal fistula, no gastrointestinal tract will be seen. Prior to proceeding with further studies, the infant should be evaluated for additional malformations. Chromosomal aberrations or fatal congenital heart disease may make aggressive therapy an exercise in dubious judgment. During evaluation, the infant should be cared for in a semi-sitting position and the upper pouch suctioned continuously via a sump tube to prevent accumulation of secretions.

TEF without atresia requires a much higher index of suspicion, and it is usual for this H-type fistula not to be diagnosed in infancy. In fact, clear identification of the H-type fistula may be difficult even at a relatively late age. Immediately prior to elective thoracotomy, endoscopic evaluation of the trachea, usually under general anesthesia, can provide a definite understanding of the pathologic anatomy, and the optical quality of newer Hopkins rod-lens endoscopes may allow identification of a tiny fistula, which often appears as a dimple on the posterior tracheal wall. During endoscopy it may also be possible to pass a small catheter through the fistula which will aid in identification of the fistula during subsequent surgery.

Surgical management of TEF has undergone an interesting 40 year evolution, resulting in variable answers to questions of *what* operation to perform, *when* to perform the operation, and *by what approach*. For TEF with distal fistula, most infants will be briefly observed and then taken to surgery for a single stage fistula division, esophageal repair, and gastrostomy. The thoracotomy will be right-sided, through the fourth intercostal space, and the dissection will be extrapleural (more tedious but ultimately more successful, especially if an anastomosis breaks down). Some surgeons will perform gastrostomy under local anesthesia early on, and this is especially helpful if thoracotomy is to be delayed for any reason (prematurity, pneumonia, etc.). If the esophageal segments cannot be mobilized sufficiently to perform anastomosis without tension on the suture line, the upper pouch will be preserved until attempts at anastomosis are repeated during a subsequent thoracotomy. The problem of the "long gap" (distance between the two esophageal segments) has been the subject of symposia and has led to remarkably ingenious therapeutic concepts, such as stretching the esophageal segments by pulsating metal "olives" in a magnetic field.

Following the final establishment of esophageal continuity, it is not unusual for these infants to experience swallowing difficulties requiring repeat esophageal dilatation under general anesthesia. The swallowing difficulty is not simply due to mechanical restriction at the anastomosis but seems to be in part due to defective peristalsis in both segments. Fortunately, this is not usually severe enough to significantly impair growth, although a period of dysphagia is probably an integral part of the recovery phase from a TEF repair.

Respiratory obstruction may appear postoperatively at any time from immediately post-extubation to months later. The immediate problem is discussed below; the cause of delayed episodes is not clear. Gastroesophageal reflux has been associated with respiratory distress, which in turn has been shown to cease following an antireflux operation. Recurrent aspiration has been cited as contributing not only to acute obstruction but also to a strikingly higher incidence of cough and bronchitis in these children. Finally, tracheal compression between the innominate artery anteriorly and a dilated atonic esophagus posteriorly has been suggested as another cause of respiratory obstruction ("reflex apnea"). Treatment has been to suture the innominate artery to the anterior chest wall to relieve tracheal compression.

On occasion, a patient presents for general anesthesia after the TEF repair for other unrelated surgery. The possibility of tracheal anatomic abnormalities, including diverticulas at the fistula site and tracheal stenosis should be kept in mind if intubation is intended.

ANESTHETIC MANAGEMENT

The preoperative visit will usually reveal a baby sitting semi-upright, receiving IV fluids, with a short length of sump tube in one nostril. For the moment, the obvious should be ignored and the "associated" searched for. Congenital heart disease, present in 15 per cent of these babies, leads the list, followed by urinary tract anomalies, anorectal maldevelopment, and, of course, the VATER association. Prematurity and chromosomal abnormalities, with or without the above associations, compound the situation, and the impact of these conditions should be determined.

In these cases there is one obvious and major preoperative question: Has the baby suffered any pulmonary insult? Although the operative dissection will probably be extrapulmonary, aspiration pneumonia can add remarkably to the morbidity of the operation and constitutes grounds to delay the procedure until the lungs have cleared. Pulmonary pathology is also an indication for stomach decompression via gastrostomy. The implications of delay of surgery are much different with the availability of hyperalimentation to support the infant preoperatively; using the gastrointestinal tract (via a "double gastrostomy") or the intravenous route for calorie supplies, the baby can continue to grow despite an interrupted esophagus. Therefore, it is possible and necessary to have optimal pulmonary status and nitrogen balance before surgery.

Premedication should consist only of atropine, administered in the operating room if desired. The usual measures contained in the first section are appropriate, with particular emphasis placed on heating and humidifying anesthetic gases to prevent depression of mucociliary transport and to prevent heat loss. The esophageal sump tube should be connected to suction and the infant intubated awake. If a gastrostomy tube is in place, it should be vented to the atmosphere. Anesthesia should then be induced utilizing spontaneous ventilation until the TEF has been divided, although it is usually possible to gently inflate the lungs, without gastric distention. Should gastric distention develop or worsen, N_2O should be eliminated from the inspired gas. Because a right thoracotomy is ordinarily performed, a midline precordial stethoscope may well be in the sterile field, while an esophageal stethoscope is obviously contraindicated. The optimal position for the stethoscope is generally on the left anterior axillary line, where heart and breath sounds can be heard well without the need for the patient's weight bearing on the device. The potential for compromise of gas exchange is extremely high during surgery; aural monitoring of ventilation is therefore vital. The endotracheal tube should be taped well clear of the nostrils, for manipulation of the sump tube will often be required intraoperatively, and avoiding the 15 mm endotracheal tube connector and associated anesthetic circuit during these maneuvers requires some consideration. Intraoperative management is that of a lateral thoracotomy possibly complicated by an unusual amount of major intraoperative airway manipulation and obstruction. Following thoracotomy closure, gastrostomy will usually be performed, if it has not been accomplished earlier.

The postoperative management of these infants is determined by the degree of preoperative pulmonary dysfunction and the possible postoperative appearance of tracheomalacia. Either severe parenchymal or tracheal disease may suggest continued intubation, although extubation is the rule in vigorous term infants. The patient should be cared for in a high humidity atmosphere for the first 24 to 48 hours postoperatively, and observed carefully for any signs of respiratory embarrassment. All involved in the care should know the depth of the esophageal anastomosis, and under no conditions should a catheter be passed to within 2 cm of this depth, even if the reason is to "suction the trachea." Suctioning should be performed only under direct vision.

The anesthetic management of repair of a small laryngotracheoesophageal cleft has changed recently with the advent of internal laryngeal surgery utilizing direct suspension laryngoscopy and an operating microscope. This involves sharing an infant's airway with the surgeon for a prolonged period, probably without the aid of an endotracheal tube because of space limitations. The patient should be anesthetized with a volatile agent in oxygen, the larynx sprayed with local anesthetic, and anesthesia maintained by insufflation into the pharynx. The anesthetic can be delivered via a laryngoscope sidearm or through a short endotracheal tube functioning as a nasal airway. A small nasotracheal tube should be inserted postoperatively and left in-situ for several days.

The management of a cleft extending the entire length of the trachea remains vexing. Several interesting techniques have been evolved and were nicely described by Ruder and Glaser in 1977. In their report, the most obvious problem, gas distention of a stomach in free communication with the airway, was prevented by inserting a number 10 Foley catheter into the stomach, inflating the balloon, and retracting it cephalad to seal the gastroesophageal junction.

In a staged procedure, the trachea could then be intubated and closed posteriorly around the endotracheal tube, while the esophagus could be closed around the Foley catheter. A second difficulty, sealing the airway distally during reconstruction, was accomplished by placing a tourniquet over the endotracheal tube. Even so, significant intermittent airway obstruction occurred during the procedure. An endotracheal tube was left in place postoperatively in this situation as well. The anesthetist faced with a complete cleft is advised to review this case report in detail prior to the procedure.

NEONATAL RESPIRATORY DISTRESS SYNDROME

The neonatal respiratory distress syndrome (RDS), which is more an expression of pulmonary immaturity rather than a true disease, accounts for over 9000 deaths per year in the U.S. Although neonatal respiratory distress syndrome is not an uncommon disease in its own right, patients with neonatal RDS who require surgery are quite uncommon. Numerous other entities (such as shock, perinatal asphyxia and meconium aspiration, transient newborn tachypnea, congenital heart disease, and streptococcal pneumonia) present similar pictures, but these are not considered here. The review of newborn physiology in the first section pointed out the numerous ways in which the term infant is anatomically and functionally immature; to this is added a brief discussion of pulmonary function when pulmonary development is foreshortened. Although term infants, especially those who have diabetic mothers, may present with RDS, the incidence of RDS with associated prematurity is so high that a combined discussion of RDS in the premature infant is appropriate.

By the end of the 26th gestational week, the canalicular lung is established. Respiratory bronchioles have emerged. An occasional capillary protrudes into an air space, and a few type I and II pneumocyte cells have appeared. The development of the terminal alveolar sac phase then begins and viability becomes possible as primitive alveoli appear. These alveoli are by no means the mature structures found in the adult, nor will they be so at birth. However, understanding of this syndrome lies not in the gross structural aberrations but in the development of type II cells. The type II cells synthesize DNA and thus produce type I cells, more type II cells, and probably surfactant. The maturation of surfactant production by the type II cells is the key to survival in RDS.

The La Place equation indicates that opening and keeping open a small alveolus requires considerable energy. Surfactant lowers alveolar lining surface tension, particularly during expiration, thus stabilizing alveoli and remarkably improving their compliance. An absence of surfactant promotes atelectasis and a lowered functional residual capacity, leaving the "flail-chest" infant with an almost insurmountable mechanical problem. The neonate's ability to maintain adequate respiration at birth depends primarily on surfactant and adequate muscle power.

The major component of this surface active material, or surfactant, is saturated phosphatidylcholine (SPC). The amount of this material increases progressively (linear with time) in the fetal lung up to 35 weeks, with a striking increase (power function with time) thereafter. Chemical analysis of amniotic fluid for surfactant was first attempted in 1972, and shortly thereafter use of the lecithin/sphingomyelin (L/S) ratio to predict RDS became widespread. However, the proportion of false negative tests in complicated pregnancies has been reported to be as high as 25 per cent. Recently a more specific test for SPC has become available and holds promise of substantially increased accuracy, especially in complicated pregnancies. Undoubtedly, considering the progress in this area in the past decade, prediction of RDS by amniotic fluid chemical analysis will be firmly and reliably established in clinical practice in the next 10 years.

Acceleration of surfactant production in utero with maternally administered glucocorticoids has been investigated but remains experimental because of the effects on the development of other fetal organs. Other drugs, such as pilocarpine, are being evaluated in animals. For the moment, active pharmacologic intervention to provoke surfactant system maturation remains beyond reach. An intriguing concept, recently successfully tried in practice, is the instillation of artificial surfactant into the lung. The small number of patients (10) in the first study prevents sweeping statements, but this is an idea that may prove useful in the future.

The clinical characteristics of RDS are usually present at birth or within hours after delivery. The majority of patients are premature and demonstrate tachypnea (respiratory rate $\geq$ 60 breaths/min) with significant retraction, nasal flaring, and expiratory "grunting." These infants will frequently be cyanotic in room air, indicating a need for supplemental oxygen. Arterial blood gas measurements will show hypoxia, hypercapnia, and acidosis. The chest x-ray will demonstrate a diffuse "ground-glass" appearance and possibly cardiomegaly. Therapy consists of supplemental O_2, continuous positive airway pressure (via head chamber, nasal prongs, face mask/chamber, or endotracheal tube), or mechanical ventilatory support (especially for patients with episodic apnea) utilizing positive end expiratory pressure.

In survivors, pulmonary compliance seems to worsen for two to three days and then improve over four to five days, probably because of accelerated maturation of surfactant synthesis in a maximally stressed infant.

Bronchopulmonary dysplasia (BPD) is a possible late complication of neonatal RDS. The clinical picture is one of a decline in pulmonary function sometime in the recovery phase of RDS. Compliance falls, shunt increases, and the infant may develop respiratory failure. The chest X-ray in BPD may show geographically alternating areas of collapse and hyperinflation. Therapy for this acute syndrome includes fluid restriction and the use of the lowest possible FI_{O_2} that insures an acceptable Pa_{O_2}. The Wilson-Mikity syndrome, a possibly related disease, was first described in 1960 as a new form of respiratory distress in premature infants. The diagnosis of this syndrome depends on a characteristic uniform "bubbly" chest x-ray, and many of these infants have pathologic changes identical to those found in adult chronic lung disease. The etiology of this disease is unknown, and the relationship of both BPD and the Wilson-Mikity syndrome to respiratory distress is unclear. Both of these syndromes are included here because they may later prove to be variants of each another, and both may be more clearly related to neonatal respiratory distress. The long-term prognosis for patients with BPD is generally good, and by 10 years of age, most will have good pulmonary function. The long-term prognosis in Wilson-Mikity syndrome is much less clear, but the abnormalities of pulmonary function described in the neonate appear to persist to at least the age of 10 years. Beyond that, little is known.

In premature infants, functional systems other than the respiratory system are also premature. Heat preservation is difficult for tiny infants, and the energy stores for calorie production are often nonexistent. Ca^{++}, Mg^{++}, and glucose homeostasis are tenuous, while intravascular volume and red cell mass are usually decreased.

Most importantly, the ductus arteriosus remains open in many prematures, with flow direction a function of pulmonary artery pressure versus aortic pressure. Pulmonary artery pressure may be near systemic pressure during the acute phase of RDS, only to fall profoundly during recovery, greatly increasing the left-to-right flow. The presence of this shunt increases the volume work of the left ventricle and may decrease lung compliance. Lastly, necrotizing enterocolitis may complicate neonatal RDS and may lead to bowel perforation, requiring colostomy. Thus, the anesthetist must be prepared to care for the critically ill patient with neonatal RDS.

ANESTHETIC MANAGEMENT

The anesthetic problems are related to the very small size of the patient, immature development of multiple organs, and respiratory distress. In some centers, the fragility of the smallest (< 1000 gm) of these infants has prompted the performance of surgery (i.e., ductal ligations) utilizing local infiltration and neuromuscular block in the newborn nursery. This eliminates transportation to the operating room. The majority of these infants, however, will be operated on outside the nursery, owing to the technical requirements of the procedure. Preoperative assessment and transportation are similar to those outlined for the term newborns, with special emphasis on certain organ systems.

Respiratory support is crucial and may vary from minimal O_2 supplementation to continuous mechanical ventilation with positive end expiratory pressure and FI_{O_2} of 1.0. A thorough review of all respiratory parameters is required prior to transport, and these should be duplicated as closely as possible in the operating room, at least initially. If the infant is intubated and breathing spontaneously, it is reasonable to establish neuromuscular blockade and controlled positive pressure ventilation prior to transport. In this way the hemodynamic impact of controlled ventilation and the adequacy of intravascular volume can be established while the infant is undisturbed. Many of these infants have been diuresed as therapy for congestive failure and will require volume expansion to tolerate continuous mechanical ventilation. This is best accomplished by utilizing packed red blood cells and fresh frozen plasma in a 2:1 ratio to maintain a hematocrit of 40 per cent.

Vascular access in the very small infant is a challenge. Many of these patients will have an umbilical arterial catheter in situ, allowing determination of central aortic pressure and a reliable pH value. PA_{O_2} measured from this catheter will be related to catheter tip location and the presence of a ductal shunt. If the ductal shunt is right-to-left, all postductal (distal to ductus) gas tensions are "falsely" low relative to the cerebral circulation. To obtain a preductal (proximal to ductus) sample, a 22 gauge catheter may be inserted (percutaneously) in the right radial artery. The right radial artery can be visualized by transilluminating the wrist with fiberoptic light source. Alternatively, the temporal artery may be catheterized. This may be also necessary when the umbilical catheter is initially satisfactory but interferes with the surgical procedure. If an arterial catheter is placed, it should be continuously infused with heparinized saline and the volume included as intake. Central venous pressure is useful in management, but is technically not easily measured. Hyperalimentation catheters, although tempting to use, should not be utilized for this purpose. A catheter tip placed in the right atrium must be thought of as being in the left atrium during any injections, because right-to-left flow across a patent foramen ovale can lead to cerebral or coronary emboli.

Utilizing a rubber band as a tourniquet, the placement of peripheral intravenous catheters can be remarkably easy early in the nursery stay but rapidly approaches the impossible after a prolonged illness. In this situation, an umbilical catheter has the advantage of providing an infusion as well as a monitoring system. Should there be no vascular access to the infant, it is wise to establish such access prior to leaving the nursery. Without an adequate means to expand intravascular volume, the induction of anesthesia in a premature child may cause a profound fall in blood pressure and cardiac output that cannot be corrected.

Once these measures have been attended to, the infant can be quickly transported to the operating room, mechanically or manually ventilated as necessary. The intravenous and arterial catheters should be continuously infused via injection pumps, or filled with heparinized saline and then occluded.

Upon arrival in the operating room, and following atropine administration, the unintubated patient should be intubated awake with O_2 supplementation and then paralyzed, since the paralyzed patient can be quickly and easily positioned, have further monitors applied, and be prepped. An initial low systolic blood pressure may obviate the use of inhalation anesthetics. Intravenous narcotics or ketamine would seem to be the drugs of choice, if anesthesia beyond local infiltration is deemed necessary.

The indications for general anesthesia in these infants may be increasing. It has been hypothesized that there is a relationship between arterial hypertension (mean BP> 50 torr) and the incidence of intracerebral hemorrhage in the premature and, furthermore, that pharmacologic prevention (i.e., general anesthesia) of hypertension is indicated. If this cause-and-effect relationship is established, there may be stronger future indications for general anesthesia in the premature.

The major intraoperative concerns for a patient with prematurity and RDS are the adjustment of ventilation for changes in compliance and of fluid therapy for intraoperative losses.

The controlled positive pressure ventilation instituted in the nursery should have established an appropriate minute ventilation and reversed hypoxemia. Further changes in ventilation can be implemented depending on the operative site (upper abdomen, lateral thoracotomy) and the measured gas tensions. If the patient is intubated in the operating room, then ventilation should commence in a fashion presented in the first section. Peak airway pressure should be closely observed and kept below 30 cm H_2O if possible. Positive end expiratory pressure is usually beneficial in these patients. Fluid therapy should consist of adequate dextrose administration (5% initially) with lactated Ringer's solution to compensate for insensible and third space losses. This rate should be decreased by 1 ml/kg/hr if anesthetic gas is heated and adequately humidified, as is strongly recommended in the premature. Blood should be replaced as lost, using red blood cells and plasma, as in the preoperative period. Every attempt to "stay even" should be made, for "catching up" through a tiny catheter may be impossible; especially if other fluids are being simultaneously infused (e.g., dextrose).

Premature infants often suffer intraventricular hemorrhages during their nursery stay. The precipitating factors are far from clear, but fluid shifts in response to osmolarity changes are frequently mentioned. Until this situation has been resolved, the osmolarity of intravenous fluids used should be carefully considered. For example, sodium bicarbonate (2000 mOsm per liter) is a potential cause of fluid compartment shifts. This can be eliminated by diluting the drug and then giving the required volume slowly.

Postoperative management of these infants depends a great deal on the severity of the underlying respiratory distress and the complexity of the surgery, and should be planned in conjunction with the follow-up physicians. Neuromuscular block can be reversed, but this may not significantly alter the postoperative course. In general, it seems reasonable to allow the block to decay spontaneously while the infant is recovering from surgery. This has the advantage of allowing the transition from mechanical ventilation with flaccidity to spontaneous ventilation with activity to occur in controlled surroundings.

This treatment plan should be modified slightly for patients with a diagnosis of bronchopulmonary dysplasia. The definition of adequate fluid therapy and acceptable FI_{O_2} in this disease is arbitrary; therefore, appropriate modification of anesthetic management for these patients is somewhat empirical. In general, they should be suspected of having a contracted intravascular volume with a large ventilation/perfusion mismatch. Massive lobar hyperinflation may be a contraindication to the use of nitrous oxide. Postoperatively, they should remain intubated and probably ventilated, at least for a short while.

The anesthetic management for patients with the Wilson-Mikity syndrome should be similar to that of an adult with emphysema, possibly including cor pulmonale as well. Oxygen toxicity is frequently mentioned as a probable cause, and FI_{O_2} should therefore be kept as low as possible yet consistent with acceptable oxygenation. Postoperative care in these patients should be similar to that described for BPD.

CONGENITAL LOBAR EMPHYSEMA (CLE)

Emphysema means a pathologic accumulation of air in an organ or tissue. In congenital lobar emphysema the air is generally confined to within one lobe of the lung, usually an upper lobe, and the lobe appears hyperinflated. Several causes of this disease have been postulated. The most frequently demonstrated etiology for the lobar sequestration of air is expiratory gas trapping due to the absence of cartilage in the bronchus to the affected lobe. Why this defect is confined to an isolated lobe is unknown; the generation of the affected bronchus may be anywhere from the mainstem bronchus to the sublobar bronchi. In other cases, multiple microscopic sections of the involved lobe have revealed a striking increase in the number of alveoli without a matching increase in number of bronchioles or pulmonary arterioles. Further, a certain percentage of cases will have clearly identifiable internal or external bronchial obstructions. The majority of cases however, have no demonstrable etiology. Except for those cases secondary to external compression, treatment is lobectomy.

The clinical picture associated with this disease is highly variable. Infants who present with congenital lobar emphysema alone most frequently demonstrate respira-

tory distress, cyanosis, wheezing, asymmetric breath sounds, displaced cardiac sounds, and tympanitic chest percussion within a few months of birth. The chest X-ray will show a hyperlucent lobe, occasionally compressing surrounding structures in a fashion difficult to distinguish from a lung cyst. Mediastinal shift should be noted, as this distortion may predict the degree of central venous obstruction present. Lobar hyperinflation also suggests foreign body aspiration, but this is an uncommon occurrence in infancy. About half of these patients will have a much longer history of frequent pulmonary infections, with intermittent respiratory distress, and failure to thrive. Such infants may require bronchoscopy to establish a firm diagnosis. Since congenital heart disease occurs commonly in conjunction with congenital lobar emphysema, patients in the chronic group may also require detailed cardiac evaluation.

Long-term followup of children who have undergone pulmonary resection for this problem in infancy shows minimal physiologic difference from normal individuals. In contrast to adults, in whom overdistention of the remaining lung occurs following pulmonary resection, infants appear to develop true hyperplasia rapidly after resection, and for clinical purposes are "normal" within a year of surgery.

ANESTHETIC MANAGEMENT

The only presentation of congenital lobar emphysema that requires relatively urgent surgery is an unusually dramatic form of tension pneumothorax not amenable to chest tube decompression. The significance of the primary disease, however, must not be allowed to overshadow many other important secondary preoperative concerns.

A preoperative review of systems is required to ascertain other developmental defects, especially congenital heart disease. Special attention should be paid to fluid balance, since respiratory distress may eliminate oral intake while tachypnea may also concomitantly increase insensible water loss. Consequently, preoperative supplemental humidification of the inspired air may be beneficial. Assessment of the degree of respiratory distress, by noting the respiratory rate and retraction, and possibly by measuring blood gas tensions, is essential.

It is important to realize that the blood pH may be adversely affected by both CO_2 retention and impaired cardiac output (decreased tissue perfusion). In these patients a decreased cardiac output may be partly due to dehydration, but, in addition, venous inflow to the right atrium may be mechanically limited due to mediastinal distortion. Fluid balance is partially correctable preoperatively; unfortunately, the mechanical restriction is not.

Premedication should consist only of atropine, and if crying aggravates the respiratory distress, it may be advisable to administer the atropine intravenously in the operating room. The surgeon should be in the room throughout the induction, prepared to intervene with thoracotomy (to relieve mediastinal distortion) if needed. Anesthesia for infants with mild to moderate hyperinflation can be induced and maintained with a volatile agent in oxygen, augmented with gentle assisted respiration (and relaxants) if necessary. The more severely distressed infant may require the support of positive pressure ventilation the most, yet tolerate it very poorly, while myocardial depression from a potent anesthetic in conjunction with central hypovolemia may cause profound hypotension. The anesthesia technique of choice for these severely affected patients may be arrived at by a process of elimination. Nitrous oxide is always contraindicated because of the danger of further expanding the trapped air mass. Muscle relaxants require controlled positive-pressure ventilation, and narcotics depress spontaneous respiration. Barbiturates can cause myocardial depression and possibly apnea. Ketamine and oxygen are viable alternatives. Oxygen should be administered preoperatively to alleviate hypoxia and possibly decrease the N_2 content of the trapped gas. Ketamine, 0.5 to 1.0 mg/kg intravenously or 6 to 8 mg/kg IM will establish anesthesia and should not cause apnea. Despite an increase in muscle tone and possibly in laryngeal reflexes, intubation should be achievable without the use of relaxants. Any positive pressure during inspiration may further distend the affected lobe; as both end-expiratory pressure and assisted inspiration are often provided by manual compression of a rebreathing bag, this is best avoided in severely distressed patients.

After intubation, the infant can quickly be positioned, further monitoring established, and lateral thoracotomy performed. Local infiltration of the incision with dilute lidocaine is helpful if the plane of anesthesia is light. Once the chest is opened and the emphysematous lobe herniates out of the chest, the procedure becomes a lobectomy complicated by the technical difficulties of dissecting and clamping the bronchus supplying the distended lung segment. Relief of the mediastinal shift allows anesthesia to continue in a more conventional fashion, usually involving potent volatile agents and controlled ventilation. If profound acidosis is suspected, the degree of cardiovascular stability during enflurane anesthesia may favor use of this drug despite extensive previous experience with halothane in chest surgery. Muscle relaxants may be used as desired. The remainder of the anesthetic and the postoperative period are generally uneventful.

The anesthetic management of congenital lung cysts shares many of the same features (e.g., a need to avoid N_2O and preserve spontaneous ventilation) as the management of congenital lobar emphysema. There is usually less hyperinflation but, unfortunately, substantially more infection, as a result of poor bronchial drainage. With congenital lung cysts, the remaining lung may be somewhat hypoplastic, resembling the situation found in congenital diaphragmatic hernia. Of interest is the fact that the arterial supply to the cyst is frequently from an anomalous systemic vessel which enters the lung away from the hilum. This unusual vascular supply has led to the theory of pulmonary sequestration, and this term is now used interchangeably with congenital cystic disease. An aortogram is required to evaluate the arterial supply completely; fatalities have been recorded from avulsion of an unsuspected anomalous vessel. Since awareness of the presence of an anomalous vessel associated with a congenital lung cyst is so critical, it is always important to consider this possibility preoperatively when treating any cystic disease of lung.

BILIARY DISEASE

Forty years ago a discussion of anesthesic considerations of neonatal biliary disease would have been so brief that a few lines would have sufficed. The removal of the "inspissated bile syndrome" as a frequent surgical diagnosis marked the beginning of an expansion in knowledge concerning unexplained jaundice in infancy. Briefly reviewing this evolution is worth while, for the final solutions to many of these problems are not in sight and the controversies are rekindled from time to time.

In 1953, Gross documented that biliary atresia, occurring in one in every 25,000 live births, was the most common cause of obstructive jaundice in infancy. As very few of these jaundiced patients could be aided by surgery, the general feeling for the next decade or so was that operative intervention was useless, and possibly harmful. A few authors fought against this, recommending early exploration with operative cholangiography in an attempt to identify infants with surgically correctable lesions prior to development of cirrhosis. In 1968, Kasai reported operative relief of "noncorrectable" biliary atresia, with successful results highly dependent on early (before 4 months of age) intervention. Success in this procedure (hepatic portoenterostomy) is defined as the re-establishment of bile flow from the liver, and occurs in approximately 50 per cent of patients. Unfortunately, resolution of liver disease does not invariably accompany a successful operation. Of those with adequate biliary drainage, about half will stabilize and the other half will continue on with progressive ascending cholangitis and cirrhosis. Although this is a depressingly low percentage of cure, it is far superior to a 1.1 per cent survival without surgery. Kasai has reported improvement in liver morphology after several years; this is a significant observation because the natural history of biliary atresia includes an associated increase in incidence of malignancy.

An alternative to the Kasai procedure may be a liver transplant, although this has been most successful for the treatment of metabolic defects. For the time being, the complexity of hepatic transplantation limits the undertaking of this procedure to only a very few special hospitals.

The differential diagnosis of neonatal jaundice includes several other entities, many of which are diagnosed only at laparotomy. Biliary hypoplasia due to minimal bile flow situations (neonatal hepatitis, intrahepatic atresia, alpha$_1$-antitrypsin deficiency) is not helped by surgery, while hypoplasia with structural abnormalities may be aided by portoenterostomy. The separation of these two categories of biliary hypoplasia usually requires operative cholangiography. Re-exploration if jaundice worsens, and portoenterostomy for hypoplasia that has become obliterative are later options for the low bile flow group. Congenital dilation of the intrahepatic bile ducts, choledochal cyst, and perforation of the extrahepatic bile ducts are other rare causes of neonatal jaundice that require surgical intervention. Lastly, some mention is necessary of the inspissated bile syndrome, which is the end result of massive neonatal hemolysis. It is unusual to see this diagnosis in an era of exchange transfusions, but exploration to irrigate the bile ducts or remove a calculus may still be necessary.

The preoperative condition of the child depends primarily on two factors — the presence or absence of cholangitis and the amount of liver disease. Cholangitis is not usually part of biliary atresia, but may be present, and commonly occurs with choledochal cysts or bile duct perforations. Liver disease is, to a variable degree, always present with biliary atresia. Although the word *atresia* implies a developmental failure, the disease suggests an ongoing inflammatory obliterative process in the bile ducts. In general, liver function worsens with time, although two infants of the same age may show great variation in measured parameters.

ANESTHETIC MANAGEMENT

The detailed etiologic evaluation of a jaundiced neonate usually commences during the second to third week of life; by five to eight weeks, two categories of patients have emerged. There is a relatively large group of non-surgical patients and a smaller diagnostic dilemma group that require exploration. The period of evaluation is significant, for the laboratory information obtained is helpful preoperatively for those requiring surgery. On occasion, other abnormalities such as heart disease are discovered, but this is rare.

In the first few weeks following delivery, the infant usually appears yellow but well. Laboratory values disclose predictable aberrations in hepatic function; PT may be elevated, but is correctable with vitamin K, while a PTT elevation may require fresh plasma. There is frequently a mild anemia, as well. It is worthwhile inquiring into glucose homeostasis and values for serum proteins, although they are usually normal.

No premedication other than atropine is required, and this may be given in the operating room if desired. The general principles stated earlier in Anesthetic Considerations in the Newborn are appropriate, with particular attention to the location of the warming mattress to prevent interference with operative cholangiography. Because of relocation, the warming mattress has a reduced effectiveness, making the use of warm, humidified gas highly desirable.

The question of what anesthetic agents to use, other than N_2O, generates an interesting response. Experts have recommended that halogenated drugs be both used and avoided, leaving the clinician in an unusual quandary. On the one hand, all such agents may have some potential for hepatic damage, and the diagnosis of biliary atresia probably implies some element of concomitant inflammatory hepatic disease. On the other hand, experience in the practice of pediatric anesthesia over the last 20 years clinically supports the use of inhalation anesthesia in general, and halothane in particular, as safe. In addition, there is no evidence linking patient outcome in biliary atresia with choice of anesthetic. The medicolegal implications of this question are beyond this discussion, but they do not seem so pressing as to demand a variation from a safe and proved method to a possibly less safe and probably less familiar alternative.

Anesthesia may be induced with intravenous thiopental, (2-4 mg/kg) followed by intravenous succinylcholine to aid intubation. N_2O/O_2/volatile agent may be used for induction and maintenance. All intravenous catheters should be in the upper extremities or neck, as the inferior vena cava may on occasion be occluded. If portoenterostomy is planned, two intravenous catheters are recommended, allowing increased flexibility to infuse glucose containing crystalloid and blood. A central venous catheter is diagnostically useful in these patients, and can also suffice as a second infusion system. Since blood loss during enterostomy can be large, and hypotension from intermittent

caval occlusion may occur, an arterial catheter may be indicated. If relaxants are administered, monitoring with a peripheral nerve stimulator is advisable.

Blood loss should be replaced with whole blood or packed red cells and fresh plasma, and if the loss is great, platelets may also be needed. Clotting studies should be obtained if replacement exceeds 75 per cent of estimated blood volume. During rapid transfusion, the ECG should be observed for a prolongation of the Q-T interval, and $CaCl_2$ (3-5 mg/kg) administered if this occurs. Obviously, the calcium should not be given into an infusion containing citrated blood.

If intraoperative efforts to maintain body temperature and blood volume have been reasonably successful, extubation can usually be performed at the close of surgery in the operating room. Before leaving the patient in the recovery room, the anesthesia record should be re-examined for clarity. These patients frequently return for reexploration, and knowledge of prior experiences can be invaluable.

CONGENITAL DIAPHRAGMATIC HERNIA (CDH)

Diaphragm development is complex and occurs coincidentally with initial lung development and the return of the gut to the abdomen. The establishment of an intact musculotendinous septum between the pleura and peritoneum occurs through mesenchymal ingrowth from several sources. During this period, the gut first elongates into the base of the umbilical cord, then returns to the abdomen in a counterclockwise manner. Should closure of the diaphragm fail to occur, or the gut return into the abdomen prematurely, the path of least resistance into the chest results in a hernia. This sequence helps to explain the high incidence of associated malrotation with CDH.

Diaphragm closure occurs slowly during the fifth to tenth week in utero, permitting or promoting several possible hernia sites. By far the most common site for the defect is through the posterolateral canal of Bochdalek. More than 80 per cent of these hernias will be left-sided, perhaps because this canal closes later in utero. The incidence of posterolateral hernia is reported to be between one in 5000 to one in 12,000 live births, with a 2:1 male to female predilection in some series. The other congenital site, accounting for 2 to 4 per cent of CDH, is through the retrosternal space of Morgagni. This hernia, caused by a failure of the lower ribs to fuse to the developing septum, is significant, primarily because of the risk of incarceration.

Eventration is a congenital developmental failure of the muscular component of the diaphragm. Many cases of eventration are asymptomatic, but severe cases may present immediately after birth with signs and symptoms identical to a Bochdalek hernia. Anesthetic management may be modified because of a thoracic rather than an abdominal surgical approach to the defect. This disease is otherwise entirely similar to CDH.

Although the first CDH was described in 1597 and the defect found in South American mummies dating from the third century A.D., the first large review of these hernias calling for early repair did not appear until 1925. Twenty years later, Gross repaired a congenital diaphragmatic hernia in a newborn and by 1953 had reported over 70 patients operated on within a few weeks of birth. Despite improvements in both surgery and anesthesia, the success reported in this first series has not been maintained, probably because of more frequent recognition and subsequent operation in terribly ill neonates. Current survival for neonates with this condition is probably about 55 per cent.

Long-term follow up of patients who have undergone repair of CDH in infancy has been generally encouraging. Conductance, compliance, and lung volume are near normal before the age of six months. Lung function tests, including spirometry and closing volume measurements, have revealed only minor abnormalities in a few patients. Unfortunately, one series reported a 10 per cent incidence of mental retardation, presumably due to hypoxia at birth.

The clinical picture is highly dependent on the type of hernia and degree of associated pulmonary dysfunction. The most severe form is a Bochdalek hernia (usually on the left). It involves most of the hemidiaphragm and allows the majority of the abdominal contents to enter the hemithorax. This results in a small abdominal cavity (scaphoid abdomen), severe compression of the ipsilateral lung, right mediastinal shift (clinically "dextrocardia"), and often marked volume reduction of the contralateral lung. There may also be associated congenital heart disease, renal defects, or central nervous system maldevelopment.

The infant begins to swallow and breathe at delivery, and symptoms present immediately after birth in severe cases. Swallowing allows air to distend the gut in the chest, worsening the mediastinal shift with an unusual form of "tension pneumothorax." The breathing pattern may reveal immediate respiratory distress and cyanosis secondary to the mediastinal shift and contralateral compression or, more ominously, to pulmonary hypoplasia. The degree of pulmonary hypoplasia holds the key to survival in these infants, for reduction of the hernia will not significantly affect survival in newborns with insufficient lung function to sustain life.

Anatomically, pulmonary hypoplasia may affect the vessels, the airways, and the parenchyma. The size of the vascular bed is decreased with an increase in arterial smooth muscle mass and a decrease in the number of vessels per unit of lung. The airways are reduced in both size and number, and there may be distortion in alveolar diameter and structure. The picture is consistent with a retardation of lung maturation at about the tenth to twelfth week in utero, and explains much of the stormy postoperative course in these babies.

The diagnosis is usually suspected from the presence of polyhydramnios (approximately one third of cases) at delivery with the newborn demonstrating respiratory distress, cyanosis, and a scaphoid abdomen. Breath sounds may be absent on the affected side or occasionally replaced by bowel sounds. In patients with left-sided defects, heart sounds may be on the right. If the diagnosis is suspected, a chest x-ray will show loops of gut in the chest. Confusion with congenital cystic adenomatoid malformation may exist, however, because of the lack of air in the gut immediately after birth. In such situations, a nasogastric tube may be passed, perhaps with a small volume of contrast material, to demonstrate an intrathoracic stomach on x-ray. Air should not be injected to confirm tube position. If an adenomatoid malformation is diagnosed, it should be managed as a case of congenital lobar emphysema, possible with accompanying pulmonary hypoplasia.

Respiratory distress, if present, should be managed by endotracheal intubation, gentle positive pressure ventilation, and possibly paralysis. Ventilation via mask is to be avoided, lest the stomach be further distended. For the infant in extremis, the FI_{O_2} should be 1.0. This may correct hypoxia and, along with positive pressure ventilation, improve acidosis. These measures may, in turn, decrease pulmonary arterial vasoconstriction and increase pulmonary blood flow. Immediate concern about a high Pa_{O_2} in the cerebral circulation should be subsidiary to concern about generalized hypoxia in this disease. The FI_{O_2} should be reduced as blood gas tensions and pH permit. Paralysis minimizes oxygen consumption in an infant in a thermoneutral environment and permits better gas exchange with minimal airway pressure. Obviously, the moribund infant will have no need for relaxants.

Following endotracheal intubation, a nasogastric sump tube should be passed and aspirated at low pressure. An umbilical, right radial, or temporal artery catheter should be inserted, along with a suitable intravenous catheter. Blood should be immediately drawn for a hematocrit, type and cross match, and gas tensions.

The urgency of surgery has been questioned recently, based on a better understanding of pulmonary hypoplasia, but immediate operation is still generally recommended. An abrupt decay in the patient's condition during the preoperative period is likely to be due to a tension pneumothorax. This should be quickly recognized and decompressed.

Through a left upper quadrant abdominal incision the hernia is reduced and the diaphragm repaired. Thoracic compliance, with the abdomen empty, is probably maximal at this time. Before this compliance is reduced by filling the abdomen, attention should be directed to intravascular volume. If adequate intravenous access was not previously established, it should be secured now. The requirement for fluid infusion may be increased significantly by improved blood flow to the previously compressed bowel. Because intra-abdominal pressure may be high postoperatively, fluids should be administered via upper extremity or neck veins.

Replacing the abdominal contents into the small abdomen may present a challenge, requiring the use of prosthetic materials to temporarily (for up to 10 days) enlarge the container. Excessive abdominal tension is especially undesirable following repair of a hemidiaphragm drawn snug by sutures. The plicated side is usually flattened and immobile, while the opposite side can be driven cephalad by pressure, losing some of its normal excursion. Also, such an increase in abdominal pressure may impede venous return from the gut and/or lower extremities. (For a discussion of prosthetic materials and abdominal closure, see Abdominal Wall Defects.)

ANESTHETIC MANAGEMENT

The guidelines in the chapter introduction are appropriate, but the time sequence may be incredibly accelerated. Little or no warning may precede the patient's arrival in the O.R. Maximal efforts should be made to maintain body temperature to minimize O_2 consumption. In this regard, overhead radiant heating and gas heat/humidification are special assets if the room is just beginning to warm. Selection of the anesthetic agents should be based on an understanding of the tremendous myocardial work load imposed by acidosis and hypoxia. The dominant right ventricle is pumping into a markedly raised resistance and is probably delivering an increased volume load because of right-to-left shunting. The non-compliant left ventricle must attempt to provide an increased output to offset hypoxia. Anesthetic myocardial depression may be intolerable in this setting. Ketamine or narcotics may be indicated if the infant is not moribund. Pulmonary artery pressure and cardiac output may fall if morphine is used, as a result of decreased pulmonary vascular resistance and a simultaneous decrease in filling pressure. Careful volume augmentation may be required to offset this. N_2O is best avoided because of slow but appreciable accumulation in the gut.

As ventilation by mask is to be avoided preoperatively so must the temptation to expand the ipsilateral lung be avoided intraoperatively. In severe cases, this is not an acutely collapsed lung but a chronically hypoplastic one; application of high airway pressure in this two-compartment model will serve to overexpand and perhaps rupture the contralateral lung. In some centers, bilateral chest tubes are inserted because of the potential for tension pneumothorax. This safety measure does not give license to raise airway pressure, however.

A frequent clinical situation is that of a child who responds to oxygen therapy, tolerates the operative procedure well, and then deteriorates hours postoperatively. It is difficult to understand why an infant with CDH should initially do well and then regress; in theory, severely hypoplastic lungs should be immediately apparent. Physiologically, however, this patient will resemble an infant with persistence of the fetal circulation (PFC), an entity recently recognized in cyanotic newborns. PFC consists of pulmonary artery hypertension with right-to-left shunting; patients with this syndrome show an increase in pulmonary muscle mass at necropsy. Therapy of PFC has been largely supportive, including fluid therapy, correction of acidosis, and mechanical ventilation. As well, vasodilators such as morphine acetylcholine and recently tolazoline have been administered with variable results. The one measure that has been successful in PFC has been hyperventilation, but an absence of parenchymal development may severely limit this modality in CDH.

This pattern of events should be remembered in planning postoperative care for these patients. Shortly after the hernia reduction and diaphragm repair, blood gas tensions and pH should be measured. A metabolic acidosis may best be treated with tromethamine (THAM) in this situation, to avoid increasing the pulmonary CO_2 excretion load. Hypoxia ($Pa_{O_2} < 80$ torr), during controlled ventilation with 100 per cent O_2 and possibly positive end expiratory pressure, is an ominous sign. A shunt of this magnitude may indicate inadequate lung function to sustain life. A Pa_{O_2} greater than 250 torr is encouraging, but it is just such a patient that may deteriorate later. Although it is possible that the infant may need little postoperative ventilatory support, the frequent late decline makes it prudent to continue with apparently successful measures until the infant has declared the direction of its clinical course. The patient should prob-

ably remain intubated in the nursery postoperatively with ventilatory support, supplemental O_2, and low positive end expiratory pressure as indicated. Transcutaneous oxygen tension monitoring should be applied to these patients. Pulmonary vasospasm secondary to hypoxia is frequently cited as the triggering event in late deterioration, and perhaps the minute-to-minute ability to detect hypoxia may prevent this. Pulmonary artery pressure measurement may be indicated to increase the meager supply of data concerning pulmonary hemodynamics in CDH patients.

The role of drug infusion and ligation of a patent ductus arteriosus are both currently unclear, as conflicting results have been published, with all suggested forms of treatment eventually entering the therapeutic picture in critical patients. If drugs are used, direct pulmonary artery infusion is probably preferable. The advisability of ductal ligation may be estimated by simultaneous measurement of pre- and post-ductal Pa_{O_2}. Equal values suggest that ligation may prove futile. Prolonged temporary support of CDH patients using extracorporeal membrane oxygenation has been suggested and, considering the rapid growth of the lungs following repair of CDH, has substantial merit. Unfortunately, the complexity of this therapeutic measure makes it improbable that it will be frequently used in most severe cases.

Future strides in CDH treatment will probably evolve in two directions. First, better methods of ventilation, perhaps utilizing high frequency positive pressure, negative pressure, or a combination of both, will be evaluated and recommended. Second, pulmonary hemodynamics in this immature lung model will become understood and drugs may become available to allow pulmonary artery tone manipulation, despite hypoxia. As in most cases of organ immaturity, any measure that buys time for growth is useful and will be pressed into service.

ABDOMINAL WALL DEFECTS

Omphalocele; Gastroschisis; Abdominal Muscle Deficiency Syndrome (Prune Belly)

Abdominal wall defects are relatively rare and are distressing in appearance. Abdominal wall and bowel development occur conjointly over the third to twelfth week in utero, while final intraperitoneal bowel fixation occurs after birth. The embryology of this nine week maturation period must be reviewed to grasp the differences among defects that may appear grossly identical.

By the third week, the embryo has developed cephalic, caudal, and lateral folds. The cephalic fold is anterior and contains the foregut as well as the site of development of the stomach and mediastinal/thoracic contents. A defect in the somatic layer of this cephalic fold causes the rare epigastric omphalocele, often with associated diaphragm, thoracic wall, and cardiac/pericardial defects.

The caudal fold, located posteriorly, is the origin of the colon, rectum, bladder, and hypogastric abdominal wall. Defects in this fold cause exstrophy of the bladder or a lower abdominal wall defect (hypogastric omphalocele).

The lateral folds form the lateral abdominal walls and the future umbilical ring. A defect in this fold results in an umbilical cord hernia or periumbilical omphalocele.

During the fourth week in utero, the growth of the gut accelerates markedly, exceeding the growth rate of the abdomen and forcing the gut into the base of the umbilical cord, where it remains until the tenth week. During the eleventh and twelfth weeks, the gut returns to the abdomen, with a counterclockwise rotation, placing the cecum in the right lower quadrant. A maturation failure in any of the folds during the third week in utero allows the gut to remain extra-abdominal but covered by peritoneum and amniotic membrane. If the defect in the abdominal wall is less than 4 cm in diameter and umbilical, it is refered to as a hernia of the cord; otherwise it is called an omphalocele.

Another periumbilical defect is gastroschisis, the probable end result of an umbilical cord hernia that ruptures in utero, allowing small intestine (with stomach, bladder, and uterus in larger defects) to present on the abdominal wall as a mass of bowel covered by fibrinous exudate, with no evidence of a hernia sac. The umbilicus is always to the left of the defect and separated from it by a bridge of skin, while the defect itself is clearly between the medial borders of the rectus muscle, rather than through the muscle, as it may grossly appear to be.

An additional similar entity is the abdom-inal musculature deficiency syndrome, referred to descriptively by Osler as the "prune belly" syndrome. The cause and embryology of this defect are unknown but, much like the previous defects, a portion of the abdominal wall is absent. In this syndrome, the missing portion is abdominal wall muscle. All patients with this defect have a non-laminated strip of muscle representing the abdominal wall; usually there is a developed rectus, although even this may be absent. Beneath the abdominal wall defect, 90 per cent of these patients have genitourinary abnormalities, usually consisting of bilateral cryptorchidism (most patients are male) with phimosis and meatal stenosis. Megaureter (implying obstruction) occurs in 85 per cent of these infants, and oligohydramnios frequently occurs. Thomas and Smith have suggested that oligohydramnios is the cause of the pulmonary hypoplasia associated with Potter's syndrome. The proposed mechanism of the pulmonary hypoplasia is a mechanical impediment to thoracic (and pulmonary) growth in utero, with results similar to that seen in diaphragmatic hernia. Similarly, severe pulmonary hypoplasia has been associated with the prune belly syndrome, especially in infants with urethral obstruction. The anesthetic implications of pulmonary hypoplasia are obvious. However, the connection between absent abdominal muscles and hypoplastic lungs is not straightforward, and an awareness of these relationships is required to avoid difficulty.

In summary, a defect into the base of the umbilical cord less than 4 cm in diameter is a hernia, while a larger defect is an omphalocele. The latter may also occur above or below the umbilicus, and a sac (as an important part of the definition) must be present, although the sac does not necessarily have to be intact. Gastroschisis is an antenatal or perinatal rupture of an umbilical cord hernia, and there is no sac present. The prune belly syndrome is well described by the title; the abdominal wall musculature is largely absent, while the abdominal contents are completely within the belly and covered by skin. The incidences are omphalocele 1 in 6000 live births, gastroschisis 1 in 20,000 to 30,000 live births, and abdominal muscle deficiency syndrome 1 in 50,000 live births.

Associated malformations were previously described for the prune belly syndrome. Such malformations may occur with the other defects as well, although much less so with gastroschisis or umbilical cord hernia than with omphalocele. Approximately 20 per cent of infants with omphalocele will have congenital heart disease, with tetralogy of Fallot being most common. Upper and lower midline defects frequently occur with nonumbilical omphaloceles, but such omphaloceles are rare. An omphalocele always occurs with Beckwith-Wiedemann syndrome (macroglossia and gigantism with neonatal hypoglycemia).

The surgical challenge caused by an intact omphalocele is a function of the amount of bowel and viscera contained in the sac and whether or not there is sufficient space in the abdomen to accept the contents of the sac. On occasion, especially if the care of other abnormalities takes precedence, conservative treatment with Mercurochrome (to form an eschar) is employed. Generally, primary single stage repair is attempted, especially if the sac contains only bowel. This involves undermining the edge of the abdominal defect to enlarge the cavity; the herniated mass can then usually be placed into the abdomen. However, respiratory compromise, inferior venal caval obstruction, and abdominal wound margin ischemia can result from such an attempt if the mass is excessively large. These problems can be avoided by suturing prosthetic material to the edges of the defect and then gradually reducing the size of the exterior viscera container every day or so. A tube gastrostomy and central vein hyperalimentation catheter are usually part of the first operation (prosthetic material attachment to abdominal wall). The abdomen enlarges with amazing rapidity as the prosthetic material is reefed, and under general anesthesia this material is eventually removed. While placement of the prosthetic material obviously solves the abdominal space problem, the placement of a foreign body may substitute sepsis in its stead. Thus, abdominal primary skin closure, if possible, is probably still the optimal treatment. Survival in uncomplicated cases is good; unfortunately many of these children have cardiac or syndrome-related defects that reduce survival to about 50 per cent.

Gastroschisis presents a different problem. In addition to having bowel outside the abdomen, it is totally exposed and must be covered emergently. The time of evisceration during gestation influences the appearance of the bowel and the size of the abdominal cavity. Prolonged exposure to amniotic fluid causes serositis with apparent shortening of the bowel and a marked increase in mass secondary to edema. The earlier in utero this occurs, the worse the bowel appears and the smaller the abdominal cavity will be. Interestingly, the smaller the defect, the worse will be the bowel condition. This is probably due to early rupture and ingrowth of the defect margin with subsequent strangulation and bowel ischemia. The matted mass of intestines can usually be placed into the abdomen, on occasion with the same technique of prosthetic enlargement to create adequate space, as in omphalocele repair. Hyperalimentation by vein is essential; however, the role of gastrostomy has been recently questioned because of a higher incidence of resultant infection. Survival with gastroschisis is probably about 80 per cent.

The prune belly syndrome encompasses a variable list of abdominal wall and genitourinary defects. Although the abdomen certainly appears bizarre, it does not require surgical correction. The urological problem requires prompt evaluation and possibly relief of obstruction. Preservation of renal function is paramount; immediate treatment is to establish urine flow. For the complete syndrome, including renal dysplasia, survival to two years of age is probably no better than 50 per cent. Recently several authors have proposed that ureteral and bladder enlargement are due to dysplasia, and have further suggested reconstruction of the bladder and distal ureter to prevent reflux. The initial results have been encouraging, but it will be a decade before final conclusions can be made.

ANESTHETIC MANAGEMENT

Preoperative evaluation of an infant with an abdominal wall defect covers a potentially large spectrum of considerations. The patient presentation may vary from a 2 kg feeble infant with a distorted mass of exteriorized bowel to a 4 kg vigorous baby with a small bulge in the base of the umbilical cord. Irrespective of the severity of the abdominal wall defect, associated problems must be evaluated. Gastroschisis has a very high incidence of prematurity (>50%), with all the associated problems (see RDS). Omphalocele often occurs with congenital heart disease or midline defect syndromes, while the abdominal musculature deficiency syndrome may include severe renal and pulmonary dysplasia. After determining the impact of associated factors, the specific defect may be addressed.

A hernia of the umbilical cord is the most straightforward situation, generally requiring only adequate exposure of the defect margin to effect repair. Larger defects, true omphaloceles, may present an abdominal cavity space problem. The developmental arrest that allowed for extra-abdominal intestine is now at least 20 weeks old. The peritoneal cavity can therefore be substantially smaller than required, and if the abdominal contents are returned and covered with skin, intra-abdominal pressure may be high. This can potentially decrease inferior venal caval flow; therefore, intravenous fluids, begun pre- or intraoperatively, must be administered by upper extremity or neck veins. Premedication should consist only of atropine, administered in the operating room if desired. The measures contained in the first section are appropriate, with emphasis on preservation of heat. Intubation should be performed with the patient awake, and anesthesia should be induced and maintained without the use of nitrous oxide, using an air/oxygen/volatile anesthetic mixture. If a nasogastric tube was not in place before, it should be inserted postintubation. For repair of a large defect, arterial gas tension monitoring is advisable. Use of the umbilical vessels for this purpose seems an improbable choice, as they are in the operative field; Filston and Izant suggested moving these vessels to the lower abdomen and this technique may prove useful.

Ventilation should be controlled during the operation. The anesthetist must be able to assess the impact of rising intra-abdominal pressure on respiration by comparing airway pressure, chest expansion, and the sound of gas exchange after repair to a previously stable baseline. Peak airway pressures over 30 to 35 cm H_2O are worrisome, while falling cardiac output and blood gas deterioration are indications that the primary closure is probably unacceptable. It must be kept in mind that a marginal

situation, consisting of a tight belly on one hand and a powerful ventilator on the other, can abruptly worsen if the lungs in between are overcompressed and rupture.

The surgical quandary revolves around the advisability of primary closure without the use of prosthetic materials. The decision is based on the anesthetist's evaluation of respiration, the presence or absence of venous obstruction in the lower body, the appearance of the wound margins, and the surgeon's past experience. Anesthetic technique may be involved in the last factor. Many experts feel that muscle relaxants are contraindicated for an omphalocele repair, feeling that they are unnecessary and fearing that their use could lead to an excessively "tight" closure upon resumption of abdominal wall muscular activity. Documentation that this has actually occurred is not available; nevertheless, variation in anesthetic technique could potentially alter the "judgment call" at a critical juncture. Neuromuscular blockade initiated prior to final closure and maintained postoperatively (with sedation and ventilaton) could be an ancillary method to help effect primary closure in a marginal situation, where the use of prosthetic materials would normally have been required. Obviously, close communication with the surgeon is paramount if such a method seems indicated.

Postoperatively the volatile agent should be discontinued and ventilation should continue to be controlled until the infant is awake. The decision to extubate is straightforward for the extreme conditions: *Yes* if the defect is small and the abdomen is adequate; *No* if the defect is large and the abdomen is tiny. The proper ventilatory management of a patient with a middle-sized defect repair and abdominal cavity is less clear. Sustained tachypnea (respiratory rate > 60-70 breaths/min) hypoxia, hypercarbia, acidosis, or the anesthetist's sense of being uncomfortable all favor continued intubation, probably utilizing continuous positive airway pressure and mechanical assistance. This is especially true if the infant has other defects, such as congenital heart disease.

If the repair requires prosthetic materials, the infant will require further surgery some time later to have the material removed. Spontaneous respiration is best for this procedure, permitting a reasonable assessment of the "end-result" prior to final closure.

Gastroschisis (or rupture of omphalocele) may present the same abdominal space problem as omphalocele, with other difficulties as well. The exposed intestines provide a large surface area, and heat loss can be quite rapid. Since the pathology involves a serous cavity, fluid loss is equally large. Finally, total serum protein and albumin levels may be significantly decreased in these infants. The time to correct these potential problems is preoperatively, but the risk of bacterial contamination is great and the press to cover the bowel is real. Fluid resuscitation should be prompt; lactated Ringer's with albumin or blood is probably best, at a rate of 10 to 20 ml per kg per hour, until blood pressure is adequate. For an infant weighing more than 2 kg, 60/35 torr is a minimal acceptable preinduction pressure (in the absence of heart disease). Intraoperative management is the same as for omphalocele repair, except for especially rigorous attention to fluid therapy and temperature maintenance. Postoperatively, the high incidence of prematurity favors continued intubation unless conditions are ideal.

Anesthetic management considerations of the abdominal muscular deficiency syndrome may simply be restricted to those for the infant with uremia. A chest X-ray is mandatory to rule out pulmonary hypoplasia. Blood gas tensions should be measured if there is any question of this diagnosis. If cystoscopy is planned as part of the evaluation of urinary obstruction, the bladder irrigating solution must be warmed, otherwise the infant will become hypothermic during the procedure. Postoperatively, these patients are somewhat analogous to patients with a high subarachnoid block, in that the absence of abdominal muscle leaves them with little ability to generate a forceful cough. The airway should be cleared of secretions prior to emergence, and if intubation was required for the procedure, the patient should be extubated awake. Postoperative care should include adequate hydration, postural drainage, and manual abdominal compression during the expiration phase in order to mimic the coughing action of the abdominal muscles. If the patient is beyond a few months of age, there may be a surprising amount of secre-

tions to deal with, much like an adult with chronic bronchitis.

REFERENCES

Anesthetic Considerations in the Newborn

Alfery, D. D., Ward, C. F., Harwood, I. R., and Mannino, F. L.: Airway management for a neonate with congenital fusion of the jaws. Anesthesiology 51:340–343, 1979.

Bennett, E. J.: Fluid balance in the newborn. Anesthesiology 43:210–224, 1975.

Betts, E. K., Downes, J. J., Schaffer, D. B., and Johns, R.: Retrolental fibroplasia and oxygen administration during general anesthesia. Anesthesiology 47:518–520, 1977.

Churchill-Davidson, H. C., and Wise, R. P.: Neuromuscular transmission in the newborn infant. Anesthesiology 24:271–278, 1963.

Cook, D. R., Wingard, L. B., and Taylor, F. J.: Pharmacokinetics of succinylcholine in infants, children and adults. Clin. Pharmacol. Ther. 20:493–498, 1976.

Cooper, L. V., Stephen, G. W., and Adjett, P. J. A.: Elimination of pethidine and bupivacaine in the newborn. Arch. Dis. Child. 52:638–641, 1977.

Dawes, G. S.: Fetal and Neonatal Physiology. Chicago, Year Book Medical Publishers, 1968.

Dreszer, M.: Fluid and electrolyte requirements in the newborn infant. Pediatr. Clin. North. Am. 24:537–546, 1977.

Eckenhoff, J.: Some anatomic considerations of the infant larynx influencing endotracheal anesthesia. Anesthesiology 12:410–420, 1951.

Edelman, C. N., and Spitzer, A.: The maturing kidney. J. Pediatr. 75:509–519, 1969.

Furman, E. B., Roman, D. G., Lemmer, L. A. S., et al.: Specific therapy in water, electrolyte and blood volume replacement during pediatric surgery. Anesthesiology 42:187–193, 1975.

Goldstein, A., Arrow, L., and Kalman, S. M.: Principles of Drug Action. New York, John Wiley and Sons, 1974.

Goudsouzian, N. H., Liu, L. N. P., and Savarese, J. J.: Metocurine in infants and children. Anesthesiology 49:266–269, 1978.

Goudsouzian, N. H., Donlon, J. V., Savarese, J. J., and Ryan, F. J.: Reevaluation of dosage and duration of action of d-Tubocurarine in the pediatric age group. Anesthesiology 43:416–425, 1975.

Goudsouzian, N. H., Ryan, J. F., and Savarese, J. J.: The neuromuscular effects of pancuronium in infants and children. Anesthesiology 41:95–98, 1974.

Gregory, G. A., Eger, E. I., and Munson, E. S.: The relationship between age and halothane requirement in man. Anesthesiology 30:488–491, 1969.

Gross, G. P., Hathway, W. E., and McGauhey, H. R.: Hyperviscosity in the neonate. J. Pediatr. 82:1004–1012, 1973.

Guyton, A. C., Jones, C. E., and Coleman, T. G.: Circulatory Physiology. Philadelphia, W. B. Saunders Co., 1973.

Hendren, W. H.: Pediatric surgery. N. Engl. J. Med. 298:456–462, 507–515, 562–568, 1973.

Kinsey, V. E., Arnold, H. J., Kalina, R. E., et al.: Pa_{O_2}

levels in retrolental fibroplasia: A report of the co-operative study. Pediatrics 60:655–668, 1977.

Kitterman, J. A., Phibbs, R. H., Tooley, W. H.: Aortic blood pressure in normal newborn infants during the first 12 hours of life. Pediatrics 44:959–968, 1979.

Krauss, A. N., Waldman, S., Frayer, W. W., and Ald, D. A.: Noninvasive estimation of arterial oxygenation in newborn infants. J. Pediatr. 93:275–278, 1978.

Lister, J.: Surgical emergencies in the newborn. Brit. J. Anaesth. 49:43–50, 1977.

Lou, H. C., Lassen, N. A., and Friss-Hanson, B.: Impaired autoregulation of cerebral blood flow in the distressed newborn infant. J. Pediatr. 94:118–121, 1979.

Miller, R. D., Agoston, S., Booij, L. D., et al.: Comparative potency in pharmacokinetics of pancuronium and its metabolites in anesthetized man. J. Pharmacol. Exp. Ther. 207:539–543, 1978.

Scarpelli, E. M.: Pulmonary Physiology of the Fetus, Newborn and Child. Philadelphia, Lea & Febiger, 1975.

Sinclair, J. C., Driscoll, J. M., Heird, W. C., and Winters, R. W.: Supportive management of the sick neonate. Pediatr. Clin. North Am. 17:863–893, 1970.

Sinclair, J. C.: Temperature Regulation and Energy Metabolism in the Newborn. New York, Grune and Stratton, 1978.

Smith, C. A., and Nelson, N. M.: The Physiology of the Newborn Infant. 4th ed. Springfield, Charles C Thomas, Publisher, 1976.

Smith, R. M.: Anesthesia for Infants and Children. 4th ed., St. Louis, C. V. Mosby Co., 1980.

Steward, D. J.: Manual of Pediatric Anesthesia. New York, Churchill Livingstone, 1979.

Tarlo, P. A., Valimaki, I., and Rautaharju, P. M.: Quantitative computer analysis of cardiac and respiratory activity in newborn infants. J. Appl. Physiol. 31:70–78, 1971.

Udkow, G.: Pediatric clinical pharmacology. Amer. J. Dis. Child. 132:1025–1032, 1978.

Walts, L. F., and Dillon, J. B.: The response of newborns to succinylcholine and d-turbocurarine. Anesthesiology 31:35–38, 1969.

Way, W. L., Costley, E. C., and Way, E. L.: Respiratory sensitivity of the newborn infant to meperidine and morphine. Clin. Pharmacol. Ther. 6:454–461, 1965.

Wingard, L. B., and Cook, D. R.: Clinical pharmacokinetics of muscle relaxants. J. Clin. Pharmacol. 2:330–343, 1977.

Winters, R. W.: The Body Fluids in Pediatrics. Boston, Little, Brown & Co., 1973.

Choanal Atresia

Carpenter, R. J., and Neel, H. B.: Correction of congenital choanal atresia in children and adults. Laryngoscope 87:1304–1311, 1977.

Caldarelli, D. D., and Griedberg, S. A.: Transnasal microsurgical correction of choanal atresia. Laryngoscope 87:2023–2030, 1977.

Healy, G. B., McGill, T., Jako, G. J., et al.: Management of choanal atresia with the carbon dioxide laser. Ann. Otol. 87:658–662, 1978.

Katlin, F. I.: Choanal atresia. In Ravitch, M. M., Welch, K. J., Benson, C. D., et al. (eds.): Pediatric

Surgery. 3rd ed. Chicago, Year Book Medical Publishers, 1979, pp. 303–304.

Winther, L. K.: Congenital choanal atresia. Arch. Otolaryngol. 104:72–78, 1978.

Pierre Robin Syndrome

Alfery, D. D., Ward, C. F., Harwood, I. R., and Mannino, F. L.: Airway management for a neonate with congenital fusion of the jaws. Anesthesiology 51:340–342, 1979.

Hanson, J. W., and Smith, D. W.: U-shaped palatal defect in the Robin anomalad: Development and clinical relevance. J. Pediatr. 87(1):30–33, 1975.

Mallory, S. B., and Paradise, J. L.: Glossoptosis revisited: On the development and resolution of airway obstruction in the Pierre Robin syndrome. Pediatrics 64(6):946–948, 1979.

Welch, K. J., and Hendren, W. H.: Pierre Robin syndrome. In Ravitch, M. M., Welch, K. J., Benson, C. D., et al. (eds.): Pediatric Surgery. 3rd ed. Chicago, Year Book Medical Publishers, 1979, pp. 327–328.

Laryngeal Papilloma

Bone, R. C., Feren, A. P., Nahum, A. M., and Winkelhake, B. G.: Laryngeal papillomatosis: Immunologic and viral basis for therapy. Laryngoscope 86:341–348, 1976.

Norton, M. L., Strong, M. S., Vaughan, C. W., et al.: Endotracheal intubation and Venturi (jet) ventilation for laser microsurgery of the larynx. Ann. Otol. 85:656–663, 1976.

Norton, M. L., and De Vos, P.: New endotracheal tube for laser surgery of the larynx. Ann. Otol. 87:554–557, 1978.

Shipkowitz, N. L., Holper, J. C., Worland, M. C., and Holinger, P. H.: Evaluation of an autogenous laryngeal papilloma vaccine. Laryngoscope 77:1047–1066, 1967.

Simpson, G. T., Healy, G. B., McGill, T., Strong, M. S.: Benign tumors and lesions of the larynx in children. Surgical excision by CO_2 laser. Ann. Otol. 88:479–485, 1979.

Snow, J. C., Kripke, B. J., Strong, M. S., et al.: Anesthesia for carbon dioxide laser microsurgery on the larynx and trachea. Anesth. Analg. 53(4):507–512, 1974.

Snow, J. C., Norton, M. L., Saluja, T. S., and Estanislao, A. F.: Fire hazard during CO_2 laser microsurgery on the larynx and trachea. Anesth. Analg. 55(1):146–147, 1976.

Vourc'h, G., Tannieres, M. L., and Freche, G.: Anesthesia for microsurgery of the larynx using a carbon dioxide laser. Anaesthesia 34:53–57, 1979.

Tracheal Esophageal Fistula

Avery, G. B., Randolph, J. G., and Weaver, T.: Gastric acidity in the first day of life. Pediatrics 37(6):1005–1007, 1966.

Berci, G.: Analysis of new optical systems in bronchoesophagology. Ann. Otol. 87:451–460, 1978.

Buker, R. H., Cox, W. A., Pauling, F. W., and Seitter, G.: Complications of congenital tracheoesophageal fistula. Amer. J. Surg. 124(6):705–710, 1972.

Chalon, J., Ali, M., Ramanathan, S., and Turndord, H.: The humidification of anesthetic gases: Its importance and control. Canad. Anaesth. Soc. J. 26(5):361–366, 1979.

Faro, R. S., Goodwin, C. D., Organ, C. H., et al.: Tracheal agenesis. Ann. Thorac. Surg. 28(3):295–299, 1979.

Greenwood, R. D., Rosenthal, A.: Cardiovascular malformations associated with tracheoesophageal fistula and esophageal atresia. Pediatrics 57(1):87–91, 1976.

Holder, T. M.: Current trends in the management of esophageal atresia and tracheoesophageal fistula. Am. Surg. 44(1):31–36, 1978.

Kluth, D.: Atlas of esophageal atresia. J. Pediatr. Surg. 11:901–919, 1976.

Koop, C. E., Schnaufer, L., and Broennie, A. M.: Esophageal atresia and tracheoesophageal fistula: supportive measures that affect survival. Pediatrics 54(5):558–564, 1974.

LaSalle, A. J., Andrassy, R. J., Ver Steeg, K., and Ratner, I.: Congenital tracheoesophageal fistula without esophageal atresia. J. Thorac. Cardiovasc. Surg. 78(4):583–588, 1979.

Miclat, N. H., Hodgkinson, R., and Marx, G. F.: Neonatal gastric pH. Anesth. Analg. 57:98–101, 1978.

Myers N. A., and Aberdeen, E.: The esophagus. In Ravitch, M. M., Welch, K. J., Benson, C. D., et al. (eds.): Pediatric Surgery. 3rd ed. Chicago, Year Book Medical Publishers, 1979, pp. 446–469.

Ruder, C. B., and Glaser, L. C.: Anesthetic management of laryngotracheoesophageal cleft. Anesthesiology 47:65–67, 1977.

Yamashita, M., Chinyanga, H. M., and Steward, D. J.: Posterior laryngeal cleft — anesthetic experiences. Canad. Anaesth. Soc. J. 26(6):502–505, 1979.

Neonatal Respiratory Distress Syndrome

Avery, M. E.: The Lung and Its Disorders in the Newborn Infant. 3rd ed., Philadelphia, W. B. Saunders Co., 1974.

Coates, A. L., Bergsteinsson, J., Desmond, K., et al.: Long-term pulmonary sequelae of the Wilson-Mikity Syndrome. J. Pediatr. 92(2):247–252, 1978.

Donat, J. F., Okazaki, H., Clienberg, F., and Reagan, T. J.: Intraventricular hemorrhages in full and preterm infants. Mayo. Clin. Proc. 52:437–441, 1978.

Farrell, P. M., and Avery, M. E.: Hyaline membrane disease. Amer. Rev. Resp. Dis. 111:657–688, 1975.

Fujiwara, T., Maeta, H., Chida, S., et al.: Artificial surfactant therapy in hyaline-membrane disease. Lancet 1:55–58, 1980.

Gregory, G. A., Kitterman, J. A., Phibbs, R. H., et al.: Treatment of the idiopathic respiratory distress syndrome with contiguous positive airway pressure. N. Engl. J. Med. 284:1331–1340, 1971.

Hack, M., Fanaroff, A. A., and Merkatz, I. R.: The low-birth-weight infant — evolution of a changing outlook. N. Engl. J. Med. 301:1162–1165, 1979.

Krauss, A. N., Levin, A. R., Grossman, H., and Auld, P. A. M.: Physiologic studies on infants with Wilson-Mikity syndrome. Ventilation perfusion abnormalities and cardiac catheterization angiography. J. Pediatr. 77(1):27–36, 1970.

Lou, H. C., Lassen, N. A., and Friss-Hanson, B.: Is arterial hypertension crucial for the development for cerebral hemorrhage in premature infants? Lancet 1:1215–1217, 1979.

Lou. H. C.. Lassen. N. A.. Tweed. W. A.. et al.: Pres-
sure passive cerebral blood flow and breakdown of the blood-brain barrier in experimental fetal asphyxia. Acta Paediatr. Scand. 68:57–63, 1979.

Northway, W. H., Rosan, R. C., and Porter, D. Y.: Pulmonary disease following respirator therapy of hyaline-membrane disease. Bronchopulmonary dysplasia. N. Engl. J. Med. 276(7):357–368, 1967.

Papeile, L., Burstein, J., Burstein, R., et al.: Relationship of intravenous sodium bicarbonate infusions and cerebral intraventricular hemorrhage. J. Pediatr. 93:834–836, 1978.

Polgar, G., and Weng, T. R.: The functional development of the respiratory system. Amer. Rev. Resp. Dis. 120:625–695, 1979.

Ross, B., Cowett, R. M., and Oh, W.: Renal function of low birth weight infants during the first two months of life. Pediatr. Res. 11:1162–1164, 1977.

Teberg, A., Hodgman, J. E., Wu, P. Y. K., and Spears, R. L.: Recent improvement in outcome for the small premature infant. Follow-up of infants with a birth weight of less than 1,500 grams. Clin. Pediatr. 16(4):307–313, 1977.

Thibeault, D. W., and Gregory, G. A.: Neonatal Pulmonary Care. Menlo Park, Addison-Wesley Publishing Co., 1979.

Thomas, D. B.: Hyperosmolarity and intraventricular hemorrhage in premature babies. Acta Paediatr. Scand. 65:429–432, 1976.

Thurlbeck, W. H., and Abell, M. R.: The Lung Structure, Function and Disease. Baltimore, Williams & Wilkins Co., 1978.

Torday, J., Carson, L., and Lawson, E. E.: Saturated phosphatidylcholine in amniotic fluid and prediction of the respiratory-distress syndrome. N. Engl. J. Med. 301:1013–1018, 1979.

Watts, J. L., Ariagno, R. L., and Brady, J. P.: Chronic pulmonary diseases in neonates after artificial ventilation: Distribution of ventilation and pulmonary interstitial emphysema. Pediatrics 60:273–281, 1977.

Wilson, M. G., and Mikity, V. G.: A new form of respiratory disease in premature infants. Am. J. Dis. Child. 99:489–499, 1960.

Congenital Lobar Emphysema

Cote, R. J.: The anesthetic management of congenital lobar emphysema. Anesthesiology 49:296–298, 1978.

Eger, E. I., II, and Saidman, L. J.: Hazards of nitrous oxide anesthesia in bowel obstruction and pneumothorax. Anesthesiology 26:61–66, 1965.

Hislop, A., and Reid, L.: New pathological findings in emphysema of childhood: I. Polyalveolar lobe with emphysema. Thorax 25:682–690, 1970.

Jones, J. C., Almond, C. H., Snyder, H. M., et al.: Lobar emphysema and congenital heart disease in infancy. J. Thorac. Cardiovasc. Surg. 49:1–10, 1965.

Martin, J. T.: Case history number 93: Congenital lobar emphysema. Anesth. Analg. 55(6):869–873, 1976.

Pierce, W. S., DeParedes, C. G.: Friedman, S., et al.: Concomitant congenital heart disease and lobar emphysema in infants: Incidence, diagnosis and operative management. Ann. Surg. 172:951–956, 1970.

Ravitch, M. M.: Congenital lobar emphysema. In Ravitch. M. M.. Welch. K. J.. Benson. C. D.. et al.

(eds.): Pediatric Surgery. 3rd ed. Chicago, Year Book Medical Publishers, 1979, pp. 524–525.

Ravitch, M. M.: Congenital cystic disease of the lung. *In* Ravitch, M. M., Welch, K. J., Benson, C. D., et al. (eds.): Pediatric Surgery. 3rd ed. Chicago, Year Book Medical Publishers, 1979, pp. 536–541.

Biliary Disease

Adelman, S.: Prognosis of uncorrected biliary atresia: An update. J. Pediatr. Surg. *13*(4):389–391, 1978.

Bill, A. H., Haas, J. E., and Foster, G. L.: Biliary atresia: Histopathologic observations and reflections upon its natural history. J. Pediatr. Surg. *12*(6):977–982, 1977.

Hood, J. M., Koep, L. J., Peters, R. L., et al.: Liver transplantation for advanced liver disease with alpha₁-antitrypsin deficiency. N. Engl. J. Med. *302*:272–275, 1980.

Howard, E. R., and Mowat, A. P.: Extrahepatic biliary atresia. Recent developments in management. Arch. Dis. Child. 52:825–827, 1977.

Kasai, M., Kimura, S., Asakura, Y., et al.: Surgical treatment of biliary atresia. J. Pediatr. Surg. *3*(6):665–675, 1968.

Kasi, M., Watanabi, I., and Ohia, R.: Follow-up studies of longterm survivors after hepatic portoenterostomy for "noncorrectable" biliary atresia. J. Pediatr. Surg. *10*(2):173–182, 1975.

Lilly, R. J., and Altman, R. P.: Biliary tree. *In* Ravitch, M. M., Welch, K. J., Benson, C. D., et al. (eds.): Pediatric Surgery. 3rd ed., Chicago, Year Book Medical Publishers, 1979, pp. 827–838.

Congenital Diaphragmatic Hernia

Berdon, W. E., Baker, D. H., and Amoury, R.: The role of pulmonary hypoplasia in the prognosis of newborn infants with diaphragmatic hernia and eventration. Amer. J. Roentgen. *103*(2):413–421, 1968.

Boix-Ochoa, J., Natal, A., Canals, J., et al.: The important influence of arterial blood gases on the prognosis of congenital diaphragmatic hernia. World J. Surg. *1*:783–787, 1977.

Bray, A. J.: Congenital diaphragmatic hernia. Anaesthesia *34*:567–577, 1979.

Dibbins, A. W., and Wiener, E. S.: Mortality from neonatal diaphragmatic hernia. J. Pediatr. Surg. *9*(5):653–662, 1974.

Eger, E. I., II, and Saidman, L. J.: Hazards of nitrous oxide anesthesia in bowel obstruction and pneumothorax. Anesthesiology 26:61–66, 1975.

Erlich, F. E., and Salzberg, A. M.: Pathophysiology and management of congenital posterolateral diaphragmatic hernias. Am. Surgeon 44:26–30, 1978.

Greenwood, R. D., Rosenthal, A., Nadas, A. S.: Cardiovascular abnormalities associated with congenital diaphragmatic hernia. Pediatrics *57*(1):92–97, 1976.

Harrison, M. R., Bjordal, R. I., Langmark, F., and Knutrud, O.: Congenital diaphragmatic hernia: the hidden mortality. J. Pediatr. Surg. *13*(3):227–230, 1978.

Holder, T. M., and Ashcraft, K. W.: Congenital diaphragmatic hernia, Ravitch, M. M., Welch, K. J., Benson, C. D., et al. (eds.): *In* Pediatric Surgery. 3rd ed., Chicago, Year Book Medical Publishers, 1979, pp. 432–435.

Kerr, A. A.: Lung function in children after repair of congenital diaphragmatic hernia. Arch. Dis. Child. 52(11):902–903, 1977.

Levin, D. L., Hyman, A. I., Heymann, M. A., and Rudolph, A. M.: Fetal hypertension and the development of increased pulmonary vascular smooth muscle: a possible mechanism for persistent pulmonary hypertension of the newborn infant. J. Pediatr. 92:265–269, 1978.

Levin, D. L.: Morphologic analysis of the pulmonary vascular bed in congenital left-sided diaphragmatic hernia. J. Pediatr. 92(5):805–809, 1978.

Levy, R. J. Rosenthal, A., Freed, M., et al.: Persistent pulmonary hypertension in a newborn with congenital diaphragmatic hernia: successful management with tolazoline. Pediatrics 60:740–742, 1977.

Merin, R. G.: Congenital diaphragmatic hernia: From the anesthesiologist's viewpoint. Anesth. Analg. 45(1):44–52, 1966.

Munizaga, J., Allison, M. J., and Aspillaga, E.: Diaphragmatic hernia associated with strangulation of the small bowel in an Atacamena mummy. Am. J. Phys. Anthrop. 48:17–19, 1978.

Murdock, A. I., Burrington, J. B., and Swyer, P. R.: Alveolar to arterial oxygen tension difference and venous admixture in newly born infants with congenital diaphragmatic herniation through the foramen of Bochdalek. Biol. Neonate 17:161–172, 1971.

Naeye, R. L., Shochat, S. J., Whitman, V., and Maisels, M. J.: Unsuspected pulmonary vascular abnormalities associated with diaphragmatic hernia. Pediatrics 58(6):902–906, 1976.

Nishibayashi, S. W., Andrassy, R. J., and Wooley, M. M.: Congenital cystic adenomatoid malformation. Clin. Pediatr. 12(18):760–761, 1979.

Peckham, G. J., and Fox, W. W.: Physiologic factors affecting pulmonary artery pressure in infants with persistent pulmonary hypertension. J. Pediatr. 93(6):1005–1010, 1978.

Priebe, C. J., and Wichern, W. A.: Ventral hernia with a skin-covered Silastic sheet for newborn infants with a diaphragmatic hernia. Surgery 82(2):569–572, 1977.

Tudehope, D. I.: Persistent pulmonary hypertension of the newborn. Med. J. Aust. *1*:13–15, 1979.

Abdominal Wall Defects

Filston, H. C., and Izant, R. J.: Translocation of the umbilical artery to the lower abdomen: An adjunct to the postoperative monitoring of arterial blood gases in major abdominal wall defects. J. Pediatr. Surg. 10:225–229, 1975.

Karamanian, A., Kravath, R., Nagashima, H., and Gentsch, H. H.: Anaesthetic management of "prune belly" syndrome. Case report. Br. J. Anaesth. 46:897–899, 1974.

Moore, T. C.: Gastroschisis and omphalocele: Clinical differences. Surgery 82(5):561–568, 1977.

Schuster, S. R.: Omphalocele, hernia of the umbilical cord and gastroschisis. *In* Ravitch, M. M., Welch, K. J., Benson, C. D., et al. (eds.): Pediatric Surgery. 3rd ed. Chicago, Year Book Medical Publishers, 1979, pp. 778–801.

Stringel, G., and Filler, R. M.: Prognostic factors in omphalocele and gastroschisis. J. Pediatr. Surg. 14(5):515–517, 1979.

Thomas, I. T., and Smith, D. W.: Oligohydramnios,

cause of the nonrenal features of Potter's syndrome, including pulmonary hypoplasia. J. Pediatr. 84(6):811–814, 1974.

Welch. K. J.: Abdominal musculature deficiency syndrome. In Ravitch, M. M., Welch, K. J., Benson, C. D., et al. (eds.): Pediatric Surgery. 3rd ed., Chicago and London, Year Book Medical Publishers, 1979, pp. 1220–1231.

Woodard, J. R.: The prune belly syndrome. Urol. Clin. North Am. 5(1):75–93, 1978.

5

Diseases of the Endocrine System

By JOHN WILLIAM PENDER, M.D.,
and LAWRENCE V. BASSO, M.D.

Parathyroid Glands
Disorders of Calcium Metabolism —
Parathyroid Gland
Abnormalities
Metabolic Bone Disease
Anesthesia for Patient with
Hyperparathyroidism
Thyroid Gland
Pathophysiology
Thyroid Function Tests
Diseases of the Thyroid Gland
Hypothyroidism
General Surgical Problems
Anesthesia for the Hyperthyroid Patient
Anesthesia for the Hypothyroid Patient
Pituitary Gland
Pathophysiology
Diseases of the Anterior Pituitary Gland
Hyperfunction of the Pituitary Gland
Diseases of the Posterior Pituitary Gland
Management of the Patient with
Panhypopituitarism Undergoing
Hypophysectomy
Anesthesia for Operations on the
Pituitary Gland

Adrenal Cortex
Pathophysiology
Adrenocortical Hypofunction (Addison's
Disease)
Adrenocortical Hyperfunction (Cushing's
Syndrome); Aldosteronism
Anesthesia for Patient with Disease of
Adrenal Cortex
Adrenal Medulla — Pheochromocytoma
Pathophysiology
Laboratory Tests
Pre- and Postoperative Management of
Patient with Pheochromocytoma
Anesthesia for Patient with
Pheochromocytoma
**Diabetes Mellitus — Management of the
Surgical Patient**
Pathophysiology
Preoperative Assessment and
Postoperative Management of the
Diabetic Patient
Surgery in the Diabetic Patient
Problems During Operation
**Hyperinsulinism — Islet Cell Tumors of the
Pancreas**
Anesthesia for the Patient with Hyperinsulinism

INTRODUCTION

The primary factor in successful surgical treatment of endocrine diseases is a complete and accurate preoperative diagnosis. Sometimes the differential diagnosis is difficult and may require the expertise of the endocrinologist, radiologist, and clinical pathologist. Armed with a complete and accurate diagnosis, the anesthesiologist and surgeon can offer the patient better relief of his symptoms and a more appealing prognosis.

PARATHYROID GLANDS

DISORDERS OF CALCIUM METABOLISM — PARATHYROID GLAND ABNORMALITIES

Physiology

Serum calcium concentration is maintained at the normal level of 9.5 to 10.5 mg per 100 ml by the effects of both parathyroid hormone (PTH) and vitamin D. When the

155

ionized calcium decreases, this acts as a potent stimulus to the release of parathyroid hormone (PTH). Parathyroid hormone increases tubular reabsorption of calcium and decreases tubular reabsorption of phosphate to raise serum calcium. A renal phosphate leak is the result of excessive PTH secretion. Calcitonin (produced in the C-cells of the thyroid gland) antagonizes the effects of PTH and is released in response to a high serum ionized calcium. Approximately 50 per cent of the serum calcium is bound to serum proteins (albumin). Forty per cent of the serum calcium is ionized, and the remaining 10 per cent is bound to such chelating agents as citrate. If the serum protein concentration decreases, the total serum calcium will also decrease. Likewise, if the serum proteins increase (such as occurs in myeloma), the total serum calcium will increase. Acidosis tends to increase the ionized calcium, while alkalosis tends to decrease it. There may be a slight tendency for the serum calcium level to drop with age, with a concomitant elevation of the serum PTH, perhaps contributing to the osteoporosis associated with the aging process.

In the last few years great strides have been made in our understanding of vitamin D metabolism. Cholecalciferol is synthesized in the skin by the effects of ultraviolet light. Cholecalciferol is hydroxylated in the liver to form 25-hydroxycholecalciferol. The 25-hydroxy derivative is further hydroxylated in the kidney to form 1,25 dihydroxy-cholecalciferol ($1,25(OH)_2D_3$). The 1,25 dihydroxy derivative is by far the most potent vitamin D compound yet discovered. $1,25(OH)_2D_3$ stimulates absorption of both calcium and phosphorus from the GI tract. Thus vitamin D provides the substrates for the formation of mineralized bone. $1,25(OH)_2D_3$ may also directly enhance mineralization of newly formed osteoid matrix in bone. Vitamin D derivatives also seem to work synergistically with parathyroid hormone in bringing about increased resorption of bone. Clinically, this is an important point because immobilization alone tends to increase bone reabsorption, and if the patient is on a vitamin D derivative, bone reabsorption may be increased further. Evidence now indicates that the hydroxylation of 25-hydroxycholecalciferol is controlled in the kidney by PTH and the phosphorus level. An elevated PTH and hypophosphatemia tend to accentuate the synthesis of $1,25(OH)_2D_3$, while low levels of PTH and high levels of phosphate will turn off the synthesis of $1,25(OH)_2D_3$ in the kidney. PTH maintains a normal calcium level in blood by increasing calcium reabsorption from bone, by promoting synthesis of $1,25(OH)_2D_3$, which, in turn, enhances calcium reabsorption from the gut, and, finally, PTH directly increases calcium reabsorption from the renal tubule.

The work-up of disorders of calcium metabolism has been greatly helped by the measurement of parathyroid hormone (PTH) in blood. But there have been several problems with the radioimmunoassay of PTH. A biologically inactive precursor of PTH known as proparathyroid hormone is cleaved in the parathyroid gland itself and forms parathyroid hormone, which is secreted directly into the blood. In the blood, at least two fragments are then formed from the native hormone. Thus, at least three parathyroid hormones exist in blood. One is the native hormone, another is the N-terminal fragment, which is biologically active and has a short half-life, and still a third is the C-carboxy fragment, which is biologically inactive and has a long half-life. Different laboratories measure different fragments, depending upon which kind of antibodies are formed in preparation for the radioimmunoassay. Many laboratories now measure the biologically inactive C-carboxy fragment accurately. Despite these problems, the PTH assay is extremely useful in evaluating patients with hypercalcemia. It is now possible to measure 25-hydroxycholecalciferol, and soon the assay for $1,25(OH)_2D_3$ should also be available.

Hypercalcemia

Patients with hypercalcemia present with a variety of symptoms that can often be nonspecific and misleading. The level of the blood calcium is often related to the degree and severity of symptoms. With calcium levels above 14 mg per 100 ml, signs and symptoms such as anorexia, nausea, vomiting, abdominal pain, constipation, polyuria, tachycardia, and dehydration may occur. Psychosis and obtundation are usually the end results of severe and prolonged hypercalcemia. Band keratopathy is a most unusual physical finding. Patients with hyperparathyroidism present commonly with a history of calcium-containing renal stones. Bone disease in hyperparathyroidism, such as subperiosteal resorption, can also be seen in x-rays of the teeth and hands. Severe bone disease in hyperparathyroidism, such as osteitis fibrosa cystica, is only very rarely seen these days. It is usually only seen in older patients who have had long-standing disease (perhaps up to 20 years). The older patient with severe osteopenia and perhaps vertebral compression fractures should also be a suspect for the diagnosis of hyperparathyroidism. Many patients with hyperparathyroidism can tolerate blood calcium levels of 12 mg per 100 ml without any symptoms whatsoever and they are often discovered accidentally on a multiphasic screening examination. Some patients with mildly elevated blood calcium (below 11.5 mg per 100 ml) will have quite vague neuromuscular complaints and present first to the rheumatologist for consultation. It was previously thought that a single parathyroid adenoma was the chief cause of the hypercalcemia of hyperparathyroidism. In recent years, however, it has been recognized that parathyroid hyperplasia, usually involving all four parathyroid glands, may be a major cause of the hyperparathyroid syndrome. Carcinoma of the parathyroid glands is extremely rare. Different institutions report varying incidences of parathyroid adenomas versus hyperplastic glands. It is conceivable that all adenomas begin as hyperplasia. Therefore, for any one patient, exactly where in the natural history of the disease an operation occurs may determine whether hyperplasia or an adenoma is found.

Patients with hyperparathyroidism have elevated calcium and low serum phosphate levels. A very mild hyperchloremic acidosis may be present. The PTH level is usually elevated. The only two situations in which hypercalcemia would be associated with a high PTH level are hyperparathyroidism and the ectopic PTH syndrome (usually a tumor of the lung or kidney that is producing a biologically active fragment of parathyroid hormone). All other causes of hypercalcemia are associated with either normal or, more appropriately, low levels of PTH. When a patient presents with an extremely high blood calcium level (above 14 mg/100 ml), this is more likely due to a distant cancer than to hyperparathyroidism. Overall, about 50 per cent of all cases of hypercalcemia are due to cancer invading bone. The technetium diphosphonate bone scan is positive in a high percentage of cancers that have metastasized to bone. Myeloma is another important cancer that is associated with hypercalcemia. The isotope bone scan is sometimes normal in this disease.

A number of other anomalies have to do with excessive absorption of calcium from the gastrointestinal tract. These abnormalities include 1) milk-alkali syndrome, which is usually due to excessive ingestion of calcium-containing antacids; 2) vitamin D intoxication; and 3) sarcoidosis, which is associated with hypersensitivity of the gastrointestinal tract to vitamin D. Hyperthyroidism is occasionally associated with increased bone resorption, and hypercalcemia may be present. Many patients with hyperthyroidism also have coexistent hyperparathyroidism. Some patients become hypercalcemic on thiazide diuretics. Thiazides increase the tubular reabsorption of calcium and may even enhance the PTH effects on the renal tubule. Most patients who have significant hypercalcemia associated with thiazide diuretics have hyperparathyroidism. An important cause of increased bone reabsorption, and occasionally mild hypercalcemia, is prolonged immobilization. Immobilization in any situation that is already associated with increased bone reabsorption, such as Paget's disease or ingestion of large quantities of vitamin D, can result in exaggerated hypercalcemia and excessive bone reabsorption. Table 5–1 lists the different causes of hypercalcemia and the appropriate laboratory studies necessary to differentiate them. In addition to the blood calcium and phosphate, the bony fraction of the alkaline phosphatase, creatinine, electrolytes, and urinary calcium level, as well as the appropriate skeletal x-rays and isotope bone scan, can all help in arriving at the correct diagnosis.

While the PTH level is elevated in both hyperparathyroidism and in patients with ectopic PTH syndrome, if the C-carboxy terminal fragment is measured, PTH levels are higher for a given serum calcium in hyperparathyroidism than in cancers associated with PTH fragment production. There have been a few case reports of some lymphoproliferative malignancies associat-

Table 5–1 *Differential Diagnosis of Hypercalcemia*

	Serum Phosphorus	Serum Alkaline Phosphatase	Creatinine	Urinary Calcium	Blood Parathyroid Hormone	Comments
Cancer						
Metastatic	N	↑	N	↑	N or ↑	Osteolytic lesion bone scan is +
Ectopic PTH production	→N	N or ↑	N	↑	↑ or N →	Cancer of lung and kidney common
Myeloma	N	N or ↑	↑	↑	→	Plasma protein ↑
Hyperparathyroidism	→	N or ↑	N	N or ↑	↑	Subperiosteal resorption, Kidney stones
Milk-alkali syndrome	N	N	↑	N	→	Alkalosis; hx CA intake
Vitamin D						
intoxication	←N	N or ←↑	←N	←↑	→→	Vitamin D levels ↑
Hyperthyroidism	N	N or ←↑	N	←↑	→	T₄ or T₃ levels ↑
Sarcoid	N	N or ←↑	N	←↑	→	Plasma proteins ↑
Thiazides	N or →	N or ←↑	N	N' or →	N or ↑	Coexistent hyperparathyroidism often
Adrenal insufficiency	N	N	N or ↑	N	→	Hyponatremia, Hyperkalemia
Immobilization	N	N	N	←↑	N	If fracture, alkaline phosphatase ↑
Paget's disease	N	↑↑	N	←↑	N	Bone scan is +

↑ = elevated.
↑↑ = markedly elevated.
N = normal.

ed with production of a prostaglandin that is in turn associated with increased bone reabsorption and hypercalcemia. Thus, cancer may produce hypercalcemia by at least three mechanisms: 1) metastasis to bone with increased bone reabsorption; 2) production by the cancer of a biologically active fragment of PTH; and 3) production of a prostaglandin that causes bone reabsorption.

Elevation of the bone fraction of alkaline phosphatase (heat labile) usually means excessive breakdown of osteoid tissue. It can be seen in any situation in which either increased bone turnover or significant unmineralized osteoid is present. Very high alkaline phosphatase is seen in Paget's disease where bone turnover is extremely high. Any state associated with excessive PTH can be associated with a high bony alkaline phosphatase, such as hyperparathyroidism or the secondary hyperparathyroidism of renal disease. However osteomalacia, in which bone turnover is extremely low but a large amount of unmineralized osteoid is present, is associated with a high rate of osteoid breakdown and therefore a high alkaline phosphatase. Urinary hydroxyproline is also a specific measure of osteoid breakdown.

A number of patients have been described with renal stones, normal blood calcium, normal to mildly elevated PTH levels, and very high urinary cyclic AMP levels. It is now thought that these patients have normocalcemic hyperparathyroidism, and many have been found to have parathyroid pathology at surgery. The high cyclic AMP levels in the urine are a reflection of PTH activity (perhaps a PTH fragment that affects only the kidney and not bone).

Treatment of Hypercalcemia. The treatment of severe hypercalcemia (especially above levels of 14–16 mg/100 ml) constitutes a medical emergency, and often treatment must be begun before the diagnosis is complete. There is no way to relate the signs and symptoms any one patient experiences to the level of the blood calcium. In an extreme situation it is possible to have one patient who is almost asymptomatic, with a calcium of 14, while another who has an identical blood calcium level will have severe polyuria, tachycardia, dehydration, and even psychosis. Age seems to be a factor; that is, for any given calcium level, the patient above age 60 will more likely be

symptomatic than will a younger patient. Tachyarrhythymias, including sinus tachycardia, are extremely common and usually out of proportion to the degree of volume depletion. Occasionally heart block will result. Extreme care must be exercised in the use of digitalis derivatives for patients with hypercalcemia. Digitalis intoxication occurs quite easily in the presence of hypercalcemia. Digitalis toxicity arrhythymias are extremely common in this setting. The Q-T interval on the ECG tends to be short but may lengthen when the calcium is above 16 mg per 100 ml.

In general, any patient with a calcium level of 16 mg per 100 ml should be considered a medical emergency. A few patients with calcium levels of 14 mg per 100 ml (especially older patients) will also qualify for emergency treatment. The most important initial step for the medical treatment of hypercalcemia is rehydration. The patient should be hydrated with normal saline or 0.5 N saline while careful monitoring of the central venous pressure is carried out. One liter may be given every three to four hours. Along with saline, furosemide 20 to 40 milligrams should be administered every 6 to 8 hours. Saline causes a calciuria, and this is augmented by furosemide. Furosemide also prevents volume overload that might result from saline administration. Simultaneous potassium infusion is important (20–30 mEq KCl per hour intravenously if renal function is normal). Hypokalemia may develop during furosemide diuresis and predispose to tachyarrhythymias. In general, patients with hypercalcemia tend to have low potassium levels even without diuretic therapy. In addition, it is reasonable to use other forms of treatment simultaneously with saline and furosemide. Corticosteroids (40–60 milligrams of prednisone) reduce the serum calcium in patients with myeloma and other lymphoproliferative diseases. Corticosteroids also are effective in the management of vitamin D intoxication and in patients with hypercalcemia associated with breast cancer. Indomethacin is said to be effective in some patients with cancer-associated hypercalcemia, probably through its prostaglandin inhibiting properties. In recent years one of the most useful drugs for the emergency treatment of hypercalcemia has been the cytotoxic antibiotic mithramycin. This drug markedly inhibits bone resorption and precipitously lowers serum calcium. It has been shown to work in nearly all known cases of hypercalcemia including hyperparathyroidism. The usual dose is 15 to 25 μg/kg as a single intravenous injection. Serum calcium usually falls within 6 to 10 hours and may remain down for as long as a week. It should be used cautiously in patients with hepatic or renal disease, as the dose may have to be reduced in these circumstances. Intravenous phosphate is no longer used as a primary treatment of hypercalcemia, since it is associated with a high incidence of metastatic calcification. Oral phosphate (Neutraphos) is sometimes useful in partially controlling hypercalcemia but up to 6 to 8 grams must be used, and at this dosage diarrhea results. Calcitonin has not proved very useful in controlling hypercalcemia because of its transient effect and the high incidence of antibody formation, which result in its ultimate ineffectiveness.

Management of the Patient with Hyperparathyroidism

The patient with hyperparathyroidism can be either followed or operated on. It is not unreasonable to observe an asymptomatic patient with a calcium of 11.5 mg per 100 ml. However, when the patient has recurrent kidney stones, neuromuscular complaints, and abdominal distress, surgery is the only alternative. Hyperparathyroidism is also associated with hypertension. There is also a tendency to hyperuricemia, mild carbohydrate intolerance, and occasionally pseudogout. The hypertension that is often associated with diminished renal function is not always reversible after successful parathyroidectomy. Even in an asymptomatic patient with a calcium of 14 mg per 100 ml, surgery is necessary, since calcium levels above 14 are associated with significant complications. The patient with hyperparathyroidism should have the calcium level reduced to or below 14 mg per 100 ml by the methods already described before operation. A single adenoma is found at least 80 per cent of the time and the surgeon is reasonably sure of the pathology at the time of surgery. The remaining 20 per cent of the time, either multiple adenomas or hyperplastic glands will be found. It is wise in these circumstances to remove at least three and one half parathyroid glands and to mark the location of the remnant of the fourth with a metal clip. Some experts advocate removing all four parathyroid glands when hyperplasia is found. A failure to remove all the pathology at the first operation will at times necessitate a second operation. Arteriography and venous localization with sampling of PTH levels in thyroidal venous beds will at times provide useful information to the surgeon in the reoperative situation. Unusual locations for parathyroid adenoma include areas behind the esophagus, in the mediastinum and intrathyroid.

Postoperative Management. If all parathyroid tissue has been removed at surgery, the blood calcium will drop precipitously within 24 hours. Even with partial parathyroidectomy, hypocalcemia will often develop quickly after surgery. Undoubtedly suppression of the remaining parathyroid tissue continues for a period of time. If the patient has significant hypocalcemia two weeks after surgery, the hypoparathyroidism is likely to be permanent and chronic vitamin D therapy becomes mandatory. There are a very few patients with hyperparathyroidism and severe bone disease (osteitis fibrosa cystica) who develop profound hypocalcemia following surgery because of marked calcium re-entry into bone following removal of the source of excessive PTH. Treatment of these patients with vitamin D preoperatively seems to prevent this postoperative hypocalcemia. The first symptoms due to acute hypocalcemia are circumoral or extremity paresthesias with associated increased neuromuscular irritability. The latter may be demonstrated by contraction of muscles supplied by the facial nerve following finger tapping over the exit of the nerve in front of the ear (Chvostek's sign) or by carpopedal spasm following occlusion of blood supply to an extremity for three minutes (Trousseau's sign). Neuromuscular irritability is increased in proportion to the degree of hypocalcemia with latent tetany present with serum calcium levels of 7 to 8 mg per 100 ml and frank tonic contractions below calcium levels of 7 mg per 100 ml. If the calcium level drops even further, generalized convulsions and laryngeal stridor may result. Prompt administration of an intravenous solution of 25 ml of 10 per cent calcium gluconate (250 milligrams of calcium) is given in 100 ml of 5 per cent dextrose in water over one hour. Subsequently, calcium gluconate can be given as a continuous intravenous drip (350 mg of calcium in one liter of dextrose in water over 12 to 24 hours) while carefully monitoring the serum calcium level. If the calcium level is still on the low side, serum potassium and magnesium levels should be checked. Both hypomagnesemia and hypokalemia augment the neuromuscular effects of hypocalcemia. Often just restoring the magnesium deficit will correct the hypocalcemia. It is preferable to use oral calcium (one or two grams four times daily of calcium gluconate) when the patient is able to take oral fluids.

During the first week or 10 days following surgery, vitamin D derivatives are avoided in order to allow the suppressed parathyroid tissue (if present) to function. Vitamin D derivatives are always started if the patient has significant hypocalcemia two weeks following surgery. The older vitamin D derivatives include vitamin D_2 (ergocalciferol) and vitamin D_3 (cholecalciferol). Of these derivatives, 40,000 units is equal to approximately one milligram. Therapy in the patient with permanent hypoparathyroidism is begun with 40,000 units daily of either vitamin D_2 or D_3. The dose is increased by 20,000 units every two weeks until the desired calcium level is attained. Vitamin D is fat soluble and the significant fat stores in adipose tissue, muscle, and liver must first be saturated before a therapeutic level is achieved.

Patients with surgical hypoparathyroidism sometimes require huge quantities of vitamin D derivatives (200,000 to 300,000 units or 5 to 7 mg daily) and thus appear to have an end-organ resistance to its effects. In the hypoparathyroid patient it is best to aim for a calcium level of 8.5 to 9.0 mg per 100 ml. While these patients will have a urinary calcium leak because of the absence of PTH, in general it is best to keep the urinary calcium level below 300 milligrams per 24 hours. If the urinary calcium level is above 300 milligrams per 24 hours, the vitamin D dose should be dropped back by 25 per cent of the patient's initial dose. Another vitamin D derivative is dihydrotachysterol (Dygratyl). Doses of 250 to 2000 micrograms of dihydrotachysterol are required to control the hypocalcemia in hypoparathyroidism.

Of great interest are the new vitamin D derivatives 25 hydroxycholecalciferol and $1,25(OH)_2D_3$. 25 hydroxycholecalciferol is 15 times more potent than the parent vitamin D_2 and $1,25(OH)_2D_3$ is about 1500 times more potent. Initial reports indicate that as little as 0.5 to 2.0 micrograms of $1,25(OH)_2D_3$ can control the hypocalcemia of hypoparathyroidism. Since PTH is a major control mechanism for the conversion of 25 hydroxycholecalciferol to $1,25(OH)_2D_3$ in the kidney, the patient with hypoparathyroidism and essentially no PTH probably has a relative lack of $1,25(OH)_2D_3$. $1,25(OH)_2D_3$ has just been released for general use under the trade name Rocaltrol and is now being investigated for use in the management of hypoparathyroid states. Along with the vitamin D preparation, the patient with hypoparathyroidism must be given an adequate amount of calcium by mouth (1 gm calcium gluconate four times daily).

The management of hypoparathyroidism is not easy, and careful follow up of patients is mandatory. A blood calcium and urinary calcium should be checked every six months following surgery. Vitamin D intoxication is an ever present danger. Eventually development of assays for the cholecalciferol derivatives will allow the physician to adjust therapy more precisely. An interesting experimental procedure involves using the diuretic chlorthalidone (50 mg daily) along with a low sodium diet. This has been reported to control hypoparathyroidism without the concomitant use of vitamin D in some cases.

Hypocalcemia

Probably the most common cause of hypocalcemia is surgical removal of the parathyroids. However, the differential diagnosis of hypocalcemia should also include chronic renal insufficiency, malabsorption syndrome, pseudohypoparathyroidism, hypomagnesemia, osteoblastic metastasis to bone, pancreatitis, and the rare autoimmune abnormality of deficiency in multiple endocrine glands. A very rare cause of hypocalcemia is thymic hypoplasia associated with hypoparathyroidism (Di George syndrome). Table 5–2 lists the differential diagnosis of hypocalcemia and some of the appropriate tests that can be used for differentiation. Measurement of PTH is not nearly as useful in differentiating the hypocalcemic states as it is in the hypercalcemic disorders. The vitamin D deficiency of the malabsorption syndrome, osteomalacia (in the adult) and

Table 5-2 *Differential Diagnosis of Hypocalcemia*

	Serum Phosphorus	Serum Alkaline Phosphatase	Creatinine	PTH	Comments
Hypoparathyroidism (usually surgical)	↑	N	N	↓ or 0	Cataract; basal ganglia calcification; other endocrine gland hypofunction
Chronic renal disease (secondary hyperparathyroidism)	↑↑	↑	↑↑	↑↑	Impaired renal 1-25 $(OH)_2D_3$ synthesis
Malabsorption syndrome Vitamin D deficiency	↓↓	↑	N	N or ↓	Vitamin D malabsorption or deficiency (osteomalacia or rickets)
Pseudohypoparathyroid variants	↑	N	N	↑	Metastatic calcification, cataracts, short stature
Hypomagnesemia	↑N	N	N	N or ↑	Malnutrition, alcoholism, malabsorption
Osteoblastic metastasis	N	N or ↑	N	N or ↑	X-ray skeletal, seen in prostatic cancer
Acute pancreatitis	N	N or ↑	N	N or ↑	Mechanism unknown
Low plasma proteins	N	N	N or ↑	N	Ionized calcium may be normal; malnutrition nephrosis

rickets (in the child), is associated with a low serum phosphorus. In all other causes of hypocalcemia the serum phosphorus tends to be elevated. It is disproportionately elevated in chronic renal failure. Cataracts and basal ganglion calcification are seen in both hypoparathyroidism and pseudohypoparathyroidism. Subperiosteal resorption (the hallmark of excessive PTH secretion) is seen mainly in chronic renal failure associated with secondary hyperparathyroidism and in some forms of pseudohypoparathyroidism. The PTH level tends to be disproportionately elevated in chronic renal failure associated with secondary hyperparathyroidism, and there are a few patients with high PTH levels in blood that develop high blood calciums (so-called tertiary hyperparathyroidism). Most of these patients following renal transplantation develop normal calciums, and only a very few turn out to have an autonomous parathyroid adenoma.

Pseudohypoparathyroidism is an unusual entity associated with short stature, round facies, and short metacarpals, as well as parathyroid hyperplasia. It represents in part an end organ resistance to the action of PTH. $1,25(OH)_2D_3$ levels are low in pseudohypoparathyroidism, and replacement of this vitamin D derivative can partially reverse the end organ resistance. Hypomagnesemia impairs PTH release and thus can cause profound hypocalcemia. Hypomagnesmia is common in patients with alcoholism, malnutrition, or chronic severe malabsorption states. The calcium level may be restored by replacing magnesium. Osteoblastic metastasis associated with increased acquisition of calcium can lower blood calcium. Relative parathyroid insufficiency may account for the persistent hypocalcemia observed in patients with acute pancreatitis.

The acute manifestations of acute hypoparathyroidism have already been discussed with postoperative management of hypercalcemia. The symptoms related to tetany seem to correlate best with the level of the ionized calcium. If alkalosis is present, it is possible for the total calcium to be normal but the ionized calcium low, and symptoms of neuromuscular irritability may result (i.e., hyperventilation syndrome). In slowly developing chronic hypocalcemia, the symptoms may be very mild despite severe hypocalcemia, and this may in part

be due to adaptive changes in the level of the ionized calcium. Even with calcium levels of 6 to 7 mg per 100 ml, minor muscle cramps, fatigue, and mild depression may be the only symptoms. Many patients with a calcium level of 6 to 6.5 mg per 100 ml are totally asymptomatic aside from some mild depression of intellectual function.

Vitamin D derivatives are used in the management of hypoparathyroidism (see preceding section), chronic renal insufficiency with secondary hyperparathyroidism, pseudohypoparathyroidism, the malabsorption syndromes, and other vitamin D deficiency states. Vitamin D deficiency states can at times be adequately managed with small amounts of D_2 or $D_3(100\mu g = 400$ units). Malabsorption syndrome associated with fat malabsorption may require an intramuscular preparation of vitamin D (2000–4000 units daily IM) if adequate oral therapy fails. A high calcium diet (2 gm elemental calcium) is indicated whenever a vitamin D preparation is used. A low phosphorus diet (including use of aluminum hydroxide) is useful in chronic renal failure, but a high phosphate diet (calcium phosphate preparation may be used) is useful in patients with malabsorption syndrome and other vitamin D deficiency states (rickets and osteomalacia. In chronic renal disease the bone abnormalities due to excessive PTH levels (subperiosteal reabsorption) are essentially reversed by 1 or 2 μg of $1,25(OH)_2D_3$ (Rocaltrol). However, the osteomalacic changes in chronic renal disease may not be totally reversed by this potent vitamin D derivative.

Pseudohypoparathyroidism and hypoparathyroidism are managed essentially in the same fashion (see preceding section). Eventually $1,25(OH)_2D_3$ may prove to be useful in both these conditions. Phenothiazines should be used with caution in patients with hypocalcemia (especially hypoparathyroidism), since they may precipitate dystonic reactions. Furosemide may enhance hypocalcemia in patients with hypoparathyroidism.

The patient going to surgery with a low total calcium, and especially a low ionized calcium, is at increased risk. Cardiac muscle irritability as well as skeletal muscle irritability may occur. A variety of arrhythmias have been reported. The characteristic finding on ECG is a prolonged Q-T interval. Hypokalemia and hypomagnesemia may potentiate the cardiac and neuromuscular irritability produced by hypocalcemia. The emergency treatment of hypocalcemia has already been discussed.

METABOLIC BONE DISEASE

The two most important metabolic bone diseases are osteoporosis and osteomalacia. Bone normally consists of a collagen matrix which is mineralized with calcium in the form of an apatite crystal. In osteoporosis there is little bone mass overall; that is, the total bone mass is less than expected for the age and sex of the patient. In osteomalacia there is failure of normal mineralization of the bone matrix, so that the ratio of bone mineral to bone matrix is much less than in either normal bone or purely osteoporotic bone. In normal bone there is a fine balance between bone formation and laying down of collagen matrix (function of the osteoblast cell) and bone resorption (function of the osteoclast cell). If bone resorption increases slightly out of proportion to bone formation, after a long period of time osteoporosis will result. In osteomalacia total bone turnover is greatly slowed down, and matrix is formed, but little or no mineralization takes place. Large areas of undermineralized matrix (called osteoid seams) accumulate, and this remains the most important characteristic of osteomalacic bone seen on bone biopsy. In hyperparathyroidism, subperiosteal resorption or, in its severest form, osteitis fibrosa cystica is a result of increased osteoclastic activity or bone resorption. Early signs of increased bone resorption in primary hyperparathyroidism can be seen in skeletal x-rays of the teeth and hands.

The differential diagnosis of osteoporosis includes the following classifications: 1) genetic, which includes osteogenesis imperfecta and homocystinuria; 2) postmenopausal and senile osteoporosis; 3) endocrine etiologies, such as hyperthyroidism or diabetes mellitus; 4) immobilization, which alone can accentuate osteoporosis enormously; 5) nutritional — scurvy or protein deficiency; 6) bone marrow replacement — myeloma and lymphoma; 7) localized osteoporosis — Sudek's atrophy; 8) drug-related — ethanol and heparin; 9) association with systemic diseases such as rheumatoid arthritis, obstructive lung disease, and chronic renal disease.

The most common causes of osteoporosis are related to aging (senile) and menopause. In a definite subset of patients menopause tends to accentuate the osteoporotic process. These patients may already have diminished bone mass, and symptoms are more likely to occur after menopause when the bone mass becomes threatened enough to result in vertebral compression fractures and fractures of the femoral neck.

Early detection of osteoporosis is not easy. The skeletal x-ray that shows classic demineralized changes in the thoracolumbar spine is already associated with at least 50 to 75 per cent loss of total bone mass. The Singh index is based on looking at the trabecular pattern of radiographs of the femoral head and neck. Certain trabecular patterns drop out early, depending upon the mechanical stress on the femoral neck. It is possible using the Singh index to grade the degree of osteoporosis. The method is, however, at best still qualitative. Photon absorption methods (Cameron-Sorenson apparatus) utilize a source of nonenergetic x-rays from an iodine-125 source. The attenuation of the photon beam as the wrist or arm is scanned can be related to the bone density. The method is reproducible and can be used to some extent to follow a patient on therapy.

What is occurring in the axial skeleton cannot always be related to the appendicular skeleton. Moreover, small changes in bone turnover are not readily discernible. Iliac crest bone biopsy is also useful, and bone mass can be roughly quantitated. Blood calcium, phosphate, and alkaline phosphatase are normal in osteoporosis.

Treatment of osteoporosis remains controversial. Most investigators believe in increasing calcium intake. This is usually given in the form of calcium gluconate, 2 grams daily. Evidence is also mounting that in the postmenopausal female estrogen definitely slows down the osteoporotic process. The use of estrogen must be weighed against the possible development of endometrial carcinoma. There is no evidence that the use of androgenic anabolic steroids, sodium fluoride, or calcitonin is helpful. Vitamin D in the patient with osteoporosis only is probably not helpful. In fact, bone resorption may even be increased by the intake of vitamin D. However, vitamin D can be used in patients with concomitant osteomalacia and osteoporosis. In the surgical patient who will be immobilized in the postoperative period, osteoporosis may be acutely accentuated. The thin, sedentary Caucasian postmenopausal female with little body muscle mass is especially prone to immobilization osteoporosis.

Osteoporosis must be differentiated from osteomalacia before appropriate therapy can be outlined. Vitamin D is definitely indicated in osteomalacia. The iliac crest bone biopsy is especially useful in this regard. The undecalcified bone specimen is fixed with an osteoid stain, and if osteomalacia is present the osteoid seams are widened. The differential diagnosis of osteomalacia includes the following disorders: 1) vitamin D deficiency (rickets in the child and osteomalacia in the adult); 2) vitamin D malabsorption, including postgastrectomy vitamin D malabsorption; 3) liver disease; 4) chronic renal disease; 5) drugs such as phenytoin, corticosteroids, diphosphonate, and fluoride; 6) phosphate depletion; 7) metabolic acidosis (renal tubular acidosis); 8) renal tubular disorders such as Fanconi syndrome; and 9) hereditary hypophosphatasia. Vitamin D deficiency and the malabsorption syndromes are managed with vitamin D and its derivatives as already outlined. Liver disease will eventually be manageable with 25 hydroxycholecalciferol, since in liver disease 25 hydroxylation of D_3 is impaired. A number of drugs have been associated with osteomalacia. Steroids result in a combination of osteoporosis and osteomalacia. Probably all patients on long-term steroid treatment could be on at least 20,000 units of vitamin D_2 twice weekly. The osteomalacia that is associated with chronic metabolic acidosis, such as renal tubular acidosis, is often markedly improved with the addition of bicarbonate to the therapeutic regimen of vitamin D. Any osteomalacic state associated with phosphate depletion or a low serum phosphate is also markedly improved by adding substantial phosphate to the diet in addition to calcium and vitamin D. The metabolic bone disease associated with chronic renal disease (renal osteodystrophy) is actually a combination of subperiosteal resorption, osteitis fibrosis (due to excessive PTH levels), and osteomalacia (due to deficient synthesis of $1,25(OH)_2D_3$) as well as osteoporosis. Further investigation in the use of $1,25(OH)_2D_3$ in renal osteodystrophy continues, but this vitamin D derivative appears to reverse most if not all the abnormalities of bone in chronic renal disease. If a patient on vitamin D is going to be immobilized, vitamin D may be synergistic with the acute bone resorption that occurs with immobilization. A 24 hour urine calcium which is above 200 to 250 milligrams is an indication for cutting back on the dose or stopping the vitamin D derivative altogether during any period of prolonged immobilization. Patients with hypercalcemia related to excess vitamin D therapy are also prone to develop renal calculi.

Paget's disease, though neither an endocrine nor a metabolic disease, is often listed in the differential diagnosis of metabolic bone diseases. Treatment consists of either diphosphonate (sodium etidronate, 5–10 mg/kg/day) or calcitonin. Calcitonin administration is associated with a high incidence of antibodies, which inactivates its effect. Bed rest or immobilization in the patient with Paget's disease often results in hypercalcemia, at times severe. Heart failure is a late and uncommon complication of Paget's disease. A small percentage of patients also develop sarcomatous changes in previously pagetoid areas of bone.

ANESTHESIA FOR PATIENT WITH HYPERPARATHYROIDISM

Agents and Methods. No anesthetic agent seems to be particularly indicated, but the anesthesiologist can contribute to the success of what may be a difficult surgical procedure. Preparation should be made for a prolonged tedious exploration of the entire anterior part of the neck, since all four parathyroid glands may have to be identified and perhaps biopsied. For a second operation, preoperative localization of hypersecreting parathyroid glands by immunoassay of venous blood from lobes of thyroid gland sometimes can reduce the complexity of the operation (Riess, 1974). Use of radionuclide and ultrasound (Crocker et al., 1979) and intravenous methylene blue (Cox et al., 1979) have been found useful in locating and identifying parathyroid glands. When the pathological glands cannot be found in the neck, the mediastinum may be explored. Reliable control of the airway with endotracheal tube under general anesthesia is necessary to allow unrestricted tissue retraction and exploration about the larynx and also to control alterations in respiration caused by possible pneumothorax.

A blood-free operative field facilitates identification of the parathyroid glands (Edis, 1979). This can be promoted by use of the head-up position of the patient, keeping in mind that this position increases the possibility of air embolism. Use of a nonflammable anesthetic agent allows use of the electric cautery in producing hemostasis. Induced hypotensive technique may be considered, or at least both arterial and venous hypertension should be prevented. Overly vigorous assisted respiraton may cause increased mean intrathoracic pressure and increased pressure in the veins of the neck. A moderate degree of extension of the neck aids surgical exposure, but marked extension can lead to compression of the veins by stretched muscles with increased bleeding in upper parts of the wound. On the other hand, vasopressor drugs and other therapy must be available for treatment of any marked arterial hypotension that may result from manipulation about the carotid sinus.

Operative Problems. CIRCULATORY. From clinical experience, circulatory complications do not seem to have been frequent or severe during removal of hyperfunctioning parathyroid glands, even in those patients with severe hypercalcemia. Theoretically, excessive serum calcium might be expected to have adverse effects on the heart. Bronsky et al. (1961) found no change in cardiac rate or rhythm in 35 patients with hypercalcemia. On the electrocardiogram the P-R interval tended to be prolonged and the Q-T interval was inversely proportional to the serum calcium level up to 16 mg per 100 ml. At levels greater than 16 mg per 100 ml, T waves were prolonged and rounded and the Q-T interval became disproportionately long. Voss and Drake (1967) reported one case of primary hyperparathyroidism exhibiting atrioventricular block, sinus arrest with ventricular rates as low as 15 per minute, and bouts of paroxysmal atrial fibrillation that were completely abolished by removal of a parathyroid adenoma. Others have described electrocardiographic changes characteristic of hyperparathyroidism (Schafer and Economou, 1970). The critical toxic level of hypercalcemia seems to be about 16 to 18 mg per 100 ml, though toxic effects vary in different patients. Digitalis in the presence of hypercalcemia in hyperparathyroidism should be used with caution, because both prolong the P-R interval and increase myocardial irritability.

RESPIRATORY. The possibility of mediastinotomy and pneumothorax has been mentioned.

NEUROMUSCULAR. No reported occurrence of altered effect of muscle relaxant drugs in the presence of hypercalcemia of hyperparathyroidism could be found. However, this might be theoretically expected because calcium ions affect membrane transport (Foldes, 1959). The gastrointestinal symptoms of hyperparathyroidism have been attributed to inhibition by calcium ions of transmission of stimuli in sympathetic ganglia, resulting in reduced intestinal neuromuscular excitability and decreased tone (Kerr et al., 1962). Also the lethargy, confusion, and psychosis associated with acute hyperparathyroidisim have been explained to be a result of the effect of calcium ions on transmission of impulses in the central nervous system.

Hypocalcemia was considered to have contributed to prolonged postoperative curarization in one patient, although this was not proved (McKie, 1969).

Postoperative Problems. HYPOPARATHYROIDISM. Most cases of hypoparathyroidism are the result of removal or injury to the parathyroid glands during thyroidectomy (Avioli, 1974). However, transient tetany has been reported in as many as 30 per cent of patients following removal of parathyroid tumors (Schafer and Economou, 1970). The first symptoms are circumoral or extremity paresthesias and increased neuromuscular irritability. The latter may be demonstrated by contraction of muscles supplied by the facial nerve following finger tapping over the exit of the nerve in front of the ear (Chvostek's sign), or by carpopedal spasm following occlusion of blood supply to an extremity for three minutes (Trousseau's sign). Neuromuscular irritability is increased in proportion to the degree of hypocalcemia, with latent tetany at a serum calcium level of 7 to 8 mg per 100 ml and frank tonic contractions below 7 mg per 100 ml. Without prompt treatment, generalized convulsions and laryngeal stridor may interfere with respiration and lead to cyanosis. Death can result. Symtpoms usually occur within the first few days after operation and may persist for up to three months until remaining parathyroid tissue is able to produce adequate parathyroid hormone. If all the parathyroid glands are removed, the condition will be permanent. To prevent life-long medication for prevention of hypoparathyroidism following removal of all glands, autotransplantation of a portion of one gland to an easily accessible location has been used. However, recurrent hyperparathyroidism has been reported to occur from activity of the transplanted gland (Brennan et al., 1978).

Treatment consists of elevation of plasma calcium concentration to approximately normal range. This can be done in an emergency by slow intravenous administration of up to 1 gm of calcium gluconate with extreme care, especially if the patient has been receiving digitalis. The dose may be repeated at intervals or given as slow intravenous drip to keep serum calcium concentration at adequate levels. As soon as oral medication can be taken, 1 gm of calcium gluconate or carbonate three or four times a day with a low phosphate diet may maintain a satisfactory serum calcium level. If the patient does not have sufficient parathyroid tissue to keep the serum calcium level within normal limits, then the problem arises of treating chronic hypoparathyroidism with low phosphate diet, large-dose calcium supplements, and vitamin D in pharmacologic doses (50,000 to 150,000 units per day). Vitamin D therapy should be avoided during the first week of postoperative tetany in order to give the patient's own parathyroid tissue a chance to resume function. The duration of action of vitamin D is measured in months, and once vitamin D therapy is started, it becomes quite difficult to determine when this therapy may be withdrawn.

THYROID GLAND

PATHOPHYSIOLOGY

Thyroid hormone biosynthesis involves four steps. They are as follows: 1) iodide trapping; 2) oxidation of iodide and iodination of tyrosine residues; 3) hormone storage in the colloid of the thyroid gland as part of the large thyroglobulin molecule; 4) proteolysis and release of hormones. All of the above steps are stimulated by pituitary

thyrotropin stimulating hormone (TSH). Proteolysis of stored hormone in the colloid is inhibited by iodide. This occurs in the normal gland but is greatly exaggerated in the thyroid gland of the patient with Graves' disease. The major circulating thyroid hormones are tetraiodothyronine (T4) and triiodothyronine (T3). Only a small amount of T3 is secreted by the normal gland. The major hormone secreted by the normal gland is T4. T4 is considered relatively inactive physiologically compared to T3, which appears to be the major biologically active hormone. In hyper- or hypothyroidism relatively more T3 is secreted than in the normal state. In peripheral tissues there exists a ubiquitous diodinase that converts T4 to T3. Thus T4 appears to be a prohormone for T3. Monodeiodinations can remove either the iodine at the 5' position to yield T3 or the iodine at the 5 position to yield reverse T3 (rT3). Reverse T3 is totally inactive biologically. In general, when T3 levels are depressed, rT3 levels are elevated. In a number of circumstances, rT3 levels are increased, such as gestation, malnutrition, chronic disease, and surgical stress (Fig. 5–1). A feedback circuit exists between the pituitary gland and the circulating thyroid hormones. High levels of thyroid hormones reduce release of pituitary TSH, while low levels result in more TSH release (Fig. 5–2). The mechanism of action of thyroid hormone is complex but involves at least two sites on the cell. Thyroid hormone appears to maintain the Na-K/intracellular-extracellular gradients via an ATPase pump linked to mitochondrial oxygen consumption. Thyroid hormone like the steroid hormones appears to have a specific nuclear receptor that can initiate transcription of genetic information.

THYROID FUNCTION TESTS

Serum T4 by Radioimmunoassay (T4-RIA). The normal plasma range of the T4-RIA is 4.5 to 10 μg/dl. The T4 is high in hyperthyroidism and low in hypothyroidism. Most of the T4 is bound to a plasma protein known as thryoid binding globulin (TBG). Changes in TBG can affect the total T4 level. Estrogens, infectious hepatitis, and genetic factors can elevate the level of the TBG and thus secondarily raise the total T4. Androgens, nephrosis, hypoprotein-

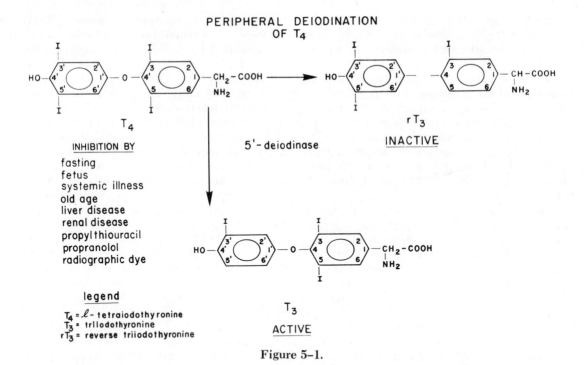

Figure 5–1.

emia, and genetic factors can lower the TBG and thus secondarily lower the total T4.

Resin Triiodothyronine Uptake (RT3U). This important in vitro test depends upon the binding of a tracer amount of radioactive triiodothyronine to an artificial resin. The amount of binding to resin is inversely proportional to the unoccupied binding sites of thyroid binding globulin (TBG). If the T4 level is high because there is an excess of TBG (i.e., estrogen administration), there will be an increase in the number of unoccupied binding sites and the resin uptake will be low. The resin uptake varies in different laboratories but the average is 20 to 25 per cent. If the resin uptake is multiplied by the total T4-RIA, an index is achieved. This index is sometimes called the "corrected T4." The corrected T4 in essence is a measure of the free T4. The "corrected T4" corrects the total T4 level for any changes in TBG concentration or changes in unoccupied binding sites on the TBG molecule. It is very difficult to assay the free T4 level directly, since it amounts to only about 0.5 per cent of the total T4 (approximately 1-2 nanograms/100 ml). The free T4 correlates directly with the metabolic status of the patient. A new radioimmunoassay that can directly measure free T4 is now being evaluated.

Serum Triiodothyronine (T3-RIA). As already discussed, most of the T3 in the normal state comes from the peripheral conversion of T4. In hyperthyroidism excessive T3 is secreted directly in high quantities from the thyroid gland. This extremely potent hormone normally is present in a concentration range of 75 to 200 nanograms per 100 ml. It is important to note that the upper limit of normal tends to drop with each decade of life. Thus, a 20-year-old patient with a level of 190 ng per 100 ml may be perfectly euthyroid while an 80-year-old patient with the same level may be hyperthyroid. The T3-RIA is particularly important in the diagnosis of hyperthyroid states. It probably correlates better with the metabolic status of the patient than the total T4.

Serum Thyroid Stimulating Hormone (TSH). In patients with primary hypothyroidism, the thyroid hormone concentration is low and the TSH level is high. Evidence is accumulating that the TSH level is the most sensitive parameter for the diagnosis of primary hypothyroidism. The TSH level may be elevated even before there are any changes in the circulating level of T4 or T3.

Radioactive Iodine Uptake. The radioactive iodine uptake (RAIU) is measured as the per cent of a tracer that is taken up by

HYPOTHALAMIC PITUITARY THYROID AXIS

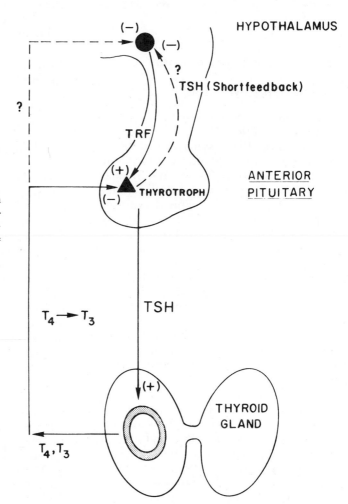

Figure 5–2. TRF = thyrotropin releasing factor; TSH = thyroid stimulating hormone; T3 = triiodothyronine; T4 = 1-tetraiodothyronine; + = stimulation; − = inhibition.

the thyroid in 24 hours. The upper limit of normal has been dropping in recent years because of the increase of iodine in the American diet. The major use of this test is to confirm the diagnosis of hyperthyroidism. The normal range is 10 to 25 per cent. Patients with hyperthyroidism have values above 25 per cent. Patients with subacute thyroiditis can be hyperthyroid but have essentially no uptake. If a patient has used inorganic iodides or dyes (e.g., gallbladder scans or intravenous pyelogram) the radioactive iodine uptake may be low.

Thyroid Scan. Iodine-123 is now used to scan instead of iodine-131. I-123 is a lower energy isotope and thus delivers less radiation to the patient. Radioactive technetium pertechnetate is also an excellent scanning agent but is not nearly as specific in deter-

mining function of the thyroid gland as the iodine isotopes. The scan is particularly useful in diagnosis of thyroid nodules. Functioning thyroid nodules are rarely malignant, while cold or hypofunctioning nodules have a greater probability for malignancy.

Other Tests. The diagnosis of pituitary or hypothalamic disease can be quite complicated. The procedure is often aided by the use of thyrotropin releasing factor. This tripeptide is the hypothalamic factor that brings about release of TSH from the pituitary. It may also be used to confirm the diagnosis of hyperthyroidism. Thyroid antibodies (antithyroglobulin and antimicrosomal) are useful in arriving at the diagnosis of Hashimoto's thyroiditis. Serum thyroglobulin levels tend to be elevated in patients with papillary cancer of the thyroid. It is a useful test with which to follow patients with thyroid cancer who have a recurrence.

DISEASES OF THE THYROID GLAND

Causes of Hyperthyroidism

Graves' disease is the most common hyperthyroid condition. As a rule, these patients have a relatively symmetrical diffusely enlarged thyroid gland. Exophthalmos may or may not be present, and in many ways seems to be independent of the metabolic status of the patient. The symptoms of hyperthyroidism are those generally associated with excessive catecholamine production, such as tachycardia, increased perspiration and heat intolerance, tremor, and weight loss. In actual fact catecholamine production in hyperthyroidism is not increased but it is postulated that the number of receptors for the catecholamines are increased. The net result is the same and thus many presenting symptoms of hyperthyroidism are much like those of a pheochromocytoma. At least one of the causes of Graves' disease is an antibody to the TSH receptor on the thyroid cell. This antibody, known as thyroid stimulating immunoglobulin (TSI), competes with TSH for the receptor and continually stimulates the thyroid cell, resulting in hyperthyroidism. The elderly patient may not always present with the typical signs and symptoms. These patients may present with extreme weakness (due to a myopathy), loss of appetite and weight loss, and personality changes. The thyroid gland may even be normal in size, and exophthalmos is often absent.

Other causes of hyperthyroidism include toxic nodular goiter. These goiters can show both hot and cold nodules on radioactive scanning. Occasionally only a single "hot" nodule which is suppressing the rest of the function of the thyroid gland (Plummer's disease) may be found on scan. Much rarer causes of hyperthyroidism include TSH secreting pituitary tumors, hydatidiform moles associated with hyperthyroidism, and factitious hyperthyroidism. Hashimoto's thyroiditis can also be associated with hyperthyroidism although much more commonly hypothyroidism results. Subacute thyroiditis is transiently associated with mild thyrotoxicosis. A newly described entity is painless thyroiditis associated with transient hyperthyroidism. This latter entity is a lymphocytic thyroiditis associated with low radioactive iodine uptake.

Preparation of the Hyperthyroid Patient for Surgery

In recent years surgery as treatment for the hyperthyroid patient has declined, especially in the patient with Graves' disease. This is probably due to the wider use and acceptance of radioactive iodine I-131 treatment. In general, the patients still considered appropriate for surgery are children, adolescents, women in whom pregnancy is associated with Graves' disease, women of child-bearing age, and patients who have extremely large thyroid glands. A number of patients will refuse radioactive iodine treatment and thereby become candidates for surgery. The traditional method for making the patient euthyroid involves giving one of the antithyroid drugs for a period of two to three months prior to surgery to inhibit thyroid hormone synthesis. The drug that is most used is propylthiouracil, since it not only inhibits thyroid hormone synthesis but also blocks the peripheral conversion of T4 to T3. The average dose is 300 mg daily in divided doses. Most patients will be euthyroid in two to three months on this dosage. If the patient is severely hyperthyroid or has an unusually large gland, larger doses may be used (up to 1 gram daily). In general, the smaller the gland, the shorter the time interval necessary to achieve euthyroidism. An alternative drug is methimazole (Tapazole). Doses of 30 to 60 mg daily are comparable to the above doses of propylthiouracil. About 10 days prior to surgery it is wise to give the patient a potassium iodide solution (10 drops daily of a saturated solution). Iodide in a patient with Graves' disease is a potent antithyroid drug, since it blocks release of stored hormone. Generally the gland will shrink considerably with iodide therapy. For years surgeons have noted that the vascularity of the gland at the time of surgery is considerably reduced by iodide. Lithium carbonate (300 milligrams four times daily) may be given in lieu of iodide, especially if there is a known allergy to iodine. Lithium carbonate, like iodide, blocks the proteolysis and release of stored thyroid hormone. There is growing evidence that the beta blocker propranolol may be an acceptable alternative to the above regimen. Not only does propranolol control the tachyarrhythmias of thyrotoxicosis but it may also have a direct antithyroid effect by blocking the peripheral conversion of T4 to T3. Propranolol in doses of 40 to 120 mg daily in divided doses two to three weeks prior to surgery may completely control all the signs and symptoms of hyperthyroidism and may be the only preoperative drug necessary. In general, the propylthiouracil-iodide method is preferred if the patient has an unusually large gland and is severely hyperthyroid. Propranolol would be used as the sole drug only in the patient who has a relatively small gland with mild to modest signs and symptoms of hyperthyroidism. Another advantage of propranolol is that it can be given intravenously. If during anesthesia tachyarrhythmias develop, 1 to 2 mg may be given as a bolus intravenously and repeated again if necessary while the patient is being monitored carefully. It is generally taught that beta blockers should not be given to patients with congestive heart failure. This rule does not apply to the patient with thyrotoxic heart disease who may be in mild congestive heart failure. If a tachyarrhythmia exists, propranolol in these situations may even be the major therapeutic intervention in the management of the patient's congestive heart failure.

Management of Thyrotoxicosis During Pregnancy

The management of the thyrotoxicosis of Graves' disease during pregnancy presents some special problems. Radioactive iodine therapy is definitely contraindicated. The physician has a choice between antithyroid drugs and surgery. Antithyroid drugs cross the placental barrier and can cause fetal hypothyroidism. This problem may be obviated on theoretical grounds by the simultaneous administration of 1-thyroxine or triiodothyronine. However, most of the evidence indicates that neither T4 nor T3 cross the placental barrier. The occurrence of fetal hypothyroidism when small doses of antithyroid drugs alone are used is quite unusual as long as the mother remains euthyroid. It is better to err on the side of undertreatment than overtreatment with antithyroid drugs. Small amounts of propylthio-uracil (50 to 100 mg per day or even every other day) are often sufficient. Chronic use of iodide in the mother is contraindicated since fetal goiter and hypothyroidism may result. The use of propranolol during pregnancy is controversial. There have been case reports that babies whose mothers had received propranolol experienced intrauterine growth retardation and low Apgar ratings. Bradycardia and hypoglycemia also have been described in these infants. The thyrotoxicosis of pregnancy tends to be quite mild and often improves in the second and third trimester. While surgery is an acceptable alternative to treatment (only after the first trimester is complete), this hardly seems necessary since the thyrotoxicosis of pregnancy usually is so easily controlled on small doses of propylthiouracil.

Following pregnancy, it is impossible to predict the outcome of the mother. While some patients remain hyperthyroid, some become hypothyroid following delivery.

The status of the neonate following delivery needs careful attention. Either hypothyroidism or hyperthyroidism may be present. Neonatal hypothyroidism is characterized by a low T4-RIA (below 7 μg/100 ml) and an elevated TSH. At times the T4 may be perfectly normal and only the TSH elevated. Experimental work indicates that measurement of reverse T3 may be useful. Amniotic fluid reverse T3 levels tends to be low in the hypothyroid fetus in the third trimester, and likewise the blood reverse T3 concentration is low after birth if hypothyroidism exists.

Management of neonatal hypothyroidism consists of the immediate replacement with 1-thyroxine in the dose range of 9 μg/kg/day. This is a relatively large dose but it is often required to normalize the TSH level and T4 concentration. Normally the T4-RIA (8-15 μg/100 ml) tends to be high in the first year of life with a slow progressive drop until after puberty. Likewise thyroid hormone replacement doses tend to be higher than in the average adult until puberty is complete.

Neonatal hyperthyroidism is most unusual and is always associated with high levels of thyroid stimulating immunoglobulins. These immunoglobulins cross the placental barrier and are probably the cause of fetal hyperthyroidism. Controlling maternal hyperthyroidism seems to prevent the development of hyperthyroidism in the infant.

If the infant is born hyperthyroid (elevated T4, T3, and reverse T3) propylthiouracil (10 mg/kg/day) should be started followed by Lugol's solution, 2 drops every 6 hours by mouth. Once the level of thyroid stimulating immunoglobulins drops, the neonatal hyperthyroidism improves. All pregnant thyrotoxic women should have thyroid stimulating immunoglobulins measured in the third trimester.

Toxic Nodular Thyroid Disease

The patient with a toxic nodular goiter who has both hot and cold nodules present on a radioactive scan is managed generally the same way as outlined above with one notable exception. These patients should never be given iodide. The excess iodide can penetrate the cold nodules of the goiter and convert a nonfunctioning nodule into a "hot" nodule and actually accentuate the hyperthyroidism (Jodbasedow effect). The patient with a single autonomous "hot" nodule can be prepared for surgery as already outlined. Iodide generally has no effect in these patients. Larger than usual doses of propylthiouracil must be used (600-1000 mg daily) because of the unusual degree of resistance that some autonomous nodules have to antithyroid drugs. In general, before sending a hyperthyroid patient to surgery the internist should make sure that both a T4-RIA and T3-RIA are in the normal range.

Thyroid Crisis

Occasionally a patient with occult hyperthyroidism may be triggered into a serious overt hyperthyroid state by another medical problem, especially an infection (e.g., pneumonia or acute appendicitis). Surgery itself may sometimes trigger this condition. Some experts refer to this as thyroid storm. This is a difficult term to define precisely. It is primarily a clinical diagnosis; the condition is characterized by fever, severe tachyarrhythmias, dehydration, and occasionally cardiac and hepatic failure. Prompt treatment is mandatory. Propylthiouracil should be given if necessary by nasogastric tube in a dosage of 200 milligrams every six hours. After the initial doses of the antithyroid drug, then sodium iodide may be started in the dosage range of 1 gram intravenously daily. Propranolol 40 to 60 milligrams p.o. every eight hours may be used. Appropriate fluid and volume replacement and antibiotics if infection exists are mandatory. If hypotension exists, adrenal cortical steroids (300 mg hydrocortisone hemisuccinate or phosphate daily) may be necessary. Occasionally this syndrome may occur during the induction of anesthesia, and the anesthesiologist must be alert to it especially in patients with a prior history of hyperthyroidism.

Following surgery, one must still be alert to the possibility of hyperthyroidism. A good deal of preformed T4 and T3 may be released into the blood by manipulation of the thyroid gland during surgery. The half-life of T3 is only about 24 hours but the half-life of T4 is of the order of two to three weeks. Postoperatively it might be necessary to continue propranolol for two to three weeks in some cases.

One should also watch for hypocalcemia, especially when a total thyroidectomy has been accomplished. At times this may just be a transient event not requiring any long-term treatment.

The long-term treatment that may be required is the management of hypothyroidism, which can have a higher incidence than expected even in the patient with a subtotal thyroidectomy. An elevated TSH level postoperatively would herald the onset of hypothyroidism. Only about 5 per cent of patients develop recurrent hyperthyroidism following surgery whereas up to 50 per cent of patients will develop hypothyroidism.

Exophthalmos

Exophthalmos remains a curious and perplexing problem. Orbital ultrasound scan has identified extraocular muscle enlargement in two thirds of patients with Graves' disease. However clinically significant exophthalmos is fortunately not common. It occurs after radioactive iodine therapy or surgery, especially the former. It may occur in patients who clinically have never been hyperthyroid. Simple forms of treatment with thiazide diuretics, artificial tear drops, taping the eyes shut at night, and sleeping with the head of the bed elevated are helpful. Some patients respond to steroids (50 mg prednisone daily p.o). Considerable success has been attained by the Stanford group with radiotherapy to the orbits. Two thousand rads is given to the orbits. This modality works best in those patients who have recent onset exophthalmos which is rapidly progressive. Despite the above measures some patients will require decompression of the orbit via a maxillary approach.

HYPOTHYROIDISM

Hypofunction of the thyroid gland can be caused by surgical ablation, radioactive iodine administration, irradiation to the neck (e.g., in Hodgkins disease), iodine deficiency or toxicity, genetic biosynthetic defects in thyroid hormone production, antithyroid drugs such as propylthiouracil, pituitary tumors, or hypothalamic disease. Perhaps the most common cause of primary thyroid hypofunction is chronic lymphocytic thyroiditis or Hashimoto's thyroiditis. The gland is usually enlarged, nontender, and extremely firm and indurated. A variety of antithyroid antibodies are found in the serum, including antithyroglobulin and antimicrosomal antibodies in high titer. Hypothyroidism seems to be the most common consequent of Hashimoto's thyroiditis and indeed is the most common cause of hypothyroidism in the adult. Patients with Hashimoto's thyroiditis are extremely susceptible to iodides and to antithyroid drugs, and overt severe hypothyroidism can be exacerbated by these maneuvers. Fullblown myxedema presents with a variety of symptoms including cold intolerance, apathy, hoarseness, constipation, retarded movement, anemia, hearing loss, and bradycardia. In contrast to Hashimoto's thyroiditis, subacute thyroiditis is characterized by a painful indurated thyroid gland and transient hyperthyroidism. Normal thyroid function is the rule after three to six months. Hypothyroidism permanently occurring after subacute thyroiditis is most unusual.

Preparation of the Hypothyroid Patient for Surgery

Hypothyroidism should be corrected in any patient who is a potential surgical candidate. For adults, adequate daily replacement is obtained with 0.1 to 0.2 mg of L-thyroxine. Synthetic thyroxine derivatives are preferred instead of desiccated thyroid preparations, since the T4 level itself can be used as a guide to therapy. Both the T4 and TSH serum level should be in the normal range in adequately treated patients. Desiccated thyroid contains small and variable quantitites of triiodothyronine (T3), and thus the T4-RIA cannot be used as a guide to therapy since the T3 contaminant will falsely lower the T4 blood level. For the same reason, preparations containing combinations of T4 and T3 are not physiologically appropriate. Moreover, T4 is completely converted in hypothyroid patients to physiological quantities of T3 by peripheral deiodinase (Fig. 5–1). Patients with significant heart disease and older patients should be treated very slowly with thyroid. It is best to begin with increments of .025 mg L-thyroxine every three to four weeks until optimal therapy is reached. Older patients seem to require less total replacement than young healthy individuals (as little as 0.1 mg L-thyroxine). Patients with coronary artery disease with angina pectoris obviously need very slow and cautious replacement. This latter group, like the older patients, are best left on lower rather than higher replacement doses. Exacerbations of angina and unstable angina may be caused by even slight overtreatment. When the TSH serum level reaches normal, adequate replacement has been attained. Following thyroidectomy, if the patient is not able to take medications by mouth, there is no immediate worry that hypothyroidism will develop. The half-life of T4 is two to three weeks. Thus the physician can wait a week or two safely (probably even up to four weeks) before exogenous thyroid hormone therapy needs to be reinstituted. Overtreatment, especially in the older patient, can be hazardous.

Myxedema Coma

Myxedema coma is a rare complication that is associated with profound hypothyroidism. It is associated with extreme lethargy, severe hypothermia, bradycardia, and alveolar hypoventilation with hypoxia, and is occasionally accompanied by pericardial effusion and congestive heart failure. Hyponatremia associated with marked decrease in free water clearance by the kidney is also often part of the syndrome. This is the one single indication for intravenous thyroxine therapy. L-thyroxine (Synthroid) is given as a single intravenous dose of 300 to 500 μg. Intravenous T3 or triiodothyronine (Cytomel) may also be given in the dose range of 25 to 50 micrograms every eight hours until the blood level of T3 is normal. Intravenous T3 probably is superior to intravenous T4, since T3 is the most physiologically active form of thyroid hormone therapy and since it bypasses the normal T4 to T3 peripheral conversion pathway, which tends to be markedly depressed in patients with serious systemic illnesses. The intravenous preparations should always be prepared fresh prior to use. It is possible to achieve a relatively euthyroid state with these preparations within three to five days.

There is some concern that the intravenous forms of thyroxine may be overused based on inappropriate interpretation of thyroid function tests in a patient who is critically ill. In the patient who is seriously ill, thyroid function tests may be quite deceptive. It is important to obtain all the necessary data. For instance, the T4 level may be quite low. One should never make a diagnosis of hypothyroidism on the basis of a T4-RIA alone. Measurement of the resin T3 uptake (RT3U) should also be done. In many critically ill patients the T4 may be low but the resin T3 uptake may be quite high, indicating that the number of thyroid binding globulin sites or the level of thyroid binding globulin itself is exceedingly low, especially in patients with chronic liver disease. The triiodothyronine level (T3) may be exceedingly low (below 50 ng/100 ml), which is a normal occurrence in severe systemic illness because of the block in conversion of T4 to T3. In reality, the "free T4" may be normal when the appropriate correction of a low T4 is made for the decreased availability of binding sites. If the TSH level is normal in the absence of pituitary disease, the patient is euthyroid. At times it may be helpful to get a direct measurement of free T4 by radioimmunoassay and a reverse T3 level. The patient is euthyroid if the free T4 is normal. However, often with systemic illness the serum T3-RIA is low but the reverse T3 is elevated if the patient is euthyroid. With true hypothyroidism T3-RIA, free T4, and reverse T3 are all low.

Adrenocortical steroids in the dosage range of 100 mg every eight hours are indicated, especially if concomitant pituitary disease with associated adrenocorticotropic hormone (ACTH) deficiency is suspected. The mortality in myxedema coma remains quite high.

Nodular Thyroid Disease

A frequent thyroid surgical candidate is the patient with suspected thyroid cancer. This occurs commonly in the situation where the thyroid scan shows a single cold or nonfunctioning nodule. In addition, many patients with a prior history of irradiation to the neck are referred to surgery, even with a multinodular gland, because of higher incidence of thyroid cancer reported 20 years or so after external radiation to the head, neck, and chest area. By far most of these patients are euthyroid prior to surgery and need no special preparation. However, if a cancer is found at surgery it is usually routine to do a total thyroidectomy. Instead of starting these patients on exogenous thyroid immediately after surgery, this should be temporarily postponed until a decision is made as to whether massive amounts of radioactive I-131 therapy are indicated. A week after 50 to 100 millicuries of I-131 is given, then exogenous replacement thyroid therapy should be instituted. Some internists prefer to start exogenous thyroid immediately after surgery, since it has a cancer suppressing effect. However, before a radioactive iodine scan or definitive therapy with radioactive iodine can be accomplished, exogenous thyroid must be stopped for at least six weeks. A good review of thyroid carcinoma can be found in the review article by Mazzaferri.

Medullary cancer of the thyroid deserves special mention because it will be referred to often in other sections as part of the multiple endocrine adenomatosis syndrome (MEA II). About 5 per cent of all thyroid cancers are of the medullary type. These cancers are the result of C-cell proliferation. Calcitonin levels are extremely elevated, and the calcitonin level can be used as a marker postoperatively to check for recurrence of the disease. Intravenous calcium or pentagastrin will stimulate calcitonin release in those cases with medullary cancer where the plasma calcitonin is normal. No release occurs in the normal state. Calcitonin would be expected to antagonize parathyroid hormone and perhaps even lower blood calcium levels. Despite enormous calcitonin levels in some patients with medullary carcinoma of the thyroid, the blood calcium is usually normal. The calcitonin level is most helpful in the early diagnosis and follow-up of patients who have recurrent disease.

Multinodular or simple goiters in a euthyroid patient sometimes require surgery because of local pressure symptoms such as dysphagia. Mild superior caval syndrome is sometimes seen with huge goiters that have substernal extension. Thyroid suppressive therapy is also sometimes useful in reducing the size of these goiters, since they may at times be TSH dependent. There are no special preoperative preparations necessary for these patients. Replacement L-thyroxine therapy should be instituted postoperatively.

GENERAL SURGICAL PROBLEMS
(Stehling, 1974)

The patient with hyper- or hypothyroidism is a greater surgical and anesthetic risk than the euthyroid patient. If possible, patients who are hyper- or hypothyroid should be brought to euthyroid status before any surgery is contemplated. For the patient who is euthyroid but has a thyroid nodule, no special preparation is necessary.

The patient with hyperthyroidism can be treated in three ways:

1. Radioactive iodine in therapeutic dose. This means of therapy is useful in the patient with a toxic nodule or diffuse toxic goiter. After such treatment these patients may not require surgery.

2. Antithyroid drugs. Propylthiouracil, 100 mg orally every six hours, or methimazole (Tapazole), 10 mg orally every six hours, can be given over a period of one to two years to keep the patient euthyroid during this time. These agents work by inhibiting thyroid hormone synthesis and thereby controlling the circulating level of thyroid hormone. In one study, duration of remission of symptoms following treatment of diffuse toxic goiter with methimazole or propylthiouracil was less than two years in 80 per cent of patients treated (Reynolds and Kotchen, 1979).

3. Subtotal thyroidectomy. The patient is treated with appropriate doses of propylthiouracil or methimazole for a period of six to ten weeks until euthyroid. At the end of that time Lugol's solution, 10 drops by mouth three times a day, is given for a period of 10 days. This results in shrinking of the gland and diminution of vascularity. Surgery can then be performed on a euthyroid patient.

The patient with hypothyroidism should be given gradually increasing doses of thyroid hormone until he is euthyroid as measured by clinical and chemical criteria. This may take three or four weeks. L-thyroxin (thyroid USP or sodium thyroxin) is a fairly slowly acting compound with a half-life of approximately 10 days. Triiodothyronine (Cytomel) is a much more rapidly acting compound with a half-life of about two days. The usual oral replacement dose of thyroid is 2 or 3 grains of desiccated thyroid per day, of sodium thyroxin 0.2 mg per day, and of triiodothyronine 75 μg per day.

ANESTHESIA FOR THE HYPERTHYROID PATIENT (Stehling, 1974)

Preferably patients suffering from hyperthyroidism are brought to a euthyroid or nearly euthyroid state by antithyroid treatment before anesthesia or operation. However, emergency procedures are occasionally necessary in nonprepared or poorly prepared hyperthyroid patients, and the anesthesiologist is then faced with their care during stressful situations that aggravate their already precarious state.

Premedication. More sedation is indicated for the hyperthyroid patient than for the euthyroid one. Apprehension aggravates the already elevated metabolic state and causes release of more catecholamines. No longer is it necessary to "steal the thyroid" by not informing the patient about the scheduled operation but instead inducing anesthesia under the guise of routine therapy, intravenous or rectal. Better drugs for sedation and preoperative preparation are now available.

Short-acting barbiturate medication to a moderate hypnotic degree helps to relieve apprehension and has some antithyroid action. Narcotics in larger than average doses decrease the metabolic rate and usually cause the patient to be less concerned about his welfare and impending events.

Anticholinergic drugs in excessive doses tend to aggravate the already present tachycardia, but small doses of scopolamine are usually indicated for sedative as well as anticholinergic effect.

Phenothiazines tend to increase the heart

rate and promote hypotension, so they should be used cautiously even though they tend to produce favorable sedation and antithyroid effects in these patients. A small test dose of a phenothiazine (Promazine, 10 mg) may be administered intramuscularly the evening before operation. If no untoward reaction occurs, a larger intramuscular dose of 25 to 50 mg for adults may be included with other premedication at least one hour before induction of anesthesia.

Prophylactic use of other agents such as reserpine, guanethidine, propranolol (Trench et al, 1978), cortisone, and intravenous iodides has been recommended during the immediate preoperative period.

Agents and Techniques. A variety of anesthetic agents and techniques have been employed for successful operation on hyperthyroid patients, and none has advantages that would exclude use of all others. Some pharmacological differences will be discussed in their practical and theoretical applications to the problems of hyperthyroidism.

Both spinal (Knight, 1945) and epidural (Brewster et al., 1956) anesthesia reduce the effects of hyperthyroidism, probably by decreasing the release of catecholamines by the adrenal medulla and at peripheral nerve endings. It was primarily the work of Brewster (1956) that led to the hypothesis that thyroxine acts by increasing the sensitivity of tissue receptors to epinephrine and norepinephrine. Whenever applicable, local and regional anesthesia are reasonable techniques. Since most hyperthyroid patients are restless and apprehensive, additional hypnosis and sedation are indicated; the dose of supplemental drugs required with regional anesthesia may approach that needed for light general anesthesia. Thyroidectomy is the most frequently performed operation on hyperthyroid patients, and even though regional anesthesia is used by some anesthesiologists and surgeons, it is not preferred by most, because there is inadequate control of the patients. Thiobarbiturates and halothane inhibit release of catecholamines. Halothane tends to further sensitize the myocardium to catecholamines and cause arrhythmias, which are among the most threatening of complications during anesthesia and operation on the hyperthyroid patients. Oyama (1973) found no change in thyroid stimulating hormone during anesthesia with diethyl ether,

halothane, methoxyflurane, thiopentone, or spinal block. Thyroxine in the serum of humans increased during anesthesia with diethyl ether and halothane but was not changed during anesthesia with thiopental, spinal block, or methoxyflurane. In later studies, isoflurane was found to have an effect similar to that of diethyl ether and halothane (Oyama et al., 1973) while althesin did not exert any hormonal influence on the thyroid gland (Oyma et al., 1975). However, Harland et al. (1974) found in patients to whom I-131 had been administered earlier that the protein bound iodine and radioactivity of plasma increased progressively during anesthesia with thiopentone, nitrous oxide, and succinylcholine. They postulated that the increased radioactivity in the plasma was due to loss of radioactivity in the liver. A single dose of thiopental may reduce thyroid activity of rats for several days, probably owing to the effects of the metabolic products that are related to the antithyroid thioureas such as prophylthiouracil. However, this property is not likely to be of much benefit during anesthesia, because the already circulating thyroid hormones remain active for several weeks.

In the past, patients with hyperthyroidism have been considered to be resistant to anesthetic agents and to require larger than average doses. This concept has not been substantiated under controlled conditions in the laboratory with anesthesia produced with pentobarbital (Prange et al., 1966), cyclopropane (Munson et al., 1968), and halothane (Babad and Eger, 1968). It is suggested that the apparent patient resistance to anesthetic agents is the result of rapid distribution of the agents as a result of increased cardiac output and rapid tissue blood flow in the hyperthyroid patient. Whatever the mechanism, induction of general anesthesia in hyperthyroid patients is usually slow, and larger doses are required.

Operative Problems. CIRCULATORY. Most life-threatening complications to the hyperthyroid patient during anesthesia are likely to be circulatory in nature. The stage is set with increased cardiac output, tachycardia, slight systolic hypertension, and increased red blood cell mass and blood volume so that cardiac work is increased. Under reasonable circumstances, compensation may be possible, but arrhythmias such as atrial fibrillation and cardiac decompensation may eventually result. Acute pulmonary edema may be the first recognized evidence of hyperthyroidism during anesthesia (Kadis et al., 1966). In hyperthyroidism, digitalization is often not helpful. Intravenous lidocaine and propranolol may be helpful in controlling tachycardia and ventricular arrhythmias. Deep anesthesia with agents known to be myocardial depressants should be avoided. Fortunately, thyroidectomy requires only light stages of general anesthesia.

HYPOXIA. Oxygen consumption is elevated, and short bouts of inadequate alveolar ventilation may result in rapid falls in oxygen tension and elevation of carbon dioxide tension in the blood. Both respiratory and metabolic acidosis occur more rapidly than in euthyroid patients. Adequate preoperative precautions must be made for assurance of an adequate airway and pulmonary ventilation with oxygen-rich gas mixture without interruption. When the thyroid is retrosternal, an endotracheal tube should be used that is long enough to extend past the area of tracheal compression but not inserted far enough to impinge on the carina or enter a bronchus. Removal of a tumor that has exerted pressure on the trachea may leave the wall of the trachea flaccid and allow it to collapse when the endotracheal tube is removed. Immediate reintubation may be lifesaving. Post-thyroidectomy paresis of both recurrent laryngeal nerves may be the cause of respiratory obstruction.

HYPERTHERMIA. Heat production is increased and the physiological mechanisms for heat loss must not be blocked. Atropine is best avoided because of its tendency to inhibit heat loss and to aggravate tachycardia. If the patient must be covered with thick surgical drapes, a cooling mattress should be installed on the operating table, especially if the surgical procedure is to be prolonged for several hours. Adequate intravenous fluids and electrolytes must be provided to allow copious perspiration and urine output. Equipment for monitoring core body temperature should be available and preferably should be attached to the patient before or soon after induction of anesthesia.

OTHER PROBLEMS. Special precautions must be taken to prevent drying or abrasion of the corneas of exophthalmic eyes. Taping of eyelids in approximation is more reliable than medication.

Postoperative Problems. RESPIRATORY

OBSTRUCTION. Since the hypermetabolic state likely will increase during the immediate postoperative period, especially after thyroidectomy, adequate pulmonary ventilation and oxygenation of tissues must be provided. The most likely cause of respiratory obstruction is pressure on the trachea by a blood clot in the neck wound, but laryngeal edema is another possibility. Equipment for opening a thyroidectomy wound for clot evaluation, passing an endotracheal tube, and performing a tracheostomy should be kept immediately available at the patient's bedside. These patients should be monitored constantly and overdosage with respiratory depressing drugs avoided. Estimation of arterial blood gases may prove useful.

THYROTOXIC CRISIS (Bobyns, 1978; Duckworth, 1978). Physiologically this complication may be viewed as a decompensated state of hyperthyroidism precipitated by the excessive release into the circulation of thyroid hormones, usually following operation on the thyroid gland. The striking features become manifest within 24 to 72 hours postoperatively, with rapid forceful sinus tachycardia or atrial fibrillation, nausea, vomiting, diarrhea, dehydration, and tachypnea. High fever, up to 107° F., may occur, along with vascular collapse. There is often marked agitation, restlessness, delirium, and prostration. Therapy of this condition consists of the following: 1) sedation with adequate doses of narcotics, barbiturates, and phenothiazines; 2) large doses of propylthiouracil to prevent further thyroid hormone synthesis (200 mg every four to six hours); 3) sodium iodide, 2 to 3 gm intravenously every 24 hours (Large doses of iodide probably suppress the release of hormone from the thyroid gland, but there is no evidence that they inhibit the peripheral action of thyroid hormone.); 4) large doses of hydrocortisone intravenously (300 mg a day); 5) cooling of the patient if the fever is very high; and 6) general supportive measures to combat nausea, dehydration, aspiration and infection. Propranolol is a very useful drug for controlling some of the symptoms of thyrotoxicosis but does not decrease the half-life of thyroxine already secreted (Lee et al., 1973), so therapy must be continued even after symptoms are controlled. The response of thyrotoxic patients to propranolol is variable (Jamison and Dive, 1979), and even preoperative preparation with propylthiouracil and/or propranolol may not prevent a thyroid storm postoperatively (Erickson et al., 1977). A dose of propranolol of 240 mg per day was not adequate when postoperative hydration and administration of iodine was discontinued too soon (Serri et al., 1978).

HYPOCALCEMIC TETANY. Removal or injury of the parathyroid glands during thyroidectomy may lead to hypocalcemia that requires calcium therapy. (See section on Parathyroid Disease.)

ANESTHESIA FOR THE HYPOTHYROID PATIENT

Mild degrees of myxedema may be overlooked when preoperative examination has been hurried, or occasionally surgical treatment may become necessary in the inadequately treated patient with hypothyroidism. Cardiovascular collapse may occur during anesthesia in such patients (Abbott, 1967). Preparation with desiccated thyroid or thyroxin by mouth may take several weeks, whereas triiodothyronine may be given intravenously with effect in a few hours. However, substitution therapy must be given slowly and cautiously under electrocardiographic control to prevent cardiac arrest from an increase in tissue metabolism more rapidly than energy can be supplied by a chronically damaged myocardium.

Premedication. Myxedematous patients are characteristically complacent and do not require large doses of sedative drugs preoperatively. Average doses of most sedative drugs are not well tolerated. Narcotics should be eliminated or reduced to a minimum. Phenothiazines are best withheld because of the danger of hypotension that is resistant to correction. Premedication should be limited to conservative doses of a short-acting barbiturate and an anticholinergic agent such as scopolamine or atropine.

Agents and Methods. Induction of anesthesia occurs rapidly, and use of the usual drug doses, concentrations, and administration rates employed for comparable euthyroid patients may easily lead to overdose. This has been attributed to increased sensitivity to depressing drugs, but other work (Prange et al., 1966; Munson et al., 1968; Babad and Eger, 1968) tends to show that this effect is the result of decreased cardiac output and tissue blood flow in these patients and hence a delayed distribution of anesthetic agents.

For the same reasons, elimination of anesthetic agents during the postoperative period will be delayed. Rapidly eliminated agents such as nitrous oxide may be preferred. Use of curare is not contraindicated and when used with nitrous oxide makes a combination that results in minimal cardiovascular disturbance.

Operative Problems. CARDIOVASCULAR. Cardiac output is low and myocardial reserve is reduced, so stress and physiologic alterations of anesthesia and operation can lead to rapid cardiac failure. Blood loss and shock are poorly tolerated, and hypotension does not respond well to therapy with vasopressors. Larger doses of vasopressors can result in ventricular tachycardia and fibrillation. Blood transfusions must be given cautiously to avoid overloading the heart. Progressive decrease in pulmonary compliance may mean that pulmonary edema is occurring. Coronary artery disease as well as general arteriosclerosis is common.

RESPIRATORY. Respiratory center response may be poor, and hypercarbia and hypoxia can occur unless pulmonary ventilation is assisted. This is somewhat abated by the decreased carbon dioxide production. Increase in mean intrathoracic pressure can further reduce an already decreased cardiac output.

BODY TEMPERATURE. Basal metabolic rate is reduced and hypothermia can occur during prolonged anesthesia unless warming measures such as a water mattress and monitoring of core body temperature are used. Hypothermia tends to aggravate circulatory and respiratory depression.

SUBSTITUTION THERAPY. During anesthesia, rapid reversal of hypothyroidism should be avoided if possible. Intravenous dose of triiodothyronine should not exceed 10 to 20 μg over a 12 hour period, at the same time the electrocardiogram should be watched for depression of the S-T segment and flattening of T waves.

Intravenous hydrocortisone should be considered in the treatment of shock resistant to moderate blood volume replacement.

Frequency of hypoglycemia, hyponatremia, anemia, and low blood volume should be kept in mind and blood values monitored when indicated so that adequate therapy can be started early.

Narcotics should be avoided or used in minimal doses to avoid respiratory depression in the postoperative period.

The complications discussed above as possible ones during anesthesia and operation are likely to extend into the postoperative period. Monitoring of circulation, respiration, temperature, and blood gasses should be continued postoperatively.

PITUITARY GLAND

PATHOPHYSIOLOGY

The pituitary gland is divided into an anterior and a posterior portion. The anterior pituitary is connected to the hypothalamus via a complex portal vascular system. Hypothalamic releasing or inhibitory factors are synthesized in the hypothalamus, secreted into the portal system, and reach the anterior pituitary gland in very high concentration. The posterior pituitary is entirely different. Specialized neurons in the hypothalamus synthesize vasopressin and oxytocin. These two hormones are then secreted through specialized axons down the stalk of the pituitary gland and are stored in the posterior pituitary gland. Some of the most exciting work done in endocrine function in recent years has been the synthesis and physiological investigation of the releasing factors of the hypothalamus. Each pituitary hormone has a specific releasing factor associated with it and in some cases a specific inhibitory factor. Except for the positive effect of thyrotropin releasing factor (TRF) on both thyroid stimulating hormone (TSH) and prolactin secretion, generally there is no overlap in function of the hypothalamic hormones except when pituitary disease exists. For instance, in acromegaly, both somatotropin releasing factor and thyrotropin releasing factor can bring about release of growth hormone. In the normal state this would not occur. Specific hypothalamic releasing hormones have been defined for thyroid stimulating hormone (TSH), corticotropin (ACTH), and the gonadotropins (both luteinizing hormone [LH] and follicle stimulating hormone [FSH]). Both a releasing and an inhibitory hypothalamic factor have been discovered for growth hormone. Prolactin is primarily associated with an inhibitory hypothalamic factor, which is probably the neurotransmitter dopamine. An additional factor involving hypothalamic control of the pituitary is the pulsatile operation of the hypothalamus, which comes about because certain periodic rhythms are linked to pituitary function. Probably the most important biological rhythm is the sleep pattern. For instance, growth hormone and adrenoadrenalcorticotropic hormones show specific nocturnal bursts. Prolactin also tends to increase in concentration in the blood immediately after sleep begins. Luteinizing hormone shows a sleep pattern especially during puberty.

The three monoamine neurotransmitters, dopamine, norepinephrine, and serotonin, all can profoundly affect hypothalamic function and all are found in high concentration in major hypothalamic centers. There is essentially no blood brain barrier in either the pituitary or the hypothalamus, and target organ products such as estrogen, testosterone, thyroid, and adrenal hormones can exert feedback at either the hypothalamic or pituitary level. Figure 5–3 depicts some of these important and complex interrelationships.

DISEASES OF THE ANTERIOR PITUITARY GLAND

Hypofunction of the Pituitary Gland

All or several of the tropic hormones may be involved in hypopituitary states. The etiology of hypopituitarism includes chromophobe adenoma, in children Rathke's pouch cysts or craniopharyngioma, necrosis following circulatory collapse due to hemorrhage following delivery (Sheehan's syndrome), surgical hypophysectomy, irradiation to the skull or brain, granulomatous disease, and hemochromatosis. Metastatic disease (especially from breast cancer) is only rarely seen. Destruction of the gland by tumor (i.e., chromophobe adenoma) is probably the most common cause of hypopituitarism. Previously chromophobe adenoma was thought to be nonfunctional. Recent data indicate that fully one third to one half of patients with chromophobe adenoma secrete excessive quantities of the hormone prolactin. Excessive secretion of prolactin may be associated with galactorrhea and gonadotropin deficiency. Hypopituitarism as a result of tumor or other states may present in a number of misleading ways, and the diagnosis may likewise be exceedingly elusive to the clinician. Amenorrhea in the female or impotence in the male may be the initial manifestation, since gonado-

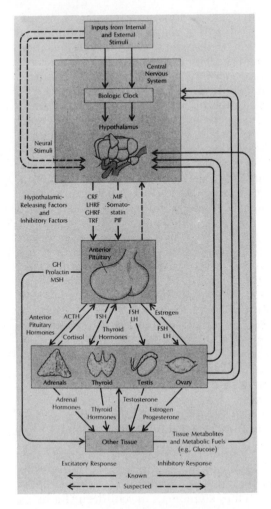

Pituitary Hormone	Hypothalamic Regulatory Hormones
Adrenocorticotropic hormone (ACTH)	Corticotropin releasing factor (CRF)
Thyroid stimulating hormone (TSH)	Thyrotropin releasing factor (TRF)
Follicle stimulating hormone (FSH) and luteinizing hormone (LH)	Gonadotropin releasing factor (GHRF)
Growth hormone (GH)	Growth hormone releasing factor (GHRF), somatostatin (inhibitory)
Prolactin	Prolactin inhibitory factor (PIF)

Figure 5–3. Basic feedback mechanisms in the neuroendocrine system.

(Used by permission of Hospital Practice, *10*: 60, 1975.)

tropins are among the first hormones to be depressed. Likewise, growth hormone deficiency in a child will result in severe growth failure. Loss of TSH or ACTH function occurs later, and then variable features related to thyroid deficiency or cortisol lack will inevitably manifest themselves. If a tumor exists, it may grow above the sella (suprasellar extension), and headaches and visual field defects, notably bitemporal hemianopsia, will occur. Single isolated deficiencies of specific pituitary hormones have been described. The most common is gonadotropin deficiency. A well known syndrome is gonadotropin deficiency associated with loss of the sense of smell (Kallmann's syndrome). This interesting hypothalamic entity is caused by failure of gonadotropin releasing factor to function appropriately.

Diagnosis of Pituitary Hypofunction. It is possible to measure by radioimmunoassay virtually all of the hormones of the anterior pituitary gland. This includes measurement of GH, TSH, LH, FSH, prolactin, and ACTH. A low LH and FSH associated with estrogen deficiency in a female or low testosterone in the male points to a hypothalamic or pituitary deficiency. Likewise a low TSH with a low T4 by radioimmunoassay also indicates either hypothalamic or pituitary deficiency. An elevated prolactin level is commonly seen associated with chromophobe adenomas.

An evaluation of the hypothalamic-pituitary-adrenal axis however can be quite difficult. The metapyrone test has long been a standard test for determination of the pituitary-adrenal axis. Metapyrone blocks the conversion of 11-deoxycortisol (compound S) to cortisol (compound F). Normally compound S is not measurable. A single oral dose of metapyrone (3 gm) is given at midnight, and plasma cortisol and 11-deoxycortisol concentrations are measured the following morning. If the 11-deoxycortisol level is greater than 10 μg per ml, this means that ACTH stimulation must have occurred and the patient has a normal pituitary-adrenal axis. If both compounds S and F are low, this means that no ACTH was stimulated and the patient has low or absent ACTH pituitary reserve. The test can also be performed using the measurement of urinary 17-hydroxycorticoids while 750 mg of metapyrone is given every four hours for six doses.

An insulin tolerance test (0.1 unit insulin

per kilogram weight intravenously) can also be used to test not only ACTH reserve but also growth hormone reserve. Hypoglycemia (blood sugar below 50 mg per 100 ml) should result in significant rises in both plasma cortisol and growth hormone if the pituitary gland is functioning normally. Failure of the plasma cortisol level to rise after intravenous insulin is an indication that ACTH reserve is low. Administration of specific releasing factors such as gonadotropin releasing factor or thyrotropin releasing factor as specific pituitary function tests has great potential but has not been widely exploited clinically.

HYPERFUNCTION OF THE PITUITARY GLAND

There are three major hyperfunctioning pituitary gland tumors: 1) prolactin secreting chromophobe adenoma; 2) an ACTH secreting tumor associated with Cushing's disease (thoroughly discussed in section on Adrenal Disease); and 3) acromegaly associated with excessive growth hormone secretion. Gonadotropin and thyrotropin secreting pituitary tumors are extraordinarily rare.

Acromegaly is a syndrome that presents with characteristic facies, weakness, enlargement of the hands and feet, thickening of the tongue, and enlargement of the nose and mandible with spreading of the teeth. The patient may even appear myxedematous. Other findings include abnormal glucose tolerance and osteoporosis. The most specific test for acromegaly is measurement of growth hormone before and after glucose. The typical acromegalic has very elevated fasting levels of GH (usually above 10 mg/ml) and the levels do not change appreciably after oral glucose. In the normal state, glucose will markedly suppress the GH level. A few patients with active acromegaly will have normal levels of fasting GH but do not suppress with glucose. The drug L-dopa, which will normally cause an elevation of GH in normal subjects, in the acromegalic has either no effect or lowers GH levels. Therapy for acromegaly is still debatable. Irradiation of pituitary (heavy particle or implants), transphenoidal hypophysectomy, and transfrontal hypophysectomy have all been tried. If suprasellar extension exists, conventional transfrontal hypophysectomy is usually indicated. For small pituitary tumors, transphenoidal hypophysectomy is rapidly becoming the treatment of choice. The dopaminergic agonist bromocriptine can lower GH levels but long-term follow-up with this drug is still lacking.

Prolactin has been one of the most interesting markers to identify patients with pituitary tumors. In the past, 30 to 50 per cent of patients that were thought to have nonfunctioning pituitary tumors actually had prolactin secreting tumors. High prolactin levels are sometimes associated with galactorrhea but not in all patients. Interference with gonadotropin function is very common in patients with pituitary tumors. Females commonly present with amenorrhea, and males present with impotence. It is important to keep in mind that certain drugs will elevate prolactin levels. Phenothiazines, methyldopa, and estrogens all can elevate prolactin levels. A high fasting prolactin level (above 150 ng/ml) is almost always due to a tumor. Therapy for prolactin secreting tumors is still being evaluated. The dopamine agonist bromocriptine can be extremely effective in controlling the prolactin level and restoring gonadotropin function. Some of these tumors are so small that they can be followed without any therapy whatsoever. Pregnancy is said to cause rapid growth of these tumors, and a surgical procedure such as transsphenoidal hypophysectomy may be necessary. Pituitary irradiation has not been uniformly successful.

Multiple Endocrine Adenomatosis Syndrome

Pituitary tumors are sometimes associated with multiple endocrine adenomatosis syndrome (MEA). Pituitary tumors are found more commonly in the MEA 1 syndrome where adenomas of the parathyroid glands and islets of the pancreas along with the Zollinger-Ellison syndrome may be associated.

DISORDERS OF THE POSTERIOR PITUITARY GLAND

Deficiency of vasopressin synthesis results in the disease known as diabetes insipidus. Clinically it manifests itself as severe polyuria. Patients with diabetes insipidus must be distinguished from compulsive water drinkers and from patients with nephrogenic resistance to the action of vasopressin.

Diabetes inspidus is commonly a sporadic disease of unknown etiology but occasionally may be familial. Very rarely trauma (basal skull fracture), encephalitis, congenital cysts, metastatic disease (mostly breast cancer), and histiocytosis X may also be possible causes. Surgical trauma, particularly with injury to the stalk of the pituitary gland during either transfrontal or transsphenoidal hypophysectomy, is also a potential cause. Nephrogenic diabetes insipidus may occur as a rare X-linked disease. It may be acquired following severe pyelonephritis, potassium depletion, or amyloidosis.

The classic test to distinguish diabetes inspidus patients from compulsive water drinkers and patients with nephrogenic diabetes insipidus is the water deprivation test. Following dehydration, patients with diabetes insipidus can only minimally concentrate their urine. When the serum osmolarity rises to 295 milliosmoles per liter (osmotic threshold), all normal patients will release vasopressin into the blood and concentrate their urine to conserve water. Simultaneous measurements of urine and plasma osmolarity are carried out as water deprivation is continued. Once the urine and plasma osmolarity have stabilized (usually with a 3-5% loss in body weight), the patient is given an injection of vasopressin (also called antidiuretic hormone, ADH). If vasopressin is being maximally secreted by the posterior pituitary, then exogenous pitressin or vasopressin will have no effect. The patient with vasopressin deficiency will never quite reach a stable plasma osmolarity and the urine osmolarity rarely gets much above 500 milliosmoles per liter. Moreover, even after severe dehydration, exogenous pitressin or vasopressin will cause significant increase in the urine osmolarity only in the patient with true diabetes insipidus. Thus, this sensitive test will even distinguish patients who have partial diabetes insipidus.

Compulsive water drinkers may at times present a diagnostic problem, since they often cannot concentrate their urine well and the water deprivation test must be carried out until the osmotic threshold is reached. Radioimmunoassay of vasopressin has now been developed and this test should be helpful if measured periodically while the water deprivation test is ongoing. Tests employing hypertonic saline as a physiological stimulus to ADH are cumbersome and difficult to interpret. It should be remembered that adrenocortical insufficiency will mask the polyuria of partial diabetes insipidus, since it lowers the osmotic threshold for vasopressin release. Institution of steroid therapy in such patients will unmask the diabetes insipidus, and severe polyuria may result.

A number of drugs have been shown to alter the release and action of antidiuretic hormone. The sulfonylurea agents, notably chlorpropamide, have been shown to augment the release of ADH. Chlorpropamide was once used in the treatment of patients with partial nephrogenic diabetes insipidus. Likewise clofibrate carbamazepine (Tegretol), vincristine, and cyclophosphamide all either release ADH or potentiate its action on the renal tubule. Ethanol as well as phenytoin (Dilantin) and chlorpromazine inhibit the action of ADH and its release. Lithium, a drug widely used to treat manic depressive disorders, can inhibit the formation of cyclic AMP in the renal tubule and probably even inhibit its synthesis of ADH directly and thus result in a diabetes insipidus–like picture. The tetracycline derivative demeclocycline produces a nephrogenic diabetes insipidus–like picture. Demeclocycline can be used to manage states associated with inappropriate ADH release. The potassium losing diuretics, such as the thiazide diuretics, can sometimes be used to treat nephrogenic diabetes insipidus. The thiazide diuretics augment the action of ADH on the renal tubule. The treatment of diabetes insipidus when essentially no ADH is present mandates the use of vasopressin. Vasopressin tannate in oil is an older agent that has largely been replaced by lypressin (8-lysine vasopressin) and more recently by DDAVP (1-deamino-8-D-arginine vasopressin). Both preparations are given intranasally. DDAVP (desmopressin) is especially useful, and 5 to 10 μg may be given only once or twice daily because its duration of action is nearly 24 hours.

For those patients who have some residual ADH function, chlorpropamide, clofibrate, or carbamazepine may be used, but even in a situation of partial ADH insufficiency DDAVP (desmopressin) may well become the agent of choice.

Management of the patient with complete diabetes insipidus during surgery usually does not present difficult problems. A very small amount of aqueous vasopressin (10-20 units per ampule) can be given as a continuous intravenous infusion. Just before surgery the patient is given an intravenous bolus of 100 milliunits aqueous vasopressin and then a constant intravenous infusion of 100 to 200 milliunits vasopressin per hour. In this situation isotonic fluids such as normal saline may be given safely and there is little danger of water depletion or hypernatremia. The plasma osmolarity should be monitored during surgery and in the immediate postoperative period. The normal range for plasma osmolarity is 283 to 285 milliosmoles per liter. Serum osmolarity can be calculated from the following formula:

$$\text{Osmolarity} = 2\ (\text{Na}^+\ \text{mEq/l}) + \frac{\text{glucose (mg/100 ml)}}{20} + \frac{\text{blood urea nitrogen (mg/100 ml)}}{3}$$

When the blood glucose and blood urea nitrogen are normal, the plasma osmolarity may be calculated by multiplying the serum sodium concentration by two. If the plasma osmolarity comes up much above 290, then hypotonic fluids should be given and the amount of aqueous vasopressin given intravenously should be increased above 200 milliunits per hour. In patients who have only partial vasopressin or ADH insufficiency, nonosmotic stimuli such as volume depletion or the stress of surgery may stimulate large quantities of ADH, and it probably is not necessary to use aqueous vasopressin unless there is a demonstrated rise in plasma osmolarity above 290 milliosmoles per liter during surgery or immediately postoperatively. Pitressin tannate in oil (5-10 units daily) may be given intramuscularly in the immediate postoperative period until the intranasal preparations can be used.

The Syndrome of Inappropriate ADH Secretion (SIADH)

Patients with the syndrome of inappropriate ADH secretion (SIADH) produce excessive quantities of ADH even when there is no physiological stimulus. The urine becomes highly concentrated and a dilutional hyponatremia develops. Blood volume, renal function, and blood pressure are normal and edema is absent. Any patient suspected of having the SIADH should be screened for the possibility of adrenal insufficiency or hypothyroidism. The diagnosis is essentially one of exclusion. Certain disorders have been associated with the SIADH, such as pneumonia, tuberculosis, central nervous system infection, head trauma, porphyria, and cancers of the lung, pancreas, thymus, and brain. A wide variety of drugs can bring about hypersecretion or augmentation of ADH and result in the syndrome of inappropriate secretion. These drugs have already been mentioned in the section on diabetes insipidus. The most common drugs that cause inappropriate secretion of ADH are chlorpropamide, clofibrate, psychotropics, thiazides, and the antineoplastic agents vincristine, vinblastine, and cyclophosphamide. Therapy is directed at managing the underlying cause and restricting the oral intake of water to less than 500 ml per day. Diuretic drugs such as furosemide may sometimes be used quite effectively in rapidly correcting the hyponatremia. Hypertonic saline in the presence of SIADH is totally ineffective, since these patients promptly secrete it in the urine. Recently both lithium and demeclocycline have been suggested for use in those patients who have chronic inappropriate ADH secretion. Demeclocycline (500–1000 mg/ daily) has been judged better than lithium.

Diagnosis in the Patient with an Abnormal Sella Turcica

The discovery of an enlarged sella turcica mandates a careful and thoughtful workup. Visual fields will help delineate whether a pituitary tumor has suprasellar extension. If bitemporal hemianopsia or a variant field defect is present, the physician can be fairly certain that suprasellar extension has occurred. If no specific endocrine disturbance can be found associated with the enlarged sella, including normal growth hormone, gonadotropins, and prolactin levels, the patient probably still has a chromophobe adenoma associated with normal pituitary function.

There are two other entities in the differential diagnosis however: an aneurysm of the carotid siphon and the so-called "empty sella" syndrome. If no endocrine disturbances are found, then the physician should consider an arteriogram to rule out an aneurysm. The empty sella syndrome is a peculiar entity associated with an enlarged sella on plain x-ray of the skull. In many patients it is merely an extension of the subarachnoid space into the sella turcica. Most patients have normal endocrine function. A few have been demonstrated to have small pituitary tumors associated with either prolactin or ACTH excess. A few patients have also been shown to have pituitary insufficiency. A pneumoencephalogram is the only way to make the diagnosis of the empty sella syndrome with any degree of certainty.

If there is a strong clinical suspicion of a pituitary tumor (e.g., the patient with gonadal insufficiency) and plain x-ray of the sella is not helpful, the physician should request that the radiologist do coned down polytomograms of the sella. This technique is often helpful in defining small pituitary tumors. The role of computerized tomography (CT) in the evaluation of pituitary disease needs further study but this is likely to become a useful modality in the future. When CT is used with contrast material, many pituitary tumors can be defined and even those with suprasellar extension may be identified. Pneumoencephalography is being used less and less but still is an excellent tool to define the exact anatomical boundaries of a pituitary lesion, especially whether or not suprasellar extension exists. The absence or presence of suprasellar extension is extremely important in deciding an appropriate therapeutic maneuver. If a patient has a pituitary tumor without suprasellar progression, then transphenoidal hypophysectomy might be considered. However, if the tumor is associated with suprasellar extension, the more complex transfrontal hypophysectomy may be the most appropriate therapy. Suprasellar extension of a pituitary tumor can be inferred by the still experimental procedure of finding significant quantities of anterior pituitary hormones such as ACTH, GH, and prolactin in the cerebrospinal fluid. Suprasellar extension of the tumor probably breaks down the blood-brain barrier, with subsequent release of anterior pituitary hormones into the cerebrospinal fluid.

MANAGEMENT OF THE PATIENT WITH PANHYPOPITUITARISM UNDERGOING HYPOPHYSECTOMY

All patients undergoing hypophysectomy should be euthyroid prior to surgery. The most serious threat to the welfare of the patient is the result of interruption of the pituitary-adrenal axis. Absence of ACTH after removal or partial removal of the anterior pituitary gland causes cessation in the secretion of cortisol. Preparation for this postoperative complication must begin in the preoperative period, as outlined in the section on hypoadrenalism. The emergence of transsphenoidal hypophysectomy as an important therapeutic procedure has greatly simplified the operative management of the patient undergoing hypophysectomy. Following transsphenoidal hypophysectomy, the patient may be tapered rather quickly to maintenance cortisol replacement therapy (see section on Cushing's disease). If the microadenoma has been completely removed and normal pituitary left behind, most patients may be completely tapered off cortisol replacement therapy within 6 to 8 weeks following transsphenoidal hypophysectomy. However, the patient who undergoes complete transfrontal hypophysectomy and has significant amounts of anterior pituitary gland removed will require higher doses of cortisol following surgery and in all probability will have to stay on replacement cortisol therapy for the remainder of his life.

The most significant complication following hypophysectomy is diabetes insipidus. In the hands of a well trained neurosurgeon, permanent diabetes insipidus is a very rare complication in the patient undergoing transsphenoidal hypophysectomy. Transient diabetes insipidus, however, is not uncommon and may last as long as six months following surgery. It can usually be managed with one of the intranasal preparations of vasopressin. DDAVP (desmopressin) is the preferable agent and may be given intranasally, 5 to 10 micrograms daily. Pitressin tannate in oil is an older agent and must be administered in the dose of 5 to 10 units intramuscularly once a day or once every other day. Permanent diabetes insipidus following transfrontal hypophysectomy is much more common, particularly if there is injury to the hypothalamus or the pituitary stalk. Moreover, patients undergoing transfrontal hypophysectomy are more likely to have suprasellar extension of the pituitary tumor, and thus the neurosurgeon will be operating very near areas such as the pituitary stalk. Therefore risk of injury to the hypothalamus and the pituitary stalk is much more common with transfrontal hypophysectomy. Diabetes insipidus may develop acutely in the postoperative period and should be managed as indicated in the section on management of diabetes insipidus.

Transsphenoidal hypophysectomy may well have a place in the management of patients with severe proliferative diabetic retinopathy and also in patients who have metastatic carcinoma of the breast with positive estrogen receptors in the breast cancer tissue. Management of diabetes before and after hypophysectomy has been outlined in the chapter on diabetic management. Following hypophysectomy, the patient with diabetes will become extremely sensitive to insulin (see section on adrenal disease and diabetes).

Replacement Hormonal Therapy for the Patient with Panhypopituitarism

Replacement therapy for the patient with panhypopituitarism has been discussed in the thyroid and adrenal section. Adrenal replacement can be easily achieved with oral cortisol (hydrocortisone) in a dosage of 15 to 20 mg in the morning and 10 to 15 mg in the late afternoon. During periods of stress the dosage may have to be increased. Patients with pituitary disease generally do not need mineralocorticoid replacement. However, hyponatremia or postural hypotension are indications for mineralocorticoid therapy (flurohydrocortisone, 0.05-0.1 mg daily p.o.). Thyroxine therapy should begin with 0.05 mg of 1-thyroxine and increased by increments of 0.025 to 0.05 mg every three to four weeks until a replacement dosage of 0.15 to 0.2 mg is reached and the serum T4 and TSH level becomes normal.

Sex hormone replacement in the male consists of testosterone enanthate, 200 to 400 mg intramuscularly monthly. Methyltestosterone, 15 to 20 mg, can be given sublingually as an alternative drug. This is a useful preparation in the prepubertal adolescent because the dose can be gradually increased by 5 mg to full replacement doses

of 20 mg. In general, the intramuscular preparations of testosterone are less toxic than the methyl substitued testosterone derivatives. Hepatotoxicity is more common with the substituted testosterones. In the female, sex hormone therapy consists of conjugated estrogens, 0.625 to 1.25 milligrams daily for 25 days of each month. On day 21 to day 25 medroxyprogesterone (Provera), 10 milligrams a day, is added to the regimen. If fertility is desired, gonadotropin therapy with a combination of an FSH preparation (Pergonal) may be tried with an LH preparation (human chorionic gonadotropin).

ANESTHESIA FOR OPERATIONS ON THE PITUITARY GLAND (Messick et al., 1978)

Anesthetic problems related to resection of the pituitary gland are those common to any craniotomy, such as provision of patent airway, adequate pulmonary ventilation, control of circulating blood volume, inhibition of increase in brain size, and effective constant monitoring for adverse complications associated with posture, anesthesia, and operation. Premedication, use of anesthetic agents and techniques, and monitoring indicated for operations on the pituitary gland are essentially those which the individual anesthesiologist prefers for operations on other parts of the brain. The effects of anesthetic agents on secretion of pituitary hormones do not constitute an important factor in the selection of agents for use during operation on the pituitary gland. The effects of various anesthetic agents on release of hormones by the normal pituitary gland have been summarized by Oyama (1973).

Resection of the pituitary was once done only for tumor but now may be considered in the treatment of a variety of pathological states, such as metastatic carcinoma of the breast, complications of diabetes mellitus, and acromegaly. This change in attitude has been made possible by the availability of reliable endocrine products for use as substitutes for the natural secretion of the endocrine glands, which are inactivated by removal of the pituitary gland.

Preoperative Considerations. The pathology of the disease for which hypophysectomy is planned as treatment greatly influences the preparation and care of the patient during the procedure. Patients with advanced cancer should be suspected of having anemia, hypovolemia, pulmonary metastases with or without pleural effusion, or pulmonary fibrosis as the result of treatment. Difficulty with tracheal intubation may be anticipated in acromegalic patients with enlarged mandibles, massive tongue and epiglottis, and thickened pharyngeal mucosa and vocal cords. Tracheostomy should be considered either preoperatively or before removal of the endotracheal tube (Kitahata, 1971; Burn, 1972; Southwick and Katz, 1979). If the patient is to lie in a head-up position, insertion of a right atrial catheter and provision for monitoring for air embolism, preferably with ultrasonic Doppler apparatus, is recommended (Newfield et al., 1978). Prior to transsphenoidal hypophysectomy, use of nose drops containing neosynephrine and bacitracin has been suggested (Wilson and Dempsey, 1978). Carbohydrate metabolism of patients with diabetes mellitus should be controlled with insulin and diet before hypophysectomy.

Postoperative Considerations. ADRENAL STEROID THERAPY. The most serious threat to the welfare of the patient is the result of the pituitary-adrenal cortex relationship. Inadequate adrenocorticotropic hormone after removal of even part of the anterior pituitary gland may cause cessation or decreased secretion of cortisol. If all the gland is removed surgically, substitution therapy will be necessary for the remainder of the patient's life in doses varying from the adult maintenance dose of cortical steroid of 25 to 30 mg a day up to 10 times this amount during periods of stress. Preparation for this postoperative complication should begin in the preoperative period, as outlined for hypoadrenocorticism.

DIABETES INSIPIDUS. The degree and duration of diabetes insipidus following hypophysectomy will depend on the degree of injury to the adjacent hypothalamus, where antidiuretic hormone is formed. In practice, it has been estimated that about 50 per cent of patients develop some polydipsia and polyuria following the operation (Pearson, 1963), but all do not require subsitution therapy with antidiuretic hormone. Urine output should be monitored accurately during the immediate postoperative period, preferably through a urinary bladder catheter. If urine output exceeds the fluid volume that conveniently can be replaced (3 to 5 liters a day), treatment with vasopressin (Pitressin) should be considered. Aqueous solutions of vasopressin have a duration of action of two to eight hours, whereas that of vasopressin tannate in oil is one to two days. Because of side effects, the dose of vasopressin should be limited to that necessary to control diuresis, especially in pregnant or coronary disease patients because of the oxytocic and coronary constrictive properties of the preparation. Chlorpropamide and thiazide diuretics might be considered as an alternate method for control of diabetes insipidus in these patients (A.M.A. Drug Evaluation, 1973). Following vasopressin therapy, fluid administration must be adapted to urinary output to avoid water intoxication.

DIABETES MELLITUS. Following hypophysectomy, no appreciable change occurs in carbohydrate metabolism in the nondiabetic patient. In adult and juvenile diabetic patients, the insulin requirement is drastically reduced postoperatively. In the adult-type diabetic, insulin may be omitted on the day of operation, and in the juvenile-type diabetic, the preoperative dose of insulin may be reduced to about one third of usual. During the postoperative period, the urines of both types of diabetic patients should be monitored for sugar, and insulin should be given as outlined in the section on diabetes mellitus.

Other Complications. Operative trauma may lead to hyperthermia. Therefore, core tempature of patients should be monitored postoperatively. Convulsive seizures may occur, and phenytoin medication may be indicated as a prophylactic measure. Pharyngeal secretions should not be removed with a suction catheter through the nose, and the patient should be closely observed for leak of cerebrospinal fluid through the nose.

Substitution therapy with thyroid and sex hormones may eventually be indicated, but not for several weeks postoperatively after more life-threatening complications have been controlled.

ADRENAL CORTEX

PATHOPHYSIOLOGY OF THE ADRENAL CORTEX

Cholesterol in the adrenal gland is converted to Δ^5 - pregnenolone. This compound is changed either to progesterone or to 17-hydroxypregnenolone. Progesterone can be converted to aldosterone, the principal mineralocorticoid, only in the zona glomerulosa of the adrenal cortex. In the zona fasciculata and zona reticularis, progesterone is made into 11-deoxycortisol and finally to cortisol, the principal glucocorticoid. Sex hormones are also synthesized in the adrenal cortex. Testosterone is the most potent sex hormone synthesized; dehydroisoandrosterone and $^4\Delta$-androstenedione are weaker androgens but at times can contribute significantly to the androgen pool. Under certain circumstances, even estradiol, the female sex hormone, can be synthesized from its precursor hormone, testosterone. Roughly 15 to 20 mg of cortisol is secreted each day by the adrenal cortex and is tightly bound by cortisol-binding globulin, transcortin. Probably it is the free cortisol that is physiologically active.

The function of cortisol is complex but in general involves 1) anti-inflammatory reactions and immune responses and 2) reactions to stress. For instance, acute stresses, such as shock, trauma, blood volume depletion, infection, surgery, and general anesthesia, may precipitate enormous surges of cortisol production from the adrenal cortex. Cortisol also has important functions in the maintenance of the blood glucose levels. It is a potent stimulator of glucose production from the liver (gluconeogenesis) and an antagonist to the function of insulin. Adrenal cortical steroids can interact directly with the genetic material of the cell via specific intracellular receptors to bring about specific enzyme induction or inhibition.

Aldosterone is the principal mineralocorticoid secreted by the adrenal cortex. One of its chief physiological functions is maintenance of the blood pressure when the patient is in the upright posture. It has profound effects in the distal renal tubule, with resulting sodium reabsorption and renal loss of both potassium and hydrogen ion.

One of the principal control mechanisms is through the renin mechanisms of the juxtaglomerular apparatus of the kidney. For instance, low extracellular volume results in renin stimulation which in turn brings about synthesis of angiotensin I. Angiotensin I is converted to angiotensin II in the lungs. Angiotensin II, in addition to being an important peripheral vasoconstrictor, is a potent stimulator of aldosterone production which in turn tends to correct the deficient extracellular volume.

Adrenal androgen production tends to increase markedly at about the age of puberty and tends to decline with advancing age. Adrenal androgens may be converted to potent androgens in the liver. For instance, androstenedione can be converted in the liver to the potent androgen testosterone. In the postmenopausal female, androstenedione can be converted peripherally to estrogen.

Cortisol and androgen production and synthesis are controlled by pituitary adrenocorticotropic hormone (ACTH). In turn ACTH is controlled by corticotropin releasing factor (CRF) present in the hypothalamus. Cortisol, through closed negative feedback loop, inhibits both ACTH and CRF.

The other important aspect of ACTH physiology is that it is secreted in a diurnal fashion. High levels are secreted in the morning, and by early evening the blood levels of ACTH are beginning to drop. Thus, plasma levels of plasma cortisol may be twice as high in the morning as in the evening. Stimuli to ACTH secretion include a dropping plasma cortisol, fever, stress, low blood sugar, and surgery. Aldosterone is normally not under control of ACTH.

ADRENOCORTICAL HYPOFUNCTION (ADDISON'S DISEASE)

Hypofunction of the adrenal gland can be divided basically into chronic and acute insufficiency. Chronic primary adrenal cortical insufficiency can be caused by granulomatosis diseases such as histoplasmosis, tuberculosis, and metastatic disease. By far the most common disease that results in hypofunction is an autoimmune disorder involving production of adrenal antibodies. Simultaneous antibodies to thyroid tissue may evolve, with a resulting thyroiditis. The combination of primary adrenalitis and primary thyroiditis is called Schmidt's syndrome. Occasionally diabetes mellitus can be part of the whole picture, as can involvement of such other endocrine glands as the parathyroids. Patients with Addison's disease present with hyperpigmentation, hypovolemia, hyponatremia, hyperkalemia, eosinophilia, and occasionally hypoglycemia.

Acute adrenal insufficiency is a critical care problem characterized by severe hypotension usually brought on by sepsis and associated with high fever. Anticoagulants such as heparin and coumadin can sometimes cause acute bleeding into both adrenal glands. Overwhelming sepsis with bacteremia can be associated with severe and acute adrenocortical insufficiency. Perhaps the most common cuase of hypofunction of the adrenal gland is pharmacologic hypothalamic-pituitary-adrenal suppression in a patient who has taken pharmacologic quantities of steroids. In general, the higher the dose of steroids used and the longer the time interval they are used, the greater is the length of time following cessation of therapy that the entire pituitary-adrenal axis will remain suppressed. However, there are documented cases in which patients were treated for only two weeks and yet demonstrated significant hypothalamic-pituitary-adrenal axis suppression for up to 8 to 12 months following cessation of therapy. Alternate day pharmacologic steroid therapy has been shown to result in less suppression of the hypothalamic-pituitary-adrenal axis. In general, it is best to give steroids to any patient going to surgery who has been treated for as short a time as two or three weeks with pharmacologic doses of steroids during the 8 to 12 months following discontinuation of therapy. When in doubt, it is better to use steroids in any borderline situation. Obviously, any patient who is on replacement cortisol therapy or is getting pharmacologic quantities of steroids should be managed as an addisonian during a surgical procedure. Until more data are available, patients on alternate day steroid should also be managed as addisonians during a surgical procedure.

Another cause of adrenal hypofunction is pituitary hypofunction. These patients are not pigmented and have relative ACTH lack or a diminished reserve of ACTH. Cortisol production is diminished, but mineralocorticoids such as aldosterone may be near normal. Extracellular volume is therefore better maintained than in primary adrenocortical insufficiency. This will be discussed further in the section on pituitary disease. Congenital or acquired enzymatic defects of either cortisol or aldosterone synthesis usually present in early infancy with volume depletion and signs of excess androgen production (virilism). The 21-hydroxylase deficiency syndrome, which in its full-blown form results in deficiency of both aldosterone and cortisol production, is the most common form of the so-called adrenogenital syndrome.

Recently a new disease has been described that results in the failure of the juxtaglomerular apparatus to secrete renin. The entire renin-angiotensin-aldosterone axis is interrupted and a relative or secondary lack of aldosterone can result. These patients frequently present with hyperkalemia and postural hypotension. This syndrome is particularly common in patients with diabetes mellitus. Patients with aldosterone deficiency alone who have adequate cortisol reserve can sometimes present with just hyperkalemia with a normal extracellular volume. Cortisol and cortisol precursors apparently can compensate because they have weak mineralocorticoid effects.

Laboratory Test for Adrenocortical Hypofunction and Management

A single plasma cortisol determination does not help in making a decision about whether or not a particular patient has hypofunction of the adrenal cortex. Both ACTH and cortisol are secreted in a pulselike fashion, and the variation in plasma cortisol can be 20 μg per ml in the early morning and as low as 5 μg per ml in the late evening. The most specific test is measurement of the plasma cortisol or the 24 hour urine 17-hydroxycorticoid excretion after parenteral administration of ACTH. A very simple recently devised test involves the use of the new synthetic derivative of ACTH (Cortrosyn). Twenty-five units are given intravenously, and plasma cortisol is measured 30 to 60 minutes later. The plasma cortisol should rise by at least 12 μg per ml from baseline if the patient is normal. In a patient who has had prolonged suppression of the hypo-thalamic-pituitary-adrenal axis, prolonged stimulation with ACTH gel (40 units intramuscularly twice daily for 5 days) may be required before appropriate urine or blood samples can be obtained. If the patient has signs of severe electrolyte problems (hyponatremia or hyperkalemia) and is volume depleted, then a potent steroid such as dexamethasone should be started immediately (0.75 mg by mouth daily). Once the patient has stabilized on this dosage, specific ACTH testing should be done. Dexamethasone is a potent steroid, and in the small doses used for replacement therapy does not significantly contribute to the 17-hydroxycorticoid urinary excretion. Thus, the urinary 17-hydroxycorticoid excretion after ACTH reflects chiefly endogenous cortisol production. The urinary 17-hydroxycorticoid excretion should be at least two to three times higher than baseline as a normal response.

In someone who is acutely ill and who is a strong suspect for adrenocorticol hypofunction, immediate testing is not indicated but immediate treatment should be undertaken, with volume replacement, intravenous glucose, and massive amounts of steroids. Acute adrenocortical insufficiency is best treated with an immediate bolus of 100 mg hydrocortisone hemisuccinate or phosphate intravenously. Thereafter it should be given in a dose of 50 mg every 4 to 6 hours. Three hundred milligrams of hydrocortisone in divided doses should be given daily for two days. Thereafter the dose may be tapered by 50 mg daily.

When the patient is stable, replacement dexamethasone may be used (0.75 to 1.0 mg daily) and appropriate ACTH testing carried out as already indicated. Replacement cortisol therapy for the patient with either chronic or acute adrenocortical insufficiency is as follows: 20 mg cortisol in the morning and 10 mg cortisol in the late afternoon. Some patients will need mineralocorticoid replacement with fluorohydrocortisone (0.05 to 0.1 mg daily). This is a potent salt-retaining hormone, and at times potassium deficiency may result. Adequate dietary potassium is important for any patient on fluorohydrocortisone. The criteria for adequate replacement therapy should include a normal blood sugar, normal blood pressure, and correction of abnormal serum electrolytes.

Overtreatment with steroids can result in the features of Cushing's syndrome with dependent edema, hypertension, and electrolyte abnormalities, especially hypokalemia. Some physicians prefer to use one of the other synthetic steroid preparations as a replacement therapy, such as dexamethasone or prednisone. In terms of simple replacement therapy, 30 mg of cortisol is equivalent to 7.5 mg of prednisone and 0.75 mg of dexamethasone. In using these preparations, the physician must keep in mind the relative biologic potencies of these drugs as well as their relative glucocorticoid and mineralocorticoid potencies and their biologic half-lives (see Table 5–3). It is very easy to overtreat patients with these potent steroids. The potent steroid analogues do not have much in the way of mineralocorticoid properties when they are used in small replacement doses only, and sometimes patients can remain significantly volume depleted. These drugs are probably best reserved for medical problems that require ongoing pharmacologic quantities of a potent anti-inflammatory drug. The long-acting steroids, however, can be used as

Table 5–3 _Relative Potencies and Biologic Half-Lives of Cortisol and Its Synthetic Analogues_

Common Name	Other Name	Estimated Potency Glucocorticoid	Mineralo-corticoid	Biologic Half-Life Hours
Cortisol	Compound F, hydrocortisone	1	1	8–12
Cortisone	Cortone	0.8	0.8	8–12
Prednisone	—	4	0.25	12–36
Methyl-prednisolone	Medrol	5	0.25	12–36
Triamcinolone	Aristocort Kenacort	5	0.25	12–36
Dexamethasone	Decadron	20–30	±	26–54
Fluorohydrocortisone	Florinef	5	200	—
Desoxycorticosterone	Percorten	0	15	—

Table 5–4   *Suggested Schedule for Preoperative and Postoperative Steroid Maintenance in the Patient with Adrenal Insufficiency*

Evening before operation	Depo-medrol 40 mg IM at 10 P.M.
Morning of operation	Hydrocortisone 100 mg IV bolus before induction of anesthesia and 100 mg IV as a continuous IV drip during surgery
Postoperatively	
Day of surgery	Hydrocortisone 50 mg IV every 6 hours
Postoperative day 1	Hydrocortisone 50 mg IV every 6 hours
Postoperative day 2	Hydrocortisone 50 mg IV every 8 hours
Postoperative day 3	Hydrocortisone 50 mg IM every 12 hours or Depo-medrol 40 mg IM
Postoperative day 4	Cortisol 50 mg p.o. A.M., 30 mg p.o. P.M.
Postoperative day 5	Cortisol 40 mg p.o. A.M., 20 mg p.o. P.M.
Postoperative day 6	Cortisol 20 mg p.o. A.M., 10 mg p.o. P.M.
	Fluorohydrocortisone 0.05–0.1 mg daily or adequate oral salt replacement

supplemental management for the patient who is going to surgery or for the patient with adrenal crisis.

Pre- and Postoperative Management of the Patient with Adrenocortical Hypofunction

The patient with adrenocortical hypofunction who is going to surgery is managed essentially the same as a patient with an acute adrenal crisis. Preoperative preparation should include blood sugar and electrolyte determinations and assessment of volme depletion. Hyponatremia or hyperkalemia would be an indication that the patient is being undertreated with corticosteroid replacement. Preoperative parenteral cortisol might in this instance be necessary. Many physicians prefer to give the patient an injection of a long-acting steroid preparation such as methyl prednisolone intramuscularly (Depomedrol) the night before surgery. It is the contention of many experts that patients on pharmacologic amounts of steroids (e.g., the patient with a connective tissue disorder on steroids) should be given a long-acting steroid preparation (Depomedrol, 40 mg daily) at least two days and sometimes three days prior to surgery. This seems to prevent an exacerbation of the patient's basic disease, which may be brought on by the surgical procedure itself.

Patients with adrenocortical deficiency tend to develop hyponatremia easily because of inability of the kidney to excrete free water. Therefore, it is wise to avoid giving these patients hypotonic fluids. During the surgical procedure and immediately postoperatively, isotonic or normal saline should be used. Because of the propensity of the addisonian to develop hypoglycemia, glucose should be included in the intravenous fluid regimen.

A convenient intravenous fluid solution is 5 per cent dextrose in normal saline. While hyperkalemia may exist preoperatively in the undertreated patient, hypokalemia may result postoperatively. Appropriate replacement with 20 mEq of potassium per hour is safe as long as renal function is normal. Table 5–4 outlines a typical steroid regimen for a patient going to surgery. A long-acting injection of steroid (Depomedrol) the evening before surgery is preferred. One hundred mg of hydrocortisone hemisuccinate (Solu-cortef) is given just before induction of anesthesia and another 100 mg is given as a constant intravenous drip during the surgical procedure itself. Two to three hundred mg of hydrocortisone is given for a day or two after surgery and thereafter the drug is tapered by about 50 mg daily until replacement doses are reached. Depomedrol is easily tolerated with essentially no pain at the injection site and has a long biologic half-life. The kind of surgery and the degree of trauma involved will determine the extent and duration of steroid treatment. For instance, an addisonian who is going to have major abdominal surgery will require several days of high doses of hydrocortisone with perhaps slower tapering than a patient going for a simple cataract operation who can be tapered quickly.

A special problem arises when a patient with adrenocortical insufficiency also has diabetes mellitus and is on insulin therapy. The section on diabetes describes just such a circumstance. In general, patients with Addison's disease are very sensitive to insulin, and the amount of insulin given during and after surgery needs careful monitoring. It is important to give intravenous glucose during the operative/postoperative period. Usually about 0.5 to 1 unit of regular insulin per hour given as a constant intravenous infusion in 5 per cent dextrose and normal saline will easily control the diabetic problem.

Sudden unexplained hypotension during surgery requires measurement of central venous pressure and often a Swan-Ganz catheter to help evaluate the volume status of the patient. The administration of a bolus of 100 to 150 mg of hydrocortisone hemisuccinate intravenously is often indicated in this situation. Corticosteroids have a permissive effect on endogenous catecholamines or exogenous vasopressor types of agents.

ADRENOCORTICAL HYPERFUNCTION

Cushing's Syndrome. Patients with excess cortisol production present with a classic constellation of signs and symptoms which in part is related to the degree and duration of the excess cortisol. The familiar picture consists of plethoric facies, thin skin, abdominal striae, easy bruisability, hypertension, hirsutism, osteoporosis, centripetal obesity, buffalo hump, supraclavicular fat pads, muscle weakness, poor wound healing, hypokalemia, and abnormal glucose tolerance. In children, impaired growth is an important aspect of the disease. By far the most common cause of Cushing's syndrome is use of pharmacologic amounts of steroids. Iatrogenic Cushing's syndrome also has a high association with beginning intracranial hypertension, cataracts, pancreatitis, and aseptic necrosis of the hips. About 80 per cent of cases of Cushing's syndrome are due to bilateral adrenal hyperplasia secondary to an ACTH secreting tumor of the pituitary gland (Cushing's disease). Adrenal adenomas and carcinomas with excess cortisol production and suppressed ACTH account for a small percentage of the total cases. Ectopic ACTH production from a cancer of the lung, pancreas, kidney, or thymus can result in an acute syndrome with almost none of the usual features of Cushing's syndrome and all of the features of mineralocorticoid excess (i.e., severe hypokalemic alkalosis). Adreno-

cortical hyperplasia can occasionally be part of the multiple endocrine adenomatosis syndrome (MEA-I).

Laboratory Tests

Plasma levels of cortisol are high in Cushing's syndrome but are not specific enough to make the diagnosis. Plasma cortisol levels may be elevated in patients on estrogens, in acute stress, and in alcoholism. However, absence of the diurnal variation is a good clue to an autonomous production of cortisol. The urinary 17-hydroxycorticosteroid excretion (17-OHS) is normally between 3 and 7 mg per gram of urinary creatinine. Urinary 17-OHS is a poor discriminator between the normal state and Cushing's syndrome, since elevated urinary levels are also found in obesity, and depressed levels are found in hepatic and renal disease. The urinary free cortisol test is a difficult laboratory procedure but an excellent discriminator between persons in the normal state and patients with Cushing's syndrome.

Perhaps the single best screening test is the short dexamethasone suppression study. This will usually distinguish obese persons from those with Cushing's syndrome in over 95 per cent of cases. One mg of dexamethasone is given by mouth at midnight. A normal response is suppression of the baseline plasma cortisol by at least 50 per cent, usually below 5 μg per 100 ml. If there is no suppression with the short dexamethasone suppression test, then the longer suppression test with collection of 24 hour urine samples for 17-hydroxycorticosteroids (17-OHS) is necessary. A baseline 24 hour urine is collected and then a low dose test with 0.5 mg of dexamethasone is given every six hours for two days. If the total urinary 17-OHS is suppressed below 3.5 mg in 24 hours, Cushing's syndrome is ruled out. If there is no suppression, then a high dose of 2 mg of dexamethasone is given every six hours for two days. Suppression on the high dose of dexamethasone but failure to suppress on the low dose helps establish the diagnosis of bilateral adrenal hyperplasia secondary to an ACTH secreting tumor of the pituitary gland. In addition, the plasma ACTH level should be mildly elevated. Failure to suppress on both the low and high dose of dexamethasone means that an adrenal tumor or the ectopic ACTH syndrome is present. The plasma ACTH level is usually quite elevated in the ectopic

ACTH syndrome but is virtually totally suppressed in the presence of an adrenal tumor.

Skull films to determine the size of the sella turcica should be obtained in all patients with bilateral adrenal hyperplasia. At times, despite careful testing, exact differentiation of all possible causes of Cushing's syndrome can be difficult. In recent years a new variant of Cushing's syndrome has been described which is associated with a paradoxical increase in cortisol production after dexamethasone. Almost all of these patients have large chromophobe adenomas.

Management of the Patient with Hypercortisolism

There have been some interesting changes in the management of Cushing's syndrome in recent years. There is increasing evidence that bilateral adrenal hyperplasia is due to ACTH secreting microadenoma of the pituitary gland (Cushing's disease). It is even possible to make a case for a hypothalamic lesion in Cushing's disease. The drug cyproheptadine, a serotonin antagonist, can inhibit secretion of ACTH in patients with Cushing's disease. Further work on long-term management with this drug is now being evaluated. The most innovative therapy for Cushing's disease is removal of pituitary adenoma or microadenoma via the neurosurgical procedure known as transsphenoidal hypophysectomy. Pituitary irradiation is a useful modality in the treatment of children with Cushing's disease but appears to have little value in the adult patient. Heavy particle irradiation may be a more useful treatment in the adult. The patient with extremely severe glucocorticoid excess and adrenal hyperplasia may still turn out to be a candidate for bilateral adrenalectomy despite the increased morbidity and mortality associated with this procedure. The precise treatment for Cushing's syndrome is still very much in doubt. It seems quite likely that transsphenoidal hypophysectomy with its low morbidity and mortality will be the treatment of choice for patients with mild disease and that bilateral adrenalectomy will be reserved as an emergency procedure for those patients with exceedingly severe disease.

Precise localization of small pituitary tumors will doubtless improve. The CT head scanner used with contrast material along with special radiographic tomographic cuts of the sella turcica can identify small pituitary tumors. Moreover, the fiberoptic equipment for performing transsphenoidal hypophysectomy will also allow precise visual localization of small tumors. As the experience of neurosurgeons improves, smaller tumors will be localized and removed. It is the feeling of many experts that use of transsphenoidal hypophysectomy will continue to increase as the primary modality for the management of patients with adrenal hyperplasia. About 10 per cent of patients with Cushing's disease who have had bilateral adrenalectomy will develop frank tumors of the pituitary (Nelson's syndrome), sometimes associated with suprasellar extension and optic nerve compression. The clinical course of these patients is characterized by severe and progressive hyperpigmentation and exceedingly high ACTH levels. This conceivably can be used as another argument against bilateral adrenalectomy for treatment of Cushing's disease.

The patient with a unilateral adenoma or carcinoma of the adrenal gland will be a candidate for surgical removal. Localization preoperatively of the tumor with an intravenous pyelogram, ultrasonic study, arteriography, or the total body scanner (CAT scanner) is obviously important.

Patients with ectopic secreting tumors and Cushing's syndrome should have the primary tumor removed whenever possible. Often, however, this is impossible. For instance, oat cell carcinoma of the lung, which is one of the more important causes of the ectopic ACTH syndrome, has usually metastasized by the time the diagnosis is made. Chemotherapy, however, is very effective in this disease. Metastatic carcinoma from the adrenal gland can sometimes be controlled by the chemotherapeutic agents aminoglutethimide and o,p,-DDD.

Pre- and Postoperative Management of the Patient with Hypercortisolism

Patients with Cushing's syndrome are extremely fragile. Significant diabetes, hypertension, electrolyte abnormalities (especially hypokalemia), and osteoporosis can all coexist. Significant elevations of blood sugar are best controlled with small amounts of insulin given intravenously (1 unit regular insulin per hour intravenously) in the operative and postoperative period, as outlined in the section on diabetes. Hypertension can often be related to significant blood volume increases associated with polycythemia and to extracellular volume increases due to salt retention. Mild congestive heart failure may coexist. The loop diuretics (furosemide) are probably the best agents to treat these latter problems during the preoperative period. It is very important, however, to be well aware of hypokalemia, which may be aggravated by diuretics. Hypokalemia can lead to muscle weakness, which can further lead to alveolar hypoventilation with restrictive lung disease. The obesity of these patients can aggravate the restrictive lung disease. Hypokalemia is best corrected by oral potassium administration, 80 to 100 mEq per day, especially if a loop diuretic is used to control hypertension. A central venous pressure line and even a Swan-Ganz catheter should be used to monitor blood volume and pulmonary arterial wedge pressure during surgery. Volume replacement must be judged accordingly.

Osteoporosis and osteomalacia often lead to vertebral compression fractures in patients with Cushing's syndrome. Prolonged immobilization in these patients is hazardous and can lead to further demineralization postoperatively. It has been suggested that all patients on high dosage steroids or with Cushing's syndrome should be on vitamin D therapy (50,000 units of calciferol twice weekly along with calcium supplementation). Following surgery, however, prolonged immobilization can even lead to hypercalcemia and renal stones. Vitamin D should probably be started when the patient is fully recovered and mobile, and not prior to surgery.

All patients going to surgery, whether for transsphenoidal hypophysectomy or bilateral adrenalectomy, should be managed as if they were addisonians. If bilateral adrenalectomy is to be done, the patient should be given 200 to 300 mg of hydrocortisone hemisuccinate or phosphate the day of surgery and the procedure outlined in Table 5-2 followed. Following surgery, it is important to taper these patients slowly. It may take several weeks before a patient with a bilateral adrenalectomy can be tapered down to a maintenance cortisol (30 mg daily) and Florinef (0.1 mg daily) replacement therapy. Rapid tapering can lead to serious hypotension and even serious psychotic and depressive episodes. Postoperative pancreatitis, probably due to surgical injury, is a potential serious complication. Pre- and postoperatively, patients with bilateral adrenalectomy are subject to strokes, myocardial infarction, intractable stress gastric ulcers, pulmonary emboli, and poor wound healing. Postoperative management should probably be carried out in the intensive care unit. Transsphenoidal hypophysectomy certainly will obviate many of the problems of bilateral adrenalectomy. Steroid replacement does not have to be as intense and may be tapered quickly. Generally, 100–200 mg of hydrocortisone hemisuccinate is given the day of surgery and the patient can be tapered completely down to replacement therapy within a week or two. Thereafter, all steroid therapy usually can be stopped if enough normal pituitary gland has been left intact.

A metapyrone test may be used to judge the integrity of the hypothalamic-pituitary-adrenal axis. There is some evidence that metapyrone may be used as a therapeutic as well as a diagnostic test. Metapyrone (11-hydroxylase inhibitor) blocks the conversion of desoxycortisol (compound S) to cortisol (compound F), the very last step in cortisol biosynthesis. It has been used in patients with adrenal hyperplasia and adrenal tumors and in the ectopic ACTH syndrome with success. It does not always work in patients with adrenal hyperplasia, since the high ACTH levels can override the effect of the 11-hydroxylase block. Theoretically the metapyrone in sufficient doses (2 or more gm/day in divided doses) may render many patients with Cushing's syndrome euadrenal prior to surgery and will have a useful role in the preoperative management of these patients. Further study of this point is necessary.

Adrenal adenomas and carcinomas are almost always unilateral, and precise localization preoperatively must be done carefully. Computerized tomography (CAT scan) will probably be the most useful modality for localizing these tumors. Operative and postoperative management is the same as already indicated. These patients must be managed as addisonians postoperatively. Generally the contralateral adrenal gland, which is normal, will have been completely suppressed by the tumor in the other adrenal. It may take several months before the suppressed adrenal is functioning following surgical removal of the tumorous adrenal gland. Following surgery, steroids should be tapered within two weeks to 30 to 40 mg of cortisol daily with fludrocortisone acetate (Florinef), 0.1 mg, if necessary. Thereafter, very slow tapering of corticosteroid therapy is indicated. Roughly 5 mg of cortisol can be tapered per month until the patient is completely off therapy and hopefully the normal adrenal gland is functioning. A metapyrone test may be useful to test the integrity of the entire pituitary-adrenal axis at this point. The metapyrone test will be discussed more extensively in the section on pituitary disease.

Primary Aldosteronism. Mineralocorticoid or aldosterone producing tumors result in sodium retention and potassium wasting, leading to hypertension and hypokalemia. The hypertension appears to be at least partially volume related. The chronic hypokalemia can lead to muscle weakness, polyuria, and abnormal carbohydrate tolerance. Excessive aldosterone secretion can result from either a functioning adrenal adenoma (Conn's syndrome) or from bilateral adrenal hyperplasia. The plasma renin level is markedly suppressed in primary aldosteronism and can be used as a good screening test. Urine potassium tends to be high in the face of a low blood potassium. The definitive test is to measure plasma aldosterone levels before and after sodium loading or after desoxycorticosterone acetate injection. Failure of the aldosterone level to be suppressed after these maneuvers is evidence that primary aldosteronism exists. It is very important to differentiate Conn's syndrome from bilateral adrenal hyperplasia because the latter condition is often not helped by surgery. Patients with functioning adrenal adenomas have lower serum potassium, lower plasma renins, and higher aldosterone production than patients with bilateral adrenal hyperplasia. Venous localization with measurement of aldosterone levels in both adrenal veins is a useful procedure. With Conn's syndrome the aldosterone level is high only in the adrenal vein draining the tumor and is suppressed on the contralateral side, while bilateral high levels indicate bilateral adrenal hyperplasia. Localization can be aided by the CAT scanner. ^{131}I-B-19 norcholesterol adrenal imaging remains an experimental procedure but has been successfully used to separate nodular hyperplasia from Conn's syndrome.

Patients with Conn's syndrome can be prepared for surgery by the use of the aldosterone antagonist spironolactone. Doses up to 300 mg daily will often reverse not only the hypertension but also the hypokalemia. Generally, these patients are normal with respect to glucocorticoid metabolism. If one adrenal gland is removed and the other is left intact, no cortisol replacement therapy is necessary. Temporary mineralocorticoid replacement therapy with Florinef (0.1 mg) might be necessary for a few weeks.

Sex Hormone Secreting Tumors of the Adrenal Gland. Hirsutism in the female may be due to either adrenal or ovarian tumor. Adrenal virilizing tumors are almost always associated with markedly elevated 17-ketosteroid urinary excretion, while functioning ovarian tumors tend to produce very potent androgens such as testosterone or dihydrotestosterone which are not measured as part of the 17-ketosteroids. At times the workup can be very confusing. There are documented cases in which adrenal tumors produced only testosterone and were stimulated by human chorionic gonadotropin. Similarly, some androgen producing ovarian tumors have been shown to respond to dexamethasone suppression. A common cause of hirsutism in females is polycystic ovarian disease, which is associated with bilaterally enlarged ovaries. Extreme feminization in males can be occasionally due to an estrogen producing tumor of the adrenal gland. Functioning sex hormone producing tumors of the adrenal gland almost always tend to be unilateral. Pelvic B-mode ultrasonography and the total body scanner are both very useful modalities for localizing lesions. Most patients do not have to be managed with glucocorticoids during or after surgery. The only exception is the patient who has associated Cushing's syndrome with cortisol excess. Then management should be as already outlined for unilateral tumors of the adrenal gland.

Adrenal genital syndrome should be ruled out as a possible cause of hirsutism. These patients are not surgical candidates. Generally, in addition to high 17-ketosteroid levels in the urine, these patients have very high urinary pregnanetriol levels and elevated 17-OH progesterone blood levels. They are generally managed with mildly suppressive doses of corticosteroids.

ANESTHESIA FOR THE PATIENT WITH DISEASE OF ADRENAL CORTEX

The relationships of adrenocortical mechanisms to anesthesia were extensively reviewed by Vandam and Moore (1960) and these concepts still are reasonably valid.

Premedication. Preoperative apprehension does not seem to elicit activation of the adrenal cortex to produce plasma cortisol levels much above the upper level of normal diurnal variations. Therefore, customary drugs and doses of premedicant agents have been employed before operation for most patients with adrenocortical dysfunction. Morphine (Briggs and Munson, 1955) and short-acting barbiturates (Vandam and Moore, 1960) have been thought to depress cortical activity, possibly through an effect at the hypothalamic level. However, in the doses used for premedication, these and other premedicant drugs exert no clinically adverse effects and do not inhibit the adrenocortical response to the stress of operation (Oyama et al., 1977). Nishioka and coworkers (1968) found that a combination of meperidine and atropine did not lower or raise plasma cortisol levels.

Anesthetic Agents and Methods. Many studies have been carried out on the effects of anesthesia on adrenocortical function. Conclusions from these studies have sometimes been contradictory, partly as a result of differences in design of the experiments and in the methods employed. Interpretation of the clinical significance of these studies has been even more confusing because there is no agreement about whether it is advantageous to employ an anesthetic method that depresses adrenal function or one that stimulates adrenal function.

The general concepts about the effect of anesthetic agents and methods will be briefly summarized. The effect of premedication agents, anesthetic agents, and muscle relaxants in cortisol production has been reviewed by Oyama (1973).

Anesthesia with thiopental and pentobarbital does not cause a rise in plasma cortisol, but increased levels following operation are not prevented. Induction of anesthesia with thiopental may decrease the degree of rise in plasma cortisol following subsequently administered inhalation agents but does not prevent the elevation entirely.

Administration of halothane leads to a rise of plasma cortisol levels but not as great as that after methoxyflurane. Halothane tends to depress the adrenal response to stress and ACTH (Nishioka et al., 1968), perhaps for as long as four hours after anesthesia has been discontinued (Carnes, 1963).

Enflurane anesthesia without operation causes a slight fall in cortisol release but does not prevent the rise caused by operation. The effect more resembles that of methoxyflurane than that of halothane and has been recommended for patients with hypercortisolism (Oyama et al., 1972).

Adequate regional anesthesia or paraplegia with transection of the spinal cord above the innervation of the operative site prevents the adrenocortical hyperfunction resulting from operation (Hume et al., 1962). After spinal anesthesia, the effects of the operation become manifest as soon as the anesthesia wears off. Johnston (1964) found plasma cortisol levels to be elevated in patients during prolonged spinal anesthesia, and believes that other afferent pathways may initiate an adrenocortical response in the presence of a spinal block. Epidural anesthesia can inhibit or prevent adrenal response to operation, depending on the level of sensory block (Enquista et al., 1977).

Hypothermia below 28° C blocks response of the adrenal cortex to both stress and ACTH. Above 30° C the response may be present but is attenuated. However, since metabolism of circulating glucocorticoids is also reduced, plasma levels may remain near normal during operations performed under hypothermia (Van Brunt and Ganong, 1963).

These changes caused by anesthetic agents and methods are insignificant when compared to the tenfold increase in secretion of cortisol that may occur during and after surgical operation. The rise seems to be in proportion to the severity of the operation; it reaches a peak six to eight hours after operation, regardless of the type of anesthesia, and persists for several days, depending on the surgical procedure and postoperative complications.

Adrenocortical Hyperfunction

Operative Problems. The problems will vary with the duration and degree of exposure to excessive glucocorticoids and to the efficacy of the preparation of the patient for operation. Problems likely to present are those related to diabetes, hypokalemia, osteoporosis, and arterial hypertension.

DIABETES. Diabetic care during operation must be coordinated with both pre- and postoperative therapy. If insulin has been required before operation, one should give half to one third the dose of long-acting insulin the morning of surgery, or else plans should be made for intravenous administration of regular insulin with monitoring of blood glucose during the operation. Glucose should be included in the intravenous fluids administered throughout the anesthesia and continued into the postoperative period until adequate carbohydrate can be taken by mouth. Postoperatively, crystalline insulin should be given every four hours, the dose determined by urine and blood sugar levels.

HYPOKALEMIA. Excess glucocorticoid secretion leads to increased reabsorption of sodium and excretion of potassium by the kidneys; low potassium stores combined with muscle wasting from increased protein catabolism may result in muscle weakness. This can interfere with adequate pulmonary ventilation unless respiration is assisted or controlled. Increased fat synthesis and fat storage on the trunk can lead to an increase in respiratory work for the "weak fat man." The hypokalemia can be relieved with supplemental oral intake of potassium chloride preoperatively.

OSTEOPOROSIS. Skeletal demineralization is widespread, so pathological fractures may occur. These patients should be moved with care.

HYPERTENSION. Polycythemia develops, total blood volume increases, and systolic and diastolic pressures rise. These changes often lead to congestive heart failure. Central venous pressure and possibly pulmonary wedge pressure monitoring should be considered during operation and the immediate postoperative period.

The atrophic skin is easily bruised, and hematomas easily develop at the sites of venipuncture and minimal trauma.

Postoperative Problems. The problems present during operation continue into the postoperative period and require continued monitoring and supportive care.

The surgical treatment for hyperfunctioning adrenal cortex is adrenalectomy or hy-

pophysectomy. The likely result will be inadequate adrenocortical secretion during the postoperative period, so substitution therapy with glucocorticoids is necessary. Such therapy should begin in the preoperative period and continue through the operation and on into the postoperative period, as outlined in the following section on acute adrenal insufficiency. Therapy may be necessary for life, depending on the amount of residual functioning adrenocortical tissue. After total adrenalectomy, substitution therapy will be necessary for the remainder of the patient's life at a dosage of approximately 30 mg a day of cortisol and 0.1 mg of Florinef daily. The dosage will have to be increased during hot humid weather, circumstances of stress, febrile episodes or intercurrent infection.

Postoperative supplements of 40 to 80 mEq of potassium chloride added to intravenous fluids daily may be needed to restore depleted body stores until food and electrolytes can be taken by mouth.

Administration of sodium salts should be kept to a minimum as long as large doses of steroids are necessary.

Postoperative pancreatitis from surgical retraction during removal of the left adrenal is a serious postoperative complication. The incidence of postoperative wound infection and slow healing is high.

Adrenocortical Hypofunction

Operative and Postoperative Problems. The status of the patient with adrenocortical insufficiency can vary widely, from the precarious asthenia of untreated severe Addison's disease to a complete lack of symptoms.

Chronic advanced hypoadrenocorticism is characterized by hyponatremia, hyperkalemia, dehydration, low blood volume, arterial hypotension, small heart, and hypoglycemia, all of which add up to a very poor risk patient in whom acute circulatory collapse is imminent. The need for extensive preoperative correction of this precarious state is evident.

On the other hand, a patient whose adreno-pituitary axis has been depressed by administration of glococorticoids in the past may have no symptoms during ordinary daily activities even without medication. However, following acute stress of operation, he may rapidly develop acute circulatory collapse and die unless treated promptly. In both states, the cornerstone of prevention and treament is the administration of cortisol.

At present, the degree and duration of adrenocortical suppression following cortisol therapy cannot be rapidly and accurately determined, although attempts at empirical predication continue (Oyama et al., 1972; Kehlet and Binder, 1973). Consequently, safe policy has been toward overtreatment, which has few sequelae when given for a short time, in preference to the risk of undertreatment, which may be fatal.

When persistent hypotension develops during anesthesia and operation, an attempt should first be made to rule out the usual causes of shock. If none can be found, central venous pressure should be measured to evaluate heart failure and establish a baseline for blood replacement. Cortisol, 100 mg may be given intravenously rapidly with occasional good results but cortisol is not the prime determinant of blood pressure during and after surgery in glucocorticoid treated patients (Kehlet and Binder, 1973). This action is explained by the need for a minimal concentration of glucocorticoid in the tissues for normal action of vasopressor drugs. Following cortisol administration, a dose of vasopressor that had previously been ineffective may produce the desired result.

Hydrocortisone acetate or methylprednisolone acetate are depot forms and are useful on the evening before surgery to make certain that the patient gets steroid treatment in the event of possible nursing error or trouble with intravenous therapy during operation. Postoperatively, the dose is decreased until maintenance therapy of 30 mg a day is reached. The largest portion of the replacement dose is given at 8:00 A.M. to mimic the normal diurnal variation in ACTH and cortisol secretion in which most cortisol is secreted between 2:00 and 6:00 A.M. It cannot be emphasized too strongly that in cortisol replacement therapy, when in doubt, GIVE IT. The complications of corticosteroid therapy are related to the total dose given over a prolonged period of time. A large dose can be given over a few days with relative impunity. However, withholding cortisol when it is needed acutely can have disastrous results.

After total adrenalectomy or prolonged adrenocortical suppression, Florinef, 0.1 mg orally (or intramuscular desoxycorticos-terone acetate in oil, 10 mg), should be given daily when the dose of cortisol has been reduced below 100 mg daily (Cahill and Thorn, 1963).

Primary Aldosteronism

Operative Problems.   Preanesthetic medication and anesthetic agents and methods for removal of an aldosterone-secreting tumor of the adrenal may be chosen as for any major operation in the upper retroperitoneal space (Finch, 1969). Whether the surgical approach is anterior through the abdomen or posterior through a subcostal incision, exposure is difficult and good muscular relaxation is necessary. This necessitates complete control of the airway by tracheal intubation and controlled respiration, since pneumothorax is always a possible complication. Usually aldosterone producing adenomas are smaller than most adrenal tumors and are more difficult for the surgeon to identify, and so more exposure and dissection may be needed. Part or all of an adrenal gland may have to be removed and serial sections made to determine the presence or absence of such small tumors. Both adrenal glands may have to be explored.

Care must be taken that circulation of the friable adrenal tissue is preserved and is not impaired by dissection or trauma in order to prevent postoperative adrenal insufficiency. The surgeon needs all the help that is possible in solving these problems.

Aldosterone promotes reabsorption of sodium by the distal renal tubules, increase in extracellular fluid, and hypertension. Loss of potassium by the kidney leads to hypokalemic alkalosis. Hypokalemia may result in muscle weakness which may lead to respiratory embarrassment and atrial and ventricular arrhythmias, even though serum potassium levels and electrocardiogram are within normal limits (Gangat et al., 1976). Preoperative repletion of potassium stores with oral administration of 2 to 6 gm per day of potassium chloride in divided doses may be indicated, even though such therapy tends to increase aldosterone secretions. Hypokalemia definitely increases the surgical risk. If potassium stores cannot readily be repleted by oral administration of potassium, spironolactone (Aldactone) can be given to diminish the aldosterone effect on the kidney tubules by competition at the effector cell membrane. A low sodium diet aids in restoring potassium deficits.

Postoperative Problems. If the aldosterone secreting tumor is completely removed, serum electrolytes rapidly return to normal. Sodium conservation by the kidney may be poor for the first month after unilateral adrenalectomy, probably as a result of the remaining adrenal not being able to secrete enough aldosterone.

Glucocorticoid secretion is usually adequate. However, if total adrenalectomy is performed or if the vascular supply to remaining adrenal tissue is damaged during partial adrenalectomy, therapy with glucocorticoid and mineralocorticoid will be required, as outlined in the section on adrenal insufficiency.

ADRENAL MEDULLA: PHEOCHROMOCYTOMA

PATHOPHYSIOLOGY

The catecholamine secreting pheochromocytoma is a rare disease characterized by hypertension that may either be sustained or paroxsymal. Contrary to previous teaching, at least one half of patients with this disease have sustained hypertension. Ninety per cent of these tumors are found in the medulla of the adrenal gland. Most tend to be unilateral, but in patients who have a familial tendency, both adrenals may be involved. Only a very small percentage of these tumors are malignant. Other locations for these tumors (less than 10%) include sites along the sympathetic chain. Most unusual sites have been reported in the thorax, bladder, brain, and the organs of Zuckerkandl. In less than 5 per cent of cases these tumors are associated with neurofibromatosis and only rarely with von Hippel-Lindau disease. The syndrome known as familial endocrine adenomatosis type II (Sipple's syndrome) consists of the association of pheochromocytoma (usually bilateral), medullary carcinoma of the thyroid, and parathyroid adenomas. One, two, or all three of these endocrine gland tumors may be found in different family members, and the genetic mode may follow an autosomal dominant pattern. A most unusual association of pheochromocytomas has been described with medullary carcinoma of the thyroid and multiple mucosal neuromata (multiple endocrine adenomatosis type III). There have been a few case reports about the rare association of pheochromocytoma with pregnancy.

The symptoms of pheochromocytoma consist of attacks of headache, palpitations, sweating, abdominal pain, nausea, visual disturbances, irritability, weight loss, angina, and fainting spells related to posture. Physical findings in addition to hypertension include postural hypotension, cardiomegaly, and mild elevation of basal body temperature. Only very rarely is a tumor palpable in the abdomen. The signs and symptoms of hypermetabolism can mimic those of thyrotoxicosis. Rarely postural hypotension can be quite severe and sometimes is the major reason the patient seeks medical attention. It may be related to the fact that occasionally the beta effects of the catecholamines may override the alpha effects. Some of these patients who present with severe postural hypotension also may have systemic hypotension and evidence of cardiomyopathy. These unusual patients have primary epinephrine secreting tumors with predominant stimulation of the beta adrenergic nervous system. By far the most common form of pheochromocytoma is associated with predominant secretion of norepinephrine relative to epinephrine. A high incidence of cardiomyopathy has been reported in pheochromocytoma associated with myocardial fibrosis.

Laboratory evaluation reveals a modestly elevated blood sugar (due to suppression of insulin secretion by beta catecholamines), a rise in hematocrit that may reflect a diminished plasma volume, and an elevated white cell count with a shift to the left. The adrenal medulla is virtually the only gland that secretes epinephrine, while norepinephrine may be secreted in both the adrenal medulla and peripherally via the postganglionic fibers of the sympathetic nervous system. Thus, the presence of epinephrine (at least 20% of the total catecholamines) and norepinephrine in excessive amounts in the urine indicates that the tumor is most likely of adrenal origin, while the secretion of excessive norepinephrine alone may indicate that the tumor has a sympathetic ganglion origin as well as an adrenal medullary origin. A high concentration of epinephrine or one of its metabolites in the urine indicates that propranolol, the beta blocker, may be effective in the management of the patient.

The turnover of both norepinephrine and epinephrine is very rapid and their half-life in the circulation is only a few minutes. This rapid removal is due partially to their metabolism by monoamine oxidase and catechol-o-methyl transferase. The metabolic end products include 3-methoxy, 4-hydroxymandelic acid (VMA) and the metanephrines. If a patient ingests a large quantity of a precursor to the catecholamines such as tyramine, which is contained in Cheddar cheese and Chianti wines, a serious hypertensive crisis may develop.

LABORATORY TESTS

By far the best tests to determine the presence of a pheochromocytoma is the measurement of 24 hour urine collections for either free catecholamines or metabolites of the catecholamines. The measurement of normetanephrine and metanephrine is probably the most reliable test. Recent evidence indicates that even a single four to six hour urine collection for the metanephrines and creatinine (using a ratio of the two parameters) is an extremely reliable screening test for pheochromocytomas. The urine VMA is less reliable and will pick up only about 80 to 85 per cent of tumors. It is very difficult to measure free urinary or plasma catecholamines, although measurement of free catecholamines in the blood may eventually be the single best screening test. A number of drugs such as methyldopa and L-dopa will interfere with the catecholamine determinations. Quinidine and tetracycline will produce interfering fluorescence in the determinations of both catecholamines and the metanephrines. Food and beverages such as citrus fruits, coffee, and chocolate have large quantities of phenolic acids that are excreted in the urine and yield a high apparent VMA. Drugs such as hydrochlorothiazide, hydralazine, reserpine, guanethidine, propranolol, or digitalis do not interfere with the urinary determinations described above. Normal values for the urinary metabolites are as follows: free catecholamines, less than 100 μg per 24 hours; metanephrines, less than 1 mg in 24 hours; VMA, less than 7 mg in 24 hours.

The phentolamine (Regitin) and histamine tests are both considered far too unreliable and dangerous. They are no longer useful diagnostic tests. Computerized tomography will shortly be the single best localizing study. Angiography probably is still necessary because it gives the surgeon a preoperative idea of where the major blood supply to the tumor is located.

PRE- AND POSTOPERATIVE MANAGEMENT OF THE PATIENT WITH PHEOCHROMOCYTOMA

Surgery is virtually the only cure for patients with pheochromocytoma. Since norepinephrine accounts for most catecholamine secretion in these tumors, an alpha blocking agent is essential. Phentolamine or phenoxybenzamine (Dibenzyline) are the two blocking agents that have been used most in the past. Oral Dibenzyline is considered presently superior to phentolamine because it can be given just once daily and tends to produce less tachycardia and postural hypotension. Treatment with Dibenzyline should begin very cautiously, with doses of 10 to 20 mg daily and slowly increased to 50 mg twice daily if necessary until control of hypertension is achieved. It is very easy to overtreat patients with this drug. Overtreatment usually manifests itself as severe postural hypotension and occasionally as severe diminution in bowel motility with almost a megacolon picture. In some cases as the disease comes under control with Dibenzyline, there may be a drop in hematocrit associated with postural hypotension. In all probability there has been an expansion of the blood volume space, which accounts for the hypotension. Plasma expanders and whole blood transfusion may be given if this happens.

Once the patient has been controlled with adequate alpha blockade, beta blockers may also be used, especially if tachyarrhythmias are a potential problem. Beta blockers should never be used before alpha blockers, since the hypertension may actually be accentuated in this circumstance. An adequate dose range for a beta blocker such as propranolol is 20 to 80 mg by mouth daily in divided doses. Arrhythmias during surgery can likewise be handled with intravenous propranolol (1-2 mg).

It is extremely important in preparing the patient with pheochromocytoma to keep him very nearly at bed rest. Excessive activity can result in wide swings in blood pressure, sometimes with an associated myocardial infarction. If a hypertensive crisis occurs preoperatively, nitroprusside (25-30 μg/min i.v.) may be used with caution and careful titration accomplished while alpha blockade with Dibenzyline is being started. Methyltyrosine, a blocker of catecholamine synthesis, has been advocated for chronic management of pheochromocytoma. In general, it has not worked well and is quite toxic. During surgery, careful management of the volume status of the patient must be carried out. Careful monitoring with a central venous line and Swan-Ganz catheter is helpful. Postoperatively, these lines probably should be left in for a period of time so that the volume status of the patient can be monitored. Control of volume postoperatively has greatly reduced the need for vasopressor therapy. If total bilateral adrenalectomy is done, the patient must be managed as an addisonian, as discussed in the section on Adrenal Hypofunction. Even if only one adrenal gland is removed, hydrocortisone, 100 to 200 mg daily intravenously, may be used especially if unexplained hypotension persists.

Postoperatively, a 24 hour urine for either VMA or metanephrine should be done to make sure that all tumorous tissue was removed. If bilateral tumors were found, then the patient must be worked up for the multiple endocrine adenomatosis syndrome type II. A careful search for a medullary carcinoma of the thyroid should be carried out (see section on nodular Thyroid Disease). About 10 per cent of patients with pheochromocytoma are malignant. The most common site for metastatic lesions is the skeleton. Palliation can be achieved with radiation therapy. The chemotherapeutic agents doxorubicin hydrochloride and cyclophosphamide have been used with some success.

ANESTHESIA FOR PATIENT WITH PHEOCHROMOCYTOMA (Pratilas and Pratila, 1979)

The patient known to have a pheochromocytoma is an increased risk for anesthesia and operation. The risk is even greater when the presence of the tumor is first suspected during anesthesia or operation and preparations for adequate care have not been made. Too frequently the diagnosis is made at autopsy (Deblasi, 1966). The first suspicion of pheochromocytoma may be made by the anesthesiologist from the reaction of the patient to the induction of anesthesia (Smith et al., 1978).

Unsuspected tumors are more likely to be encountered during emergency operations than during operations following adequate preoperative examination when a high degree of suspicion exists. Out of 11 autopsy diagnoses reported by Scott and co-authors (1965), four patients had died during or following operative procedures, all but one of which was an emergency operation.

Pregnancy seems to precipitate the symptoms of pheochromocytoma, and the diagnosis may not be suspected because the condition mimics toxemia. Too often the diagnosis is made in the delivery room or at autopsy. Before the availability of effective drugs to control the pathophysiology, mortality in pregnancy with pheochromocytoma was reported to range from 25 to 50 per cent (Humble, 1967).

The immediate cause of death is most frequently cerebrovascular accident, congestive heart failure with pulmonary edema, or ventricular fibrillation (Scott et al., 1965). The most important cause of death in children during the operative and immediate postoperative period is the presence of a second, undisclosed tumor.

The periods of greatest danger occur during induction of anesthesia, during tracheal intubation, while positioning of the patient on the operating table, during surgical manipulation of the tumor, and after ligation of venous drainage from the tumor. In the well prepared patient the prognosis for successful removal of a pheochromocytoma has steadily improved in recent years as a result of the introduction of drugs to control the effects of the catecholamines liberated from the tumor. This has made possible the reporting of removal of a pheochromocytoma in series of 46 (Deoreo et al., 1974) and 80 (Desmonts, 1977) patients without a death.

Premedication. Atropine is generally considered to be contraindicated. The reasons given for avoiding the use of atropine are mostly hypothetical and include tachycardia, central nervous system stimulation, and potentiation of vasopressor activity of catecholamines.

Use of narcotics has been suspected of inciting tumor activity through their histamine-like effects or by depression of respiration (Deblasi, 1966). Other surgical teams have used narcotics as part of patient preparation without noticeable ill effects.

Chlorpromazine may aggravate the arterial hypotension that occurs after removal of the pheochromocytoma, but other phenothiazines have been recommended for premedication (Deblasi, 1966).

Cooperman et al. (1967) did not find the anxiety supposed to be characteristic of patients with functioning chromaffin tumors to be important and achieved adequate preoperative sedation with an oral dose of barbiturate only. This effect was attributed in part to careful explanation to the patient about the procedures to be followed.

Monitoring. Because of the rapid sudden changes in circulation caused by released catecholamines, accurate constant monitoring is an absolute necessity in order for the magnitude of the changes to be controlled with antagonists. Modes to be included are electrocardiogram, central venous pressure, pulmonary artery wedge pressure, mean arterial pressure with radial artery catheter, and urinary output. In order for the monitoring information to be used effectively two large bore peripheral intravenous catheters should be available, one for blood and intravenous fluids and one for administration of drugs.

Anesthetic Agents and Methods. Most anesthetic agents and methods in common use have been recommended by some authors for removal of pheochromocytomas and avoided as unsatisfactory by other authors. Probably most would agree that the choice of anesthetic agents is less important than the understanding with which they are used. Smooth induction of anesthesia and avoidance of hypoxia and hypercarbia are important. Most reports indicate that some form of general anesthesia is preferable to regional anesthesia, but better-than-average muscular relaxation must be available for adequate exposure of the retroperitoneal tumor with minimal manipulation and retraction of the tumor. Deep general anesthesia tends to inhibit release of catecholamines by the tumor but aggravates the hypotension that occurs after removal of the tumor. Induction of anesthesia with intravenous barbiturate is almost universal, but rapid administration may stimulate secretion by the tumor as a result of induced hypotension or hypoventilation (Deblasi, 1966).

Endotracheal techniques seem to have been used universally along with general anesthesia. The necessity for muscle relaxants or deep anesthesia to achieve adequate operating conditions has made assisted or controlled respiration necessary to prevent respiratory acidosis and hypoxia.

Halothane sensitizes the myocardium to catecholamines but has enjoyed wide use because of its tendency to inhibit sympathetic activity. Its tendency to potentiate arrhythmias probably limits its use.

Neurolept anesthesia with pancuronium for muscle relaxation has proven satisfactory. The theoretical advantages are that droperidol reduces blood pressure response to catecholamines and raises the threshold to epinephrine induced arrhythmias, while fentanyl does not cause histamine release as does morphine. Pancuronium does not lead to histamine release as does tubocurarine (Clarke et al., 1974; Csanky-Treels et al., 1976).

Enflurane has proven to be useful, since it does not sensitize the myocardium to epinephrine-induced dysrhythmia to the same extent as does halothane (Ortiz and Diaz, 1975; Kreul et al., 1976).

Succinylcholine seems to have been the most popular muscular relaxant for tracheal intubation. However, Stoner and Urbach (1968) report a patient with pheochromocytoma who developed ventricular bigeminy on each of four consecutive trials immediately after an intravenous drip of succinylcholine was begun. After removal of the tumor, no arrhythmia followed administration of succinylcholine, as was the case when the same patient was anesthetized later. Advisability of the use of tubocurarine has been questioned because of its histamine-like effect, since histamine has been used as a diagnostic test for provoking secretions by a pheochromocytoma. In clinical practice these apprehensions seem to have been exaggerated, and tubocurarine has been used to good advantage.

Operative Problems. More patients are overtreated than are undertreated during removal of a pheochromocytoma. The anesthesiologist's objective is not to try to maintain constant physiologic homeostasis, since such is practically impossible when catecholamine blood levels are fluctuating widely. The objective should be only to dampen the effects of the catecholamines and keep them within limits that are safe for the individual patient.

HYPERTENSION. Although pheochromocytomas vary in relative amounts of epinephrine and norepinephrine secreted, in general, the ratio found in the secretion of tumors is norepinephrine 85 per cent and epinephrine 15 per cent, which is a reversal of the ratio secreted by the normal gland. Release into the circulation of large amounts of these potent amines results in marked and dangerous elevations in blood pressure. Efforts to decrease catecholamine synthesis by administration of agents such as alpha methyl tyrosine (Desmonts et al., 1977) have resulted in indifferent success. The best results have come from attempts to neutralize the effects of the circulating catecholamines on the target cells. Phenoxybenzamine (Dibenzyline) and phentolamine (Regitine) have been the most useful drugs in controlling hypertension. Both are alpha receptor blocking agents, but phenoxybenzamine has a longer duration of action and is more convenient for control of hypertension during the preoperative period.

Because of its rapid onset and short duration of action, phentolamine is a useful drug for control of hypertension during anesthesia and operation. The initial intravenous dose is 1 to 5 mg at intervals of 30 to 45 seconds until blood pressure is controlled. Such use is usually followed by a refractory tachycardia. An intravenous infusion of 0.01 per cent phentolamine may be used and smaller supplemental doses given as needed. Its use should be discontinued 30 to 40 minutes prior to ligation of venous drainage of the tumor to prevent aggravation of the hypotension that follows.

Continuous administration of sodium nitroprusside solution allows even more rapid and accurate control of hypertension. One hundred mg in 500 ml. of 5 per cent glucose can be administered with an infusion pump at rates varying with the elevation of blood pressure. When infusion is stopped, recovery from the nitroprusside effect occurs in a few minutes. This helps to alleviate the hypotension that occurs so frequently when the venous drainage from the tumor has been severed. The search for multiple tumors is enhanced because the hypertension that follows manipulation of second tumors is not masked by residual effects of drugs previously administered to control hypertension. Sodium nitroprusside is effective in patients resistant to phentolamine (Nourok et al., 1963).

Epidural anesthesia has been used to control release of catecholamines during general anesthesia for removal of pheochromocytoma (Cousins and Rubin, 1974).

Wide fluctuations in blood pressure can be tolerated without harm by most patients, but cerebrovascular accidents and congestive heart failure with acute pulmonary edema may be precipitated by hypertension.

HYPOTENSION. Since the half-life of epinephrine and norepinephrine in blood is extremely short, their concentration falls rapidly when the tumor source is removed. If blood pressure does not decrease sharply at this time, suspicion is justified that the tumor is multiple and that secreting tumor tissue still persists; a search for it is indicated at this stage in the operation. Hypotension was once considered the result of a type of tachyphylaxis whereby receptors in smooth muscle had partially adjusted to high blood concentrations of epinephrine and norepinephrine and were not activated when concentrations suddenly decreased to normal or below. The logical therapy was to raise the blood concentration by administration of norepinephrine (Levophed) for 24 to 36 hours with a continuous intravenous drip. The drip was continuously regulated to maintain blood pressure at a desired minimum until the patient could be "weaned" from the drip and get his own autoregulated secretion established. Although this theory has been superseded, a continuous intravenous drip of 8 mg of norepinephrine in 1000 ml of glucose or electrolyte solution should be prepared before anesthesia is induced and kept ready for attachment to a reliably patent intravenous catheter. It then is available for rapid alleviation of hypotension, should this occur to a degree that threatens adequate perfusion of tissue when all the pheochromocytoma has been removed. Since extravenous infiltration or even intravenous infusion into a superficial vein of 0.1 per cent norepinephrine has resulted in slough of tissues, the solution can be more safely administered through a central venous catheter whose internal end is in the superior vena cava. In addition to infusion of norepinephrine, such a catheter may be used to monitor central venous pressure and thereby prevent too rapid administration of fluids, plasma, or blood, which otherwise might lead to pulmonary edema. Phenylephrine (Neosynephrine) and metaraminol (Aramine), as a dilute intravenous solution, have been recommended as a continuous drip in place of the norepinephrine solution.

A more acceptable explanation of the hypotension that occurs following separation of a pheochromocytoma from the circulation is that the prolonged preoperative hypertension has caused or masked a decreased blood volume. Preoperative prevention of hypertension with phenoxybenzamine or phentolamine for several days will let the blood volume be restored toward normal. During operation, blood loss should be accurately monitored and replaced with perhaps more than has been lost by about 500 ml, provided that central venous pressure does not rise above 12 cm of water. The hypotension that does occur following tumor removal should be treated with rapid administration of whole blood, plasma, albumin, or electrolyte solution to restore blood volume and maintain a systolic blood pressure of about 100 mm mercury. During such rapid administration, central venous pressure should be monitored to prevent overloading a damaged heart.

To effect such treatment, adequate venous catheters are necessary. In addition to the central venous catheter, at least two other large bore intravenous catheters should be placed and secured in a thick-walled peripheral vein before the operation is allowed to begin.

CARDIAC ARRHYTHMIA. The beta-receptor stimulating properties of high concentrations of epinephrine, and of norepinephrine to some degree, lead to chronotropic effects on the heart and to arrhythmias. Continuous electrocardiographic monitoring is essential for diagnosis and evaluation of these arrhythmias. Ventricular fibrillation, a frequent cause of death during the operative and postoperative periods, is better prevented than treated. Serious arrhythmias may so impair cardiac output that a paradoxical hypotension occurs in spite of markedly elevated peripheral resistance, and cardiac failure may result.

The beta-receptor blocking agent propranolol (Inderal) has been a valuable addition to the armamentarium of the anesthesiologist for the treatment and prevention of ventricular arrhythmias. Its effect on supraventricular arrhythmias is less certain. Although preoperative use of oral doses of 20 to 120 mg has been advocated in conjunction with alpha-blocking agents, some authors do not believe that prophylactic use of beta blockers is necessary. Most authors agree that intravenous doses of 1 to 5 mg of propranolol during operation are useful for controlling ventricular arrhythmias and tachycardia. The duration of action of propranolol is 30 to 45 minutes. Relative contraindications to its use are heart failure and asthma. Ross and co-workers (1967) have questioned the use of beta-blocking agents without concomitant use of alpha-blocking agents because of the otherwise unopposed hypertensive effect of epinephrine. Tachyphylaxis following repeated administration of alpha-blocking drugs can be alleviated by concomitant use of beta-blocking agents (Salem and Ivankovic, 1969). Intravenous lidocaine in 50 to 100 mg intravenous doses to treat ventricular arrhythmias during removal of pheochromocytomas is preferred by many anesthesiologists but was not found to be as effective as propranolol by others (Cooperman et al., 1967).

Postoperative Problems. Control of blood volume has greatly reduced the need for vasopressor therapy. However, blood pressure must be carefully monitored for 24 to 36 hours after operation. Hypotension is the most frequent cause of death in the immediate postoperative period. Intra-arterial, central venous, pulmonary artery, and peripheral venous catheters should be left in place at the end of the operation, and norepinephrine solution should be kept available during postoperative monitoring.

If adrenalectomy is performed as part of the surgical procedure, 100 mg of hydrocortisone as the soluble succinate or phosphate salt every four to six hours for one or two days may be indicated as a prophylactic measure. Even if adrenalectomy is not done, an empirical dose of hydrocortisone may be useful when response to blood volume replacement and vasopressor therapy does not seem adequate.

Summary of Special Preparations. Before induction of anesthesia for removal of a pheochromocytoma, preparation of the following materials and equipment should be considered, in addition to the usual anesthetic drugs and supplies: propranolol ampules, phentolamine ampules, metaraminol,

80 mg in 500 ml, or norepinephrine, 8 mg in 1000 ml of intravenous solution, cross-matched blood, hydrocortisone, intra-arterial catheter and strain gauge, central venous catheters, Swan-Ganz catheter, one or more large-bore peripheral venous catheters, electrocardiograph, core temperature recording apparatus, and water mattress for children.

DIABETES MELLITUS — MANAGEMENT OF THE SURGICAL PATIENT

DEFINITION

Diabetes mellitus is a chronic metabolic disorder characterized by abnormal carbohydrate metabolism which results in inappropriately high blood sugars. Diabetics are commonly divided into two main categories, those who require insulin (juvenile type) and those who do not (maturity onset diabetes). The term juvenile diabetic may be a misnomer, since many older patients also fall into the same category. Most children and adolescents who are diabetic have the juvenile type; that is, they require insulin to prevent ketoacidosis. The maturity onset diabetic is usually older and tends to be overweight. This type of patient can be controlled with either oral sulfonylurea drugs or with diet alone. These patients tend to have relative insulin insensitivity rather than insulin deficiency. The genetics of the disease is slowly being worked out. In identical twins, maturity onset diabetes is concordant; that is both twins have the disease. However only a 50 per cent concordance occurs in identical twins with the juvenile type. Thus, there must be causative factors other than genetic ones. It has recently been shown that human leucocyte antigen HLA-B8, which is controlled on chromosome 6, has a much higher prevalence in patients with juvenile type diabetes mellitus.

PATHOPHYSIOLOGY

If insulin deficiency is severe, such as occurs in the juvenile onset diabetic, amino acids are released from skeletal muscle and free fatty acids are released from adipose tissue. Hepatic uptake of both amino acids and free fatty acids is markedly increased, and the liver begins to produce glucose and ketone bodies. The levels of both rise and this leads to the classic signs and symptoms of diabetes, including polyuria, dehydration, and ketoacidosis. In the juvenile diabetic the beta cell of the islets fails, with resulting insulin deficiency, while the alpha cell actually appears to oversecrete glucagon. The excess glucagon levels may contribute to the hyperglycemia by stimulating hepatic glucose production (glucogenesis). The reason for the failure of the beta cell in the juvenile diabetic remains purely speculative. A current hypothesis holds that a viral infection initiates an autoimmune response in which the beta cells are destroyed by antibody. The pathophysiology of the maturity onset diabetic is also complicated. There certainly appears to be a strong genetic component from the identical twin studies. There appears to be both a relative deficiency of insulin along with delayed release from the beta cell. The problem is made worse by relative insulin resistance, which is always a result of obesity. Obesity seems to unmask the predisposition to diabetes. One theory holds that as the adipose tissue enlarges because of excess stored triglyceride, the receptor for insulin is modified and the actual number of receptors is decreased. Insulin levels rise with resulting elevated blood levels of insulin. Thus, an insulin resistant state develops.

Complications

There is a wide body of evidence accumulating that strongly suggests that microangiopathy (disease of small blood vessels) correlates with the degree and duration of the blood sugar elevation. The basement membrane of the blood vessels appears to thicken. Abnormalities of the red blood cells and platelets along with elevated fibrinogen levels lead to sludging of blood and contribute to hypoxia in the smaller blood vessels. The thickened basement may predispose to the tendency of these blood vessels to leak. The leading cause of new blindness in the U.S. and Europe today is diabetes. After 20 years of diabetes, about 75 per cent of diabetics will have significant retinopathy. About 20 per cent will have serious proliferative retinopathy. Laser photocoagulation has been shown to slow down the progression of retinopathy. Vitrectomy, in which blood is removed from the vitreous, remains an unproven technique for restoring vision. Approximately half of all juvenile diabetics will develop renal failure after 20 to 30 years of diabetes. Death as a result of myocardial infarction, hypertension, or congestive heart failure is often associated with significant uremia. Neuropathy is a somewhat different complication and is not necessarily related to the level of the blood sugar. One hypothesis holds that sorbitol, a by-product of glucose metabolism, accumulates in nerve cells. The associated decrease in inositol levels may damage the nerve. Atherosclerosis or macroangiopathy may appear at an early age in the diabetic. Strokes and myocardial infarction are about 5 to 10 times more common in the diabetic than in the general population. Elevated blood lipids (cholesterol and triglyceride) and hyperglycemia are factors involved in the premature development of atherosclerosis in the diabetic but are not the sole factors. The development of significant vascular disease manifests itself very commonly in the feet. Macro- and microangiopathy as well as neuropathy can lead to ulcerations in the feet. Secondary infection is quite common at this point and immediately puts the diabetic in a precarious position. This is a very common reason for hospitalizing the diabetic patient.

DIAGNOSIS

The disease is diagnosed by demonstrating abnormal carbohydrate metabolism. It is not necessary to perform further tests when the fasting blood sugar is clearly elevated. In the presence of normal blood glucose, a glucose tolerance test is the next step. Individuals with a normal glucose tolerance test for all practical purposes do not have diabetes mellitus. Age should always be taken into account in the evaluation of carbohydrate tolerance. The insulin response to carbohydrate stimulus diminishes with each decade of life. Thus, part of the aging process itself may lead to a diabetic state, which in turn leads to mild hyperglycemia, and this in turn leads to atherosclerosis.

Secondary causes of carbohydrate intolerance should always be considered in the differential diagnosis. Disease entities such as pancreatitis, hemochromatosis, pheochromocytoma, and hyperthyroidism should be ruled out. Primary disturbances of lipid metabolism, such as primary hyperlipidemia, can result in secondary carbohydrate intolerance. All patients with mild hyperglycemia without evidence of ketosis should be investigated for possible hypertriglyceridemia. Children with diabetes develop polyuria, thirst, and, as insulin deficiency worsens, frank diabetic ketoacidosis and coma. The maturity onset diabetic however usually does not get as ill. Failing vision because of a refractive error of the lens due to hyperglycemia may bring him or her to the ophthalmologist. The dentist may see chronic severe periodontal problems as the first manifestation of diabetes. Hyperglycemia may lead to minor soft tissue infections that may lead the patient's doctor to the diagnosis. Likewise, the gynecologist may see a patient with recurrent monilial vaginal infections and become suspicious of the diagnosis. Often a routine annual checkup may reveal an elevated blood sugar in an otherwise asymptomatic individual. Recently, measurement of the glycolated hemoglobin (Hb A_{1c}) has been proposed as a way of monitoring long-term control. Concentrations of Hb A_{1c} are believed to reflect mean blood glucose levels during the preceding several weeks.

The sulfonylurea agents in recent years have stimulated a major controversy in the field of diabetes research. This stems partly from the University Group Diabetes Project (UGDP). This large multicenter study showed that sudden deaths were more frequent in patients using these oral drugs. Actually, only one oral drug was studied (tolbutamide). It still seems reasonable at the present time to use these drugs in certain situations. The obese maturity-onset diabetic who cannot lose weight and still has significant symptomatic hyperglycemia and glycosuria remains a good candidate for oral sulfonylurea agents. Some patients on oral drugs going to surgery should be managed with insulin during anesthesia and immediately postoperatively.

Intensive research into new methods for delivering insulin is now underway. Electronically driven implantable insulin delivery systems and transplanted islet cells are among the methods now being explored.

PREOPERATIVE ASSESSMENT AND POSTOPERATIVE MANAGEMENT OF THE DIABETIC PATIENT

Preoperative evaluation of the diabetic patient going to surgery should include an evaluation of the cardiovascular system and renal function. The anesthesiologist should evaluate the age of the patient by adding to the chronological age the number of years the patient has had diabetes. For instance if the patient is chronologically 30 years old and has had diabetes for 20 years, the patient for practical purposes should be considered 50 years old. Preoperatively, the patient should have a blood glucose and electrolyte determination, especially serum potassium. Hypokalemia during the induction of anesthesia may be a major responsible factor in the development of cardiac arrhythmias. Serum creatinine is a better gauge of renal function than blood urea nitrogen. The cardiovascular system should be evaluated with an electrocardiogram. Oral drugs should be stopped well in advance of surgery. The oral drug Diabinese has a long half-life and should be stopped at least 36 hours before surgery. In general, it is best to manage patients who have been on oral drugs with insulin during the operative and postoperative course of the surgical procedure. Blood lipids (cholesterol and triglyceride) are important cardiovascular risk factors in the diabetic; another important risk factor in the diabetic is autonomic insufficiency. Autonomic insufficiency in the diabetic manifests itself in its earliest form as a lack of cardiac beat-to-beat variation. Diabetics with autonomic insufficiency tend to have higher heart rates and a significant lack of normal sinus arrhythmia. The heart rate may not vary by more than four or five beats from one minute to the next. These patients have been shown to have a significant incidence of sudden arrhythmias during surgery, especially sudden cardiovascular arrest.

Certain drugs should be mentioned for their ability to produce or contribute to hyperglycemia. The thiazide diuretics and loop diuretics (e.g., furosemide) are commonly used in diabetics and can contribute significantly to hyperglycemia. Both drugs are excellent antihypertensives. In no way should their hyperglycemic properties obviate their use in a hypertensive emergency. Furosemide especially is quite useful in the management of hypertension in the diabetic. Dilantin can cause mild hyperglycemia by decreasing beta cell function in the islets of Langerhans. Diazoxide is a potent antihypertensive drug when given rapidly intravenously but it also can produce profound hyperglycemia. It probably should be avoided altogether in the diabetic. Alternative drugs for managing hypertensive crisis should be used, such as nitroprusside. Of course, steroids can also markedly elevate the blood sugar. In patients with adrenocortical insufficiency or following hypophysectomy, replacement adrenocorticoid therapy is indicated. This point has been discussed in the section on adrenal disease. Immunosuppressive drugs are also known to produce mild hyperglycemia.

One drug that deserves special mention is the beta blocker propranolol. Propranolol itself does not change the blood sugar but it occasionally can modify and blunt the symptoms related to an insulin reaction by blocking the effects of the rapid catecholamine release induced by an insulin reaction. Thus the patient may not be aware that his blood sugar is low. Theoretically it also may inhibit insulin release from the islets. Both of these potential effects have not turned out to be clinically significant, and propranolol remains an excellent drug for the management of hypertension in the diabetic.

In recent years it has been recognized that insulin can be given in small amounts as a continuous intravenous infusion in the management of diabetic ketoacidosis. As little as 5 to 7 units of regular insulin per hour given as a continuous intravenous drip for a few hours can break even severe ketoacidosis. Thus only 50 to 75 units of regular insulin may be given totally, whereas with the older intermittent bolus method, up to 400 units of regular insulin may have been required to break a ketoacidosis state. Moreover, by the continuous intravenous method, less hypoglycemia and hypokalemia result. Ketoacidosis can no longer be considered a truly insulin resistant state.

In the case of the diabetic patient going to surgery who is ketosis free, a continuous infusion of intravenous regular insulin can be begun preoperatively and continued through the period of anesthesia and into the postoperative period. Even if the patient is going to surgery later in the day (say at 12 noon), the intravenous infusion may be started at 8 or 9 o'clock and continued. One to two units of regular insulin per hour given intravenously continuously is sufficient to maintain the blood sugar between 150 and 250 mg per 100 ml. Usually, preoperatively 15 units of regular insulin is put in one liter of 5 per cent dextrose and water and given at the rate of 100 cc per hour. Approximately 30 to 40 per cent of the insulin sticks to the bottle and IV tubing and is not available to the patient. Obviously this must be taken into account when mixing the IV solutions. Depending upon the patient's daily insulin requirements, more insulin may have to be used. Some anesthesiologists become quite concerned about giving insulin during the period of anesthesia itself. Blood sugar should be determined one or two times during the anesthetic period. This can be done quite simply in the operating room using the Ames reflectometer and the dextrostix method. Dextrostix are glucose oxidase impregnated paper strips that turn purple in proportion to the concentration of blood sugar. The Ames reflectometer (Eyetone)* is a simple spectrophotometer that quickly indicates the blood sugar concentration.

In the postoperative period, intravenous insulin may be continued but in somewhat higher concentrations, usually closer to 2 units per hour. This protocol may have to be continued until the patient is able to take fluids by mouth. For the patient who has had a vitrectomy, this period of time will generally be about 12 hours. However, patients who have correction of a retinal detachment generally have a great deal of pain, and a longer period of treatment with both intravenous fluids and insulin will be required (about 48 hours). The choice of intravenous fluids after surgery depends somewhat upon the patient's renal and cardiovascular status. Generally 1 liter of 0.45 per cent saline in 5 per cent dextrose with 40 mEq of KCl per liter can be started postoperatively and given at the rate of 100 cc per hour. If renal failure and/or cardiovascular disease exists, obviously the

amount of salt and potassium given will have to be modified. A low serum phosphate is an indication for adding potassium hydrogen phosphate to the intravenous fluids. If ketosis develops following surgery, the old "sliding scale" is still useful. It can be used every four to six hours in the following way. If the urine shows 1 per cent or 2 per cent glucose, then an extra 5 units to 10 units of regular insulin is given subcutaneously. If the urine acetone is moderate or large an extra 5 units of regular insulin is given in addition to the amount required to cover the glucosuria. It should be noted that urine glucose is in no way a measure of blood glucose. The sliding scale must always be adjusted by appropriately correlating the urine glucose with an occasional blood sugar determination. Table 5–5 summarizes the fluid and intravenous insulin therapy in the operative and postoperative periods. In general, patients who require more than 50 units of insulin daily will require somewhat more insulin at surgery (1.5–1.8 units/hr) than the patient whose daily insulin requirement is less than 50 units daily.

Management of the diabetic who also has adrenocortical insufficiency or who has undergone a transsphenoidal hypophysectomy can be difficult. It is important to remember that patients with adrenocortical insufficiency can be exquisitely sensitive to insulin. The schedule given in Table 5–5 should be modified somewhat for this unusual situation. Instead of 1 to 2 units per hour of regular insulin, no more than one half to 1 unit of insulin should be given as a continuous intravenous infusion. Hypoglycemia can develop precipitously, and these patients must be watched carefully. Hydrocortisone, 100 mg, should be given intravenously just before induction of anesthesia, and thereafter 50 mg can be given every four to six hours. About 300 mg of hydrocortisone should be given the day of surgery. Thereafter the dose may be tapered by 50 mg a day until replacement therapy is attained (about 30 mg daily). Normal saline should be given in place of 0.45 per cent saline, since these patients can also become salt depleted owing to absence of mineralocorticoids.

Hypertension in the diabetic during anesthesia and immediately postoperatively can be managed with furosemide or nitroprusside. Clonidine (Catapres), prazosin (Mini-

---

*Ames Company, Division Miles Laboratories, Elkhart, Indiana 46514.

Table 5–5   *Fluids and Continuous I.V. Insulin in the Operative and Postoperative Period**

		Pre-op	Post-op
		5% D/W 100 cc/hr	1 Liter 5% D/W 0.5 Normal** Saline-50 mEq. KCl: 100 cc/hr
Subcutaneous insulin			
	daily requirements < 50 U	15 U regular insulin in 1 liter ≃ 1 U/hr†	20 U regular insulin in 1 liter ≃ 1.3 U/hr†
	daily requirements > 50 U	25 U regular insulin in 1 liter ≃ 1.5 U/hr†	30 U regular insulin in 1 liter ≃ 1.8 U/hr†

*Modify if renal failure exists.
**If serum PO_4 is low, consider intravenous K_2HPO_4.
†About 30 to 40 per cent insulin sticks to bottle and IV tubing.

press), minoxidil (Loniten), and methyldopa (Aldomet) are useful antihypertensive drugs if renal failure exists. Clinical deterioration of diabetic patients with precipitous development of ketoacidosis following surgery can be due to a "silent" myocardial infarction. Probably because of autonomic insufficiency, diabetics do not develop the typical symptoms or pain normally seen with myocardial infarction. Another potential complication related to autonomic insufficiency in the diabetic is a neurogenic bladder with subsequent urine retention and occasionally serious urinary tract infections with resulting ketoacidosis.

Recently a glucose controlled insulin infusion system, the Biostator, has been developed by Life Sciences Instruments (Miles Lab.).* This remarkable instrument is equipped with a glucose electrode that continuously senses the blood sugar. This information is fed to a computer that continuously displays the blood sugar concentration and is programmed to maintain normal blood sugars by infusing either glucose or insulin. The level of blood sugar desired can be selected and the computer automatically makes the appropriate adjustments. The cost of the instrument is at present prohibitive, and for most routine problems it probably is not necessary. Further improvement of this technology should, however, prove interesting.

As a rule, 24 hours after surgery, if good diabetic control has been attained (i.e., absence of ketonuria) one half to three fourths of the usual long-acting insulin dose may be given and supplemented throughout the day with 5 to 20 units of regular insulin. The actual dose depends upon the degree of glycosuria, and the previously mentioned sliding scale may be used (i.e., 10 units for 4+ and 5 units for 3+ glycosuria). Patients undergoing minor elective surgery (e.g., cataract removal under local anesthesia) receive three fourths of their usual dosage of either insulin or oral hypoglycemic agents. To avoid the possibility of hypoglycemia, 1 liter of 5 per cent glucose and water should be given during the surgical procedure.

Emergency surgery in an uncontrolled diabetic represents a serious problem. If significant ketoacidosis is present, surgery is contraindicated until the acidosis is controlled. Usually a period of 8 to 12 hours is all that is required to correct major electrolyte fluid and acid-base problems. Continuous intravenous insulin, 5 to 7 units per hour, is begun after an appropriate loading dose is given rapidly intravenously (1 to 2 units per kg body weight). It is important to give enough insulin during this period of time to correct the ketoacidosis in a reasonable period of time. A combination of the bolus method every three hours and the continuous intravenous method is best. Blood glucose and serum ketone dilutions should be done every two to three hours, and an appropriate amount of insulin should be given. If the ketosis has not been significantly broken by three to four hours, then double the amount of the initial insulin bolus should be given. For instance, if 50 units (1 unit/kg) was the initial bolus used, and if the serum ketone test was positive in the 1:16 dilution initially and had not changed four hours later, then 100 units of regular insulin should be given intravenously at this time. Alternatively, the con-

*Miles Laboratory, Elkhart, Indiana 46514.

tinuous intravenous infusion of insulin may be increased from 5 units per hour to 10 units per hour.

The patient should be on strict record of intake and output of fluids, and in addition blood should be checked for creatinine and electrolytes (Na, K, Cl, HCO_3). An arterial pH will determine the severity of the acidosis. Administration of 0.9 per cent sodium chloride (isotonic) should be undertaken immediately on admission. Extracellular volume depletion may be 10 per cent of total body weight. Hypotonic solutions should be avoided because they can precipitously reduce plasma osmolarity and thereby secondarily lead to cerebral edema. Alkalinizing solutions such as sodium bicarbonate should be reserved for patients with arterial pH levels below 7.2. Inadvertent excess of bicarbonate administration may paradoxically lower the pH of cerebrospinal fluid and lead to further central nervous system depression.

Patients with obvious circulatory collapse should be given blood, plasma, or a plasma volume expander such as dextran. The potassium deficit in body stores on admission may be considerable (up to 5 mEq per kg body weight) even though hyperkalemia exists. By the third or fourth hour of treatment hypokalemia may develop and potassium chloride infusion should be begun. If renal function is normal, up to 40 mEq of potassium chloride in 5 per cent dextrose and water may be given safely every hour until the potassium deficit is corrected. If hypokalemia is present on admission, potassium chloride infusion should begin immediately but cautiously. Urine output should be monitored carefully during the period of potassium chloride infusion. By the third or fourth hour of treatment, carbohydrate metabolism is accelerated by insulin and blood glucose begins to fall and hypoglycemia may develop. Obviously glucose (5% dextrose) should be given at this point.

At times significant ketonemia may still be present despite low blood sugars. There are several reasons for giving glucose at this point: 1) in order to continue to give insulin to correct the ketonemia, 2) glucose itself has an antiketogenic effect, and 3) deficient glycogen stores are repleted. Once ketonemia has been corrected, serious consideration may be given to major surgery. Pre-

and postoperative management is the same as already outlined.

SURGERY IN THE DIABETIC PATIENT

The objectives of good management of the diabetic patient during surgery are 1) prevention of diabetic acidosis and 2) prevention of severe fluid loss and hypoglycemia, especially during the period of anesthesia. For elective major surgery in the controlled diabetic patient three general methods have been used in the past.

1. On the morning of surgery no long- or intermediate-acting insulin is given. Instead, 2 liters of 5 per cent glucose with 10 to 15 units of crystalline regular insulin added to each liter is given during the surgical procedure. This method, although empiric, seems to work reasonably well. It is important to note that there is no clear quantitative relationship between the amount of insulin injected and the amount of carbohydrate utilized.

2. In the second method, the usual type and dose of insulin is given in the morning. Of course, on the morning of surgery the patient is given nothing by mouth; instead, 50 gm of intravenous glucose (500 ml of 10% glucose or 1000 ml of 5% glucose) is substituted for each missed meal. This method may be continued in the immediate postoperative period until the patient is able to take fluids. The amount of postoperative care is minimal with this method. Anesthesiologists have been critical of this method because of the possibility of hypoglycemia. In the experience of many who use this method, hypoglycemia is virtually never a problem, presumably because the surgical stresses cause hyperglycemia and increase insulin needs.

3. The third method is perhaps the most widely used. If the operation is scheduled for the morning, one half of the usual daily dose of insulin is given that morning. One or 2 liters of 5 per cent glucose and water is given during the surgical procedure. If the operation is scheduled for later in the day, one third of the usual daily dose of insulin is given that morning. Nothing is given by mouth. One liter of 5 per cent dextrose and water is given prior to the operation. Every four to six hours following the initial insulin

dosage, additional regular or short-acting insulin (5–15 units) may be given, depending upon the degree of glucosuria. No insulin should be given two hours prior to the operation. During the surgical procedure, at least 1 liter of 5 per cent dextrose and water should be given. This method avoids hypoglycemia during surgery but increases the need for careful postoperative care.

In the postoperative period the clinical situation must be evaluated at four- to six-hour intervals. Fluid, electrolyte balance, and degree of glucosuria should be closely evaluated. Mild glucosuria is a more desirable objective than a glucose-free urine. Hypoglycemia should be avoided. If glycosuria is heavy and persistent, short-acting or regular insulin should be administered subcutaneously (5 to 10 units every six hours). At times, sudden hypoglycemia may develop in the postoperative period, especially when a previous stressful problem has been relieved. For instance, removal of an intra-abdominal abscess may at times reduce insulin requirements by as much as 50 per cent in the first 24 hours after surgery. In the very sick patient, ketonuria may develop postoperatively. If the ketonuria is only mild or moderate, associated with heavy glucosuria without significant ketonemia or acidosis, 10 to 30 units of regular insulin is given subcutaneously and the situation is re-evaluated in four to six hours. Severe ketosis with significant lowering of the plasma bicarbonate will require greater amounts of insulin (50 or more units). Careful follow-up of acid-base balance and fluid status is mandatory. Electrolytes and plasma ketone bodies must then be checked every four hours and the proper adjustments made. As a rule, 24 hours after surgery, if good diabetic control has been attained (i.e., absence of ketonuria), one half to three fourths of the usual insulin dose may be given and supplemented throughout the day (every six to eight hours) with 5 to 15 units of regular insulin. The actual dose depends upon the degree of glucosuria. If the Clinitest method is used to measure urine glucose, the following scale will be practical and useful:

Urine Glucose	Regular Insulin Dose
Trace	No insulin
1/4%	5 units
1/2%	8 units
1%	10 units
2%	15 units

It should be noted that the urine glucose is in no way a measure of the blood glucose. The blood glucose for any given degree of urine glucose will vary greatly from one patient to another, depending upon the maximal renal tubular reabsorptive capacity for glucose. Blood sugar determinations should be obtained at least twice daily for at least two to three days postoperatively and correlated with the urine glucose. The "sliding scale" should be adjusted accordingly.

If the patient is receiving oral drugs, they should be stopped at least 24 hours before operation. One exception is chlorpropamide, which has an exceptionally long half-life and for which a 48 hour period of discontinuance is required. Then, in the preoperative period, the patient may be switched to 5 to 10 units of a long-acting insulin preparation such as NPH or lente insulin. Thereafter any of the three methods previously described can be used. Most patients who receive oral drugs for diabetic control are mild diabetics of the adult-onset variety who are *not* ketosis prone. Often if hyperglycemia is extremely mild (i.e., fasting or postprandial blood sugars are under 150), it is possible to avoid the use of insulin entirely in both the pre- and postoperative periods. However, if ketosis is present, insulin therapy is mandatory. Although ketosis is usually absent in the mild diabetic on oral agents in the preoperative period, the sudden stress of surgery may induce significant ketonuria and at times ketonemia. Insulin should then be administered in the fashion already outlined for postoperative management.

Patients undergoing elective minor surgery (e.g., a cataract removal under local anesthesia) receive three fourths of their usual dosage of either insulin or oral hypoglycemia agents. To avoid the possibility of hypoglycemia, 1 liter of 5 per cent glucose and water should be given during the surgical procedure.

PROBLEMS DURING OPERATION
(Alberti and Thomas, 1979)

Both anesthesia and the stress of the surgical procedure tend to aggravate the carbohydrate metabolism defect of the patient with diabetes mellitus. In order to achieve the advantages of operation, the disadvantages must be accepted, but a determined attempt can be made to minimize them. The anesthesiologist can best accomplish this by being informed about the patient, the status of the diabetes, and all associated complications. An internist can best prepare the diabetic patient for operation and control the diabetes during the postoperative period, but during the operative period, care of the patient is the primary responsibility of the anesthesiologist. Communication and understanding between internist and anesthesiologist are necessary for smooth coordination as patient care changes from one physician to the other.

Premedication and Preparation

Withholding oral administration of all food and fluids is of as much or more importance for diabetic patients as for nondiabetic ones. The former custom of allowing glucose solution by mouth within a few hours of anesthesia induction in order to prevent hypoglycemia following preoperative administration of insulin is to be condemned. If glucose is needed during the preoperative period, it should be given intravenously and the patient's stomach kept as empty as possible.

As a general statement, preoperative medication for diabetic patients may be the same as would be used if the same patient were not diabetic. Narcotics tend to cause hyperglycemia in some animals, but in man the doses of narcotics used as premedication cause no rise in blood sugar and do not inhibit the hyperglycemia that follows administration of anesthetic agents such as ether (Greene, 1963). Atropine in premedication doses does not inhibit ether hyperglycemia.

Since reduction of postanesthetic nausea and vomiting is especially desirable in the diabetic patient, in order to reduce ketosis and promote early oral intake of carbohydrate it has been recommended that the dose of preoperative narcotic be reduced.

Both thiobarbiturates and oxybarbiturates in anesthetic doses are capable of inhibiting the hyperglycemia following ether anesthesia, but there is no evidence that the sedative dose of oxybarbiturate usually given as premedication has such an effect consistently (Greene, 1963; Henneman and Bunker, 1961).

Anesthetic Agents and Methods

Some agents used to produce anesthesia also cause alteration in carbohydrate metabolism, but their actions and sites of action are far from clear. Many observations made in animals have been arbitrarily applied to man. Studies made in man have been limited largely to measurements of changes occurring in peripheral blood that may or may not accurately reflect the changes occurring in cells. Bunker (1963) well summarized the present understanding in this statement: "A variety of 'metabolic' effects of anesthesia have been reported but much of the data is fragmentary or poorly controlled. Any postulated direct effects of anesthesia on intermediary metabolism are obscured by the marked metabolic consequences of endocrine, renal and respiratory disturbances in acid-base balance." Hyperglycemia caused by surgery is probably due to increase in cortisol, growth hormone, and sympathetic stimulation, so is not limited to the duration of anesthesia but persists for several days into the postoperative period (Clarke, 1973). Some changes caused by anesthetic agents are listed below.

Diethyl Ether. Because it was introduced early and found to produce marked changes in peripheral blood, the effects of diethyl ether have been studied more extensively than those of any other anesthetic agent. Administration of diethyl ether to animals and man has been followed to some degree in most subjects, but not all, by the following: hyperglycemia and increase in lactic acid, pyruvic acid, excess lactate-pyruvate ratio, citrate, ketoglutamate, ketone bodies, and serum inorganic phosphate.

Greene (1967) divides the changes produced by ether anesthesia into indirect and direct effects. The hyperglycemia is an indirect effect from increased sympathetic activity causing an increase in glycogenolysis in the liver. It is not known whether the stimulation is via the sympathetic fibers going to the liver or whether it is more indirectly caused by the release of epinephrine into the blood, which follows general sympathetic stimulation. Other indirect effects are caused by increase in plasma corticosteroids, changes in renal blood flow and function, stress of surgical procedure, and changes in tissue gas tensions. Increase in tissue carbon dioxide leads to marked changes in carbohydrate metabolism as the result of either altered tissue blood flow or tissue oxygen consumption or both (Greene, 1961).

The direct effects of ether itself on carbohydrate metabolism are less certain. They are hypothesized to be related either to an inhibition of the effect of insulin on transport of glucose across plasma membranes (cell and mitochondrial membranes) or to inhibition of phosphorylation of glucose in the mitochondria.

In spite of such evidence about alteration of carbohydrate metabolism by diethyl ether, Greene (1967) concludes that ether is not definitely contraindicated as an anesthetic agent for the diabetic patient, provided that rapid return to consciousness and a low incidence of postoperative nausea and vomiting are promoted.

Halothane. Measurements of blood changes indicative of altered carbohydrate metabolism during halothane have been variable. The mild hyperglycemia reported might have been associated with other variables such as operation, premedication, pulmonary ventilation, and use of other medications, but progressive hypoglycemia has also been reported in dogs (Galla and Wilson, 1964). Since little change occurs in lactate and pyruvate, and no excess lactate is present, the conclusion has been drawn that halothane may be administered without occurrence of anaerobic metabolism (Lowenstein et al., 1964). Lack of increase in diabetogenic growth hormone or blood glucose or decrease in insulin has resulted in halothane being a satisfactory anesthetic agent for diabetic patients (Oyama and Takazama, 1971; Greene, 1974). There is evidence that part of the negative inotropic effect of halothane on the heart is the result of interference with glucose uptake or metabolism prior to the phosphofructokinase step (Paradise and Ko, 1970). In vitro studies indicate that halothane inhibits the release of insulin in response to hyperglycemia, but this does not seem to affect the plasma insulin levels during anesthesia (Greene, 1974; Bruner, 1974).

Thiopental. When combined with inhalation of 70 per cent nitrous oxide and 30 per cent oxygen, Henneman and Bunker (1961) found that thiopental caused no change in blood glucose, a decrease in blood lactic, pyruvic, citric and alphaketoglutaric acid, and a slow increase in serum inorganic phosphorus. However, in spite of these minimal changes in peripheral blood, glucose tolerance was depressed. Oyama and co-workers (1971), in a later different study, could find no evidence of glucose intolerance during thiopental-nitrous oxide anesthesia. Subsequent investigations have found that thiopental-nitrous oxide anesthesia without operation does not cause any significant changes in blood glucose, insulin, cortisol, or growth hormone (Clarke, 1973; Greene, 1974), and there is some evidence that this type of anesthesia partly inhibits or delays the effects of operation on metabolism (Mehta, 1972).

Enflurane. Without surgery, enflurane anesthesia leaves glucose, insulin, cortisol, and growth hormone almost unaffected (Clarke, 1973) and there is no change in insulin:glucose ratio (Greene, 1974).

Isoflurane. Alveolar concentrations of 1.3 MAC isoflurane in oxygen without operation in man caused a significant increase in growth hormone and glucose levels in blood but no significant change in insulin or cortisol (Oyama et al., 1975).

Regional Anesthesia. Properly conducted local anesthesia has no effect on carbohydrate metabolism (Wylie and Churchill-Davidson, 1966). Since arteriosclerosis is a frequent complication of diabetes, a large percentage of the surgical procedures on these patients is required because of vascular insufficiency in the lower extremities. For these operations, subarachnoid and epidural anesthesia are satisfactory and without undue complication. Greene (1967) does not consider diabetic neuropathy a contraindication to the use of spinal anesthesia.

Epidural anesthesia is more effective than general anesthesia in ameliorating the changes in blood glucose, growth hormone, and cortisol caused by operation (Brandt et al., 1976). Increased blood lactate during epidural anesthesia was explained as possibly being due to decreased blood flow in muscle (Cooper et al., 1979).

Patient Care in the Operating Room

Selection of anesthetic agent or agents does not seem to be a major factor in the safe conduction of a surgical procedure on a diabetic patient. No agent is specifically beneficial for diabetes, and no agent is categorically contraindicated. Too much emphasis has been placed on the production of hyperglycemia by some anesthetic agents, because it is generally agreed that mild hyperglycemia in itself is not dangerous in the diabetic patient (Wylie and Churchill-Davidson, 1966; Moore, 1959). In a study of the postoperative course of a large number of diabetic patients, no difference in blood sugar concentrations could be correlated with the anesthetic agents employed during operation. The most significant factors influencing postoperative blood sugars were intensity of stress of operation, length of administration of anesthesia, and nutritional state of the patient (Galloway and Shuman, 1963). However, because of minimal effects on carbohydrate metabolism, a combination of thiopental, nitrous oxide, and a muscle relaxant has been considered to have advantages for producing general anesthesia in the diabetic patient.

The important objectives are prevention of acidosis, acetonemia, and hypoglycemia. Acetonemia and hypoglycemia are prevented by adequate administration of glucose and insulin in proper proportions of dosage and method as determined by consultation between internist and anesthesiologist.

Respiratory acidosis is best prevented by adequate pulmonary ventilation and carbon dioxide elimination. No harmful effect of mild overventilation (e.g., respiratory alkalosis) on diabetes mellitus has been demonstrated. Reliable facilities for adequate assisted respiration should be available during any anesthesia for operation on a diabetic patient and mandatory if any metabolic acidosis persists.

Metabolic acidosis is prevented or corrected by administration of fluids and electrolytes, as indicated by determination of serum electrolytes and blood gases, prevention of hypoxemia, promotion of adequate blood flow in tissues, and avoidance of anesthetic agents that tend to cause changes in acid-base balance.

These are the same objectives routinely sought during any anesthesia for patients without systemic complications, but the diabetic patient has a decreased reserve for maintaining homeostasis, so the anesthesiologist must be better informed about biochemical changes occurring in his diabetic patient than in the good risk, high reserve patient.

HYPERINSULINISM — ISLET CELL TUMORS OF THE PANCREAS

Of the multiple causes of either fasting or postprandial hypoglycemia, only two may pose significant problems for the anesthesiologist. The only important cause of fasting hypoglycemia that can cause serious problems during surgery is an insulin secreting tumor of the pancreas. Islet cell tumors can at times be exceedingly difficult to evaluate, and at times the diagnosis may remain in doubt. A patient with a persistently low blood sugar (below 50 mg/100 ml) should immediately become suspect for the diagnosis. Overnight fasting glucose and insulin measurements and the calculation of the ratio $\frac{\text{INSULIN} \, \mu\text{U/ml}}{\text{GLUCOSE mg/100 ml}}$ should be carried out. Patients with functioning islet cell tumors have a ratio that is consistently above 0.3 and often greater than 0.4. If normal ratios are still present after an overnight fast, a prolonged fast of up to 24 to 48 hours may be necessary before the ratios are repeated. Exercise may at times cause these tumors to secrete tremendous amounts of insulin. If the above tests are still normal under the above conditions, then a stimulation test with either tolbutamide, leucine, or glucagon should be carried out. These stimulatory tests must be monitored carefully, since profound hypoglycemia may be induced. If the insulin-glucose ratio remains normal despite the above maneuvers, a thorough search should be made for a noninsulin secreting tumor such as retroperitoneal fibroma or sarcoma. If all the tests are indicative of an islet cell tumor, celiac angiography should be utilized to localize the site of the tumor in the pancreas. About 50 per cent of tumors can be isolated in this fashion. An isotope liver scan should be done preoperatively to make sure that liver metastases are not present before surgery is contemplated.

Extracts of functioning islet cell tumors contain variable quantities of proinsulin in addition to insulin, and variable quantities of proinsulin may be secreted along with insulin. C-peptide is the protein link between the two insulin chains that form the proinsulin molecule. Before insulin is secreted, the C-peptide is cleaved from proinsulin and is secreted along with the insulin molecules. C-peptide can now be measured by a specific immunoassay and can be used to differentiate the patient who is giving himself or herself exogenous insulin from the patient with a true insulin secreting tumor of the pancreas. Exogenous insulin contains no C-peptide. Once the diagnosis of insulinoma has been established, the physician should look for other endocrine functioning tumors, such as adenomas of the pituitary and parathyroid glands. Insulinomas may be part of the so-called multiple endocrine adenomatosis syndrome type I, which at times may be an autosomal dominant disease. Insulinomas are usually benign, but occasionally they are malignant with spread to the liver. In malignant disease, the primary, and at times solitary, metastasis in the liver may be surgically removable. In widespread metastatic disease, palliative therapy with diazoxide is indicated. This drug specifically blocks insulin release from the pancreas. Streptozotocin is a cytotoxic drug that has specific activity against the pancreatic beta cell and has been used with some success in insulinomas.

Surgical excision is indicated for all benign insulinomas. Only two thirds of all such tumors can be localized at surgery. When the tumor cannot be palpated by the surgeon, small pieces of pancreas should be selectively removed and carefully examined by the pathologist. Administration of glucose during the surgical procedure is not considered mandatory, probably because the stress of surgery induces secretion of counterinsulin hormones such as adrenocatecholamines and adrenocorticosteroids. However, the blood sugar needs to be carefully monitored at frequent intervals during surgery. Hypoglycemia during surgery must be corrected immediately by rapid infusion of 5 to 10 per cent dextrose. It takes the clinical laboratory in most hospitals at least 20 to 25 minutes to do a standard blood glucose by the glucose oxidase method and this may not be satisfactory. The Dextrostix* method is rapid but may be quite inaccurate in the very low or very high blood sugar ranges. The new Ames Eyetone Reflectometer* is a small spectrophotometer that can accurately measure the purple color of the Dextrostix from 50 to 400 mg per 100 ml of blood in 60 seconds. It can be kept in the operating room and requires little technical skill to manipulate. It has been used successfully for many patients during surgery for removal of insulinomas. The anesthesiologist can help the surgeon by informing him of the blood sugar measurement. An abrupt rise in blood sugar during the surgical procedure may be good presumptive evidence that the tumor has been excised in

toto. If no definitive tumor is found and the surgeon is removing small amounts of pancreas, a sudden rise in the blood sugar may be the only objective evidence that one or more functioning adenomas have been removed.

A recently published report documents the successful use of the Biostator during surgery for removal of an insulinoma. This instrument has been developed by Life Sciences Instruments* (see Fig. 5–4). It is equipped with a glucose electrode that continuously monitors the venous blood sugar and gives a continuous reading. This information is fed into a computer that can be programmed to maintain a relatively normal blood sugar. The computer automatically directs the infusion of either glucose or insulin, depending upon the level of the blood sugar. The continual readout of the blood sugar is of enormous help to the surgeon in helping him to decide whether all the tumor has been removed. Considering the rarity of insulinomas in general and the enormous expense of the Biostator, it is doubtful that most community hospitals will be able to afford one. However, this instrument may also have great application in the management of the diabetic patient during surgery, and thus deserves consideration.

After surgical removal of an insulin secreting tumor, frank diabetes may develop during the postoperative period. Blood sugars may become high enough to require administration of insulin. Unless as much as 90 per cent of the pancreas has been removed, hyperglycemia following operation is generally transient. Hypoglycemia following surgery is good evidence that the tumor was not found or that metastatic nodules were present, usually in the liver.

ANESTHESIA FOR HYPERINSULINISM

During resection of a hyperfunctioning islet cell tumor the main problem of the anesthesiologist is to recognize and treat hypoglycemia. Use of some rapid type of blood sugar analyzer, either continuously or intermittently, is ideal but may not always be available. Use of clinical signs of hypoglycemia during general anesthesia then becomes necessary. Increased sympathetic

---

*Ames Company, Division of Miles Laboratories, Elkhart, Indiana 46514.

*Miles Laboratory, Elkhart, Indiana.

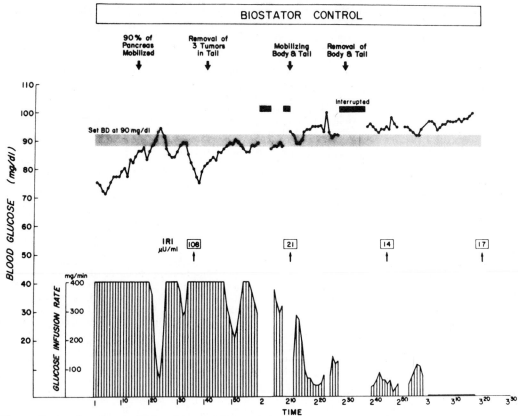

Figure 5–4. Continuous monitoring of blood glucose with feedback-controlled dextrose infusion during exploration and removal of insulin-secreting tumor of the pancreas. BD refers to the preselected blood glucose level of 90 mg/dl, which the Biostator was programmed to maintain. Serum immunoreactive insulin measured during the procedure is represented by the boxed inserts. (From Karam, J., et al. Amer. J. Med. *66*:675, 1979.)

outflow caused by hypoglycemia may be evidenced by sweating, tachycardia, hypertension, and/or dilated pupils. Decreased cerebral metabolism may lead to slowing of electroencephalogram or arterial hypotension (Hargadon and Ormston, 1963). Based on the occasional need for intravenous 50 per cent glucose during nitrous oxide–narcotic-relaxant anesthesia, Colella and Vandam (1972) elected to use diethyl ether as the anesthetic agent for removal of an insulinoma and were successful in maintaining a stable blood sugar throughout.

REFERENCES

Disorders of Calcium
Metabolism — Parathyroid Gland
Abnormalities

De Luca, H. F.: Vitamin D Endocrinology. Ann. Intern. Med. 85:367, 1976.

Hecht, A., Gershberg, H., et al.: Primary hyperparathyroidism: Laboratory and clinical data in 73 cases. J.A.M.A. 233:519, 1975.

Shaw, J. W.: Urinary cyclic AMP analyzed as a function of the serum calcium and parathyroid hormone in the differential diagnosis of hypercalcemia. J. Clin. Invest. 59:14, 1977.

Benson, R. C., Riggs, B. C., Pichard, B. M., and Arnaud, C. D.: Radioimmunoassay of parathyroid hormone in hypercalcemic patients with malignant disease. Am. J. Med. 56:882, 1974.

Davis, D. R., et al.: Selective venous catheterization and radioimmunoassay of parathyroid hormone in the diagnosis and localization of parathyroid tumors. Lancet 1:1079, 1973.

Haussler, M. R., and McCain, T. A.: Basic and clinical concepts related to vitamin D metabolism and action. N. Engl. J. Med. 297:974, 1031, 1977.

Schneider, A. B., and Sherwood, L. M.: Pathogenesis and management of hypoparathyroidism and other hypocalcemic disorders. Metabolism 24:871, 1975.

Chase, L. R., Nelson, G. L., and Aurbach, G. D.: Pseudohypoparathyroidism, defective excretion of 3'5' AMP in response to parathyroid hormone. J. Clin. Invest. 48:1832, 1969.

Stogmann, W., et al.: Pseudohypoparathyroidism: Disappearance of the resistance to parathyroid extract during treatment with vitamin D. Am. J. Med. 59:140, 1975.

Murray, T. M., Peacock, M., et al.: Nonautonomy of hormone secretion in primary hyperparathyroidism. Clin. Endo. 1:235, 1972.

Seihi, W. N., Jium, J. J., et al.: Acute treatment of hypercalcemia with furosemide. New Engl. J. Med. 283:836, 1970.

Kaye, M., Chatterjee, G., et al.: Arrest of hyperparathyroid bone disease with dihydrotachysterol in patients undergoing chronic hemodialysis. Ann. Intern Med. 73:225, 1970.

Fournier, A. E., Arnaud, C. D., et al.: Etiology of hyperparathyroidism and bone disease during chronic hemodialysis. J. Clin. Invest. 50:599, 1971.

Aldinger, K. A., and Samoan, N. A.: Hypokalemia and hypercalcemia. Ann. Intern. Med. 87:571, 1977.

Paloyon, E., Lawrence, A. M., and Straus, F. H.: Hyperparathyroidism. New York, Grune & Stratton, 1973.

Esselstyn, C. B., Jr., Levin, H. S., et al.: Reappraisal of parathyroid pathology in hyperparathyroidism. Surg. Clin. North Am. 54:443, 1974.

Purnele, D. C., et al.: Hyperparathyroidism due to single gland enlargement. Arch. Surg. 112:369, 1977.

Schneuder, A. B., and Sherwood, L. M.: Calcium homeostasis and the pathogenesis and management of hypercalcemic disorders. Metabolism 23:975, 1974.

Thomson, D. L., and Frame, B.: Involutional osteopenia: Current concepts. Ann. Intern. Med. 85:789, 1976.

Rasmussin, H., and Bordier, : The Physiological and Cellular Basis of Metabolic Bone Disease. Baltimore, Williams & Wilkins, 1974.

Mundy, G. R.: Differential diagnosis of osteopenia. Hosp. Pract. 1 Nov. 65–72, 1978.

Schneider, A. B., and Sherwood, L. M.: Calcium homeostasis and the pathogenesis and management of hypercalcemic disorders. Metabolism 23:975, 1974.

Anesthesia for Patients with
Hyperparathyroidism

Reiss, E.: Hyperthyroidism: Current perspectives. Adv. Int. Med. 19:287, 1974.

Crocker, E. F., Jellins, J., and Freund, J.: Parathyroid lesions localized by radionuclide substraction and ultrasound. Radiology 130:215, 1979.

Cox, R. J., Moore, D. B., and Wolfman, E. F., Jr.: Localization of the parathyroid gland by intraoperative methylene blue staining. Surg. Gynecol. Obstet. 148:769, 1979.

Edis, A. J.: Prevention and management of complications associated with thyroid and parathyroid surgery. Surg. Clin. North Am. 59:83, 1979.

Bronsky, D., et al.: Calcium and the electrocardiogram. Electrocardiographic manifestations of hyperparathyroidism and marked hypercalcemia from various other etiologies. Am. J. Cardiol. 7:833, 1961.

Voss, D. M., and Drake, E. H.: Cardiac manifestations of hyperparathyroidism with presentation of a previously reported arrhythmia. Am. Heart J. 73:235, 1967.

Schafer, M., and Economou, S. C.: Ode to an Indian rhinoceros, or the evaluation and preparation of patients for parathyroid surgery. Surg. Clin. North Am. 50:227, 1970.

Foldes, F. F.: Factors which alter the effects of muscle relaxants. Anesthesiology 20:464, 1959.

Kerr, W. H., Currie, D. J., and Welsh, W. K.: Surgical aspects of primary hyperparathyroidism: A review. Canad. J. Surg. 5:422, 1962.

McKie, B. D.: Hypoglycemia and prolonged curarization. Brit. J. Anaesth. 41:1091, 1969.

Avioli, L. V.: The therapeutic approach to hyperparathyroidism. Am. J. Med. 57:34, 1974.

Brennan, M. F., et al.: Recurrent hyperparathyroidism from an autotransplanted parathyroid adenoma. N. Engl. J. Med. 299:1057, 1978.

Thyroid Gland

Thyroid Function Tests

Britton, K. E. et al.: A strategy for thyroid function test. Br. Med. J. 8:350, 1975.

Larsen, P. R.: Thyroidal tri-iodothyronine and thyroxine in Graves' disease: Correlation with presurgical treatment, thyroid status and iodine content. J. Clin. Endocrinol. Metab. 41:1098, 1975.

Hamilton, C. R., and Maloof, F.: Unusual types of hyperthyroidism. Medicine 52:195, 1973.

Harbach, H., and Avioli, L. V.: Hyperthyroidism in Graves' disease: current trends in management and diagnosis. Arch. Intern. Med. 136:725, 1976.

Chopra, I. J.: Reciprocal changes in serum concentrations of reverse T_3 and T_4 in systemic illness. J. Clin. Endocrinol. Metab. 41:1043, 1975.

Carlsen, H. E., Hershman, J. M.: The hypothalamic pituitary axis. Med. Clin. North Am. 59:1045, 1975.

Abuid, J., and Larsen, P. R.: Triiodothyronine and thyroxine in hyperthyroidism: Comparison of the acute changes during therapy with antithyroid drugs. J. Clin. Invest. 54:201, 1974.

Evered, D.: Thyroid function after subtotal thyroidectomy for hyperthyroidism. Br. Med. J. 1:25, 1975.

Brown, J., et al.: Thyroid physiology in health and disease. Ann. Intern. Med. 81:68, 1974.

Refetoff, S.: Thyroid hormone therapy. Med. Clin. North Am. 59:1147, 1975.

Vagenahis, A. G.: Recovery of pituitary thyrotrophic function after withdrawal of prolonged thyroid suppression therapy. New Engl. J. Med. 293:681, 1975.

Wood, L. C., and Maloaf, F.: Thyroid failure after potassium iodide treatment of diffuse toxic goiter. Trans. Assoc. Am. Physicians 88:235, 1975.

The National Cancer Institute: Information for physicians on irradiation-related thyroid cancer. Cancer 26:150, 1976.

Mazzaferri, E. L., et al.: Papillary thyroid carcinoma. Impact of therapy in 675 patients. Medicine 56:171, 1977.

McDougall, I. R., and Kriss, J. P.: Management of the eye manifestations of thyroid disease. Pharmacol. Ther. 2:95, 1977.

Reviews

Ingbar, S. H.: The thyroid gland. In Williams, R. H. (ed.): Textbook of Endocrinology. 5th ed., W. B. Saunders Co., Philadelphia, 1974, p. 95.

Larsen, P. R.: Tests of thyroid function. Med. Clin. North Am. 59:1063, 1975.

General Surgical Problems

Stehling, L. C.: Anesthetic management of the patient with hyperthyroidism. Anesthesiology 41:585, 1974.

Reynolds, L. R., and Kotchen, T. A.: Antithyroid drugs and radioactive iodine. Arch. Intern. Med. 139:651, 1979.

Trench, A. J., et al.: Propranolol in thyrotoxicosis. Cardiovascular changes during thyroidectomy in patients pretreated with propranolol. Anaesthesia 33:535, 1978.

Knight, R. T.: Use of spinal anesthesia to control sympathetic overactivity in hyperthyroidism. Anesthesiology 6:225, 1945.

Brewster, W. R., Jr., Isaacs, J. P., Osgood, R. F., and King, T. L.: The hemodynamic and metabolic interrelationships in the activity of epinephrine, norepinephrine, and the thyroid hormones. Circulation 13:1, 1956.

Oyama, T.: Endocrine responses to anaesthetic agents. Brit. J. Anaesth. 45:276, 1973.

Oyama, T., Lato, P., Holaday, D. A., and Chang, H.: Effects of isoflurane anaesthesia and surgery on thyroid function in man. Canad. Anaesth. Soc. J. 22:474, 1975.

Oyama, T., Maeda, A., Fin, F., Satone, T. A., and Kudo, M.: Effect of althesin on thyroid-adrenal function in man. Brit. J. Anaesth. 47:837, 1975.

Harland, W. A., et al.: Release of thyroxine from the liver during anaesthesia and surgery. Brit. J. Anaesth. 46:818, 1974.

Prange, A. J., Jr., Lipton, M. A., Shearin, R. B., and Love, G. N.: The influence of thyroid status on the effects and metabolism of pentobarbital and thiopental. Biochem. Pharmacol. 15:237, 1966.

Munson, E. S., Hoffman, J. C., and Difazio, D. C.: The effects of acute hypothyroidism and hyperthyroidism in cyclopropane requirement (MAC) in rats. Anesthesiology 29:1074, 1968.

Babad, A. A., and Eger, E. I.: The effects of hyperthyroidism and hypothyroidism on halothane and oxygen requirements in dogs. Anesthesiology 29:1087, 1968.

Kadis, L. B., Bennett, E. J., Dalal, F. V., and Zauder, H. L.: Anesthetic management of thyrotoxicosis. Anesth. Analg. (Cleve.) 45:145, 1966.

Dobyns, B. M.: Prevention and management of hyperthyroid storm. World J. Surg. 2:293, 1978.

Duckworth, W. C.: Thyroid crisis. South. Med. J. 71:195, 1978.

Lee, T. C., et al.: The use of propranolol in the surgical treatment of thyrotoxic patients. Ann. Surg. 177:643, 1973.

Jamison, M. H., and Dive, H. J.: Postoperative thyrotoxic crisis in a patient prepared for thyroidectomy with propranolol. Brit. J. Clin. Pract. 33:82, 1979.

Erickson, M., Rubenfelds, S., Garbera, T., and Kohler, P. O.: Propranolol does not prevent thyroid storm. N. Engl. J. Med. 296:263, 1977.

Serri, O., Gagnon, R. M., Goulet, Y., and Somma, M.: Coma secondary to apathetic thyrotoxicosis. Canad. Med. Assoc. J. 119:605, 1978.

Abbott, T. R.: Anaesthesia in untreated myxedema. Brit. J. Anaesth. 35:510, 1967.

Pituitary Gland

Reichlin, S.: Regulation of the hypophysiotropic secretions of the brain. Arch. Intern. Med. 135:1350, 1975.

Jenkins, J. S., Gilbert, C. J., and Ang, V.: Hypothalamic pituitary function in patients with craniopharyngiomas. J. Clin. Endocrinol. Metabol. 43:394, 1976.

Weisberg, L. A., Zimmerman, E. A., and Frantz, A.

G.: Diagnosis and evaluation of patients with an enlarged sella. Am. J. Med. 61:590, 1976.

Spiger, M., Jubiz, W., and Meikle, A. W.: Single dose metyrapone test: review of a 4 year experience. Arch. Intern. Med. 135:698, 1975.

Carmalt, M. B., et al.: The treatment of Cushing's syndrome by transsphenoidal hypophysectomy. Quart. J. Med. 46:119, 1977.

Williams, R. A., Jacobs, H. S., et al.: The treatment of acromegaly with special reference to transsphenoidal hypophysectomy. Quart. J. Med. 44:79, 1975.

Chang, R. T., et al.: Detection, evaluation and treatment of pituitary microadenomas in patients with galactorrhea and amenorrhea. Am. J. Obstet. Gynecol. 128:356, 1977.

Jacobs, H. S.: Prolactin and amenorrhea. N. Engl. J. Med. 295:954, 1976.

Spark, R. F., et al.: Complete remission of acromegaly with medical treatment. J.A.M.A. 241:573, 1979.

Daughaday, W. H., and Oyer, P. E.: Growth hormone hypersecretion and acromegaly. Hosp. Pract. 13(8)75, 1978.

Jordan, R. M., et al.: Cerebrospinal fluid hormone concentration in the evaluation of pituitary tumors. Am. J. Int. Med. 85:49–55, 1976.

Jordan, R. M., and Kendall, J. W.: The primary empty sella syndrome. Am. J. Med. 62:569, 1977.

Cohen, K. L.: Metabolic, endocrine and drug-induced interference with pituitary function tests: A review. Metabolism 26:1165, 1977.

Reviews

Frohman, L. A.: Neurotransmitters as regulators of endocrine function. Hosp. Pract. 10:54, 1975.

Kleischer, N., and Guiellemin, R.: Clinical applications of hypothalamic releasing factors. Adv. Int. Med. 18:303, 1972.

Maffly, R. H.: Diabetes insipidus. Disturbances in body fluid osmolarity. In Andoreale, T. E (ed.): Disturbances in Body Fluid Osmolarity. American Physiological Society, Bethesda, Maryland, 1977.

Daughaday, W. H.: The adenohypophysis. In Williams, R. H., (ed.): Textbook of Endocrinology, 5th ed. Philadelphia, W. B. Saunders Co., 1974, pp. 31–79.

Anesthesia for Operations on the Pituitary Gland

Messick, J. M., et al.: Anesthesia for transsphenoidal surgery of the hypophyseal region. Anesth. Analg. (Cleve.) 57:206, 1978.

Oyama, T.: Endocrine responses to anaesthetic agents. Brit. J. Anaesth. 45:276, 1973.

Kitahata, L. M.: Airway difficulties associated with anaesthesia in acromegaly. Brit. J. Anaesth. 43:1187, 1971.

Burn, J. M. B.: Airway difficulties associated with anaesthesia in acromegaly. Brit. J. Anaesth. 44:413, 1972.

Southwick, J. P., and Katz, J.: Unusual airway difficulty in the acromegalic patient: Indications for tracheostomy. Anesthesiology 51:72, 1979.

Newfield, P., et al.: Transsphenoidal hypophysectomy (letter to the Editor). Anesth. Analg. (Cleve.) 57:142, 1978.

Wilson, C. B., and Dempsey, L. C.: Transsphenoidal microsurgical removal of 250 pituitary adenomas. J. Neurosurg. 48:13, 1978.

Pearson, O. H.: Endocrine consequences of hypophysectomy. Anesthesiology 24:563, 1963.

Antidiuretics, A.M.A. Drug Evaluations. Chicago, American Medical Association, 1973, pp. 453–456.

Adrenal Cortex

Krueger, D. T., et al.: Cyproheptadine-induced remission of Cushing's disease. New Engl. J. Med. 293:893, 1975.

Melby, J. C.: Systemic corticosteroid therapy; pharmacology and endocrinologic considerations. Ann. Intern. Med. 81:505, 1974.

Tyler, F. H.: Laboratory evaluation of disorders of the adrenal cortex. Am. J. Med. 53:664, 1972.

Liddle, G. W., and Shute, A. M.: The evolution of Cushing's syndrome as a clinical entity. Adv. Intern. Med. 15:155, 1969.

Meikle, A. W., and Tyler, F. H.: Potency and duration of action of glucocorticoids. Am. J. Med. 63:200, 1977.

Koch-Weser, J.: Withdrawal from glucocorticoid. N. Engl. J. Med. 295:30, 1976.

Haynes, R. C., and Larner, J.: Adrenocorticotrophic hormone. In Goodman, L. S., and Gilman, A. (eds.): The Pharmacological Basis of Therapeutics. 5th ed., New York, Macmillan, 1975, pp. 1472–1506.

Orth, D. N.: Metapyrone is useful only as adjunctive therapy in Cushing's disease. (Editorial) Ann. Intern. Med. 89:128, 1978.

Melby, J. C.: Identifying the adrenal lesion in primary aldosteronism. (Editorial) Ann. Intern. Med. 76:1039, 1972.

Plonk J., et al.: Modification of adrenal function by the antiserotonin agent cyproheptadine. J. Clin. Endo. Met. 42:291, 1976.

Liddle, G. W.: Pathogenesis of glucocorticoid disorders. Am. J. Med. 53:638, 1972.

Daughaday, W. H.: Cushing's disease and busaphilic microadenoma. (Editorial) N. Engl. J. Med. 298:793, 1978.

Mattingly, D., and Tyler, C.: Overnight urinary 11-hydroxycorticoid estimations in diagnosis of Cushing's syndrome. Br. Med. J. 2:668, 1976.

Gwinup, G., and Johnson, B.: Clinical testing of the hypothalamic-pituitary-adrenocortical system in states of hypo- and hypercortisonism. Metabolism 24:777, 1975.

Spechart, P. F., et al.: Screening for adrenocortical insufficiency with cosyntropin. Arch. Intern. Med. 128:761, 1971.

Tyorell, J. B., et al.: Cushing's disease. Selective trans-sphenoidal resection of pituitary microadenomas. N. Engl. J. Med. 298:753, 1978.

Sachar, E. J.: Hormonal changes in stress and mental illness. Hosp. Pract. 10(7):49, 1975.

Fauci, A. S., et al.: Glucocorticoid therapy: mechanism of action and clinical considerations. Ann. Intern. Med. 84:304, 1976.

Braws, J. J., et al.: Plasma electrolytes, renin, and aldosterone in the diagnosis of primary hyperaldosteronism. Lancet 2:55, 1968.

Odell, W. D., et al.: Adrenal Medulla. Catecholamines. A Symposium. Calif. Med. 117:32, 1972.

Gittes, R. F., and Bendixen, H.: Pheochromocytoma tumor localization and surgical management. Calif. Med. 118:1, 1973.

Vliet, P. D., et al.: Focal myocarditis associated with pheochromocytoma. N. Engl. J. Med. 274:1102, 1966.

Drasin, H.: Treatment of malignant pheochromocytoma. West. J. Med. 128:106, 1978.

Griffith, M. I., et al.: Successful control of pheochromocytoma in pregnancy. J.A.M.A. 229:437, 1974.

Palmer, R. F., and Lassetor, K. C.: Sodium nitroprusside. N. Engl. J. Med. 292:294, 1975.

Page, L. B., and Roher, J. W.: Pheochromocytoma with predominant epinephrine secretion. Am. J. Med. 47:648, 1969.

Kaplan, N. M., Kramer, N. J., et al.: Single voided urine metanephrine assays in screening for pheochromocytoma. Arch. Intern. Med. 137:190, 1977.

Stewart, B. H., et al.: Localization of pheochromocytoma by computed tomography. N. Engl. J. Med. 299:460, 1978.

Reviews

Liddle, G. W., and Melmox, K. L.: The Adrenals. In Williams, R. H., (ed.): Textbook of Endocrinology. 5th ed. Philadelphia, W. B. Saunders Co., 1974, pp. 233–322.

Anesthesia for Patient with Disease of Adrenal Cortex

Vandam, L. D., and Moore, F. D.: Adrenocortical mechanisms related to anesthesia. Anesthesiology 21:531, 1960.

Briggs, F. N., and Munson, P. L.: Studies on mechanism of stimulation of ACTH secretion with aid of morphine as blocking agent. Endocrinology 57:205, 1955.

Oyama, T., Toyota, M., Schinozaki, Y., and Kudo, T.: Effects of morphine and ketamine anesthesia and surgery on plasma concentrations of luteinizing hormone, testosterone, and cortisol in man. Brit. J. Anaesth. 49:983, 1977.

Nishioka, K., Levy, A. A., and Dobkin, A. B.: Effect of halothane and methoxyflurane anesthesia in plasma cortisol concentration in relation to major surgery. Canad. Anesth. Soc. J. 15:441, 1968.

Oyama, T.: Endocrine responses to anaesthetic agents. Brit. J. Anaesth. 45:276, 1973.

Carnes, M. A.: Anesthetic considerations in adrenocortical disease. In Jenkins, M. T. (ed.): Anesthesia for Endocrine Diseases. Philadelphia, F. A. Davis Co., 1963, p. 141.

Oyama, T., Matsuki, A., and Kudo, M.: Effect of ethrane anaesthesia and surgical operation on adrenocortical function. Canad. Anaesth. Soc. J. 19:394, 1972.

Hume, D. M., Bell, C. C., and Barter, F.: Direct measurement of adrenal secretion during operative trauma and convalescence. Surgery 52:174, 1962.

Johnston, I. D. A.: Endocrine aspects of the metabolic response to surgical operation. Ann. Roy. Col. Surg. 35:270, 1964.

Enquista, A., Brandt, M. R., Fernandes, A., and Kehlet, H.: The blocking effect of epidural analgesia on the adrenocortical and hyperglycemic responses to surgery. Acta Anaesth. Scand. 21:330, 1977.

Van Brunt, E. E., and Ganong, W. T.: The effects of preanesthetic medication, anesthesia and hypothermia on the endocrine response to injury. Anesthesiology 24:500, 1963.

Kehlet, H., and Binder, L.: Adrenocortical function and clinical course during and after surgery in unsupplemented glucocorticoid-treated patients. Brit. J. Anaesth. 45:1043, 1973.

Cahill, C. F., Jr., and Thorn, G. W.: Preoperative and postoperative management of adrenal cortical hyperfunction. Anesthesiology 24:472, 1963.

Finch, J. S.: Primary aldosteronism. Review of the anaesthetic experience in sixty patients. Brit. J. Anaesth. 41:880, 1969.

Gangat, Y., Turner, L., Baer, L., and Puchner, P.: Primary aldosteronism with uncommon complications. Anesthesiology 45:542, 1976.

Adrenal Medulla: Pheochromocytoma

Anesthesia for Patient with Pheochromocytoma

Pratilas, V., and Pratila, M. G.: Anaesthetic management of pheochromocytoma. Canad. Anaesth. Soc. J. 26:253, 1979.

Deblasi, S.: The management of the patient with pheochromocytoma. Brit. J. Anaesth. 38:740, 1966.

Smith, D. S., Aukberg, S. J., and Levitt, J. D.: Induction of anesthesia in a patient with undiagnosed pheochromocytoma. Anesthesiology 49:368, 1978.

Scott, H. W., Riddell, D. H., and Brockman, S. K.: Surgical management of pheochromocytoma. Surg. Gynec. Obstet. 120:707, 1965.

Humble, R. M.: Pheochromocytoma, neurofibromatosis and pregnancy. Anaesthesia 22:296, 1967.

Deoreo, G. A., Stewart, B. H., Tarazi, R. C., and Gifford, R. W.: Preoperative blood transfusion in the safe surgical management of pheochromocytoma: A review of 46 cases. J. Urol. 111:715, 1974.

Desmonts, J. M., le Hoveller, J., Remond, P., and Duvaldestin, P. R.: Anesthetic management of patients with pheochromocytoma. Brit. J. Anaesth. 49:991, 1977.

Cooperman, L. H., Engelman, K., and Mann, P. E. G.: Anesthetic management of pheochromocytoma employing halothane and beta adrenergic blockade. Anesthesiology 28:575, 1967.

Clarke, A. D., Tobias, M. A., and Challen, P. D.: The use of neurolept analgesia during surgery for pheochromocytoma. Brit. J. Anaesth. 44:1093, 1974.

Csanky-Treels, J. C., Lawick Van Pabst, W. P., Brands, J. W. J., and Stamenkovic, L.: Effects of sodium nitroprusside during excision of pheochromocytoma. Anaesthesia 31:60, 1976.

Ortiz, F. T., and Diaz, P. M.: Use of enflurane during resection of a pheochromocytoma. Anesthesiology 42:495, 1975.

Kreul, J. F., Dauchot, P. J., and Anton, A. H.: Hemodynamic and catecholamine studies during pheochromocytoma resection under enflurane anesthesia. Anesthesiology 44:265, 1976.

Stoner, T. R., Jr., and Urbach, K. T.: Cardiac arrhythmias associated with succinylcholine in a patient with pheochromocytoma. Anesthesiology 29:1228, 1968.

Nourok, D. S., Gwinup, G., and Hamlui, G. T.: Phentolamine resistant pheochromocytoma treated with sodium nitroprusside. J.A.M.A. 183:841, 1963.

Cousins, M. J., and Rubin, R. B.: The intraoperative management of pheochromocytoma with total epidural sympathetic blockade. Brit. J. Anaesth. 46:78, 1974.

Ross, E. J., Prichard, B. N. C., Kaufman, L., Robertson, A. I. G., and Harries, B. J.: Preoperative and operative management of patients with phaeochromocytoma. Brit. Med. J. 1:191, 1967.

Salem, M. R. and Ivankovic, A. D.: Management of phentolamine-resistant pheochromocytoma with beta-adrenergic blockade. Brit. J. Anaesth. 41:1087, 1969.

Diabetes Mellitus

Creutzfeldt, W., Kabberling, J., and Neel, J. V.: The Genetics of Diabetes Mellitus. New York, Springer-Verlag, 1976.

Cahue, G. F., Etzweler, D. D., and Frunkel, N.: Control and diabetes. N. Engl. J. Med. 294:1004, 1976.

Cahue, G. F.: Physiology of insulin in man. Diabetes 20:785, 1971.

Anderson, O. O., Dechert, T., and Nerup, J.: Immunological aspects of diabetes mellitus. Acta Endocrinol. (Kbh) 83, 1976.

Archer, J. A., Gorden, P., and Roth, J.: Defect in insulin binding to receptors in obese man. J. Clin. Invest. 55:166, 1975.

Williamson, J. R., and Kilo, C.: Current status of capillary basement membrane disease in diabetes mellitus. Diabetes 26:65, 1977.

Shapiro, F. L., Kjellstrand, C. M., and Goetz, F. C.: End stage diabetic nephropathy. Kidney Inter. 6(Suppl. 1), 1974.

Shen, S. W., and Bressler, R.: Clinical pharmacology of oral and antidiabetic agents. N. Engl. J. Med. 296:493, 1977.

University Group Diabetes Program: A study of the effects of hypoglycemic agents in vascular complications in patients with adult onset diabetes mellitus. Diabetes 19 (Suppl. 2) 747, 1970.

Kitabchi, A. T., Ayyagari, V., and Guerra, S. M. O.: The efficacy of low-dose versus conventional therapy of insulin for treatment of diabetic ketoacidosis. Ann. Intern. Med. 84:633, 1976.

Madison, L. L.: Low-dose insulin: a plea for caution. N. Engl. J. Med. 294:393, 1976.

Posner, J. B., Swanson, A. G., and Plum, F.: Acid base balance in cerebrospinal fluid. Arch. Neurol. 12:479, 1965.

Kreisberg, R. A.: Diabetic ketoacidosis. New concepts and trends in pathogenesis and treatment. Ann. Intern. Med. 88:681, 1978.

McGarry, J. D., and Foster, D. W.: Regulation of ketogenesis and clinical aspects of the ketotic state. Metabolism 21:471, 1972.

Ewing, D. J., Campbell, I. W., and Clarke, B. F.: Mortality in diabetic autonomic neuropathy. Lancet 1:601, 1976.

Kitabchi, A. E., et al.: The efficacy of low-dose versus conventional therapy of insulin for treatment of diabetic ketoacidosis. Ann. Intern. Med. 84:633, 1976.

Problems During Operation

Alberti, K. G. M. M., and Thomas, D. J. B.: The management of diabetes during surgery. Brit. J. Anaesth. 51:693, 1979.

Greene, N. M.: Inhalation Anesthetics and Carbohydrate Metabolism. Baltimore, Williams & Wilkins Co., 1963.

Henneman, D. H., and Bunker, J. P.: Effects of general anesthesia on peripheral blood levels of carbohydrate and fat metabolites and serum inorganic phosphorus. J. Pharmacol. Exp. Ther. 133:253, 1961.

Bunker, J. P.: Neuroendocrine effects on carbohydrate metabolism. Anesthesiology 24:515, 1963.

Clarke, R. S. J.: Anaesthesia and carbohydrate metabolism. Brit. J. Anaesth. 45:237, 1973.

Greene, N. M.: Carbohydrate metabolism and anesthesia. Internat. Anesth. Clin. 5:411, 1967.

Greene, N. M.: Lactate, pyruvate and excess lactate production in anesthetised man. Anesthesiology 22:404, 1961.

Galla, S. J., and Wilson, E. P.: Hexose metabolism during halothane anesthesia in dogs. Anesthesiology 25:96, 1964.

Lowenstein, E., Clark, J. D., and Villareal, Y.: Excess lactate production during halothane anesthesia in man. J.A.M.A. 190:110, 1964.

Oyama, T., and Takazama, T.: Effects of halothane anaesthesia and surgery on human growth hormone and insulin levels in plasma. Brit. J. Anaesth. 43:573, 1971.

Greene, N. M.: Insulin and anesthesia. Anesthesiology 41:75, 1974.

Paradise, R. R., and Ko, K.: The effect of fructose on halothane depressed rat atria. Anesthesiology 32:124, 1970.

Bruner, E. A.: Anesthesia and the endocrine pancreas. Anesthesiology 41:1, 1974.

Mehta, S.: The influence of anesthesia with thiopentone and diazepam on the blood sugar level during surgery. Brit. J. Anaesth. 44:75, 1972.

Oyama, T., Latto, P., and Holaday, D.: Effect of isoflurane anesthesia and surgery on carbohydrate metabolism and plasma cortisol levels in man. Canad. Anaesth. Soc. J. 22:696, 1975.

Wylie, W. D., and Churchill-Davidson, H. C.: A Practice of Anesthesia. 2nd ed., Chicago, Year Book Medical Publishers, 1966.

Brandt, M., Kehlet, H., Binder, C., Hagen, C., and McNeilly, D. S.: Effect of epidural analgesia on glucoregulatory endocrine response to surgery. Clin. Endocrinol. 5:107, 1976.

Cooper, G. M., Holdcroft, A., Hall, G. M., and Alaghband-Zadeh, J.: Epidural analgesia and the metabolic response to surgery. Canad. Anaesth. Soc. J. 26:381, 1979.

Moore, F. D.: Metabolic Care of the Surgical Patient. Philadelphia, W. B. Saunders Co., 1959, pp. 638–645.

Galloway, J. A., and Shuman, L. R.: Diabetes and surgery, a study of 667 cases. Am. J. Med. 34:177, 1963.

Hyperinsulinism — Islet Cell Tumors of the Pancreas

Merimee, T. J.: Spontaneous hypoglycemia in man. Adv. Intern. Med. 22:301, 1977.

Schnell, N., Malmar, G. D., and Ferris, D. O.: Circulating glucose and insulin in surgery for insulinoma. J.A.M.A. 217:1072, 1971.

Karan, J. H., et al.: Feedback-controlled dextrose infusion during surgical management of insulinomas. Am. J. Med. 66:675, 1979.

Koutras, P., and White, R. R.: Insulin-secreting tumors of the pancreas. Surg. Clin. North Am. 52:299, 1972.

Kitabchi, A. E.: Proinsulin and C-peptide. A review. Metabolism 26:547, 1977.

General Reference

Bondy, P. K.: Disorders of carbohydrate metabolism. In Bondy, P. K. (ed.): Ducan's Diseases of Metabolism. 7th ed., Philadelphia, W.B. Saunders Co., 1975.

Anesthesia for Hyperinsulinism

Hargadon, J. J., and Ormston, T. O.: Anesthesia for excision of islet-cell tumour of the pancreas. Brit. J. Anaesth. 35:807, 1963.

Colella, J. J., and Vandam, L. D.: Diethyl ether anaesthesia for a patient with hyperinsulinism. Anesthesiology 37:354, 1972.

6

Pulmonary Diseases

By DAVID D. ALFERY, M.D.,
and JONATHAN L. BENUMOF, M.D.

Introduction
General Considerations
  History
  Physical Examination
  Signs of Increased Pulmonary Vascular
    Resistance
  Radiography
  Pulmonary Function Testing
  Specialized Tests
  Preoperative Preparation
  Intraoperative Monitoring

Specific Diseases
  Vascular Conditions
  Infiltrative-Alveolar Disorders
  Multisystem Diseases with Pulmonary
    Involvement
  Fibrotic Lung Diseases
  Obstructive Pulmonary Diseases
  Bullous Disease of the Lung
  Isolation Precautions for the Patient with
    Active Tuberculosis

INTRODUCTION

This chapter discusses uncommon diseases that produce significant pulmonary damage and thus require specific anesthetic considerations. Conditions that have multiorgan system involvement which are not primarily pulmonary and/or produce only mild lung injury have been omitted; similarly, diseases that are commonly seen, such as chronic bronchitis and asthma, are not discussed. Several conditions, such as sarcoidosis and Wegener's granulomatosis, that have been included are not truly "pulmonary" diseases but have pulmonary pathology as a major manifestation. In addition, several systemic illnesses are discussed insofar as their pulmonary involvement is concerned.

The first section of this chapter discusses clinical findings (history, physical, roentgenographic, etc.) of pulmonary pathology. In addition, the progression of signs from pulmonary hypertension to right ventricular hypertrophy and cor pulmonale is described. Although this progression is not seen in all the conditions that are later discussed, it does occur to some degree in most of them. In addition, pulmonary function tests, intraoperative monitoring requirements, and preoperative therapeutic options are discussed as they relate to lung disease. Thus, the first section serves as a framework upon which specific diseases may be described.

The second section of this chapter deals with individual diseases. While some repetition exists in the discussion of anesthetic considerations, each section is in context, permitting easier full access to any specific disease entity. Each specific condition is organized into two parts. The first part discusses the definition, incidence, etiology, pathology, clinical features, roentgenologic and laboratory findings, treatment, and prognosis of the condition. The second part contains the anesthetic considerations that are relevant to the disease.

GENERAL CONSIDERATIONS

HISTORY

Dyspnea. Dyspnea is a term used to indicate the subjective awareness of disturbance of breathing. Dyspnea may be divided clinically into four main categories:

1. The commonest use refers to a sense of discomfort on breathing, as in patients with airway obstruction due to chronic bronchitis or asthma, restrictive lung disease, or left ventricular failure, or those with mechanical embarrassment such as pleural effusion or pneumothorax. Thus the disturbance of breathing is perceived as difficulty in breathing (shortness of breath). In chronic diseases, it is common to find that the patient begins to complain of dyspnea only after his respiratory reserve is quite severely impaired.

2. In dry pleurisy dyspnea is due to pain on breathing.

3. In such conditions as metabolic acidosis or anemia the patient may be aware of more rapid or deeper respiration without actual discomfort.

4. Occasionally, patients suffering from neurosis become conscious of the normally unconscious process of breathing; they may feel difficulty in "getting air down into the lung," and indulge in frequent sighing respirations.

Cough. Cough is possibly the most common manifestation of respiratory disease. It is so common among cigarette smokers that many of them regard a morning cough as "normal." The cough reflex can be initiated by a wide variety of stimuli. The commonest stimulus to cough is the formation of sputum in the respiratory tract, and the cough process is an essential element in keeping the tract clear. Sensitivity is increased by inflammation of the mucous membrane.

Occasionally a bout of paroxysmal coughing may be so prolonged that the raised intrathoracic pressure seriously interferes with the venous return to the heart. At the same time, the intracranial pressure is elevated, causing increased cerebral vascular resistance. Both effects are maximal at the end of the paroxysm and may result in hypoxia of cerebral tissue and "cough syncope," which is sometimes accompanied by tonic and clonic spasms resembling epilepsy.

Sputum. The normal adult produces about 100 ml of mucus from the respiratory tract in a day. When excess mucus is formed it may accumulate, stimulate the mucous membrane, and be coughed up as sputum. Sputum may be formed in response to physical, chemical, or infective insult to the mucous membrane of the airways.

Mucoid sputum is clear or white. Black sputum may be mucoid sputum flecked with detritus of cigarette smoke or atmospheric smoke. Coal miners' sputum may contain coal dust, and patients with coal miners' penumoconiosis may occasionally cough up tarry material derived from areas of progressive massive fibrosis. Purulent sputum may contain a variable amount of pus mixed with mucus. Purulent sputum is usually yellow but if it has been stagnant it may be green, owing to the action of verdoperoxidase derived from neutrophils. Blood-stained sputum varies from small streaks to gross hemoptysis and always warrants investigation. An acute hemorrhagic exudate in the alveoli, as in pneumonia, may result in brown particles of altered blood, so-called "rusty sputum." Plugs or casts may be found in the sputum from asthmatic patients. In chronic conditions such as chronic bronchitis or bronchiectasis, measurement of the amount of sputum produced each 24 hours, or in the first hour after waking, is a useful means of comparing patients and estimating progress.

Chest Pain. The most important form of chest pain due to respiratory disease is pleuritic pain. It is characteristically worse on breathing and coughing, and can usually be accurately localized by the patient.

Generalized complaints that often accompany these common symptoms of respiratory disease include weakness, lethargy, fatigue, weight loss, and anorexia.

PHYSICAL EXAMINATION

General Observation. The patient may be observed to be breathless, either at rest or after mild effort. If the patient has chronic bronchitis or emphysema, breathing may be through pursed lips or grunting in nature. In restrictive or painful conditions, respiration may be rapid and shallow, and there may be a sudden catch in breathing if the patient takes a deep breath, due to pleuritic pain. Sweating, cyanosis of the nailbeds or lips, coarse tremor or twitching, mental confusion, drowsiness, or coma may be observed in patients who are hypoxemic and/or hypercapnic.

Inspection of the Chest. The chest should be inspected for rate and type of respiration and symmetry of chest wall movement. Undue flattening or indrawing beneath one of the clavicles may indicate longstanding fibrosis at the apex. A sunken and immobile hemithorax, the so-called "frozen chest," may indicate immobilization of a lung by grossly thickened pleura. In chronic airway obstruction, contraction of accessory muscles may be observed along with inspiratory indrawing of the suprasternal and supraclavicular fossae as a result of high negative intrathoracic pressure. There may also be expiratory filling of the jugular veins due to elevated intrathoracic expiratory pressure. In chronic bronchitis, emphysema, and asthma, the chest is often barrel shaped because of the overinflation of the lungs caused by airway obstruction. Overall diaphragmatic function can be assessed grossly by simply watching the rise in the abdominal wall with inspiration and fall with expiration during spontaneous quiet breathing. Hoover's sign, the indrawing rather than flaring of the anterior rib margins with inspiration, is a reliable sign of lung hyperinflation; it is caused by horizontal rather than downward contraction of the diaphragm. Scars from previous thoracotomy should be noted.

Palpation of the Chest. The position of the trachea should be identified. Deviation of the trachea is the main indication of lateral shift of the upper mediastinum, while deviation of the apex beat and cardiac dullness are the main indications of shift of the lower mediastinum.

Percussion of the Chest. Percussion over normal lung has a resonant quality; this can be modified by the density of the overlying tissue (muscle, fat). Percussion over consolidated, atelectatic and fibrotic lung, and pleural fluid will dampen the reflected sound and the note will be perceived as dull (short and nonmusical). Percussion over organized fluid is completely dampened and termed flat. Percussion over air (pneumothorax) results in a sound that is hyperresonant or tympanitic. It is important to determine the upper level of the liver dullness, which is most easily done in the midclavicular line on the right side. With quiet breathing and the patient supine, liver dullness normally lies at the level of the sixth rib. Deviation of the liver dullness downward may be caused by excessive lung inflation.

Vocal Fremitus. The only value of this crude sign is to help to distinguish dullness on percussion due either to underlying consolidation or to pleural effusion. Fremitus is decreased in pleural effusion and increased in consolidation.

Normal Breath Sounds. The type, location, pitch, loudness, and description of normal breath sounds are presented in Table 6-1.

Abnormal Breath Sounds. Absent or diminished breath sounds occur in emphysema and pneumothorax. Rales, rhonchi, and wheezes are abnormal and are examples of adventitious sounds. These may be generated from a variety of mechanisms but usually indicate constriction of airways or abnormal fluid in airways, or both. The

Table 6-1. *Normal Breath Sounds*

Type	Location(s) Where Typically Heard	Pitch	Amplitude (Loudness)	Inspiration Expiration Ratio	Description
Vesicular	Over most of the chest except over major airways	Low	Moderate	3:1	"Breezy" (sound of wind in trees)
Tracheal	Over trachea	Very high	Very great	5:6	Loud and harsh, "tubular"
Bronchial	Over major central airways	High	Great	2:3	Hollow, "tubular"
Bronchovesicular	Over major central airways	Medium	Moderately great	1:1	"Breezy," "tubular," "tent-shaped"

character of these sounds is influenced by the size of the airway, with smaller airways resulting in a finer and more high-pitched sound. The nature of the moisture also influences the resultant sound, with thinner and more fluid moisture resulting in a drier sound.

A friction rub is usually a low pitched, repeatedly interrupted sound, much like that heard when leather surfaces creak together. It is often repeated in the same phase of respiration (both inspiration and expiration) when purely pleural in origin, with the heart beat when pericardial based, and with both respiration and heart beat when arising from both pleura and pericardium.

An outline of the physical findings in different pathologic conditions is presented in Table 6–2.

SIGNS OF INCREASED PULMONARY VASCULAR RESISTANCE

As a result of pathologic alterations in the pulmonary vasculature, the resistance within the vessels frequently increases so that the pressure in the pulmonary artery rises. Although such factors as obstruction or obliteration of the pulmonary vascular bed may be prominent in pulmonary disease, hypoxic pulmonary vasoconstriction plays an important part, and the level of pulmonary hypertension usually correlates well with the degree of oxygen desaturation. Any accompanying chronic hypercapnia may also contribute to pulmonary vasoconstriction. Examination of the lungs themselves provides no indication of the presence of pulmonary hypertension. Signs indicative of this abnormality are found during examination of the heart.

Pulmonary Hypertension. The auscultatory signs of pulmonary hypertension are an increase in the pulmonary component of the second heart sound, loss of the normally present split in the second heart sound, the appearance of a high pitched early systolic ejection click, and the presence of a fourth heart sound. Other signs suggestive or indicative of pulmonary hypertension include dilatation of the main pulmonary arteries and fullness of the apical vessels on ordinary chest radiography, electrocardiographic evidence of right ventricular hypertrophy (RVH), and, most definitively, direct

demonstration of high pulmonary pressures during cardiac catheterization. In a few patients, development of pulmonary hypertension causes right-to-left flow through a patent foramen ovale that was of no functional consequence when right ventricular pressures were normal. The superimposition of anatomic shunting from this mechanism on the physiologic shunting resulting from the underlying lung disease may lead to severe refractory hypoxemia.

Right Ventricular Hypertrophy. An increased pulmonary vascular resistance places a heavy burden on the right ventricle in that it must work harder to force blood through the pulmonary vascular bed. As a result, the ventricle frequently hypertrophies. The earliest evidence of right ventricular hypertrophy is usually electrocardiographic and consists of clockwise rotation, right axis deviation, large and dominant R wave in lead V_1, decreasing amplitude of R wave and increasing amplitude of S wave from leads V_2 to V_6, inverted T wave in leads V_1 to V_6, and depressed ST segments in leads V_2 to V_6. With chronicity of pulmonary disease, right atrial hypertrophy may manifest as tall, peaked P wave in leads II and III and a large diphasic P wave in lead V_1. A prominent pulsation along the right border of the sternum, associated with conspicuous retraction over the left ventricle giving the anterior chest a rocking motion synchronous with the heart beat, is suggestive of right ventricular hypertrophy.

Cor Pulmonale. When right ventricular failure develops from chronic pulmonary disease, the condition is called cor pulmonale. The signs of cor pulmonale may include all of those of pulmonary hypertension and right ventricular hypertrophy. In addition, there may be a pulmonic diastolic murmur, a third heart sound, chronic dependent edema, enlargement and/or tenderness of the liver, ascites, distention or pulsation (large A waves) of neck veins, and an increased venous pressure.

RADIOGRAPHY

Examination of the P-A Chest Film. It is important to study a posterior-anterior (P-A) or anterior-posterior (A-P) chest film in an orderly manner. The position of the patient

Table 6–2. *Physical Findings that Occur with Pulmonary Pathology*

	Inspection and Palpation	Percussion	Fremitus	Breath Sounds	Adventitious Sounds	Other
Normal	Equal rib and diaphragm movement	Resonant	Present	Vesicular	None	"Bronchophony" in normal spoken voice
Consolidation	Slight restriction of motion on side affected	Dull	Increased	Bronchial	Rales	"Egophony" (E to A) and whispered pectoriloquy
Pleural effusion or empyema	Reduced movement on side affected	Dull or flat	Absent	Diminished or absent	Friction rub early	Mediastinal shift away
Pneumothorax	Slightly enlarged and restricted movement	Hyper-resonant	Absent	Diminished or absent	None	Mediastinal shift away
Fibrothorax	Small and very restricted movement	Dull	Present	Reduced to absent	None	Mediastinal shift toward
Cavity	Normal	Usually normal	Usually present	Amphoric	Coarse rales	Coin sign
Major atelectasis	Slightly small and restricted on side affected	Dull	Normal	Diminished	Rales after deep breath or cough	Tracheal and mediastinal shift toward
Bronchial asthma	Normal or enlarged	Hyper-resonant	Reduced	Diminished with prolonged expiratory phase	Wheezes	Distress
Bronchitis	Normal	Normal	Normal	Vesicular with prolonged expiration	Rhonchi with coarse rales	Cyanotic (blue bloater)
Diffuse pulmonary fibrosis; interstitial lung disease	Symmetrically diminished	Normal	Normal	Harsh vesicular with prolonged expiration	Coarse rales uninfluenced by coughing	—
Pulmonary edema	Normal	Normal	Normal	Bronchial if interstitial; vesicular if alveolar	Moist rales	Distress
Emphysema	Enlarged and restricted bilaterally	Hyper-resonant	Normal or reduced	Diminished with prolonged expiratory phase	Occasional rhonchi; often fine rales late in inspiration	Hoover's sign; high clavicle; muscular wasting (pink puffer)

should be ascertained first. The distance between the vertebral spine (or lateral edge of the vertebral body) and the medial end of the clavicle should be noted on each side. This will show if there is rotation to one side which may make a normal hilar opacity appear unduly prominent or explain an apparent deviation of the mediastinum or an apparent difference in transradiancy in the two lung fields. A reasonable system and order for viewing the P-A chest film is as follows: bones and soft tissues, apical to basal mediastinum, heart, hila, pleura, and finally lungs.

Alveolar Infiltrates. Processes that flood the alveolar air spaces with fluid or cells produce patchy, confluent, ill-defined lung densities. Pneumonia, edema, hemorrhage, and some forms of tumor are examples. Air-filled bronchi become visible when surrounded by infiltrated or consolidated tissue; this picture has been called the air bronchogram.

The silhouette sign is another helpful finding in recognizing small infiltrates. Normally the profile of the heart, mediastinum, and diaphragm can be seen because a tissue of different density (i.e., aerated lung) is situated next to them. If that bit of lung becomes infiltrated with water-density material (pus, for example), the silhouette, or visible edge, is lost.

Interstitial Infiltrates. Pathologic processes that primarily involve the interlobar connective tissue and spare the alveoli produce a linear or nodular pattern. As the interstitial process progresses toward fibrosis, the X-ray appearance changes from nodular to reticular. Finally, the lines may be arranged transversely, or they may interdigitate to produce a "honeycomb" appearance. The infiltrating material may be fibrous (pneumoconiosis or collagen disease), edematous (the pre-alveolar phase of congestive heart failure), neoplastic (permeation by metastatic neoplasm), or inflammatory.

Correlation of clinical and radiologic features such as cardiomegaly, pulmonary venous congestion, pleural effusion, or hilar adenopathy makes the interstitial process more understandable. Similarly, a history of occupational exposure, multisystem disease, or antecedent tumor has obvious implications. Lung biopsy is sometimes required and usually, but not always, is diagnostic.

Atelectasis. Discoid or platelike subsegmental atelectasis appears as coarse transverse linear densities, usually at the lung bases. Occlusion of a lobar bronchus will cause collapse and atelectasis of an entire lung lobe. Direct signs of lobar atelectasis include displaced fissures, compacted vessels, crowded air bronchograms, and increased lobar density. Indirect signs of lobar atelectasis may be easier to appreciate and include mediastinal shift, diaphragmatic elevation, narrowed rib spaces, and compensatory overexpansion of other lobes. Etiologies of lobar collapse include endobronchial obstruction by tumor, mucus plugs, or aspirated foreign material. Extrinsic bronchial compression can produce the same picture, classic examples being adenopathy effects on the right middle lobe and gross left atrial enlargement effects on the left lower lobe. Failure to correct atelectasis may result in infection.

Pleural Effusion. When searching for pleural fluid, there are several clues concerning its distribution that often prove useful. The posterior costophrenic recess is deeper than the lateral one; therefore, in the upright position a very small effusion is best seen on lateral projection. A subpulmonic pleural effusion may accumulate between the diaphragm and the undersurface of the lung in the upright position. On the left side, it will show as a soft-tissue space between aerated lung and the gastric air bubble. On the right, it can mimic an elevated diaphragm. In either case, a lateral decubitus film taken with the affected side down will demonstrate the effusion as the fluid rolls out into a visible position. Fluid in a fissure (interlobar effusion) can be mistaken for a lung mass on P-A projection. A

lateral view shows the characteristic location and biconvex configuration. There are usually, but not always, other evidences of pleural abnormality. When a pleural effusion has a straight, rather than a laterally upcurved, surface coexistent pleural air (hydropneumothorax) may be present.

Pneumothorax. A pneumothorax most often appears as a strip of radiolucency external to the lung surface and devoid of vascular markings. In the supine position the air layers anteriorly, and a P-A or A-P film may not demonstrate a small pneumothorax. If the patient is placed in the lateral decubitus position with the unaffected side down, a P-A or A-P film shows the air between the visceral and parietal pleura at the lateral margins of the non-dependent lung (vertically the highest position available). In the upright position, a P-A or A-P film reveals a pneumothorax apically. A pneumothorax under tension causes a mediastinal shift and compression of both contralateral and ipsilateral lung.

Emphysema. The classic radiologic signs of emphysema are an increased A-P chest diameter, low flat diaphragms, highly radiolucent and expanded lung fields, and the presence of bullae. However, there are patients who have severe airway obstruction but only modest overexpansion in whom chest films look quite innocuous in the face of profound physiologic impairment.

Pulmonary Embolus. There are several radiologic features that may be present singly or in combination which suggest a pulmonary embolus. These include pleural fluid, triangular, wedged, or pie shaped parenchymal densities, distended hilar vessels, prominent main pulmonary artery, and hypovascular peripheral lung segments.

PULMONARY FUNCTION TESTING

Obstructive Pattern. Slow ventilatory rate with reduced expiratory rates, normal or reduced vital capacity, reduced maximal voluntary ventilation, increased residual and closing volume, and increased functional residual and total lung capacity characterize an obstructive pattern in pulmonary function testing.

Restrictive Pattern. This type of abnormality is evidenced by rapid ventilatory rate with reduced tidal volume, reduced vital capacity, normal expiratory flow rates, normal maximal voluntary ventilation, decreased residual volume, decreased functional residual and total lung capacity, and decreased lung compliance.

SPECIALIZED TESTS FOR PULMONARY DISEASE

Other techniques of laboratory investigation of pulmonary disease include fluoroscopy, tomography, sputum examination, bronchoscopy (with biopsy) and bronchography, serologic tests for antibodies, ventilation and perfusion scans, computerized axial tomography, percutaneous needle lung biopsy, pulmonary angiography, and blood gas analysis.

PREOPERATIVE PREPARATION

In addition to thorough preoperative evaluation, optimal medical management of treatable conditions should be attempted before surgery. This includes any of the following options: patients should always discontinue smoking; sputum should be collected for culture and sensitivity testing and active infections treated; chest physical therapy and hydration may mobilize secretions; breathing and coughing exercises should be taught; patients can be instructed in the use of the incentive spirometer; bronchodilators should be given for reversible airway obstruction, and in severe cases therapeutic levels of theophylline are assured by laboratory testing; cor pulmonale is treated with diuretics and digitalis.

INTRAOPERATIVE MONITORING

Extensive pulmonary disease requires special intraoperative monitoring. Airway pressure measurement is necessary in conditions that produce decreased static compliance. In this situation, high inflation pressures are generally required, but they may be minimized by utilizing low tidal volumes and rapid ventilatory rates. Thus, the potential hazards of bullous rupture and decreased cardiac output are decreased by minimizing inflation pressure. An indwelling arterial cannula should be considered if multiple intraoperative blood gas analyses are anticipated.

Normally, the central venous pressure provides adequate information of intravascular status and cardiovascular performance. With progressive pulmonary disease, however, obliteration of pulmonary vasculature causes eventual elevation first of pulmonary vascular resistance and later of pulmonary artery pressures. When this occurs, the left- and right-sided cardiac circulations must be assessed separately, since the central venous pressure may no longer reflect left-sided filling pressures. In addition, the pulmonary artery diastolic pressure, which normally approximates the pulmonary artery capillary wedge pressure, will be elevated and a significant diastolic-to-wedge pressure gradient will be present. In this situation, only the wedge pressure can be relied upon to reflect left-sided cardiac performance and intravascular volume status. For these reasons, the use of a pulmonary artery catheter should be considered if pulmonary hypertension and/or cor pulmonale is present, especially if large fluid shifts are anticipated. The use of a pulmonary artery catheter with thermistor allows repeated and rapid determination of cardiac output and calculation of pulmonary vascular resistance and cardiac work indices.

SPECIFIC DISEASES

VASCULAR CONDITIONS

Pulmonary Embolism

General Description. Pulmonary thromboembolism is a complication of venous thrombosis and has been estimated to be the cause of 50,000 deaths in the United States per year. Since well under 10 per cent of pulmonary emboli are lethal, at least 500,000 people suffer a pulmonary embolic event each year. However, only a very small minority of patients who have recently suffered a detectable pulmonary embolism must undergo surgery; the indications for surgery are related to their pulmonary insult (embolectomy or inferior vena cava plication) or heparin therapy (bleeding ulcer).

Venous thrombosis is prerequisite for pulmonary thromboembolism. Vascular factors that enhance thrombogenesis are blood flow stasis, vessel wall damage, and abnormalities in blood coagulation (including congenital deficiency of antithrombin III). Patient disease risk factors include obesity, diabetes, marked peripheral arterial disease, the presence of any malignancy, varicose veins, and advancing age. The clinical situations in which combinations of blood flow stasis, coagulation alterations, and venous injury are associated with a high incidence of venous thrombosis and pulmonary embolism include the postoperative period, post-trauma, post-body burns, the postpartum period, protracted right or left ventricular failure, and any condition that requires bedrest or immobility for a prolonged period. The vast majority of pulmonary emboli arise from venous thromboses of the lower extremities and pelvis; rarely, they originate from superficial veins or the upper extremities.

Resolution of a venous thrombus depends on two processes: fibrinolysis and organization. Fibrinolysis is the initial mechanism; when it is incomplete, the slower process of organization completes the resolution sequence, incorporating the residual thrombus into the vessel wall. The fibrinolytic-organization sequence is usually complete in seven to 10 days.

The diagnosis of venous thrombosis of the lower extremities depends upon detection of vessel wall inflammation and venous obstruction. Laboratory diagnostic methods include radiofibrinogen techniques, impedance phlebographic and Doppler ultrasound methods, and contrast phlebography. However, more than 50 per cent of venous thrombi escape clinical detection, and it is therefore not surprising that routine autopsy data often show a 20 to 30 per cent incidence of pulmonary emboli. When special attention is given to the pulmonary vascular bed, the incidence may be as high as 60 per cent.

A pulmonary embolus has immediate vascular and airway physiologic effects. First, a large embolus in a major vessel will cause an increased pulmonary artery pressure. Increased pulmonary artery pressure can have multiple effects: 1) the formation of pulmonary edema in non-embolized regions of the lung; 2) loss of vasoconstriction in hypoxic regions of the lung; 3) creation of right-to-left transpulmonary shunts through arteriovenous anastomoses and anatomically present foramen ovale (potentially possible in 20% of patients); 4) decreased cardiac output due to increased pulmonary vasculature resistance. The second major physiologic effect of a pulmonary embolus is the release of serotonin if the embolus contains platelets. Serotonin can cause additional pulmonary changes: increased pulmonary artery pressure, increased pulmonary capillary permeability, and generalized bronchoconstriction. Third, a major embolus causes a large alveolar dead space. Subsequent regional hypocapnic bronchoconstriction minimizes the size of the alveolar dead space compartment. Fourth, loss of surfactant may occur in the embolized regions of the lung, causing embolized lung pulmonary edema and alveolar collapse. A pulmonary embolus that occurs in the presence of any disorder that has substantially reduced the pulmonary vascular bed, the functional capability of the right ventricle, or the adequacy of pulmonary gas exchange will cause a degree of cardiopulmonary compromise that is excessive in terms of the extent of the occlusion alone.

A major embolus is usually pushed peripherally shortly after impaction by vigorous right ventricular contractions, and many of the acute mechanical effects of the embolus are removed. However, initially transudated fluid will take days to clear. In addition, impaired regeneration of surfactant may occur subacutely and contribute to continued embolized lung pulmonary edema and alveolar collapse. Finally, as emboli begin to resolve, reperfusion of these poorly and nonventilated embolized regions of the lung may cause continued hypoxemia.

Since the pulmonary artery, the bronchial artery, and the airways supply the lung with oxygen, very few pulmonary emboli result in pulmonary infarction. Experimentally, it appears that compromise of at least two of the three oxygen sources is necessary to cause infarction. The rarity of infarction also reflects the fact that the total occlusion of a vessel by an embolus is uncommon. Although infarction is often read on chest x-ray after pulmonary embolus, the radiographic densities that do appear usually represent areas of pulmonary edema and atelectasis.

Once pushed peripherally, pulmonary emboli, like venous thrombi, tend to resolve rather rapidly and in a manner similar to that of venous thrombosis: by fibrinolysis and organization. Even massive emboli, which remain relatively centrally located, usually resolve in a period of days to weeks. This is particularly true in young persons without pre-existing cardiopulmonary disease. Thus, perfusion defects rarely remain beyond six weeks.

The first requisite for the diagnosis of pulmonary embolism is a high index of suspicion. The only consistently occurring symptom is nonspecific dyspnea, and the majority of patients have no other complaint. Other symptoms that may occur are those related to venous thrombosis and those related to large emboli, such as syncope, chest pain, and hemoptysis. The only consistently occurring physical signs are nonspecific tachypnea and tachycardia. When pulmonary infarction occurs, a pleural friction rub and fever may be present.

Laboratory tests aid considerably in making the diagnosis. In most cases of pulmonary embolus, the chest x-ray is normal; positive findings that may appear include an enlarged pulmonary artery contour, a patchy parenchymal density, pleural effusion, oligemia of the lung zone, and elevation of a hemidiaphragm. Arterial hypoxemia is often present, but its absence does not exclude the diagnosis. The electrocardiogram and vectorcardiogram show right ventricular strain after large emboli. Pulmonary perfusion and ventilation scintiphotography and pulmonary angiography are tests with high reliability and specificity in diagnosing pulmonary embolism. Pulmonary angiography, if performed with a catheter in the pulmonary artery, offers the special diagnostic advantage of assessing the hemodynamic status of the patient.

The drug of choice in the treatment of acute deep venous thrombosis and pulmonary embolism is heparin. Therapeutic thrombolysis may be attempted with streptokinase or urokinase in patients with massive emboli and marked cardiopulmonary compromise. Arterial hypoxemia is treated with oxygen. If hypotension is present, a pressor agent is necessary. Patients who are at risk of recurrent deep venous thrombosis or pulmonary embolism and those whose repeat perfusion scans show continued defects attributable to embolism warrant long-term anticoagulation.

Emergency pulmonary embolectomy and vena caval interruption are two surgical procedures that are performed infrequently today. Pulmonary embolectomy is usually futile because the embolus is quickly pushed peripherally; if not, death will occur. In addition, aggressive medical therapy is usually quite successful. Inferior venal caval interruption prevents large emboli from reaching the lungs, but the development of large collateral circuits may allow further pulmonary emboli to occur. It is the policy in many institutions to perform caval interruption only as a life saving measure in a closely defined group of patients, namely those with recurring massive, acute embolic obstruction. These patients may undergo caval interruption because heparin therapy cannot protect them against embolic recurrence during the first few days of therapy. Because an additional embolus during this interval could be fatal, the operation is warranted in spite of its limitations. A second group of patients for whom caval interruption warrants consideration are those in whom significant embolization occurs and heparin therapy cannot be employed safely. Occasionally, other surgical procedures must be performed on patients who have recently had a pulmonary embolus. For example, massive gastrointestinal hemorrhage may occur as a result of anticoagulation in a patient with an undiagnosed duodenal ulcer.

Anesthetic Considerations. Patients undergoing vena caval interruption or embolectomy following a massive pulmonary embolus are critically ill. Physical, electrocardiographic, and roentgenologic evidence of right heart failure should be sought. Arterial blood gases must be measured. If angiography has been performed, the pulmonary pressures recorded at the time of testing should be checked for the presence of elevated pulmonary artery pressures. If elevated pressures are noted, a pulmonary artery catheter with pulmonary artery capillary wedge pressure monitoring may prove helpful intraoparatively to guide anesthetic and fluid management. In each case, the benefits from such monitoring must be weighed against the difficulty in placing the catheter in the face of systemic anticoagulation and partial obstruction in the pulmonary arterial tree. If heart failure is present, digitalis should be considered. These patients should have an indwelling arterial cannula placed in order to monitor blood gases and continuously record blood pressure. The use of agents that cause significant cardiac depression should be minimized. High oxygen concentrations should be used if hypoxemia exists preoperatively. Inotropic agents should be available for immediate use if cardiac decompression occurs. If pulmonary embolectomy is performed, cardiopulmonary bypass must be utilized. After the pulmonary artery has been opened, vigorous inflation of the lungs may help to push clots back toward the surgeon and aid in their removal.

Primary Pulmonary Hypertension

General Description. Primary pulmonary hypertension is a progressive disease in which severe pulmonary hypertension results from increased pulmonary arterial resistance. Although the etiology of primary pulmonary hypertension is unknown, genetic factors probably play a role. Primary pulmonary hypertension has been reported in twins, in five members of three generations in one family, and in a father and his two children. These data suggest an autosomal dominant mode of genetic transmission with variable penetrance. The finding of a plasmin inhibitor in 10 members of a kindred with this condition indicates that in some cases the disease may be due to an inherited inability to lyse pulmonary microemboli. Ingestion of certain drugs has been implicated in the genesis of this disease as well. In the 1960's a twenty-fold increase in the incidence of pulmonary hypertension was found in European patients treated with the anorexic drug aminorex fumarate. In most patients, symptoms of exertional dyspnea and syncope developed less than a year after ingestion of the drug, and elevated pulmonary pressures were documented by cardiac catheterization. Withdrawal of the drug from the market resulted in a dramatic decrease in the incidence of the disease. In addition, an animal model for the production of pulmonary hypertension exists, with the ingestion of pyrrolizidine alkaloids from plants that are readily available for human consumption.

Characteristic pathologic findings are usually seen. The arterioles develop muscular thickening and intimal proliferation that may progress to total occlusion of the vessel lumen. The intima of the pulmonary trunk and large elastic vessels becomes atherosclerotic, and the media of these vessels become thickened by muscular hyperplasia. These changes can result in systolic pulmonary pressures of 65 to 90 torr and a pulmonary vascular resistance of up to eight times normal. Cardiac output is characteristically low. Since pulmonary artery capillary wedge pressure is usually low, a significant pulmonary artery diastolic-to-wedge pressure gradient exists. A variable drop in pulmonary vascular resistance occurs when infusing various vasodilator drugs such as tolazoline, acetylcholine, and isoproterenol, indicating a labile resistance component. The lability is more apparent in young patients and earlier in the course of the disease.

Roentgenographically, the lungs show evidence of diffuse oligemia, with the peripheral pulmonary arteries being narrow and inconspicuous. The main pulmonary arteries are prominent and taper rapidly distally; increased amplitude of pulsation of the main pulmonary artery may be seen fluoroscopically. Later, right ventricular enlargement is seen.

The female to male disease prevalence ratio is 3:1. The disease appears most often between the ages of 20 and 40, although it has been reported in an age range from 1 to 68. Most of the symptoms that occur are brought on by exercise and consist of dyspnea (almost all patients), syncope, angina, and hemoptysis. Right ventricular physical findings progress from those of enlargement to failure. Giant jugular A waves, third heart sound, right sternal heave, accentuated pulmonary heart sound, and tricuspid regurgitation have all been described. Cyanosis may be present, and a low cardiac output may be reflected by a weak pulse and cold extremities.

Useful tools for diagnosing primary pulmonary hypertension in addition to a familial tendency, clinical findings, and chest X-ray are electrocardiograms and cardiac catheterization. Right atrial and ventricular hypertrophy with right axis deviation is commonly seen. Arrhythmias that occur include atrial fibrillation, atrial and ventricular extrasystoles, and supraventricular tachycardia. Catheterization of the right side of the heart reveals pulmonary artery hypertension, a normal pulmonary capillary wedge pressure, high pulmonary vascular resistance, and, in cases of right ventricular failure, low cardiac output. Pulmonary function may be completely normal; however, in more severe cases there is decreased arterial oxygen saturation and diffusing capacity. The arterial PCO_2 is usually reduced by hyperventilation. Fatalities have been reported in patients with primary pulmonary hypertension undergoing lung scan, and this procedure is seldom employed in the evaluation of such patients; death presumably resulted from occlusion of an already compromised pulmonary artery circulation by particles of microaggregated albumin. Similarly, patients with this disease have a propensity to sudden death during other diagnostic procedures that are well tolerated by other patients — angiography, catheterization, and lung biopsy.

Until recently, there has been no satisfactory treatment for the disease. However, two recent reports indicate that hydralazine and diazoxide may cause significant and possibly long-lasting reductions in pulmonary vascular resistance in patients with this disease. Anticoagulant therapy has been used to diminish the possibility of thromboembolic disease and to retard thrombosis in the pulmonary vasculature. Heart failure is treated by conventional methods.

The prognosis in this condition has been extremely poor. However, the recent introduction of successful short term (6 months) vasodilator therapy may considerably improve the prognosis in the future. Although some patients have been reported to survive for up to 18 years following diagnosis, the average duration of life from onset of symptoms is less than five years. Patients with clearly familial pulmonary hypertension sometimes have a more prolonged course.

Anesthetic Considerations. The most important consideration in the preoperative evaluation of these patients is the assessment of cardiac status. The signs and symptoms of right heart failure as described above should be sought. If heart failure exists, optimum medical treatment with cardiac glycosides and diuretics should be undertaken prior to elective operative procedures. If the patient has been on this therapeutic regimen for a prolonged period, the serum K^+ must be measured. Evaluation of pulmonary function is usually not necessary unless severe symptoms or signs of hypoxemia are present. If there is evidence that pulmonary emboli have contributed to the development of pulmonary hypertension, or if the opera-

tive condition subjects the patient to an increased threat of pulmonary embolus, minidose heparin administration should be considered.

The presence of right heart failure is a relative contraindication to drugs that cause moderate to severe cardiac depression. A regional technique is preferable for extremity or lower abdominal surgery. However, if minidose heparin has been given, the prothrombin time and partial thromboplastin times should be checked immediately prior to administering a regional block. For extensive procedures wherein large fluid shifts are anticipated in patients with significantly elevated right-sided cardiac pressures, pulmonary artery catheter monitoring is necessary. The pulmonary artery wedge pressure must be followed in this situation, since a pulmonary artery diastolic-to-wedge pressure gradient will exist. Excessive increases in right-sided pressures are treated with vasodilators such as nitroglycerin or by decreasing anesthetic-induced myocardial depression.

Pulmonary Arteriovenous Fistula

General Description. The most common type of congenital pulmonary arteriovenous fistula consists of an abnormal vascular communication from the pulmonary artery to the pulmonary vein. A congenital pulmonary arteriovenous fistula is usually fed by a single distended afferent artery and drained by a single distended efferent vein. Occurring less often are complex malformations that are fed by multiple pulmonary arteries; these lesions may involve the entire blood supply to a lobe. The complex type of communication is the type most commonly associated with a clinical picture of cyanosis, clubbing of the digits, and polycythemia. Less common, although still classified as arteriovenous fistula, is pulmonary sequestration; in this condition, a systemic high pressure vessel directly communicates with relatively thin-walled low pressure pulmonary vessels.

One third of patients have multiple arteriovenous communications within the lungs. Approximately 50 per cent of patients with pulmonary fistulas have abnormal communications in other organs; this condition is called Rendu-Osler-Weber's disease or hereditary hemorrhagic telangiectasia. This latter condition is a genetic disease with a dominant, nonsex-linked mode of inheritance. Not all patients with this disease have pulmonary communications, and involvement is then limited to the skin, mucous membranes, and other organs.

The classic roentgenologic picture is that of a round or oval homogeneous mass of consistent density, slightly lobulated in contour but sharply defined, ranging from less than 1 to several centimeters in diameter. The fistulas are seen most commonly in the lower lobes. Tomograms may be helpful in identifying feeding and draining vessels. Fluoroscopic examination may show pulsation of the hilar vessels, indicating a preponderance of blood flow to the side containing the fistula. Angiography may be required to confirm the diagnosis; it is mandatory in all cases where resectional surgery is contemplated.

Approximately 10 per cent of pulmonary arteriovenous fistulas are identified in infancy or childhood; the majority are not diagnosed until early middle age to middle age. Symptoms are extremely variable, and many patients have no complaint at all. The most common presenting symptom is hemoptysis, while dyspnea occurs in approximately one half of patients. Transient cerebral symptoms occur in some patients; their etiology is unknown, but they may be due to hypoxemia or cerebral embolus. Signs of this condition include cyanosis, finger clubbing, and a continuous murmur or bruit over the fistula. Very large fistulas can cause high output cardiac failure. Telangiectasis of the mucous membranes suggests Rendu-Osler-Weber's disease.

Laboratory investigation reveals polycythemia in cyanotic patients. Conversely, repeated hemorrhages from nose or lung fistulas may cause anemia in others. Cardiac catheterization demonstrates increased cardiac output with normal pulmonary artery pressures. The electrocardiogram is usually normal.

Pulmonary arteriovenous fistulas are usually operated on after diagnosis is made. They are surgically removed because of their tendency to increase in size and because of the risk of massive hemorrhage. For most cases, a wedge resection or lobectomy is performed.

Anesthetic Considerations. The cardiac status of the patient must be assessed preoperatively because a patient with a large communication may be in a state of high output cardiac failure. The use of agents that cause significant myocardial depression should be minimized if this condition is present.

Consultation with the surgeon may disclose problems anticipated with the resection. A large fistula that may be difficult to remove requires the placement of an extra large-bore intravenous cannula and adequate blood available for transfusion. Care must be taken to avoid air from entering the circulation, since the potential for systemic embolization exists. A double lumen endotracheal tube should be used if the surgeon feels it would significantly facilitate the resection or avoid hemorrhage to the contralateral lung. If anemia exists, the patient should be transfused preoperatively.

The presence of a large right-to-left shunt will interfere with oxygenation. An adequate inspired oxygen concentration must be delivered in order to ensure that all blood delivered to ventilated regions will be as completely saturated as possible. A right-to-left shunt will also interfere with the uptake of anesthetic gases; thus induction with volatile agents may be prolonged. Recovery from anesthesia should not be prolonged because the shunt will no longer be present. Similarly, any heart failure that exists preoperatively should be improved following the operation.

INFILTRATIVE-ALVEOLAR DISORDERS

Pulmonary Alveolar Proteinosis and Pulmonary Alveolar Microlithiasis

General Description. PULMONARY ALVEOLAR PROTEINOSIS. Pulmonary alveolar proteinosis is a disease of unknown etiology characterized by deposition within the air spaces of the lung of a granular material high in lipid and protein content. The disease was first reported as recently as 1958, and most cases since then have come from the United States.

Pathological changes are confined to the lungs. Post mortem, the lungs are heavy and firm with the gross architecture preserved. Microscopically, early pathologic changes are confined to the alveolar space, as the alveolar epithelial lining and interstitial tissue remain normal until pulmonary fibrosis develops late in the disease. The alveoli are filled with a granular lipoproteinaceous material. The origin of the material is not certain, although it is probably related to the observed presence of swollen type II alveolar cells and macrophages. It has been postulated that the material represents an accumulation of a modified surfactant produced by type II alveolar cells or the inability of macrophages to properly clear normal surfactant.

The contribution to the development of alveolar proteinosis from infection and immunologic mechanisms is uncertain. *Pneumocystis carinii* infection has been associated with this condition. Alveolar proteinosis has been described in infants and has usually been associated with lymphopenia, immunoglobulin deficiency, or thymic lymphoplasia. There also appears to be an increased incidence in patients with hematologic malignancy or lymphoma.

The male to female disease prevalence ratio is 2:1, and the diagnosis is usually made between 20 and 50 years of age. Approximately one third of cases of pulmonary alveolar proteinosis are asymptomatic. The remainder manifest a variety of symptoms, most commonly shortness of breath on exertion, usually progressive in severity. Cough is often present and usually is nonproductive; however, cough may occasionally be associated with gelatinous or even purulent expectoration. Fatigue, weight loss, pleuritic pain, fever, and hemoptysis may also be present. Physical signs are limited to coarse and fine rales, clubbing of the digits, and cyanosis in severe cases.

The roentgenographic pattern of pulmonary alveolar proteinosis is similar to that of pulmonary edema. Since the process is one of air space consolidation, the basic lesion is an acinar shadow. Confluence of acinar shadows is the rule, with the production of irregular, poorly defined, patchy areas scattered bilaterally in the lung fields. While the "bat's wing" pattern of pulmonary edema may be seen, the cardiac enlargement, interstitial edema, and streaking of the upper lobes are absent. Kurley B lines may be present and probably represent lymphatic obstruction. Lymph node enlargement at the hilum or mediastinum is not seen, nor is pleural effusion. Resolution may be complete or partial, leaving a spotty, asymmetrical picture of air space consolidation in areas not previously affected. Patients with progressive disease eventually develop pulmonary fibrosis.

Laboratory investigation reveals the white blood cell count to be normal or slightly elevated. Polycythemia is common; less often hyperglobulinemia, hyperlipidemia, and an increase in serum lactate dehydrogenase are seen. Severe cases show hypoxemia on room air arterial blood gas analysis, reflecting a ventilation-perfusion inequality. Abnormalities in pulmonary function studies parallel the clinical symptomatology; a reduction in lung compliance, diffusing capacity, and vital capacity occur as the disease progresses. Definitive diagnosis must be made from examination of material obtained during fiberoptic bronchoscopy, lung lavage, or lung biopsy.

Massive irrigation of the tracheobronchial tree has been employed with good success as a means of removing the lipoproteinaceous material from severely infiltrated alveoli. Saline is used as the irrigant, and one lung is lavaged at a time, with ventilation maintained to the other lung. Chest percussion during lavage enhances removal of the offending material. Following lung lavage, arterial blood gases and symptoms improve for months at times. In rare, severe cases in children, bilateral pulmonary lavage has been done with patients on partial cardiopulmonary bypass. Other treatments that have been tried with less favorable results include corticosteroids, potassium iodide, and various enzymes.

As many as one half of symptomatic patients (one third of all patients) will spontaneously improve or recover. Pulmonary alveolar proteinosis is fatal in about a third of cases, with death resulting from respiratory failure and/or superimposed opportunistic infection by *Nocardia, Aspergillus, Cryptococcus,* and *Pneumocystis carinii.*

PULMONARY ALVEOLAR MICROLITHIASIS. There are fewer than 100 reported cases of this disease, which is characterized by the presence of myriad tiny calculi within the alveoli. The majority of cases probably begin in early life but are not diagnosed until early adulthood. There is no sex predominance. A familial occurrence has been detected in more than half the reported cases. Although its etiology is unknown, it has been theorized that microlithiasis may result from some undefined alteration in the alveolar lining membrane or in alveolar secretions, which promote alkalinity at the alveolar interface and predispose to the development or precipitation of calcium phosphate and calcium carbonate within the alveoli.

The intra-alveolar microliths are composed mainly of calcium and phosphorus in a composition similar to that of bone. Although they are found almost exclusively within the alveoli, there is evidence that they may be formed within the alveolar walls and then extrude into the air spaces. In the early stages of the disease, the alveolar walls appear normal. In the later stages, the walls are thickened as a result of interstitial fibrosis and giant cell formation. Blebs and bullae may form, especially in the lung apices. In severe cases, pulmonary hypertension and cor pulmonale may result from obliteration of normal pulmonary vasculature.

The majority of patients are asymptomatic when the disease is first discovered. The diagnosis is often made after a screening chest x-ray or during investigation of persons whose siblings are known to have the disease. Patients usually remain asymptomatic until a far advanced picture is seen on chest x-ray. The first symptom that develops in advanced cases is dyspnea on exertion. As the disease progresses further, some patients complain of hemoptysis and cough. Cyanosis, finger clubbing and signs of right heart failure are seen late. In some patients, however, the disease becomes static and further deposition of microliths ceases. In a few patients, spontaneous rupture of bullae results in pneumothorax.

Although considerable variation occurs from patient to patient, the fundamental chest x-ray pattern is characteristic and diagnostic. A fine, sandlike micronodulation diffusely involving both lungs is seen. On close examination, the individual deposits can be identified with sharply defined borders, usually less than 1 millimeter in diameter. The opacities appear to predominate in the lower lungs as a result of increased lung thickness in this region. Pleural thickening is often read roentgenographically,

but it probably represents exceptionally heavy deposition of microliths in the subpleural parenchyma. Pulmonary function testing reveals a wide variety of results depending upon the state of the disease. Some studies have found a decrease in lung volumes and diffusion capacity. Ventilation-perfusion inequalities occur in later stages of the disease. Blood gas analysis reveals hypoxemia only in far advanced cases. Lung biopsy is diagnostic but is seldom necessary.

The diagnosis of pulmonary alveolar microlithiasis is made from the classic chest x-ray pattern associated with the disease in conjunction with the striking lack of physical complaints. The course of the disease is prolonged over many years, and death may result from pulmonary insufficiency or cor pulmonale. Only symptomatic treatment exists for this condition.

Anesthetic Considerations. Patients who are hypoxemic on room air require high inspired oxygen concentrations during anesthesia. Adequacy of oxygenation should be checked intraoperatively by blood gas analysis. When pulmonary function testing reveals a restrictive defect, higher than normal inflation pressures are required during controlled ventilation; consequently, small tidal volumes and a rapid respiratory rate should be used in order to minimize inflation pressures.

If right heart failure is present, treatment with cardiac glycosides and diuretics may be necessary preoperatively. Anesthetic agents should be selected with regard to their potential for producing myocardial depression. If significant pulmonary hypertension is present and large fluid shifts are anticipated, a pulmonary artery catheter is necessary in order to measure pulmonary artery capillary wedge pressure.

Therapeutic bronchopulmonary lavage is performed on severe cases of *pulmonary alveolar proteinosis*. A left-sided double-lumen endotracheal tube is chosen for intubation because it is easier to ensure complete ventilation of the left lung than the right. In addition, the endobronchial cuff inflates symmetrically on the left side, providing added assurance of the ability to produce an adequate seal. After a sleep dose of thiopental and paralysis with succinylcholine, the tracheobronchial tree is topicalized with a local anesthetic. The endotracheal tube is placed into the left mainstem bronchus and anesthesia is maintained with halothane or enflurane in oxygen. We prefer a disposable, clear plastic tube for this procedure because correct placement of the endobronchial lumen is vital to the success of the lavage; the clear plastic allows direct visualization of the endobronchial cuff with a flexible pediatric bronchoscope. When in the proper location, the cuff is inflated until the wall of the endobronchial tube begins to invaginate; then 1 ml of air is withdrawn. This usually corresponds to a balloon seal pressure of approximately 60 cm H_2O. The high balloon seal pressure is required because peak inspiratory pressure and lavage fluid pressures are high. After direct visualization, the tube position is also confirmed with an intraoperative chest x-ray.

Baseline values for left and right dynamic lung compliances as well as arterial blood bases are measured. Prior to the performance of pulmonary lavage, ventilation is maintained with 100 per cent oxygen for 10 minutes to allow denitrogenation of the lung. One lung lavage is performed with normal saline, instilling volume until a pressure of 30 cm H_2O is reached. Percussion is applied to the filled lung in order to loosen the proteinaceous material. The fluid is then allowed to drain out under gravity pressure. The procedure is repeated, typically 10 to 20 times, until the lavage fluid clears, indicating that most of the proteinaceous material has been removed. During the lung lavage period frequent auscultation of the ventilated lung is necessary in order to detect accidental bilateral lavage due to endotracheal tube movement or cuff failure (should this occur, the procedure must be terminated prematurely). Throughout the lavage period frequent blood gases should monitor the adequacy of ventilation and oxygenation. Since blood flow is reduced to the lavaged (hypoxic) lung primarily when it is filled with saline, the period when the fluid is drained is particularly hazardous. An indwelling arterial catheter facilitates frequent blood gas sampling, and allows constant monitoring of systemic blood pressure.

After the lavage is complete, the entire lung should be intermittently suctioned, ventilated, and sighed until dynamic compliance returns to pre-lavage values. Most patients can be extubated following the procedure since their pulmonary function will be improved. After a few days' rest and recovery they are returned to the operating room to have the opposite lung lavaged.

Eosinophilic Lung Disease

General Description. LOEFFLER'S SYNDROME. A syndrome of pulmonary consolidation and blood eosinophilia may exist without any identifiable causative factor or may have its onset in relation to infections, parasitic infestations, or drug therapy. The term "Loeffler's syndrome" should be reserved for conditions in which the etiology is unknown. Biopsy specimen of areas of pulmonary consolidation reveal interstitial and alveolar edema containing a large number of eosinophilic leukocytes. Although Loeffler's syndrome appears to have a predilection for patients with a history of atopy, the alveolar capillary walls and basement membranes are devoid of immune deposits.

The clinical course usually lasts less than a month. Signs and symptoms are extremely varied, from asymptomatic patients to those with high fever, dyspnea, and cough. Daily roentgenograms reveal migratory areas of consolidation that are characteristically homogeneous in density but ill-defined, peripheral, and nonsegmental. Laboratory investigation reveals leukocytosis composed of a high percentage of eosinophils.

If pulmonary parenchymal involvement is extensive, pulmonary function testing may reveal a restrictive pattern in association with lowered arterial PO_2 and a decrease in diffusing capacity. Loeffler's syndrome occasionally develops in patient with bronchial asthma, and in these patients pulmonary function testing shows a mixed obstructive/restrictive pattern.

The majority of patients with Loeffler's syndrome recover within a month. Treatment is limited to administering corticosteroids to patients with severe cases, asthma, and atopy.

CHRONIC EOSINOPHILIC PNEUMONIA. Chronic eosinophilic pneumonia is quite similar to Loeffler's syndrome, except that it runs a more protracted and severe course. The etiology is unknown, although there appears to be an increased incidence in patients who have undergone desensitization treatment to a variety of allergens. As in Loeffler's syndrome, an atopic background is frequently seen. Women are affected slightly more frequently than men.

Biopsy specimens in this illness typically show massive infiltration of alveolar walls and sacs by white blood cells; eosinophils predominate among macrophages, histiocytes, lymphocytes, and polymorphonuclear granulocytes. Mild angiitis occurs in some cases. In addition, granuloma formation with or without necrosis and cavitation has been described.

In general, the clinical symptoms are much more severe than those seen in Loeffler's syndrome and consist of high fever, malaise, weight loss, and dyspnea. Hemoptysis occurs rarely. The roentgenographic pattern of chronic eosinophilic pneumonia is identical to that seen in Loeffler's syndrome, except that in this illness the lesions often persist unchanged for days to weeks unless steroid therapy is given.

Laboratory investigation usually reveals eosinophilia. Many patients are hypoxemic on room air. As in Loeffler's syndrome, pulmonary function tests may reveal a restrictive defect and lowered diffusing capacity.

The disease has a dramatic beneficial response to corticosteroid therapy. Consequently, an early diagnosis may abort an otherwise lengthy and incapacitating illness. Severe cases require oxygen therapy before steroid therapy brings about improvement.

EOSINOPHILIC LUNG DISEASE OF SPECIFIC ETIOLOGY. A variety of agents have been identified as causes of pulmonary disease in association with eosinophilia. Drugs that have been associated with a Loeffler's-like syndrome include penicillin, the sulfonamides, tricyclic antidepressants, hydrochlorothiazide, and chromium sodium.

Nitrofurantoin administration has also been associated with pulmonary disease and eosinophilia. In contrast to Loeffler's syndrome, some of these patients have a serious clinical course that results in pulmonary fibrosis. This syndrome is described in detail in the section on drug-induced pulmonary disease.

Numerous parasitic infestations (*Ascaris lumbricoides, Strongyloides stercoralis, Ancylostoma duodenale, Necator americanus,* *Wuchereria bancrofti, Toxocara canis, and Schistosoma haematobium*) have caused a Loeffler's-like illness. The illness is thought to be due to larvae passing through the lungs. Usually the illness is transient; treatment with drugs specific for the organism resolves it.

Anesthetic Considerations. With the exception of chronic eosinophilic pneumonia, these conditions are usually not protracted. Elective operations should be delayed until the acute illness is over or until improvement results from the use of steroids. In patients chronically taking steroids, the possibility of adrenal suppression exists and perioperative steroid coverage is necessary.

In patients with evidence of respiratory compromise from the history and physical examination, preoperative room air blood gas analysis and pulmonary function testing should be done. Although a restrictive defect most often results from fibrosis, an obstructive component may arise from the simultaneous presence of asthma. Medical management with bronchodilators is necessary in these patients. When severe fibrosis is present, controlled ventilation with a small tidal volume and rapid respiratory rate is utilized in order to minimize the high inflation pressures that are required. High inspired oxygen concentrations are needed to provide adequate oxygenation. Intraoperatively, arterial blood gas analysis should confirm the presence of adequate oxygenation.

MULTISYSTEM DISEASES WITH PULMONARY INVOLVEMENT

Wegener's Granulomatosis

General Description. Wegener's granulomatosis is a rare, usually fatal disease that has been variously classified as an autoimmune disease, an eosinophilic lung disease, a granulomatous disease, a collagen disease, or a vascular disease depending on the presumed basic pathologic process. The disease characteristically has a triad of findings: necrotizing giant-cell granulomatosis of the upper respiratory tract and lung, widespread necrotizing vasculitis of small arteries and veins, and glomerulonephritis. Although the etiology of Wegener's granulomatosis is unknown, both the immunologic and pathologic manifestations suggest a fulminant hypersensitivity or auto-allergic process. No specific antigen has been identified for this condition.

Biopsy of the involved tissue in the nose and nasopharynx reveals granulomatous tissue (midline granuloma) containing Langerhans and foreign-body giant cells with epithelioid cells. Renal, pulmonary, and skin biopsies show inflammatory perivascular exudate and fibrin deposition in small arteries, capillaries, and venules. Renal disease manifests as focal or generalized glomerulonephritis.

The age distribution ranges from infancy to old age, with the mean age at diagnosis approximately 40 years. Although the clinical presentation varies somewhat, the classical presenting features are complaints referable to the upper respiratory tract. These include severe rhinorrhea, paranasal sinus pain and drainage, and nasal ulcerations. Paranasal sinusitis often leads to severe deformity; secondary bacterial infection, most commonly with *Staphylococcus aureus,* occurs frequently. Destructive lesions of the epiglottis and larynx may occur, resulting in narrowing of the airway lumen. Often, pulmonary symptoms such as cough, hemoptysis, and pleuritis accompany the upper respiratory complaints. Pulmonary infiltrates occur frequently and can take many forms. They are often seen on the chest x-ray as bilateral with no characteristic lobar localization, while cavitation is quite common. Total occlusion of the pulmonary arteries by vasculitis can result in increased dead space. Bronchial obstruction and destruction can result in increased transpulmonary shunt.

The renal disease seen with Wegener's granulomatosis is progressive and is responsible for 90 per cent of deaths. The urinary findings are those of acute glomerulonephritis, with proteinuria, hematuria, and erythrocyte casts. Renal failure is inevitable if treatment is not instituted.

The cardiovascular effects of this illness are due to cardiac involvement with both granuloma and vasculitis. Coronary vasculitis and pancarditis are typical findings. Conduction defects may result in arrhythmia and have been reported as the cause of sudden death in several patients. In the peripheral vasculature, digital arteritis and infarction of the tips of the fingers may occur.

Nervous system involvement is seen in up to 50 per cent of patients. Manifestation consists primarily of cranial and peripheral nerve involvement. In addition, cerebral aneurysms, cerebral arteritis, and pseudotumor cerebri have all been reported.

The skin is involved in about 50 per cent of patients, with ulceration caused by acute necrotizing angiitis of dermal vessels. More than half of the patients have polyarthralgia as a manifestation of joint involvement. Joint involvement is usually transient and mild, although frank arthritis develops in some patients. Ophthalmic complications include conjunctivitis, granulomatous keratitis, pseudotumor of the orbit, and proptosis. Middle ear involvement with otitis media and hearing loss is seen frequently. Nonspecific complaints of fever, weight loss, and anorexia occur as well. Thus, Wegener's granulomatosis can involve virtually any organ system with vasculitis or granulomas, or both.

Typical laboratory findings include anemia, leukocytosis, hyperglobulinemia, and elevated sedimentation rate. Peripheral eosinophilia is rare. Antinuclear antibody and lupus erythematosus cell preparation tests are negative.

Until recently, the clinical course was one of progressive deterioration, with death usually occurring within six months from renal insufficiency, occasionally from respiratory failure, and rarely (and suddenly) from cardiac arrest. In recent years, therapy with cytotoxic drugs, either alkylating agents or purine antagonists, not only has resulted in clinical remission of the disease but also has led to apparent cures, even in patients with renal involvement. In patients who develop renal failure in spite of control of the active disease with immunosuppressive therapy, renal transplantation has been successfully performed without subsequent development of glomerulonephritis. Most treatment regimens utilize long-term steroid therapy in addition to cytotoxic agents. Therapy is tapered and then often discontinued if a patient has been free of all traces of the disease for a year; follow-up evaluation is necessary in order to determine relapses and the need for further therapy.

Anesthetic Considerations. Anesthetic considerations for patients with Wegener's granulomatosis begin with an assessment of the drug therapy they are receiving. If steroids have been used chronically and the possibility of adrenal suppression exists, exogenous perioperative steroid coverage will be necessary. The side effects of immunosuppressive therapy, such as anemia, thrombocytopenia, and liver dysfunction, should be noted.

Anesthetic considerations are based on organ system involvement. The upper airway manifestations of nasal ulceration, deformity, and sinusitis contraindicate the use of nasal intubation in most cases. The larynx, epiglottis, and subglottic area may also be involved in destructive lesions. Careful preoperative evaluation is imperative; indirect laryngoscopy and laryngeal tomograms may be helpful. Since hemorrhage or dislodging of friable tissue is very possible during laryngoscopy and intubation, extraordinary gentleness and caution are required. Thus, an awake, locally anesthetized or spontaneously breathing patient under general anesthesia may be preferred for intubation. If paralysis is required (to enhance gentleness and/or vision), the airway should be tested by positive pressure ventilation via mask before instrumentation. Several small endotracheal tubes should be avilable in case the tracheal lumen is narrow. Because of the pulmonary parenchymal involvement, a high inspired oxygen concentration may be necessary. Intraoperative blood gas analysis will confirm the adequacy of gas exchange. Intra- and postoperatively, these patients must be watched closely for airway obstruction by friable and necrotic material that was loosened by the trauma of laryngoscopy, intubation, head movement during positioning, and positive pressure ventilation.

Possible renal impairment requires quantification by urinalysis, BUN, serum creatinine, and creatinine clearance. The complications that accompany significant renal failure, such as anemia, hypertension, and coagulation defects, should be identified and minimized preoperatively. The presence of renal impairment dictates caution in selecting agents which rely primarily on the kidney for excretion. Similarly, fluid and electrolyte balance must be ensured.

Cardiovascular involvement may be apparent with the presence of left ventricular hypertrophy or ischemia. When these are present, care must be taken to maintain a favorable myocardial oxygen supply/demand ratio. The presence of peripheral arteritis will influence aggressiveness in the placement of arterial lines and repeated arterial punctures.

In light of the above problems, consideration should be given to the use of regional techniques whenever possible. However, central nervous system involvement, present in 50 per cent of patients, dictates that a thorough preanesthetic neurologic examination be performed and documented in the chart prior to the administration of any regional block.

Sarcoidosis

General Description. Sarcoidosis is a disease of unknown etiology that is characterized pathologically by noncaseating granulomas in the lung, liver, spleen, lymph nodes, bone, eyes, and skin. Although the etiology is not known with certainty, there is a good deal of evidence indicating that immunologic mechanisms may be involved. Decreased T-cell (a lymphocyte modified by the thymus) function is evidenced by the findings of decreased cutaneous delayed hypersensitivity to recall antigens (anergy) and decreased numbers of total circulating T cells. These patients frequently have a polyclonal hypergammaglobulinemia, rheumatoid factor, and increased antibody titers against several viral antigens. In addition, B-cells (lymphocytes which cause a humoral response to antigens) are often found in sarcoid granulomas, while immune complexes are found circulating in the serum. It has been postulated that the etiologic agent enters the body via the lungs, and from there disseminates to virtually any organ in the body. Then perhaps a loss of regulatory T-cell function leads to an overactive B-cell system, which results in an immune complex mediated granulomatous response in the various involved organs.

In the United States, the disease is more prevalent in rural areas, especially affecting women who are black. Fifty per cent of patients are diagnosed between 20 and 50 years of age. Approximately 50 per cent of patients with sarcoidosis are asymptomatic; most of these patients are diagnosed after a screening chest X-ray reveals a bilateral enlarged lobulated contour of the hilar lymph nodes without evidence of pulmonary parenchymal involvement. When symptoms occur, such as a dry cough and shortness of breath (20 to 30%), they are insidious and may mask other organ system involvement. Pulmonary function changes are common even in the absence of x-ray evidence of pulmonary parenchymal involvement. Early in the disease a restrictive defect occurs. Vital capacity and functional residual capacity are reduced, the alveolar-arterial oxygen tension gradient is increased, diffusion capacity is decreased, and ventilation/perfusion abnormalities are present. With progression of the disease, the chest x-ray may show nodular and acinar infiltrative patterns. In 20 per cent of these patients, the signs and symptoms and chest x-ray findings further progress to those of pulmonary fibrosis. Compliance is gradually reduced as fibrosis develops. An obstructive component to the disturbance in lung function occasionally occurs late in the disease. Severe cases will evidence additional changes consistent with pulmonary hypertension and cor pulmonale.

Widespread lymph node enlargement occurs in the majority of cases. Microscopic involvement of the liver is present in three fourths of all patients, and it can be of a sufficient degree to impair function. A similar incidence of splenic involvement is found; occasionally splenectomy is required because of hypersplenism or its effect as a space-occupying mass. Ocular involvement is manifested as uveitis and is present in about 20 per cent of patients. Cutaneous involvement presents as slightly raised dermal nodules or plaques in one third of patients. Necropsy evidence indicates a 20 per cent involvement of the heart, although serious clinical manifestations are present in only about 5 per cent of patients. In these patients, however, complete heart block, heart failure, and paroxysmal arrhythmias such as premature ventricular beats and ventricular tachycardia may result in death. Bone and joint involvement is manifested by arthritis. Central nervous system involvement is characterized by cranial nerve palsies. The larynx is involved in 2 per cent of patients and may be severe enough to require tracheostomy. Twenty per cent of patients may have interstitial sarcoid nephritis.

Laboratory investigation reveals a hemoglobin level below 11 gm per 100 ml in up to 20 per cent of patients, and thrombocytopenia and leukopenia may accompany the anemia. Serum alkaline phosphatase levels are elevated in a third of patients. Hypercalcemia appears in some patients with the disseminated form of the disease. One half of all patients have elevated levels of serum globulins during the active phase of the disease. The presence of rheumatoid factor (38%) correlates with the degree of pulmonary involvement.

The diagnosis of sarcoidosis can be made with certainty with tissue biopsy and positive Kveim test. The biopsy specimens are usually obtained from supraclavicular nodes during mediastinoscopy, or transbronchially via the fiberoptic bronchoscope. The Kveim test consists of the intradermal injection of a saline suspension of sarcoid tissue obtained from the spleen of affected patients. The test site is biopsied four to six weeks after injection; a positive reaction is the development of a sarcoid granuloma in the injection area. Not all patients with sarcoidosis will have a positive Kveim test.

The majority of patients with sarcoidosis are asymptomatic and remain so throughout the course of the illness. Some degree of permanent disability occurs in 20 to 25 per cent of patients, the majority from pulmonary fibrosis. The overall mortality rate is from 5 to 10 per cent and is most often due to cardiac decompensation as a result of cor pulmonale secondary to pulmonary fibrosis. Other causes of death include respiratory failure, cardiac arrhythmia, or central nervous system disease. Widespread and progressive involvement of organ systems constitutes indications for treatment of sarcoidosis. Anti-inflammatory agents, such as chloroquin and oxyphenbutazone, and steroids constitute the most effective agents used. Immunosuppressive drugs are tried when there has been inadequate response to corticosteroid therapy.

Anesthetic Considerations. In the majority of patients who are diagnosed with sarcoidosis after a screening chest x-ray, symptoms of the disease will not be present. Extensive evaluation and unusual precautions are not necessary in this patient population.

For patients with physical symptoms and signs of the disease, preoperative evaluation involves multiple organ systems. The degree of pulmonary impairment is assessed by room air blood gas analysis and pulmonary function testing. The presence of rheumatoid factor often correlates with the degree of pulmonary involvement. The presence of a restrictive defect necessitates high inspired oxygen concentrations, and, if ventilation is controlled, small tidal volumes and a rapid respiratory rate are utilized in order to minimize inflation pressure.

Cardiac involvement is assessed by examination for the presence of cor pulmonale or conduction disturbances. If cor pulmonale is present, it should be treated with conventional measures, and anesthetic agents must be selected with regard to their potential to produce myocardial depression. Severe pulmonary hypertension dictates the use of a pulmonary artery catheter to monitor cardiovascular dynamics and left-sided cardiac filling pressures if an extensive procedure is anticipated. Preoperative arrhythmia, especially premature ventricular contractions, necessitates increased vigilance for arrhythmia in the operating room.

Since the larynx is involved in 2 per cent of cases, the airway should be evaluated carefully. Temporomandibular joint involvement from arthritis associated with sarcoidosis may also be present. If the airway is compromised, obvious precautions are needed.

Preoperative liver function tests should be obtained. Abnormal results are helpful in selecting drugs that either do not depend primarily on the liver for metabolism and excretion or do not have the potential to cause liver damage. Impaired renal function requires strict attention to fluid and electrolyte status. Bone marrow involvement may result in anemia that may require preoperative transfusion. Finally, patients maintained on chronic steroid therapy require perioperative coverage with additional steroids to prevent complications resulting from adrenal suppression.

Collagen or Connective Tissue Diseases of the Lung

General Description. Connective tissue is made up of cells and fibrils. The fibrils, composed of elastin, collagen, and reticulum, lie embedded within a proteinaceous gel called ground substance. The collagen vascular diseases are a group of disorders whose common pathologic feature is fibrinoid necrosis of connective tissue caused by alterations in the chemical composition and physical characteristics of the ground substance. When the fibrinoid necrotic connective tissue surrounds blood vessels, a vasculitis also results. The collagen diseases that will be discussed include systemic lupus erythematosus, progressive systemic sclerosis (scleroderma), and rheumatoid pleuropulmonary disease. Dermatomyositis and polymyositis evidence pulmonary involvement in only a small minority of patients and are not included; the anesthetic considerations in these illnesses are similar to those in other fibrotic lung diseases. Wegener's granulomatosis, while occasionally classified as a collagen or vascular disease, has distinct features not usually associated with the conditions listed above; it is discussed on pages 236–238.

SYSTEMIC LUPUS ERYTHEMATOSUS (SLE). At present, evidence indicates that immunologic mechanisms play a prominent role in the pathogenesis of SLE. Patients with SLE may show a variety of serologic abnormalities, including a positive Coombs' test, falsely positive reaction to the Wassermann test, and antibodies to blood clotting factors and to a number of nuclear materials. Good correlation exists between the amount of DNA antibody and circulating DNA-anti-DNA complexes, and activity and severity of idiopathic SLE; similarly, a reduction in the number of these antibodies and complexes with immunosuppressive therapy and plasmapheresis correlates well with clinical remission. The antigen-antibody complex engulfed by polymorphonuclear neutrophils is the basis of the in vitro lupus erythematosus cell test. The hemotoxylin body is the in vivo equivalent of the in vitro LE cell; it represents nuclear damage of cells caused by antinuclear antibodies. It is formed in the tissues of affected organs and has a characteristic staining picture of a purple globule.

Although the final common pathway for the genesis of this disease probably involves immunologic mechanisms, genetic influences may determine whether the disease will develop in response to antigenic stimuli. Viruses, for example, may promote autoantibody formation by altering or stimulating tissue or cell antigen. In addition, a familial tendency has been noted. Lastly, certain drugs (hydralazine and procaine amide, for example) may possibly act as antigens and induce a lupus syndrome almost identical to the idiopathic form.

Systemic lupus erythematosus characteristically affects women during childbearing age, with a female-to-male predominance of approximately 10 to 1. The clinical course is usually prolonged, with frequent remissions and exacerbations; the onset of the disease and subsequent relapses may be precipitated by drugs, emotional upset, infection, or exposure to sunlight.

The lungs and pleura are involved in 30 to 70 per cent of patients with SLE. Pleural involvement consists of a fibrinous pleuritis that results in bilateral pleural effusions. Pericardial effusion may be observed on chest x-ray as an increase in the size of the cardiac silhouette. Pulmonary lesions include interstitial pneumonitis, acute vasculitis, arteriosclerosis, focal alveolar hemorrhage, and bronchopneumonia. Symptoms of this disease are often protean and consist of dyspnea, cough, pleural pain, and rarely hemoptysis. Roentgenographic changes in the chest are often minimal and many dyspneic SLE patients have a normal chest x-ray. Pulmonary function tests usually show a degree of impairment out of proportion to the rather mild changes indicated by the clinical and roentgenologic picture. A restrictive defect with reduction in the lung volumes is typically observed. Flow rates are normal, while diffusing capacity is reduced. Room air arterial blood gases show arterial oxygen desaturation with low or normal PCO_2. Lung compliance is reduced as a result of fibrosis.

The most common organs involved with SLE other than the lung are the skin, upper respiratory tract, joints, kidney, and serosal surfaces. Thus the clinical picture varies considerably. Arthritis and arthralgia are observed in over 90 per cent, cutaneous manifestations in 80 per cent, and Raynaud's phenomenon in 20 per cent of patients. Neuropsychiatric complaints, seizures, or psychotic episodes eventually occur in up to one-half of all patients with SLE. A similar number develop renal disease, with some requiring chronic hemodialysis.

The most specific laboratory tests for diagnosing SLE are the demonstration of antibodies to DNA and circulating DNA-anti-DNA complexes. The LE cell test and the detection of antinuclear antibodies are also useful. Other findings frequently incude anemia, leukopenia, a positive direct Coombs' test, a false-positive Wassermann test, positive rheumatoid factor, and thrombocytopenia.

Steroid administration constitutes the basic treatment for SLE, in addition to symptomatic measures such as salicylates for fever. In severe cases immunosuppressive and antimalarial drugs are added. The usual clinical course is chronic with an occasional acute exacerbation. Death occurs in a minority of patients over a 10 year period from renal failure, CNS involvement, and myocardial infarction.

DIFFUSE SYSTEMIC SCLEROSIS (SCLERODERMA). Diffuse systemic sclerosis is a collagen disease characterized by the atrophy and sclerosis of many organ systems. Autoimmune mechanisms may play a role in the pathogenesis of diffuse systemic sclerosis, although the evidence is less convincing than for most of the other collagen diseases. Antinuclear antibodies are present in about half of afflicted patients, but a positive LE cell test is present in less than 5 per cent. Rheumatoid factor has been identified in a third of patients, and some have mild degrees of hypergammaglobulinemia. The pathologic changes seen in this disease consist of edema and cellular infiltration of the connective tissues of the body in the early stages. Later this reaction is replaced by a proliferation of fibrous tissue and eventual atrophy.

Females are affected three times more often than men. The disease is usually diagnosed during middle age. There are a variety of ways in which these patients present, but most involve complaints referable to the skin, gastrointestinal tract, joints, or lungs. The disease usually begins insidiously; weakness, malaise, weight loss, diffuse stiffness and aching, polyarticular arthritis, edema of the hands, and Raynaud's phenomenon are common initial manifestations. Cutaneous involvement usually precedes visceral involvement.

Pulmonary manifestations occur in up to 90 per cent of patients. The pulmonary pathologic process is diffuse interstitial fibrosis. The histologic characteristics are indistinguishable from those of chronic idiopathic interstitial fibrosis. Initially, pulmonary involvement may cause a slightly productive cough and dyspnea on exertion. With progression of the disease dyspnea worsens. Pulmonary function tests almost invariably show abnormalities in these patients, even when the chest x-ray is normal. A restrictive ventilatory defect occurs with decreased vital capacity and residual volume, the latter diminishing progressively with increasing fibrosis. Both the diffusing capacity and lung compliance are decreased, and ventilation-perfusion inequalities are usually demonstrable. Timed vital capacity, maximum breathing capacity, and forced expiratory volumes are reduced only in proportion to the reduction in vital capacity unless the patient is a cigarette smoker. Room air arterial blood gases often reveal hypoxemia with exercise and sometimes at rest, without CO_2 retention. Roentgenologically, involvement in the lungs appears as a reticular or reticulonodular pattern, depending upon the stage of the disease. The lower lung zones are affected most severely. Over the course of several years, serial x-rays may reveal considerable loss of lung volume. Small cysts are occasionally seen near the lung periphery, and rupture of these cysts may cause pneumothorax. Pleural involvement is uncommon in this disease. There is an increased incidence of lung cancer in patients with progressive systemic sclerosis.

Other organ involvement accompanies the lung changes. Almost all cases have skin changes eventually, and most often these changes occur early. Classically, the skin is taut, thickened, or edematous, bound tightly to subcutaneous tissues, especially in the face and hands. Esophageal dysfunction is demonstrated by the presence of dysphagia and impaired motility. Arthritis occurs in about one half of patients and may lead to impaired mobility and deformity. Cardiac involvement may be indicated by conduction abnormalities such as bundle-branch block or a prolonged P-R interval. Cardiac decompensation may result from cor pulmonale, sclerosis of the cardiac muscle, or a combination of the two. The development of significant albuminuria, pyuria, and casts in the urine is associated with renal involvement or malignant hypertension.

In contrast to systemic lupus erythematosus, steroids and immunosuppressive therapy have not been shown to be beneficial in treating patients with progressive systemic sclerosis. Anti-inflammatory agents are used when there is evidence of inflammation. Alpha blockers, reserpine, and stellate ganglion block are used to treat Raynaud's phenomenon. Conventional antihypertensive therapy is used for elevated blood pressure, but progressive renal disease may result in continued hypertension; renal transplant is necessary in some patients. D-Penicillamine and potassium p-aminobenzoate are two other agents that are sometimes used to treat patients with this disease. The prognosis is unfavorable; five-year survival may be as low as 50 per cent. The cause of death is usually cardiovascular, pulmonary, or renal.

RHEUMATOID DISEASE OF THE LUNGS AND PLEURA. Extra-articular problems occur in more than 50 per cent of patients with rheumatoid arthritis. These include subcutaneous nodules, pulmonary fibrosis, digital vasculitis, skin ulceration, lymph node enlargement, neuropathy, splenomegaly, episcleritis, and pericarditis. Estimates of the incidence of pleuropulmonary disease in patients with rheumatoid arthritis vary considerably, ranging from 1 to 25 per cent, with most series reporting 5 per cent or less. The pulmonary manifestations of rheumatoid disease may be considered under five categories: diffuse interstitial fibrosis, pleural effusion, necrobiotic nodules, Caplan's syndrome, and pulmonary arteritis with pulmonary hypertension.

It has been estimated that about one fifth of all cases of pulmonary interstitial fibrosis are caused by rheumatoid disease. In its most severe form it leads to a pathologic picture of "honeycomb lung." The roentgenographic manifestations include medium to coarse reticulation, often more prominent at the bases, and a "honeycomb" picture. Associated symptoms consist of dyspnea on exertion, and occasionally cough and pleuritic pain. Pulmonary function tests show a restrictive defect along with a reduction in diffusing capacity.

Pleural abnormalities make up the most common manifestations of rheumatoid disease in the thorax; they may occur in up to 20 per cent of patients. Pleural effusion is seen twice as commonly in males, and most patients are middle-aged at the time of occurrence. The pleural fluid is an exudate with a high protein and lactate dehydrogenase level and a low sugar level. The only unique roentgenologic feature of these effusions is the tendency to remain unchanged for many months or even years. The great majority of the effusions are unilateral and are the only x-ray abnormality present. Effusions in these patients typically cause no pulmonary symptoms or only minor ones.

The necrobiotic nodule is a well-circumscribed nodular mass in the lungs, pleura, or pericardium that is pathologically identical to a subcutaneous rheumatoid nodule. The pulmonary nodules occur rarely, usually in association with advanced rheumatoid disease and multiple subcutaneous nodules elsewhere. The roentgenologic appearance is typically that of several well-circumscribed masses, ranging from 3 mm to 7 cm in diameter, situated in the periphery of the lung. Cavitation is common, and reactive pleural effusion may coexist. When several nodules appear, they may be confused with pulmonary metastases. When appearing singly, a pulmonary rheumatoid nodule may be misdiagnosed as a primary carcinoma. Unless extremely large or involved with infection, these nodules cause no symptoms. A blood eosinophilia occurs in up to one half of patients.

Caplan's syndrome is characterized by single or multiple well-defined 0.5 to 5 cm spherical opacities in the lungs that occur in conjunction with various pneumoconioses. These pulmonary lesions are commonly associated with coal miner's pneumoconiosis, although they may also occur with chronic exposure to silica, asbestos, or aluminum powder. The etiology of this syndrome appears to be a hypersensitivity reaction to irritating dust particles in the lungs of rheumatoid patients who are already hyperimmune. Although there are differences microscopically, the chest x-ray appearance of the nodular lesions of Caplan's syndrome is identical to that of the necrobiotic nodules of rheumatoid arthritis without pneumoconiosis. The nodules tend to develop rapidly and appear in groups; they may remain unchanged, calcify, cavitate, fibrose, or regress. There is no apparent relationship between the severity of the arthritis and the extent and type of roentgenographic changes in the lungs. Opacities may appear before, coincident with, or after the clinical onset of arthritis. Pulmonary symptoms eventually develop and are primarily due to the pneumoconiosis.

The last type of pleuropulmonary involvement seen in rheumatoid arthritis patients is arteritis involving the pulmonary vessels. Arteritis may represent the only manifestation of pulmonary involvement or may occur with any of the other forms of pulmonary pathology described above. The arteritis is similar to that seen in other diseases, such as Wegener's granulomatosis, with a fibroelastoid intimal proliferation. Narrowing of the lumen of the pulmonary vessels secondary to the arteritis may lead to pulmonary hypertension and eventually to cor pulmonale. The roentgenologic, clinical and laboratory presentation of this condition is similar to that of primary pulmonary hypertension with the exception that in rheumatoid arthritis other forms of pulmonary involvement may coexist.

Anesthetic Considerations. The discussion of anesthetic considerations for the collagen vascular diseases will be limited to the management of pulmonary problems. Since there are several organ systems involved in all three diseases, reference should be made to other chapters for consideration of problems related to other specific organ systems.

Since the physical signs and symptoms and chest x-ray often do not reflect the amount of pulmonary impairment found in these patients, preoperative evaluation of pulmonary function tests and analysis of room air arterial blood gases should be performed. When significant restrictive disease with decreased lung compliance and diffusing capacity is present, a high inspired oxygen concentration is necessary to avoid hypoxemia. If ventilation is controlled, small tidal volumes with a relatively rapid respiratory rate should be used in order to minimize excessive inflation pressure. Regional techniques may be preferable for extremity and lower abdominal surgery if severe pulmonary disease is present.

Patients with progressive systemic sclerosis often present an additional upper airway problem; the skin around the mouth may be extremely taut, thereby limiting the size of the opening. This may preclude oral intubation and necessitate blind nasal or fiberoptic nasal intubation.

Oral intubation may also be hindered in the conditions described above by the arthritic involvement of the temporomandibular joint. Rheumatoid arthritics may have extensive involvement of the cervical spine that limits neck mobility. In addition, rheumatoid disease may affect the cartilaginous portions of the larynx and result in a narrow laryngeal aperture. Severe small-sized endotracheal tubes should be available when intubation is planned in a patient with rheumatoid arthritis.

If cor pulmonale exists, consideration should be given to preoperative digitalization and to the selection of anesthetic drugs that cause minimal myocardial depression. A pulmonary artery catheter is useful if significant pulmonary hypertension exists and large fluid shifts are expected. Since a pulmonary artery diastolic-to-wedge pressure gradient can be expected in this setting, the pulmonary artery capillary wedge pressure should be used to assess vascular volume status.

Histiocytosis X

General Description. Histiocytosis X, also called reticuloendotheliosis, histiocytic reticulosis, and eosinophilic xanthomatous granuloma, is a multisystem disease that may involve lymph nodes, lung, skin, central nervous system, liver, spleen, stomach, intestine, kidney, and bone. Pulmonary lesions are characterized morphologically by the granulomatous infiltration of the alveolar septa and bronchial walls by histiocytes. Scattered among the infiltrating histiocytes are eosinophils and giant cells. The early histologic appearance resembles inflammation; later stages of the disease are characterized by fibrosis. The "X" in the title was originally added to denote a lack of knowledge of the etiology of this disease, and ignorance of its cause persists to this day.

Histiocytosis X may be subdivided into three diseases possessing a similar histologic picture. The distinction between the three varieties depends chiefly on the clinical presentation and course of the disease and less on age of onset and organs involved. Letterer-Siwe's disease occurs in infants and children and is characterized by widespread dissemination and a fulminating fatal course. Hand-Schüller-Christian disease becomes manifest during childhood or adolescence. Part of or all of a triad of physical signs of exophthalmos, diabetes insipidus, and osteolytic lesions of the skull may be present. Eosinophilic granuloma, the third subdivision, presents during adult life. It is usually localized to the lungs and/or bones, although it may be disseminated throughout the body.

Histiocytosis X cannot always be assigned with confidence to one of these three categories. Since eosinophilic granuloma has predominant pulmonary involvement, the following discussion focuses on this disease.

Eosinophilic granuloma occurs mainly in young adult white males and is extremely uncommon. A genetic mechanism has been suggested as at least partially causative in that a father and son have been reported to have this disease. Presently, definitive diagnosis of this diffuse pulmonary disease is facilitated by use of open lung biopsy.

In addition to the usual involvement of the bone marrow, involvement of the lungs is often widespread. During the early or active stages of the condition, the lungs show widespread granularity or nodularity, with individual foci up to a few millimeters in diameter. These foci consist of aggregates of histiocytes, giant cells, eosinophils, lymphocytes, and polymorphonuclear cells. The granulomatous lesions that are found are quite vascular and occur mainly in the peribronchial and perivascular interstitial tissues. As the disease progresses, fibrosis replaces the early picture of eosinophilic granuloma. With advanced disease, gross disorganization of pulmonary architecture leads to formation of multiple cysts that tend to give the lung a honeycomb appearance.

The x-ray picture varies with the stage of the disease, but it is characteristically symmetrical and diffuse. The granulomatous or active stage of the disease is manifested by multiple nodules 1 to 10 mm in diameter, which are more extensive in the upper zones of the lung. In the latter stages, as fibrosis develops, the picture changes to a reticular-nodular pattern. The end stage disease results in a coarse reticular appearance that may include a cystic, honeycomb pattern, particularly in the apices. Lymph node involvement and pleural effusions are uncommon, although pneumothorax occurs frequently.

About a third of patients with eosinophilic granuloma are asymptomatic when first diagnosed, the disease being discovered by screening chest x-ray. Nonspecific symptoms, including fever, weight loss, and fatigue, occur in 30 per cent of patients. A slightly higher percentage complain of dyspnea, while more than half have a nonproductive cough. Chest pain occurs in a fourth of patients, and diabetes insipidus occurs in about 20 per cent. Physical findings are usually of little help in making the diagnosis.

Early in the active form of the disease pulmonary function remains close to normal, as deterioration with fibrosis begins to occur. A restrictive defect eventually develops, as evidenced by a decreased lung volume and normal flow rate during pulmonary function testing. Low diffusing capacity and ventilation-perfusion inequalities are seen as well. Lung biopsy is required to make the diagnosis.

Large doses of corticosteroids may afford dramatic objective and subjective relief in some patients. However, the overall prognosis for eosinophilic granuloma is poor. The disease usually progresses slowly, resulting in eventual respiratory insufficiency and death in many of the patients.

Anesthetic Considerations. Many of these patients are asymptomatic, and no unusual anesthetic problems exist in this setting. Those with signs and symptoms of pulmonary disease require preoperative investigation of pulmonary function and room air arterial blood gas analysis. The presence of ventilatory restriction and hypoxemia dictates the use of high inspired oxygen concentrations and intraoperative blood gas analysis. If ventilation is controlled, small tidal volumes with rapid respiratory rates are required in order to minimize inflation pressure.

FIBROTIC LUNG DISEASES

Idiopathic Pulmonary Fibrosis: Hamman-Rich Syndrome

General Description. A syndrome of progressive, rapidly fatal diffuse pulmonary fibrosis was first described in 1935 by Hamman and Rich and has since been termed the "Hamman-Rich syndrome." Since their original description, it has become increasingly apparent that the Hamman-Rich syndrome represents the end of a spectrum of diseases now termed idiopathic pulmonary fibrosis. In the past 45 years a number of syndromes have been described which have varied histological features, but all involve a diffuse interstitial pneumonia, which commonly results in diffuse pulmonary fibrosis. These conditions have been termed diffuse fibrosing alveolitis, usual interstitial pneumonia, bronchiolitis obliter-

ans with diffuse interstitial pneumonia, desquamative interstitial pneumonia, and lymphoid interstitial pneumonia. Although many investigators have abandoned these specific designations, they remain important as probably representing various stages in the development of idiopathic pulmonary fibrosis. For convenience, pulmonary fibrosis is now categorized as idiopathic (unassociated with any known disorder) or as associated with a collagen vascular disorder. This section discusses idiopathic pulmonary fibrosis.

Although this condition is termed idiopathic, there is considerable evidence that the pathologic changes result from an immunologic reaction to a variety of stimuli. Immunofluorescent studies of lung biopsies from some patients with idiopathic pulmonary fibrosis have demonstrated tissue-bound immune complexes implicating T-cell mediated processes directed against collagen. The presence of elevated levels of IgG, antinuclear antibody, rheumatoid factor, and cryoimmunoglobulins in some patients also offers evidence of immune mechanisms being involved. Histologic observations show that alveolar inflammation predominates in the early stages of the disease; gallium scan results also show that the lung parenchyma has areas of active neutrophilic inflammation. Bronchoalveolar lavage results in fluid with elevated levels of IgG and neutrophils.

The major histologic abnormality seen with this condition is an increase in the amount of fibrous tissue in the alveolar septa. Inflammatory cells, mainly lymphocytes, macrophages, and plasma cells occur within these areas of increased fibrous tissue. In many areas where alveolar septa are thickened, the air side is lined by large cuboidal cells, often associated with collections of free cells in the alveolar sacs. The former cell type change has been referred to as "cuboidalization of alveolar lining cells" and the latter cell type change as "desquamation." Electron microscopy has shown that many of these desquamated cells are macrophages. The amount of desquamation varies not only from patient to patient but also within the same limited area of the biopsy specimen. This finding strengthens the concept that "desquamative interstitial pneumonitis" and "usual interstitial pneumonitis" are simply part of the same disease rather than specific disease entities, with "desquamative interstitial pneumonitis" representing a more advanced stage of the disease. In addition to involvement of the alveoli, most biopsy specimens include peribronchiolar fibrosis, and many of the airway lumens contain cellular debris. The airways are narrowed in the majority of patients. Finally, most patients show thickening of the walls of the muscular pulmonary arteries by both medial hypertrophy and fibrinous intimal proliferation.

The chest x-ray appearance depends on the stage of the disease. The lower lung zones often show predominant involvement. Early in the course of the disease, the chest x-ray shows localized linear, nodular, or ill-defined densities or a ground glass pattern, probably representing the alveolitis stage of the disease. Later, as fibrosis occurs, reticular and reticulonodular patterns begin to appear. The proximal pulmonary arteries may be dilated. Terminal stages usually show coarse reticulation, often associated with cystic lesions and bullae.

Although the age range is broad, idiopathic pulmonary fibrosis occurs most often during middle age, with symptoms occurring for several years prior to diagnosis. Once diagnosis is made, the disease usually runs a fairly rapid course. The onset of idiopathic pulmonary fibrosis is associated with breathlessness, especially during exercise. A nonproductive cough, weight loss, and easy fatigability are also early symptoms of this illness. Physical findings progress from minimal early in the disease to the appearance of tachypnea, harsh dry rales at the lung bases, clubbing of the fingers, and findings consistent with pulmonary hypertension late in the disease.

The majority of patients with idiopathic pulmonary fibrosis are hypoxemic at rest and worsen with exercise. Over 90 per cent have an elevated sedimentation rate, and many demonstrate circulating cryoimmunoglobulins, rheumatoid factor, antinuclear antibodies, and other abnormal gamma globulins. Fiberoptic bronchoscopy with bronchoalveolar lavage yields free floating macrophages and neutrophils, and is now an important diagnostic tool in the evaluation of these patients.

Pulmonary function tests reveal significant reductions in both total lung capacity and diffusing capacity, while airflow rates remain normal. The decreased diffusing capacity signifies a reduction of available alveolar-capillary surface area. However, the most important cause of the hypoxemia in these patients is ventilation-perfusion mismatching. Over 50 per cent of patients have an increase in physiological dead space which clinically results in tachypnea. Physiologic shunt is usually significantly increased late in the disease. Thus, measurement of the alveolar-arterial oxygen gradient on exercise is considered particularly useful in following patients receiving therapy. Finally, patients with idiopathic pulmonary fibrosis have a volume-pressure curve that is shifted downward and to the right.

In summary, idiopathic pulmonary fibrosis most likely begins as an alveolitis (ground glass or nodular appearance on x-ray; inflammatory cells and "desquamation" seen histologically) and gradually develops into alveolar septal fibrosis (reticular or reticulonodular appearance radiographically; increasing alveolar fibrosis seen microscopically). The process may be reversible in the alveolitis stage, but once septal fibrosis occurs, the anatomical parenchymal derangements are permanent.

The evidence implicating the immune process in the pathogenesis of idiopathic pulmonary fibrosis provides the basis for treatment. Steroids are administered to most patients, and many are treated with immunosuppressive drugs as well. The course of the disease is somewhat variable, but progressive pulmonary involvement and hypoxemia are the rule. Patients treated early in the course of the disease do better than those treated after fibrosis has occurred. Although some patients may live up to 15 years after diagnosis is made, the average life span of a patient with idiopathic pulmonary fibrosis is only 4 years after the onset of symptoms. Twenty per cent of patients die from right heart failure; most succumb to primary respiratory failure, often precipitated by infection.

Anesthetic Considerations. The most useful tests for evaluating the clinical course of these patients are lung volumes, chest x-ray, diffusing capacity, and resting arterial oxygen tension. Since right heart failure and cor pulmonale account for 20 per cent of deaths due to this illness, the functional status of the right ventricle should be assessed and, if necessary, treated by conventional methods (digitalis and diuretics).

If chronic steroid therapy has been employed, perioperative coverage with exogenous steroids is necessary. If immunosuppressive therapy has been utilized, possible bone marrow depression (anemia, thrombocytopenia) should be recognized. In addition, susceptibility to infection may be enhanced, and scrupulous aseptic techniques should be employed.

Since ventilation-perfusion inequalities and a decrease in diffusing capacity make the possibility of intraoperative hypoxemia more likely, high inspired oxygen concentrations and frequent blood gas analysis are necessary. If ventilation is controlled and excessive inflation pressure is to be minimized (decreased compliance and lung volume), a small tidal volume with a rapid respiratory rate should be used (perhaps quite rapid in view of the increase in physiological dead space). If significantly elevated pulmonary artery pressures are suspected and large intraoperative fluid shifts are anticipated, the pulmonary artery wedge pressure should be monitored, since a pulmonary artery diastolic-to-wedge pressure gradient will be present. If right ventricular failure is present as well, agents should be selected with regard to their propensity to cause myocardial depression.

The Pneumoconioses

General Descriptions. Diseases caused by the inhalation of inorganic dust, often termed the pneumoconioses, are in large measure occupational diseases. The reaction of the lung to inhaled particles depends upon several factors. The chemical nature of inhaled dust is a major determinant of the type of reaction that occurs. Size is an important consideration; nearly all particles 20 microns or more in diameter are deposited in the nasopharynx, trachea, and bronchi, whereas the great majority of particles that penetrate the alveoli measure 5 microns or less. Other factors that contribute to determining the extent of lung reaction are the intrapulmonary distribution of inhaled dust particles, the concentration and duration of exposure to the dust, individual susceptibility, and individual ability to clear dust particles. The last factor involves two mechanisms: mucociliary escalator transport and lymphatic drainage. It is probable that variations in the efficiency of these defense mechanisms account for some of the individual susceptibility to the pneumoconioses.

Pneumoconiosis can be defined as the accumulation of dust in the lungs and the tissue reaction to its presence. Pulmonary tissues react to inhaled dust in two general ways: 1) a desmoplastic reaction resulting in permanent scarring (the collagenous pneumoconioses such as silicosis and asbestosis) and 2) a minimal stromal reaction consisting mainly of the formation of reticulin fibers (the noncollagenous pneumoconioses such as siderosis, stannosis, and baritosis). The above definition excludes other occupational disease such as byssinosis, berylliosis, and the hypersensitivity pneumonitides in which particles do not accumulate in the lungs. They are discussed in other sections of this chapter.

SILICOSIS. The development of silicosis depends on the inhalation of respirable free silica particles under 10 microns in size. The size range for maximal alveolar deposition is 1 to 3 microns. Workers at risk for developing silicosis include foundry workers, sand blasters, granite workers, and pottery workers.

The pathogenesis of silicosis involves the inhalation of silica particles, their penetration of the lung periphery, ingestion of the particles by macrophages, death of the macrophages, and release of the contents of the killed cells, including silica particles. The cycle of macrophage ingestion of free silica and subsequent death is continued by other macrophages, resulting in the gradual accumulation of debris and the eventual production of connective tissue. The connective tissue is deposited around the silica in a laminated "onion-skin" fashion resulting in characteristic 2 to 3 mm diameter nodules. Autoimmunity may play a role in the development of silicosis, in that silicotics have an increased incidence of autoantibodies and autoimmune disease. Immune reactions may aid in supplying a large and continuing supply of macrophages to the areas of reaction.

Three types of tissue reaction to silica have been distinguished: chronic, in which moderate exposure extends over a period of 20 to 40 years; accelerated, with increased particle doses for a period of five to 15 years; and diffuse, in which there is a heavy alveolar deposition of particles for a period of less than five years.

Silicosis is most often a chronic process, and the symptoms develop late; it is unusual for the chest x-ray to become positive before 20 years of exposure. The earliest symptoms in chronic cases are cough and expectoration. Dyspnea on exertion is the principal symptom of established silicosis and is almost always associated with significant x-ray changes. Hemoptysis and chest pain are not uncommon. Weight loss is a characteristic finding of silicotuberculosis and other infective pneumoconioses. Severe disease can result in respiratory failure. Respiratory failure may be further aggravated by pneumothorax that resists successful treatment because of the difficulty in sealing the air leak in the poorly retractile tissue and in obtaining re-expansion of the fibrotic lung once a seal has been achieved.

In the majority of patients with accelerated silicosis the major features of the pulmonary disease are identical to the chronic form, but the overall course of deterioration is much faster. Mycobacteriosis affects 25 per cent of these patients, with half of the infections due to atypical organisms. Approximately 10 per cent of patients with the accelerated form of the disease develop connective tissue disorders, including progressive systemic sclerosis (scleroderma), rheumatoid arthritis, and systemic lupus erythematosus. In these patients, the pulmonary disease usually has a more rapid progression of roentgenographic and functional abnormalities. In some of these cases, treatment with adrenal corticosteroids may be helpful.

Silicoproteinosis is the name applied to the diffuse type of disease that results from heavy exposure to silica. The diffuse reaction produces so much pulmonary fibrosis that few characteristic nodules are seen. Dyspnea on exertion may appear within six months of first exposure. There is associated weakness and weight loss, and in severe cases, cyanosis and diffuse rales. Progressive deterioration may be temporarily and partially suppressed by corticosteroids; death results from intractable hypoxia.

The diagnosis of silicosis usually depends on historical and roentgenographic evidence. A history of significant exposure to silica is required. X-ray changes provide the evidence that exposure has produced pulmonary disease. In the simple chronic form of the disease small nodules are seen and are usually more prominent within the upper lung fields. In the complicated forms,

massive densities predominate. The acute diffuse form of the disease is characterized by extensive interstitial fibrotic changes, and nodules are poorly defined. The lungs appear small and the diaphragms are high. Lung biopsy is usually not required to make the diagnosis. When lung biopsy is required, an open chest procedure is usually performed.

For patients with silica-produced pneumoconiosis, lung function is extremely variable because the disease itself has several forms, infections and immune reactions may compound the disease in some patients, there may be exposure to multiple dusts, and changes due to cigarette smoking may be superimposed. Despite these complex factors, the following generalizations can be made: 1) in simple cases, clinical tests of ventilatory function are often normal; 2) symptomatic silicotics can demonstrate pulmonary restriction, obstruction, and mixed patterns of ventilatory impairment; 3) complicated cases demonstrate reduced diffusing capacity and exercise-induced hypoxemia; and 4) terminal cases have severe restrictive impairment and hypoxemia.

Current therapy is directed entirely at the complications of silicoses. Anti-tuberculosis drugs should be given if suspicion of mycobacterial infection arises and should not wait for confirmation by cultures. The high proportion of atypical mycobacterial infection dictates the initial use of three anti-tuberculosis drugs, including rifampin. When autoimmune diseases complicate silicosis, corticosteroids should be tried. When obstruction forms part of the functional impairment, bronchodilator therapy may result in significant improvement. Heart failure is treated with digitalis and diuretics. Supplmental oxygen must be administered in the preterminal stages of the disease.

ASBESTOSIS. There are two major sources of exposure to asbestos dust: 1) primary occupations of asbestos mining and its processing in a mill and 2) secondary occupations such as insulation, textile manufacturing, construction work, and shipbuilding. Pulmonary disease secondary to asbestos inhalation differs from other pneumoconioses in that larger particles, up to 100 microns in length, may cause the lung damage.

Asbestos causes pulmonary fibrosis, a high incidence of mesothelioma, and increased susceptibility to bronchogenic carcinoma. The mechanism of these changes is unknown. Possibilities include direct physical irritation, a response to released silicic acid and metallic ions, or an autoimmune reaction resulting from antigens liberated through the interaction of macrophages and asbestos fibers. Evidence for an autoimmune contribution to the pathophysiology of this disease is the finding of circulating rheumatoid and antinuclear factors in over a fourth of asbestos workers with abnormal roentgenograms. As with other pneumoconioses, the development of the disease depends in large measure on the duration and degree of exposure. Clinical manifestations usually do not appear until 20 to 40 years after exposure; host susceptibility may play a role in patients evidencing the disease more quickly.

Asbestos fibers that reach alveoli initiate a macrophage response in a manner similar to that seen in silicosis. Asbestos bodies are formed by the deposition of ferritin on the asbestos fibers within macrophages, first as a smooth coating and then in the form of beading as the macrophages shrink and rupture. Varying degrees of fibrosis result, occurring first in lower, then middle, and eventually upper lobes. Conglomerate lesions of massive fibrosis, comparable to the progressive massive fibrosis of silicosis, are uncommon in asbestosis. Pleural involvement is usually present and is manifested by the appearance of pleural thickening, plaques, mesothelioma, and/or effusions. Pleural effusion is almost always found with an accompanying mesothelioma. Necrobiotic nodules are occasionally seen in patients with combined asbestosis and rheumatoid disease.

The great majority of patients with pleuropulmonary asbestosis have no symptoms. Symptoms seldom develop before 20 to 30 years of exposure; a more rapid appearance is seen in patients who are cigarette smokers. Dyspnea is almost invariably associated with serious interstitial fibrosis, although widespread pleural thickening may contribute to its appearance. Dyspnea is usually progressive, despite removal of patients from asbestos exposure. Other symptoms include cough, production of sputum, and pleural pain. Basal crepitation, signs of pleural effusion, and clubbing of the digits may be evident. Asbestos bodies are invariably found in the sputum of patients with x-ray evidence of the disease.

Cor pulmonale may develop late in the disease.

The roentgenographic changes in asbestosis may be both pleural and parenchymal, although the former is usually more striking. Three types of pleural changes have been observed: pleural plaques (most common), pleural calcifications, and pleural effusion. Each of these changes may occur alone or in combination with the others. Parenchymal x-ray changes consist of various sized opacities. Small opacities may form a nodular and/or reticular pattern. Large opacities occur infrequently and are invariably associated with widespread interstitial fibrosis.

Patients with interstitial fibrosis caused by asbestos exposure usually show a restrictive pattern of pulmonary function, with decreased vital capacity, residual volume, and diffusion capacity, while airway resistance remains relatively normal. Pulmonary compliance is usually significantly reduced. Hypoxemia may be seen on exercise, but the arterial PCO_2 remains normal or low. Patients who are cigarette smokers often manifest a mixed obstructive/restrictive pattern on pulmonary function testing.

Asbestosis has the highest incidence of associated neoplasia of all the non-neoplastic pulmonary diseases, with a risk factor 10 times that seen in the general population. The risk associated with exposure to both asbestos and cigarette smoking is considerably more than additive and is probably multiplicative. The neoplasias that these patients develop include bronchogenic, gastrointestinal, and laryngeal carcinoma, and mesothelioma. Although mesothelioma is not invariably associated with asbestos, approximately 80 per cent of patients with this malignancy have been exposed to asbestos. Although the mesotheliomas are most often pleural, an increased incidence of peritoneal mesotheliomas occurs as well. The prognosis for patients with mesothelioma is extremely poor, survival seldom exceeding two years from the time of diagnosis. Some patients exposed to asbestos may die of cor pulmonale or ventilatory failure in the absence of neoplasia.

COAL-WORKERS' PNEUMOCONIOSIS. Coal miners are susceptible to a variety of pulmonary diseases, including coal-worker's pneumoconiosis, emphysema, silicosis, chronic bronchitis, and tuberculosis. By far the most common form of respiratory disease in this patient population is simple coal-worker's pneumoconiosis (CWP), which is caused by the inhalation of large quantities of carbon dust. Complicated pneumoconiosis, or progressive massive fibrosis (PMF), is a less common, although often more serious type of illness, and exposure to silica has been incriminated in its etiology. In addition, continued exposure of patients with simple CWP to coal dust may lead to the development of PMF. In all coal miners, the prevalance of CWP is approximately 10 per cent, of which only 0.4 per cent is PMF. Despite the general relationship between years spent underground and the dust levels to which patients have been exposed, there are marked regional differences in prevalence that cannot be explained by exposure to dust alone. Thus, it appears that the physical and chemical composition of the coal dust is an important determinant of the nature and severity of the disease. In general, coal miners have a normal life expectancy; the excess deaths due to complicated pneumoconiosis are counterbalanced by a lower death rate from lung cancer and coronary artery disease.

Inhaled dust particles larger than 5 microns in diameter are deposited in the conducting system and removed by mucociliary transport. Injury that follows inhalation of smaller particles shares a mechanism similar to that of other pneumoconioses. Maccrophages phagocytize deposited particles and carry them to the terminal bronchioles, where they are in turn removed by ciliary transport. If the dust load is excessive, this mechanism is overwhelmed, and the macrophages begin to aggregate in the respiratory bronchioles and alveoli. Fibroblasts appear, and a thin layer of reticulin is laid around the stationary fibroblasts to produce collagen. The respiratory bronchioles and alveoli gradually accumulate a mass of dying macrophages, coal dust, and fibroblasts. This aggregation of debris and collagen leads to the formation of the coal macule, the primary lesion of CWP. The macules have a predilection for the upper lobes. As they enlarge, the respiratory bronchioles dilate, the end result being an area of focal emphysema. Simple CWP does not produce cor pulmonale unless there is coincident bronchitis. In contrast, the PMF lesions may be massive, obliterate pulmonary vessels, and cause pulmonary hypertension. The etiology of this type of pneumoconiosis

(PMF) remains unclear. Tuberculosis infection may play a role, since atypical acid-fast bacilli are often isolated from patients with PMF. The presence of rheumatoid, antinuclear, and antilung antibodies, particularly in the more advanced cases of PMF, suggests an immunologic mechanism.

Coal-workers' pneumoconiosis is subdivided into simple and complicated pneumoconiosis (PMF) according to the appearance of the chest x-ray. The diagnosis of complicated pneumoconiosis requires pulmonary opacities to be larger than 1 cm in diameter.

Unlike patients with silicosis, coal workers with simple CWP suffer little clinical disability and seldom demonstrate evidence of their disease if removed from their dust-ridden environment. The presence of severe shortness of breath in a patient with simple CWP is virtually always related to a non-occupationally related disease, such as chronic bronchitis or emphysema, rather than to coal mining. Symptoms usually develop only when the disease becomes complicated by PMF. When symptoms do appear, they include cough, mucoid expectoration, dyspnea on exertion, frequent attacks of acute purulent bronchitis, and expectoration of black sputum. Chest pain and hemoptysis rarely occur. The signs of PMF are those of consolidation and collapse of the affected area. In advanced PMF, signs of pulmonary hypertension and right ventricular hypertrophy may develop along with congestive heart failure.

The results of pulmonary function testing in coal workers are variable, owing to differences in the populations studied. Respiratory symptoms in these patients are associated with a decrease in ventilatory capacity, but smoking is by far the most important factor in producing respiratory dysfunction. The contribution of simple CWP and years spent underground to decrease in ventilatory capacity are slight in comparison. Thus, diffusion capacity is decreased in patients with simple CWP who smoke, while it remains normal in coal miners who do not smoke. In contrast, patients with severe PMF have extremely abnormal pulmonary function tests and often develop marked pulmonary hypertension.

Caplan's syndrome or rheumatoid pneumoconiosis is CWP in association with rheumatoid arthritis. The chest x-ray contains 0.5 to 5 cm rounded opacities that appear in the course of a few weeks along with joint manifestations of rheumatoid arthritis. A high incidence of rheumatoid factor is found in the serum of these patients as well as in those with PMF.

Other less common pulmonary diseases found in coal miners are industrial bronchitis, emphysema, and silicosis. Bronchitis becomes more prevalent in these patients as exposure to dust increases. Industrial bronchitis, for the most part, affects the larger airways and is due to the deposition of non-respirable particles larger than 6 microns in diameter. If exposure is long and heavy, a small decrease in ventilatory capacity develops in some workers as a result of overloading the mucociliary transport system. There are usually no radiographic signs present. Simple CWP or coal mining per se does not lead to the development of disabling emphysema in the absence of PMF. Finally, both simple and complicated silicosis are occasionally seen in coal miners, but seldom before 20 years of exposure. Simple silicosis causes little in the way of signs and symptoms, but the conglomerate lesions cause widespread tissue destruction and thus the appearance of expected pulmonary-related findings.

OTHER PNEUMOCONIOSES. There are many other pulmonary diseases that are caused by the inhalation of dust particles. For the most part, the pathophysiology is similar to that of the other pneumoconioses described above; the inability of defense mechanisms to clear materials leads eventually to varying degrees of interstitial fibrosis and conglomeration.

Graphite pneumoconiosis is caused by the inhalation of mixed dust particles containing carbon and varying quantities of free silica. This may occur in workers utilizing graphite in the manufacture of steel, lubricants, lead paints, and electrodes. The pathologic lesions are quite similar to those seen in coal-workers' pneumoconiosis, and symptoms do not differ significantly from other fibrotic pneumoconioses. Pulmonary function abnormalities have been reported to be both restrictive and obstructive.

Silicosiderosis develops from prolonged inhalation of silica mixed with iron oxide. It is seen in foundry workers and those associated with the steel industry. Again, the roentgenographic and pathologic picture is similar to that seen in coal workers. In contrast, however, the incidence of broncho-genic carcinoma is higher in these patients than in the general population.

Stannosis is a pneumoconiosis caused by the inhalation of tin oxide. Again, pathologic findings resemble coal-workers' pneumoconiosis. Baritosis results from the inhalation of particulate barium sulfate. In contrast to the other pneumoconioses, roentgenographic abnormalities characteristically regress after removal from the dust-filled environment. Other dusts that have caused pulmonary disease are silver, antimony, aluminum, fiber glass, and tungsten carbide. Both the incidence and pathology produced by these conditions are mild compared with those produced by asbestos, silica, and coal dust.

Anesthetic Considerations. The diagnosis of pneumoconiosis is presumed by obtaining a history of exposure and symptoms of respiratory difficulties and is largely confirmed by chest x-ray. Preoperative room air arterial blood gas analysis and pulmonary function testing should be performed.

A history of cigarette smoking considerably complicates the clinical picture. Thus, chronic bronchitis, emphysema, and fibrotic restrictive disease may coexist. If pulmonary function testing reveals an obstructive component to lung disease, the patient should be tested for reversibility of obstruction. Bronchodilators should be considered if a reversible component exists. Preoperative pulmonary toilette is important in this population of patients.

Many patients with pneumoconiosis, particularly those with silica-induced pneumoconiosis or progressive massive fibrosis secondary to inhalation of coal dust, have active tuberculosis. If active tuberculosis is suspected, a multiple drug regimen should be begun. If operation is imperative, appropriate precautions should be taken to prevent contamination with mycobacterial organisms (see pp. 264 to 265 for a description of isolation precautions for patients with active tuberculosis).

Most patients with severe fibrotic lung disease have evidence of both arterial hypoxemia when breathing room air and a restrictive defect in ventilation. High inspired oxygen concentrations and intraoperative blood gas analysis may be required. Controlled ventilation requires low tidal volumes with higher rates, which in turn minimizes increases in inflation pressures caused by decreased lung compliance.

If significant airflow obstruction exists, an increased expiratory time may be necessary.

Severe cases of pneumoconiosis may have cor pulmonale, which requires preoperative treatment with cardiac glycosides and diuretics. Anesthetic agents should be considered with regard to their propensity to cause cardiac depression. Central venous or pulmonary artery pressure monitoring is helpful in assessing intraoperative cardiac dynamics. If large intraoperative fluid shifts are anticipated and significant pulmonary hypertension exists, it is necessary to monitor volume status with the pulmonary artery capillary wedge pressure, since a pulmonary artery diastolic-to-wedge pressure gradient is present.

Drug-Induced Pulmonary Disease

General Description

PHARMACOLOGIC AGENTS. *Toxic Antineoplastic Drug Reactions.* Toxic pulmonary reactions to therapeutic antineoplastic agents are usually true effects of some pharmacologic action of the drug. Toxic reactions are typically dose dependent and can be produced in a large percentage of patients if a sufficient amount of the drug is administered. Important drugs included in this category are busulfan, cyclophosphamide, bleomycin, and chlorambucil.

Busulfan is an alkylating drug that is used primarily for treatment of chronic myelogenous leukemia. Symptoms may occur after three or four years of chronic therapy and include the gradual onset of fever, chills, weakness, cough, and shortness of breath. Chest X-ray studies reveal a diffuse interstitial and intra-alveolar process. The histologic abnormality consists of an organizing fibrinous edema with bizarre, atypical type II granular pneumocytes. The pathologic process is a chemically induced alveolitis with proliferation of granular pneumocytes followed by fibrosis of alveolar walls. The process of intra-alveolar fibrosis is often reversible in the early stages; discontinuing the drug and giving high doses of steroids may help. When fibrosis has occurred, however, pulmonary function testing shows a restrictive defect with lowered diffusing capacity. Some patients may die of "busulfan lung" rather than leukemia.

Cyclophosphamide, another widely used antineoplastic drug, may also produce lung toxicity. Cases resemble "busulfan lung" radiographically, histologically, and in their clinical course, and a similar mechanism of injury has been proposed. A restrictive ventilatory defect results from eventual fibrosis if the process is allowed to continue.

Pulmonary lung toxicity is a major factor in limiting the use of bleomycin against epidermoid carcinoma, lymphoma, and other types of neoplasm. The pulmonary injury induced by this agent is also similar to that of busulfan. The toxic pulmonary insult of bleomycin consists of a decrease in the number of type I pneumocytes and hyperplasia and metaplasia of type II pneumocytes. With continued stimulation, the type II cells are shed into the alveolar spaces. A serofibrinous reaction occurs, and intra-alveolar material accumulates. Interstitial edema develops, and reticular and collagen deposition takes place in the alveolar septa. Eventually, the organized alveolar masses are incorporated into the thickened alveolar walls, producing extensive fibrosis. The clinical course of bleomycin toxicity is varied. Some patients develop rales, rhonchi, or pleural rubs; others have a normal clinical examination but develop pulmonary infiltrates on chest x-ray. In about half of the patients in whom early lung toxicity is noted on physical examination, the physical findings regress over one to two months' time after discontinuing the drug. In patients in whom x-ray abnormalities are found, however, regression of these abnormalities and clinical findings occurs more slowly. The incidence of bleomycin-induced pulmonary injury is unknown but may approach 50 per cent of patients treated. Lung toxicity has been noted at all dosage levels, but risk of injury increases with a total dose above 450 mg. The combination of bleomycin and radiation therapy may cause an accelerated fibrotic pulmonary reaction when compared with the fibrotic reaction that occurs when either agent is used alone. Several respiratory failure deaths have been reported following only a moderate dose of bleomycin and a course of radiotherapy.

Chlorambucil and melphalan are two other alkylating drugs that have been associated with fibrotic pulmonary disease. The appearance of pulmonary toxicity with these agents is quite uncommon.

Hypersensitivity (Allergic) Antineoplastic Drug Reactions. Hypersensitivity reactions to antineoplastic drugs occur in only a small percentage of patients. The reactions are neither dose dependent nor a true effect of some pharmacologic action of the drug. An allergic hypersensitivity reaction requires previous exposure to the drug, an induction period in order to produce antibodies, and re-exposure to small amounts of the offending agent to elicit the response. True allergic reactions are seen with asparaginase and procarbazine.

L-asparaginase is most frequently used in the treatment of acute lymphocytic leukemia. One series of children receiving chemotherapy with this drug reported a 33 per cent incidence of hives and dyspnea. Another series reported shortness of breath (22%), urticaria (65%), hypotension (18%), and facial edema (11%). Treatment with antihistamines and steroids usually controls symptoms, but in some cases further therapy with asparaginase must be withheld.

Procarbazine, a monoamine oxidase inhibitor, is an important drug used for therapy of Hodgkin's disease, small-cell carcinoma of the lung, lymphoma, and central nervous system malignancies. Several cases of acute allergic pneumonitis have been attributed to therapy with this agent. Symptoms consist of cough, fever, and shortness of breath. Pulmonary infiltrates and pleural effusion appear on chest x-ray. The histological picture consists of a proliferative alveolar reaction including interstitial leukocyte infiltration, occasional eosinophils, and alveolar septal edema. Fibrosis is not present. Recovery should be complete when administration of the drug is discontinued.

Azathioprine has also been implicated in one case report as a cause of allergic pneumonitis. After six weeks of oral therapy, symptoms of respiratory distress appeared along with bibasilar infiltrates on chest x-ray. Pulmonary function testing revealed a pronounced decrease in forced expiratory volume and forced vital capacity. Discontinuing azathioprine and administering steroids resulted in prompt clinical improvement. After three months, findings on chest x-ray and pulmonary function studies had returned to normal.

Antineoplastic Drug Reactions—Mechanism Unknown. Methotrexate is an antimetabolite used primarily in the treatment of acute lymphocytic leukemia. Symptoms of fever, cough, and dyspnea can occur 10 days to four months after the start of therapy. X-ray studies of the chest in these patients show diffuse, bilateral interstitial infiltrates. Pleural effusions are rare. Eosinophilia may occur concomitantly, often in association with infection by *Pneumocystis carinii*. Interestingly, leukemic patients treated with methotrexate are usually in remission when the respiratory illness occurs. In this circumstance leukemic infiltration of the lungs must be ruled out.

Histologic changes are somewhat similar to those seen with busulfan toxicity; however, the atypical, bizarre cells are absent, and poorly defined, noncaseating granulomas containing multinucleated giant cells may be present.

If the drug is discontinued, most of the pathologic process may be reversible. A course of steroid treatment may hasten improvement of the patient's pulmonary condition.

The mechanism of pulmonary injury resulting from treatment with methotrexate is controversial. Simple direct pulmonary toxicity or hypersensitivity phenomena do not explain the common findings that continuation of methotrexate therapy during acute illness fails to aggravate the condition and that re-exposure to methotrexate is rarely associated with pneumonitis. It has been suggested that the timing of drug administration appears to affect the frequency of pulmonary reactions, with more frequent doses resulting in a higher rate of pulmonary toxicity.

Antibiotics. Nitrofurantoin and the sulfonamides have been associated with pulmonary injury. There are two types of reaction to nitrofurantoin: acute and chronic. The acute reaction is a pneumonitis and is felt to be caused by a cell-mediated immune process. Fever, chills, dyspnea, and cough may begin two hours to 10 days after a course of nitrofurantoin therapy is started. A diffuse alveolar or alveolar-interstitial infiltrate and pleural effusions can be seen on chest x-ray which clears within 24 to 48 hours after the drug is withdrawn.

The chronic reaction is a distinct clinical entity and occurs less commonly than the acute reaction. There is no fever, pleural effusion, or eosinophilia with this form of illness. In addition, there seems to be no relationship between the acute and chronic stages. The chronic form begins insidiously, six months to six years later, with cough and dyspnea. The chest roentgenogram shows a diffuse interstitial fibrosis. The fibrosis is at least partially reversible when the drug is withdrawn and corticosteroids are administered.

The sulfonamides have been implicated in the causation of vasculitis. In addition, a pulmonary infiltration with eosinophilia has been attributed to sulfonamide therapy.

Vasoactive Drugs. Methysergide is the only drug that can produce a chronic pulmonary effusion. The pulmonary injuries that have been described have involved the parenchyma as well as the pleural lining. Parenchymal damage has been due to aortic and mitral insufficiency, interstitial pneumonitis, and pulmonary fibrosis. Pleural changes consist of inflammation and fibrosis. The chest x-ray picture of pleural fibrosis consists of a fine, ground-glass haze over the lungs.

The onset of pulmonary complications is ordinarily insidious, with the patient having taken the drug for six months to several years before cough and dyspnea begin. In the early stage, the interstitial pneumonitis can regress if the drug is discontinued. Fibrotic changes, however, are nonreversible. Steroids may be tried if improvement following drug withdrawal does not occur.

RADIATION INJURY. Pulmonary radiation causes a pulmonary parenchymal reaction. Radiation therapy results in damage to those cells in the lung which reproduce most rapidly: capillary, endothelial, bronchial, and type II alveolar cells. Regeneration of these cells is impeded, and eventually fibrosis distorts the pulmonary architecture.

The severity of the reaction is influenced by the volume of the lung tissue radiated, the radiation dose-time product, the radiation dose-time quotient (rate of radiation), and the type of radiation administered. Radiation pneumonitis rarely occurs with a dose of less than 2000 rads, while doses in excess of 6000 rads given over five to six weeks will almost invariably lead to severe pneumonitis. Other variables that influence pulmonary damage include re-treatment, associated chemotherapy, and corticosteroid withdrawal.

The combination of all factors results in a 5 to 15 per cent incidence of respiratory symptoms in patients undergoing standard radiation therapy. When symptoms develop they usually occur from two to six months after therapy is completed. Symptoms of acute radiation pneumonitis usually consist of nonproductive cough, weakness, fever, and dyspnea. Shortness of breath is usually mild, but in some cases death can occur from respiratory insufficiency. Acute radiation pneumonitis may persist for up to a month and then either resolve or progress to chronic fibrosis. In a minority of patients, fibrosis develops insidiously without an acute phase being recognized.

Respiratory symptoms may occur without roentgenographic changes. X-ray changes that do appear occur from several weeks to two years following treatment. Acute radiation pneumonitis is manifested roentgenographically by consolidation of lung parenchyma, usually with loss of volume. The late or chronic stages of radiation damage are characterized by fibrosis. Extensive thickening of the pleura may also be present. Radiation fibrosis, if it occurs, is usually well established and stable nine to 12 months after the completion of radiation therapy.

Pulmonary function studies may be a more sensitive index of pulmonary damage than roentenographic evaluation. The major impairment in function is restrictive in nature; vital capacity and flow rates are reduced, the former to a proportionately greater degree. Diffusing capacity is decreased when a large volume of lung is involved; it may return to normal as the acute process subsides but more commonly remains decreased as fibrosis develops.

Anesthetic Considerations. Thorough preoperative assessment is necessary in this group of patients, since there is often a poor correlation between physical symptoms, the chest x-ray, and the results of pulmonary function testing. For specific agents such as x-ray treatment or bleomycin therapy, the amount or dose administered may give an indication of the likelihood of pulmonary damage being present. For other drugs, such as those associated with hypersensitivity, damage should begin to resolve once therapy has been discontinued. Procarbazine, a monoamine oxidase inhibitor, should be discontinued for at least two weeks preoperatively if at all possible. Since most of the drugs discussed above are used to treat neoplastic disease, a recent chest x-ray should be obtained to assess signs of pulmonary injury as well as evidence of metastatic disease or active infection. When significant pulmonary disease is suspected (by history) or evident (by clinical examination and chest x-ray), pulmonary function testing should be done, along with room air arterial blood gas analysis. If the patient has been receiving chronic steroid treatment and the possibility of adrenal suppression exists, exogenous steroids must be provided during the perioperative period. Finally, preoperative assessment should include other organ systems that might be affected by treatment with these drugs. For example, anemia and thrombocytopenia may be present as a result of bone marrow suppression.

Intraoperatively, most of these patients, if currently taking immunosuppressive agents, will be at increased risk of developing infection; strict adherence to aseptic techniques is therefore mandatory. Hypoxemia is avoided by using high inspired oxygen concentrations and monitoring arterial blood gases, when appropriate. If restrictive lung disease is present and ventilation is controlled, small tidal volumes with a rapid rate should be used in order to minimize inflation pressure. However, because of a decrease in lung compliance, relatively high inflation pressures may still be required to deliver even a small tidal volume. If cor pulmonale and pulmonary hypertension are present and large fluid shifts are expected, a pulmonary artery catheter may be necessary in order to monitor left-sided cardiac filling pressures. Anesthetic agents should be selected with regard to their potential to produce myocardial depression in this setting.

Patients treated with bleomycin deserve special comment. The incidence of pulmonary failure and death is increased in patients treated with bleomycin and radiation therapy even without operation. In a recent report on patients undergoing esophageal resection after receiving combined therapy of bleomycin and radiation, an alarmingly high incidence of postoperative respiratory failure leading to death was noted. The respiratory failure appeared from immediately after operation to as long as two weeks postoperatively (after some patients had been discharged from the hospital). At autopsy, pathological examination revealed severe interstitial pneumonitis. Other patients who received the same preoperative therapy but had only exploratory surgery did not experience postoperative pulmonary complications. The authors speculated that a possible mechanism of the pulmonary complications was that the preoperative therapy may have sensitized the lungs, while the subsequent surgical trauma triggered a reaction in the lungs leading to respiratory failure.

In another report, five patients received bleomycin without radiation therapy preoperatively, and all died shortly after surgery from respiratory failure secondary to interstitial pneumonia. The operation performed was not precisely stated. The patients who died were compared with a group of patients who received bleomycin without radiation therapy preoperatively but who underwent surgery without complications. In the patients who died, the intraoperative inspired oxygen concentration was 40 per cent, whereas in the patients who survived the intraoperative inspired oxygen concentration averaged 24 per cent. The authors theorized that bleomycin may sensitize the lungs to increased inspired oxygen concentrations (40%) and result in an "oxygen toxicity" response. The report further implies that survivors had more aggressive monitoring (pulmonary artery catheter intraoperatively) and stricter attention to fluid status than did nonsurvivors. At the present time it seems reasonable to place patients who have received bleomycin in therapy preoperatively, especially when combined with radiation therapy, in a high risk category. In addition to thorough preoperative evaluation, pulmonary artery catheter monitoring should be undertaken if fairly large fluid shifts are anticipated. The lowest inspired oxygen concentration necessary to avoid hypoxemia should be utilized and arterial blood gases monitored. The surgeons should attempt to minimize physical trauma to the lungs when working in the thorax. Postoperatively, patients should be watched closely in an intensive care unit for signs of developing adult respiratory distress syndrome.

Goodpasture's Syndrome and Idiopathic Hemosiderosis

General Description. Goodpasture's syndrome is a rare disease characterized by repeated episodes of pulmonary alveolar hemorrhage in association with glomerulonephritis. The disease occurs in young adults and has a striking male predominance. It has been reported in brothers, suggesting a familial occurrence.

Goodpasture's syndrome is an autoimmune disease. Patients with this disease have circulating antibodies against glomerular and alveolar basement membrane, and immunofluorescent studies have demonstrated deposition of IgG and complement in glomeruli and alveoli. The pulmonary lesions in Goodpasture's syndrome are caused by an antiglomerular basement membrane antibody that cross-reacts with lung basement membrane. Thus, bilateral nephrectomy usually, but not always, results in cessation of pulmonary hemorrhage in these patients and suggests that the kidneys play a primary role in the etiology of the disease.

The pathological picture is one of intra-alveolar hemorrhage that is typically confined to the peripheral air spaces. Other pathologic changes depend upon whether episodes of a similar nature have occurred previously. With repeated hemorrhages, some degree of organization of intra-alveolar blood may be present; interstitial fibrosis is apparent in most cases. Alveolitis and alveolar necrosis are absent unless secondary pneumonitis has been superimposed. Vasculitis, when present, is minor. As a result of hemorrhage, large quantities of iron in the form of hemosiderin may accumulate in the lungs, and an iron-deficiency anemia may result. In the kidneys, a proliferative type of glomerulonephritis is found.

X-ray changes that are seen depend in large measure on the extent of hemorrhage that has previously occurred. Early in the disease the pattern is one of diffuse mottled opacities representing patchy air space consolidation. The opacities are confluent in many areas, and air bronchograms may be observed in areas of major involvement. X-rays obtained over the several days after an acute episode characteristically show the fluffy deposits of acinar consolidation to be gradually replaced by a reticular pattern in the same distribution, indicating clearing of the air spaces of macrophages. Within two weeks, the x-ray returns to normal. With repeated episodes and increasing deposition of hemosiderin, progressive interstitial fibrosis is produced, as indicated by the persistence of a fine reticular pattern. Hilar lymph nodes may be enlarged; pleural effusion and pneumothorax are rare.

Hemoptysis is the most frequent presenting symptom. Exertional dyspnea, cough, weakness, fatigue, and lassitude occur late, along with hematuria. Substernal chest pain unrelated to activity may also occur. Physical findings are generally related to anemia and hypertension and include pallor, a systolic ejection murmur, hepatosplenomegaly, retinal hemorrhage, and edema. Signs and symptoms of renal and pulmonary involvement are not always present at the same time, and hemoptysis commonly precedes the clinical manifestations of renal disease by several months.

Laboratory investigation reveals anemia with a normal bone marrow examination. Urinalysis is usually abnormal, with proteinuria, hematuria, and cellular and granular casts. The white blood cell count is elevated in 50 per cent of cases, accompanied by a differential count showing a shift to the left. Azotemia eventually develops in most cases.

Pulmonary function tests are normal early in the disease, but as fibrosis occurs, they demonstrate a restrictive pattern. Diffusing capacity is reduced, and resting arterial PO_2 may be normal or low. Severe cases result in elevated pulmonary artery pressure with exercise.

Corticosteroid therapy has been employed widely in the treatment of Goodpasture's syndrome, although results have been disappointing in most cases. Cytotoxic and immunosuppressive drugs appear to be more promising therapeutic agents, particularly if therapy is instituted before severe impairment of renal function becomes manifest. A number of reports have documented disappearance of the pulmonary manifestations of Goodpasture's syndrome after hemodialysis or renal transplantation. Plasmapheresis has been employed to remove the pathogenic antibody.

The prognosis in Goodpasture's syndrome is poor. The mean duration of survival following diagnosis has been less than one year. However, individual case reports have documented prolonged survival for as long as 12 years when such techniques as renal transplantation or plasmapheresis are combined with cytotoxic therapy.

Idiopathic pulmonary hemosiderosis (IPH) is a disease of unknown etiology which has a pulmonary lesion similar to that which occurs in Goodpasture's syndrome. However, IPH differs from Goodpasture's syndrome in that renal disease and the demonstration of antiglomerular basement membrane antibody on immunofluorescence staining must be absent. Thus, immune mechanisms have not been incriminated in the etiology of IPH.

IPH is typically diagnosed in children below the age of 10; in this age group there is no sex predominance. When the disease appears in older patients, it occurs twice as often in men as in women. The pulmonary presentation of IPH is similar to that seen in Goodpasture's syndrome. Hemoptysis is the earliest symptom, and it is followed by dyspnea, lethargy, weakness, and cough. Some authors recognize two types of IPH: 1) recurrent acute episodes of intra-alveolar hemorrhage associated with the above symptoms, leading to progressive finger clubbing, hepatosplenomegaly, and icterus; and 2) a more insidious process, with more prolonged illness and milder exacerbations in which hemoptysis is manifested by intermittent blood streaking, and complete remissions are common. Myocarditis develops in a minority of patients. Results of the chest x-ray findings in IPH and Goodpasture's syndrome are similar. In addition, however, eosinophilia and cold agglutinins are seen in some patients with IPH.

Definitive diagnosis of IPH in young patients may require special techniques. Examinations of sputum for hemosiderin-laden macrophages provides supportive evidence. Radioactive chromium-labeled red blood cells may be injected and observed to accumulate within lung parenchyma. Lung biopsy may be obtained percutaneously, by transbronchial techniques, or by limited thoracotomy.

The prognosis of IPH is variable. Although steroids have been used to treat this illness, there is no specific therapy available. The average interval from onset of symptoms until death is less than three years; however, individual cases have survived for up to 20 years. Death has resulted from either massive hemoptysis, respiratory failure, or cor pulmonale.

Anesthetic Considerations. The anesthetic considerations in Goodpasture's syndrome begin with the preoperative evaluation of lung and kidney function and the detection of anemia. Room air arterial blood gas analysis, pulmonary function tests, urinalysis, electrolytes, BUN, serum creatinine, and complete blood count should be obtained.

Since pulmonary involvement may be episodic, elective operations should be performed when active hemorrhage is not present. If interstitial fibrosis has occurred, a restrictive defect to ventilation will be present. High inspired oxygen concentrations, small tidal volumes, and rapid respiratory rates will minimize but not prevent high inflation pressures during controlled ventilation. Intraoperative blood gas analysis should ensure adequate oxygenation.

Anemia, if severe, should be corrected preoperatively by blood transfusion. Although these patients have chronic anemia that may be compensated by an increased cardiac output, the presence of pulmonary disease puts them at a higher risk for inadequate oxygenation during surgery.

Renal considerations are discussed in the chapter on renal disease. Obviously, fluid and electrolyte status, the need for renal excretion of drugs, hypertension, coagulation defects, and other problems which accompany renal disease must be carefully considered.

If chronic steroid therapy has been utilized, perioperative coverage with exogenous steroids must be given. Immunosuppressive drug therapy dictates care in preventing infection by strict adherence to aseptic techniques.

The anesthetic considerations for patients with idiopathic pulmonary hemosiderosis are the same as those for Goodpasture's syndrome with the exception of the renal considerations, since the kidneys are normal in these patients.

Hypersensitivity to Organic Dusts — Extrinsic Allergic Alveolitis

General Description. Since "farmer's lung" was first described in 1924, a number of terms have described alveolar hypersensitivity to specific antigens contained in a wide variety of organic dusts, and include hypersensitivity pneumonitis, respiratory membrane hypersensitivity, and interstitial granulomatous pneumonitis. Similarities exist among the clinical, pathologic, and roentgenologic features of all of these diseases.

The development of alveolar hypersensitivity depends upon small antigenic particles (usually spores) reaching the alveoli in numbers sufficient to sensitize the patient, with production of antibodies that subsequently elicit an alveolitis. Identification of the major source of allergen (antigen) in farmer's lung (the spores of the thermophilic actinomyces, *Micropolysopa faeni*, found in moldy hay) has led to the discovery of an increasing number of similar diseases. The major examples are bagassosis, caused by the spores of *Thermoactinomyces vulgaris* in moldy sugarcane residue; mushroom-worker's lung, caused by the spores of both

T. vulgaris and *M. faeni* in mushroom compost; and malt-worker's lung, caused by the spores of *Aspergillus clavatus* and *Aspergillus fumigatus* in moldy barley and malt dust. Other related illnesses that have been described include bird-fancier's lung, maple bark disease, cheese-worker's lung, grain-weevil hypersensitivity, wood pulp-worker's lung, and detergent-worker's lung. The spores involved in all of these diseases are of the order of 6 microns or less in size, enabling them to penetrate the alveoli.

Pulmonary injury following exposure to organic dust antigens is caused by an immune-complex mechanism. Most patients suffering from these diseases have high titers of precipitating antibodies directed against the offending agents. Unexplained is the fact that many asymptomatic workers have the antibodies as well.

There are three pathologic stages recognized in these diseases. The acute stage consists primarily of bronchiolitis. Immuno-fluorescent study of the lung tissue reveals high concentrations of antibodies in the walls of involved bronchioles. The subacute stage, which occurs one to two months later, consists of noncaseating bronchial histiocytic granulomas closely resembling those seen in sarcoidosis, which cause obstructive bronchiolitis and alveolitis. A striking interstitial pneumonitis may also develop. In the chronic state, which occurs over the next several months, granulomas disappear, the lesions become nonspecific, and fibrosis supervenes. The end result is a variable mixture of scarring, pneumonitis, and emphysema.

The chest x-ray appearance parallels the severity of the disease. In the subacute state granular or nodular mottling is scattered diffusely throughout both lung fields. Acute exacerbations during this stage reveal acinar shadows and air space consolidation. If the patient is removed from the antigen, the chest x-ray may return to normal in several weeks. If exposure is continued or repeated, the diffuse nodular pattern is replaced by a medium to coarse reticular pattern indicative of parenchymal fibrosis. A "honeycomb" pattern is compatible with late fibrosis.

Symptoms usually develop within six to eight hours of exposure to organic dusts, and they commonly occur in the evening after a day's work close to the offending agent. Fever, chills, malaise, and generalized non-pleuritic chest pain are characteristic, together with a dry irritant cough and respiratory distress. Weight loss is common. In a small number of patients, usually those with a history of allergy, the clinical picture may suggest asthmatic bronchitis; the acute asthmatic episode develops within a few minutes of exposure, subsides slowly, and may be repeated as a "late" response some four to six hours after the initial episode of bronchospasm. Chronic exposure to the antigens in any of these patients results in progressive dyspnea, pulmonary hypertension, right heart strain, and failure.

Pulmonary function testing is helpful in diagnosing extrinsic allergic alveolitis, in that an aerosol "challenge" with the suspected antigen may cause an abrupt deterioration in these tests and thereby simulate the naturally occurring "acute" or provocative allergic response. In established disease with fibrosis, a nonreversible restrictive pattern develops, with reduced lung volumes, static compliance, and diffusing capacity.

Treatment of these diseases consists primarily of the removal of the patient from the environment that contains the offending agent. Acute stage changes are for the most part reversible, and adrenal corticosteroids are often helpful in hastening remission. Avoidance of re-exposure is of prime importance in preventing progression of the disease to chronic fibrosis.

Anesthetic Considerations. A restrictive pattern of pulmonary impairment is often present which, during controlled ventilation, requires the use of small tidal volumes and rapid ventilatory rates in order to minimize inspiratory pressure. However, ventilatory pressures should still be expected to be higher than normal owing to reduced lung compliance. High inspired oxygen concentrations should be used intraoperatively, and oxygenation should be monitored with blood gas determination.

If right heart failure exists, optimal management with cardiac glycosides and diuretics should be obtained preoperatively. In these patients, the need to minimize cardiac depression versus the need for a high inspired oxygen concentration will dictate the choice between a narcotic-based general anesthetic and a volatile anesthetic. Use of a pulmonary artery catheter is helpful in monitoring cardiovascular dynamics in response to anesthesia and surgery. In addition, pulmonary artery capillary wedge pressures are needed in patients with significant pulmonary hypertension when large intraoperative fluid shifts are anticipated.

OBSTRUCTIVE PULMONARY DISEASES

Cystic Fibrosis

General Description. Cystic fibrosis is the most common lethal genetic syndrome among white children. Most of the mortality in cystic fibrosis is due to pulmonary pathology, which also accounts for much of the chronic progessive pulmonary disease encountered in children. Approximately 5 per cent of most white populations are carriers of the cystic fibrosis gene. The incidence of cystic fibrosis in the United States among whites is approximately 1:2000; incidence in the non-white population is much lower. Nationally, there are believed to be 15,000 to 20,000 patients, and approximately 2000 of these are adults.

Evidence indicates that cystic fibrosis is transmitted as an autosomal recessive trait, suggesting a discrete biochemical or structural defect. However, to date no single lesion has been identified to account for all the pathophysiologic phenomena of cystic fibrosis. Obstruction of exocrine gland ducts or the passageways into which exocrine gland secretions are discharged is common to all patients with cystic fibrosis. Lack of water, alterations of electrolyte content, and abnormal organic constituents (especially mucous glycoproteins) have all been implicated in the pathogenesis of inspissated secretions. For example, cystic fibrosis secretions from several types of glands are relatively dehydrated, and sodium and chloride concentrations in the sweat are markedly elevated.

Mucociliary transport is a major pulmonary defense mechanism whereby natural debris, inhaled particulate matter, and bacteria are removed from the lung. Although a causal relation between impairment of mucociliary transport and the development of obstructive lung disease is difficult to prove, this assumption forms the basis for many of the therapeutic modalities employed in treating cystic fibrosis. The mechanism by which mucociliary transport is impaired in this syndrome is not yet known. Immunoglobin function appears to be normal in patients with cystic fibrosis; however, almost all these patients eventually develop chronic pulmonary infection. This implies a defect in local rather than systemic defense mechanisms. Impaired mucociliary transport undoubtedly contributes to increased bacterial colonization and eventual infection in the lung.

Since the diagnosis of cystic fibrosis rests on clinical criteria, it is more appropriate to classify it as a syndrome than as a disease. The manifestations of cystic fibrosis involve many organ systems, and the pattern of presentation is variable. Abnormalities of the respiratory gastrointestinal, genitourinary systems, and sweat glands account for the clinical picture.

Cystic fibrosis patients have normal lungs at birth. The earliest pulmonary lesion is hypertrophy and dilatation of bronchial glands and goblet cells; this is followed by mucous plugging of peripheral airways which, in turn, is followed by the development of bronchitis and bronchiolitis. A vicious cycle of obstruction, chronic infection, and continued tissue destruction develops. Bronchiolitis, bronchiectasis, fibrosis, and airway obstruction cause progressive loss of pulmonary function and eventually result in death. In many patients, bronchiectasis results in the development of a right peribronchial vascular network. The increased bronchial blood flow empties into the pulmonary venous circulation, resulting in right-to-left shunting and further compounding the problems of uneven distribution of ventilation and perfusion. Infection or trauma to this rich peribronchial vascular network can result in hemoptysis. The pulmonary involvement in cystic fibrosis is usually diffuse but is frequently worse in the lung apices. An occasional patient may develop severe bronchiectasis in a single lobe and benefit from lobectomy.

The most prominent and constant symptom of pulmonary involvement is cough. The cough is initially dry and hacking, but with progression of the disease it becomes productive. Decreased exercise tolerance and an increased respiratory rate occur with increasing severity of the disease. Airway obstruction with air trapping leads to increased anteroposterior diameter of the chest. Rales and rhonchi and signs of increased work of breathing (such as retractions and the use of accessory breathing muscles) are seen. Digital clubbing often accompanies respiratory involvement. Although the course of pulmonary disease is highly variable and greatly influenced by therapy, it tends to be progressive. Once bronchiectasis develops, the course usually accelerates with more frequent exacerbations, and the disease eventually culminates in respiratory failure, cor pulmonale, and death.

The upper airway is often involved in cystic fibrosis; chronic pansinusitis occurs in almost all patients. Nasal polyps are seen in 10 to 15 per cent and are a common cause for performing surgery. Mouth breathing in this situation is common and may interfere with the normal humidification of inspired air.

Gastrointestinal problems occur frequently in patients with cystic fibrosis, although they are usually overshadowed by the pulmonary pathology. From 7 to 25 per cent of patients with cystic fibrosis develop meconium ileus at birth. After the newborn period, malabsorption and manifestations of pancreatic insufficiency occur in 80 to 90 per cent of patients. Biliary disease of varying degree is found in a third of patients. Focal biliary cirrhosis with eosinophilic concretions in the intrahepatic ducts is present in approximately 25 per cent of patients. Older patients have an increased chance to develop diffuse cirrhotic changes, and some may evidence elevations of hepatic enzymes. Severe complications of liver disease, including liver failure and portal hypertension, occur in 2 to 3 per cent of patients.

Genitourinary manifestations of cystic fibrosis include a high rate of sterility in men and a low pregnancy rate for women. Sweat gland abnormalities are the most constant clinical finding in cystic fibrosis and result in a high rate of salt loss; excessive losses of salt and fluid may lead to severe dehydration in hot weather. Adults with cystic fibrosis have lower mean systolic and diastolic blood pressures, presumably due to chronic salt losses.

Pulmonary function testing closely reflects the pathophysiology of the disease. The earliest manifestation of pulmonary dysfunction in cystic fibrosis is an increased alveolar-arterial oxygen difference, which results from uneven distribution of ventilation perfusion and later from peribronchial shunting. As airway involvement progresses, large airway obstruction becomes manifest with decreases in maximal mid-expiratory flow, forced expiratory volume, and large airway closure during forced expi-

ration. Air trapping and loss of elastic recoil result in elevation of residual volume and functional residual capacity. The earliest radiologic signs of pulmonary disease due to cystic fibrosis are bronchial thickening and irregular areas of hyperinflation. Segmental or lobar atelectasis, cyst formation, extensive bronchiectasis, and extensive infiltrates are seen in advanced disease.

There are four criteria for the diagnosis of cystic fibrosis: 1) a positive sweat test (sweat chloride > 60 mEq per liter); 2) chronic obstructive pulmonary disease of varying degree, which is seen in a large majority of patients; 3) exocrine pancreatic insufficiency, noted in 80 to 90 per cent of patients; 4) family history, which is helpful but not always present. Most authorities require at least two of the above criteria for a diagnosis, and the diagnosis is rarely made in the absence of a positive sweat test.

Because pulmonary involvement leads to most of the morbidity and mortality resulting from cystic fibrosis, treatment centers on the lung. Annual influenza vaccination, protection from unnecessary exposure to infection, and avoidance of smoking are minimal preventive measures. Pulmonary infections are treated aggressively, with relatively long periods of antibiotic therapy after appropriate culture and sensitivity studies have been done. In some patients, continuous antimicrobial therapy is necessary. At present, *Pseudomonas* is the most common pathogen isolated from cystic fibrosis patients, although *H. influenza* is found frequently as well. Allergic aspergillosis and tuberculous infection are other pulmonary complications that occur. Mist-tent therapy, hydration, expectorant drugs, and intermittent aerosol therapy with phenylephrine, bronchodilators, and mucolytic agents have all been used with varying success to aid in mucociliary transport and productive coughing. Segmental postural drainage, assisted by chest clapping, vibration, and coughing, has gained widespread acceptance for the treatment of airway obstruction in patients with cystic fibrosis. These maneuvers may increase sputum production twofold over coughing alone and increase vital capacity and expiratory flow rates in selected patients. Treatment aimed at other organ involvement in this disease includes pancreatic enzyme replacement and vitamin and nutritional supplementation.

Several very aggressive treatments of the pulmonary disease in cystic fibrosis have been used. First, treatment of obstructive airway disease can include tracheobronchial suctioning and lavage. Bronchopulmonary lavage may be done via either a bronchoscope or a double-lumen endotracheal tube. At this time, bronchopulmonary lavage is a controversial treatment for this disease. (Anesthetic considerations for therapeutic bronchopulmonary lavage utilizing one lung anesthesia are discussed under pulmonary alveolar proteinosis, on pages 234–235.) Second, lobectomy may benefit some patients with severe lobar bronchiectasis. The other frequent indication for thoracic surgery in cystic fibrosis is recurrent pneumothorax. Third, respiratory failure is seen late in the course of the disease and is heralded by increased dyspnea, cyanosis, sputum production, and retention of CO_2. Short-term ventilatory support may usefully prolong life when acute infection is superimposed on only moderately severe respiratory disease. Although the endotracheal tube provides a route for suctioning, positive pressure ventilation may impact secretions in the smaller airways. Many physicians caring for patients with cystic fibrosis feel that endotracheal intubation is contraindicated in treating respiratory failure with advanced pulmonary involvement. Fourth, cor pulmonale may be seen late in the disease; treatment is aimed at relief of hypoxemia and cardiac support with diuretics and possibly digitalization.

Early diagnosis and the treatment regimen described above have resulted in longer life spans for patients with cystic fibrosis. The national survival rate is now 50 per cent at 16 years, and many special centers for cystic fibrosis report a 50 per cent patient survival well into the 20's. It appears that males have better survival rates than females, and the progression of their disease may be less rapid than that of females. Reasons for these differences are not known.

Anesthetic Considerations. Preoperative evaluation of patients with cystic fibrosis is important in minimizing postanesthetic morbidity. Optimal care is dependent upon cooperation between the pulmonologist, surgeon, and anesthesiologist. An attempt should be made to quantitate the severity of pulmonary disease present. The physical impairment that the patient suffers and the amount of sputum production are especially noteworthy. In most cases, pulmonary function testing should be undertaken and, when significant impairment is found, room air arterial blood gas analysis should be performed. If an extensive procedure is planned that could result in a prolonged postoperative course, the results of a preoperative sputum culture may aid in differentiating postoperative pulmonary infection from colonization. If hepatic involvement due to cystic fibrosis is suspected, liver function studies should be performed. If a nasal intubation is indicated, the patient should be evaluated for the presence of nasal polyps. Premedication should be individualized; anticholinergic drugs, which could cause inspissation of secretions in some patients, are probably best avoided unless strongly indicated. Glycopyrrolate has a greater drying effect than scopolamine or atropine. We favor light premedication or avoid it all together in order to hasten recovery from general anesthesia. If possible, the patient should receive chest physiotherapy immediately preceding the operation.

Intraoperative consideration begins with the type of anesthesia to be administered. Conduction techniques are indicated for extremity and perineal surgery. The types of general anesthetic agents utilized are determined in large part by the amount of pulmonary disease present and the potential need for high inspired oxygen concentrations. Halogenated volatile agents permit the use of a high inspired oxygen concentration, and, if the pulmonary disease is moderate, induction and recovery from general anesthesia should be rapid. On the other hand, if advanced pulmonary disease is present, induction and recovery may be prolonged by using inhalation techniques. If short-term postoperative ventilatory support is planned, deep balanced anesthesia with nitrous oxide and narcotics facilitates patient acceptance of an endotracheal tube postoperatively. If a lengthy operation is performed, an endotracheal tube should be inserted in order to facilitate intraoperative suctioning of secretions. Ventilation can be assisted or controlled to maintain lung expansion and minimize atelectasis. All anesthetic gases should be heated and humidified. At the conclusion of prolonged procedures in nonphysiological positions, appropriate postural drainage and tracheal suction should be performed in positions that counteract the possible intraoperative deleterious effects of gravity.

The ideal postoperative course consists of rapid emergence from anesthesia, early mobilization, and early resumption of chest physiotherapy. During or following thoracotomy, intercostal nerve blocks can be performed to aid in postoperative coughing and mobilization of secretions. All patients should be carefully monitored for signs of respiratory insufficiency. If a complicated course is encountered in the postoperative period, sputum or tracheal aspirate should be cultured frequently and daily chest x-rays obtained in order to aid in eary detection and treatment of pulmonary infection.

Alpha₁-antitrypsin Deficiency

General Description. Alpha₁-antitrypsin deficiency, first described in 1964, accounts for approximately 1 per cent of patients with emphysema. The disease is inherited by an autosomal codominant gene. It has been estimated that 4.7 per cent of the population are heterozygotes (carriers) and only 0.06 per cent homozygotes.

Alpha₁-antitrypsin is a glycoprotein that is synthesized in the liver and released into the serum in order to neutralize circulating proteolytic enzymes and thus prevent tissue damage. Alpha₁-antitrypsin deficiency results in the inability to avoid pulmonary elastolysis by proteolytic enzymes.

In these patients, emphysema occurs at an earlier age and is more severe than that seen from other causes. In emphysema associated with a normal alpha₁-antitrypsin level, alveolar destruction is most severe in the upper lobes. In severe alpha₁-antitrypsin deficiency, however, destruction of the lower lobes predominates. The clinical signs and symptoms of emphysema that occur with or without a deficiency of the enzyme are similar. Overinflation and hyperlucency of the parenchyma, flattening of the diaphragms, and obliteration of the pulmonary vasculature are seen on chest x-ray. Pulmonary function testing reveals loss of elastic recoil, air trapping, obstruction to air flow, and increased total lung volume and residual volume.

Anesthetic Considerations. Inherited alpha₁-antitrypsin deficiency should be suspected when severe clinical signs and symptoms of emphysema appear at an early age, especially in the absence of a history of smoking. The diagnosis can be supported by a family history and a roentgenologic picture showing predominantly lower lobe involvement. The diagnosis is confirmed by analysis of the serum level of alpha₁-antitrypsin. Preoperative evaluation should include room air arterial blood gas analysis and pulmonary function tests. Since obstruction to air flow is usually seen, the potential reversibility of this problem should be evaluated with the use of bronchodilators. If a reversible component exists, bronchodilator therapy should be considered. Therapeutic theophylline levels should be assured by serum analysis in very severe cases.

If ventilation is controlled, small tidal volumes and rapid respiratory rates should be used. Adequate oxygenation should be achieved with high inspired oxygen concentrations and confirmed by blood gas analysis.

Hypersensitivity to Organic Dusts — Aspergillosis and Byssinosis

General Description. The greatest incidence of fungus-induced hypersensitivity disease of the lung is caused by *Aspergillus fumigatus*; this illness is termed hypersensitivity bronchopulmonary aspergillosis. The majority of patients with this condition also have asthma and peripheral eosinophilia. There is an inverse relationship between the severity of the illness and the age of onset of asthma prior to the development of aspergillosis. There is no known sex or age predilection.

Inspissated mucoid impaction is the most common morphologic abnormality seen with this condition; it consists of the plugging of one or more orders of bronchi distal to the lobar bronchus, with resultant poststenotic dilation and distortion. Anatomic distribution shows bilateral upper lobe predominance.

The pathogenesis is not fully understood, but it appears likely that the primary abnormality is a constitutional defect that results in inspissated bronchial secretions. Immunologic mechanisms account for a good deal of the pathophysiology. *Aspergillus fumigatus* can grow in the secretions of the respiratory tract and release antigens that can be systemically absorbed without actual invasion of tissue by the fungi. Reaginic and precipitating antibodies are then produced against the aspergillus antigens. Local hypersensitivity reactions mediated by both antibodies result in sputum, peribronchial and systemic eosinophilia, inspissated secretions, and pulmonary infiltrates. Changes in the bronchi are often permanent, with replacement of respiratory epithelium by squamous epithelium.

The clinical features of this illness include fever, chills, malaise, weight loss, and productive cough. Wheezes and dyspnea are present in many patients. A surprising feature of the clinical picture is the comparatively mild symptomatology, sometimes associated with apparent (chest x-ray) extensive pulmonary disease. Indeed, some patients have no symptoms referable to the chest.

The dilated mucus-filled bronchi produce a distinctive roentgenographic pattern: homogeneous finger-like opacities of equal density situated in a bronchial distribution. When several bronchi in one lobe are involved, a grapelike appearance may be seen. Tomographic evaluation is useful in evaluating the extent and location of pulmonary involvement.

Laboratory evaluation reveals both sputum and serum eosinophilia. Pulmonary function testing shows an obstructive pattern along with decreased diffusing capacity.

Byssinosis is an occupational disease that occurs in workers involved in processing cotton, retted flax, and hemp fibers. Most of the reported cases have come from the United Kingdom. The incidence of the disease in the population at risk varies widely and is largely dependent upon the dust size and particle number that the workers are exposed to. In contrast to patients with hypersensitivity bronchopulmonary aspergillosis, a family history of atopy is unusual in these patients.

It is likely that some fraction of the offending dusts causes the nonantigenic release of histamine and perhaps other pharmacologically active substances; these substances, in turn, cause bronchoconstriction, cough, tightness in the chest, and breathlessness. These symptoms initially appear only occasionally on return to work after a weekend, with subsequent improvement during the working day. With progression of the disease the symptoms persist throughout the week, indicating irrevers-

ible ventilatory insufficiency. Finally, the disease becomes clinically indistinguishable from chronic bronchitis and emphysema and may eventually cause cor pulmonale.

Some patients demonstrate airflow obstruction even in the absence of symptoms; expiratory flow rates are always diminished in the presence of clinical disease. There are no specific radiologic abnormalities associated with byssinosis. Chest roentgenologic findings late in the illness are compatible with those seen in chronic bronchitis and emphysema.

The control of byssinosis lies in removal of the patient from the offending agent. Cigarette smoking aggravates symptoms in these patients and should be discontinued. Antihistamines may improve flow rates in byssinosis without necessarily providing subjective relief. In chronic cases, measures of value in the treatment of pulmonary emphysema and chronic bronchitis are indicated.

Anesthetic Considerations. An obstructive pattern of lung disease predominates in these conditions. Since there is often poor correlation with the chest x-ray, pulmonary function testing should be carried out preoperatively. Optimum medical management of any associated pulmonary conditions, such as asthma or chronic bronchitis, is necessary prior to surgery. Preoperative pulmonary toilette may improve lung function in cases where bronchial plugging is present. Antihistamines may be helpful in byssinosis.

The need for high inspired oxygen concentrations is dictated by the results of pre- and intraoperative blood gas analysis. Since the airways are often quite reactive, especially if asthma is present, manipulation of the airway should be minimized. When intubation is necessary, topicalization with lidocaine and the use of potent volatile halogenated agents decreases the response to this maneuver. The humidification and warming of anesthetic gases facilitates removal of mucus plugs by endotracheal tube suctioning.

BULLOUS DISEASE OF THE LUNG

General Description. A bulla is an air-filled, thin-walled space within the lung that results from destruction of alveolar tissue. The walls of bullae are formed by pleura, connective tissue septa, or compressed lung parenchyma. A bulla represents a local end stage area of emphysematous destruction.

The diagnosis of bullous disease of the lungs depends upon the roentgenologic identification of local thin-walled, sharply demarcated areas of avascularity in the chest. The walls characteristically appear as hairline shadows, but since the air cysts are most often at or near the lung surface, usually only a portion of the wall is visible. They tend to occur more frequently in the upper lobes of the lung. Tomography may provide improved visibility of a bulla already identified and may reveal bullae not even suspected on plain chest x-ray. Pulmonary arteriography occasionally permits even finer resolution of the disease.

In the majority of cases bullae enlarge progressively, although the rate of enlargement is not predictable. Occasionally, infection or hemorrhage into a bulla is apparent on chest x-ray by a fluid level within an air sac. Rarely, hemorrhage may be so massive as to require emergency surgery. Spontaneous pneumothorax commonly occurs in association with small apical blebs; less often, pneumothorax develops from large bullae involving the lower lobes.

Patients with bullae are often classified into two types: those with obstructive pulmonary disease and those with normal pulmonary parenchyma. The majority of bullae must be diagnosed by x-ray, since most do not cause symptoms or physical signs. However, the appearance of a single bulla in a severely dyspneic patient indicates that the bulla is accompanied by diffuse obstructive emphysema.

Primary bullous disease usually causes only minimal abnormality in pulmonary function, with airway resistance, vital capacity, and flow rates at near normal. Diffusing capacity may be decreased if adjacent lung parenchyma is severely compressed. In the majority of patients with primary bullous disease there is no clinical disability, and hence surgery is not indicated. Bullectomy is performed in severe cases wth depressed pulmonary function in order to allow healthy lung to expand into the area occupied by the bullae. In these cases, pulmonary function testing often reveals significant improvement postoperatively.

Patients with bullae and chronic obstructive pulmonary disease are not different clinically from patients with chronic lung disease without bullae. Thus, pulmonary function studies show reduction in flow rates, increased functional residual capacity and residual volume, impaired mixing efficiency, and decreased diffusing capacity. Pulmonary artery pressures generally increase in these patients during exercise (in contrast to the normal pressures seen in the bullous disease patients without chronic lung disease). In this group of patients, surgical intervention does not often result in dramatic clinical improvement, although favorable changes in pulmonary function tests and arterial blood gases should occur.

Anesthetic Considerations. Specific anesthetic consideration will vary, depending on the presence or absence of underlying lung disease. In bullous disease associated with chronic obstructive pulmonary disease a high inspired oxygen concentration is needed. When ventilation is controlled, prolonged expiratory time may be necessary to permit emptying of alveoli.

Some large bullae may communicate with a bronchus. When exposed to positive pressure ventilation these bullae may enlarge via a ball-valve mechanism or rupture, causing a pneumothorax. Either an expanding bulla or tension pneumothroax could impair venous return to the heart and cause circulatory impairment in addition to further compromising ventilation. Thus it is best, if possible, to avoid positive-pressure ventilation until the chest is open. Intubation, then, should be performed while the patient is spontaneously breathing, either anesthetized or awake with the airway topicalized. A potent inhalation agent will allow the use of a high inspired concentration of oxygen. If disease is confined to one hemithorax, a double-lumen endotracheal tube can be utilized to isolate the affected lung and provide positive-pressure ventilation if necessary. Because of the rapidity with which closed air spaces take up nitrous oxide and expand in size, this gas should be avoided in patients with large noncommunicating lung air cysts.

ISOLATION PRECAUTIONS FOR THE PATIENT WITH ACTIVE TUBERCULOSIS

It is not within the scope of this chapter to discuss pulmonary infections. However, occasionally a patient is brought to the operating room requiring an anesthetic who has suspected or known tuberculosis that is only partially treated. Because cross infection from the patient to the population at large poses a serious risk, a discussion of the anesthetic consideration for isolation of patients with *active* tuberculosis is included here.

Conservative guidelines dictate three weeks as a safe interval of combined chemotherapy prior to the abandonment of respiratory isolation precautions. After this period, patients are considered noninfectious even though bacilli may still be seen in smears and grown in cultures. In general, precautions that are used in dealing with patients with active tuberculosis include a combination of the use of disposable equipment, bacterial filters, disinfection of nondisposable equipment after use, and minimizing patient contact with non-essential items.

Although it constitutes an added expense, the easiest and surest way of minimizing the spread of bacilli to other patients is the use of disposable anesthetic equipment. A disposable circle system composed of inspiratory and expiratory tubes, Y-piece connector, endotracheal tube, CO_2 absorber, and mask are available commercially and should be utilized. Bacterial filters (0.22 μ pore size) should be inserted on the patient side of the unidirectional valves if a disposable CO_2 absorber is not available. The ventilation can be protected by a filter on the hose leading to it. The use of bacterial filters increases the resistance in the breathing circuit progressively with time; filters should be changed if the operation lasts over eight hours. After the operation is over, all disposable equipment used should be immediately placed into airtight plastic bags.

If disposable equipment is not available, a system that is easily disassembled and sterilized, such as a Magill circuit, should be employed. Although bacterial filters may also be used, prevention of contamination of nondisposable items cannot be guaranteed. Consequently, all items that are to be reused must be disinfected individually after the operation. Immediately after use and while still in the operating room, articles should be submerged in a fresh solution of an alkaline detergent-germicide and soaked for 30 minutes. The articles should then be hand dried and packaged by a gowned and gloved worker. Complete sterilization is then carried out either by heat or gas techniques. Glass and metal parts can be either autoclaved or gas sterilized. Items that are not heat stable, such as electrical equipment, suction apparatus, endoscopy equipment, and rubber and plastic items, must be gas sterilized with ethylene oxide. Adequate aeration (24 hours) is necessary before these items are reused. An alternative for gas or heat sterilization is disinfection by soaking in a gluteraldehyde solution for 30 minutes after cleaning. Surfaces that have not had direct exposure, such as the anesthesia machine, anesthesia cart, gas tanks, and monitoring equipment, must be cleaned with a chemical disinfectant. Solutions that may be used include iodophors, ethyl and isopropyl alcohol, synthetic or substituted phenols, and quaternary ammonium compounds combined with alcohol. Seventy per cent ethyl alcohol is the most commonly used disinfectant.

General measures aimed at minimizing patient exposure to non-essential items should be attempted. All unnecessary equipment should be removed from the operating room prior to the patient's arrival. The patient should wear a mask whenever possible. If a regional technique is feasible, it may save considerable work in cleaning equipment. If a general anesthetic is administered, intraoral manipulation should be kept to a minimum. Everthing that comes in contact with the patient should be placed individually in a disposable plastic bag or germicide solution. Finally, all personnel in the operating room should wear disposable gloves, gown, hat, and shoe covers and leave them in the operating room at the end of the operation. A double mask for the anesthesiologist affords added protection from wetting by sweating, saliva, or patient secretions. Finally, the scrub suit should be changed prior to taking care of other patients.

REFERENCES

Pulmonary Embolism

Moser, K. M.: Pulmonary embolism. Am. Rev. Resp. Dis. 115:829, 1977.

Alpert, J. S., Smith, R., Carlson, J., et al.: Mortality in patients treated for pulmonary embolism. J.A.M.A. 236:1477, 1976.

Alpert, J. S., Smith, R. E., Ockene, I. S., et al.: Treatment of massive pulmonary embolism: The role of pulmonary embolectomy. Am. Heart J. 89:413, 1975.

Primary Pulmonary Hypertension

Tsagaris, T. J., and Tikoff, G.: Familial primary pulmonary hypertension. Am. Rev. Resp. Dis. 97:127, 1968.

Sleeper, J. C., Orgain, E. S., and McIntosh, H. D.: Primary pulmonary hypertension. Review of clinical features and pathologic physiology with a report of pulmonary hemodynamics derived from repeat catheterizations. Circulation 26:1358, 1962.

Walcott, G., Burchell, H. B., and Brown, A. L., Jr.: Primary pulmonary hypertension. Am. J. Med. 49:70, 1970.

Klinke, W. P., and Gilbert, J. A. L.: Diazoxide in primary pulmonary hypertension. N. Engl. J. Med. 302:91, 1980.

Rubin, L. J., and Peter, R. H.: Oral hydralazine therapy for primary pulmonary hypertension. N. Engl. J. Med. 302:69, 1980.

Arteriovenous Fistula of the Lung

Gomes, M. M. R., and Bernatz, P. E.: Arteriovenous fistulas: A review and ten-year experience at the Mayo Clinic. Mayo. Clin. Proc. 45:81, 1970.

Ellman, P., and Hanson, A.: Pulmonary arteriovenous aneurysm. Br. J. Dis. Chest 53:165, 1959.

Björk, V. O., Intoni, F., Aletras, H., et al.: Varieties of pulmonary arteriovenous aneurysms. Acta Chir. Scand. 125:69, 1963.

Pulmonary Alveolar Proteinosis

Genereux, G. P.: Lipids in the lungs: Radiologic-pathologic correlation. J. Canad. Assoc. Radiol. 21:2, 1970.

Busque, L.: Pulmonary lavage in the treatment of alveolar proteinosis. Canad. Anaesth. Soc. J. 24:380, 1977.

Lippman, M., Mok, M. S., and Wasserman, K.: Anesthetic management for children with alveolar proteinosis using extra-corporeal circulation. Br. J. Anaesth. 49:173, 1977.

Blenkarn, G. D., Lanning, C. F., Kylstra, J. A.: Anesthetic management of volume controlled unilateral lung lavage. Canad. Anaesth. Soc. J. 22:154, 1975.

Eosinophilic Lung Disease

Chusid, M. J., Dale, D. C., West, B. C., et al.: The hypereosinophilic syndrome: Analysis of fourteen cases with review of the literature. Medicine 54:1, 1975.

Carrington, C. B., Addington, W. W., Goff, A. M., et al.: Chronic eosinophilic pneumonia. N. Engl. J. Med. 280:787, 1969.

Wegener's Granulomatosis

Wolff, S. M., Fauci, A. S., Horn, R. G., et al.: Wegener's granulomatosis. Ann. Intern. Med. 81:513, 1974.

Israel, H. L., and Patchefsky, A. S.: Wegener's granulomatosis of lung: diagnosis and treatment. Ann. Intern. Med. 74:881, 1971.

Fauci, A. S., and Wolff, S. M.: Wegener's granulomatosis: Studies in eighteen patients and review of the literature. Medicine 52:535, 1973.

Lake, C. L.: Anesthesia and Wegener's granulomatosis: Case report and review of the literature. Anesth. Analg. 57:353, 1978.

Sarcoidosis

Schatz, M., Patterson, R., and Fink, J.: Immunologic lung disease. N. Engl. J. Med. 300:1310, 1979.

James, D. G.: Modern concepts of sarcoidosis. Chest 64:675, 1973.

Levinson, R. S., Metzger, C. F., and Stanley, N. N.: Airway function in sarcoidosis. Am. J. Med. 62:51, 1977.

James, D. G., Neville, E., and Walker, A.: Immunology of sarcoidosis. Am. J. Med. 59:388, 1975.

Mitchell, D. N., and Scadding, J. G.: Sarcoidosis. Am. Rev. Resp. Dis. 110:774, 1974.

Collagen or Connective Tissue Diseases of the Lung

Huang, C. T., and Lyons, H. A.: Comparison of pulmonary function in patients with systemic lupus erythematosus, scleroderma, and rheumatoid arthritis. Am. Rev. Resp. Dis. 93:865, 1966.

Matthay, R. A., Schwartz, M. I., Petty, T. L., et al.: Pulmonary manifestations of systemic lupus pneumonitis. Medicine 54:397, 1975.

Popper, M. S., Bogdonoff, M. L., and Hughes, R. L.: Insterstitial rheumatoid lung disease. A reassessment and review of the literature. Chest 62:243, 1972.

Weaver, A. L., Divertie, M. B., and Titus, J. L.: Pulmonary scleroderma. Dis. Chest 54:490, 1968.

Lewis, G. B. H.: Prolonged regional analgesia in scleroderma. Canad. Anaesth. Soc. J. 21:495, 1974.

Jenkins, L. C., and McGraw, R. W.: Anesthetic management of the patient with rheumatoid arthritis. Canad. Anaesth. Soc. J. 10:407–415, 1969.

Walker, W. C., and Wright, V.: Diffuse interstitial pulmonary fibrosis and rheumatoid arthritis. Ann. Rheum. Dis. 28:252, 1969.

Histiocytosis X

Zinkham, W. H.: Multifocal eosinophilic granuloma, natural history, etiology, and management. Am. J. Med. 60:457, 1976.

Enriquez, P., Dahlin, D. C., Hayles, A. B., et al.: Histiocytosis X: A clinical study. Mayo Clin. Proc. 42:88, 1967.

Carlson, R. A., Hattery, R. R., O'Connell, E. J., et al.: Pulmonary involvement by histiocytosis X in the pediatric age group. Mayo Clin. Proc. 51:542, 1976.

Laios, N. C., and Lovelock, F. J.: Eosinophilic granuloma of the lung. Am. Rev. Resp. Dis. 83:394, 1961.

Idiopathic Pulmonary Fibrosis: Hamman-Rich Syndrome

Crystal, R. G., Fulmer, J. D., Roberts, W. C., et al.: Idiopathic pulmonary fibrosis: Clinical, histologic, radiographic, physiologic, scintigraphic, cytologic, and biochemical aspects. Ann. Intern. Med. 85:769, 1976.

Liebow, A. A., Steer, A., Billingsley, J. G.: Desquamative interstitial pneumonia. Am. J. Med. 39:369, 1965.

Carrington, C. B., Gaensler, E. A., Coutu, R. E., et al.: Usual and desquamative interstitial pneumonia. Chest 69 (Suppl.):261, 1976.

Pneumonoconiosis

Ziskind, M., Jones, R. N., and Weill, H.: Silicosis. Am. Rev. Resp. Dis. 113:643, 1976.

Gaensler, E. A., Carrington, C. B., Coutu, R. F., et al.: Pathological, physiological, and radiological correlations in the pneumoconioses. Ann. N.Y. Acad. Sci. 200:574, 1972.

Kleinfield, M., Messite, J., and Shapiro, J.: Clinical, radiological, and physiological findings in asbestosis. Arch. Intern. Med. 117:813, 1966.

Morgan, W. K. C., and Lapp, N. L.: Respiratory disease in coal miners. Am. Rev. Resp. Dis. 113:531, 1976.

Drug-Induced Pulmonary Disease

Rosenow, E. C.: The spectrum of drug-induced pulmonary disease. Ann. Intern. Med. 77:977, 1972.

Green, M. R.: Pulmonary toxicity of antineoplastic agents (Medical Progress). West. J. Med. 127:292, 1977.

Ansell, G.: Radiological manifestations of drug-induced disease. Clin. Radiol. 20:133, 1969.

Prato, F. S., Kurdyak, R., Saibil, E. A., et al.: Physiological and radiological assessment during the development of pulmonary radiation fibrosis. Radiology 122:389, 1977.

Cooper, G., Jr., Guerrant, J. L., Harden, A. G., et al.: Some consequences of pulmonary irradiation. Am. J. Roentgenol. 85:865, 1961.

Gross, N. J.: Pulmonary effects of radiation therapy. Ann. Intern. Med. 86:81, 1977.

Goldiner, P. L., and Schweizer, O.: The hazards of anesthesia and surgery in bleomycin-treated patients. Semin. Oncol. 6:121, 1979.

Nygaard, K., Smith-Erichsen, N., Hatlevoll, R., et al.: Pulmonary complications after bleomycin, irradiation, and surgery for esophageal cancer. Cancer 41:17, 1978.

Goodpasture's Syndrome and Idiopathic Pulmonary Hemosiderosis

Proskey, A. K., Weatherbee, L., Easterling, R. E., et al.: Goodpasture's syndrome: A report of five cases and review of the literature. Am. J. Med. 48:162, 1970.

Repetto, G., Lisboa, C., Emparanza, E., et al.: Idiopathic pulmonary hemosiderosis. Pediatrics 40:24, 1967.

Lockwood, C. M., Rees, A. J., Peterson, T. A., et al.: Immunosuppression and plasma-exchange with treatment of Goodpasture's syndrome. Lancet 1:711, 1976.

Hypersensitivity to Organic Dusts

Gilbert, T. M., and Patterson, R.: Pulmonary allergic aspergillosis. Ann. Intern. Med. 72:395, 1970.

Hargreave, F. E. (Review Article): Extrinsic allergic alveolitis. Canad. Med. Assoc. J. 108:1150, 1973.

Cystic Fibrosis

Wood, R. E., Boat, T. F., and Doershuk, C. F.: Cystic fibrosis. Am. Rev. Resp. Dis. 113:833, 1976.

Landau, L. I., and Phelan, P. D.: The spectrum of cystic fibrosis. A study of pulmonary mechanics in 46 patients. Am. Rev. Resp. Dis. 108:593, 1973.

Beier, F. R., Renzitti, A. D., Mitchell, M., et al.: Pulmonary pathophysiology in cystic fibrosis. Am. Rev. Resp. Dis. 94:430, 1966.

Salanitre, E., Klonymus, D., and Rackow, H.: Anesthetic experience in children with cystic fibrosis of the pancreas. Anesthesiology 25:801, 1964.

Schwachman, H., and Smith, R. M.: Case history: Cystic fibrosis, problems of management. Anesth. Analg. 44:140, 1965.

Doershuk, C. F., Reyes, A. L., and Regan, A. G.: Anesthesia and surgery in cystic fibrosis. Anesth. Analg. 51:413, 1972.

Alpha₁-antitrypsin Deficiency

Stevens, P. M., Hnilica, V. S., Johnson, P. C., et al.: Pathophysiology of hereditary emphysema. Ann. Intern. Med. 74:672, 1971.

Lieberman, J.: Heterozygous and homozygous alpha₁-antitrypsin deficiency in patient with pulmonary emphysema. N. Engl. J. Med. 281:270, 1969.

Hepper, N. G., Black, L. F., Gleich, G. J., et al.: The prevalence of alpha₁-antitrypsin deficiency in selected groups of patients with chronic obstructive lung disease. Mayo Clin. Proc. 44:697, 1969.

Bullous Disease of the Lung

Tinker, J., Vandam, L., and Cohn, L. H.: Tension lung cyst as a complication of postoperative positive pressure ventilation therapy. Chest 64:518, 1973.

Eger, E. I. II, and Saidman, L. J.: Hazards of nitrous oxide anesthesia with bowel obstruction and pneumothorax. Anesthesiology, 26:61, 1965.

Isenhower, N., Cucchiara, R. F.: Anesthesia for vanishing lung syndrome: Report of a case. Anesth. Analg. 55:750, 1976.

Viola, A. R., and Zuffardi, E. A.: Physiologic and clinical aspects of pulmonary bullous disease. Am. Rev. Resp. Dis. 94:574, 1966.

Lopex-Majano, V., Kieffer, R. F., Jr., Marine, D. N., et al.: Pulmonary resection in bullous disease. Am. Rev. Resp. Dis. 99:554, 1969.

Isolation Precautions for the Patient with Active Tuberculosis

The expert's opine. Surv. Anesth. 22:587, 1978.

Johnston, R. F., and Wildrich, K. H.: The impact of chemotherapy on the care of patients with tuberculosis. Am. Rev. Resp. Dis. 109:638, 1974.

Lumley, J.: Decontamination of anesthetic equipment and ventilators. Br. J. Anaesth. 48:3–8, 1976.

7

Cardiac Diseases

By JAMES L. BROOKS, Jr., M.D.,
and JOEL A. KAPLAN, M.D.

Introduction
Cardiomyopathies
  General Classification
Coronary Artery Disease
  Review of Physiology of Coronary Artery
    Disease and Its Modification by
    Unusual Disease
Pulmonary Hypertension and Cor
  Pulmonale
  Pulmonary Hypertension
  Cor Pulmonale
Constrictive Pericarditis and Cardiac
  Tamponade

Constrictive Pericarditis
Cardiac Tamponade
Valvular Lesions
  Aortic Stenosis
  Pulmonic Stenosis
  Aortic Insufficiency
  Pulmonic Insufficiency
  Mitral Stenosis
  Tricuspid Stenosis
  Mitral Regurgitation
  Tricuspid Insufficiency
Conclusion

INTRODUCTION

The anesthetic management of uncommon cardiovascular disease states differs in no fundamental way from the management of the more familiar ones, since it rests on the same precepts of management. These include: 1) understanding the disease process and how it manifests itself in the patient; 2) a thorough understanding of anesthetic and adjuvant drugs, including their cardiovascular effects; 3) the proper use of monitoring; and 4) an understanding of the requirements of the surgical procedure.

Certainly, the most common major cardiovascular diseases encountered are arteriosclerotic coronary artery disease, rheumatic valvular disease, and essential hypertension. Experience with these disease states has made the anesthesiologist familiar with both the pathophysiology and the management of cardiac patients. While the disease states discussed in this chapter are not often encountered, we have endeavored to show not how unusual these uncommon diseases are but rather how, in many circumstances, they can be reduced to very familiar patterns of physiology and pathophysiology.

The principle of understanding a disease state and how it manifests itself in a patient remains the same whether the disease is common or uncommon. An evaluation of the degree of cardiovascular involvement using available clinical and laboratory information is necessary to make a rational assessment of the disease state in each individual patient. A thorough understanding of the cardiovascular effects of the anesthetic and adjuvant drugs to be employed allows the patient to be managed using a rational anesthetic plan. Recent advances in understanding of the cardiovascular pharmacology of anesthetic drugs and new techniques of circulatory support (e.g., afterload reduction) have provided great flexibility in the management of the patient with impaired cardiovascular function. The use of hemodynamic monitoring provides the best guide to intra- and postoperative treatment of patients with uncommon cardiovascular diseases. Monitoring is certainly no substitute for an understanding of physiology and pharmacology or clinical judgment, rather the monitoring provides information that facilitates clinical decisions. Since the diseases to be discussed are rarely seen, extensive knowledge of their pathophysiology, particularly in the anesthetic and surgical setting, is largely lacking, and monitoring helps bridge this gap. An understanding of the requirements of the surgical procedure is necessary in all operations in order to anticipate intraoperative problems, but especially in the diseases considered here. The anesthesiologist must communicate with the surgeon during the procedure, since the surgeon himself may be encountering the disease for the first time.

This section does not provide an exhaustive list or consideration of all the uncommon diseases that affect the cardiovascular system, though it covers a wide range. Rather than an encyclopedic treatment of every disease that could affect the cardiovascular system, we have made the assumption that no matter how bizarre a disease entity is, it can only affect the cardiovascular system in a limited number of ways. It can affect the myocardium, the coronary arteries, the pulmonary circulation, and/or the valves, or it can impair cardiac filling. Subsections in this chapter follow this basic pattern. Under each section are lists of uncommon diseases that may produce a cardiomyopathy, coronary artery disease, pulmonary hypertension, or other cardiac disorder, along with various comments and *caveats* for each disease. This method of presentation provides a reasonable approach to any uncommon disease, how to consider it, and how to prepare for its anesthetic management.

CARDIOMYOPATHIES

GENERAL CLASSIFICATION

Diseases of the myocardium can be classified in a number of ways. On an etiologic basis, they are usually thought of as primary myocardial diseases, in which the basic disease locus is the myocardium itself, and secondary myocardial disease, in which the myocardial pathology is associated with some systemic disorder. On a pathophysiologic basis, myocardial disease can be bro-

ken down into three categories: congestive, obstructive and restrictive. Unfortunately, there is often not a sharp division among these three pathophysiologic states, and a particular patient may have features suggestive of any or all three of the categories. Congestive cardiomyopathy encompasses both inflammatory and noninflammatory forms, and its most prominent clinical feature is myocardial failure manifested as ventricular dilatation, elevated filling pressure, and pulmonary edema. This, for example, is the usual response in cases of severe myocarditis. The obstructive form of myocardial diseases consists of hypertrophy of the myocardial muscle and it occurs in two forms: 1) a familial form of *concentric* hypertrophy, usually of the entire left ventricle, and 2) a sporadic form of *asymmetric* hypertrophy, usually of the left ventricular septal wall. The asymmetric type is the so-called idiopathic hypertrophic subaortic stenosis (IHSS). Restrictive cardiomyopathy usually results from an infiltration of the myocardium by fibrous tissue or some other substance that decreases the compliance of the ventricle and impedes filling. It usually presents a picture that mimics the physiology of constrictive pericarditis, often coupled with myocardial failure due to loss of muscle mass.

Congestive Cardiomyopathy

Congestive cardiomyopathy exists in both an inflammatory and a noninflammatory form (Tables 7-1 and 7-2).

The *inflammatory* variety, or myocarditis, is usually the result of infection or parasitic infestation. Myocarditis presents the clinical picture of fatigue, dyspnea, and palpitations usually in the first weeks of the infection, progressing to overt congestive heart failure with cardiac dilatation, tachycardia, pulsus alternans, and pulmonary edema. Between 10 and 33 per cent of patients with infectious heart diseases will have at least electrocardiographic evidence of myocardial involvement. Mural thrombi often form in the ventricular cavity and may result in systemic or pulmonary emboli. Supraventricular and ventricular arrhythmias are common. Complete recovery from infectious myocarditis is the rule, but there are exceptions such as myocarditis associated with diphtheria or Chagas' disease. Occasionally, acute myocarditis may even pro-

Table 7-1 *Cardiomyopathies (Congestive)*

Disease Process	Mechanism	Associated Circ. Problems	Misc.
Inflammatory (Myocarditis)			
1. Bacterial			
a. Diphtherial	Endotoxin competitive analogue of cytochrome B	Arrhythmias, ST-T wave changes 1. Conduction system, especially BBB 2. Rare, valvular endocarditis	Temporary pacing often required
b. Typhoid	Inflammatory changes* with fiber degeneration	1. Arrhythmias 2. Endarteritis, endocarditis, pericarditis, ventricular rupture	
c. Scarlet fever β hemolytic strep	Inflammatory changes	Conduction disturbances and arrhythmias	
d. Meningococcus	Inflammatory changes and endotoxin, generalized and coronary thrombosis	1. Disseminated intravascular coagulation 2. Peripheral circulatory collapse (Waterhouse-Frederickson)	
e. Staphylococcus	Sepsis, acute endocarditis	Endocarditis, pericarditis	
f. Brucellosis	Fiber degeneration and granuloma formation		
g. Tetanus	Inflammatory changes, cardiotoxin	Severe arrhythmias	Apnea
h. Melioidosis	Myocardial abscesses		
2. Spirochaetal Leptospirosis a. Syphilis	Focal hemorrhage and inflammatory changes	1. Severe arrhythmias 2. Endocarditis and pericarditis	Temporary pacing
3. Rickettsial a. Endemic typhus b. Epidemic typhus	Inflammatory changes Symptoms secondary to vasculitis and hypertension	ECG changes, pericarditis Arrhythmia Vasculitis	
4. Viral a. Cocksackie B	Inflammatory changes	Usually only ECG abnormality 1. Constrictive pericarditis 2. AV-nodal arrhythmias	
b. Echovirus Mumps Influenza Infectious mononucleosis Viral hepatitis Rubella Rubeola	Inflammatory changes 1. Primary atypical pneumonia — associated Stokes-Adams attacks 2. Herpes simplex — associated with intractable shock 3. Arbovirus — constrictive pericarditis is reported sequela	1. Arrhythmia 2. Heart block 3. Pericarditis	

Rabies
Varicella
Lymphocytic choriomeningitis
Psittacosis
Viral encephalitis
Cytomegalovirus
Variola
Herpes zoster

5. Mycoses
  a. Cryptococcosis
    Blastomycosis
    Actinomycosis
  b. Coccidioidomycosis
	Usually obstructive symptoms
	Reported congestive heart failure
		Valvular obstruction
		Constrictive pericarditis	

6. Protozoal a. Trypanosomiasis (Chagas' disease — see text)	1. Inflammatory changes 2. Neurotoxin of *T. cruzi*	1. Severe arrhythmia secondary to conduction system degeneration 2. Mitral and tricuspid insufficiency secondary to cardiac enlargement	Pacing often required
b. Sleeping sickness	Inflammatory changes		Unusual manifestations of disease
c. Toxoplasmosis	Inflammatory changes	Cardiac tamponade	
d. Leishmaniasis Balantidiasis	Inflammatory changes		Unusual manifestations
7. Helminthic Trichinosis	Inflammatory changes Usually secondary to adult or ova infestation of myocardium or coronary insufficiency second to same		
Schistosomiasis Filariasis	Cor pulmonale — secondary pulmonary hypertension	Arrhythmias	

*Inflammatory type usually has myofiber degeneration, inflammatory cell infiltration, edema.

Table 7-2 *Cardiomyopathies (Congestive)*

Disease Process	Mechanism	Associated Circ. Problems	Misc.
Non-Inflammatory Congestive Cardiomyopathy			
1. Nutritional disorders			
a. Beriberi	Thiamine deficiency Inflammatory changes	1. Peripheral A-V shunting with low SVR 2. Usually high output failure with decreased SVR, but low output with normal SVR may occur	
b. Kwashiorkor	Protein deprivation	Degeneration of conduction system	
2. Metabolic disorders			
a. Amyloidosis	Amyloid infiltration of myocardium	1. Associated with restrictive and obstructive forms of cardiomyopathy 2. Valvular lesions 3. Conduction abnormalities	
b. Pompe's disease Glycogen storage disease type II	Alpha glucuronidase deficiency Glycogen accumulation in cardiac muscle	Septal hypertrophy	
c. Hurler's syndrome	Accumulation of glycoprotein in coronary tissue and parenchyma of heart	Mitral regurgitation	
d. Hunter's syndrome	Same	Similar but milder than Hurler's	
e. Primary xanthomatosis	Xanthomatosis infiltration of myocardium	1. Aortic stenosis 2. Advanced coronary artery disease	
f. Uremia	Multiple metastatic coronary calcifications Hypertension Electrolyte imbalance	1. Anemia 2. Hypertension 3. Conduction defects 4. Pericarditis and cardiac tamponade	Most cardiac manifestations dramatically improve after dialysis
g. Fabry's disease	Abnormal glycolipid metabolism secondary to ceramide trihexosidase with glycolipid infiltration of myocardium	1. Hypertension 2. Coronary artery disease	
3. Hematologic diseases			
a. Leukemia	Leukemic infiltration of myocardium	1. Arrhythmias 2. Pericarditis	
b. Sickle cell	Intracoronary thrombosis with ischemic cardiopathy	1. Coronary artery disease 2. Cor pulmonale	Usually resolve with successful therapy

Disease	Mechanism	Cardiac Manifestation	Comments
4. Neurologic disease			
a. Duchenne's muscular dystrophy	Muscle fiber degeneration with fatty and fibrous replacement	Conduction defects possibly secondary to small vessel coronary artery disease	50% incidence of cardiac involvement
b. Friedreich's ataxia	Similar to Duchenne's with collagen replacement of degenerating myofibers	1. Conduction abnormalities 2. ? IHSS	
c. Roussy-Lévy hereditary polyneuropathy	Similar to Friedreich's		
d. Myotonia atrophica	Similar to above	Conduction abnormalities, possibly Stokes-Adams attacks	
5. Chemical and toxic			
a. Ethyl alcohol (see text)	Myofiber degeneration secondary to direct toxic effect of ETOH and/or acetaldehyde		
b. Beer drinker's cardiomyopathy	Probably secondary to the addition of cobalt sulfate to beer with myofiber dystrophy and edema		
c. Cobalt intoxication	Similar to beer drinker's cardiomyopathy	Cyanosis	Acute onset and rapid course
e. Phosphorus	Myofiber degeneration secondary to direct toxic effect of phosphorus, which prevents amino acid incorporation into myocardial proteins		
f. Fluoride	1. Direct myocardial toxin 2. Severe hypocalcemia secondary to $[F]^-$ binding of calcium ion		
g. Lead	1. Secondary to nephropathic hypertension 2. Direct toxin	Hypertension	
h. Scorpion venom	Sympathetic stimulation with secondary myocardial changes		CNS symptoms and aspiration pneumonitis are usually the predominant symptoms. Relatively unresponsive to adrenergic agents. Adrenergic blockade probably indicated
i. Tick paralysis	?		
6. Radiation	Hyalinization and fibrosis due to direct effect of x-radiation	Toxic myocarditis 1. Conduction abnormalities secondary to sclerosis of conduction system 2. Coronary artery disease 3. Constrictive myo- and pericarditis	

Table continued on the following page

Table 7-2 *Cardiomyopathies (Congestive)*—(Continued)

Disease Process	Mechanism	Associated Circ. Problems	Misc.
7. Miscellaneous systemic syndromes			
a. Rejection cardiomyopathy	Lymphocytic infiltration and general rejection phenomena	Arrhythmias and conduction abnormalities	After heart transplantation
b. Senile cardiomyopathy	Unrelated to coronary artery disease		
c. Rheumatoid arthritis	1. Rheumatoid nodular invasion 2. Secondary to coronary arteritis	1. Mitral and aortic regurgitation 2. Coronary artery disease 3. Constrictive pericarditis	
d. Marie-Strumpell (ankylosing spondylitis)	Generalized degenerative changes	Aortic regurgitation	
e. Cogan's syndrome (non-syphilitic interstitial keratitis)	Fibrinoid necrosis of myocardium	1. Aortic regurgitation 2. Coronary artery disease	
f. Noonan's syndrome (male Turner's)	? (No detectable chromosome abnormality)	1. Pulmonary stenosis 2. Obstructive and non-obstructive cardiomyopathy	
g. Pseudoxanthoma elasticum (Grönblad-Strandberg)	Connective tissue disorder with myocardial infiltration and fibrosis	1. Valve abnormality 2. Coronary artery disease	
h. Trisomy 17–18	Diffuse fibrosis		
i. Scleredema of Buschke	Myocardial infiltration with acid mucopolysaccharides		
j. Wegeners granulomatosis	Panarteritis and myocardial granuloma formation	1. Mitral stenosis (?) 2. Cardiac tamponade	
k. Periarteritis nodosa	1. Panarteritis 2. Changes secondary to hypertension	1. Conduction abnormalities 2. Coronary artery disease	
8. Post-partum cardiomyopathy	Mechanical impairment of cardiac function		? Viral etiology Self-limited with good prognosis
9. Neoplastic diseases			
a. Primary mural cardiac tumor		Obstructive symptoms	
b. Metastases — malignant (especially malignant melanoma)			
10. Sarcoidosis	1. Cor pulmonale secondary to pulmonary involvement 2. Sarcoid granuloma leading to ventricular aneurysms	1. Cor pulmonale 2. ECG abnormalities and conduction disturbances 3. Pericarditis 4. Valvular obstruction	

gress to a recurrent or chronic form of myocarditis, resulting ultimately in a restrictive type of cardiomyopathy secondary to fibrous replacement of the myocardium.

In the bacterial varieties of myocarditis, isolated electrocardiographic changes or pericarditis are common and usually benign, whereas congestive heart failure is unusual. Diphtheritic myocarditis is generally the worst form of bacterial myocardial involvement, since, in addition to inflammatory changes, its endotoxin is a competitive analogue of cytochrome-B and can produce severe myocardial dysfunction. The conduction system is especially affected in diphtheria, producing either right or left bundle-branch block, which is associated with a 50 per cent mortality. When complete heart block supravenes, the mortality rate approaches 80 to 100 per cent. Syphilis and leptospirosis represent two examples of spirochaetal myocardial involvement. Tertiary syphilis is associated with multiple problems, including arrhythmias, conduction disturbances, and congestive heart failure. Viral infections manifest themselves primarily with electrocardiographic abnormalities including P-R prolongation, Q-T prolongation, ST and T-wave abnormalities, and arrhythmias, though each viral disease produces slightly different electrocardiographic changes, with complete heart block being the most significant. Most of the viral diseases have the potential to progress to congestive heart failure if the viral infection is severe. Especially noteworthy in this regard is the Coxsackie-B virus which most commonly produces severe viral heart disease. Presenting as fulminating cardiac failure with severe A-V nodal involvement and respiratory distress, viral myocarditis is common in nursery epidemics of Coxsackie-B infection. Recovery from Coxsackie-B myocarditis is usual, but the condition may progress to a constrictive pericarditis. Primary atypical pneumonia has the unusual feature of producing Stokes-Adams attacks secondary to A-V node involvement. Mycotic myocarditis has protean manifestations that depend on the extent of mycotic infiltration of the myocardium and may present as congestive heart failure, pericarditis, electrocardiographic abnormalities, or valvular obstruction. Of the protozoal forms of myocarditis, Chagas' disease, or trypanosomiasis, is the most significant, and the

most common cause of chronic congestive heart failure in South America. Electrocardiographic changes of right bundle branch block and arrhythmias occur in 80 per cent of patients. In addition to the typical inflammatory changes in the myocardium that produce chronic congestive failure, a direct neurotoxin from the infecting organism, *Trypanosoma cruzi*, produces degeneration of the conduction system, often causing severe ventricular arrhythmias and heart block with syncope. The onset of atrial fibrillation in these patients is often an ominous prognostic sign. Helminthic myocardial involvement may produce congestive heart failure, but more commonly symptoms are secondary to infestation and obstruction of the coronary or pulmonary arteries by egg, larval, or adult forms of the worm. Trichinosis, for example, produces a myocarditis secondary to an inflammatory response to larvae in the myocardium, even though the larvae themselves disappear from the myocardium after the second week of infestation.

The *noninflammatory* variety of congestive cardiomyopathy also presents the picture of myocardial failure, but in this case secondary to degenerative or infiltrative processes in the myocardium (see Table 7–2). Alcoholic cardiomyopathy is a typical hypokinetic noninflammatory cardiomyopathy associated with tachycardia and premature ventricular contractions that progresses to left ventricular failure with incompetent mitral and tricuspid valves. This cardiomyopathy is probably due to a direct toxic effect of ethanol or its metabolite acetaldehyde, which releases and depletes cardiac norepinephrine. In chronic alcoholics, acute ingestion of ethanol produces decreases in contractility, elevations in ventricular end-diastolic pressure, and increases in systemic vascular resistance. Alcoholic cardiomyopathy is classified in three hemodynamic stages. In Stage I, cardiac output, ventricular pressures, and left ventricular end-diastolic volume are normal, but the ejection fraction is decreased. In Stage II, cardiac output is normal, though filling pressures and end-diastolic volume are increased, and ejection fraction is decreased. In Stage III, cardiac output is decreased, filling pressures and end-diastolic volume are increased, and ejection fraction is severely depressed. Generally speaking,

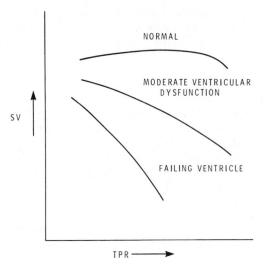

NORMAL

MODERATE VENTRICULAR
DYSFUNCTION

SV

FAILING VENTRICLE

TPR ⟶

Figure 7–1. Stroke volume (SV) as a function of total peripheral resistance (TPR) for a normal left ventricle, for a left ventricle with moderate dysfunction, and for a failing left ventricle.

all of the noninflammatory forms of congestive cardiomyopathy probably undergo a similar progression.

Both the inflammatory and noninflammatory forms of congestive cardiomyopathy present a picture identical to that of the congestive heart failure produced by severe coronary artery disease, even to the extent that, in some conditions, the coronary arteries are also involved by the process that has produced the cardiomyopathy. The pathophysiologic considerations are familiar ones. As the ventricular muscle begins to fail, the ventricle will dilate in an effort to take advantage of the increased force of contraction that results from increasing myocardial fiber length. As the ventricular radius increases, however, ventricular wall tension rises, increasing both the oxygen consumption of the myocardium and the total internal work of the ventricular muscle. As the myocardium fails and the cardiac output falls, a compensatory increase in sympathetic activity occurs in an effort to maintain both blood pressure and cardiac output. One feature of the failing myocardium is the loss of its ability to maintain stroke volume in the face of increased arterial impedance to ejection. Figure 7–1 shows that with increasing left ventricular dysfunction, stroke-volume becomes more and more dependent on arterial impedance. In the failing ventricle, stroke volume falls

almost linearly with increases in impedance. The increased sympathetic outflow that accompanies left ventricular failure initiates a vicious cycle of increased resistance to forward flow, decrease in stroke volume, decrease in cardiac output, and further sympathetic stimulation in an effort to maintain circulatory homeostasis. The key hemodynamic features of congestive cardiomyopathy are elevated filling pressures, a failure of myocardial contractile strength, and a marked inverse relationship between arterial impedance and stroke volume. The clinical picture of congestive cardiomyopathy falls into the two familiar categories of "forward" failure and "backward" failure. The features of "forward" failure, such as fatigue, hypotension, and oliguria, are related to decreases in cardiac output with reduced organ perfusion, particularly reduced perfusion of the kidney, which is thus stimulated to increase the effective circulating blood volume through sodium and water retention. "Backward" failure is related to the elevated filling pressures required by the failing ventricle and manifests itself in the form of orthopnea, paroxysmal nocturnal dyspnea, pulmonary congestion, and pulmonary edema.

Anesthesia and Monitoring. Electrocardiographic monitoring is essential in the management of patients with congestive cardiomyopathy, particularly in those with myocarditis. Ventricular arrhythmias are common, and complete heart block, which can occur from these conditions, requires rapid diagnosis and treatment. The electrocardiogram is also useful in monitoring ischemic changes when coronary artery disease, from whatever cause, is associated with the cardiomyopathy, as in amyloidosis. Direct intra-arterial blood pressure monitoring during surgery provides continuous blood pressure information and a convenient route for obtaining arterial blood gases. Any patient in congestive heart failure with a severely compromised myocardium who requires anesthesia and surgery should have left-sided filling pressures monitored, if at all possible. Monitoring right-sided filling pressures is of equal importance in patients in whom the cardiomyopathy exists along with pulmonary hypertension or cor pulmonale. In addition to measuring filling pressures, a thermodilution pulmonary artery catheter can be used to obtain cardiac outputs and the calculation of systemic and pulmonary vascular resistances, which allow serial evaluation of the patient's hemodynamic status. Recent technical advances in catheter design have incorporated pacing wires into some pulmonary artery catheters, which may be a distinct advantage in managing the patient with myocarditis and associated heart block.

Once considered the ideal technique for all cardiac diseases, the avoidance of myocardial depression still remains the goal of anesthetic management for patients with congestive cardiomyopathy. All of the inhalational anesthetic drugs are known myocardial depressants, and for this reason these agents are probably best avoided in this group of patients. An anesthetic based on a combination of narcotics, tranquilizers, and nitrous oxide can be employed instead. For the patient with a severely compromised myocardium, fentanyl may be a useful narcotic, since cardiovascular changes associated with its use are minimal. For peripheral or lower abdominal surgical procedures, the use of a regional anesthetic technique is a reasonable alternative, provided filling pressures are carefully controlled and the hemodynamic effects of the anesthetic are monitored. In planning the anesthetic management of the patient with congestive cardiomyopathy, one should also consider associated cardiovascular conditions, such as the presence of coronary artery disease, valvular abnormalities, outflow tract obstruction, and constrictive pericarditis.

Patients with congestive heart failure often require circulatory support intra- and postoperatively. Inotropic drugs such as dopamine and dobutamine have been shown to be effective in low output states and have the further advantage that in low doses they produce modest changes in systemic vascular resistance. In severe failure, more potent drugs such as epinephrine or isoproterenol may be required. As noted above, in the failing ventricle, stroke volume is inversely related to impedance to forward flow, and reduction of left ventricular afterload with drugs such as nitroprusside is effective in increasing cardiac output. In addition, in patients with myocarditis, especially of the viral variety, support of the circulation with transvenous pacing may be required should heart-block occur.

Obstructive Cardiomyopathy

Obstructive cardiomyopathy usually results from hypertrophy of ventricular muscle and occurs in either concentric or asymmetric forms (Table 7–3). Other conditions can also produce a picture of obstructive cardiomyopathy due to massive infiltration of the ventricular wall, as in Pompe's disease, where a massive accumulation of cardiac glycogen in the ventricular wall produces obstruction to ventricular outflow.

Asymmetric septal hypertrophy (ASH), or idiopathic hypertrophic subaortic stenosis (IHSS), is a variant form of an idiopathic hypertrophic cardiomyopathy. However, it presents a picture that is typical of the

Table 7–3 *Cardiomyopathies (Obstructive)*

Disease Process	Mechanism	Associated Circ. Problems
I. Idiopathic concentric hypertrophy	Symmetrical hypertrophy of left ventricle and outflow tract (usually non-obstructive)	
II. Idiopathic hypertrophic sub-aortic stenosis (IHSS or asymmetric septal hypertrophy)	(See text)	
III. Infectious		
A. Tuberculosis	Granulomatous obstruction to outflow tract	
B. Syphilis	Gumma in outflow tract or interference with aortic valve function	
C. Actinomycosis	Mycotic mass in outflow tract	
IV. Systemic syndromes		
A. Sarcoid	Like tuberculosis	1. Cor pulmonale 2. Congestive cardiomyopathy 3. Valve malfunction
B. Glycogen storage disease Type II (Pompe's)	Glycogen infiltration of septal walls	1. Congestive cardiomyopathy 2. Coronary artery disease
C. Noonan's syndrome	Left ventricular outflow obstruction	Pulmonary stenosis
D. Lentiginosis	Right and left AV-septal hypertrophy	
V. Cardiac tumors	Obstruction depends on location and size	

problems encountered in virtually all forms of obstructive cardiomyopathy, including the concentric hypertrophic form. The salient anatomic feature of IHSS is hypertrophy of ventricular muscle at the base of the septum in the left ventricle below the aortic valve. Pathologically, this is a disorganized mass of hypertrophied myocardial cells extending from the left ventricular septal wall, often involving the papillary muscles. Obstruction to left ventricular outflow is caused by this hypertrophic muscle mass, and mitral regurgitation at the end of systole results from papillary muscle involvement. The outflow tract obstruction can result in hypertrophy of the remainder of the ventricular muscle, secondary to increased pressures in the ventricular chamber. As the ventricle hypertrophies, ventricular compliance falls, and passive filling of the ventricle during diastole is decreased. For this reason, the stiffened ventricle becomes increasingly reliant on the presence of atrial contraction to increase ventricular end-diastolic volume. Occasionally, IHSS is associated with a right ventricular outflow tract obstruction as well.

The determinants of the functional severity of the ventricular obstruction in IHSS are: 1) the systolic volume of the ventricle, 2) the force of ventricular contractions, and 3) the transmural pressure distending the outflow tract. Large systolic volumes in the ventricle distend the outflow tract and reduce the obstruction, whereas small systolic volumes narrow the outflow tract and increase the obstruction. When ventricular contraction is vigorous, the hypertrophied septum contracts and bulges into the outflow tract, increasing the obstruction. When aortic pressure is high, there is an increased transmural pressure that distends the left ventricular outflow tract, but as aortic pressure falls, this distending force is decreased, narrowing the outflow tract. This results in marked falls in cardiac output and even mitral regurgitation as the mitral valve becomes the relief point for ventricular pressure.

Anesthesia and Monitoring. Patients with IHSS can be extremely sensitive to slight changes in ventricular volume, heart rate and rhythm, and changes in blood pressure. Accordingly, monitoring should be established that allows continuous assessment of these three parameters, particularly in patients in whom the obstruction is severe. In patients with IHSS coming to surgery for septal myomectomy, the electrocardiogram, an indwelling arterial catheter, and a pulmonary artery catheter are necessary monitors. In patients with lesser degrees of obstruction coming for other procedures, monitoring should provide at least some indication of ventricular volume, force of ventricular contraction, and transmural pressure distending the outflow tract.

In the anesthetic management of patients with IHSS, special consideration should be given to those features of the surgical procedure and anesthetic drugs that can produce changes in intravascular volume, ventricular contractility, and transmural distending pressure of the outflow tract. Volume depletion, for example, can be produced by blood loss, sympathectomy secondary to spinal anesthesia, the use of nitroglycerin, or the position of the patient. Ventricular contractility can be increased by a tachycardia occurring during and/or after endotracheal intubation or by sympathetic stimulation at the time of skin incision. Transmural distending pressure can be decreased by hypotension secondary to anesthetic drugs, hypovolemia, or positive pressure ventilation. In addition, increases in heart rate are poorly tolerated by patients with IHSS. Not only does a tachycardia increase contractility but it also decreases systolic ventricular volume, increases turbulent flow across the obstruction, and results in a narrowed outflow tract. Halothane is probably the most popular anesthetic drug in the management of this condition. Halothane decreases the force of ventricular contraction and, when coupled with adequate volume replacement and a slow heart rate, tends to minimize the severity of obstruction. Morphine, on the other hand, is often difficult to use due to the venodilatation and hypovolemia that occur. Fentanyl produces minimal vascular side effects and a slight decrease in heart rate, and thus may be a useful anesthetic agent in these patients in conjunction with continued preoperative propranolol therapy. Figure 7–2 summarizes the anesthetic and circulatory management of IHSS.

Restrictive Cardiomyopathy

Restrictive cardiomyopathies are usually the end stage of myocarditis or of an infiltra-

Clinical Problem	Treatment	Relatively Contraindicated
1) ↓ Preload	Volume Replacement Phenylephrine	Vasodilators Spinal, Epidural
2) ↑ Heart Rate or ↑ Contractility	Halothane Enflurane Propranolol	Ketamine Sympathomimetics
3) ↓ Afterload	Phenylephrine	Vasodilators Spinal, Epidural

Figure 7–2. Clinical features of IHSS.

tive process of the myocardium such as amyloidosis or hemochromatosis (Table 7–4). When a restrictive cardiomyopathy occurs, it mimics constrictive pericarditis coupled with myocardial dysfunction. Pulsus alternans, for example, occurs in restrictive cardiomyopathy and constrictive pericarditis. Restrictive cardiomyopathy is characterized by impairment of ventricular filling and poor ventricular contractility. Cardiac output is maintained in the early stages by elevated filling pressures and an increased heart rate, but, in contrast to constrictive pericarditis, an increase in myocardial contractility to maintain cardiac output is usually not possible. Diseases such as endocardial fibroelastosis appear similar to a restrictive cardiomyopathy in that there is impairment of diastolic ventricular filling, but differ in that contractility is not usually impaired.

Anesthetic and monitoring considerations in restrictive cardiomyopathies are virtually identical to those of constrictive pericarditis and cardiac tamponade with the additional feature of poor ventricular function. The combination of a restrictive and a congestive cardiomyopathy results in a more precarious situation than usually exists either alone or with constrictive pericarditis or cardiac tamponade where ventricular contractility is normal. The reader is referred to the section on constrictive pericarditis for a fuller treatment of the physiology and management of restrictive ventricular filling; and to the section on congestive cardiomyopathy for the management of impaired ventricular function. The anesthesiologist must tailor his anesthetic management for whichever feature, restrictive physiology or heart failure, is dominant in a particular patient.

CORONARY ARTERY DISEASE

The most important aspects of coronary artery disease remain the same no matter what the etiology of the obstruction of the coronary arteries is (Table 7–5). Like coronary artery disease produced by arteriosclerosis, the coronary artery disease produced by an unusual disease retains the same key clinical features. Physiologic considerations remain essentially the same, as do treatment and anesthetic management.

In the preoperative assessment, one should inquire about the symptoms produced by the coronary artery disease. The obvious symptoms to look for in the history are angina, the patient's exercise limitations, and symptoms of myocardial failure, such as orthopnea or paroxysmal nocturnal dyspnea. The physical examination retains its importance, especially when quantitative data regarding cardiac involvement are not available. Physical findings such as S_3 and S_4 heart sounds are important, as are auscultatory signs of uncommon conditions such as cardiac bruits, which might occur in a coronary arteriovenous fistula. If catheterization data are available, the specifics of coronary artery anatomy and ventricular function, such as end-diastolic pressure, ejection fraction, and the presence of wall motion abnormalities are all useful. After ascertaining the extent of coronary insufficiency, the special aspects of the specific disease entity producing the coronary insufficiency should be considered. As an example, in ankylosing spondylitis coronary insufficiency is produced by ostial stenosis, yet valvular problems often coexist and even overshadow the coronary artery disease. In rheumatoid arthritis, on the other hand, airway problems may be the most

Table 7-4 *Cardiomyopathies (Restrictive — Including Restrictive Endocarditis)*

Disease Process	Mechanism	Associated Circ. Problems	Misc.
I. End-stage of acute myocarditis	Fibrous replacement of myofibers		
II. Metabolic			
A. Amyloidosis	Amyloid infiltration of myocardium	1. Valvular malfunction	
B. Hemochromatosis	Iron deposition and secondary fibrous proliferation	2. Coronary artery disease Conduction abnormalities	
III. Drugs — Methysergide (Sansert)	Endocardial fibroelastosis	Valvular stenosis	Similar to changes in carcinoid syndrome
IV. Restrictive endocarditis	Picture very similar to constrictive pericarditis		
A. Carcinoid	Serotonin-producing carcinoid tumors — but serotonin is apparently not causative agent for fibrosis	1. Pulmonary stenosis 2. Tricuspid insufficiency and/or stenosis 3. Right-sided heart failure	
B. Endomyocardial fibrosis	Fibrous obliteration of ventricular cavities	Mitral and tricuspid insufficiency	
C. Loeffler's disease	Fibrosis of endocardium with decreased myocardial contraction	Subendocardial and papillary muscle degeneration and fibrosis	
D. Becker's disease	Similar to Loeffler's	Similar to Loeffler's	

significant part of the anesthetic challenge. Hypertension, which frequently coexists with arteriosclerotic coronary artery disease, is also a feature of the coronary artery disease produced by Fabry's disease. Another feature to consider is whether metabolic disturbances exist along with the coronary artery disease, as indeed they might where systemic lupus erythematosus produces both coronary artery disease and renal failure.

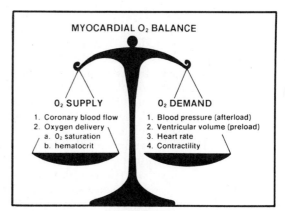

Figure 7–3. Myocardial O_2 supply and demand balance.

REVIEW OF THE PHYSIOLOGY OF CORONARY ARTERY DISEASE AND ITS MODIFICATION BY UNUSUAL DISEASES

The key to the physiology of coronary artery disease is the balance of myocardial oxygen supply and demand (Fig. 7–3). Myocardial oxygen supply depends on the patency of the coronary arteries, hemoglobin concentration, P_{O_2}, P_{CO_2}, and the coronary perfusion pressure. The same factors determine supply in uncommon diseases, but the specific manner in which an uncommon disease modifies any or all of the factors of supply either directly in the coronary arteries or indirectly through involvement of other systems should be sought. A knowledge of the anatomy of the coronary circulation and how arterial patency can be affected by the disease process is a useful starting point. This information is usually gained from coronary angiography in arteriosclerotic disease, but in a number of uncommon diseases, for example the ostial stenosis associated with ankylosing spondylitis, certain general assumptions can be made about coronary artery anatomy (see below). In assessing the patency of the coronary arteries, one should also consider the viscosity of the blood, since flow is a function both of the size of the conduit and the nature of the fluid in the system. In disease processes such as thrombotic thrombocytopenic purpura, sickle-cell disease, or polycythemia vera, the altered blood viscosity can assume critical importance. While hemoglobin concentration is usually not a limiting factor in the supply of oxygen to the myocardium, in diseases like leukemia, anemia may be a prominent feature, and the myocardial oxygen supply may be reduced accordingly. Similarly, the P_{O_2} is usually not a limiting factor, but in conditions where coronary artery disease exists concomitantly with cor

pulmonale, as in schistosomiasis or sickle-cell disease, the inability to maintain adequate oxygenation may limit the myocardial oxygen supply. In fact, in sickle-cell disease it may be the key feature, since the failure to maintain an adequate P_{O_2}, secondary to repeated pulmonary infarctions, further increases the tendency of cells containing hemoglobin-S to sickle, compromising myocardial oxygen delivery through sludging in the coronary microcirculation.

The main factors determining myocardial oxygen demand include heart rate, ventricular wall tension, and myocardial contractility. Tachycardia and hypertension after endotracheal intubation, skin incision, or other noxious stimulation are common causes of increased oxygen demand during surgery. In addition, complicating factors of an unusual disease may also produce increases in demand. Increases in rate may occur as a result of tachyarrhythmias secondary to S-A or A-V node involvement in amyloidosis or in Friedreich's ataxia. Increases in wall tension, for example, may occur in severe hypertension associated with systemic lupus, periarteritis nodosa, or Fabry's disease. Outflow tract obstruction with increased ventricular work can occur in primary xanthomatosis or in tertiary syphilis; and an increase in the diastolic ventricular radius with increased wall tension can occur in situations such as the aortic regurgitation associated with ankylosing spondylitis.

Modern cardiac anesthesia practice should attempt to tailor the anesthetic management to the problems posed by the peculiarities of the coronary anatomy. For example, knowledge of the presence of a lesion in the left main coronary artery dictates great care during anesthesia to avoid even relatively modest hypotension or tachycardia. Lesions of the right coronary artery are known to be associated with an increased incidence of atrial arrhythmias, and steps must be taken either to treat these or to compensate for their cardiovascular effects. In diseases such as primary xanthomatosis or Hurler's syndrome, the infiltrative process that produces coronary artery disease usually involves the coronary arteries diffusely, but some diseases may have features that can mimic either isolated left main coronary artery disease or right coronary artery disease. The Bland-White-Garland syndrome, which is the anomalous origin of the left coronary artery from the pulmonary artery, or coronary ostial stenosis produced by an aortic valve prosthesis may behave as left main coronary artery disease. A similar syndrome could be produced by bacterial overgrowth of the coronary ostia, ankylosing spondylitis, a dissecting aneurysm of the aorta, or Takayasu's arteritis. Right coronary artery disease could be mimicked by the syndrome of the anomalous origin of the right coronary artery from the pulmonary artery, or infiltration of the S-A or A-V nodes in amyloidosis or Friedreich's ataxia. Consider also that in small artery arteritis, which occurs in periarteritis nodosa or systemic lupus, the small arteries supplying the S-A or A-V node may be involved in the pathologic process, producing ischemia of the conduction system.

In Table 7–5 the diseases that produce coronary artery disease have been divided into those that produce coronary artery disease associated with good left ventricular function and those that produce coronary artery disease in conjunction with poor left ventricular function. These are the usual presentations of the disease processes, and this division further corresponds to the usual way of thinking about coronary artery disease. In any of the diseases ventricular function can regress from good to poor. In some conditions, the coronary artery disease progression and ventricular function deterioration occur at the same rate, and left ventricular function is eventually severely depressed. In other situations, coronary insufficiency is primary, and left ventricular dysfunction eventually occurs after repeated episodes of ischemia and/or thrombosis. Ventricular function must usually be evaluated by clinical signs and symptoms, since it is unlikely that cardiac catheterization will have been performed in these patients. The

Table 7–5 *Uncommon Causes of Coronary Artery Disease*

I. Coronary artery disease associated with cardiomyopathy (poor left ventricular function)
  A. Pathologic basis — infiltration of coronary arteries with luminal narrowing
    1. Amyloidosis — valvular stenosis, restrictive cardiomyopathy
    2. Fabry's disease — hypertension
    3. Hurler's syndrome — often associated with valvular malfunction
    4. Hunter's syndrome — often associated with valvular malfunction
    5. Primary xanthomatosis — aortic stenosis
    6. Leukemia — anemia
    7. Pseudoxanthoma elasticum — valve abnormalities
  B. Inflammation of coronary arteries
    1. Rheumatic fever — in acute phase
    2. Rheumatoid arthritis — aortic and mitral regurgitation, constrictive pericarditis
    3. Periarteritis nodosa — hypertension
    4. Systemic lupus erythematosus — hypertension, renal failure, mitral valve malfunction
  C. Embolic or thrombotic occlusion of coronary arteries
    1. Schistosomiasis ⎱ –cor pulmonale depending on
    2. Sickle cell anemia ⎰ length and extent of involvement
  D. Fibrous and hyaline degeneration of coronary arteries
    1. Radiation
    2. Duchenne's muscular dystrophy
    3. Friedreich's ataxia — ? associated with IHSS
    4. Roussy Lévy — hereditary polyneuropathy
  E. Anatomic abnormalities of coronary arteries
    1. Bland-White-Garland syndrome (left coronary artery arising from pulmonary artery) — endocardial fibroelastosis, mitral regurgitation
    2. Ostial stenosis secondary to ankylosing spondylitis— aortic regurgitation

II. Coronary artery disease usually associated with normal ventricular function
  A. Anatomic abnormalities of coronary arteries
    1. Right coronary arising from pulmonary artery
    2. Coronary A-V fistula
    3. Coronary sinus aneurysm
    4. Dissecting aneurysm
    5. Ostial stenosis — bacterial overgrowth, syphilitic aortitis
    6. Coronary artery trauma — penetrating or non-penetrating
    7. Spontaneous coronary artery rupture
  B. Embolic or thrombotic occlusion
    1. Coronary emboli
    2. Malaria and/or malarial infested red blood cells
    3. Thrombotic thrombocytopenic purpura
    4. Polycythemia vera
  C. Infections
    1. Miliary tuberculosis—intimal involvement of coronary arteries
    2. Arteritis secondary to salmonella or endemic typhus (associated with active myocarditis)
  D. Infiltration of coronary arteries
    1. Gout — conduction abnormalities, possible valve problems
    2. Homocysteinuria
  E. Miscellaneous
    1. Thromboangiitis obliterans (Buerger's disease)
    2. Takayasu's arteritis

converse of severe arterial disease coupled with relatively good left ventricular function is the picture of a cardiomyopathy associated with almost incidental coronary artery disease, as occurs in Hurler's syndrome, amyloidosis, or systemic lupus. Most anatomical lesions, such as coronary A-V fistula or coronary insufficiency produced by trauma, usually are associated with good left ventricular function. There is, predictably, a clinical gray zone in which coronary artery disease and poor left ventricular function coexist but without either process clearly predominating. These can only be characterized by the extent of involvement of the coronary arteries and the myocardium in the disease process, as in tuberculosis or syphilis. The important point is that ventricular function be assessed in light of the known disease and that the anesthetic management be prepared accordingly. (See pages 269–279 for the management of poor left ventricular function associated with these disease processes.)

Anesthesia and Monitoring. The functional impairment of the myocardium and coronary circulation dictates the extent and type of monitoring to be employed. The type of electrocardiographic (ECG) monitoring is dictated, to some extent, by knowledge of the coronary anatomy. Those diseases in which the pathophysiology of the left coronary artery disease is mimicked are best monitored using the V_5 precordial lead, whereas in those in which right coronary artery disease is simulated, standard ECG leads used to assess the inferior surface of the heart, such as leads II, III, or AVF are preferable. Knowledge of ventricular filling pressures is especially important in diseases associated with poor ventricular function. The use of a Swan-Ganz pulmonary artery catheter is preferable to central venous pressure monitoring in the assessment of left ventricular function, and, in the case of coronary artery disease, the pulmonary artery catheter can give early evidence of ischemia-induced changes in ventricular compliance, which may precede electrocardiographic evidence of myocardial ischemia. Urine output is another important parameter, and is especially significant in diseases associated with nephropathy, such as longstanding sickle-cell disease or systemic lupus. Where severe cardiomyopathy associated with coronary artery disease exists, monitoring cardiac output and systemic vascular resistance is useful in evaluating both the effects of anesthetic drugs and therapeutic interventions. An indwelling arterial catheter for monitoring arterial blood gases is important, especially where pulmonary disease or cor pulmonale complicates the clinical picture, as in schistosomiasis or sickle-cell disease. One *caveat* should be noted in the use of intra-arterial monitoring: When peripheral arterial monitoring is used in cases of generalized arteritis, such as Takayasu's arteritis or Buerger's disease, or in cases of sludging in the microcirculation, as in sickle-cell disease, one should be particularly meticulous in assessing the adequacy of collateral blood flow prior to cannulation of the peripheral artery, and the area distal to the cannulated artery should be checked frequently for signs of arterial insufficiency.

The anesthetic employed in these conditions should be tailored to the degree of myocardial dysfunction. In cases of pure coronary insufficiency with good left ventricular function, anesthetic management is aimed at decreasing oxygen demand by decreasing myocardial contractility and blood pressure, as is done in patients who have coronary arteriosclerotic disease with normal ventricular function. Techniques commonly employed include the combination of a volatile anesthetic agent, such as halothane or enflurane, with nitrous oxide, or a nitrous-narcotic technique that employs the intermittent use of vasodilators such as nitroprusside or nitroglycerin for blood pressure control. In patients with poor ventricular function, the anesthetic technique attempts to maintain what are often tenuous hemodynamics by avoiding drugs that produce significant degrees of myocardial depression. The narcotic-nitrous oxide technique has been found to be effective, specifically the use of morphine or fentanyl in combination with sedative-hypnotic drugs such as diazepam.

Just as the anesthetic technique should be tailored to the degree of ventricular dysfunction, so measures designed for support of the circulation will be determined by associated cardiovascular conditions. In periarteritis nodosa or Fabry's disease, hypertension is often associated with poor left ventricular function; and in such a situation, one would probably elect to employ a vasodilator such as sodium nitroprusside or nitroglycerin to control the hypertension rather than a volatile anesthetic. The principles for the management of intraoperative arrhythmias remain the same as for the treatment of arrhythmias in the setting of arteriosclerotic coronary artery disease.

PULMONARY HYPERTENSION AND COR PULMONALE

PULMONARY HYPERTENSION

Pulmonary hypertension is defined as an elevation of the pulmonary artery pressure above the accepted limit of normal, for whatever cause. The accepted upper limit of normal is about 35/15 torr, or a mean pulmonary artery pressure of 13 to 18 torr. Pulmonary hypertension has been further subdivided into mild, moderate, and severe forms by some authors.

The normal pulmonary vasculature changes from a high resistance circuit in utero to a low resistance circuit in the newborn secondary to several concomitant changes: 1) the relief of hypoxic vasoconstriction that occurs with the first spontaneous breath; 2) the stinting effect of air-filled lungs on the pulmonary vessels, which increases their caliber and decreases their resistance; and 3) the functional closure of the ductus arteriosus, secondary to an increase in the Po_2, which increases blood flow through the lungs and thus produces an increase in the open capillary cross-sectional area. The muscular media of the fetal pulmonary arterioles normally involutes in postnatal life. Assuming there is no severe active vasoconstriction, pulmonary artery pressure remains low owing to the numerous parallel vascular channels that accept increased blood flow as pulmonary blood volume is increased. For this reason, pressure·is not normally increased in the pulmonary circuit, since the containing space for the pulmonary blood volume increases instead.

Three general pathologic conditions can occur that will convert this normally low resistance circuit into a high resistance circuit. A high resistance circuit will develop from 1) increases in capillary or pulmonary venous pressures; 2) decreases in the cross-sectional area of the vasculature; or 3) increases in pulmonary arterial blood flow. Table 7–6, which lists causes of pulmonary

Table 7–6 Conditions Producing Pulmonary Artery Hypertension (PAH)

I. PAH produced by elevations of capillary and pulmonary venous pressure
   A. Mitral stenosis, mitral regurgitation, left atrial myxoma
   B. Hypertension, left ventricular failure
   C. Aortic stenosis or insufficiency

II. PAH produced by increases in pulmonary artery blood flow
   A. Congenital lesions: patent ductus arteriosus, atrial septal defect, ventricular septal defect, total anomalous venous return with right atrial or superior vena cava drainage, single ventricle, transposition of great vessels
   B. Acquired lesions: post-myocardial infarction ventricular septal defect

III. PAH produced by loss of arterial cross-sectional area
   A. Chronic hypoxia*
     1. Emphysema, chronic bronchitis, cystic fibrosis
     2. High altitude — mild PAH is a normal response — Monge's disease — chronic mountain sickness
     3. Chest and airway problems
       a. Pickwickian syndrome
       b. Kyphoscoliosis
       c. Chronic hypoxia secondary to enlarged adenoids
   B. Pulmonary fibrosis — produces fibrous occlusion and obliteration of small pulmonary arterioles with dilatation of large pulmonary arteries
     1. Massive pulmonary fibrosis — silicosis and other pneumoconioses
     2. Interstitial fibrosis (fibrosing alveolitis) — abnormalities of alveoli and bronchi that extend to incorporate the pulmonary arterioles in the fibrotic process
       a. Collagen diseases
         1) Scleroderma
         2) Dermatomyositis
       b. Metals
         1) Berylliosis
         2) Cadmium
         3) Asbestosis
       c. Primary pulmonary disease
         1) Hamman-Rich
         2) Sarcoidosis
       d. Iatrogenic
         1) Radiation
         2) Busulphan therapy
       e. Miscellaneous
         1) Letterer-Siwe
         2) Hand-Schuller-Christian
   C. Pulmonary emboli
     1. Recurrent
       a. Thromboemboli
       b. Parasitic
         1) Bilharzia
         2) Schistosomiasis
       c. Fat and tumor emboli
       d. Sickle cell
     2. Solitary emboli
       a. Massive thromboembolism
       b. Amniotic fluid
       c. Air
   D. "Primary" pulmonary hypertension — idiopathic
     1. Primary pulmonary arterial hypertension
     2. Primary pulmonary venous hypertension
   E. Dietary causes
     1. Crotalaria labrunoides seeds
     2. Aminorex fumarate — European appetite suppressant
     3. Oral contraceptives
   F. Hepatic cirrhosis — possibly secondary to development of plexiform and angiomatoid lesions in the lung
   G. Filariasis — adult worms in pulmonary circulation*
   H. Foreign body granulomas

*Conditions producing cor pulmonale.

hypertension, is arranged according to these three pathophysiologic mechanisms.

Increases in capillary or pulmonary venous pressure may be caused by conditions such as left ventricular failure, mitral regurgitation, or mitral stenosis. In addition to the passive increase in pulmonary blood volume, active vasoconstriction also occurs in the pulmonary vascular bed. Hypoxic vasoconstriction induced by ventilation-perfusion mismatching or reflex constriction occurring with the passive stretching of the muscular media of the pulmonary arterioles may be the basis of this phenomenon.

A decrease in pulmonary arterial cross-sectional area results in increased pulmonary vascular resistance, as dictated by Poiseuille's law, which states that resistance to flow is inversely proportional to the fourth power of the radius of the vessels. Very small decrements in pulmonary cross-sectional area can result in striking increases in resistance. There are a number of causes of decreased pulmonary arterial cross-sectional area. Filarial worms, the eggs of *Schistosoma mansoni,* or multiple small thrombotic emboli are typical of embolic causes of pulmonary hypertension. Primary deposition of fibrin in the pulmonary arterioles and capillaries is another cause of decreased cross-sectional area; and this, in fact, may be the mechanism of primary, or idiopathic, pulmonary hypertension. Whatever the initiating cause of fibrin formation in this condition, there is increased thrombogenesis in the pulmonary arterioles and/or pulmonary capillaries which can produce striking decreases in the total cross-sectional area. This also may be the cause of the pulmonary arterial hypertension associated with the use of oral contraceptives, which are known to increase thrombogenesis. Arterial medial hypertrophy can occur if there is increased flow or pressure in the pulmonary circulation early in life. In this situation, the muscular media of the pulmonary arterioles undergo hypertrophy rather than the normal postnatal involution. As the muscle hypertrophies, there is increased reflex contraction in response to the elevations in pulmonary arterial pressure. This raises the pulmonary arterial pressure even higher by further reducing cross-sectional area. If this pulmonary arterial pressure elevation is long-standing, it results in intimal damage to the pulmonary arterioles

followed by fibrosis, thrombosis, and sclerosis with an irreversible decrease in cross-sectional area of the arterial bed, as often occurs in long-standing mitral valve disease or emphysema. Pulmonary hypertension can also be caused by primary vasoconstrictors, such as the seeds of the crotalaria plant, or by hypoxia associated with high altitude or pulmonary parenchymal disease.

Pulmonary hypertension resulting from increases in pulmonary arterial flow is usually associated with various congenital cardiac lesions, such as atrial-septal defect, ventricular-septal defect, patent ductus arteriosus, or, in adult life, the ventricular-septal defect occurring after a septal myocardial infarction. Usually, however, pulmonary arterial pressure in these conditions remains normal, and slight degrees of hypoxia are needed to convert the pulmonary circulation to a high pressure system. Evidence for this contention includes the observation that there is an increased incidence of pulmonary hypertension in infants with congenital left-to-right shunting and increased pulmonary blood flow who were born at high altitudes compared with similar infants born at sea level. Long-standing increases in flow with intimal damage may result in fibrosis and sclerosis, as noted above. An increase in pulmonary arterial pressure in these cases ultimately may result in the Eisenmenger syndrome, in which the increased pulmonary arterial pressure results in a conversion of left-to-right shunting to right-to-left shunting with the development of cyanosis.

Like systemic arterial hypertension, pulmonary hypertension is characterized by a prolonged asymptomatic period. As pulmonary vascular changes occur, an irreversible decrease in pulmonary cross-sectional area develops, and cardiac output becomes fixed as a result of the fixed resistance to flow. This results in the symptoms of dyspnea, fatigue, syncope, and chest pain. The diagnostic dilemma presented by pulmonary hypertension is in differentiation of primary pulmonary hypertension from secondary hypertension, due to another condition such as left ventricular failure or mitral stenosis. Usually, in these circumstances, the symptoms of the primary condition are the most prominent, and the pulmonary hypertension is of secondary significance. When pulmonary hypertension exists alone, the key feature of its pathophysiology is a fixed cardiac output. Right ventricular hypertrophy commonly occurs in response to pulmonary hypertension, which may progress to right ventricular dilatation and failure.

COR PULMONALE

Cor pulmonale is usually defined as right ventricular hypertrophy, dilation, and failure secondary to pulmonary arterial hypertension *that is due to a decrease in the cross-sectional area of the pulmonary bed.* This excludes, therefore, right ventricular failure, which occurs after increases in pulmonary arterial pressure secondary to increases in pulmonary blood flow, pulmonary capillary, or venous pressure. Both increases in pulmonary blood flow and passive increases in pulmonary venous and capillary pressure can produce right ventricular failure, but they do not, strictly speaking, produce cor pulmonale. Fortunately, the physiologic and anesthetic considerations in cor pulmonale and in right ventricular failure from other causes are similar. Given this restriction, though, there are still numerous causes of cor pulmonale including pulmonary parenchymal disease, chronic hypoxia, and primary pulmonary arterial disease.

Cor pulmonale is divided into two types: acute and chronic. Acute cor pulmonale is usually secondary to a massive pulmonary embolus, resulting in a 60 to 70 per cent decrease in the pulmonary cross-sectional area associated with cyanosis and acute respiratory distress. With acute cor pulmonale there is a rapid increase in right ventricular systolic pressure to 60 to 70 torr, which slowly returns towards normal secondary to displacement of the embolus peripherally with increased blood flow past the embolus, lysis of the embolus, and increases in collateral blood flow. These changes often occur within two hours of the onset of symptoms. Massive emboli may be associated with acute right ventricular dilatation and failure, elevated central venous pressure, and cardiogenic shock. Another feature of massive pulmonary emboli is that the pulmonary vasoconstrictive response to embolization may be so intense that it persists after the pulmonary hypertension progresses to acute right ventricular failure, even in the absence of an angiographically demonstrable pulmonary embolus.

Chronic cor pulmonale presents with a rather different picture. It is associated with right ventricular hypertrophy and a change in the normal crescentic shape of the right ventricle to a more ellipsoidal shape that is consistent with a change from volume work, which the right ventricle normally performs, to a ventricular geometry more appropriate to the pressure work required by a high afterload. Curiously, left ventricular dysfunction may occur in association with right ventricular hypertrophy that cannot be related to any obvious changes in the loading conditions of the left ventricle. Chronic cor pulmonale is usually superimposed on long-standing pulmonary arterial hypertension.

Chronic bronchitis is probably the most common cause of cor pulmonale in adults, and its pathophysiology will be examined as a guide to understanding and managing cor pulmonale from all causes. Initially, the pulmonary vascular resistance in chronic bronchitis is normal or slightly increased because cardiac output increases. Later, there is an increase in pulmonary vascular resistance or an inappropriately elevated pulmonary vascular resistance for the amount of pulmonary blood flow. Recall that in the normal situation there is a slight decrease in the pulmonary resistance when pulmonary blood flow is increased, which is probably secondary to an increase in pulmonary vascular diameter and in flow through collateral channels. In chronic bronchitis, the absolute resistance of the pulmonary circulation may not change, owing to the inability of the resistance vessels to dilate. A progressive loss of pulmonary parenchyma occurs and, because of dilatation of the terminal bronchioles, there is an increase in pulmonary dead space that causes progressively more severe mismatching of pulmonary ventilation and perfusion. In response to the ventilation-perfusion mismatch, the pulmonary circulation attempts to compensate by decreasing blood flow to the areas of the lung that have hypoxic alveoli. This occurs at the expense of a decrease in pulmonary arteriole cross-sectional area and an elevation in pulmonary arterial pressure.

Long-standing chronic bronchitis results in elevations in pulmonary arterial pressure, with resulting right ventricular hypertrophy. In any form of respiratory embarrassment, whether it be infection or simply progression of the primary disease, further increases in pulmonary vascular resistance increase pulmonary arterial pressure, and right ventricular failure supervenes. With the onset of respiratory problems in the patient with chronic bronchitis, a number of changes occur that can make pulmonary hypertension more severe and can precipitate right ventricular failure. A respiratory infection produces further abnormalities of the blood gas values, with declines in PO_2 and elevations in PCO_2. Generally the pulmonary artery pressure is directly proportional to the PCO_2, though the pulmonary circulation is more sensitive to changes in PO_2. With a fall in PO_2 there is usually an increase in cardiac output in an effort to maintain oxygen delivery to tissues. This increased blood flow through the lungs may result in further elevations in the pulmonary artery pressure due to the fixed decreased cross-sectional area of the pulmonary vascular bed. In addition, patients with chronic bronchitis and long-standing depression of PO_2 values often have compensatory polycythemia. The polycythemic blood of the chronic bronchitic produces an increased resistance to flow through the pulmonary circuit because of its increased viscosity, and attempts to increase cardiac output during respiratory compromise simply make the situation worse.

The patient with chronic bronchitis normally has an increase in airway resistance made worse during acute respiratory infection as a result of secretions and edema that further decrease the caliber of the small airways. These patients also have a loss of structural support from degenerative changes in the airways and from a loss of the stenting effect of the pulmonary parenchyma. For these reasons, the patient's small airways tend to collapse during exhalation and there is a rise in airway pressure due to this "dynamic compression" phenomenon. In chronic bronchitis and emphysema the decrease in cross-sectional area of the pulmonary vessels results not from fibrotic obliteration of pulmonary capillaries or arterioles but rather from a hypertrophy of the muscular media of the pulmonary arterioles. The vessels become compressible but not distensible, so that with exhalation and an increase in intrathoracic pressure, airway compression results in a further increase in pulmonary vascular resistance and an increase in pulmonary arterial pressure. The hypertrophied muscular media prevents the resulting increase in pulmonary arterial pressure from distending the pulmonary

vessels and maintaining a normal pulmonary artery pressure. With the onset of respiratory embarrassment in the chronic bronchitic, there are increases in pulmonary artery pressure, afterload, and the work requirement of the right ventricle that may result in right ventricular failure. A similar pattern may be observed in other forms of pulmonary disease, since the compensatory mechanisms are much the same as in chronic bronchitis. Chronic bronchitis, however, is somewhat more amenable to therapy, since the acute pulmonary changes are often reversible. Relief of hypoxia, for example, may be expected to afford some amelioration of the pulmonary hypertension. In pulmonary hypertension and cor pulmonale secondary to pulmonary fibrosis, relief of hypoxia probably has little to offer the pulmonary circulation, since the increase in pulmonary vascular resistance is due not to vasoconstriction of muscular pulmonary arterioles but rather to a fibrous obliteration of the pulmonary vascular bed.

Anesthesia and Monitoring. Monitoring for patients with pulmonary hypertension and cor pulmonale should provide a continuous assessment of pulmonary arterial pressure, right ventricular filling pressure, right ventricular myocardial oxygen supply/demand balance, and some measure of pulmonary function. The electrocardiogram allows for the monitoring of arrhythmias, and in the setting of right ventricular hypertrophy where there is an increased possibility of coronary insufficiency, it allows observation of the development of ischemia or acute strain of the right ventricle, seen in leads II, III, or AVF. Pulmonary artery pressure monitoring provides an indication of the work load imposed on the right ventricle in cor pulmonale. The Swan-Ganz catheter affords the potential for monitoring the pulmonary artery pressure and also for monitoring the central venous pressure as an indication of the right ventricular filling pressure. Further, the Swan-Ganz catheter allows a distinction to be made between right and left ventricular failure by comparison of the right atrial pressure and the pulmonary capillary wedge pressure (left atrial pressure). It can also aid in the distinction between left ventricular failure and respiratory failure. In left ventricular failure, an elevated pulmonary artery pressure occurs with an elevated pulmonary capillary wedge pressure, whereas in respiratory failure, there is often an elevation of pulmonary artery pressure with a normal pulmonary capillary wedge pressure. The use of the thermodilution Swan-Ganz pulmonary artery catheter allows for the determination of cardiac output and pulmonary vascular resistance. It is important to follow the pulmonary artery pressure in this setting, since an increase in pulmonary artery pressure is often the cause of acute cor pulmonale, and serial measurements of pulmonary artery pressure and the pulmonary vascular resistance allow one to evaluate the effects of therapeutic interventions. Monitoring of arterial blood gases seems to be the most uncomplicated way of assessing pulmonary function. The use of an indwelling arterial catheter facilitates the obtaining of arterial blood samples and reduces patient discomfort. However, calculation of intrapulmonary venous admixture by using mixed venous blood samples obtained from the pulmonary artery is a more sensitive indicator of pulmonary dysfunction than arterial PO_2 values alone. In the future, in situations of marked abnormalities of ventilation and perfusion secondary to cor pulmonale, continuous monitoring of blood gas tensions and pH may be useful.

In the anesthetic management of patients with pulmonary hypertension and cor pulmonale, special consideration must be given to the degree of pulmonary hypertension, those factors that improve or worsen it, and the functional state of the right ventricle. For example, if pulmonary hypertension is coexistent with hypoxia in the patient with chronic bronchitis, administration of oxygen may afford significant relief of the pulmonary hypertension. If, however, the pulmonary hypertension is secondary to massive pulmonary fibrotic changes, one would expect little relief of pulmonary hypertension by the administration of oxygen. If the patient has an increase in blood viscosity, as in the polycythemia of chronic hypoxia, moderate hemodilution may be of some benefit in reducing the pulmonary vascular resistance if oxygen delivery can be maintained. When pulmonary hypertension is present without right ventricular failure, volatile anesthetics that decrease hypoxic vasoconstriction may be the anesthetic drugs of choice. One should be aware, however, that with the relief of hypoxic vasoconstriction, there may be a resultant fall in the PO_2. Halothane may also be indicated if pulmonary hypertension exists in patients who have pulmonary parenchymal disease with a significant bronchospastic component. In contrast to the volatile anesthetic agents, nitrous oxide can increase pulmonary artery pressure and should be used cautiously in this setting.

When pulmonary hypertension coexists with cor pulmonale one should attempt in the anesthetic management to preserve right ventricular function. The same anesthetic drugs that may have been useful in pure pulmonary hypertension are now probably contraindicated because of their myocardial depressant effects. The primary concern is the maintenance of right ventricular function in the face of an elevated right ventricular afterload. In this setting, a technique employing narcotics such as fentanyl or sedative-hypnotic drugs such as diazepam probably provides the best cardiovascular stability.

Circulatory supportive measures in the setting of right ventricular failure do not differ in theory from measures employed in managing left ventricular failure (Table 7–7). Concern should be directed at ventricular preload, the inotropic state of the ventricle, and ventricular afterload. Right ventricular preload can be assessed by measurement of the central venous pressure, preferably as part of full hemodynamic monitoring with a Swan-Ganz catheter. Preload can be augmented by judicious fluid infusion or purposely decreased with a vasodilator such as nitroglycerin that primarily affects venous capacitance in low doses. Ventricular preload can also be reduced by the initiation of positive pressure ventilation. The right ventricular contractile state can be estimated by the cardiac output, in addition to observing the right ventricular response to volume (Frank-Starling function curve). Inotropic support is often required in the setting of right ventricular failure with chronic cor pulmonale, and these patients usually come to surgery after having been treated with a digitalis preparation. If further inotropic support is required, an inotropic agent should be selected only after considering its pulmonary effects, and the effects of the inotropic intervention should be monitored. For example, in the setting of right ventricular failure, norepinephrine dramatically increases pulmonary artery pressure and pulmonary vascular resistance and is probably contraindicated. On the other hand, isoproterenol or dobutamine tend to reduce pulmonary artery pressure and pulmonary vascular resistance, and would probably be the inotropic drugs of choice in right ventricular failure. Just as in left ventricular failure, where the reduction of left ventricular afterload can produce an increase in stroke volume and cardiac output, so in right ventricular failure, reduction in right ventricular afterload can produce similar effects. Vasodilators that have been found effective in reducing the afterload of the right ventricle include phentolamine, sodium nitroprusside, and nitroglycerin.

As noted previously, the use of positive pressure ventilation may produce falls in right ventricular preload and, in addition, may produce an increase in pulmonary artery pressure by physically reducing the cross-sectional area of the pulmonary vasculature during the positive phase of ventilation. In a similar fashion, the use of positive end-expiratory pressure (PEEP) may be quite detrimental to the patient in right ventricular failure secondary to pulmonary hypertension. PEEP, like intermittent positive pressure ventilation, may produce a fall in venous return and right ventricular preload and can also increase pulmonary vascular resistance and pulmonary artery pressure. Before instituting PEEP, it must be remembered that the functional residual capacity is already increased in patients with chronic obstructive pulmonary disease, and the use of PEEP may have little to offer in terms of improving ventilation-perfusion matching.

In patients with chronic bronchitis, in whom a significant degree of bronchospasm exists, anesthetic drugs such as halothane,

Table 7-7 *Abbreviated Pulmonary Vascular Pharmacopeia*

Drug	PA Pressure	PCWP	Pulmonary Blood Flow	SAP	HR	PVR
α and β agonists						
1. Norepinephrine 0.10–0.20 μg/kg/min	↑	↑ to ↑↑	---**	↑↑	↓	NC* to ↑
2. Methoxamine 5–10 mg	↑	↑	---	↑↑	↓↓	---
3. Phenylephrine 50–100 μg	↑↑	---	↓	↑↑	↓↓	↑↑
4. Epinephrine 0.05–0.20 μg/kg/min	↑	NC or ↓	↑	↑↑	↑	↑
5. Dopamine 2–10 μg/kg/min	NC	NC or ↓	↑	NC or ↑	↑	NC
6. Dobutamine 5–15 μg/kg/min	---	↓	↑↑	NC or ↑	↑	↓
7. Isoproterenol .015–0.15 μg/kg/min	SL† ↓	↓	↑↑	↓	↑↑	↓
β-antagonist Propranolol 0.5–2 mg	---	NC to ↑	NC to ↓	NC to ↓	↓	NC to ↑
α-antagonist Phentolamine 1–3 μg/kg/min	↓	↓	↑	↓	↑	↓
Smooth muscle dilators						
1. Aminophylline 500 mg	↓	↓	---	---	↑	↓
2. Sodium nitroprusside 0.5–3 μg/kg/min	↓	↓	↑↑	NC to ↓	↑	↓
3. Nitroglycerin 0.5–5 μg/kg/min	↓↓	↓↓	NC to ↑	↓	↑	↓

*NC = No change.
**--- = Data unavailable.
†SL = Slight.

which decrease bronchial smooth muscle tone, can be advantageous. Bronchospasm can also be treated intraoperatively by the use of bronchodilators such as aminophylline or terbutaline. Though aminophylline occasionally produces a mild tachycardia and has an arrhythmogenic potential, it is especially useful in the setting of pulmonary hypertension and right ventricular failure, since it is also a direct pulmonary arterial dilator, which in combination with its effect of relieving hypoxia produced by bronchospasm, tends to reduce pulmonary artery pressure.

CONSTRICTIVE PERICARDITIS AND CARDIAC TAMPONADE

Normal Pericardial Function

The pericardium is not essential to life, as is demonstrated from the benign results of pericardiectomy, but the pericardium normally provides resistance to overfilling of the ventricles; for example, in tricuspid regurgitation, mitral regurgitation, or hypervolemic states. The intrapericardial pressure reflects intrapleural pressure and is, therefore, a determinant of ventricular transmural filling pressure. The pericardium also serves as an accessory to the action of negative pleural pressure in helping to maintain venous return to the heart during spontaneous ventilation.

CONSTRICTIVE PERICARDITIS

Constrictive pericarditis results from fibrous adhesion of the pericardium to the epicardial surface of the heart (Table 7–8). Its key feature is a resistance to normal ventricular diastolic filling. Constrictive pericarditis is a chronic condition that is usually well-tolerated by the patient until symptoms are severe. Cardiac tamponade, in contrast, is a syndrome in which the onset of restrictive symptoms is rapid and dramatic.

A number of characteristic hemodynamic features accompany constrictive pericarditis. The normal slight respiratory variation in blood pressure is virtually abolished in constrictive pericarditis. In contrast, dramatic respiratory variations in blood pressure occur with cardiac tamponade. With adequate blood volume, the right atrial pressure in constrictive pericarditis is usually equal to or greater then 15 torr and usually equals the left atrial pressure. Early in the disease, cardiac output is normal, but with progression the cardiac output falls. Most symptoms are related to this fall in cardiac output or to the elevated venous pressure that develops in response to the decreased cardiac output and restriction of right ventricular filling. The pulmonary artery systolic pressure is usually less than 40 torr, which helps to distinguish pericarditis from cardiac failure. Both constrictive pericarditis and cardiac tamponade demonstrate a diastolic "pressure plateau." The right atrial pressure equals the right ventricular end-diastolic pressure, pulmonary artery diastolic pressure, and left atrial pressure. Constrictive pericarditis often resembles restrictive cardiomyopathy and occasionally presents a diagnostic dilemma; however, in contrast to constrictive pericarditis, cardiac output in restrictive cardiomyopathy is decreased from the beginning, left atrial pressure is increased, mean pulmonary artery pressure is increased, and there is a normal respiratory variation in arterial blood pressure.

Since constrictive pericarditis restricts ventricular diastolic filling, normal ventricular end-diastolic volumes are not obtained and stroke volume is decreased. In an effort to maintain cardiac output in the face of a decreased stroke volume, compensatory mechanisms include an increase in heart rate and contractility, which usually occur secondary to an increase in endogenous catecholamine release. This maintains cardiac output in the face of the restricted stroke volume until the decrease in ventricular diastolic volume is quite severe. As cardiac output falls, there is decreased renal perfusion. This results in increased liberation of aldosterone, providing for a compensatory increase in extracellular volume. The increase in extracellular volume increases right ventricular filling pressure, which eventually becomes essential for maintaining ventricular diastolic volume in the face of severe pericardial constriction.

CARDIAC TAMPONADE

Cardiac tamponade, like constrictive pericarditis, also restricts ventricular diastolic filling, but it is caused by extrinsic conpression of the ventricular wall from fluid in the pericardium. Symptoms of cardiac tamponade are usually rapid in onset but depend on the rate and volume of pericardial fluid accumulation. With rapid fluid accumulation in the pericardium, a small volume can produce symptoms. With a more gradual accumulation of fluids, the pericardium stretches slightly, and larger pericardial volumes are tolerated before symptoms occur. Once symptoms begin, however, they proceed rapidly because of the sigmoidal relationship of pressure and volume in the pericardial sac. As the limit of pericardial distensibility is reached, small increases in volume produce dramatic increases in intrapericardial pressure. Removal of volume from the pericardium follows only a slightly different compliance curve, and removal of small volumes in a situation of severe cardiac tamponade can produce very dramatic relief of symptoms as a result of a rapid fall in pressure.

The features of cardiac tamponade result from restriction of diastolic ventricular filling and increased pericardial pressure. An increase in pericardial pressure produces a fall in the diastolic ventricular volume, which results in a decrease in stroke volume. The increased pericardial pressure is transmitted to the ventricular chamber, which prevents a fall in ventricular pressure in diastole, decreasing the atrial-to-ventricular pressure gradient, and impeding ventricular filling. Increased intraventricular pressure decreases coronary perfusion

pressure (the arterial diastolic pressure minus the ventricular end-diastolic pressure) and also results in early closure of the tricuspid valve, limiting diastolic flow and reducing ventricular volume. Figure 7–4 provides a diagrammatic summary of the pathophysiology of cardiac tamponade. The compensatory mechanisms in cardiac tamponade are similar to those in constrictive pericarditis. A fall in cardiac output results in an increase in endogenous catecholamines. The consequent increases in heart rate and contractility help maintain cardiac output in the face of a decreased stroke volume. Increased contractility increases the ejection fraction, allowing more complete ventricular emptying. Two features to consider in the compensatory mechanisms of cardiac tamponade are the opposing tendencies in the oxygen supply/demand balance. The increased heart rate increases oxygen demand, both through an increase in contractility and in the number of ventricular activations per minute. It also decreases the diastolic time for coronary perfusion. On the other hand, the increased contractility and heart rate produce more complete ventricular emptying, which may decrease wall tension and decrease the oxygen demand. Elevation in blood pressure that may result from an increase in cardiac output and contractility may raise arterial diastolic pressure, thus increasing coronary perfusion pressure and oxygen supply. There is no way to tell beforehand which of these two opposing tendencies will be predominant.

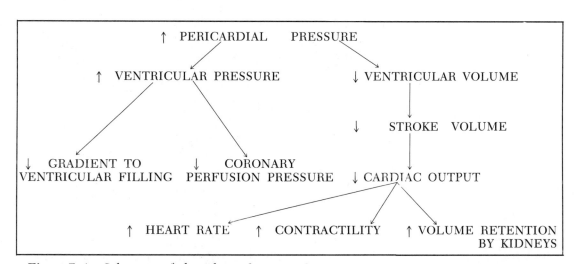

Figure 7–4. Schematic of physiology of tamponade.

Table 7–8 *Conditions Producing Constrictive Pericarditis and Cardiac Tamponade*

	Associated Cardiac Conditions
I. Constrictive pericarditis	
A. Idiopathic	
B. Infectious	
1. Can be sequela of most acute bacterial infections that produce pericarditis	Chronic myocarditis
a. Tularemia	1. Cardiomyopathy
b. Tuberculosis	2. Valvular malfunction
2. Viral — especially arbovirus, coxsackie B	
3. Mycotic	
a. Histoplasmosis	Valvular obstruction
b. Coccidioidomycosis	
C. Neoplastic	
1. Primary mesothelioma of pericardium	
2. Secondary to metastases — especially malignant melanoma	1. Cardiomyopathy
	2. Coronary artery disease
D. Physical causes	
1. Radiation	
2. Post-traumatic	1. Cardiomyopathy
3. Post-surgical	2. Coronary artery disease
E. Systemic syndromes	
1. Systemic lupus	1. Cardiomyopathy
	2. Coronary artery disease
	3. Aortic stenosis
2. Rheumatoid arthritis	1. Cardiomyopathy
	2. Cardiac tamponade
3. Uremia	
II. Cardiac tamponade	
A. Infectious	Myocarditis
1. Viral — most	1. Cardiomyopathy
2. Bacterial — especially tuberculosis	2. Valve malfunction
3. Protozoal	
a. Amebiasis	
b. Toxoplasmosis	
4. Mycotic infection	Valvular obstruction

B. Collagen disease
  1. Systemic lupus   1. Cardiomyopathy
                                            2. Coronary artery disease
                                            3. Constrictive pericarditis
  2. Acute rheumatic fever
  3. Rheumatoid arthritis   1. Cardiomyopathy
                                            2. Coronary artery disease
                                            3. Aortic stenosis

C. Metabolic disorders
  1. Uremia   Low cardiac output
  2. Myxedema
D. Hemorrhagic diatheses
  1. Genetic coagulation defects
  2. Anticoagulants
E. Drugs
  1. Apresoline (Hydralazine)
  2. Procainamide (Pronestyl)
  3. Diphenylhydantoin (Dilantin)
F. Physical causes
  1. Radiation   1. Cardiomyopathy
                                          2. Coronary artery disease
                                          3. Constrictive pericarditis
  2. Trauma
    a. Surgical manipulation
    b. Intracardiac catheters
    c. Pacing wires
G. Neoplasia
  1. Primary — mesothelioma
                 — juvenile xanthogranuloma
  2. Metastatic
H. Miscellaneous
  1. Post-myocardial infarction — ventricular rupture
  2. Pancreatitis
  3. Reiter's syndrome
  4. Behcet's syndrome
  5. Loeffler's syndrome — endocardial fibroelastosis with eosinophilia   Aortic regurgitation
  6. Long-standing congestive heart failure   Restrictive cardiomyopathy

The hemodynamics of cardiac tamponade are similar to those of constrictive pericarditis in that both have a diastolic pressure plateau where the right ventricular end-diastolic, pulmonary capillary wedge, and left atrial pressures are equivalent. In contrast to constrictive pericarditis, the cardiac output is usually depressed from the outset in cardiac tamponade. A paradoxical pulse of at least 20 torr is very common in cardiac tamponade; whereas it is usually absent in constrictive pericarditis. Another subtle difference between cardiac tamponade and constrictive pericarditis is that usually in cardiac tamponade there is an inspiratory augmentation of venous return; whereas in constrictive pericarditis there is no augmentation or only minimal augmentation of venous return during inspiration.

Anesthesia and Monitoring. Monitoring should be aimed at the compensatory mechanisms in constrictive pericarditis and cardiac tamponade. The electrocardiogram should be observed for heart rate and ischemic changes, since the myocardial oxygen supply/demand ratio can be altered by the pathologic process (e.g., the high ventricular filling pressure) and also by therapeutic interventions. Filling pressures should also be assessed. The decision between the use of a Swan-Ganz pulmonary artery catheter or a central venous pressure catheter is based on the following: 1) the state of ventricular function; 2) the surgical procedure; and 3) the postoperative monitoring requirements. Central venous pressure monitoring is indicated in the following instances: 1) if cardiac tamponade is superimposed on an otherwise normal ventricle, as in trauma; 2) if the surgical procedure is merely drainage of the tamponade fluid and an exploration of the pericardium in an effort to determine the cause of the tamponade (here the CVP will adequately indicate the relief of cardiac tamponade); and 3) if postoperative monitoring is only aimed at following the potential reaccumulation of pericardial fluid. The central venous pressure is probably more sensitive than the pulmonary capillary wedge pressure in diagnosing reaccumulations of pericardial fluid (Fig. 7-5). The right ventricle has a very steep Starling curve with a relatively narrow range of filling pressures, which are lower than those of the left ventricle. In addition, filling pressures that would indicate reaccumulation of pericardial fluid

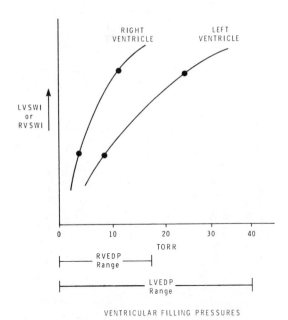

Figure 7-5. Right and left ventricular function curves where left or right ventricular stroke work index (LVSWI or RVSWI, respectively) is plotted as a function of right or left ventricular end-diastolic pressure (RVEDP or LVEDP, respectively).

are more widely divergent from the normal right ventricular filling pressures than they are from the filling pressures of the left ventricle. Accordingly, monitoring right ventricular filling pressures is a more sensitive indicator of developing tamponade. On the other hand, in cardiac tamponade produced by radiation or uremia, coupled with a cardiomyopathy, or in constrictive pericarditis of any cause, the Swan-Ganz catheter probably provides more information. During a pericardiectomy, the Swan-Ganz catheter is useful in assessing myocardial depression occurring secondary to cardiac manipulation or to the kinking of coronary arteries when the heart is lifted out of the pericardial sac and in assessing the volume status of the patient. Postoperative monitoring must address both the problems of reaccumulation of pericardial fluid and of the development of overt ventricular failure in patients with an underlying cardiomyopathy. The decision to employ intra-arterial monitoring of the blood pressure is made by considerations similar to those used in selecting appropriate monitoring for filling pressures. In uncomplicated cardiac tamponade, auscultatory blood pressure measurements are probably adequate, but if ventricular compromise is present or if considerable manipulation of the heart, as in a pericardiectomy, is anticipated, intra-arterial monitoring is probably the only reasonable way to follow beat-to-beat changes in cardiac output and blood pressure.

Since the symptoms of cardiac tamponade and constrictive pericarditis both result from impedance to diastolic filling, the initial measures of circulatory support for these conditions are similar. Cardiovascular support may be required prior to definitive therapy in either condition, but especially in cardiac tamponade. Circulatory therapy should be directed toward the three main compensatory mechanisms in these conditions: 1) maintenance of adequate ventricular filling; 2) maintenance of heart rate; and 3) maintenance of myocardial contractility. Intravascular volume maintenance is critical in these conditions, and falls in filling pressures can result in dramatic decreases in cardiac output. Because an increased heart rate maintains the cardiac output in the face of a decreased stroke volume, beta-stimulators such as isoproterenol or dobutamine are probably the inotropic drugs of choice, since they increase the heart rate and usually decrease the systemic vascular resistance. Drugs such as phenylephrine or methoxamine are contraindicated, since they increase systemic vascular resistance and usually decrease heart rate reflexly secondary to increases in blood pressure. With the use of inotropic drugs, such as isoproterenol and dobutamine, myocardial contractility is also maintained, contributing to homeostasis by increasing ejection fraction.

The first step in the anesthetic management of cardiac tamponade is to assess its severity. The anesthesiologist needs to decide whether induction of anesthesia can be tolerated. This is assessed, primarily, by noting the arterial blood pressure. If the arterial blood pressure is low, for example 70/50 torr, pericardiocentesis or a pericardial window under local anesthesia is needed prior to induction of anesthesia, since even minimal myocardial depression under these circumstances will probably result in major hemodynamic decompensation. After the relief of severe cardiac tamponade, one should reassess cardiac function. Usually after complete relief of tamponade, the situation is one of a normal ventricle in which normal diastolic filling and blood pressure

have been restored. If this is the case, then one can proceed with a careful intravenous barbiturate induction followed by a volatile anesthetic agent or a narcotic-nitrous oxide anesthetic technique. If the tamponade is not completely relieved, or if ventricular function is still depressed, general anesthesia can be managed with fentanyl and diazepam or with intravenous ketamine. Morphine, under these circumstances, is relatively contraindicated, since it may produce a fall in filling pressures associated with histamine release and venous dilation. If the patient initially presents with relatively mild cardiac tamponade, the anesthetic technique employing fentanyl and diazepam or ketamine can be used from the outset. In this setting, an increase in the heart rate associated with the use of some muscle relaxants, such as pancuronium or gallamine, may be advantageous in maintaining circulatory homeostasis. In the presence of restricted ventricular diastolic filling, the initiation of positive pressure ventilation may severely decrease venous return. When this occurs, intravascular volume must be increased in an effort to increase the ventricular filling pressure. After the relief of tamponade the physiologic situation tends to revert to normal, and further anesthetic requirements will then depend on the degree of cardiac manipulation by the surgeon in exploration of the pericardium if, for example, bleeding from a coronary graft is the cause of the tamponade. In this case, there will be continuing hemorrhage that must be handled by blood replacement in the usual manner.

Though both constrictive pericarditis and cardiac tamponade restrict ventricular filling, constrictive pericarditis tends to be chronic in nature, and acute circulatory support is usually not needed. In constrictive pericarditis, the altered physiology remains throughout most of the surgical procedure, whereas in cardiac tamponade the altered physiology is often rapidly relieved by opening the pericardium. The features of anesthetic management are similar to those of unrelieved cardiac tamponade: maintaining the intravascular volume, heart rate, and myocardial contractility. In this setting, similar anesthetic techniques are also used, but a number of special problems may arise in the patient who comes to surgery for pericardiectomy. Arrhythmias, often requiring a continuous lidocaine infusion, are quite frequent with the dissection of the adherent pericardial sac away from the ventricular epicardial surface. Rapid changes in filling pressures with cardiac manipulation occur, and many times there is literally a beat-to-beat change in blood pressure along with changes in filling pressure and cardiac output. Thus, it is important for the anesthesiologist to be in constant communication with the operating surgeon concerning the hemodynamic response to the various manipulations of the heart. During pericardiectomy with frequent episodes of hypotension, it is often difficult to distinguish relative hypovolemia and transient myocardial depression, which occur with cardiac manipulation, from incipient myocardial failure. Here the Swan-Ganz catheter is particularly useful in distinguishing between hypotension due to hypovolemia and hypotension secondary to myocardial failure. Pericardiectomy is frequently associated with bleeding and coagulation problems. During the procedure there is a continued oozing of blood from the raw pericardial and epicardial surfaces requiring transfusion of whole blood and fresh-frozen plasma. If the patient will not tolerate the severe cardiac manipulation, cardiopulmonary bypass with systemic heparinization is required for circulatory support during the procedure, particularly during the dissection on the posterior cardiac surface. If cardiopulmonary bypass and heparinization are required, then the coagulation problems become very complex, requiring multiple transfusions of fresh-frozen plasma and platelets. These bleeding problems often continue after heparin reversal by protamine. Even without the use of cardiopulmonary bypass, postoperative mechanical ventilation is usually the easiest method of managing the postpericardiectomy patient until multiple intraoperative problems such as continued bleeding, arrhythmias, and myocardial injury and depression are resolved.

VALVULAR LESIONS

The normal function of the cardiac valves is to maintain one-way forward flow and the integrity of the cardiac chambers during contraction. Valvular lesions interfere with this function either by producing obstructions to forward flow or by failing to maintain chamber integrity and allowing varying degrees of backward flow. This section will consider the pathophysiology of uncommon causes of valvular lesions and how these diseases affect cardiac compensatory mechanisms. The cardiac dysfunction caused by valvular lesions can be more easily understood in the light of normal valvular function. Taking the left ventricle as a model, there is an initial passive filling of the ventricle from the left atrium when the atrial pressure exceeds the left ventricular diastolic pressure. With atrial contraction there is increased diastolic filling and, as the ventricular volume increases, the mitral valve leaflets begin to drift together. Ventricular contraction is divided into two phases: isovolumic and isotonic. With isovolumic contraction the pressure in the ventricle increases. The mitral valve snaps closed, and left ventricular pressure rises until it equals the aortic diastolic pressure. At this point, the aortic valve opens and blood is ejected during the isotonic phase of left ventricular contraction until the left ventricular pressure falls below the aortic pressure, at which time the aortic valve closes. The left ventricular chamber pressure falls during the phase of isovolumic relaxation until the pressure in the ventricle is below the pressure in the left atrium. At this point, the mitral valve opens and blood from the left atrium again enters the left ventricle.

Lesions producing valvular stenosis are usually graded on the basis of valve area according to the Gorlin formula, which states that flow across the stenotic valve is directly proportional to the square root of the difference in transvalvular pressure. This relationship states that the valve area is the key factor in determining flow across an obstruction. Flow is also influenced by such factors as blood viscosity and turbulence across the valve. Regurgitant lesions are usually evaluated on an angiographic basis on a scale of 1 to 4+ depending on the rate of dye clearance.

Rheumatic valvular lesions often exist as isolated defects in a relatively normal cardiovascular system, and they can be present for extended periods without symptoms. In contrast, the uncommon diseases considered here produce valvular lesions that are usually not associated with an otherwise normal circulatory system; since these lesions frequently occur in the setting of cardiomyopathy, pulmonary hypertension, cor pulmonale, or coronary artery disease. The asymptomatic period in rheumatic lesions is related to the effectiveness of intrinsic cardiovascular compensatory mechanisms, and symptoms begin only when these compensatory mechanisms fail. With the diseases considered in this section, the normal methods of compensation are often severely compromised, and anesthetic management begins with a consideration of alterations in the compensatory mechanisms. Since anesthetic management of valvular lesions is directed at preserving the compensatory mechanisms, it is essential to understand how these diseases interfere with compensation and how anesthetic manipulations interact with them.

AORTIC STENOSIS (Table 7–9A)

Aortic stenosis results from a narrowing of the aortic outflow tract, with a pressure gradient across this narrow orifice. The obstruction to flow is proportional to the cross-sectional area of the obstructed outlet for which the left ventricle compensates by increasing the transvalvular pressure to maintain flow. The ventricle undergoes concentric hypertrophy in order to force blood across the stenotic valve but as a result suffers a decrease in compliance and a loss of part of its ability to dilate. As a result of hypertrophy, ventricular wall tension per unit area is decreased, but total ventricular oxygen demand is increased because of an increase in left ventricular mass. Another method of compensation for aortic stenosis is an increase in ventricular ejection time that decreases the turbulent flow across the valve, thus decreasing flow resistance and allowing for more complete ventricular emptying. As ventricular compliance falls, passive filling of the ventricle during diastole is decreased and the ventricle becomes increasingly reliant on atrial augmentation of ventricular diastolic volume. In this setting, the atrial "kick" may add as much as 30 per cent to the left ventricular end-diastolic volume. In aortic stenosis, ventricular filling pressures increase, related both to decreased ventricular compliance, where the same filling volume produces an increase in filling pressure, and to a real increase in intravascular volume. Left ventricular hypertrophy in aortic stenosis results in a decreased wall tension overall,

but the increased intraventricular systolic pressure virtually eliminates systolic coronary flow. Diastolic subendocardial blood flow also falls as a result of a decrease in transmural pressures; and for this reason, perfusion pressures must remain elevated in order to provide adequate myocardial blood flow.

In light of the foregoing, it should now be considered how a disease process might affect compensatory mechanisms. First, a disease could potentially interfere with the compensatory mechanism of concentric hypertrophy and increased ventricular contractility. In Pompe's disease, left ventricular hypertrophy occurs but is secondary to massive myocardial glycogen accumulation, and for this reason, the ventricular strength is not increased to compensate for the outflow tract obstruction that commonly occurs in this disease. Another example would be amyloidosis where aortic stenosis is coupled with a congestive cardiomyopathy. Here, as in Pompe's disease, there is an inability to increase either ventricular muscle mass or contractility. A disease process may also interfere with the critical atrial augmentation of ventricular end-diastolic volume as, for example, in sarcoidosis or Paget's disease. Diseases of this type infiltrate the cardiac conduction system, resulting in arrhythmias or heart block with the loss of synchronous atrial contraction. The requirement for elevated ventricular diastolic filling pressure may be compromised in a situation such as methysergide toxicity, which can produce mitral stenosis coupled with aortic stenosis. This reduces both passive ventricular filling and ventricular filling resulting from atrial contraction. Diseases that affect the conduction system in addition to producing loss of atrial contraction can also produce tachyarrhythmias which decrease ventricular ejection time and increase turbulent flow across the valves. Table 7–9 lists causes of aortic stenosis and key features of pathophysiology that can adversely affect cardiac compensatory mechanisms.

PULMONIC STENOSIS (Table 7–9A)

As in aortic stenosis, the valve area is the critical determinant of transvalvular blood flow. Pulmonic stenosis produces symptoms that are similar to the classic clinical fea-

Table 7-9A Uncommon Causes of Valvular Lesions

Disease	Features Affecting Compensatory Mechanisms		
	Atrial Transport and Rhythm	Contractility and Hypertrophy	Associated Problems
A. Aortic stenosis (A.S.)			
1. Congenital and degenerative diseases			
a. Congenital			
1) Valvular			
2) Discrete subvalvular			
3) Supravalvular			Coarctation of aorta, polycystic kidneys
b. Biscuspid valve			
c. Degenerative			
1) Senile calcification			
2) Mönckeberg's sclerosis			
2. Infectious diseases			
a. Syphilis		Congestive and obstructive cardiomyopathy	
b. Actinomycosis		Congestive and obstructive cardiomyopathy	
3. Infiltrative diseases			
a. Amyloidosis	S-A and A-V nodal infiltration	1. Congestive cardiomyopathy 2. Coronary artery disease	
b. Pompe's disease		1. Obstructive cardiomyopathy 2. Congestive cardiomyopathy	
c. Fabry's disease		Cardiomyopathy	Hypertension
d. Primary xanthomatosis	Atrial arrhythmias with rapid rate	1. Congestive cardiomyopathy 2. Coronary artery disease	
4. Miscellaneous			
a. Sarcoid	Arrhythmias and inflammation of conduction system	1. LV dyssynergy with aneurysm 2. LV infiltration and cardiomyopathy	
b. Endocardial fibroelastosis		1. Restriction of ventricular filling 2. Interference with subendocardial blood flow with decreased oxygen delivery to myocardium	1. Mitral valve malfunction with stenosis producing poor ventricular filling 2. Regurgitation decreasing LV pressure development
c. Methysergide		Restriction of ventricular filling secondary to endocardial fibrosis	Similar to endocardial fibroelastosis
d. Paget's disease	1. Arrhythmias with loss of atrial kick 2. Complete heart block		Possible mitral stenosis and poor ventricular filling

B. Pulmonary stenosis (P.S.)		
1. Congenital		
a. Valvular		
b. Infundibular		
c. Supravalvular with peripheral coarctation		
2. Genetic — Noonan's syndrome	Cardiomyopathy — obstructive and non-obstructive	Aortic regurgitation
3. Infiltrative		Aortic stenosis and outflow tract obstruction
a. Pompe's	Arrhythmias secondary to conduction system infiltration	
	Congestive cardiomyopathy	
b. Lentiginosis	Massive A-V septal hypertrophy Cardiomyopathy	Cor pulmonale
c. Sarcoid	Arrhythmias secondary to conduction system involvement	Tricuspid insufficiency Pulmonary insufficiency
4. Infectious		
a. SBE	Heart block	
b. Tuberculosis		
c. Rheumatic fever	Usually associated with other valvular lesions	
5. Neoplastic		
a. Mediastinal tumors	Rhythm or cardiomyopathic complications will depend on extent of wall involvement in the neoplastic process	
b. Primary tumors		
1) Sarcoma		
2) Myxoma		
c. Malignant carcinoid syndrome	Endocardial fibrosis	1. Pulmonary hypertension 2. Pulmonary regurgitation 3. Tricuspid regurgitation and/or stenosis
6. Physical — extrinsic causes		
a. Aneurysm of ascending aorta or sinus of Valsalva		Dependent on cause
b. Constrictive pericarditis	Picture of restrictive cardiomyopathy but usually with good ventricular function	
c. Post-surgical banding		Often associated with other congenital cardiac anomalies

tures of aortic stenosis: fatigue, dyspnea, syncope, and angina. The compensatory mechanisms in pulmonic stenosis are similar to those in aortic stenosis. Initially, under the stress of right ventricular outflow obstruction, the right ventricle dilates but eventually undergoes concentric hypertrophy and changes from a crescent-shaped chamber best suited to handle volume loads to an ellipsoidal chamber best suited to handle a pressure load. Secondly, there is an increase in ejection time, maintained with a slow heart rate. Thirdly, increases in ventricular filling pressure occur as a result of an increase in intravascular volume and of a change in the compliance of the right ventricle. The presence of angina, which occurs occasionally in pulmonary stenosis, should especially be noted. Usually, the right ventricle is a thin-walled chamber with low intraventricular pressures. This normal situation results in a high transmural perfusion pressure and good subendocardial blood flow that limits development of ischemia of the right ventricle. Concentric hypertrophy increases both right ventricular mass and right ventricular pressures, increasing potential for ischemia of the right ventricle, since right ventricular oxygen requirements are increased and coronary perfusion pressure may be decreased. Cyanosis can occur with severe pulmonic stenosis accompanied by a low, fixed cardiac output. When right ventricular pressure rises, fetal intracardiac shunts may reopen, producing right-to-left intra-atrial shunting. Usually, isolated pulmonic stenosis is well-tolerated for long periods until compensatory mechanisms fail. When a second valvular lesion coexists with pulmonic stenosis, the potential effects of this lesion on compensatory mechanisms should be considered.

Compensatory mechanisms in pulmonic stenosis can be altered in much the same way as in aortic stenosis. Decreases in right ventricular contractility occur in infiltrative diseases of the myocardium, such as Pompe's disease or sarcoidosis. The loss of the atrial "kick" and the development of tachyarrhythmias have the same implications for cardiac function in pulmonic stenosis as in aortic stenosis. In subacute bacterial endocarditis, tricuspid insufficiency may coexist with pulmonic stenosis, producing an impairment of pressure development in the right ventricle, especially when right ventricular failure supravenes. With the increase in right ventricular mass and the increased requirement for oxygen delivery to the right ventricle, the possibility should be considered that oxygen supply may be compromised, as in the coronary artery pathology of Pompe's disease.

AORTIC INSUFFICIENCY (Table 7–9B)

The primary problem in aortic insufficiency is a decrease in net forward blood flow from the left ventricle due to diastolic regurgitation of blood back into the left ventricular chamber. The first question to ask in the setting of aortic insufficiency is whether the condition is acute or chronic, since this is often the main determinant of the degree of compensation when the patient is first seen. Aortic insufficiency represents an almost pure volume overload of the left ventricular chamber. The left ventricle responds initially with dilation to maximize the effects of increases in fiber length. Acutely, this may result in heart failure, since the increased ventricular diameter increases wall tension and oxygen demand. An acute increase in ventricular volume may also compromise the anchoring of the mitral valve by changing the geometric relationship of the papillary muscles, resulting in mitral regurgitation and pulmonary edema. In chronic aortic insufficiency, however, a number of compensatory changes minimize the degree of diastolic regurgitation. The first compensatory mechanism is changes in the left ventricle itself. The left ventricle increases chamber size with eccentric hypertrophy (i.e., hypertrophy in the setting of chamber enlargement). The left ventricular compliance is increased, which produces an increase in ventricular volume at the same or a lesser ventricular filling pressure, thus reducing ventricular wall stress. The increase in ventricular volume allows full use of the Frank-Starling mechanism, whereby the strength of ventricular contraction is increased with increasing fiber length and the ejection fraction is maintained, since both stroke volume and ventricular end-diastolic volume increase together. Despite these compensatory mechanisms, however, a number of studies have shown that ventricular contractility does tend to be slightly depressed. In contrast to aortic stenosis, the supplementation of ventricular end-diastolic volume by the atrial contraction is not essential to ventricular compensation in aortic insufficiency. A rapid heart rate seems to be advantageous in aortic insufficiency as opposed to a slow rate in aortic stenosis, since the rapid heart rate in aortic insufficiency reduces the time for diastolic filling and helps prevent diastolic overdistension of the ventricle from regurgitant flow. In aortic insufficiency the amount of regurgitant flow increases as systemic vascular resistance increases; thus the third major compensatory mechanism in aortic insufficiency is the maintenance of a low peripheral resistance, since forward flow in aortic insufficiency is inversely proportional to the systemic vascular resistance.

The increase in chamber size and eccentric hypertrophy, which help maintain cardiac function in aortic insufficiency, can be compromised in such conditions as ankylosing spondylitis in which myocardial fibrosis limits the increase in chamber size to the degree that this disease produces a restrictive picture. Cogan's syndrome produces a generalized cardiomyopathy with coronary artery disease and can alter the compensatory mechanism by decreasing both the ability of the left ventricle to hypertrophy and that of the coronary arteries to deliver oxygen to the ventricle. Increases in left ventricular compliance could be prevented in such situations as aortic insufficiency produced by methysergide, which produces an endocardial fibrosis and thus decreased ventricular compliance. The usual ability of the left ventricle to maintain the ejection fraction in aortic insufficiency could be compromised by the cardiomyopathy of amyloidosis where, rather than being maintained, the ejection fraction will fall as ventricular dysfunction increases. The aortic insufficiency produced by acute bacterial endocarditis is occasionally associated with complete heart block, resulting in a slow heart rate with ventricular overdistension and a decrease in cardiac output. Aortic insufficiency due to conditions such as systemic lupus associated with systemic arterial hypertension and increased peripheral resistance can increase the regurgitant fraction in the face of the incompetent aortic valve.

PULMONIC INSUFFICIENCY (Table 7–9B)

Pulmonic insufficiency usually occurs in the setting of pulmonary hypertension or cor pulmonale but may exist as an isolated lesion, as in acute bacterial endocarditis in heroin addicts. Pulmonary insufficiency is extremely well tolerated for long periods of time. Like aortic insufficiency, it represents a volume overload on the ventricular chamber, but the crescentic right ventricular geometry is such that volume loading is easily handled. Compensatory mechanisms for pulmonic insufficiency are the same as for aortic insufficiency: an increase in right ventricular compliance, rapid heart rate, and low pulmonary vascular resistance. The right ventricle is normally a highly compliant chamber, and with its steep filling pressure-stroke volume curve it functions very well in the presence of volume increases. The degree of pulmonic regurgitation is determined by the pulmonary-arterial-diastolic-to-right-ventricular-end-diastolic pressure gradient. For this reason, low pulmonary vascular resistance and concomitant low pulmonary diastolic pressure are essential to maintaining forward flow. In general, there is less increase in ventricular-end-diastolic volume than in aortic insufficiency. The ejection fraction, however, is not as well maintained in pulmonic insufficiency as it is in aortic insufficiency. With severe pulmonic regurgitation, as in aortic insufficiency, eccentric hypertrophy of the ventricular chamber occurs.

Disease states can interfere with the compensatory mechanisms of the right ventricle in several ways. Diseases that produce pulmonary insufficiency, such as the malignant carcinoid syndrome, also produce an endocardial fibrosis that decreases the ability of the right ventricular chamber to dilate in response to volume loading. Increases in pulmonary vascular resistance increase both right ventricular afterload and the regurgitant fraction. This is especially true when pulmonary insufficiency is secondary to pulmonary hypertension. Hypoxia from any cause can increase pulmonary vascular resistance as, for example, the hypoxia which results from pulmonary vascular dysfunction in carcinoid syndrome. It is unusual for cardiomyopathy to exist alongside isolated pulmonary insufficiency, thus the potential for eccentric hypertrophy is usual-

Table 7-9B *Uncommon Causes of Valvular Lesions*

Disease	Features Affecting Compensatory Mechanisms			Associated Cardiovascular Abnormalities
	LV Compliance and Contractility	Heart Rate and Rhythm	Vascular Resistance	
A. Aortic regurgitation (A.R.)				
1. Infiltrative disease				
a. Amyloidosis	Congestive and restrictive cardiomyopathy	Arrhythmias with infiltration of conduction system		1. Coronary artery disease 2. Stenosis or insufficiency of other valves
b. Morquio's c. Schere's	Usually isolated aortic insufficiency with mild mucopolysaccharidosis			
d. Pseudoxanthoma elasticum	Congestive cardiomyopathy			
2. Infectious disease				
a. Bacterial endocarditis		Complete heart block		Insufficiency of other valves
b. Syphilis	Congestive or restrictive cardiomyopathy	Infiltration of conduction system		1. Aortic stenosis 2. Aortic aneurysm
c. Rheumatic fever				
3. Congenital valve disease				
a. Bicuspic aortic valve	Usually intact compensatory mechanisms			
b. Aneurysm of sinus of Valsalva				
c. Congenital fenestrated cusp				
4. Degenerative				
a. Marfan's	Normal	Normal	Cystic medial necrosis of aorta with dissection	Pulmonary insufficiency
b. Osteogenesis inperfecta	Normal	Normal	Cystic medial necrosis	Mitral regurgitation
5. Inflammatory				
a. Relapsing polychondritis				Mitral regurgitation
b. System lupus erythematosus	Pericarditis and effusion		Hypertension secondary to renal disease	Mitral regurgitation
c. Reiter's syndrome				
d. Rheumatoid arthritis	Congestive cardiomyopathy	Complete heart block		1. Aortic stenosis 2. Mitral stenosis and/or insufficiency 3. Constrictive pericarditis 4. Cardiac tamponade

Lesion	Hemodynamic consequences	Conduction effects	Vascular effects	Associated lesions
6. Systemic syndromes				
a. Ankylosing spondylitis	1. Coronary artery disease 2. Congestive cardiomyopathy	Complete heart block		Aortic dissection
b. Cogan's syndrome			Generalized angiitis	
c. Noonan's syndrome	Cardiomyopathy			Pulmonic stenosis
d. Ehlers-Danlos				Spontaneous vascular dissection
7. Miscellaneous causes	Interference with compensation depends on cause, e.g., syphilis, Marfan's, traumatic			
a. Aortic dissection				Mitral valve stenosis and/or insufficiency
b. Methysergide	Endocardial fibrosis — restriction of LV filling			
c. Traumatic rupture	Acute dilatation and failure			
B. Pulmonic regurgitation (P.R.)				
1. Congenital				
a. Isolated	Usually tolerated as isolated lesion			
1) Hypoplastic				
2) Aplastic				
3) Bicuspid				
b. Associated with other congenital cardiac lesions	Toleration of P.R. depends on degree of myocardial dysfunction induced by other cardiac lesions			
2. Acquired				
a. Syphilitic aneurysm of P.A.	Congestive cardiomyopathy	Infiltration of conduction system	Luminal narrowing	
b. Rheumatic	Tolerated well in isolation			
c. Bacterial endocarditis	Endocardial fibrosis	Complete heart block		Endocarditis of other valves
d. Echinococcus cyst	Endocardial fibrosis			Tricuspid valve malfunction
3. Malignant carcinoid syndrome				Tricuspid valve malfunction
4. Physical				
a. Traumatic				
b. After valvotomy for pulmonic stenosis	Decreased ventricular compliance if RV hypertrophic from PS			
5. Functional — secondary to pulmonary hypertension	Ventricular hypertrophy with decreased compliance		Elevated pulmonary resistance due to pulmonary hypertension	1. Chronic obstructive pulmonary disease 2. Mitral stenosis 3. Primary pulmonary hypertension

ly left intact. However, syphilis could present a situation in which cardiomyopathy exists along with pulmonic insufficiency, though this would depend on the extent of syphilitic involvement of the myocardium.

MITRAL STENOSIS (Table 7–9C)

The primary defect in mitral stenosis is a restriction of normal left ventricular filling across the mitral valve. As in other stenotic lesions, the area of the valve orifice is the key to flow; and, as the orifice gets smaller, turbulent flow increases across the valve, and total resistance to flow increases. The valve area usually cannot be altered without surgery. The important features in compensation of mitral stenosis are 1) increasing the pressure gradient across the valve, and 2) minimizing turbulent flow. The mechanisms whereby compensation is accomplished in mitral stenosis include: 1) dilation and hypertrophy of the left atrium, 2) increases in atrial filling pressures, and 3) a slow heart rate, or at least not a rapid heart rate, to allow sufficient time for diastolic flow and to decrease the turbulent flow. Usually decompensation in rheumatic mitral stenosis occurs when atrial fibrillation occurs with a rapid ventricular rate, resulting in a loss of the atrial contraction, which helps maintain diastolic transvalvular flow, and an increase in pulmonary vascular engorgement due to decreased flow across the mitral valve. Thus, altered left ventricular function is usually not the limiting factor in the ability of the heart to compensate for mitral stenosis. The observation has been made that cardiac index is decreased for between 48 to 72 hours after mitral valve replacement, which may be secondary to either trauma to the left ventricle involved in excising the mitral valve or to chronic depression of left ventricular function, which occurs in mitral stenosis, even though the left ventricle is "protected."

As in other valvular lesions produced by uncommon diseases, one should look for coexistent cardiovascular problems that interfere with compensatory mechanisms. Diseases such as sarcoidosis or amyloidosis can infiltrate atrial muscle, preventing left atrial hypertrophy or dilation and interfering with atrial transport during diastole. Amyloidosis, gout, and sarcoidosis can also affect the conduction system of the heart,

resulting in heart block, tachyarrhythmias, or atrial fibrillation.

TRICUSPID STENOSIS (Table 7–9C)

Tricuspid stenosis is usually associated with mitral stenosis as a sequela of rheumatic fever. Usually the other valve lesions associated with tricuspid stenosis determine heart function and the tricuspid stenosis often exists as an almost incidental lesion. Isolated tricuspid stenosis is very rare. The problems in tricuspid stenosis are similar to those in mitral stenosis. There is a large right-atrial-to-right-ventricular diastolic gradient, and flow across the stenotic tricuspid valve is related to valve area. The compensatory mechanisms in tricuspid stenosis are also similar to those in mitral stenosis. First, an increase in right atrial pressure maintains flow across the stenotic valve, and occasionally this is associated with peripheral edema. Second, the heart compensates with right atrial dilatation and hypertrophy, increases in the strength of atrial contraction, and improvement in atrial transport of blood across the stenotic valve. The implications of slow heart rate in tricuspid stenosis are the same as in mitral stenosis, and, as in mitral stenosis, ventricular contractility is usually well-maintained but may be depressed. The onset of atrial fibrillation in tricuspid stenosis is a less crucial event than in mitral stenosis. In tricuspid stenosis it may produce symptoms such as cyanosis or an increase in peripheral edema, while in mitral stenosis it may produce a dramatic increase in pulmonary congestion, respiratory distress, and signs of left-sided failure.

Diseases can interfere with cardiac compensation for tricuspid stenosis in much the same way as they can interfere with cardiac compensation for mitral stenosis. Dilatation and hypertrophy of the right atrium can be compromised by an associated cardiomyopathy in systemic lupus. There may be further restriction of right ventricular filling in conditions such as malignant carcinoid syndrome that produce an endocardial fibrosis which further limits right ventricular filling. Frequently, tricuspid stenosis coexists with pulmonic stenosis in the carcinoid syndrome, resulting in an extremely severe restriction of cardiac output. Diseases that interfere with the conduction system of the

Table 7–9C *Uncommon Causes of Valvular Lesions*

Disease	Features Affecting Compensatory Mechanisms			Associated Conditions
	Rhythm	Atrial Transport	LV Function	
A. Mitral stenosis (M.S.)				
1. Inflammatory				
a. Rheumatic fever				
b. Rheumatoid arthritis	Heart block	1. Pericardial constriction 2. Cardiac tamponade	Congestive cardiomyopathy	1. Aortic stenosis and insufficiency 2. Mitral insufficiency
2. Infiltrative				
a. Amyloidosis	1. Heart block 2. Infiltration of conduction system	Atrial dilatation and hypertrophy	Congestive and restrictive cardiomyopathy	Malfunctioning of other valves
b. Sarcoidosis	Infiltration of conduction system			
c. Gout	Infiltration of conduction system		Congestive cardiomyopathy	1. Pulmonary hypertension 2. Cor pulmonale
3. Miscellaneous				
a. Left atrial myxoma				
b. Parachute mitral valve	Normal compensatory mechanism			
c. Concentric ring of left atrium				
d. Methysergide				
e. Wegener's granulomatosis	Arrhythmias secondary to myocardial vasculitis	Myofiber degeneration	Endocardial fibrosis Congestive cardiomyopathy	Mitral insufficiency
B. Tricuspid stenosis				
1. Inflammatory				
a. Rheumatic fever	Usually associated with other valvular lesions			
b. Systemic lupus	Arrhythmias secondary to pericarditis			
2. Fibrotic				
a. Carcinoid syndrome		Fibrosis evolving to hypertrophy and dilatation	1. Pulmonary hypertension with increased RV afterload 2. Endocardial fibrosis	Pulmonary stenosis
b. Endocardial fibroelastosis	Similar to carcinoid syndrome			
c. Methysergide	Similar to carcinoid syndrome			
3. Miscellaneous				
a. Hurler's	Infiltration of conduction system	Infiltration of atrial wall	Congestive cardiomyopathy	Mitral and aortic valvular abnormality
b. Myxoma of right atrium		Usually normal compensatory mechanisms		Aortic stenosis

heart can produce arrhythmias, particularly tachyarrhythmias, which have the same implications in tricuspid stenosis as they do in mitral stenosis.

MITRAL REGURGITATION (Table 7–9D)

Mitral regurgitation, like aortic regurgitation, results from failure of the affected valve to maintain chamber integrity during the cardiac cycle. Mitral regurgitation occurs by one of three basic mechanisms: 1) damage to the valve apparatus itself; 2) inadequacy of the chordae tendineae-papillary muscle support of the valvular apparatus; or 3) left ventricular dilation and stretching of the mitral valve annulus with a loss of the structural geometry required for valvular closure during systole. Mitral regurgitation represents a volume overload of both the left atrium and the left ventricle, producing as much as a four- to fivefold increase in ventricular end-diastolic volume. In mitral regurgitation, ventricular contractility is usually well preserved because of the parallel unloading circuit through the open mitral valve, which allows a rapid reduction of wall tension in the ventricle during systole. Ironically, mitral regurgitation serves as its own protective afterload reduction system. Compensatory mechanisms in mitral regurgitation include ventricular dilatation, elevations in ventricular filling pressure, and the maintenance of low peripheral resistance. As in the situation of volume overloading in aortic insufficiency, ventricular dilatation allows maximum advantage to be gained from the Frank-Starling mechanism, maintaining ejection fraction and cardiac output. Again, as in aortic insufficiency, forward flow from the ventricle is inversely related to the systemic vascular resistance. A low peripheral resistance maintains forward flow, whereas increases in peripheral resistance increase the degree of regurgitant flow through the mitral valve. In mitral regurgitation the heart tends to benefit from a relatively rapid heart rate, since a slow rate is associated with an increased ventricular diastolic diameter that may distort the mitral valve apparatus even further and result in increased regurgitation, in addition to increasing oxygen demand by an increase in wall tension.

A number of diseases can be cited that interfere with the compensatory mechanisms in mitral regurgitation. When mitral regurgitation is secondary to amyloid infiltration of the mitral valve, ventricular dilatation is compromised by coincident amyloid infiltration of the ventricular myocardium, which restricts ventricular diastolic filling. Amyloid infiltration of the conduction system can cause heart block and bradycardia, resulting in increased mitral regurgitation for reasons noted above. In mitral regurgitation associated with left ventricular failure there is, in addition to poor left ventricular function, an elevation of endogenous catecholamine activity, which increases peripheral vascular resistance, resistance to forward flow, and regurgitant flow.

TRICUSPID INSUFFICIENCY (Table 7–9D)

Triscuspid insufficiency is mechanically somewhat similar to mitral insufficiency. The most common cause of tricuspid insufficiency, however, is right ventricular failure. Even in this setting, tricuspid insufficiency is usually well tolerated, just as it is well-tolerated when it exists in isolation. Tricuspid insufficiency represents a volume overload of both the right ventricle and the right atrium, but because of the high compliance of the systemic venous system, pressure in the right atrium is usually not elevated as it sometimes is in the left atrium in mitral insufficiency. This remains true until the right ventricle loses its compliance, as it might when faced with a high pressure afterload, as in pulmonary hypertension resulting in right ventricular hypertrophy and failure, and in tricuspid insufficiency. The main compensatory mechanism in tricuspid insufficiency is adequate filling of the right ventricle. Since the right ventricle is constructed to efficiently handle a volume load, with adequate filling, cardiac output is usually maintained. An increase in venous return, which occurs as a result of the negative intrapleural pressure resulting from spontaneous ventilation, helps maintain adequate right ventricular filling even in the presence of tricuspid insufficiency. The main reason tricuspid insufficiency is well tolerated is that it is usually superimposed on a normal right ventricle that continues to function with good contractility as long as

Table 7-9D *Uncommon Causes of Valvular Lesions*

Disease	Features Affecting Compensatory Mechanisms			
	Rate	LV Function and Compliance	Vascular Resistance	Associated Conditions
A. *Mitral regurgitation (M.R.)*				
1. Conditions producing annular dilatation				
a. Aortic regurgitation		Usually in failure at this stage	Elevated with low output	
b. Left ventricular failure		LV failure	Usually elevated	
2. Conditions affecting the chordae and papillary muscles				
a. Myocardial ischemia	Associated arrhythmias, especially bradyarrhythmias	Often poor	Normal or elevated if cardiac output decreased	
b. Chordal rupture				
c. IHSS		Hyperkinetic with low ventricular compliance	Usually elevated	
3. Condition affecting the valve leaflets				
a. Marfan's / Ehlers Danlos / Osteogenesis inperfecta		Usually intact — these conditions also affect connective tissue of chordae tendineae		
b. Rheumatic fever			Aortic stenosis may be present	Other associated valve abnormalities
c. Rheumatoid arthritis	Heart block	Congestive cardiomyopathy	Aortic regurgitation	Coronary artery disease
d. Ankylosing spondylitis	A-V dissociation			Coronary artery disease
e. Amyloid	S-A and A-V nodal infiltration	Restrictive and congestive cardiomyopathy		
f. Gout	Urate deposits in conduction system	Usually normal		
B. *Tricuspid regurgitation*				
1. Annular dilatation				
a. RV failure		RV in failure	Often secondary to pulmonary hypertension	
b. Pulmonary insufficiency		RV in failure or extremely dilated	Often secondary to pulmonary hypertension	
2. Leaflets, chordae and papillary muscles				
a. Epstein anomaly				
b. Acute bacterial endocarditis				
c. Rheumatic fever		Compensation intact		

right ventricular filling is maintained. Usually, only conditions that result in right ventricular failure, such as pulmonary hypertension, will cause tricuspid insufficiency to become hemodynamically significant. In this situation, the loss of integrity of the right ventricular chamber due to the incompetent tricuspid valve results in an increase in regurgitant flow at the expense of forward flow through the pulmonary circulation, decreasing the volume delivered to the left ventricle, with a resulting decrease in cardiac output.

Anesthesia and Monitoring. Perioperative problems will arise from valvular lesions when compensatory mechanisms acutely fail. Monitoring should be selected to give a continuing assessment of the status of these compensatory mechanisms. Certain aspects of monitoring should be considered common to all valvular lesions. First, the electrocardiogram is essential for monitoring cardiac rhythm and ischemic changes. Filling pressures should certainly be monitored, employing either the Swan-Ganz catheter or a central venous pressure catheter, as appropriate to the specific lesion. Blood pressure can best be monitored with an indwelling arterial catheter. Sphygmomanometric monitoring is less desirable, particularly when lesions are severe, since blood pressure and cardiac output may be very labile and continuous assessment is required. In addition, an arterial line provides for the monitoring of blood gases, which is important when pulmonary function is compromised.

In lesions such as aortic or pulmonic stenosis, where high pressure chambers have developed, monitoring of V_5 or limb lead II, respectively, is mandatory for assessing ischemia. Monitoring of rate and rhythm is especially important in regurgitant lesions and in mitral and tricuspid stenosis for the reasons noted above. The reason for aggressive monitoring of filling pressures is clear if one recalls that many lesions, mitral stenosis for example, are exquisitely sensitive to preload. In tricuspid and pulmonic stenosis, the Swan-Ganz catheter may be difficult, if not impossible, to pass but, fortunately, right-sided filling pressures indicate loading conditions, and these can be monitored with a central venous pressure line. In right-sided regurgitant lesions, however, the Swan-Ganz catheter can usually be passed if regurgitant

flow is not so great that it interferes with the forward movement of the balloon-tipped catheter. If the chest is to be opened in patients in whom it was not possible to pass a Swan-Ganz catheter, and in whom one anticipates ventricular compromise postoperatively, a pulmonary artery pressure line and thermistor can be inserted under direct vision for intra- and postoperative determination of cardiac outputs. A left-sided atrial pressure line may also be inserted to follow left-sided filling pressures. In left-sided valvular lesions, a Swan-Ganz catheter is indicated for monitoring both filling pressures and cardiac output. With the Swan-Ganz catheter in place, vascular resistances for both the pulmonary and the systemic circulations can be calculated, allowing an assessment of therapeutic interventions, as has been mentioned before. Further, changes in wave forms of the PCWP or CVP trace can often indicate increases in regurgitation or the development of regurgitation in situations of ventricular overdistention.

The anesthetic management of valvular lesions must avoid significant depression of contractility, since virtually all valvular lesions depend on good contractility as a major compensatory mechanism. This is especially true if the valve lesion is coexistent with a cardiomyopathy in which minor decreases in contractility can result in major cardiac decompensation. In valvular lesions, a narcotic technique probably represents the least trespass on physiologic reserves. Fentanyl produces the fewest cardiovascular changes of any narcotic studied, although bradycardia and chest wall rigidity occasionally occur. Both of these problems are usually easily handled by the use of a muscle relaxant such as pancuronium, which reduced chest rigidity and corrects the bradycardia by increasing heart rate. The use of morphine occasionally causes falls in preload secondary to its histamine-releasing properties, but when morphine is given slowly, (5 mg/min or less), this is usually not a major problem. Nitrous oxide is a traditional supplement to narcotic analgesia, but it should be recalled that nitrous oxide is to some degree a myocardial depressant and has the property of slightly increasing both pulmonary and systemic vascular resistance. This is usually not of great significance, but it may be important in severe regurgitant lesions when it may serve to increase regurgitant flow. Ketamine is probably not an unreasonable anesthetic in regurgitant lesions, owing to its slight sympathetic stimulating properties, but it is probably contraindicated in stenotic lesions because of the problem of an increase in heart rate. Muscle relaxants, when used in valvular lesions, should probably be selected according to their autonomic properties. For example, pancuronium or gallamine may be useful in aortic insufficiency owing to the increase in heart rate produced by both of these muscle relaxants. In mitral stenosis, on the other hand, dimethyltubocurarine may be the appropriate muscle relaxant, since it apparently has the fewest autonomic side effects and will not result in a detrimental increase in heart rate. In a similar manner, adjuvant drugs for sedation and amnesia can be selected on the basis of analogous considerations. Drugs such as the phenothiazines or the butyrophenones, which have mild alpha-adrenergic blocking properties, may be usefully employed in lesions such as aortic or mitral insufficiency where decreases in systemic vascular resistance can have a beneficial effect on forward flow. Diazepam has been shown to decrease left ventricular filling pressure in congestive failure and could possibly be usefully employed here. Where sympathetic tone is increased and is important in maintaining cardiovascular homeostasis or where elevated ventricular filling pressures are critical, one should employ these adjuvant drugs with care, since the loss of sympathetic outflow with sleep or the onset of alpha-blockade may be detrimental.

CONCLUSION

Although the main focus of each of these sections has been on the cardiovascular pathology encountered in uncommon diseases, the clinician should remember that very few of these diseases have isolated cardiovascular pathology. Many of the diseases discussed are severe multi-system diseases, and an anesthetic plan must also consider the needs of monitoring dictated by other systemic pathology (e.g., measurements of blood sugar in diabetes secondary to hemochromatosis) and the potential untoward effects of drugs in unusual metabolic disturbances (e.g., the use of drugs with histamine releasing properties such as curare, morphine, or thiopental in the malignant carcinoid syndrome).

Certainly, it cannot be stated dogmatically that one anesthetic technique is absolutely superior to all others in the management of any particular lesion, particularly those due to the often bizarre conditions discussed here. The key to the proper anesthetic management of any uncommon disease lies in an understanding of the disease process, particularly the compensatory mechanisms involved in maintaining cardiovascular homeostasis, the cardiovascular effects of anesthetic drugs, and monitoring of the effects of anesthetic and therapeutic interventions.

REFERENCES

Cardiomyopathies

Fowler, N. O.: Classification and diagnosis of myocardial diseases. *In* Fowler, N. O. (ed): Myocardial Diseases. New York, Grune & Stratton, 1973, pp. 25–37.

Abelman, W. H.: Clinical aspects of viral cardiomyopathy. *In* Fowler, N. O. (ed): Myocardial Disease. New York, Grune & Stratton, 1973, pp. 253–280.

Wigle, E. D., Felderhof, C. H., et al.: Hypertrophic obstructive cardiomyopathy. *In* Fowler, N. O. (ed.): Myocardial Diseases. New York, Grune & Stratton, 1973, pp. 297–318.

Perloff, J. K.: The myocardial disease of heredofamilial neuromyopathies, *In* Fowler, N. O. (ed.): Myocardial Diseases. New York, Grune & Stratton, 1973, pp. 319–336.

Segel, L. D., and Mason, D. T.: Alcohol and the heart. *In* Advances in Heart Disease. New York, Grune & Stratton, 1977, pp. 481–489.

Wenger, N. K.: Myocarditis. *In* Hurst, J. W.: The Heart. 4th ed., New York, McGraw-Hill, 1978, pp. 1529–1955.

Braunwald, E.: Cardiomyopathy. *In* Hurst, J. W.: The Heart. 4th ed., New York, McGraw-Hill, 1978, pp. 1560–1566.

Mason, D. T., Spann, J. F., et al.: Alterations of hemodynamics and myocardial mechanics in patients with congestive heart failure. Prog. Cardiovasc. Dis. *12*:502, 1970.

Dodge, H. T., and Baxley, W. A.: Hemodynamic aspects of heart failure. Am. J. Cardiol. *22*:24, 1968.

Mason, D. T.: Regulation of cardiac performance in clinical heart disease. *In* Mason, D. T.: Congestive Heart Failure, Yorke Med Bks, 1976, pp. 111–128.

Tonkin, M. J., Rosen, S. M., et al.: Renal function and edema formation in congestive heart failure. *In* Mason, D. T.: Congestive Heart Failure, Yorke, Med Bks, 1976, pp. 169–182.

Rubin, E.: Alcoholic myopathy in heart and skeletal muscle. N. Engl. J. Med. *301*:28, 1979.

Bing, R. J.: Cardiac metabolism: Its contributions to alcoholic heart disease and myocardial disease. Circulation 58:965, 1978.

Maron, B. J., Cardiac metabolism: Its contributions to

alcoholic heart disease and myocardial disease. Circulation 58:965, 1978.

Maron, B. J., and Epstein, S. E.: Hypertrophic cardiomyopathy: A discussion of nomenclature. Am. J. Cardiol. 43:1242, 1979.

Rosing, D. R., Kent, K. M., et al.: Verapramil therapy: A new approach to the pharmacologic treatment of hypertrophic cardiomyopathy. I: Hemodynamic effects. Circulation 60:1201, 1979.

Mikulik, E., Cohn, J. N., et al.: Comparative hemodynamic effects of inotropic and vasodilator drugs in severe heart failure. Circulation 56:528, 1977.

Matlof, H. J., and Harrison, D. C.: Acute haemodynamic effects of practolol in patients with idiopathic hypertrophic subaortic stenosis. Br. Heart J. 35:152, 1973.

Leier, C. V., Heban, P. T., et al.: Comparative systemic and regional hemodynamic effects of dopamine and dobutamine in patients with cardiomyopathic heart failure. Circulation 58:466, 1978.

Hug, C. C., Kaplan, J. A.: Pharmacology: Cardiac drugs. In Kaplan, J. A.: Cardiac Anesthesia, New York, Grune & Stratton, 1979, pp. 39–70.

Chatterjee, K., and Parmley, W. W.: The role of vasodilator therapy in heart failure. Prog. Cardiovasc. Dis. 19:301, 1977.

Goldberg, L. I., Hirsh, Y., and Resenkov. L.: New catecholamines for treatment of heart failure and shock: An update on dopamine and a first look at dobutamine. Prog. Cardiovasc. Dis. 19:327, 1977.

Coronary Artery Disease

Sonnenblick, E. H., and Skelton, C. L.: Myocardial energetics: Basic principles and clinical applications. N. Engl. J. Med. 285:668, 1971.

Sonnenblick, E. H., Ross, J., and Braunwald, E.: Oxygen consumption of the heart: Newer concepts of its multifactorial determination. Am. J. Cardiol. 22:328, 1968.

Waller, J. L., Kaplan, J. A., and Jones, E. L.: Anesthesia for coronary revascularization. In Kaplan, J. A.: Cardiac Anesthesia, New York, Grune & Stratton, 1979, pp. 241–280.

Kaplan, J. A.: Electrocardiographic monitoring. In Kaplan, J. A.: Cardiac Anesthesia. New York, Grune & Stratton, 1979, pp. 117–66.

Bigger, T. J., Dresdale, R. J., Heissenbuttel, R. H., et al.: Ventricular arrhythmias in ischemic heart disease: Mechanism, prevalence, significance, and management, Prog. Cardiovasc. Dis. 19:255, 1977.

Hoffman, J. I., and Buckberg, G. D.: The myocardial oxygen supply-demand ratio. Am. J. Cardiol. 41:327, 1978.

Klocke, F. J.: Coronary blood flow in man. Prog. Cardiovasc. Dis. 19:117, 1976.

Wenger, N. K.: Rare causes of coronary artery disease. In Hurst, J. W.: The Heart. 4th ed., McGraw-Hill, 1978, pp. 1345–1361.

Forrester, J. S., Diamond, G., McHugh, T. J., et al.: Filling pressures in the right and left sides of the heart in acute myocardial infarctions. N. Engl. J. Med., 285:190, 1971.

Swan, H. J. C., Ganz, W., Forrester, J. S., et al.: Catheterization of the heart in man with the use of a flow directed balloon-tipped catheter. N. Engl. J. Med. 283:447, 1970.

Bland, J. H. L., and Lowenstein, E.: Halothane-induced decrease in experimental myocardial ischemia in the non-failing canine heart. Anesthesiology 45:287, 1976.

Lowenstein, E., Hallowell, P., and Levine, F. H.: Cardiovascular response to large doses of intravenous morphine in man. N. Engl. J. Med. 281:1389, 1969.

Stanley, T. H., and Webster, L. R.: Anesthetic requirements and cardiovascular effects of fentanyl-oxygen and fentanyl-diazepam-oxygen anesthesia in man. Anesth. Analg. 57:411, 1978.

Smith, R. R. C., and Hutchins, G.: Ischemic heart disease secondary to amyloidosis of intramyocardial arteries. Am. J. Cardiol. 44:413, 1979.

Bharati, S., Lev, M., et al.: Infiltrative arrhythmias: Electrophysiologic and pathologic correlation. Am. J. Cardiol. 45:163, 1979.

Perloff, J. K.: Myocardial disease of heredofamilial neuromyopathies. In Fowler, N. O. (ed.): Myocardial Disease, New York, Grune & Stratton, 1973, pp. 319–335.

Gerry, J. L., Buckley, B. H., and Hutchins, G.: Clinicopathologic analysis of cardiac dysfunction in 52 patients with sickle cell anemia. Am. J. Cardiol. 42:211, 1978.

Conti, C. R., Selby, J. H., et al.: Left main coronary artery stenosis: Clinical spectrum, pathophysiology, and management. Prog. Cardiovasc. Dis. 22:73, 1978.

Hillis, L. D., and Braunwald, E.: Myocardial ischemia. N. Engl. J. Med. 296:971, 1034, 1093, 1977.

Pulmonary Hypertension and Cor Pulmonale

Blount, S. G., and Grover, R. F.: Pulmonary hypertension. In Hurst, J. W.: The Heart. 4th ed., New York, McGraw-Hill, 1978, pp. 1456–1476.

Dexter, L., and Dalen, J. E.: Pulmonary embolism and acute cor pulmonale. In Hurst, J. W.: The Heart. 4th ed., New York, McGraw-Hill, 1978, pp. 1472–1484.

Feldman, N. T., and Ingram, N. T.: Chronic cor pulmonale. In Hurst, J. W.: The Heart. 4th ed., New York, McGraw-Hill, 1978, pp. 1485–1496.

Harris, P., and Heath, D.: Causes of pulmonary arterial hypertension. In The Human Pulmonary Circulation. New York, Churchill Livingstone, 1977, pp. 226–242.

Harris, P., and Heath, D.: The pulmonary vasculature in emphysema. In The Human Pulmonary Circulation. New York, Churchill Livingstone, 1977, pp. 504–521.

Harris, P., and Heath, D.: Pulmonary haemodynamics in chronic bronchitis and emphysema. In The Human Pulmonary Circulation. New York, Churchill Livingstone, 1977, pp. 522–546.

Harris, P., and Heath, D.: The pulmonary vasculature in fibrosis of the lung. In The Human Pulmonary Circulation. New York, Churchill Livingstone, 1977, pp. 626–634.

Harris, P., and Heath, D.: Pharmacology of the pulmonary circulation. In The Human Pulmonary Circulation, New York, Churchill Livingstone, 1977, pp. 182–210.

Krayenbuehl, H. P., Turina, J., and Hess, O.: Left ventricular function in pulmonary hypertension. Am. J. Cardiol. 41:1150, 1978.

Stein, P. D., Babbah, H. N., Anbe, D. T., and Maryilli, M.: Performance of the failing and non-failing right ventricle of patients with pulmonary hypertension. Am. J. Cardiol. 44:1050, 1979.

Baum, S. L., Schwartz, A., et al.: Left ventricular function in chronic obstructive lung disease. N. Engl. J. Med. 285:361, 1971.

West, J. B.: Blood flow to the lung and gas exchange. Anesthesiology 41:124, 1974.

Benumof, J. L., and Wahrenbrock, E. A.: Local effects of anesthetics on regional hypoxic pulmonary vasoconstriction. Anesthesiology 43:525, 1975.

Webb-Johnson, D. C., and Andrews, J. L.: Bronchodilator therapy (Part I). N. Engl. J. Med. 297:476, 1978.

Webb-Johnson, D. C., and Andrews, J. L.: Bronchodilator therapy (Part II). N. Engl. J. Med. 297:758, 1978.

Constrictive Pericarditis and Cardiac Tamponade

Shabetai, R., Mangiardi, V., et al.: The pericardium and cardiac function. Prog. Cardiovasc. Dis. 22:107, 1978.

Hancock, E. W.: Constrictive pericarditis. J.A.M.A. 232:176, 1975.

Field, J., Shiroff, R. A., et al.: Limitations in the use of the pulmonary capillary wedge pressure with cardiac tamponade. Chest 70:451, 1976.

Morgan, B. C., Guntheraeth, W. G., et al.: Relationship of pericardial to pleural pressure during quiet respiration and cardiac tamponade, Circ. Res. 16:493, 1965.

Pories, W. J., and Gaudiani, V. A.: Cardiac tamponade. Surg. Clin. North Am. 55:573, 1975.

Shabetai, R., Fowler, N. O., et al.: The hemodynamics of cardiac tamponade and constrictive pericarditis, Am. J. Cardiol. 26:480, 1970.

Brown, D. F., and Older, T.: Pericardial constriction as a late complication of coronary bypass surgery. J. Thorac. Cardiovasc. Surg. 74:61, 1977.

Kaplan, J. A., Bland, J. W., et al.: The perioperative management of pericardial tamponade. South. Med. J. 69:417, 1976.

Berger, R. L., Loveless, G., et al.: Delayed and latent postcardiotomy tamponade, Ann. Thor. Surg. 12:22, 1971.

Valvular Lesions

Reddy, P. S., Curtiss, E. L., et al.: Cardiac tamponade: Hemodynamic observations in man. Circulation 58:265, 1978.

Thomas, S. J., and Lowenstein, E.: Anesthetic management of the patients with valvular heart disease. Int. Anesth. Clin. 17:67, 1979.

Schlant, R. C., and Nutter, D. O.: Heart failure in valvular heart disease. Medicine 50:421, 1971.

Chambers, D. A.: Acquired valvular heart disease. *In* Kaplan, J. A.: Cardiac Anesthesia, New York, Grune & Stratton, 1979, pp. 197–240.

Miller, G. A. H., Kirklin, J. W., and Swan, H. J. C.: Myocardial function and left ventricular volumes in acquired valvular insufficiency. Circulation 31:374, 1965.

Kelly, D. T., Spotnitz, H. M., et al.: Effects of chronic right ventricular volume and pressure loading on left ventricular performance. Circulation 44:403, 1971.

McCullough, W. H., Covell, J. W., and Ross, J.: Left ventricular dilatation and diastolic compliance changes during chronic volume overloading. Circulation 45:943, 1972.

Jose, A. D., Taylor, R. R., and Bernstein, L.: The influence of atrial pressure on mitral incompetence in man. J. Clin. Invest. 43:2094, 1964.

Braunwald, E.: Mitral regurgitation. N. Engl. J. Med. 281:425, 1969.

Brodeur, M. T. H., Lees, M. H., et al.: Right ventricular volume in pulmonic valve disease. Am. J. Cardiol. 19:671, 1967.

Ross, J., and McCullagh, W. H.: Nature of enhanced performance of the dilated left ventricle in the dog during chronic volume overloading. Circ. Res. 30:549, 1972.

Meerson, F. Z., and Kapelko, V. I.: The contractile function of the myocardium in two types of cardiac adaptation to a chronic load. Cardiology 57:183, 1972.

Roberts, W. C., and Perloff, J. K.: Mitral valvular disease. Ann. Intern. Med. 77:939, 1972.

Smith, J. A., and Levine, S. A.: The clinical features of tricuspid stenosis. Am. Heart J. 23:739, 1942.

Morgan, J. R., Forker, A. D., et al.: Isolated tricuspid stenosis. Circulation 44:729, 1971.

Yu, P. N., Harken, D. E., et al.: Clinical and hemodynamic studies of tricuspid stenosis, Circulation 13:680, 1956.

Kitchin, S., Turner, R.: Diagnosis and treatment of tricuspid stenosis. Brit. Heart J., 26:354, 1964.

Keefe, J. F., Walls, J., et al.: Isolated tricuspid valvular stenosis. Am. J. Cardiol. 25:252, 1970.

Morgan, J. R., and Focker, A. D.: Isolated tricuspid insufficiency. Circulation 43:559, 1971.

Hansing, C. E., and Rowe, G. C.: Tricuspid insufficiency. Circulation 45:793, 1972.

Seymour, J., Emanuel, R., et al.: Acquired pulmonary stenosis. Brit. Heart J. 30:776, 1968.

Johnson, L. W., Grossman, W., et al.: Pulmonic stenosis in the adult. N. Engl. J. Med. 287:1159, 1972.

Hamby, R. L., and Gulotta, S. J.: Pulmonic valvular insufficiency: Etiology, recognition, and management. Am. Heart J. 74:110, 1967.

Price, B. O.: Isolated incompetence of the pulmonic valve. Circulation 23:596, 1961.

Fowler, N. O., and Duchesne, E. R.: Effect of experimental pulmonary valvular insufficiency on the circulation. J. Thorac. Cardiovasc. Surg. 35:643, 1958.

Holmes, S. C., Fowler, N. O., et al.: Pulmonary valvular insufficiency. Am. J. Med. 44:857, 1968.

Rees, J. R., Epstein, E. J., et al.: Haemodynamic effects of severe aortic regurgitation, Brit. Heart J. 26:412, 1964.

Judge, T. P., Kennedy, J. W., et al.: Quantitative hemodynamic effects of heart rate in aortic regurgitation. Circulation 44:355, 1971.

Miller, R. R., Vismara, L. A., et al.: Afterload reduction therapy with nitroprusside in severe aortic regurgitation: Improved cardiac performance and reduced regurgitant volume. Am. J. Cardiol. 38:564, 1976.

Bolen, S. L., and Alderman, E. L.: Hemodynamic consequences of afterload reduction in patients with chronic aortic regurgitation. Circulation 53:879, 1976.

Stewart, S. R., Robbins, D. C., et al.: Acute fulminant aortic and mitral insufficiency in ankylosing spondylitis. N. Engl. J. Med. 299:1448, 1978.

Heller, S. J., and Carleton, R. A.: Abnormal left ventricular function in patients with mitral stenosis. Circulation 42:1099, 1970.

Kroetz, F. W., Leonard, J. J., et al.: The effect of atrial contraction on left ventricular performance in valvular aortic stenosis. Circulation 35:852, 1967.

Yoran, C., Yelling, E. L., et al.: Mechanism of reduction of mitral regurgitation with vasodilator therapy. Am. J. Cardiol. 43:773, 1979.

Yoran, C., Yellin, E. L., et al.: Dynamic aspects of acute mitral regurgitation, Circulation 60:170, 1979.

8

Hematologic Diseases

By J. ANTONIO ALDRETE, M.D., M.S.
and FRANK GUERRA, M.D.

Megaloblastic Anemias
    Vitamin B_{12} Deficiency (Pernicious
      Anemia)
    Folate Deficiency
Blood Loss Anemia
Anemia Due to Renal Failure
Anemia Due to Hepatic Failure
Aplastic Anemia
Sideroblastic Anemias
Hemolytic Anemias
    Hereditary Spherocytosis
    Hereditary Elliptocytosis
    Other Congenital Hemolytic Anemias
    Hemoglobinopathies
    Autoimmune Hemolytic Anemias
    Drug-Induced Hemolytic Anemias
    Spur Cell Anemia
    Microangiopathic Hemolytic Anemia
    March Hemoglobinuria
    Gaucher's Disease
    Felty's Syndrome

Hemochromatosis
Erythropoietin
    Relation of 2,3-DPG to Hemoglobin
      Function
Diseases of the White Cell Elements
    Agranulocytosis
    Cyclic Neutropenia
    Myeloproliferative Diseases
Disorders of Hemostasis
    Abnormalities of Platelet Function and/or
      Capillary Vessels
    Abnormalities of Blood Coagulation
    Disorders Affecting Vessel and/or Platelet
      Function and Blood Coagulation
Transfusion Reactions
    Allergic Reactions
    Febrile Reactions
    Pyrogen Reactions
    Hemolytic Reactions
    Other Effects of Transfusion

This chapter deals with the blood, the alterations of its cellular elements, and the many biochemical functions of its intracellular fragments, enzymes, and molecular components. It reviews the current concepts of diseases of the hematopoietic and reticuloendothelial systems, from congenital aberrations to acquired malignancies, as well as extrinsic factors such as local or systemic disease and drug toxicity that can produce either depletion (pancytopenias, anemias, agranulocytosis) or abnormal proliferation (polycythemias, leukemias) of formed elements.

The considerations that anesthesiologists must keep in mind when managing patients with hematologic disorders are discussed, as are the various related diseases. Recent advances in the molecular basis of hemoglobinopathies are considered, as is the importance of the role that organic phosphate compounds such as 2,3-diphosphoglycerate and adenosine triphosphate have on the transport of oxygen by hemoglobin. The experimental work dealing with the depressant effects of anesthetic agents on the bone marrow is reviewed. Finally, possible therapeutic implications and potential professional hazards involved in chronic exposure to minute concentrations of anesthetic (gaseous and volatile) agents are elaborated upon. In his classic description of leukemia or "white blood," Virchow stated in 1845, "I have presented these observations only with the purpose of showing that such a remarkable and unusual case may have so many relationships with further investigations, and so many suggestions for explaining other questions, but it remains a rather uncertain subject for positive proof and conclusion so long as it itself remains unexplained." Nearly the same could have been said of every hematologic disorder. Since then, significant advances have been made, and in the process Virchow's prediction has been proved true in many entities.

To facilitate the understanding of some of the terminology, the various generations of blood cells as they germinate from the stem cells of the bone marrow are schematized in Figure 8–1.

MEGALOBLASTIC ANEMIAS

More than 95 per cent of the cases of megaloblastic anemia are caused by a deficiency of either vitamin B_{12} or folate.

The hematologic findings include anemia, granulocytopenia, and thrombocytopenia. The thrombocytopenia is usually not so severe as to cause spontaneous bleeding. Peripheral blood and bone marrow show macrocytes (oval, egg-shaped, or tear-drop forms), and poikilocytes. Granulocytes are hypersegmented, and four-lobed eosinophils may be present.

VITAMIN B_{12} DEFICIENCY (PERNICIOUS ANEMIA)

Vitamin B_{12} deficiency is the result of glandular atrophy of the stomach, with impaired production of gastric intrinsic factor.[2] Strictly speaking, pernicious anemia is one of a number of causes of vitamin B_{12} deficiency, with its attendant megaloblastic anemia. Other causes include partial gastrectomy, sprue, cancer, dietary deficiency of vitamin B_{12}, congenital deficiency of intrinsic factor, selective vitamin B_{12} malabsorption, blind loop syndromes, cancer, fish tapeworm, thyroid disease (Hashimoto's thyroiditis with thyroid antibodies, myxedema), lupus erythematosus, drugs (colchicine, para-aminosalicylic acid, alcohol, phenformin, anticonvulsants and neomycin — mild interference with vitamin B_{12} absorption), regional ileitis, hypoadrenalism, hypoparathyroidism, pregnancy, severe chronic pancreatitis, and moniliasis.[3, 4] A very rare variety is the congenital form of pernicious anemia, in which case the gastric mucosa is normal, with impaired acid secretion seen in siblings born from consanguineous unions.[2, 3] Occasionally, pernicious anemia may also be present in patients with diverticulosis and intermittent bowel obstruction.[5, 6]

Dietary deficiency of vitamin B_{12} is rare in the United States, except in people with unusual dietary habits, such as pure vegetarians. It is more common in areas of the world where animal protein is rarely consumed.[7]

Clinical findings in vitamin B_{12} deficiency may include such symptoms as dyspnea on exertion, anorexia, weight loss, weakness, easy fatigability, palpitations, syncope, headache, and angina pectoris, any or all of which may be symptoms of anemia. Other, more specific complaints include sore tongue, limb paresthesias, ataxic gait, bowel and bladder motor disturbances, and defects in memory. Neurological effects in patients with a megaloblastic anemia strongly suggest vitamin B_{12} deficiency. These effects may become irreversible if they persist untreated over extended periods of time.

On physical examination, the complexion is typically lemon-yellow as a result of combined anemia and jaundice. There may be lingual papillary atrophy or glossitis. Liver and spleen may be enlarged. Congestive heart failure, cardiac arrhythmias, and murmurs may be noted.

Laboratory examinations revealing hypersegmented granulocytes and a mean corpuscular volume greater than 100 $c\mu$ in the presence of severe anemia may suggest the diagnosis. This can be confirmed by a low serum vitamin B_{12} level, performed either by radioisotope dilution methods or by microbiological assays. Measurement of the amount of radioactive B_{12} absorptive capacity may be useful in the differential diagnosis of megaloblastic anemias. Serum unconjugated bilirubin and lactic dehydrogenase may be elevated, owing to an increased production and destruction of erythroblasts and granulocytes.[8]

Of particular interest to anesthesiologists is the literature on the interaction between nitrous oxide and vitamin B_{12}.[9] Nitrous oxide oxidizes cob(I)balamin to cob(II)balamin. This destroys the normal activity of vitamin B_{12}.[10] Lassen et al[11] showed that four of six patients who had been receiving prolonged nitrous oxide as part of a treatment regimen for tetanus developed leukopenia and megaloblastic anemia. Ames et al[12] showed that 50 per cent nitrous oxide given to a patient for six hours produces a mild megaloblastic depression of bone marrow. Twenty-four hours of administration produces severe changes. Vitamin B_{12} partially reverses this effect, as does the withdrawal of nitrous oxide. This effect is probably of no great clinical significance and certainly does not suggest the need to limit the use of nitrous oxide under ordinary clinical circumstances.

FOLATE DEFICIENCY

Folate deficiency is an entity usually secondary to sociopsychological illnesses such as alcoholism, poverty, or food faddism. Since folate is also absorbed in the upper two thirds of the small intestine, it is associated with the diseases of the small bowel previously listed. Proportionally, infants and children have a greater requirement for folate than do adults; this is probably related to the greater demand for active cell growth and division in the former.[7] Since body stores of folate are small, dietary inadequacy of folic acid is rapidly reflected clinically.

Megaloblastic anemia caused by folate deficiency has been documented by Sullivan et al[13] in infants fed almost exclusively on goat's milk, which is poor in folate content.

In adults, folate deficiency is quite common in alcoholics, in whom ethanol appears to impair hematopoiesis by affecting folate metabolism.[14, 15] An increased folate requirement has been documented in pregnancy, hemolytic anemia, and hyperthyroidism.[2, 3] It has been shown that diphenylhydantoin[16] and estrogen-containing contraceptives[17] may produce folate deficiency by inhibiting the activity of intestinal conjugase.[18] Folic acid antagonists used for cancer chemotherapy (e.g., methotrexate) are another cause of drug-induced folate deficiency.

The history of intake of a folate-deficient diet usually suggests the diagnosis, with or without alcoholic antecedents. A smooth tongue, lack of subcutaneous fat, hyperpigmentation, organomegaly, and ankle edema are the most frequent physical findings; they may or may not be accompanied by peripheral neuropathy (glove-stocking type) or hepatic encephalopathy. Neurological findings are due to alcoholism or liver disease, and not to folate deficiency per se.

Folate deficiency anemia is of the macrocytic type, accompanied by hypersegmental granulocytes and oval macrocytes that are difficult to distinguish from those seen in vitamin B_{12} deficiency. Serum folate is lower than the normal range.

The specific treatment recommended for these megaloblastic anemias is the adminis-

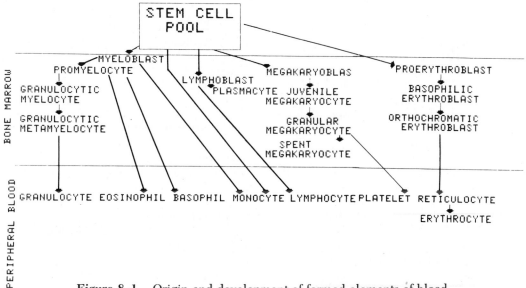

Figure 8–1. Origin and development of formed elements of blood.

tration of the deficient factor, either vitamin B_{12} parenterally or folic acid orally. In general, a well-balanced diet rich in animal protein is also advised.[7]

In the preparation of these patients for elective surgery, the aforementioned measures may be sufficient. Transfusions may be indicated only for patients with cardiovascular symptoms, such as angina pectoris, syncope, and postural hypotension. Transfusions should be administered with great caution, since these patients often have an increased blood volume and may develop congestive heart failure.

Patients with megaloblastic anemia who are in shock, who have congestive heart failure with pulmonary edema or septicemia, and who in addition face emergency surgery, must be treated vigorously. Large doses of vitamin B_{12} and folic acid are given parenterally. The hemoglobin may be brought to normal levels by transfusion, as long as blood with low hemoglobin content is removed from the opposite arm simultaneously, to avoid overloading the circulation. This is probably best regulated by monitoring the central venous and arterial pressures. Massive doses of antibiotics are required in the face of infection. Because of the multiple systemic manifestations of megaloblastic anemia, there are many considerations. Anemia results in an increase in 2,3-diphosphoglycerate (2,3-DPG), which decreases the affinity of oxygen for hemoglobin. This mechanism alone is not enough to compensate for decreased oxygen carrying capacity with severe anemia.

The presence of liver disease in these patients must be evaluated. Hepatic dysfunction may result in altered drug matabolism due to enzyme deficiencies, altered drug distribution and efficacy due to changes in serum proteins, bleeding disorders as a result of deficiencies in hepatically synthesized clotting factors, and systemic and pulmonary shunting causing hypoxia and a hyperdynamic cardiovascular state.

Neurological sequelae may preclude the use of conduction anesthesia. Succinylcholine might be contraindicated if clinically significant muscle wasting has supervened.

Elective surgery should not be undertaken in the patient with untreated, symptomatic megaloblastic anemia. Great caution should be exercised in anesthetizing these patients for emergency surgery.

BLOOD LOSS ANEMIA

During the preoperative evaluation of surgical patients, anemia of moderate degree may be unexpectedly encountered in an otherwise apparently healthy patient. In most instances, the operative procedure can be postponed until a complete work-up of the patient is achieved, but in a few cases the situation has to be evaluated immediately and diagnosed and acted upon promptly.

Since the stability of peripheral hemoglobin levels is maintained by the balance of blood production on one side and destruction on the other, chronic blood loss is the most common cause of anemia; but in the event that the iron stores of the body are insufficient to meet the requirements of the compensatory demand, an iron deficiency type of anemia develops.

After hemorrhage, there is little change in the blood picture until the blood volume has been restored, usually within 36 to 48 hours. Serial hematocrit shows that full equilibration, characterized by a decrease in hematocrit and restoration of normal blood volume, is not achieved until the fourth or fifth day. The replacement of red cells lags behind that of the blood volume. The marrow liberates large numbers of reticulocytes.

The anemia is normochromic and normocytic with mild leukocytosis (10,000 to 20,000) and with few myelocytes or metamyelocytes. The platelet count is usually not altered, except in severe hemorrhage, in which counts of 50,000 to 100,000 may be seen. This is even more apparent when massive transfusions of blood containing a low number of platelets have recently been given.

If iron stores are plentiful, the bone marrow compensates adequately for chronic blood loss; however, iron stores may be rapidly depleted, and then the red cells produced are hypochromic.

The classic experiments performed in volunteers by Moore and associates[19] demonstrated the typical metabolic and cardiovascular changes that occur after sudden hemorrhage, detailed description of which is beyond the scope of this chapter.

In the event of chronic blood loss, blood volume may be normal while hematocrit may be significantly diminished. If hemoglobin levels are below 10 gm per 100 ml, transfusion should be considered preoperatively, especially if the patient is debilitated and symptomatic of anemia. Certainly, if blood loss is anticipated during operation, blood replacement should be meticulous and compulsive.

The acutely bleeding patient should have blood volume and red cells replaced prior to the induction of anesthesia, if at all possible. Volume replacement can be monitored by improvement in symptoms of weakness, dizziness, and postural light-headedness, and signs of postural hypotension and tachycardia. Central venous and Swan-Ganz pressure measurements give very useful data about the patient's volume status.

Often, because of rapid life-threatening bleeding, the patient may need to be operated upon while still volume depleted. Choice of anesthetics for induction and maintenance of anesthesia must take this life-threatening situation into account. Ketamine and pancuronium have been suggested as useful under these circumstances, because of their stimulation of the cardiovascular system. While these agents may be good in specific cases, the further stimulation of an already maximally stimulated cardiovascular system may have disastrous effects, especially in elderly patients.

Hypovolemia will, furthermore, cause a maldistribution of pulmonary blood flow and make a patient who already has a decreased oxygen carrying capacity even more hypoxic.[20] Noble[21] has shown that there is an increase in lung water and a decrease in myocardial performance in dogs after hemorrhagic shock.

Hypovolemia has been shown to exaggerate the depressant effects of trichloroethylene and enflurane in combination with propranolol.[22, 23] This effect was not seen with isoflurane, which apparently has B-receptor activating properties.[24] Tanifuji and Eger[25] have shown that hypotension from a combination of blood loss and trimethaphan decreased the MAC of halothane by 20 to 58 per cent. The decrease in MAC was directly proportional to the decrease in blood pressure. This effect seems to relate to the decrease in volume. In an earlier study,[26] Cullen and Eger demonstrated no change in the MAC of halothane with acute isovolemic anemia.

ANEMIA DUE TO RENAL FAILURE

The anemia of chronic renal failure is normochromic and normocytic. There is often a reticulocytosis. The severity of the anemia may vary with the degree and duration of renal failure, but mild renal failure may be associated with severe anemia. This is basically due to three factors: decreased erythropoiesis, retention of toxins, and hemolysis. The effect on erythropoiesis is related to the decrease in renal mass and hence decreased ability to respond to a drop in red blood cell mass with increased erythropoietin production.[27] Uremia may also impair the responsiveness of the bone marrow to erythropoietin.[28] This in turn is reflected in bone marrow hypoplasia and decreased iron utilization, both of which occur in uremia. In addition, a decreased intestinal absorption of iron and its reduced incorporation into red cells have been demonstrated. The iron deficiency may be exacerbated by bleeding, as a result of platelet dysfunction.[29] Blood may also be lost in the dialysis coil and as a result of blood removal for laboratory studies.[30]

Folic acid deficiency may occur as a result of loss of folate in dialysate and as a result of decreased dietary intake.[31]

Satisfactory chronic hemodialysis is associated with a gradual but slowly progressive improvement in hematopoiesis.[30] Red blood cell survival as measured with Cr^{51} varies inversely with the level of azotemia. In some patients with acute renal insufficiency, there may be a predominance of hemolysis. However, in more chronic cases of renal failure, there is impaired erythropoiesis. Consequently, anemia develops gradually with a compensatory expansion of plasma volume. Attempts to bring the hematocrit to normal levels by rapid transfusions may be not only futile but even dangerous.

Under other circumstances, the markedly low hematocrit levels seen in uremia may be unacceptable; however, in our experience with patients undergoing kidney transplantation[32] and in that of others,[33] patients with chronic anemia tolerate anesthesia remarkably well, probably because they have a normal or higher than normal plasma volume. It is therefore recommended not to set a specific rule as to an acceptable hematocrit, but rather to evaluate each patient individually.

ANEMIA DUE TO HEPATIC FAILURE

Chronic severe liver insufficiency is also associated with anemia, which may or may not be related to deficiency of folic acid or bleeding from esophageal varices, gastritis, or duodenal or gastric ulcers. Bleeding may be exacerbated by thrombocytopenia or decreased levels of bleeding factors. The degree of anemia is usually related to the degree of liver damage. Again red cell mass is decreased by abnormal red cell maturation and an element of hemolysis,[34] leaving a concomitant increase of plasma volume to which hyperaldosteronism and hypoproteinemia may contribute.[35] Alcoholics with cirrhosis may have a decreased intake of folic acid and may have a megaloblastic anemia. Bone marrow response to anemia is diminished in these patients.[4]

As in patients with renal insufficiency, the presence of low hematocrit levels in patients with chronic liver disease does not contraindicate the administration of anesthesia; neither should blood transfusions have to be instituted preoperatively in an effort to bring the hematocrit to normal levels. Slow induction, titrating the dosages of ultra-short-acting barbiturates, may be undertaken without undue hazards. However, blood loss should be promptly replaced and the loss of ascitic fluid compensated for by the infusion of electrolyte and colloid solutions.[36]

APLASTIC ANEMIA

In this type of anemia, the bone marrow fails to produce normal numbers of erythrocytes, in spite of adequate amounts of all hematopoietic factors.

Injury to blood-forming tissues resulting in a defective erythropoiesis is the mechanism for this entity. Neutropenia and thrombocytopenia may occur. Drugs and chemicals causing aplastic anemia include antimicrobials, analgesics, anticonvulsants, antihistamines, anti-inflammatory agents, tranquilizers, antithyroid drugs, hypoglycemics, and chemicals such as benzene, carbon tetrachloride, and glue. Also associated with aplastic anemia is viral hepatitis,[37, 38] an almost universally irreversible and fatal condition. As mentioned in a separate section, prolonged inhalation of nitrous oxide and other anesthetic agents may also result in the same effects. The 10 most common offenders have been recorded in the Registry on Blood Dyscrasias of the American Medical Association.[39] The distinct mechanisms by which these drugs or chemicals produce marrow hypoplasia have not been clarified for all agents. Nevertheless, a defect in an enzyme system, whether acquired or inherited, seems to be responsible for at least the aplastic anemia produced by chloramphenicol, in which a defect in DNA metabolism has been implicated by Nagao and Mauer.[40] Associated with deficient erythropoiesis is intramedullary hyperhemolysis, which is exacerbated when patients receive transfusion therapy.

The onset of the disorder is gradual, and symptoms are usually related to the degree of anemia; pallor of the skin and mucous membranes is striking, suggesting abnormal bleeding. There are ecchymoses, petechiae, epistaxes, and gingival bleeding.[8] Infection as a result of granulocytopenia and monocytopenia may be the first manifestation. Pancytopenia is the most common feature, but anemia and/or leukopenia may be the only characteristics. The bone marrow may be normal, hypercellular, or hypocellular, with an increase of mononuclear cells resembling leukocytes and of plasma cells and reticulum cells. Serum iron is elevated, with a saturated iron-binding capacity, even before blood transfusions are received.[41, 42]

The avoidance of potentially incriminated drugs is perhaps the best prophylactic therapy. If patients are given these compounds, repeated blood counts should be performed at regular intervals and preferably the drugs interrupted as soon as evidence of depression of hematopoiesis is noted. Once the disorder is established, treatment is unsatisfactory. Antibiotics, blood transfusions, steroids, cobaltos chloride, and androgens may be resorted to. Specifically, corticosteroids are helpful in cases of associated thrombocytopenia. The mortality rate is extremely high.

Occasionally, in patients with aplastic

anemia, splenectomy and thymectomy have been employed in treatment, but only a few patients responded well to either of these procedures. Adequate preparation with fresh blood transfusions, platelet infusions, and stepped-up dosages of steroids should be achieved before surgical intervention is contemplated in case of emergency.

SIDEROBLASTIC ANEMIAS

Defects in hemoglobin synthesis and red cell formation as well as accumulation of iron in the bone marrow are typical of this group of anemias, which are present in a number of different conditions.

They are either inherited, such as that seen in thalassemia, or acquired, of which the most descriptive are those observed in pyridoxine-responsive states, leukemias, and myeloid metaplasia as well as in patients on isoniazid (INH) therapy.[43] Other conditions associated with sideroblastic anemia include cancer, rheumatoid arthritis, myxedema, and megaloblastic anemia.

The bone marrow is usually hypercellular, with ineffective erythropoiesis and normo- or megaloblastic maturation. Evidence of defective iron metabolism may be obtained by demonstrating iron granules in the normoblasts of the bone marrow smear. Excessive iron accumulation may also be seen in the liver, spleen, or lungs. Some

patients with this syndrome have been shown to metabolize tryptophan abnormally. INH interferes with pyridoxine metabolism, and sideroblastic anemia may complicate the treatment of tuberculosis.

Although unpredictable, pyridoxine therapy may reverse the condition temporarily or for a long period of time.[44] Occasionally, androgens have also been shown to be of value.

If the anemia is severe, these patients may require multiple transfusions, leading to iron overload in the tissues. Some patients develop acute myelocytic leukemia. It is not known whether sideroblastic anemia is an early manifestation of leukemia or whether this anemia occurs as a result of a leukemic predisposition.

HEMOLYTIC ANEMIAS

An essential feature in hemolytic anemias is a reduction in the life span of the erythrocytes. These anemias have been placed under various classifications — none of them general enough to encompass all — the most accepted classification being congenital and acquired forms of hemolytic anemias. The hemolytic anemias may also be classified in terms of whether the deficit causing the hemolysis is intracellular or extracellular (see Table 8–1). What follows is a discussion of the most important of these entities.

HEREDITARY SPHEROCYTOSIS

This is a mendelian dominant disorder of the red cell membrane without geographic or ethnologic confinements, but it is most frequent in Europeans. It is not sex linked. Although present from infancy, it is often not recognized until adulthood.[45] The association with other abnormalities, such as brachycephaly, polydactyly, brachydactyly, and eye defects with spherocytosis has been noted.

The typical clinical triad is acholuric jaundice, mild to moderate anemia, and a palpable spleen. Less frequent is the occurence of gallstones and leg ulcers.

At examination, the erythrocytes are more spheroidal and less disclike, with a smaller diameter but greater thickness than normal corpuscles. The hemoglobin content of

---

Table 8–1 *Hemolytic Disorders*

Intracellular
  Membrane abnormalities
    Hereditary spherocytosis (elliptocytosis, stomatocytosis)
    Paroxysmal nocturnal hemoglobinuria
  Enzyme defects
    G-6-PD deficiency
    Pyruvate kinase deficiency
  Hemoglobinopathies
    Thalassemias
    Hemoglobin S and C disease
    Unstable hemoglobins
Extracellular
  Immune hemolytic disease
    Cold antibody type
    Warm antibody type
  Fragmentation hemolytic disease
    Mechanical (valvular)
    Microangiopathic
  Clostridial toxemia
  Hypersplenism

Adapted from Lichtman, M.A. (Ed.) *Hematology for Practitioners.* Boston: Little, Brown, & Co., 1978, p. 135.

spherocytes is normal, but the concentration is slightly above the normal range. The reticulocyte count is markedly elevated, between 2 and 20 per cent. There is also increased osmotic fragility typical of spherocytes; this can be further confirmed by incubation fragility and spontaneous lysis tests at 37° C after mechanical trauma.[46]

The erythrocyte lifespan ranges from 20 to 30 days, increasing by 50 to 70 per cent after splenectomy. Atypical spherocytosis and compensated spherocytosis are minor variants of the hereditary form. As in other hemolytic anemias, aplastic crises can result from marrow aplasia.[47]

The bone marrow is hyperplastic, with subsequent skeletal deformities; erythropoiesis is normoblastic, with an increased number of mitotic figures. The spleen and liver may also be involved. As treatment, splenectomy has been successful for patients with chronic hemolytic anemia and a history of aplastic crisis. Splenectomy significantly decreases the rate of hemolysis.[48] It should not be done before the age of four because of the increased risk of infection in splenectomized children.[49] In adult patients undergoing splenectomy, the gallbladder should be examined carefully and concurrent cholecystectomy should be performed in the event of cholelithiasis. Blood transfusions have been palliative only. Steroid therapy is indicated only when autoimmune hemolytic anemia coexists with spherocytosis.

Hereditary Elliptocytosis

This hereditary anemia is characterized by the presence of elliptical erythrocytes inherited following a dominant mendelian pattern.[50] It exists as a nonclinical trait, found incidentally in a routine blood test. A more severe variety is clinically indistinguishable from spherocytosis.[51] This condition should be distinguished from iron deficiency, thalassemia, myelopathic anemia, megaloblastic anemia, and sickle cell disease, which may also exhibit elliptocytes.

The degree of elliptocytosis varies from patient to patient, sometimes involving 90 per cent of the cells, which may be markedly elongated or merely oval. Poikilocytes, microcytes, and cell fragments are frequently seen in cases of severe hemolysis. Although no biochemical abnormality of hemoglobin has been demonstrated, coexistence with Hb S or Hb C has been documented.[52] Osmotic fragility may or may not be increased, but increased mechanical fragility can be expected. The longevity of elliptocytes is normal or near normal.

Clinically significant hemolysis occurs in 10 to 15 per cent of patients and is characterized by splenomegaly, jaundice, gallstones, hemolytic crisis, and aplastic anemia. In cases of severe hemolytic elliptocytosis, splenectomy affords some benefit.

OTHER CONGENITAL HEMOLYTIC ANEMIAS

These include *nonspherocytic hemolytic anemia* and miscellaneous or atypical forms of hemolytic anemias. Of the latter, erythropoietic porphyria and congenital Heinz body anemias are variants.

These disorders are rare, but not as rare as the scanty reports in the literature would suggest. *Erythropoietic porphyria* is the association of congenital hemolytic anemia with porphyria. In such patients the administration of barbiturates may exacerbate the disease.[53]

Heinz body anemia either is transient, affecting premature babies, or persists into later childhood, associated with too large doses of vitamin K, although it is certainly caused by a congenital defect of the erythrocytes.[54] The three red cell defects associated with this disorder are 1) metabolic abnormalities such as G-6-PD deficiency, 2) the thalassemias, and 3) unstable hemoglobins.[55] Heinz bodies are globin precipitates that shorten the life span of the red cell. The result may be a chronic hemolytic anemia of varying severity. Signs include pallor, jaundice, splenomegaly, dark urine, and cholelithiasis. Oxidant drugs may exacerbate hemolysis.

Glucose-6-phosphate dehydrogenase deficiency is a relatively common hereditary red blood cell metabolic defect with the hallmark of erythrocyte destruction by certain drugs or stresses. Nearly 10 per cent of American Negro men are affected, the defect being an X chromosome-linked recessive trait with variable penetrance.[56] Women may also manifest hemolysis, as some of their red blood cells will be affected. Agents that precipitate hemolysis in this disorder include aspirin, phenacetin, chloramphenicol, isoniazid, primaquine, quinine, sulfonamides, fava beans, naphthalene, probenecid, and vitamin K. Diseases include alcoholic hepatitis, diabetic acidosis, malaria, pneumonia, renal acidosis, septicemia, and viral hepatitis. Patients with G-6-PD deficiency are unable to reduce methemoglobin produced by sodium nitrate, hence the administration of sodium nitroprusside or prilocaine is contraindicated.

Since erythrocytes are anucleated, they depend upon the glycolytic cycle for their source of energy, and about 10 per cent of the glucose metabolized is oxidized through the hexose monophosphate shunt. G-6-PD serves as a donor of hydrogen ion to triphosphopyridine nucleotide (TPN); this when reduced provides H^+ ion to reduce glutathione (GSH), methemoglobin, and hydrogen peroxide. Absence of G-6-PD allows for accumulation of products of oxidation, precipitation of hemoglobin, and lysis of red cells.[53, 56, 57]

Siniscalco and collaborators[58] found a trend for G-6-PD to be accompanied by color blindness and hemophilia in certain population groups. The same group of investigators also noted a balance polymorphism with malaria, suggesting certain protection from the parasitic infestations, just as shown in sickle cell anemia.

Symptoms appear two to five days after the beginning of ingestion of the offending agents, with a sudden hemolytic reaction, fall in hemoglobin, and hemoglobinuria. Clinical findings include abdominal pain, hemoglobinuria, and icterus. The history of Mediterranean or African heritage and the recent exposure to oxidant agents should make the clinician suspicious.

The disorder is diagnosed by demonstrating Heinz bodies in the patient's blood during the hemolytic process, and by the finding of low GSH concentration and/or instability in erythrocytes spectrophotometrically. There are specific assays for G-6-PD available. Assay must be done at a time remote from the time of hemolysis when enzyme deficient red cells are present in the circulation. The treatment usually consists of discontinuance of the causative agent and occasionally blood transfusions. Hemolysis is usually self-limited even in the presence of the responsible agent. The same process in the eye is associated with the failure of soluble lens protein synthesis and cataract formation. Therefore the report of patients with cataracts, seizures, and G-6-PD deficiency is not surprising, although the relation to neurologic symptoms such as convulsions is not clear.[59]

HEMOGLOBINOPATHIES

A special section of this chapter dealing with rare diseases is devoted to those conditions characterized by abnormal hemoglobins. This specific interest should not surprise anyone, since as anesthesiologists we are concerned with the maintenance of homeostasis, including the integrity of respiratory function. However, increased and decreased ventilation are not infrequently produced under anesthesia, and we have learned to avoid or use these deviations from normal to our advantage.

An adequate supply of oxygen and efficient removal of carbon dioxide are goals sought by every anesthetist. In a review of hematologic diseases, the importance of the delivery of oxygen to the tissues as the intermediate step in tissue respiration cannot be overlooked.

Patients with hemoglobinopathies deserve special consideration when an anesthetic technique is contemplated in which hypoxia, hypo- or hypercarbia, or metabolic or respiratory acidosis may develop, because any of these pathologic conditions may alter the biochemical affinity of hemoglobin for oxygen.

With the advent of modern laboratory methodology and our greater knowledge in genetics, some diseases that were previously considered isolated entities have been found to have certain common pathophysiologic bases. This is the case with the hemoglobinopathies, which are clinical syndromes caused by defective hemoglobin synthesis resulting from genetically determined abnormalities in the formation of the globin moiety of the molecule. These disorders can be divided into *qualitative* hemoglobinopathies, characterized by the production of structurally abnormal hemoglobin molecules, and *quantitative* hemoglobinopathies, those typified by a deficient production of normal hemoglobin. Occasionally, these alterations may coexist.[52]

Normal Globin Synthesis. Before entering a discussion of the abnormal hemoglobin states, a brief description of the structure of the hemoglobin molecule and the genetic factors influencing globin synthesis is in order.

Hemoglobin is structured by globin, a colorless protein, and four heme radicals (Fig. 8–2), which give it a red color; its molecular weight is 64,458. Globin is composed of four polypeptide chains made up of 141 amino acids, forming two alpha and 146 amino acids in two beta peptide chains in the adult (hemoglobin A). There is also present a low concentration of hemoglobin A_2, which has two alpha and two delta chains.

The heme groups of the hemoglobin molecule are metal complexes with an iron atom in the center of a porphyrin structure, consisting of 4 pyrrole rings attached by methane linkages. The iron atom contained in the heme radical is hexavalent. Four of these coordination valences are attached to the four nitrogen atoms of the pyrrole rings, the fifth is bound to a globin polypeptide chain (most likely to the imidazole group of the histidine residue), and the sixth bond combines reversibly with oxygen.

Erythrocyte precursors synthesize porphyrin and globin components in the bone marrow. Porphyrins are formed from simple substances, glycine and succinyl-coenzyme A. The first step in this synthetic process requires pyridoxol phosphate (vitamin B_6). Uroporphyrin and coproporphyrin are not intermediate compounds in the direct synthetic pathway; however, they are by-products of protoporphyrin synthesis, and small quantities are normally present in the feces and urine. Normal red cells contain a minimal amount of free protoporphyrin (20 to 40 μg/100 ml of erythrocytes) and of free coproporphyrin.[60]

The final step in the biosynthesis of hemoglobin involves the combination of iron, protoporphyrin, and globin. Precise details of this reaction are not clarified as yet, but it is commonly assumed the Fe^{++} is inserted into the porphyrin nucleus to form ferroprotoporphyrin 9, type III or heme, which then combines with one of the globin peptide chains. Although iron uptake begins in the most immature erythrocytic precursors, the actual formation of the hemoglobin molecule per se takes place for the most part in the more mature precursors, including the reticulocytes.

Role of Hemoglobin in Respiration. The primary functions of the red cells are to transport oxygen to the tissues and to assist in the removal of carbon dioxide. In a normal adult human subject at rest, approximately 250 ml of oxygen is consumed each minute, whereas about 200 ml of carbon dioxide is produced in the same period. Hemoglobin permits the transport of about 100 times more oxygen than could be handled by the plasma alone, if the gases existed in physical solution only in the latter. The iron atoms contained in the hemoglobin molecule possess the attribute of reversible oxygenation; that is, they can facilitate the binding and release of oxygen without changing their valence. When oxygen combines with hemoglobin, its two unpaired electrons are paired with those of iron; consequently, oxygen is unable to accept electrons in transfer and cannot act as an

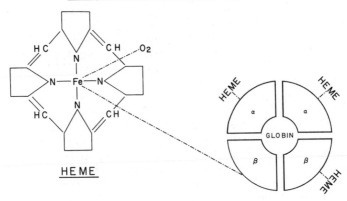

Structure of Hemoglobin A Molecule

HEME

Figure 8–2.

oxidizing agent. Hemoglobin combines reversibly with oxygen according to the following equation:

$$Hb + 4O_2 \rightarrow Hb\,(O_2)_4$$

This equation is truly a measure of the degree of interaction between hemes, so each heme as it is in the molecule facilitates the interaction of oxygen with the next heme molecule (see Fig. 7–2). Oxygen is added sequentially to the two α-chains and subsequently to the two β-chains. After the addition of the first two oxygen molecules, 2,3-DPG is released from the hemoglobin molecule, thus increasing its affinity for the remaining oxygen molecules.[4]

The association and dissociation of oxygen and hemoglobin are complex and depend on several factors, including oxygen tension, pH, carbon dioxide tension, electrolytes, temperature, and levels of 2,3-DPG. The normal sigmoidal oxyhemoglobin dissociation curve (Fig. 8–3) provides an important physiologic advantage; at low oxygen tension, minor changes in PO_2 bring about the association with, or dissociation from, hemoglobin of large quantities of oxygen. At one given time, the four atoms of iron in a molecule of hemoglobin may be bound to none, one, two, three, or four molecules of oxygen. When one heme group joins with oxygen, the affinity for oxygen of the other heme moieties is raised. Thus hemoglobin in venous blood with a PO_2 of approximately 35 to 40 torr is ideally suited to accept oxygen in the lungs, where

alveolar air has a tension of about 100 torr. Similarly, hemoglobin in arterial blood with a PO_2 of 90 torr readily gives oxygen to the tissues, where oxygen tensions are around 50 torr or less. It has also been noted that hemoglobin combines with carbon monoxide even more readily than with oxygen (210-fold) to form carboxyhemoglobin.

In addition to their vital role in the transport of oxygen, hemoglobin and the erythrocytes have other functions. These include the transport of carbon dioxide from the tissues to the lungs, where it is given up and eliminated in the expired air. Although CO_2 is carried in the cells and in the plasma, the large majority is included as 1-carbonic acid,2-carbamino-bound CO_2, in combination with hemoglobin and 3-bicarbonate in combination with the cations sodium or potassium. The carbon dioxide in hemoglobin is about 20 per cent of the total blood CO_2 and is important because of the relatively high rapidity of the reaction:

$$Hb \cdot NH_2 + CO_2 \rightarrow Hb \cdot NH \cdot COOH$$

where $Hb \cdot NH_2$ represents a free amino group of hemoglobin capable of combination with CO_2 to form the carbamino compound.[61]

Although the rate at which the aforementioned reaction would attain equilibrium is too slow, it accounts for approximately 70 per cent of the CO_2 carried in the blood as bicarbonate. This apparent paradox is explained by the action of the enzyme carbonic anhydrase, which is associated with hemoglobin and catalyzes the removal of CO_2 from H_2CO_3; since the reaction is reversible

Figure 8–3. Hemoglobin saturation curves in various abnormal hemoglobins.

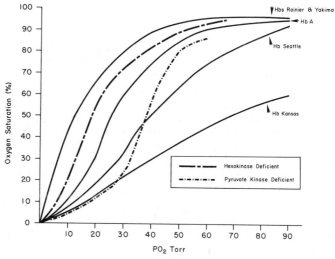
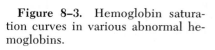

at the tissue level, the formation of H_2CO_3 from CO_2 and H_2O is also accelerated by the same enzyme.

Changes in Molecular Structure Seen in Hereditary Hemoglobinopathies

Hereditary diseases involving the structure of hemoglobin are of particular interest to anesthesiologists. These entities present significant problems in some geographical areas of the world and usually, though not consistently, follow ethnologic patterns. Advances in biochemistry as applied to hematology have allowed us to identify the specific abnormality of hemoglobin synthesis as well as to selectively pinpoint the precise alteration in the genetic mechanism producing it. These concepts have revealed that in some instances abnormal molecular structure can be related to abnormal function and, in turn, to the clinical symptoms observed in each case.

There are several general mechanisms by which abnormal hemoglobins are produced. These are:

1. Change of one DNA nucleotide for another, resulting in a substitution of one amino acid for another.
2. The addition of extra amino acids to the polypeptide chain of hemoglobin.
3. Chromosome crossover resulting in mixed hemoglobin chains.
4. The addition or deletion of a single DNA nucleotide, which results in a shift of the amino acid sequence. Depending on where in the hemoglobin structure the substitution occurs, there may result decreased hemoglobin solubility (e.g., hemoglobin S), hemoglobin instability with hemolysis (e.g., hemoglobin Köln, stabilization of heme iron in the ferric state (hemoglobin M).
5. Substitutions at α and β chain contact points with increased oxygen affinity (hemoglobin Chesapeake) or decreased oxygen affinity (hemoglobin Kansas).[4]

Each individual amino acid has a specific position in the chain and is identified by a "code" related to the sequence of three of the nucleotides of messenger RNA; thus, a change in a single nucleotide will result in a different amino acid.[60] A typical example is observed in sickle hemoglobin, in which a change in a purine base makes valine instead of the glutamic acid molecule in the sixth amino acid of the beta chain.[62] Similar

changes account for most of the inherited aberrations of hemoglobin. Less frequently, two amino acid substitutions occur in a single polypeptide chain, as in the Hb C_{Harlem} with two independent mutations taking place within the same gene.

In two other cases, amino acid residues are actually missing or deleted from a polypeptide chain (Hb$_{Freiburg}$ and Hb$_{Gun\ Hill}$). In case of hereditary persistence of fetal hemoglobin, there is complete deletion of two closely linked genes. Homozygotes with this disease synthesize neither of the two normal hemoglobins of the adult, and their hemoglobin is exclusively fetal in type. Other abnormalities in hemoglobin structure are produced by substitutions, deletions, and added linkages of their respective amino acid chains.[63]

In thalassemias, hemoglobin synthesis is abnormal and one or the other polypeptide chain is produced at a retarded rate but has a normal structure; although the precise cause for this retardation has not been identified, it is suspected of being related to insufficiency of messenger RNA. When insufficient alpha chains are produced, the beta chains accumulate and combine to form Hb$_{H\beta}$.[4, 60]

The clinical manifestations of hemoglobinopathies are determined by both the quantity and the quality of molecules produced. As previously mentioned, the particular fashion in which the globin chains and their heme rings are bonded together lends unusual stability to the molecule. If these precise stereochemical relationships are disturbed, abnormal oxygen binding and decreased stability may result. For example, although the β-chains accumulated in excess in thalassemia are individually normal, the structure of the molecule is deranged, with Hb H possessing a high affinity for oxygen, so high that it cannot be released to the tissues. In this case, the hemoglobin is nonfunctional and unstable, tending to precipitate within the erythrocytes, resulting in their premature destruction.[63, 64]

Although some amino acids are substituted without apparent consequences, others appear to be essential. Therefore, significant abnormalities occur at some of these sites. This is the case with the Hb M syndrome, in which four of the five hemoglobins M are produced when the histidine residue is substituted on either side of the iron atom of the heme ring. Ordinarily, this atom is in the ferrous state, allowing reversible binding of oxygen; it changes to the ferric form, and then cannot combine reversibly with oxygen, except that enzymes contained within the erythrocytes reverse this process, so that nearly all hemoglobin iron is in the ferrous state. Substitution of tyrosine for histidine renders ferric iron so stable that the erythrocyte enzymes are unable to reduce it. The homozygote condition has not been reported and is presumably incompatible with life[63] (Tables 8–2 and 8–3).

In a similar example, methemoglobinemia is conditional rather than absolute in Hb$_{Zurich}$, in which histidine is replaced by arginine. Heterozygotes most often show no unusual symptoms, except for a slightly shortened life span of the red blood cells. However, methemoglobinemia may suddenly appear if these patients have received sulfonamides or other oxidant drugs; moreover, hemoglobin may denature and precipitate fulminant hemolytic anemia. Presumably, these patients will be even more likely to develop this complication with conventional doses of the local anesthetic prilocaine hydrochloride.

The affinity of hemoglobin for oxygen may vary in some of these conditions. Hemoglobins Chesapeake and Rainier, and even more so Hb H, have an increased affinity for oxygen, resulting in a loss of the normal sigmoidal shape of the oxygen dissociation curve[17] (Fig. 8–3). This phenomenon in turn affects the Bohr effect (change of oxygen affinity produced by variations of pH), so that by increasing the affinity of

blood for oxygen, it causes a decreased release of the gas to the tissues, thus eventually simulating a compensatory erythropoiesis, resulting in polycythemia.[61] Efforts to offset this process by bleeding may indeed prevent the advantage of this built-in protective mechanism.

Although we are dealing in this chapter with rare hematologic diseases, special mention must be made of perhaps the most common, but still rare, hemoglobin inherent aberrations: sickle cell disease and the thalassemias.

Sickle Cell Anemia

The entity caused by Hb S presence is perhaps the best understood of these conditions, although it is not a true intramolecular dysfunction; it is perhaps better explained as an abnormal reaction between molecules of Hb S in the erythrocytes of homozygotes, resulting in sickle cell anemia.

Although the disorder was first noted by J. B. Herrick in 1904[65] while examining a black student, it was not until 1927 that Hahn and Gillespie demonstrated that sickling was produced by reduction of oxygen tension and pH in blood, and that hemoglobin was the incriminating factor when erythrocyte "ghosts," from which the hemoglobin had been extracted, would not sickle.[66] By using electrophoresis, Pauling et al.[67] showed the differences between normal and sickling hemoglobin to be related to molecular structure, and subsequently demonstrated this difference to be a specific

Table 8–2   *Substitutions under Different Pathologic Conditions in the Alpha Chain of Globin's Amino Acids*

Normal Amino Acid	1 Val	16 Lys	23 Glu	30 Glu	43 Phe	57 Gly	58 His	68 Asp	87 His	92 Arg	116 Glu	136 Leu
Type of Hb:												
Hb I		Asp										
Hb Memphis			Gln									
Hb G Honolulu				Glu NH$_2$								
Hb Torino					Val							
Hb Norfolk						Asp						
Hb M Boston							Tyr					
Hb G Philadelphia								Lys				
Hb M Iwate									Tyr			
Hb J Capetown										Gln		
Hb Chesapeake										Leu		
Hb O											Lys	
Hb Bibba												Pro

Table 8-3　Changes in the Beta Chain of Globin's Amino Acids Occurring in Different Hemoglobinopathies

	1 Val	6 Glu	7 Glu	23 Val	26 Glu	28 Leu	35 Tyr	42 Phe	63 His	63 His	67 Val	67 Val	88 Leu	92 His	92–96 —	98 Val	99 Asp	99 Asp	102 Asn	121 Glu	130 Tyr	145 Tyr
Hb S		Val																				
Hb C		Lys																				
Hb G San Jose			Gly																			
Hb Freiburg				Deleted																		
Hb E					Lys																	
Hb Geneva						Pro																
Hb Philadelphia							Phe															
Hb Hammersmith								Ser														
Hb Zurich									Arg													
Hb M Saskatoon										Tyr												
Hb Sydney											Ala											
Hb M Milwaukee												Glu										
Hb Santa Ana													Pro									
Hb M Hyde Park														Tyr								
Hb Gun Hill															Deleted							
Hb Köln																Met						
Hb Kempsey																	Asn					
Hb Yakima																		His				
Hb Kansas																			Thr			
Hb D Punjab																				Gln		
Hb Wien																					Asp	
Hb Rainer																						His

substitution of an amino acid in the beta chain (Table 8–3).

Epidemiologic studies have suggested why the trait is so common among the black population. It is most prevalent in West and Central Africa, where most of the slave trade was carried on during colonial times, and correlation studies have implied an inverse ratio of Hb S to the malignant falciparum form of malaria. It has since become apparent, but has not always been understood, that the heterozygote's sickle cell trait is advantageous in these regions, because it protects the erythrocytes against invasion by the parasitic organism. This protection is most effective in infants, who then have greater chances of tolerating their first attack of malaria, thus explaining the existence of an otherwise disadvantageous mutation. This may be the reason why black population groups survived and thrived in an environment intolerable to other people.

Sickle cell trait has also been observed in Mediterranean peoples, although with a much lower incidence. Specifically, it has been noted in Sicily, Turkey, and some of the Arab countries, where malaria was endemic, but it may also reflect the migration of ethnic groups originally from Africa toward the Mediterranean countries, Central Europe, North America, and the West Indies.

Under anoxic conditions, the Hb S molecules stack up in long aggregates, forming liquid crystals or tactoids which are truly polymerized hemoglobin chains twisted as cable elements when sickled cells are examined by electron microscopy.

Molecularly, the substitution of valine in the sixth position of each of the beta chains provides two reactive sites; when oxygen desaturation occurs, Hb S molecules tend to concentrate together by bonding with each other at the reactive sites, forming tactoids.[62]

Clinical manifestations and laboratory evidence of this hemoglobinopathy have been noted in heterozygotes under anesthesia, in patients with cyanotic heart disease, only to disappear after its correction, and in acute alcoholism, probably resulting from hypoventilation with its attendant hypoxia and acidosis. Alterations of peripheral blood flow, such as those produced by hemorrhagic, septic, and/or cardiogenic shock, tourniquet application, or aortic occlusion, by affecting regional oxygen tensions and pH may also elicit sickling.

Sickle cell disease is clinically considered to have two forms:

Sickle cell trait is observed in heterozygotes of the Hb S gene, with an approximate incidence of 10 per cent in the black American population. Approximately 30 to 50 per cent of the hemoglobin in erythrocytes is Hb S, the remainder being Hb A.[68] The life span of the red blood cells is normal; thus most of the patients are usually asymptomatic. In the laboratory, sickling can be demonstrated in vitro by exposing blood to a reducing agent.[69] Sickle crisis may occur in these individuals if they are exposed to a hypoxic environment. Acute illness may be assumed to be the result of sickling in these individuals when in fact it is not. McCormick[70] reports that 22 of 135 patients with sickle "trait" had postmortem visceral infarcts. Dalal and colleagues report that the critical PO_2 for sickling is 30 torr in homozygotes and 20 to 30 torr in patients with sickle cell trait.[71] Harris[72] points out that erythrocytes in trait are more resistant to acidosis than are homozygous erythrocytes. Open heart surgery has been successfully performed in these patients, with a decrease in the level of hemoglobins from 41 to 10 per cent as a result of dilution.[73]

Sickle cell anemia is the homozygous state of the Hb S gene, found in about 0.5 to 1 per cent of American blacks. The cells contain predominantly Hb S, with small amounts of Hb F. In patients with this variety, the longevity of the erythrocytes is shortened as a result of their increased fragility; sickling can occur in vivo and is easily demonstrated in vitro.

Patients with sickle cell anemia have disorders involving various organ systems. In evaluating these patients preoperatively, the anesthesiologist must bear in mind that sickling of the cells with occlusion of vessels and hemolysis is the original lesion responsible for the clinical and histologic manifestations of this disease, and that these patients are at constant risk during anesthetic management as well as during the postoperative period.

The symptoms of this disease may begin during the first year of life.[74] The earliest sign in children under three years of age is often pain and swelling of the hands and feet. Patients with this disease may have cardiomegaly, probably resulting from cor pulmonale secondary to repeated small pulmonary emboli.[75] The cardiac output is increased to compensate for the low hemoglobin content, and the plasma volume is greater than normal.[76]

In the lungs, a loss of functional pulmonary tissue and a diffusion defect may result in decreased arterial oxygen saturation which is exacerbated by exertion.[77] Despite the low hemoglobin, these patients may have a chronically expanded pulmonary capillary bed as a compensatory mechanism to maintain an appropriate level of membrane diffusing capacity.[78]

There is a shift of the oxygen dissociation curve to the right in cases of sickle cell anemia, but not in the sickle cell trait; as previously mentioned, this aberration facilitates the liberation of oxygen from hemoglobin into tissues.[79]

From the liver there is greater demand to metabolize the hemolyzed blood; not infrequently it is enlarged, and function tests may or may not be abnormal, depending on the degree of hepatic involvement. Jaundice and/or cholelithiasis can coexist, and in advanced cases iron deposited as hemosiderin can eventually lead to cirrhosis.[75]

During acute crisis, thrombi may form in every parenchymal organ; lung, kidney, or brain involvement is most likely to result in serious complications.[78]

Sickling Crises. The chronic hemolytic anemia is exacerbated by crises resulting from exposure of Hb S containing erythrocytes to low oxygen tensions that can even occur normally in venous blood. Because of their odd shape, sickling cells are vulnerable to destruction by the spleen phagocytes and reticuloendothelial cells. In an attempt to compensate, the bone marrow activates erythropoiesis, but this balance is incomplete, resulting in a hemoglobin level around 8 gm per 100 ml.

By the mechanisms previously mentioned, excessive sickling results in acute crises that may have a variety of pathophysiologic and clinical manifestations.

Hematologic crises are of the sequestration type when the primary triggering episode results in an increase in the number of sickling erythrocytes that will eventually be trapped in the reticuloendothelial system with an acute loss of circulating cells (Fig. 8–4). This sequestration is responsible for many deaths in the postpartum period and even perhaps in the postoperative surgical stage.

Hemolytic type. When the destruction of sickled erythrocytes is accelerated, the hemolytic anemia is exacerbated.

Aplastic type. On occasion, probably because of termination of folic acid supply, the bone marrow enters an aplastic phase, with a short life span and no erythropoiesis; subsequently, rapid fall of hemoglobin takes place.[75]

Painful crises. Triggered by hypoxemia and/or acidosis and favored by sluggish circulation, viscosity of the blood is increased, aggravating the decreased flow to compromised peripheral tissues. Eventually, if the process advances, complete vascular occlusion results, manifested mostly by severe pain localized to the involved area, frequently the extremities and abdomen.[75, 80]

Patients with sicklemia may present in the operating room for various procedures. They may undergo skin grafting of chronic leg ulcers, cholecystectomy owing to pigment stones, relief of persistent painful priapism, curettage of osteomyelitic bone cavities, or splenectomy because of hypersplenism.

Preoperative Preparation. Under elective conditions any effort to improve the patient's general condition is warranted. Treatment of infections is mandatory. However, the most important factor is the evaluation of the hematologic state.

The logistics of blood transfusions has evolved from heroic measures to more common ones. Mostly in adults, severe reactions, including death, have been reported following the administration of blood. Recently, symptomatic crises of sicklemia have been treated successfully with limited exchange transfusions of buffy coat-free, packed erythrocytes, resulting in a rise in the oxygen-carrying capacity of the blood.[81, 82] By this method, near complete removal of hemoglobin S can be achieved in a few hours, whenever surgical emergencies demand prompt preparation. In addition, the prophylactic administration of folic acid has been recommended to treat superimposed megaloblastic anemia. Efforts to eliminate any localized or systemic infections are justified, because sickling crises are often initiated by febrile illnesses.

The anesthetic technique elected should carry no risk of hypoxia, acidosis, stasis, and

REDUCED OXYGEN TENSION

ACIDOSIS

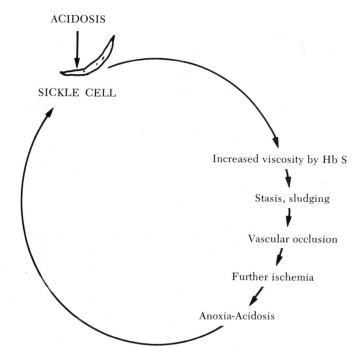

SICKLE CELL

Figure 8–4. Physiopathologic vicious circle acting in the development of crisis in sickle cell anemia.

Increased viscosity by Hb S

Stasis, sludging

Vascular occlusion

Further ischemia

Anoxia-Acidosis

cooling. To prevent hypoxia, the rules for safe anesthetic practice must be adhered to. The preoperative medication should not depress respiratory function. Elegbeleye et al.[83] have shown that patients who are homozygous for sickle hemoglobin have a normal sensitivity to carbon dioxide as determined by CO_2 response curves. Special care must be exercised to prevent airway obstruction and/or arterial hypotension during induction of and recovery from anesthesia. Inhaled oxygen concentrations of at least 30 per cent provide arterial oxygen tensions that are normal or slightly higher than normal in patients devoid of cardiopulmonary disease. However, whenever serious cardiac or respiratory function disorders are present, or in patients undergoing thoracotomy, concentrations greater than 45 per cent are needed to ensure safe levels of arterial oxygenation.[82] Moreover, adequate alveolar volume ventilation and normal cardiac output must be preserved in order to avoid ventilation-perfusion ratio alterations, even in the presence of the recommended inhaled oxygen concentrations.

The desirability of avoiding acidosis in sickle cell anemia may perhaps justify the prophylactic administration of alkaline buffer infusions.[84] Similarly, pulmonary hyperventilation, as long as it is not carried to extremes, affords relative protection.

Although Gilbertson[85] used the Esmarch tourniquet in 12 sicklemic patients without untoward effects, positional changes and tourniquets are undesirable because of the likelihood of intravascular stasis. Incidental fall of body temperature in air-conditioned operating rooms or deliberate hypothermia is to be avoided, because metabolic acidosis, stasis, and increased blood viscosity are commonly found in most patients with sickle cell anemia. Fluid and electrolyte administration must be done with care to prevent overloading or electrolyte imbalances. Furthermore, because a certain degree of liver damage is not rare in these patients, and because Hilkowitz and Jacobson[86] reported low levels of serum cholinesterase activity in five of a group of 14 patients with hemoglobin SC disease, titrated doses of succinylcholine are recommended.

Most authors[87, 88, 89, 90] are of the opinion that any anesthetic technique is acceptable for the management of sickle cell disease patients so long as the aforementioned complications are avoided. Guinee et al.,[91] using repeated determinations of the percentage of sickled erythrocytes and blood acid-base before, during, and after well-conducted anesthesia and surgery, found in every case that the blood oxygen tension increased during anesthesia and that the percentage of sickled cells was markedly reduced. This effect persisted in all cases for 24 hours, and in one patient for 96 hours, after anesthesia.

After surgery, the greatest threats to sicklemic patients appear to be episodes of hypoxemia and respiratory infections. It has been shown that low arterial oxygen tensions can develop even two minutes after extubation,[92] and also may be seen six days postoperatively[93] in patients without apparent respiratory distress or previous lung disorder. The emphasis on continuous oxygen inhalation, even before patients leave the operating room, and on monitoring of oxygenation of arterial blood in patients with sickle cell disease is therefore justified because even minimal and evanescent falls of Pa_{O_2} may elicit a sickling crisis.[94]

Most reports in the literature[86, 87, 88, 95] concerning patients with sickle cell disease who undergo surgery and anesthesia disclose a considerable incidence of respiratory infections in the postoperative period. Deaths have resulted from this complication. Because of the fact that decreased oxygen tensions are the rule in severe pulmonary infections, great efforts must be made to avoid this complication. Such efforts may include prophylactic intermittent positive pressure breathing with bronchodilators, chest physiotherapy, and early institution of the "stir up" philosophy of early ambulation.

Treatment.   Many treatments have been tried for sickle crisis, including alkalinization, anticoagulants, dextran, carbon monoxide, nitrites, phenothiazines, vasodilators, and defibrination, with little success.[4] Alkalinization of the blood does not relieve sickling, once it has taken place.[94] Because of the vasodilating effects of magnesium sulfate and the prolongation of clotting time caused by it, Anstall and his collaborators[96] suggested it as a means to prevent thrombus formation and sludging of erythrocytes.

Lehman and Huntsman[60] proposed its use in the treatment of sickle cell crises or prophylactically during surgery; however, the potentiation of muscle relaxant drugs by the magnesium ion is not to be forgotten,[7] and the doses of neuromuscular blocking drugs should be curtailed accordingly.

Preliminary clinical studies suggested that low molecular weight dextran, by preventing sludging, might be useful in the treatment of patients with bone pain; however, intravenous infusion of 5 per cent dextrose solution was found to be as beneficial as dextran.[98] Nevertheless, dextran can be resorted to in the event of uncontrollable crises. Its value as a preventive of vascular thrombosis in sickle cell disease has not been clarified.

Although the spleen plays a small role in the course of complications of sickle cell anemia, in mixed hemoglobinopathies the spleen may be enlarged. Isolated cases of marked improvement have been reported[99, 100] after splenectomy in patients with sickle cell anemia. This has been explained by exclusion of an enlarged organ where a larger than normal number of erythrocytes would be trapped and eventually destroyed. A basis for this contention may be the sequence of events that occurs in the hypersplenic syndrome, as demonstrated by Jandl and Aster,[101] who described a slowed transit of red blood cells, establishing a slow-mixing vascular compartment, consumption of available glucose, and premature death of mature erythrocytes.

Many other measures have been suggested in the treatment of crises and specific localizations of sickling and thrombosis. To relieve painful persistent priapism, continuous epidural block has been used with a certain amount of success by some authors.[102] Ketamine was successful in producing detumescence in seven children with priapism.[103] Also, preliminary studies suggest that indomethacin may be effective in the treatment of thrombotic crises.[104] Even more recently, the intravenous administration of urea appeared quite promising, not only in the prevention of crises by stabilizing the erythrocyte-plasma membrane, but also in the treatment of crises by improving the circulation to sequestered areas.[105, 106] The bulk of current evidence indicates that this is of no value[4]. Great care must be exercised in large obstetric services where accidental hypoxemia may occur among unsuspected heterozygous mothers and their homozygous newborns, in whom sickling is of serious consequence.[107, 108] Oral ingestion of sodium citrate has been successful in treating painful crises.[109]

Hemoglobin S is not the only hemoglobin that sickles. Hemoglobin C$_{Harlem\ 1}$, Hemoglobin C$_{Georgetown}$, and Hemoglobin I all sickle at low oxygen tensions.[4]

In agreement with other authors,[85, 95, 110, 111] we suggest that greater efforts be made to screen patients with either the trait or the anemia forms of sickle cell disease in areas where it is endemic or where, because of ethnologic migrations of susceptible individuals, it has become common.

Thalassemia

This disease is also known as Cooley's anemia, Mediterranean anemia, or target cell anemia. It is a recessively inherited condition in which there is an abnormality of hemoglobin synthesis, pronounced marrow hyperplasia with considerably ineffective erythropoiesis, an unusual composition of hemoglobins in the red cells, and a mild hemolytic state.

Thalassemia is widely distributed in subtropical regions in the Mediterranean coastal areas, Central Africa, and Asia. Genetically it is transmitted by a recessive gene with varying degrees of expression; when it is homozygous it is called thalassemia major or T. disease, whereas the heterozygous form is termed thalassemia minor or T. trait.[112]

Biochemically, it is thought that a block of Hb A production causes a compensatory increase of fetal hemoglobin (Hb F).[60] From this point of view there is a β-thalassemia with defective β-chain synthesis that interacts with other hemoglobinopathies (i.e., Hb S, Hb C) and that is rare in black people,[113] and a γ-thalassemia with a defect on γ-chain synthesis that has no association with other β-chain hemoglobinopathies and is common in blacks.[112] There are α-thalassemias as well that result from abnormalities in α-chain synthesis. There are three forms: α-thalassemia trait, intermediate, and major. The intermediate form is called hemoglobin H disease and is characterized by an abnormally large amount of insoluble β-chains. Anemia may be moderately severe, with hemolysis increased by oxidant drugs. In the homozygous major

form, there are no α-chains synthesized. This syndrome results in fetal death because of ineffective oxygen transport to tissues.[8]

Hyperplasia of bone marrow occurs, with subsequent skeletal deformities such as prominent maxilla, sunken nose, and thickened skull, resembling mongolism. Typically, the hemoglobin ranges from 5 to 7 gm, with hypochromic, microcytic and anisocytic erythrocytes and target and nucleated cells present, as well as an increase of Hb F. Because the red cells are so thin, there is a greater resistance than normal to hypotonic saline and their longevity is reduced to 70 days.[114] In contrast to sickle cell disease, the cause of hemolysis in thalassemia is not clear.

There are three clinical types of thalassemia: severe, intermediate, and mild, according to the degree of anemia. Usually, it presents with an apparent hemolytic anemia in infancy, with pallor and/or jaundice and splenomegaly. The severe homozygous state is incompatible with life, and the fetus is born dead. In the intermediate state, there is a mild hypochromic anemia, resistant to iron therapy. These patients may develop cholelithiasis, chronic liver disease, osteoporosis, and siderosis as they get older.[6] On incubation with methyl violet, intracellular inclusion bodies and an excess of Hb H may be found. In the mixed heterozygous condition, an association with a gene of a different abnormal hemoglobin is found, resulting in each gene being derived from one parent and thus having thalassemia-Hb S and thalassemia-Hb C.[45, 115] In the mild form, thalassemia minor, there is a minimal hypochromic, microcytic anemia that may be confused with iron deficiency.

Even rarer varieties of thalassemia have been given specific terms. In hemoglobin Lepore, the γ-chains are normal but the β-chain amalgamates with Δ-chains. The condition called hemoglobin "Barts" is seen mostly in infants and is due to defective synthesis of γ-chain amino acids.[60, 115]

Repeated blood transfusion is the most effective, although not innocuous, treatment. Splenectomy is useful only in cases of hypersplenism. It is perhaps at this time that anesthesiologists may be faced with this problem. Optimal preparation of these patients is attained by transfusion until a level of 10 gm per 100 ml of hemoglobin is reached. The concomitant administration of a chelating agent such as desferrioxamine has been advocated. Plasma volume may be higher than normal, and care must be exercised to avoid circulatory overload.

In addition to the concern for the hematologic abnormalities observed in patients with thalassemia, a peculiar facial deformity with overgrowth of the maxillae may make visualization of the glottis quite difficult at the time of laryngoscopy. Therefore, assurance of airway patency must be attained before rendering these patients apneic.[116]

As in many similar conditions, a variety of systems may be involved, including liver, kidneys, cardiovascular, central nervous, and immune. As a result, careful study and search for dysfunction must be done prior to anesthesia with efforts made to correct abnormalities when possible and to choose appropriate anesthetic techniques as necessary. De Laval et al[73] report open heart surgery on three patients with β-thalassemia minor without difficulty.

Hemoglobin SC Disease

This is the most severe hemoglobinopathy after hemoglobin SS (sickle cell disease). It results from the inheriting of hemoglobin S from one and hemoglobin C from the other parent.[117] Anemia, splenomegaly, jaundice, aseptic necrosis of the femoral head, retinal disease, bone marrow infarction, hepatic disease, and splenic infarction occur.

There is an increased risk of eclampsia, abortion, stillbirth, heart failure, infection, and sudden death among parturients.[118] Eclampsia may be difficult to distinguish from intracerebral sickling, which may result from anemia of pregnancy, increased oxygen consumption, sedatives, anesthesia, blood loss, or intravascular coagulation. Precautions are the same as for sickle cell anemia.

AUTOIMMUNE HEMOLYTIC ANEMIAS

These disorders are characterized by premature destruction of erythrocytes with antibody bound to the cell surface. The antibody is demonstrated by a positive direct antiglobulin (Coombs') test, but it is not necessarily associated with hemolysis. The immunity is produced by an underlying systemic disease or exogenous stimulus. The diseases associated with autoimmune states are lymphocytic leukemia, lymphoma, Hodgkin's disease, connective tissue disorders and hypersensitivity states,[119] bacterial infections, mononucleosis, and tumors of the ovary or breast.[8]

The multisystemic aspect of these entities is demonstrated by an increased frequency of serum antibodies directed against white cells, platelets, thyroid, and deoxyribonucleic acid (DNA). In essence, they are the hemolytic manifestation of an altered immune response.[120]

Although there is no apparent genetic or racial predisposition, certain susceptibility has been observed in some families. Most case reports have been of patients of European origin, with a relative frequency in individuals of blood group O. The clinical picture is that of chronic anemia, with anisocytosis, macrocytosis, and a moderate increase of reticulocytes. Splenomegaly is the common feature, with congestion and hyperplasia of the reticulum cells. Similar lesions are found in the hepatic parenchyma in terminal cases. Renal tubular damage and hemosiderosis may also be seen. Dacie[121] classified autoimmune hemolytic anemias into three types: idiopathic, secondary, and paroxysmal.

The idiopathic or primary autoimmune hemolytic anemia, also called antiglobin-positive hemolytic anemia, is caused by autoantibodies present in the blood. Coombs, Mourant, and Race[122] first showed that erythrocytes synthesized by incomplete forms of Rh isoantibodies were agglutinated by anti-human-globulin serum prepared by immunizing rabbits against human serum proteins.

The antibody may be a lysin or an agglutinin, and it may be active at body temperature or below. The presence of agglutinins may be recognized by clumping of the blood during collection, or in the red cell counting chamber. Warm antibodies act best at 37° C, and their potency is not enhanced at lower temperatures. Cells coated with an incomplete antibody give a positive Coombs test. With high titers, agglutination may be demonstrated in vitro. Cold antibodies are demonstrable in vitro. They may be lysins or agglutinins and are effective only at low temperatures or when active at temperatures near 37° C. Their power is enhanced at lower temperatures. Occasionally, leukopenia and thrombocytopenia coexist as complicating factors in cases of severe autoimmune hemolytic anemias.[121]

Paroxysmal Cold Hemoglobinuria (Cold Antibody Type)

This rare condition, also called Marchiafava-Micheli syndrome, is triggered by exposure of the whole body or part of the body to cold, usually about 20° F; although the hemolytic process is chronic, there is marked exacerbation during acute attacks. The most frequent cause is congenital syphilis, but cases of unknown etiology have also been reported.[123, 124] There is also an association with infectious mononucleosis and *Mycoplasma pneumoniae* pneumonitis.

The clinical features of cold agglutination disease are related to stasis with pain, mottling of skin, cyanosis, necrosis, and ulceration in fingers, toes, and face.[8] Acute exacerbations are manifested by backache, hemoglobinuria, fall in hemoglobin, and splenomegaly. At this time, the antiglobulin test is positive and the existence of cold hemolysin can be demonstrated by the Donath-Landsteiner reaction. Antisyphilitic treatment may cure this disease whenever positive serologic reactions are present. Vasomotor phenomena have been noted, even progressing to the extreme of gangrene in isolated cases. The paroxysm or attack consists of constitutional symptoms and evidence of hemoglobin in the urine after exposure to cold[125]. Lysis in vitro may be enhanced by increases of carbon dioxide or falls of pH. Whether these mechanisms also act in vivo is not known.

Whenever lues is proved, specific treatment must be instituted. Antihistaminic drugs, ACTH, and vitamin C have been recommended, but perhaps the most important feature is the avoidance of cold and damp exposure. Glucocorticoids, anticoagulants, cytotoxic drugs, and splenectomy have not been very effective in this illness. Transfusion of blood should be avoided, since the cold agglutinin reacts with an antigen that is present in almost all adult red blood cells.

In patients who are known to have cold antibodies, blood should be warmed with an appropriate device during transfusion. It should not be necessary to mention this injunction, since *all* blood should be warmed prior to transfusion.

"Warm Type" of Autoimmune Hemolytic Disease

This disorder can be observed in patients suffering from chronic lymphatic leukemia and lymphosarcoma, diffuse lupus erythematosus, or ulcerative colitis, or patients who are receiving therapy with quinine, methyldopa, penicillin, para-amino salicylic acid, acetophenacitin, quinidine, or other drugs.

Methyldopa and penicillin act as antigens, stimulating the formation of a red cell antibody that may show Rh specificity; the other drugs appear to produce antibody only after interacting with the red cell surface without showing antigenic specificity.

Normocytic normochromic anemia is present, with spherocytes having an increased osmotic fragility. Bone marrow hyperplasia is consistent, producing reticulocytosis, and occasionally normoblasts are released into the circulation. Leukopenia and thrombocytopenia are also frequent. Red cell survival is markedly reduced, with a mean cell life of less than 10 days.[126]

The disease appears most commonly in middle-aged patients with insidious anemia, jaundice, and hemoglobinuria. It is diagnosed simply by the antiglobulin test. Since splenectomy has been shown to be a valuable form of treatment, these patients may come to the operating room after having received considerable doses of corticosteroids and/or immunosuppressive drugs such as mercaptopurine or azathioprine. Ideally, the operation is undertaken after the hemolytic process has been controlled and appropriate steroid coverage has been instituted. Occasionally, prolonged apnea of unexplained origin may occur postoperatively. This may be related to an interaction between muscle relaxants and other drugs the patient may be taking. Means for continuous assistance of ventilation should be available.[127]

Autoimmune Hemolytic Anemias Secondary to Other Diseases

Patients suffering severe viral infections frequently develop cold autoantibodies manifested as hemolysis, usually developing at a late stage of the disease and occasionally complicated by venous thrombosis and, more rarely, pulmonary emboli. Of the viral infections, those most commonly incriminated are viral pneumonia, infectious mononucleosis, measles, varicella, encephalitis, herpes simplex, and those produced by Coxsackie virus.[128]

With the exception of advanced cases, the degree of anemia is moderate, and because most of these patients have the disease for prolonged periods, it is not unlikely that certain compensation of the blood volume has been made. Of great danger would be contemplation of surgery and anesthesia in patients with unsuspected autoimmune hemolytic anemia, because theoretically some of them may be prone to paroxysms of hemolysis with changes of body temperature, falls of pH, hypercarbia, or blood transfusion, depending on the type of "sensitization" they had developed.[127]

DRUG-INDUCED HEMOLYTIC ANEMIAS

These nonimmune disorders may occur in all patients receiving large doses of some drugs and in only a proportion of patients who have received usual dosages. Irregular and distorted erythrocytes, methemoglobinemia or sulfhemoglobinemia, and the presence of Heinz bodies or punctate basophilia are some of the hematologic alterations that suggest drug-induced hemolysis.

Lead produces anemia partly by hemolysis and partly by inhibition of hemoglobin synthesis[129], which is characterized by chronic hypochromic normocytic or microcytic anemia in patients exposed to chemicals containing lead, most frequently paints. Red cell lifespan may be decreased as a result of the effect of lead on the cell membrane[130]. In latent forms, a high count of stippled cells is very suggestive of the disease. This results from a peculiar interaction between lead and hemoglobin.[129] Clinically it is manifested by gastrointestinal symptoms, colicky pains, constipation, and vomiting. Eventually, chronic nephritis, arteriosclerosis, and encephalopathy may also develop.

The diagnosis is confirmed by the presence of stippled cells in excess of 0.3 per cent and excretion in the urine of δ-aminolevulinic acid above 0.6 mg per 100 ml or coproporphyrin III above 100 μg per liter.[131, 132] The identification of fluorescent erythrocytes rapidly confirms the diagnosis.[133]

Prophylaxis is perhaps the best treatment.

Removal of the cause of lead toxicity is usually all that is necessary in mild cases. Chelating agents such as EDTA or penicillamine may hasten the removal of lead deposited in tissues. Occasionally these patients may undergo craniotomy, and instances of hyperthermia have occurred under anesthesia.[134]

Exposure to high concentrations of *benzene* is likely to occur when it is used as a solvent in industry, resulting in aplastic hemolytic anemia. The condition of the bone marrow varies from true aplasia to marked hyperplasia with a failure of maturation.[135] A leukemoid picture may occasionally supervene.[136] Feedings of *hexachlorobenzene* to rats will result in a similar disorder,[137] which can be ameliorated by the administration of adenosine monophosphate.[138]

Phenylhydrazine, although used extensively in the past to reduce the red cell mass in patients with polycythemia, is seldom used currently. The mechanism for hemolysis is by oxidative denaturation of hemoglobin.

Sulfones used in the treatment of some dermatologic disorders may lead to hemolytic anemia after about 10 days of treatment.

More rarely, hemolytic anemia may result from therapy with or accidental ingestion of other pharmacologic agents, such as phenothiazine, phenylsemicarbazide, acetophenetidin, sulfonamides, and chlorates.[139]

Hemolysis can also develop during severe infections or in a more protracted manner during certain parasitic infestations. It occurs almost invariably in infections produced by *Clostridium welchii* and Bartonella bacilliforms, and less frequently in β-hemolytic streptococci, *Escherichia coli*, and staphylococcal septicemias. Malarial infestations are always accompanied by mild hemolysis, produced by the invading parasite, and eventually by concomitant hypersplenic lytic trapping.

SPUR CELL ANEMIA

This hemolytic process, characterized by red cells resembling acanthocytes, has been reported in patients with alcoholic cirrhosis of the liver. The spur cells have a strong morphologic similarity to the erythrocytes seen in acanthocytosis. Nevertheless, certain definite differences exist between the two conditions; the neurologic involvement, typical retinitis pigmentosa, and associated lipid abnormalities seen in acanthocytosis are absent in spur cell anemia.[140]

The spur cells are more clearly identified in isotonic saline solution, and in acid media they tend to "smooth out," probably by swelling. The patient's erythrocytes treated with plasma of patients suffering from the disease have an increased cholesterol content. By electron microscopy, the spurs projecting from the main red cell mass have been demonstrated,[141] with a certain disorganization of the membrane into very fine lines interpreted as an alteration of the outermost protein portion of the membrane.

The abnormal plasma factor is presumably related to hepatic disease, most likely a protein or protein-bound compound and hence not dialyzable, that injures the red cells, causing spur formation and susceptibility to hemolysis.

MICROANGIOPATHIC HEMOLYTIC ANEMIA

This is a peculiar syndrome that has been noted to be present in patients with a variety of clinical conditions. It consists of hemolysis, burr cell poikilocytosis, thrombocytopenia, hepatic and reticuloendothelial siderosis, and in some cases[142] extramedullary hematopoiesis. The condition seems to be due to mechanical trapping and fracturing of red blood cells in small blood vessels.[143]

It has been associated with postpartum renal failure,[144] hemangioendothelioma of the liver,[142] carcinoma of the stomach,[145, 146] hemangiomas,[142] and cirrhosis of the liver.[147] Other causes include collagen-vascular diseases (lupus erythematosus, polyarteritis nodosa), carcinomatosis, malignant hypertension, pre-eclampsia, rejection of renal transplants, and thrombotic thrombocytopenic purpura.[8]

Disseminated intravascular coagulation (DIC) has been proposed as a causative factor in some of the cases reported, with the initial event being perhaps red cell lysis, followed by platelet agglutination, and finally activation of coagulation factors.[148] Abruptio placentae may be the precipitant for DIC. However, viral etiology has also been suggested by Gianantonio et al.[149] who isolated Coxsackie virus, and by others who reported an outbreak.[150]

Heparinization and steroid administrations have been reported as useful in the treatment of this condition.[144]

MARCH HEMOGLOBINURIA

This is a rare hemolytic condition in which hemoglobinemia and hemoglobinuria occur in certain individuals after severe exertion.[151] The red cells are morphologically and functionally normal but appear to be lysed by trauma during circulation through the feet, in which there is some mechanical defect that can be relieved by the simple expedient of wearing cushion insoles or by abstaining from extreme exercise.[152]

Low plasma haptoglobin is usually secondary to the presence of free plasma hemoglobin and appears to be related to a "renal threshold" for hemoglobin and the eventual occurrence of hemoglobinuria.[153] Absence of severe myalgias and the rise in hemoglobinemia clearly distinguish this condition from myoglobinuria. A case of acute tubular necrosis after an episode of march hemoglobinuria has been reported,[154] probably caused by repeated excessive erythrocyte lysis with eventual renal tubular injury.

GAUCHER'S DISEASE

This rare familial disorder of cerebroside metabolism was first described by Gaucher in 1882. It results from the lack of the enzyme β-glucocerebrosidase with accumulation of cerebrosides in the histiocytes. It affects all age groups and is characterized by an insidious onset, a prolonged course, and organomegaly, of which the most significant is splenomegaly, sometimes of massive proportions. Other less defined features are pingueculae (brown, wedge-shaped conjunctival thickenings at the lateral scleral margins) and brownish skin pigmentation.[155]

Hematologically, this disease is distinguished by anemia, neutropenia and/or thrombocytopenia in the presence of normal or increased marrow precursors. The diagnosis is confirmed when foam cells (atypical histocytes loaded with cerebrosides) are demonstrated in the bone marrow, spleen, or liver.

In patients with marked hypersplenism, prompt and sustained hematologic improvement has resulted after splenectomy.[156] Anesthetists may then see these patients in the operating room; adequate preparation is desirable, but transfusion to achieve near normal hemoglobin levels is not always necessary, because most often the plasma volume is normal.

FELTY'S SYNDROME

This clinical syndrome is characterized by chronic rheumatoid arthritis, splenomegaly, hepatomegaly, adenopathy, anemia, and leukopenia — this last being due to a relative or absolute neutropenia.[157] Bone marrow smears reveal granulocytic hyperplasia with "maturation arrest" at the myelocyte-metamyelocyte level. The etiology is obscure, but the protein abnormalities along with presence of the rheumatoid factor suggest an immunologic mechanism.

These patients, who may be very debilitated,[158] represent a significant anesthetic risk.

Some patients respond favorably to corticosteroid therapy, but splenectomy is followed by marked improvement, mainly in those patients with profound neutropenia and frequent infections. Infections, including those of the respiratory system, occur in 50 per cent of patients.[157] Ideally, splenectomy may be undertaken when complete control of the infective process is achieved and under steroid drug coverage.[159] This operative procedure is the most effective treatment for the syndrome. Patients may also appear in the operating theater for debridement or incision and drainage of infections.

HEMOCHROMATOSIS

This condition is characterized by iron overload, with fibrosis of the parenchymal organs, chiefly the liver and pancreas. The most common form, primary hemochromatosis, is an excessive and uncontrolled tendency to absorb iron from the gastrointestinal tract, possibly inherited as a recessive character.[160]

Secondary hemochromatosis can appear in other diseases in which excessive iron storage is typical, such as repeated and prolonged blood transfusions in intractable anemia, prolonged administration of parenteral iron, and chronic ingestion of a diet rich in iron.

The clinical features of hemochromatosis are hepatosplenomegaly resulting from cirrhosis of the liver, cardiac arrhythmias, skin pigmentation, diabetes mellitus, portal hypertension, and testicular atrophy. Laboratory confirmation is attained by demonstrating a fully saturated iron-binding capacity and a raised serum iron; iron deposition in the liver is confirmed at biopsy.

Potentially, these patients are prone to develop thrombosis and/or congestive heart failure when subjected to surgical procedures.

This disease is amenable to rational treatment when instituted in the early stages of the process. The most effective therapeutic maneuver has been repeated venesection; considering that 550 ml of blood removes about 250 mg of iron, it would take approximately four years to deplete the average hemochromatosis patient entirely of iron at the rate of 550 ml of blood weekly. However, the frequency of venesection is usually regulated by the serum iron level. With the exception of desferrioxamine, chelating agents have proved unsatisfactory in the treatment of this disease.

In addition to iron deposition in the liver and kidney as well as functional impairment of these organs, the heart may also be involved. Heart block and atrial arrhythmias are common manifestations of cardiac involvement. The deposition of iron pigments in the myocardium appears to spare the sinus node and the walls of the coronary arteries. With heavy deposition, necrosis and edema of the atrioventricular node occur. The reasons for this selectivity are not clear, but a difference in local tissue metabolism was suggested by James.[161] This contention is further supported by the observation that patients with hemochromatosis may have xanthine oxidase deficiency.[162] The effects that drugs such as cardiac glycosides, sympathomimetic amines, and anesthetics have on this type of cardiac conduction defect remain to be shown.

ERYTHROPOIETIN

The story of the discovery of the control of the differentiation of the formed elements of blood from stem cells is fascinating. On the basis of observations of increased blood hemoglobin in animals and humans living at high altitude, there was presumed to be a factor within the bone marrow that regulates red blood cell production and differentiation. However, objective proof of this contention was lacking until 1950, when Reissmann,[163] using parabiotic rats (i.e., rats with crossed circulations), provided the expected evidence. Following exposure of one of the partners to hypoxic atmospheres, both animals were observed to develop polycythemia and erythroid hyperplasia of the bone marrow. Thus, there appeared to be a substance capable of passing through small capillaries that might be responsible for stimulating erythropoiesis in the nonhypoxic rat. A confirmation of this study in animals was made in humans by Stohlmann,[164] who observed a patient with a reversed-flow shunt through a patent ductus arteriosus. This patient had oxygenated blood flow in the upper part of the body, and unsaturated blood irrigated the infradiaphragmatic areas; red cell hyperplasia was found in both sternal and iliac marrow aspirates, indicating that marrow hypoxia is not a prerequisite for increased erythropoiesis.

Three conclusions can be derived from these observations. (1) Hypoxia or severe anemia induces the release of a factor that stimulates erythropoiesis. (2) This plasma-contained factor may generate erythropoiesis without intermediary lower-than-normal oxygen saturation of the blood. (3) The chief anatomic source of this factor in man is below the diaphragm.

Reduced marrow activity can be produced by hypertransfusion, hypophysectomy, starvation, and induction of polycythemia by chronic hypoxia. Some of these stimuli have been utilized to develop an experimental model for assay methodology of erythropoietin. More recently, in vitro methods utilizing bone marrow cultures and a quantitative immunologic assay have been proposed for this purpose.[165]

From whatever studies have been performed, erythropoietin appears to be a glycoprotein with an electrophoretic mobility similar to that of a γ-globulin. Its approximate molecular weight is 36,000. Although it seems weakly antigenic, specific antibodies that inhibit erythropoietin activity have been prepared.

The primary action of erythropoietin is to effect differentiation of stem cells into red cell precursors. The exact mechanism of this process is not completely known, but Stohlmann[164] suggested that enzyme induction relevant to hemoglobin synthesis is involved. Erythropoietin appears to have no other important physiologic action outside the marrow. Under intense erythropoietin stimulation, the red cell precursors extrude their nuclei and leave the marrow earlier, shortening the maturation processes and skipping some of the mitotic divisions; thus macrocytes or stress erythrocytes enter the circulation prematurely, but they appear to have a shorter life span.

The kidney appears to be the chief site of production of erythropoietin, on the basis of Jacobson's observation[166] that bilateral nephrectomy results in the cessation of erythropoietin production (Fig. 8–5). Hypernephromas, renal infarcts, hydronephrosis, and renal cysts have been associated with increased production of erythropoietin.[167] Usually, however, renal injury is associated with decreased erythropoietin production and an attendant anemia. Current theory suggests that erythropoietin is inactivated by an inhibitor that somehow becomes inactivated itself in the conditions mentioned above, with resultant release of free erythropoietin. There also appear to be extrarenal sites of erythropoietin production, including the liver and macronuclear macrophages. Nathan and his associates[168] showed that in anephric humans erythropoiesis continues, though at a reduced rate.

It has been estimated that erythropoietin levels in blood averaged 0.02 μg per milliliter. These levels rise 10 to 30 hours after exposure to hypoxia. Renal tissue oxygenation appears to be a mediator in the physiological regulating mechanism of red cell homeostasis, because tissue oxygenation is influenced by endocrine, pulmonary, and cardiovascular factors that may increase or decrease the amount of circulating red cells by altering erythropoietin production.[169]

Accelerated production may be observed in patients with arterial desaturation or with

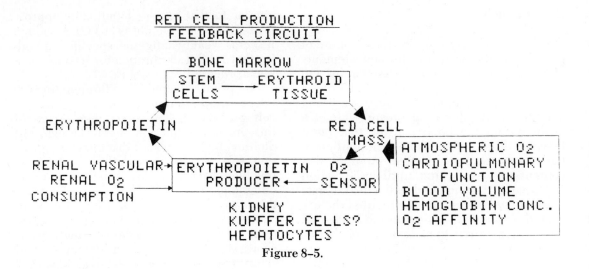

Figure 8–5.

anemia of diverse types. Some neoplasms with associated polycythemia, such as cerebellar hemangioblastoma, ovarian tumors, uterine fibroids, hepatoma, pheochromocytoma, and renal tumors, especially hypernephroma, have been shown to elicit elevated erythropoietin activity. Administration of cobalt salts, by producing hypoxia at the cellular level, results in the same effect. On the other hand, decreased production of erythropoietin has been observed in anemic patients with advanced renal disease.

The role of erythropoietin in the hematopoiesis of the embryo is not fully understood. Maternal blood has low normal levels, but cord blood has considerable activity, even higher when taken from anoxic infants. Furthermore, large amounts of erythropoietin have been measured in the amniotic fluid of women whose pregnancies are complicated by erythroblastosis, thus strongly suggesting an active erythropoietin mechanism in utero.[165] Important knowledge about the mechanisms involved in red cell production will be attained when full understanding of the release, activity, and fate of erythropoietin is attained.

RELATION OF 2,3-DPG TO HEMOGLOBIN FUNCTION

The red cells of man and other mammals contain high concentrations of the organic phosphate 2,3-diphosphoglycerate, about 4.5 μ moles per milliliter. By spectrophotometric methods, Benesch and Benesch demonstrated that the removal of 2,3-DPG

from hemoglobin resulted in a gradual "shift to the left" of the oxygen dissociation curve, indicating a subsequent increased affinity of hemoglobin for oxygen.[170] Other organic phosphates had less influence on this function.

Since then, further correlation of 2,3-DPG as the influential factor in the affinity of hemoglobin for oxygen has been reported. Valtis and Kennedy[171] showed that blood stored in acid citrate dextrose (ACD) had an increased oxygen affinity, indicating a shift to the left of the dissociation curve. This finding was reiterated by other authors,[172, 173] who noted a prompt fall of 2,3-DPG, which could be considerably delayed by the addition of inosine. Schweizer and Howland[174] have shown that citrate-phosphate-dextrose stored blood maintains higher levels of 2,3-DPG.

This phenomenon may occur more often than expected in the operating room. After massive transfusion of stored blood low in 2,3-DPG, and thus with a high oxygen affinity, the amount of oxygen unloaded to the tissues may be compromised in spite of an apparent adequate Pa_{O_2}. Replenishment of 2,3-DPG in the depleted transfused erythrocyte can take place in about 24 hours in vitro and four hours in vivo; however, it may not be rapid enough in the critically ill patient with concomitant respiratory complications.[175, 176]

Abnormal levels of 2,3-DPG have also been observed in newborn infants and in persons with certain metabolic disorders.[177] Moreover, low levels have been noted in carbon monoxide poisoning, septic shock, and hypothyroidism,[178] and in patients with hexokinase deficiency, whereas considerable elevation has been seen in patients with hyperthyroidism[179] and pyruvate kinase deficiency.[180] In sickle cell anemia, the "shift to the right" of the oxygen equilibrium curve may be explained by elevated levels of 2,3-DPG associated with anemia.[181]

There have also been indications that variations of intracellular 2,3-DPG may play a role in the adaptation to chronic hypoxia. Under these circumstances, the oxygen hemoglobin dissociation curve shifts to the right, with a greater amount of oxygen delivered, an obvious advantage in the hypoxic patient. This mechanism may influence the adaptation to low oxygen tension at high altitudes, suggesting that red cell metabolism is exquisitely sensitive to hypoxic stimuli by changing levels of 2,3-DPG and thus appropriately adjusting the oxygen dissociation curve.[182] There are, however, conflicting data suggesting that adaptation to high altitudes may be associated with *increased* hemoglobin affinity for oxygen.[183]

2,3-DPG is produced enzymatically from 1,3-DPG by the action of a mutase. There is an inhibition of this enzyme by 2,3-DPG. This inhibition is released when 2,3-DPG binds to desaturated hemoglobin under hypoxic conditions. The shift of the oxygen dissociation curve may be quantified by the use of the P_{50} or the partial pressure at which 50 percent of hemoglobin is saturated. A shift to the right implies an increased P_{50}, while a shift to the left implies a decrease.

Concentrations of 2,3-DPG appear to be regulated by several mechanisms. Endogenous factors such as intracellular pH changes, thyroid hormone,[184] and ATP-ADP ratio appear to be important determinants of 2,3-DPG concentration.[185] Oxidant compounds released during exercise may be responsible for the observed rapid rise of 2,3-DPG in this physical condition.[186] Propranolol appears to shift the hemoglobin dissociation curve to the right. The role of 2,3-DPG in this reaction is still a matter of debate.

DISEASES OF THE WHITE CELL ELEMENTS

A considerable number of rare and other, less uncommon, diseases of the leukocyte series, whether or not they have specific relation to anesthesia, will be dealt with in this section, so as to serve as a readily available reference for anesthesiologists who wish a brief description of such diseases and who wish to determine if certain precautions must be observed when managing one of these patients.

AGRANULOCYTOSIS

This entity was thought to be an infectious disease until it was demonstrated that the primary factor was reduction of the granulocytes in blood, which lowered resistance and led to bacterial infection. The drugs that were the most common offenders contained a known leukocyte depressant in their molecule, in the form of a benzene ring, which appears to have a detrimental effect on granulopoiesis.[187] However, the well-conducted experiments of Moeschlin and Wagner[188] have further suggested the presence of leukocyte antibodies in the plasma, probably caused by the incriminated drug.

Immunologic reactions are responsible for the appearance of agranulocytosis with drugs such as aminopyrine;[189] however, the agranulocytosis observed after the administration of sulfa and chloramphenicol[190] implies at least one other mechanism, because the onset of the disease is rarely seen during therapy and usually appears later.

The possibility of an intrinsic abnormality resulting from a genetically determined defect has been proposed. This appears to consist of an inherited metabolic defect, perhaps DNA replication, that eventually leads to reduced marrow growth, whether producing agranulocytosis or, less selectively, producing aplastic anemias.[191] This finding, in fact, has restricted the use of chloramphenicol to very specific, limited cases of typhoid fever or severe gram-negative septicemia, when no other antibiotic is effective.

The following drugs may produce agranulocytosis:[192, 193, 194, 195, 196]

Anticonvulsants: methylphenylethylhydantoin, trimethadione.
Antihistaminics: phenothiazines, ethylenediamines.
Antimicrobial agents: arsenobenzol, chloramphenicol, sulfonamides, thiosemicarbazone, streptomycin, oxytetracycline,

chlortetracycline, carbenicillin, cephalosporins.

Antithyroid agents: thiouracils, methimazole.

Sedatives: urethane, amidopyrine, phenacemide, chlorpromazine, barbiturates.

Others: phenothiazines, procainamide, gold preparations, phenylbutazone, nitrophenols, mercurial diuretics, quinidine, quinacrine HCl, mercury, amphetamines.

Pisciotta has done a complete review of drug-induced leukopenia, to which readers are referred for details.[197] Neutropenia is also associated with such illnesses as systemic lupus erythematosus,[198] rheumatoid arthritis (Felty's syndrome),[199] and hematologic malignancies. Radiation or chemotherapy may result in severe neutropenia.[200] Bacterial, viral, fungal, protozoal, and rickettsial infections may be associated with severe neutropenia.

Without limitations of sex or age, after a prodromal period patients usually complain of sore throat, fever, and dysphagia, progressing to mental confusion and stupor. In peripheral blood the most significant findings are leukopenia and granulocytopenia without anemia or thrombocytopenia. In the bone marrow, the cells of the granulocytic series are greatly reduced and toxic granulations are seen in the younger cells.

In the preantibiotic era the mortality from this complication was nearly 100 per cent. The mortality continues to be high, especially if agranulocytosis is of abrupt onset.[201, 202] The most important aspect of treatment is withdrawal of the offending drug and administration of an antibiotic agent to combat the superimposed infection. Adequate hydration and maintenance of normal body temperature are also of value. Isolation techniques should be employed as prophylaxis against infection, but they should not be so rigid as to compromise patient care. Granulocyte transfusions may be attempted in severe or prolonged cases. Glucocorticoids have been used.[203] Although still controversial, they may be of use in situations in which an immune mechanism is postulated as etiologic.

Although there are no good data currently, it is clear that patients with agranulocytosis are at risk for postoperative infections should they require surgery (i.e., splenectomy for Felty's syndrome). Whether general anesthetics add to the immune incompetence of these individuals is still open to debate and further study.

CYCLIC NEUTROPENIA

This is a well-established but poorly understood rare familial entity[204] that may occur at any age. It is characterized by the regular decrease of the neutrophilic granulocytes, progressing to total disappearance in the circulation at approximately 21-day intervals.[205] The neutropenia is due to cyclic arrest of production of the entire neutrophilic series. During this time, patients may have fever, malaise, and oropharyngeal ulceration, accompanied by arthralgia, headache, and lymphadenopathy.

Steroid therapy has a temporary beneficial effect; splenectomy appears to produce a more lasting benefit. Antibiotics may be used to treat active infections, but should not be used prophylactically.[206]

MYELOPROLIFERATIVE DISEASES

These disorders are characterized by uncontrolled proliferation of all or individual bone marrow elements, and may or may not involve organs other than the bone marrow.

Leukemia

With the signs of most malignant neoplastic processes, this entity encompasses the diseases presenting with an infiltrative and destructive proliferation of one individual group of cells.

Several factors are in controversy as to the etiology of these conditions. Evidence continues to accumulate incriminating viruses as the cause of some forms of leukemia. In fowl and mice, the disease is transmissible; viruses and mycoplasma have been isolated from leukemic cells in man, but thus far they have not been proved to transmit the disease.[207]

Epidemiologic studies have shown seasonal and local variations in sporadic series of cases of acute leukemia, thus suggesting an infective origin.

Exposure to radiation also appears to be a causative factor. This contention has been based on the high incidence of this disease among radiologists, when safety measures were not yet established,[208] and supported by the frequency of leukemia observed in infants whose mothers had radiologic examinations during pregnancy. After the atomic explosions in Hiroshima and Nagasaki, the incidence rose fourfold there in 10 years.[209] Furthermore, anesthesiologists exposed to radiation and anesthetic vapors may have a statistically significant higher chance of dying from reticuloendothelial malignancies,[210] a point that obviously deserves further study, since it appears to constitute a professional hazard. Pharmacologic (benzene) and genetic (with chromosomal abnormalities) factors have also been incriminated as causing certain types of leukemia.[211]

Pathologically, in leukemia there is a disorganized proliferation either of the primitive "blast" cells of the marrow or lymph glands, or of the more mature cells. The increase of one particular strain of cells in the marrow does not necessarily imply an increased production, but rather, in some instances, a failure of some marrow cells to mature. The most frequently involved organs are the liver, spleen, kidneys, lymph glands, skin, lungs, brain and meninges. In late stages, the progressive infiltration of the bone marrow leads to anemia that is normocytic or macrocytic and normochromic and eventually to thrombocytopenia. Occasionally, the bone marrow becomes megaloblastic owing to relative folate deficiency.

In acute leukemias, granulocytopenia frequently occurs, making patients more susceptible to infections; this is also seen in chronic lymphatic leukemia caused by a disturbed antibody synthesis and resultant hypogammaglobulinemia.

Isolated cases of unexplained increased intracranial pressure, later found to be leukemia, have suggested that intracranial hypertension may be an early sign of this disease. Although cerebrospinal fluid pleocytosis is common once the entity is physically established, these reports suggest an early involvement of the central nervous system, which perhaps varies in degree from patient to patient.[212]

The chronic course of myeloblastic, lymphoblastic, and monoblastic leukemias may go on for years, with occasional acute exacerbations; however, the illness may begin as acute leukemia, or this form may be the terminal event. In the acute phase, anemia results from blood loss through hemorrhage, decreased blood production, and increased hemolysis.[213] Immature white cells enter the circulation in considerable numbers and provide the identification of the type of leukemia. Leukemoid reactions occurring in infections can be differentiated by the proportionately lower number of immature circulating elements.

Acute leukemia usually runs a short course, being more severe in small children. Among the therapeutic agents used in acute leukemias, folic acid, purine antagonists, and adrenocorticosteroids, in series or in various combinations, afford palliative benefit only. Blood transfusions are also temporarily helpful.[214] Of the antimetabolites, 6-mercaptopurine, amethopterin, vincristine, cyclophosphamide, rubidomycin, and busulfan are more commonly used.[215]

Its usual modes of presentation may be facial or buccal ulceration, anemia, hemorrhage, and/or fever. In peripheral blood smears blast cells occur in excess of 50 per cent of the total leukocyte count, which may vary from 20,000 to 100,000, along with low hemoglobin concentration and erythrocyte count. Anisocytosis and punctate basophilia may be present in the red cells. It is in this form of leukemia that nitrous oxide appears to lower the elevated white blood cell counts when inhaled continuously for several days.[216] The myelodepressant property of this anesthetic gas deserves further investigation.

Chronic Myeloid Leukemia. Chronic myeloid leukemia (CML) occurs mostly in adult patients between the ages of 30 and 50 years.

The diagnosis may be suggested by the combination of anemia and splenomegaly in a person of appropriate age. Hepatomegaly, lymphadenopathy, ecchymoses, and sternal tenderness may be present. Symptoms include easy fatigability, malaise, sweating, heat intolerance, early satiety, and abdominal fullness. The blood smear shows normocytic normochromic anemia of moderate degree associated with a highly elevated leukocyte count. The predominant cell is the granulocyte, with 20 to 30 per cent myelocytes and absent blast forms. Leukocyte alkaline phosphatase is absent, thus distinguishing CML from leukemoid reactions or other myeloproliferative disorders.[8] There is an 80 per cent incidence of the

Philadelphia chromosome, which is a translocation of the long arms of chromosomes 22 and 9.[217] Vitamin B_{12} serum levels and binding capacity are increased as a result of increased neutrophil production of transcobalamin I, a B_{12}-binding protein.[218]

For the treatment of this disease, either radiotherapy or chemotherapy may be resorted to. Remissions are usually induced by localized radiation of the spleen and occasionally of the spine, or by the administration of radioactive phosphorus.[215] Busulfan, a derivative of nitrogen mustard, is perhaps the most effective chemotherapeutic agent available now. Important side effects of busulfan that are of consequence to anesthesiologists are bone marrow aplasia, pulmonary fibrosis, and an addisonian syndrome.[219] Although still controversial, steroids may be combined with an antimitotic agent with beneficial effect.[216] Specifically, testosterone enanthate and fluoxymesterone have been effective in the treatment of the anemia seen in this disease.

Lymphocytic Leukemia. The beginning of this form of leukemia is insidious, and the disease usually runs a chronic course. It is manifested by enlargement of superficial lymph nodes. Symptoms are usually generated by the hematologic picture — fatigue, exertional dyspnea, and weakness appearing if anemia is severe, whereas bleeding gums and petechiae are caused by a depressed platelet count.[220] Anemia occurs in half of the patients initially.[8] There may be an associated autoimmune hemolytic anemia.[221] There is hypogammaglobulinemia with increased susceptibility to infection.[222] Also, a variety of skin lesions occur in lymphocytic leukemia, varying from exfoliative dermatitis to herpes zoster and infiltration of the skin by leukemic cells. In addition to the markedly generalized lymph node enlargement, hepatosplenomegaly is usually found, and many times patients can be diagnosed by the dermatologic changes described above. Examination of peripheral smears shows leukocytosis with an increased absolute lymphocyte count. These lymphocytes are small in size, and some of them are in the blast form.

Of significant interest to anesthesiologists is the reported increased metabolic rate, up to 20 to 40 per cent, in these patients. Compensatory oxygen flows must be supplied during and after anesthesia whenever these patients undergo surgical procedures, usually for diagnostic purposes or to relieve obstructive symptoms resulting from uncontrolled proliferation of lymph nodes.[223]

The survival time in patients with chronic leukemia varies from one to nine years. Severe anemia and thrombocytopenia indicate a poor prognosis.[224] Although this disease is incurable, alkylating agents, radiotherapy, and adrenocortical steroids[225] can be combined to prolong the lives of these patients and make them comfortable. In vitro studies suggest that the cytocidal action of colchicine may be of benefit in the chronic form of this disease.[226] Granulocytopenia and hypogammaglobulinemia predispose these patients to infection, which may complicate a postoperative course. Since these patients are generally elderly, they may come to surgery for a variety of ailments unrelated to their leukemia. Thrombocytopenia, if severe and associated with excessive bleeding, may require platelet transfusions.

Monocytic Leukemia. This form of leukemia is considered a separate and well-defined entity, with chronic and acute phases. The acute form has an insidious onset, with symptoms similar to those observed in the other varieties of leukemia. Often the most striking abnormality is a marked swelling of the gums, which eventually become ulcerated and necrotic, making instrumentation of the upper airway difficult. With certain frequency, patients develop perirectal abscesses that may require drainage under anesthesia.[227]

Laboratory examination discloses a severe monocytic leukemia with a high leukocyte count, of which monocytes constitute from 30 to 90 per cent including mature, blast, and promonocyte forms. There may also be nucleated erythrocytes, and the platelet count is usually reduced. The bone marrow is hypercellular, with blast and older cells of the monocytic series predominating.[228]

In the chronic form of monocytic leukemia, severe anemia is a prevailing feature of the clinical picture; it is more frequently seen in middle-aged patients, mostly males. Splenomegaly sometimes reaches enormous dimensions, and the skin presents infiltrative and hemorrhagic lesions distributed all over the body.

The acute phase has a rapid course, usually terminating in two or three months. The treatment of both forms of monocytic leukemia is unsatisfactory. Radiation and splenectomy are of no value; the alkylating agents and the antimetabolic drugs produce little if any benefit. Transfusions are usually necessary for the anemia, which is refractory to other measures.[229]

Hairy Cell Leukemia. This is a peculiar type of leukemia characterized by the proliferation of a cell with morphologic aspects and clinical features different from other leukemias. This entity was previously termed leukemic reticuloendotheliosis and has been described mostly in adult males who presented with weakness, fatigue, and bleeding episodes. On physical examination hepatosplenomegaly prevails. Lymphadenopathy is rare. Skin rashes have frequently been seen.[230] The associated anemia is of the normocytic normochromic type, with nucleated red blood cells in peripheral blood, as well as moderate thrombocytopenia. Pancytopenia is usually present. If the white blood count is elevated, it is due to the presence of the atypical cells. Peculiar cells noted in the marrow and blood smears may be as large as lymphocytes, with a round shape and windblown appearance resembling pseudopods.

The course of hairy cell leukemia is considerably more benign than that of similar conditions such as reticulum cell sarcoma. Survival may range from months to years. Antimetabolites, steroids, and blood transfusions provide palliation. Splenectomy may improve the cytopenias.[8]

Erythroleukemia. This rare disorder is also known as DiGuglielmo's disease. It presents as a leukemia-like process, affecting erythropoiesis. It may occur at all ages, although it is most frequently seen in middle-aged patients. The presenting symptoms are usually vague, consisting of weakness, fatigue, dyspnea, and weight loss. Bleeding in skin and mucous membranes and muscle pains may also occur.

The bone marrow shows intense hyperplasia. There are severe megaloblastic changes. Gigantoblasts, which are multinucleated erythroid precursors, are seen. Extramedullary foci may be present in the liver and spleen, which are usually enlarged. Nevertheless, anemia is present, indicating that erythropoiesis, although very active, is ineffective.[231] Leukopenia, increased reticulocyte count, and normal platelet counts are common. Scrutiny of the peripheral blood discloses nucleated red cells and myeloblasts.[232]

Initially, it was noted that the administration of folic acid or vitamin B_{12} failed to improve the anemia; this was later confirmed by the observation that serum vitamin B_{12} levels are unusually high in erythroleukemia.[233]

The prognosis for patients with DiGuglielmo's disease is poor, and most patients succumb within one year of the appearance of the first symptoms, although isolated cases of survivals for 10 years or longer have been reported.[234]

A drug-induced etiology of DiGuglielmo's disease has been suggested by Kotlarek-Haus et al.,[235] who attributed a case of erythemic myelosis to chronic ingestion of phenacetin.

Multiple Myeloma

Generalized proliferation of a primitive type of plasma cell characterizes this disease. This proliferation, predominantly seen in the bone marrow, has all the features of a malignant process. It occurs most frequently in middle-aged individuals, and is twice as common in males as in females. Myeloma cells have an appearance similar to plasma cells, but usually have a more triangular shape and a pseudopodial outline. Simultaneously, there is a characterized abnormality of the plasma proteins, with a sharp peak of γ-globulin (60 per cent of cases) and β-globulin (25 per cent of cases). One fourth of patients have no monoclonal protein spike and show only Bence Jones proteinuria with hypogammaglobulinemia. With the use of in vitro preparations, it has been proved that the aberrant proteins and the typical Bence Jones protein found in plasma and urine are produced by myeloma cells.

Since as much as 20 or 30 gm of protein may be excreted in the urine each day and there are from 70 to 90 gm of protein available in a normal diet, a considerable portion of the protein is taken from the metabolic needs. However, in this disease the levels of plasma proteins are increased mostly at the expense of the globulin fraction, specifically the γ-globulin, but in some instances the alpha and beta fractions are also involved. In spite of this quantitative advantage of γ-globulin, patients with multiple myeloma respond poorly to the antigenic challenge.[236]

The qualitative difference in plasma proteins may bring about a proportionally lower than normal albumin contentration, which in turn may result in alterations of the binding process essential for distribution. Greater amounts of the drug may remain unbound and thus exert an unexpected depressive effect in some systems while being ineffective in others.

Another example of the profound alterations of protein metabolism in this disease is the occasional occurrence in the serum of a cold precipitable globulin called cryoglobulin that can also be present in other diseases. In addition, a form of amyloidosis may be present in about one tenth of these patients; the distribution of the amyloid material is widespread and may be indirectly related to products of the abnormal proteins deposited in various tissues.

A peculiar feature of myelomatosis is hypercalcemia, sometimes as high as 16 or 18 mg per 100 ml without significant alteration of a serum phosphorus or alkaline phosphatase. Moderate elevations of serum calcium levels may produce gastrointestinal disturbances, weakness, apathy, polydipsia, and polyuria; excessively high values may cause electrocardiographic changes, vascular collapse, and ventricular fibrillation. What effect high serum calcium concentrations may have on the clinical action of muscle-relaxing drugs has not been studied, but it is known that acetylcholine release by the nerve endings is enhanced in a Ca^{++} rich medium.[237]

The usual presenting symptom is pain, often disabling and difficult to control, which is due to bone involvement and pressure on the adjacent nerves. Pathologic fractures of the ribs, femur, sternum, humerus, and other long bones are likely. In other patients, the prominent feature is recurrent attacks of fever or pneumonia that may coincide with greatly elevated serum globulin levels; whether these pulmonary lesions are manifestations of small infarctions or localized pneumonitis is uncertain; however, clinical and radiologic signs strongly suggest an infectious process.[238]

Hyperviscosity syndrome relates to the presence of monoclonal proteins. Symptoms include headache, heart failure, vertigo, visual disturbance, and alterations in consciousness including coma.[239]

Radicular pain secondary to vertebral compression fractures may make spinal puncture extremely difficult; furthermore, the occurrence of peripheral neuritis may be a relative contraindication to this form of regional anesthesia.

Renal insufficiency occurs in multiple myeloma and may be a dominant and terminal feature of it, resulting probably from dehydration and stasis of urine flow and precipitation of Bence Jones protein in the renal tubules. A peculiar characteristic of kidney failure secondary to multiple myeloma is the presence of azotemia without hypertension, which should strongly arouse the suspicion of myelomatosis. Renal failure is one of the common causes of death.

Radiologically, typical "punched-out" lesions, varying in diameter from 1 mm to 12 cm, are seen in the absence of osteoblastic reaction and may occur in several bones but are most easily observed in flat bones. The peripheral blood examinations may reveal anemia, usually normocytic. The leukocyte count is generally normal, and the diagnosis may be suggested by the presence of increased numbers of plasma cells or any other abnormal mononuclear cells found in the bone marrow. Marrow aspiration may show myeloma cells, some appearing as vacuolated "moth cells" and others containing protein particles.[240] Finally, the diagnosis is confirmed by electrophoretic examination of the serum proteins and the finding of Bence Jones protein in the urine.

Patients with multiple myeloma may be given anesthesia when further documentation of the diagnosis by bone biopsy is necessary. Ideally, serum calcium levels should be brought to normal limits by administering adrenal corticosteroids or resorting to more heroic measures such as titrated intravenous infusion of potassium- or magnesium-containing solutions.[241] Special concern must be given to postoperative respiratory care, because there is an increased susceptibility of those patients to pulmonary infection, probably owing to the high serum protein values, causing an increase in blood viscosity and leading to thrombosis of small pulmonary vessels. Lung infections may also be favored by the subnormal antibody response and pulmonary hypoventilation produced by painful fractures of the ribs or vertebrae.[238]

Myeloma patients may be severely dehydrated secondary to vomiting. This may result in acute renal failure. Fluid status should be corrected prior to anesthesia. It is suggested that overnight fasting without intravenous fluid infusion may be dangerous.[8] Positioning on the operating table must be done with caution to avert the possibility of iatrogenic fractures.

No one specific therapeutic agent is available for this disease. Only palliative measures are recommended, consisting of immobilization of fractures, body braces, and analgesic drugs for the patient's comfort. If anemia is severe, blood transfusions may be required. Decompression laminectomies are sometimes required to alleviate pain from compression fractures or to restore motion in paralyzed muscle groups. Most chemotherapeutic agents have been proved inefficient; however, urethane, chlorambucil, melphalan, and cyclophosphamide have been used in the treatment of multiple myeloma with limited success. Localized radiation may be directed toward specifically painful lesions, and spontaneous fractures may heal more rapidly.

Myelofibrosis (Myeloid Metaplasia)

Although resembling myeloid leukemia in some aspects, this proliferative disease tends to involve several marrow cells. Its cause has not yet been determined. There are proliferation of fibroblasts and excessive collagen synthesis in the bone marrow.[243]

Clinically, this entity may be difficult to differentiate from myeloid leukemia, except for the occasional occurrence of polycythemia. However, metaplasia is not limited to the spleen, for the liver and lymph glands are also enlarged. In peripheral blood there are polycythemia, leukocytosis, and thrombocytopenia, but the characteristic feature is leukoerythroblastic anemia.[244]

Symptoms are related to anemia, thrombocytopenia, and splenomegaly. They include easy fatigability, bruisability, bone pain, sweating, and abdominal fullness.[8] Anesthesiologists may be consulted for evaluation of these patients when splenectomy is indicated because of hypersplenism; adequate preoperative preparation should consist of maintenance doses of steroids, which may be increased just before surgery, and the administration of fresh blood transfusions. Since there may be a considerable expansion of plasma volume with trapping of red cells in the spleen, the continuous monitoring of central venous pressure is advisable so as to avoid overloading of the circulation. Furthermore, depending on the degree of hepatic involvement, the metabolic degradation of some of the anesthetic drugs may be impaired, and therefore agents devoid of this problem are desirable. Portal hypertension may occur.[245] Distortion of the gastroesophageal junction by the enlarged spleen may cause reflux.[8] Management of anesthetic induction with cricoid pressure and endotracheal intubation is probably indicated.

Average survival is six years. Death occurs as a result of infection, cardiovascular disease, and/or bleeding. One fifth of patients develop acute myelogenous leukemia terminally.

Megakaryocytic Myelosis

This is a variation of myeloid metaplasia in which megakaryocyte proliferation tends to predominate, although it may be associated with thrombocytemia. The platelets, although present in excessive numbers, are defective in constitution and produce a hemorrhagic tendency. The platelet abnormality may be demonstrated by the thromboplastic generation test or by demonstrating either a deficiency in the production of platelet Factor II or failure of agglutinability with adenosine diphosphate.

Temporary control of the bleeding tendency has been achieved by administration of radioactive phosphorus or busulfan. Thrombophoresis (removal of platelets by centrifugation followed by the return of the remaining blood to the patient) has also been recommended. The possibility of disseminated intravascular clotting occurring in a patient with megakaryocytic myelosis under stress conditions has not been defined, but it may not be remote, considering the platelet abnormalities present.

Waldenström's Macroglobulinemia

This rare entity occurs most often in elderly patients, with an incidence approximately similar to that of multiple myeloma. A history of recent weight loss, weakness, and frequent infections accompanied by hepatosplenomegaly and moderate lymphadenopathy is common.[246] Occasionally, retinal hemorrhages and a bleeding tendency may be present. Radiologically, generalized demineralization of the bones is seen. Specific renal lesions, consisting of amyloidosis and deposits on the endothelial aspect of the basement membrane large enough to occlude the capillary lumen, have been reported; examination of these thrombi show them to contain IgM.[247]

Bone marrow aspirates may reveal infiltration of bizarre cells called lymphoplasmacytic cells that possess cytoplasm similar to that observed in plasma cells, but with a nucleus of a lymphocyte. These cells are also found in the lymph nodes, spleen, and liver, and rarely in peripheral blood. Total plasma proteins are increased, associated with an elevated sedimentation rate and serum viscosity. Immunoelectrophoresis may reveal a dense γM band. The Sia test, which is based on the insolubility of macroglobulins in distilled water, is often positive, and 5 to 10 per cent of the patients will have Bence Jones proteins in the urine.[248] A definite diagnosis is given by the finding of significant concentrations of high molecular weight globulins at the ultracentrifugation of the serum.[249]

The high concentration of macroglobulins in Waldenström's disease results from an increased protein synthesis by β-lymphocytes. This in turn is believed to slow the flow of blood, eventually resulting in vascular stasis, thrombosis, and hemorrhage in the retina as well as in vessels in other parts of the body.[250] Cryoglobulins may cause Raynaud's phenomenon, cold urticaria, and vascular occlusion.[251] Hemorrhagic diathesis is thought to occur from inhibition of production of platelet Factor III, resulting from coating of the platelets with macroglobulins. By the process of plasmapheresis, macroglobulins may be removed from blood or they may be reduced by depolymerization, after the administration of penicillin or penicillamine. More effective has been treatment with chlorambucil, melphalan, and cyclophosphamide.

Heavy γ-Chain Disease

This rare myeloproliferative disorder results from the aberrant production of myeloma-type protein with a specific chemical characteristic but without Bence Jones protein. Clinically, there are generalized lymphadenopathy, hepatosplenomegaly, anemia, fever, eosinophilia, and a tendency to infection. The bone marrow usually shows an excess of plasma cells and lymphocytes.[252]

All reported patients with heavy chain disease have been males between 40 and 75 years of age. Again, the decrease in immunoglobulins seen in these patients probably accounts for their marked susceptibility to bacterial infection.[253]

External radiation, steroids, and antimitotic drugs have produced short-term improvement, but no definite treatment is currently available.

Burkitt's Lymphoma

This disorder, first described by Burkitt in 1958, is seen mostly in children. It is characterized by rapidly growing tumors located in the mandible, salivary glands, adrenals, liver, heart, and retroperitoneum; superficial lymph nodes are seldom involved.[254] Most reports have come from Africa and a few from the United States. Radiation produces limited regression of the tumors, but chemotherapy is of little benefit.[255]

Owing to the location of these tumor masses, difficult intubation of the trachea may be foreseen whenever their anatomic configuration would make laryngoscopy difficult. Blind nasotracheal intubation may be attempted, following the breathing sounds as a guide or the protrusion of the catheter in the neck.[256] If this is of no avail, a polyethylene catheter may be threaded in a retrograde direction, inserting it percutaneously into the trachea and securing it through the mouth; then an endotracheal tube can be inserted around the catheter.[257]

Polycythemia

Meaning an increase in the total blood cell mass, polycythemia really signifies an increase in hemoglobin concentration, total red cell count, and packed cell volume; in addition, the peripheral hematocrit is increased as a result of contraction of plasma volume.

In general, three forms of this disease are considered: primary polycythemia; secondary polycythemia; and pseudo- or relative polycythemia.

Primary Polycythemia. This disorder,

also called polycythemia rubra vera, is of unknown origin but is considered a manifestation of a myeloproliferative disorder with hyperplasia of the erythropoietic elements.

This proliferation leads to an anatomic and functional disorganization of the bone marrow. The essential change in blood is an increase in hemoglobin content, with the red cell count varying from six to ten million per cubic millimeter, and the hematocrit between 50 to 75 per cent. Subsequently there is an increase in blood viscosity and capillary dilatation, which increases their fragility.[258]

Hence the blood flow slows, resulting in a prolonged circulation time and peripheral cyanosis. Concomitantly, there is an increased incidence of thrombotic and hemorrhagic complications that are markedly exacerbated during the postoperative period. Some serum enzymes have been noted to be elevated in polycythemia vera; serum muramidase lysozyme is markedly elevated, reflecting a proliferative granulocytic process.[259]

The disease mainly affects middle-aged men and women, with vague symptoms presenting in individuals with plethoric facies. There are also typical retinal changes with mild splenomegaly. If arterial hypertension is present, this has been regarded as a separate entity termed Gaisböck's disease.[260] The most satisfactory long-term treatment of polycythemia is radioactive phosphorus, although it usually takes two months before obvious improvement is obtained.[261] In emergency circumstances, such as threatening thrombosis or hemorrhage or when one of these patients has to be prepared for emergency surgery, venesection may be resorted to. Repeated venesections, although used as long-term treatment, are not satisfactory, because they provide only temporary control and further stimulate marrow activity.[262] During surgical procedures it is important to avoid extreme venostasis due to positioning as well as prolonged bouts of hyper- and hypotension.[263] The risk of complications is high.[264] These include hemorrhage and thrombosis. Mortality related to surgery is 15 per cent. Reduction of hematocrit lowers morbidity. The prognosis in this form of polycythemia is reasonably good so long as the increase in the red cell mass is controlled; otherwise

patients may succumb to cerebrovascular or cardiovascular accidents.

Secondary Polycythemia. Secondary polycythemia is usually a complication of a primary disorder such as hypoxia from living at high altitudes, chronic cardiac and/or pulmonary disease, or methemoglobinemia and sulfhemoglobinemia. Other causative disorders have been discussed in detail in dealing with the subject of erythropoietin.[260]

The bone marrow is usually hyperplastic, with an increased red cell count, whereas the leukocyte and platelet counts are almost invariably normal. There is an increased formation of uric acid from the elevated nucleic acid turnover, and patients may develop gout. The direct effects of chronic hypoxia are the dominant clinical features, and cyanosis may be pronounced; clubbing of the fingers is very common. Treatment is usually directed to the primary condition, but in the presence of an excessively high hematocrit the same measures discussed under primary polycythemia may be used.

Pseudopolycythemia. This condition is found as a result of marked decrease in plasma volume. The most common cause is dehydration, which is readily corrected by administration of intravenous fluids. Another type of pseudopolycythemia is occasionally seen in adult men and has an obscure cause. Patients are usually asymptomatic, and their hematocrit may be moderately raised in peripheral blood, but the total red cell mass is normal, whereas the plasma volume is reduced. In essence, it is a disorder of plasma volume regulation, probably caused by poorly defined endocrinologic changes. Expansion of the plasma volume by infusion produces a transient fall of the hematocrit.[258]

DISORDERS OF HEMOSTASIS

Gradually, the mystery and complexity of hemostasis has been unraveled. Currently it is thought to be a phenomenon initiated by vascular injury, leading to a buildup of a mechanical plug composed of platelets, followed by activation of the coagulation mechanism. The generation of thrombin leads to the deposition of fibrin that strengthens the friable platelet plug. Eventually a series of reactions limits the distribution of thrombin only to the site of vascular injury, thus creating a firm mechanical barrier that prevents the escape of blood. However, all these events can occur only in constricted blood vessels, since the unhampered blood flow would easily disrupt the forming plug. This vasoconstriction is mediated by locally released hormonal factors.

The trend of events described above is an oversimplification of a much more complicated process that is exemplified in a diagrammatic fashion in Figure 8–6, indicating the rate and interaction of the initially required insult, the participation of collagen, platelets, and thrombin in the eventual clot formation.[265] However, it must be realized that this primary hemostatic mechanism is sufficient only to produce temporary cessation of bleeding; definite hemostasis requires the participation of the whole coagulation system to stabilize the hemostatic clot.

The crucial reaction in the coagulating mechanism is the conversion of prothrombin to thrombin, a proteolytic enzyme that cleaves fibrinogen to form fibrin. Two pathways lead to this event: a) the *intrinsic blood clotting system*, so called because all its participants circulate in blood, is activated by vascular injury and has as its first component Factor XII, which is enzymatically activated and in turn attacks Factor XI and simultaneously activates the fibrinolytic system. A chain of reactions culminates with the formation of thromboplastin, which eventually participates in the conversion of prothrombin to thrombin (Fig. 8–7). A similar end is achieved by b) the *extrinsic blood clotting system,* in which a circulating clotting factor (Factor VII) can directly cleave Factor X through a series of steps involving proteins released by endothelial cells and other tissues. Vitamin K is required for the formation of one of Factor VII's precursors.

A number of disorders affect hemostasis at different levels of the hemostatic phenomenon. In order to comply with the current concept of blood coagulation and for the sake of discussion, these entities will be considered in three categories.

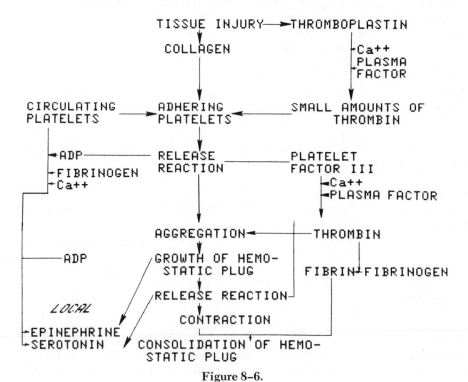

Figure 8–6.

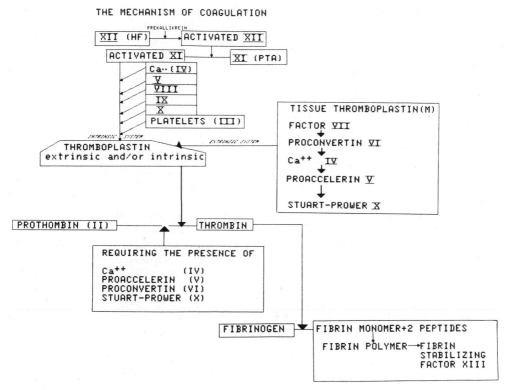

Figure 8–7.

Abnormalities of Platelet Function and/or Capillary Vessels

Thrombocytopenic Purpura

This disease is characterized by a decreased number of circulating thrombocytes, accompanied by spontaneous bleeding. It appears that adenosine diphosphate (ADP) released from injured tissues or from platelets is responsible for the aggregation of platelets at the site of injury.[265] Thromboplastin activity depends on the quantity as well as quality of available platelets, eventually influencing clot retraction by their interference with fibrin, and this in turn depends on the presence of ADP as an energy source (Fig. 8–6).[266]

Thus, when a significant decrease of platelets exists, at least one or two of the stages of blood coagulation are impeded.[265-268] In addition, the plasma factor contributing to the maintenance of vascular integrity is supplementary to the mechanical role of the platelets in clot formation.[266] When platelets are diminished, both factors would be affected.

Clinically, thrombocytopenic purpura develops over a period of weeks, becoming apparent by a noticeable increase of bruises after minor trauma, menorrhagia, or epistaxis; eventually petechiae appear as a result of tiny extravasations of blood from the arteriolar end of the capillary loop in the skin or mucosa. Bleeding through gastrointestinal and urinary tracts may also occur, progressing to a considerable amount of blood loss.[269]

Thrombocytopenia may reflect decreased marrow production, increased peripheral destruction, increased sequestration of platelets in the spleen, or dilution by transfusion of blood products depleted of viable platelets.[265]

The degree of thrombocytopenia is not necessarily related to the clinical manifestations, and anemia may or may not be present, depending on the amount of blood recently lost. Clot retraction is delayed and occasionally nonexistent after 24 hours. The tourniquet test is consistently positive. In bone marrow aspirates, the megakaryocytes are usually increased but immature, containing two or four separate nuclei with few granules in their cytoplasm. Two forms of thrombocytopenic purpura have been described (Table 8–4).

Idiopathic Thrombocytopenic Purpura. (ITP) This entity has no known cause, although hereditary and familial trends have been reported, occurring mostly in adolescents and young adults. An abnormal immunologic mechanism has been proposed but not yet proved; nevertheless, there are indications for the existence of platelet antibodies, and thus the spleen would remove the sensitized platelets[270] as well as produce platelet agglutinins, thus suppressing megakaryocyte function in the bone marrow.[271] The course of the disease may be permanent or unpredictably silent for years, with occasional sudden reappearances; but in most cases death results from recurrences even after many years of remission.

Acute ITP is primarily a disease of children; profound thrombocytopenia begins abruptly, two to three weeks after a viral infection. A circulating 7S gammaglobulin, specific for platelets, is present and may be transplacentally transmitted to the fetus if a pregnant woman develops ITP.[265]

High dosages of corticosteroids have been shown to be effective, probably because they decrease antigen-antibody reactions and protect the vascular endothelium.[272] The administration of platelet concentrates may be indicated shortly before or immediately after splenectomy, which is reserved only for those cases not controllable by steroids. Whole blood transfusions are used to replace blood lost in life-threatening hemorrhage. Therapeutic agents that modify platelet adhesiveness may be indicated.[273]

Secondary Thrombocytopenic Purpura. This disorder is related to a primary agent or disease and may be caused by invasion of the marrow with subsequent suppression or destruction, such as that seen in some malignancies, granulomatous diseases, and severe acute bacteremia or viremia.[274]

Direct suppression of marrow elements can also be caused by radiation or treatment with antimetabolite and alkylating agents. Some susceptible patients have developed secondary thrombocytopenic purpura after chronic ingestion of analgesics,[275] antipyretics,[39, 276] or antibiotics,[190, 191] after eating certain foods, or after exposure to insecticides and organic dyes.

Peripheral destruction of platelets can occur when excessive demands are made owing to abnormal coagulation, hypersplenism, hypothermia, heat stroke, hemangioendothelioma, incompatible blood transfusion, and some collagen disorders.[277] In most of these disorders, absence of the plasma factor required for normal platelet production has been described; however, specific mechanisms have been proposed for each of the previously listed causes. At any rate, the immunologic nature of the mech-

Table 8–4 *Laboratory Diagnostic Characteristics of Idiopathic Thrombocytopenic Purpura*

Laboratory Diagnostic Characteristics	Acute ITP	Chronic ITP
Peripheral blood		
Platelet count	5000–20,000/mm³	40,000–200,000/mm³
Platelet morphology	Normal platelets	Larger, bizarre platelets
Eosinophilia	Often	0
Lymphocytes	Often	0
Anemia	Normochromic with reticulocytosis	Normochromic with reticulocytosis*
Platelet agglutinins	Rare	In about 50% of cases
Bone marrow	Normoblastic + myeloid hyperplasia	Hyperplasia present*
Platelet survival time	1–6 hours	12–24 hours
Bleeding time	Prolonged	Prolonged
Coagulation time	Normal	Normal
Clot retraction	Poor to absent	Poor to absent
Tourniquet test	Positive	Positive
Prothrombin consumption test	Abnormal	Abnormal

*Present only if active bleeding is present.
Abstracted from Platt, W.R.: Color Atlas and Textbook of Hematology, J.B. Lippincott Co., 2nd ed., Philadelphia, 1979, p. 380.

anism of this form of thrombocytopenic purpura has been demonstrated, and the sensitivity has been passively transferred.[270]

Identification of the etiologic agent is the most important factor leading to treatment of the disease by its suppression. Agents used for treatment of idiopathic thrombocytopenic purpura have also been useful in these cases; specifically, transfusion of fresh platelet concentrates may be life-saving in arrest of severe hemorrhagic episodes.[278]

Neonatal Thrombocytopenic Purpura. This form of thrombocytopenic purpura may affect both mother and baby or either of them alone. The infant may appear normal at the time of delivery only to develop purpura several hours later. It is likely that Rh sensitization may be important, because maternal isoagglutinins may form, cross the placenta, and destroy the fetal platelets.[268] Other authors believe that a platelet depressing factor present in the mother's plasma can gain access to the fetal circulation, resulting in a decreased number of platelets.[268]

Steroid therapy is indicated, and a splenectomy may be of value when the former therapy fails.

Thrombotic Thrombocytopenic Purpura. Also called Moschcowitz's disease, thrombotic thrombocytopenic purpura occurs most commonly in females 10 to 40 years old and is accompanied by hemolytic anemia, neurologic degeneration, and renal disease.

This entity is related to the collagen diseases and is primarily the result of a vascular lesion mostly in arterioles and capillaries of practically any organ.[279] Most patients have a dramatically fulminating course, but a few have chronic or relapsing forms. Massive doses of steroids and splenectomy can prevent rapid deterioration.

Nonthrombocytopenic Purpuras

Having all the hemorrhagic features of other forms of purpura, these patients have platelet counts within normal limits.

Allergic purpura, also known as the Schönlein-Henoch syndrome, is characterized by intermittent bouts and marked variability of cutaneous lesions.[276] In addition, there is gastrointestinal involvement, with diarrhea, colicky pain, and vomiting. Nephritis, joint pain, and hemarthrosis may also be present.[280] Occasionally, the upper respiratory tract is also affected, and diffuse infiltration of blood into tissues occurs. When this lesion involves the submucosa of the glottis, it places the airway in jeopardy. Intubation of the trachea under these circumstances may be difficult, and tracheostomy is sometimes necessary.

Some cases of ITP are mediated by *immunological mechanisms*; that is, quinidine induces the formation of an antiquinidine antibody that may bind to platelet surfaces; complement is fixed and the platelet is injured, resulting in its prompt removal by the spleen.

Post-transfusion purpura is a rare cause of thrombocytopenia. In addition to the common tissue-specific (HLA) antigens, platelets have specific antigens, among which PI^{A1} is present in 98 per cent of the population. A PI^{A1} negative donor receiving PI^{A1} positive platelets may develop severe thrombocytopenia, since the developed antibodies form complexes that coat the recipient's PI^{A1} negative platelets, causing their destruction.

Increased capillary permeability allows the escape of blood cells into the surrounding tissue. This can be triggered by hypersensitivity to certain drugs or foods and occasionally coexists with streptococcal infection.[271] Treatment is largely supportive, with little improvement from steroid therapy.

Infectious purpura is a finding in advanced forms of infectious disorders such as Rocky Mountain spotted fever, typhus, meningitis, and bacterial endocarditis; occasionally it is also seen in chickenpox or smallpox. The mechanism of this type of purpura is related to vascular endothelial injury, but a pathognomonic histologic lesion has not been observed.

Treatment should be directed to the underlying disease, and steroids may be indicated except in those infections that are usually exacerbated by them.[281]

Anesthetic Considerations in Patients with Purpuras

Preoperative preparation is essential and may consist of transfusions of whole blood or its fractions. Platelet concentrate infusions may be required shortly before and during surgery in patients with thrombocytopenia. In most instances, steroid therapy may augment the number of platelets, correct the delayed bleeding time, and increase capillary resistance.[282]

Below 100,000 platelets per μl bleeding increases linearly with decreases in platelet count according to the following formula:

$$\text{Bleeding time (in min.)} = 30.5 - \frac{\text{Platelet count}/\mu l}{3850}$$

No specific premedicants are preferred, but those that can produce secondary thrombocytopenic purpura should be avoided. The anesthetic techniques preferred have generally been by inhalation and/or by intravenous agents. Local and regional nerve blocks have been considered with reservations, because of the probability of injuring vessels that may be in the vicinity. This contention is even more appropriate in the case of lumbar puncture to achieve spinal or peridural blocks. Spinal hematomas, although rare, may have disastrous consequences, and their likelihood is increased in these patients; therefore, use of lumbar puncture is discouraged.

The choice of anesthetic agents is secondary, and, as in many other problems, the way it is done is far more important than what is given. Jacoby, Hamelberg, and Jones[283] expressed concern over the mucosal lesions that laryngoscopy and endotracheal intubation may produce in patients with platelet counts lower than 50,000 per milliliter. However, Touvet and his coworkers[284] did not encounter this problem in their experience, so long as these procedures were performed atraumatically.

During sugery, special care must be devoted to the prevention of hypotension from anesthetic overdose and the acute onset of adrenal insufficiency.

In the postoperative period, mainly after splenectomy, left pleural effusion and bleeding from the splenic pedicle must be kept in mind as possible complications.[285] Hyperthermia may occur even if no apparent cause is diagnosed. Thromboembolic complications are not uncommon, and prophylactic measures should be taken. Frequent blood counts, including platelets, are desirable in order to abort episodes of hyperplaquetosis. Pulmonary emboli may also be seen in these cases, although they are usually secondary to a poorly managed condition.

Hereditary Hemorrhagic Telangiectasia

This disease is genetically transmitted by either sex and usually runs an asymptomatic course until the cutaneous lesions appear in the second or third decade; these are red or purple, and pinpoint in size; they blanch with pressure. Recurrent hemorrhages and telangiectasia may follow after slight trauma to skin or mucous membranes.

No abnormalities are observed in the coagulation studies. The striking laboratory findings are those of anemia. Mechanical methods have controlled some of the accessible lesions; but otherwise loss of blood may prove difficult or impossible to control in inaccessible areas.[286]

Allergic vasculitis or purpura is caused by immune mechanisms that produce vascular necrosis resulting in local bleeding into affected organs. Another type of vascular defect reflects an intrinsic abnormality of the connective tissue supporting blood vessels. Vascular fragility may be due to inherited disorders of connective tissues, or it may reflect the consequences of prolonged steroid therapy or of vitamin C deficiency (scurvy).

ABNORMALITIES OF BLOOD COAGULATION

Hemophilia

Hemophilia is a deficiency of Factor VIII, or antihemophilic factor (AHF), passed from one generation to the next as a sex-linked recessive trait. Ordinarily, the female is the carrier without suffering the disease, although there has been confirmation of deficient Factor VIII in some females who are offspring of a female carrier and a man with Factor VIII deficiency.[287, 288] The mating of a male and a female both deficient in Factor VIII has probably never occurred, except in laboratory animals, with all the offspring having the clinical entity (Fig. 8–8).[289]

Occurrence is one in 10,000 to 25,000 persons, the exact prevalence being difficult to estimate because of the wide variation in Factor VIII levels in the normal population.

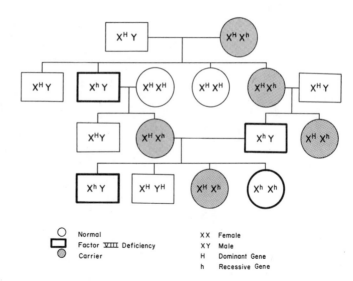

Figure 8–8. Schematic diagram of the inbred genetic possibilities in hemophilia (Factor VIII deficiency), with hypothetical combinations expressed in one family.

Hemophilia is one of the oldest recognized bleeding disorders. In the past, many affected children died in early infancy or childhood, but now, with the availability of transfusion therapy and specific plasma factors, mildly affected hemophiliacs may reach adult life before serious bleeding occurs. More severely affected individuals may have repeated episodes of bleeding from cutaneous surfaces, gastrointestinal, respiratory, and genitourinary tracts, and intra-articular cavities, the latter resulting in painful hemarthroses and permanent ankylosis.

Patek and Taylor[290] first proposed that the disorder was produced by the deficiency of a globulin. In the absence of this globulin, the first phase of coagulation is impeded. There is a direct relationship between the quantitative deficiency of AHF and the severity of bleeding. The level of Factor VIII in any one patient is remarkably constant throughout life, but levels below 3 per cent are usually found in symptomatic patients, although bleeding diatheses may occur in patients with levels as high as 20 per cent.[291]

Not all hemophiliacs are severe bleeders; spontaneous bleeding occurs in patients with less than 1 per cent of normal clotting activity. Those with levels between 3 and 5 per cent bleed spontaneously only rarely; while those having 10 to 15 per cent of their clotting activity may escape detection until exposed to surgical or dental procedures or to severe injury.[292]

Antihemophilic factor is needed in the development of blood thromboplastin activity; in its absence, the only effective hemostatic defense left to a patient is that supplied by the vascular phase of hemostasis and the extrinsic system. For an injury to larger vessels, the defenses are not sufficient to achieve hemostasis, and extensive and profuse bleeding ensues.

Previously, the diagnosis of hemophilia was made only when it could be demonstrated in vitro that plasma from the patient in question failed to clot that of a patient with known "hemophilia." This concept has been shown to be incorrect, because there are a variety of coagulation disorders that can mimic the clinical picture of hemophilia. The platelet count, tourniquet test, and bleeding time are normal, because they depend on capillary integrity. Clot retraction is likewise normal, because fibrin and platelet functions are adequate.[293] As the determination of prothrombin time does not depend on the factor deficient in hemophilia, this test is also normal (Table 8–5).

The coagulation time is usually prolonged owing to a decrease in the generation of thromboplastin activity, although it may also be normal even in severe depression of AHF. The thromboplastin generation test can be used to identify the specific defect in these cases, and, by simple modifications, the same measurement would provide the determination of the percentage of Factor VIII activity present in the suspect plasma. Recently the partial thromboplastin time has also been used for this purpose.[293]

Table 8-5   *Laboratory Characteristics of Clotting Factor Deficiencies*

Deficiency	Tourniquet Test	Clotting Time	Clot Retraction	Platelet Count	Bleeding Time	Prothrombin Consumption	Prothrombin Time	Partial Thromboplastin Time	Thromboplastin Generation Test
Fibrinogen (I)	—	Prolonged	Normal	Normal	Normal	—	Abnormal	—	—
Prothrombin II	—	Normal	Abnormal	Normal	Normal	—	Abnormal	Abnormal	—
Thrombocytopenia	+	Normal	Abnormal	Decreased	Normal	Abnormal	Normal	Normal	Abnormal corrected by normal platelets
Factor (V)	—	Normal	Normal	Normal	—	Abnormal	Abnormal	Normal	—
Factor (VII)	—	Normal	Normal	Normal	Normal	Normal	Abnormal	Abnormal	—
AHG (VIII) mild	—	Normal	Normal	Normal	Normal	Abnormal	Normal	Abnormal	Abnormal corrected by plasma
AHG (VIII) severe	—	Prolonged	Normal	Normal	Normal	Abnormal	Normal	Abnormal	Abnormal corrected by plasma
Plasma thromboplastin component (IX)	—	Prolonged	Normal	Normal	Normal	Abnormal	Normal	Abnormal	Abnormal corrected by serum
Stuart-Power (X)	—	Normal	Normal	Normal	Prolonged	Abnormal	Abnormal	Abnormal	Abnormal corrected by serum
Plasma thromboplastin antecedent (XI)	—	Normal	Normal	Normal	Normal	Normal	Normal	Abnormal	Abnormal corrected by plasma and serum
Hageman's trait (XII)	—	Prolonged	Normal	Normal	Normal	Normal	Normal	Abnormal	Abnormal corrected by plasma and serum
Pseudohemophilia A (von Willebrand's disease)	±	Normal	Normal	Normal	Normal or prolonged	Normal	Normal	Normal	Normal
Pseudohemophilia B	Rarely	Normal or prolonged	Normal	Normal	Prolonged	Abnormal	Normal	Abnormal	Abnormal corrected by plasma
Normal:	<5 petechiae	5–10 min	Complete in 24 hrs	150,000 to 400,000	3 min or less	>15 sec	12 sec	40–80 sec	7–12 sec

Lately, the immunological detection of Factor VIII aberrations and quantitative measurements have aided in the differential diagnosis of hemophilia and von Willebrand's disease[294] and in the identification of hemophilia carriers as well as the prenatal diagnosis of the disease.[295] The use of specific antibodies has facilitated the application of radioimmunoassay and bio-assay techniques for this purpose.

For centuries all surgery was denied to these patients, and a procedure as simple as a dental extraction represented a major threat to life. Until recently, conditions that made surgery imperative were catastrophic. Now, however, it is possible to prepare for such emergencies with a reasonable possibility of success, and even semi-elective operations have been undertaken prophylactically, thus preventing later operations under more disadvantageous conditions.

Modern blood banking methods have made available large quantities of blood and plasma for use in the treatment of severe hemorrhage. But perhaps the most promising treatment is the highly potent biological preparations, human and from other sources, of Factor VIII. Moreover, concentrates of human AHF (35 per cent), although quite costly, allow the maintenance of more acceptable Factor VIII levels — the final goal of this therapy being to increase Factor VIII activity to a hemostatic level.[296]

Factor VIII Preparations and Concentrates. Ever since the differentiation of blood groups and the introduction of transfusions, this therapeutic tool has been used to treat bleeding hemophiliacs. In the 1940's, the administration of fresh-frozen plasma (FFP) became the accepted therapy for control of hemorrhage in these patients.

What level of AHF activity must be attained to abort a hemorrhage in a hemophiliac? This is a difficult question to answer, but usually it depends upon the clinical nature of the bleeding episode encountered. For the common hemarthroses and intramuscular hematomas, a plasma activity of 10 to 25 per cent is frequently enough to control them. This level produces a partial thromboplastin time of 110 seconds. When severe traumatic injury occurs or when surgical procedures are performed, considerably higher levels are essential, and concentrations ranging from 35 to 50 per cent are necessary to assure hemostasis.[293]

The amount of Factor VIII contained in the infused material and its volume influence the effectiveness of replacement therapy; finally the blood space in which exogenous AHF is diluted will also affect its concentration, being in man twice that of the circulating plasma. Children have an approximate plasma volume of 45 ml per kilogram of weight; the half-life of Factor VIII being 10 to 15 hours, the following formula has been suggested: $N = 0.45 \times$ patient's weight in kilograms $\times$ required therapeutic activity, where N is the number of units of Factor VIII required. The different therapeutic preparations, volumes required, and results in improvement of Factor VIII activity in the recipient are depicted in Table 8–6.

Lyophilized plasma is available with an activity comparable to that of normal plasma. When fresh plasma prepared from ACD blood is quickly frozen, most of the Factor VIII is preserved; when administered at a rate of 15 ml per kg every 12 hours, the patient's Factor VIII level rises to 10 to 20 per cent.[291] Larger volumes may result in circulatory overload.

Cohn's fraction I consists of a considerable proportion of fibrinogen which also contains Factor VIII. When reconstituted in 200 ml of water, a unit of fraction I is equivalent to 200 ml of fresh plasma, and its infusing results in hyperfibrinogenemia, high sedimentation rate, and, occasionally, hemolysis.[297] Using this preparation, there

Table 8–6 *Available Biological Preparations Containing Factor VIII*

Preparation	Volume (ml)	Factor VIII Units	Total Protein (gm)	Initial Dose (ml/kg)	Factor VIII Activity
Normal plasma	200	200	14	15	30%
Fresh frozen plasma	200	140	14	15	20%
Fraction I	200	200	2.0	23	50%
Glycin precipitate	30	300	1.2	2.25	50%
Cryoprecipitate	13	100	0.42	3.0	50%

is a possibility of contamination with homologous serum hepatitis virus, because it is made from pooled plasma from many donors; moreover, its extremely high cost makes it impractical. Highly concentrated fractions have also been prepared, providing four times the activity of regular fibrinogen.[298]

Rich antihemophilic factor precipitates may result from the addition of aliphatic amino acids such as glycine to plasma concentrate. When reconstituted to a volume of 30 ml, it is equivalent to 300 ml of fresh plasma. A danger of serum hepatitis, similar to that seen with fibrinogen, is possible.[299]

Cryoprecipitate fractions, obtained from fresh frozen plasma and allowed to thaw slowly, may yield 50 per cent of the original Factor VIII. It is dissolved in 10 ml of citrated saline, making a total volume of 13 ml containing approximately 7.7 ml of Factor VIII activity per milliliter of suspension. It is relatively easy to prepare and is feasible for all large, active blood banks, at an acceptable cost.[300]

Extremely highly concentrated Factor VIII preparations have been made from porcine and bovine plasma by British investigators.[301] AHF concentrations of 1000 times or more than human plasma have been reported, although their administration to patients has resulted in immunologic responses such as allergy, thrombocytopenia, and fever. Moreover, the remote but actual possibility of transmission of hoof and mouth disease has made their use very limited. Nevertheless, this type of preparation may be the only life-saving resource in some instances of severe hemorrhage for which other preparations have failed.

Factor VIII concentrates have been evaluated in the treatment of minor bleeding episodes on an outpatient basis. Of these preparations, the Courtland concentrate appears to have a shorter in vivo recovery time and a longer half-life than others.

Several precautions must be observed in the use of these concentrates; first, a diagnosis of hemophilia must be confirmed and other similar disorders ruled out. Repeated estimations of Factor VIII assay must be performed in order to monitor the effect of the therapy instituted.

A significant decrease in bleeding episodes has been observed when AHF concentrate was given prophylactically in a fixed schedule to adults with severe hemophilia. As reported by Kasper and collaborators,[302] when 500 Factor VIII units were given daily to known hemophiliacs, bleeding episodes occurred about one fourth as often as during baseline control periods.

Prophylactic infusion therapy has been advocated to promote hemorrhage control[303] in patients contemplating surgery, or with persistent single joint hemarthrosis or recurrent head trauma, or in need of physical therapy and rehabilitation. These programs usually consist of either cryoprecipitate (1 bag = 125 U) or commercial concentrate (250–1250 U/vial).[304]

In spite of the aforementioned advances, nonimperative surgical procedures are to be avoided in these patients. Whenever operation must be performed, the proper preparation of these patients is mandatory. A near normal Factor VIII plasma level can be attained by administration of some of the fractions already listed. By repeated monitoring of AHF plasma concentration, the ideal time to sustain the operative procedure is determined, and the operation is given preference over other cases. A concentration of at least 35 per cent of Factor VIII must be obtained.[293, 301]

A recently published report including anesthetic procedures for 21 male hemophiliacs having multiple operative procedures revealed that most were between 20 and 40 years of age.[305] The majority of the operations were orthopedic and required correction of Factor VIII deficiency within two hours prior to surgery. In the postoperative period, the patients received factor concentrate every eight hours for the subsequent three to five days, then every 12 hours until discharge from the hospital. General anesthesia was given by mask in 29 instances, and endotracheal intubation was performed in 11 cases without apparent complications due to the anesthetic procedure itself. Two patients received brachial plexus blocks through the axillary approach without undue sequelae. No excessive bleeding was noted intraoperatively, but there were five instances of postoperative bleeding at the incision site.

Expertise and team effort are absolutely necessary in these cases. A definite plan must be adhered to by hematologist, anesthesiologist, and surgeon. Large intravenous indwelling catheters must be secured, and unnecessary aggravation to the skin must be avoided. Management of airway patency must be done atraumatically because lesions to the oral or pharyngeal mucosa can result in massive submucosal hematoma and hemorrhage. If the airway is compromised, an endotracheal tube is inserted and tracheostomy avoided if possible, as it increases the danger to the patient. Drainage of hematoma in these areas is usually impractical and impossible because it does not localize, but diffuses through the fascial planes. Superficial hemorrhage can be controlled by application of continuous pressure while the infusion of fresh plasma or concentrates is started. After elevation of AHF is obtained, pressure should be released to allow blood with adequate Factor VIII to replace the AHF-deficient blood in the blocked vessels and then reapplied.

Similar precautions must be carried out for dental extractions; ideally prophylaxis by dental hygiene is carried out in these patients. The use of dental splints of acrylic resin to protect the gums has been proposed, in order to prevent the dislodgment of a clot once it has formed, thus avoiding the use of sutures.[306] Also the administration of high doses of steroids has been reported to reduce bleeding after dental extractions in hemophiliac patients.[307]

In an interestingly designed clinical study, Sinclair found that the blood loss after tooth extraction in adequately treated hemophiliac patients was significantly less than in normal patients treated conventionally.[308] This observation points out once more the need for excellent control of the bleeding disorder before undertaking even minor surgical procedures. Strangely enough, hemorrhage-free dental extractions have been reported with hypnosis, without the use of blood or plasma, using protective splints and carefully packing the socket.[309]

Utilizing a combination of ischemic tourniquet and cooling, surgical procedures have also been performed on the extremities of hemophiliac patients.[310] At any rate, it appears that proper preparation by AHF concentrates is of the utmost importance.[311]

Finally, the treatment of pain in patients afflicted with this disease deserves special mention. The residual effects of hemarthroses and hemorrhages into soft tissue produce pain of various intensity. Amino-

salicylic acid and other salicylate preparations, in addition to their untoward effects on the gastric mucosa and the renal tubules, also impair platelet function, as discussed elsewhere in this chapter. These lesions may produce severe gastrointestinal or renal hemorrhages that may be fatal to patients with hemophilia.[312, 313] For joint pain, immobilization and muscle relaxant drugs can be used, followed by restoration of function by gradual mobilization and physiotherapy.[314]

Teractan, phenoperidine, diazepam, and dextromoramide in combination with local cold application may relieve pain without the adverse effects of salicylates.[315]

Christmas Disease

Also called hemophilia B and plasma thromboplastin component or Factor IX deficiency, Christmas disease has in the past been confused with hemophilia, and not without reason. It is clinically indistinguishable from hemophilia, and, although it is transmitted as a sex-linked recessive character, symptoms can also appear in female heterozygotes.[316]

It occurs in 1 in 100,000 persons; the offspring of a Factor IX-deficient male and a normal female would be two normal sons and two carrier daughters. The offspring of a carrier female and a normal male would be a normal son, one Factor IX-deficient son, one carrier daughter, and one normal daughter. Therefore, all daughters of affected males are carriers, but only half of the sons are affected.

Since Factor IX takes part in the first phase of coagulation, its deficiency impedes the development of thromboplastin activity (see Table 8–5).[317] Manifestations of hemorrhagic diathesis may appear at birth and throughout life; minor trauma may produce tremendous hemorrhages. As in hemophilia, the coagulation time is often prolonged, but it also may be normal. Definite identification is made by the thromboplastin generation test.[318]

Synthesis of Factor IX occurs mostly in the liver and is influenced by vitamin K. Although it is less frequent than true hemophilia, it is probably the second most common inherent coagulation defect. Hemophilia B Layden,[319] an intriguing variant of Christmas disease, is a familial disease in which family members have very low Factor IX during childhood that rises to between 20 and 60 per cent in older members; symptoms ameliorate after puberty.

Carriers of this disease may have a reduced level of coagulation-active factor IX and they may be identified by performing a prothrombin time with bovine thromboplastin. There is no immunoassay method for detection of carriers.

Treatment is perhaps more difficult than in Factor VIII deficiency. The introduction of a concentrate containing plasma Factors II, VII, IX, and X, which has allowed elective surgical procedures in patients with hemophilia B, has given rise to enthusiasm.[320-323]

Stuart Factor (Factor X) Deficiency

This disease is transmitted by an incompletely recessive autosomal gene; it is most severe in the homozygote but is still manifested in the heterozygote and carriers.[324] Interestingly enough, temporary Stuart factor deficiency has been reported after exposure to an insecticide. In addition to the previously mentioned aberrant coagulation test results, the one-stage prothrombin time is prolonged, because Factor X is essential for optimal development of thromboplastin activity (see Table 8–5).[325]

Transfusion of whole blood is generally effective in relieving symptoms; since Factor X is stable, fresh material is not necessary. Small amounts of normal serum may also correct this disorder and stop bleeding episodes.

Congenital Fibrinogen Deficiency

In this congenitally transmitted, sex-linked recessive disease seen in siblings of consanguineous marriages, absence of fibrinogen prevents the coagulation process from completing its final phase; that is, the conversion of fibrinogen to the fibrin clot is impeded. The main defect is a decrease in synthesis of fibrinogen, rather than an increase in its destruction.[326] Bleeding may occur at birth, resembling Factor VII deficiency but less severe. Minor trauma usually generates severe hemorrhages, but crippling hemarthroses do not occur in this disease.[327]

The blood clotting time, one-stage prothrombin time, and thrombin time are usually abnormal. Quantitative determination of fibrinogen reveals only minute amounts or total absence.[328, 329]

The administration of fibrinogen corrects the deficiency, although half of it is lost within 48 hours. Owing to distribution and equilibration of circulating plasma proteins with those contained in the interstitial space, the first dose of administered fibrinogen will have less effect than will subsequent comparable doses.[330]

Dysfibrinogenemia is characterized by the production of abnormal fibrinogen molecules that react slowly with thrombin or that polymerize slowly after fibrinopeptides have been released. There is prolongation of the thrombin time as well as the PTT and PT.

Fibrinogen Deficiency

Fibrinogen, or Factor I, arises from the liver or reticuloendothelial system, being a globulin with a molecular weight of 450,000, and is associated with an elevated sedimentation rate in which α and β globulin are altered and albumin is depressed. Fibrinogen is decreased below 100 mg/100 ml when large amounts of thromboplastin appear in the blood stream. Congenital deficiency is a non-sex-linked recessive trait frequently associated with consanguineous intermarriage. In one type of abnormality, the plasma level of fibrinogen is very low, reflecting insufficient production. Dysfibrinogenemia is characterized by the production of abnormal fibrinogen molecules that react slowly with thrombin. There is prolongation of the thrombin time as well as PTT and PT.

Acquired fibrinogen deficiency is by far more common in operating and delivery rooms than is the congenital form. Decidual and placental extracts are both rich sources of thromboplastin activity, and widespread intravascular clotting may follow. The details of its pathophysiology and treatment are discussed elsewhere.

Factor VII Deficiency

This is an inherited disease; the gene appears to be an autosomal recessive.[331] Patients can have a normal clotting time and thromboplastin generation test. Since Fac-

Table 8–7 *Characteristics of Clotting Factors*

Factor	I	II*	V*	VII	VIII	IX	X	XI	XII	XIII
Name	Fibrinogen	Prothrombin	Proaccelerin	Proconvertin	Antihemophilic Factor	Christmas Factor	Stuart Factor	PTA	Hageman Factor	Fibrin Stabilizing Factor
Normal Range	150–350 mg%	70–130 mg%	70–130 mg%	70–150 mg%	50–200 mg%	70–130 mg%	70–130 mg%	70–130 mg%	40–150%	50–200%
Requirements for Surgical Hemostasis	70 mg%	20 mg%	5 mg%	20 mg%	30 mg%	20 mg%	10 mg%	20 mg%	None	1%
Half-life of Transfused Factor	4 days	2–5 days	12 hours	300 min.	17 hours	40 hours	40 hours	60 hours	-----	12 days
Stability on Storage at 4°C for 21 Days	φ	φ	7 days	φ	7 days	φ	φ	7 days	φ	φ
Stability at −30°C for 1 Year	φ	φ	φ	φ	φ	φ	φ	φ	φ	φ
Concentrates Available	Cohn Fraction I	Commercial multi-factor	None	Commercial multi-factor**	Cryoprecipitate comm. multi-factor**	Commercial multi-factor**	Commercial multi-factor**	None	None	None
Genetic Pattern in Congenital Deficiencies	Autosomal recessive	Autosomal recessive	Autosomal recessive	Autosomal recessive	Males affected, females are carriers	Males affected, females are carriers	Autosomal recessive	Autosomal recessive	Autosomal recessive	Autosomal recessive, some sex linked

*Factor III is thromboplastin, Factor IV is calcium, Factor VI is now known as activated Factor V.
φ = No change.
**Contains Factors II, VII, IX, X.

tor VII is thought to be formed in the liver and is vitamin K dependent, it may be decreased in severe liver disease and is the earliest factor reduced during coumadin therapy.

These patients may show abnormal bleeding from childhood; the tourniquet test and platelets are normal, but the one-stage prothrombin time is prolonged.[332]

Administration of fresh blood or plasma to patients with congenital defect of Factor VII temporarily improves the condition and may help stop bouts of bleeding.[333] Plasma or plasma concentrate infusions have been noted to stop uncontrollable bleeding in Factor VII deficient patients undergoing surgical procedures. Factor VII deficit has also been noted after hepatectomy in the dog.[334] Because the half-life of Factor VII is about 12 hours, blood or plasma transfusions must be given daily for its deficiency. When this defect is produced by liver disease or anticoagulant therapy, parenteral administration of vitamin K reverses the condition in four to six hours (Table 8–7).

Factor XIII (Fibrin Stabilizing Factor) Deficiency

Also called Laki-Lorand factor, this is a plasma globulin activated by thrombin that participates in clot formation, cementing together fibrin filaments. The acquired deficiency may be associated with liver disease or fibrinolysis.[335]

The disorder may also appear at birth or may not become noticeable until childhood.[336] It occurs in either sex and is related to consanguinity. Usually, the defect is corrected by administration of small volumes of whole blood.[337]

Differentiation from hemophilia is important. Laboratory tests are all normal except the polymerization and formation of stable fibrin.

DISORDERS AFFECTING VESSEL AND/OR PLATELET FUNCTION AND BLOOD COAGULATION

Von Willebrand's Disease

This hemorrhagic familial disease is transmitted as an autosomal dominant with varying degrees of expressivity, producing prolonged bleeding concomitant with a decrease of Factor VIII (AHF). Abnormal platelet function, a capillary abnormality, and deficiency of specific plasma factor have been incriminated.[338] The concentration of antihemophilic protein is diminished; therefore, the coagulant and platelet adherence promoting activities are suppressed. This latter deficiency may be corrected by administration of fraction 1-0 of normal plasma, thus bringing the bleeding time within normal limits.[339, 340]

This disorder is usually apparent in the first few weeks and persists throughout life; there is an unpredictable variability of bleeding, but rarely do these patients succumb from an episode of bleeding.[341] Similarly, there is little consistency in the laboratory findings from patient to patient, or even in the same patient from one examination to the next. The platelets are quantitatively normal, but with a marked decrease of platelet adhesiveness, resulting in a prolonged bleeding time.[342] The coagulation time is also delayed, and the thromboplastin generation test is normal.[343]

Variants of Factor VIII globulin between hemophilias and von Willebrand disease patients are readily detected by immunological techniques as well as by the ristocetin-induced platelet aggregation method.[295]

Fresh whole blood, fresh plasma, and fresh frozen plasma have been effective in the control of bleeding.[340] Any surgical procedure is hazardous and should be avoided whenever possible. If surgery is unavoidable under emergency circumstances, the patient should be prepared by the infusion of fresh plasma, repeated every second day until healing is completed.[344, 345]

A definite warning for the avoidance of aspirin or any other salicylate therapy in patients with this type of bleeding disorder has been advocated by Quick,[346, 347] who demonstrated prolongation of bleeding time after aspirin ingestion. Perkins[348] believes that the cryoprecipitate[153] used in the treatment of hemophilia as described by Pool and Shannon[300] also contains an antibleeding factor that is responsible for the defect observed in von Willebrand's disease. A definite challenge to anesthesiologists is the anesthetic management of one of these patients when bleeding comes from an intrapulmonary site. Bowes[349] reported a case with hemoptysis and hemothorax that required thoracotomy and was prepared by cryoprecipitate, fresh blood, and plasma.

Thrombasthenia

Thrombasthenia is a hereditary autosomal recessive disorder. Also termed Glanzmann's disease, it is characterized by prolonged bleeding time, poor clot retraction, and failure of platelets to aggregate in the presence of ADP,[349] or any other aggregating agent.

At least two main biochemical disorders have been implicated in the production of this disease. First, deficiency of glyceraldehyde-3-phosphate dehydrogenase and pyruvate kinase observed in some patients resulted in a 50 per cent reduction of platelet ATP, thus affecting the contractile protein of the platelet and in turn its function.[350]

Second, in other patients with normal platelet glycolytic cycles and ATP levels, the nonutilization of platelet ATP is probably due to reduced Mg^{++} and ATPase levels. Platelets appear unable to release phospholipid, and thus perhaps the structural abnormality is located in the platelet membrane.[351]

Thrombopathia

Thrombopathia is a deficiency of platelet Factor III, resulting in failure to produce normal thromboplastin activity, manifested by an abnormal thromboplastin generation test.[352] In the presence of calcium ions, thromboplastin brings about the conversion of prothrombin to thrombin; however, it requires activation by accessory Factors V, VII, and X for optimal function. All other tests of hemostasis are normal, but patients may have moderate symptoms of abnormal bleeding, sometimes unexpectedly found in the operating field.

Deficiencies of blood thromboplastin are associated with classic hemophilia and hemophilia A, Christmas disease, vitamin K deficiencies and liver disease, thrombocytopenias, thrombasthenia, and the postpartum period.

Thrombocytosis

An increase in the number of circulating platelets, over 1,000,000 per μl can be either reactive or autonomous. In *reactive thrombocytosis* there is also an elevated number of megakaryocytes with a smaller size and ploidy occurring in chronic infection, non-hematological malignancies, and mild iron deficiency anemia. What stimulates the increased formation of platelets is unknown. Rarely is there bleeding or thrombotic episodes; therefore, therapy is not required.

Autonomous thrombocytosis is a primary marrow disorder in which megakaryocytes are enlarged with increased cytoplasmic mass and ploidy. The platelets do not aggregate in response to epinephrine and ADP. Bleeding and thrombotic episodes are frequent and subside when the number of platelets is reduced by the administration of alkylating agents. This disorder may accompany polycythemia vera.

Disseminated Intravascular Coagulation

This complex coagulation disorder has received great attention and has been the subject of many investigations during the last decade. Although thrombosis and hemorrhage have been considered to be diametrically opposed conditions in the scale of blood clotting, both are present in this syndrome characterized by bleeding resulting from increased intravascular blood coagulation.

In reality, this syndrome appears in a group of hemorrhagic diatheses of acute onset, with a clinical picture dominated by circulatory collapse.[353] Although these diatheses have been coded into several terminologies, the most appropriate, to our present knowledge, is that of "consumption coagulopathies" because the hemorrhagic tendency appears to be closely related to an acute activation of the clotting mechanism, resulting in intravascular use of plasma clotting factors. This phenomenon, probably triggered by the action of intravascular thrombin, results in the following changes: decreased fibrinogen levels, thrombocytopenia and low levels of prothrombin, Factor V (ACG), and Factor VIII (AHG).[353, 354]

For the sake of grouping, four classes of disseminated intravascular coagulation have been considered.

1. Generalized Shwartzman reaction, occurring after a previous sensitization, can be accompanied by massive intravascular pre-

cipitation of fibrin. Within a few hours, the level of prothrombin falls to about 20 per cent and that of ACG to 50 per cent. In addition, the platelets are reduced not only in quantity but also in quality,[355] because the remaining circulating thrombocytes show impaired procoagulation.

This entity has been noted in severe infections produced by *Escherichia coli, Pseudomonas aeruginosa,*[356] *Proteus vulgaris, Neisseria meningitidis, Aerobacter aerogenes,* and *Serratia marcescens.*[357] These infectious processes may occur more frequently in obstetric (infected abortions) and genitourinary surgery (from manipulations). Similar clinical pictures have been reported from hyperacute rejection of renal homografts,[358] in purpura fulminans and necrotica, the Waterhouse-Friderichsen syndrome, and thrombotic thrombocytopenic purpura,[359] and after advanced infectious mononucleosis complicated by hepatic cirrhosis.[360] During septicemia, extensive fibrin deposition has been noted, probably by activation of the Hageman factor (XII) and release of platelet Factor III by the corresponding endotoxin.[357, 361]

These reactions can be blocked by anticoagulants,[355, 362, 363] and by the opportune exogenous activation of fibrinolysis the lesion can be reversed in some instances.[353]

2. Other groups of diseases encompass those in which the activation of the clotting system is triggered by autoinfusion of tissue procoagulants. The severity of the clinical picture depends on the amount of the material entering the circulation and its intrinsic activity, because each tissue has different thromboplastin activity.

In abruptio placentae,[364] eclampsia and toxemia of pregnancy,[365] the hemorrhagic accidents have great similarities. Fibrinogen and platelets play important roles in the clotting episode, which is usually triggered by tissue thromboplastin. Almost simultaneously, enhanced fibrinolysis complicates the picture as a secondary phenomenon. It is of interest that renal lesions are common to these three conditions.

Definite evidence of the thromboplastic activity of amniotic fluid has been provided by Reid et al.[366] Fortunately this is low in comparison with that produced by placental extracts, and the clinical picture may be dominated by acute cor pulmonale caused by fetal debris lodging in the pulmonary circulation. Similar thromboplastic properties have been shown in some snake venoms, but a marked "defibrinogenation" is typical of these cases.[367] Also, slow release of procoagulants into the blood stream has been seen in patients with neoplasms of lung,[368] prostate, and pancreas. Here, although thrombolytic and fibrinolytic disorders are present, intravascular clotting appears to be the dominant feature.[369]

In the hemolytic-uremic syndrome, the erythrocytes appear to possess thromboplastic properties, and hemolysis results in intravascular activation of the clotting system;[370] this is followed by jaundice, hemorrhagic diathesis, and renal failure. A closely related mechanism has been proposed in Marchiafava-Micheli anemia.

3. Experimental and clinical observations have demonstrated that during fat embolization, procoagulant action is seen, mostly manifested by localized petechial hemorrhages in various organs.[361] It appears that by activating Factor XII (Hageman factor) or Factor XI (PTA), fatty acids released into the circulation initiate a series of events leading to intravascular clotting.[371] The liberation of fibrin degradation products mediates this event.

4. The Kasabach-Merritt syndrome is characterized by marked thrombocytopenia and hypofibrinogenemia, occurring in infants with large hemangiomas.[359, 372] It has been suggested that platelets are "consumed" in the stagnated blood contained in the hemangioma, resulting in constant activation of the clotting system. Radiotherapy has been reported to be successful; it is much preferred to surgical excision, which in these cases may present the threat of triggering disseminated intravascular coagulation.

Coagulopathy with resultant oozing has been noted in massive injuries.[373] DIC has been thought to be a contributing factor, since there is consumption of coagulation factors and decrease in fibrinogen and platelets. Fibrinolysis may or may not be present, and this factor alone should not be considered pathognomonic. The consumption of coagulating factors appears acutely and shortly after injury and is not an ongoing process.[373, 374] In addition, qualitative and quantitative platelet deficiencies may coexist.

During hypovolemic shock, thrombin and fibrin thrombi are deposited in the microcirculation, thus activating the fibrinolytic system, lysing the excessive fibrin. This process has been called *primary fibrinolysis* in contrast to secondary fibrinolysis, which has been reported to occur during multiple blood transfusion. In this latter case, an excessive amount of plasmin or other fibrinolytic activator is released, which lyses clots and fibrin.

When thrombocytopenia, hypofibrinogenemia, and clot lysis occur within two hours, DIC is likely. Even when hypofibrinogenemia is present without lysis of the clot, DIC may be suspected.[375]

Many investigators have reported altered hemostasis following multiple trauma. In a recent study, Attar and his collaborators[376] showed that an oscillatory pattern of alternating phases of hyper- and hypocoagulability occurred after severe trauma. Specifically, patients with cerebral injuries exhibited more persistent increased coagulation, probably because of hypothalamic lesions. Fibrinolytic activity was increased in practically every major injury, and the vasoactive polypeptide bradykinin apparently contributed to the production of shock in these patients.[377]

The euglobulin lysis time has also been noted to be decreased during hemorrhagic shock.[334] Clot retraction may be measured semiquantitatively as percentage according to the formula:

$$\frac{\text{Volume of expressed serum} \times 100}{\text{Volume of whole blood}}$$

or quantitatively as the percentage of expressed serum in the total preformed serum:

$$\frac{\text{ml serum} \times 50}{100 - \text{hematocrit}}$$

Therapy. As paradoxical as it may seem, the adequate and timely administration of anticoagulants has appeared successful in the treatment of some of these hemorrhagic conditions.

Heparin is indicated in the initial phase when intravascular coagulation is taking place, in order to stop the consumption of clotting factors and the intravascular deposition of fibrin.[355, 358, 378, 379] Obviously, if fibrinogen is given during this phase of hypercoagulability, the outcome may be fatal. The amount of heparin required is relatively small, and it is perhaps better to titrate the selected dose. To start, 50 units per kg of heparin is given intravenously. Platelet count and fibrinogen level should be determined again in two to three hours and be the guidelines for subsequent doses. Heparin has been noted to neutralize the inhibitory effect of a prostaglandin (PGI_2) on platelet aggregation without losing its anticoagulant action.[382] With excessive dosages of heparin, hemorrhage increases. On the other hand, if fibrinogen is given, greater depositions of fibrin will occur; but both will take place if nothing is done.

In the late phase, there is still deposition of fibrin, but the clotting system is in the process of recuperation because of the enormous potential turnover of clotting factors. At this point, use of heparin is contraindicated, and fibrinogen can be hazardous because there is prompt replacement from endogenous sources.[364, 381] It is then that the enhancement of fibrinolysis seems appropriate.[379, 384, 385] Successful treatment with epsilon-aminocaproic acid has been reported when it is used alone in a late phase of disseminated intravascular coagulation or after heparin.[384, 386] This is specifically the case when fibrinolysis has been activated endogenously, as in autoinfusion of tissue activators, such as in multiple trauma.[376]

Heparin has also been useful in the treatment of disseminated intravascular coagulation occurring in toxemia,[378] the Shwartzman reaction,[355, 358, 362] purpura fulminans, and the Moschcowitz syndrome.[385] The ideal condition for use of heparin is in the Kasabach-Merritt syndrome.[359, 372]

Under anesthesia, this disorder of coagulation may be encountered in obstetrics, extensive lung and prostatic resections, cardiopulmonary bypass, major vascular surgery, resuscitation of polytraumatized patients, intracranial operations, transplantation, and many other instances when large volumes of blood are lost and replaced (Table 8–8). The favorable or antagonistic effect that anesthetic drugs may have in disseminated intravascular coagulation has been insinuated,[386, 387] but thus far there is little objective evidence for withholding or using a specific drug or technique on this basis. Perhaps a drug hypersensitivity reac-

Table 8-8 *The Three Tube Simple Diagnostic Test Can Be Performed and Interpreted in the Operating Room*

Tube	Changes in Tube	Possible Diagnosis
#1 (oxalate)	Free hemoglobin ⟶ Hemolytic (red serum) Decreased platelets ↘ Incompatible ↗ cross match ↘ Thrombocytopenia Transfusional hemorrhagic diathesis	
#2 (Clotting Tube)	Poor clot retraction ↗ Prolonged ⟶ Circulating anticoagulants clotting time ⟶ Thromboplastin deficiency ⟶ Hypoprothrombinemia ⟶ Fibrinolysin ↗ Clot lysis ↗	
#3 (Topical Thrombin)	Poor clot with ⟶ Hypofibrinogenemia thrombin	

The three tube test can be performed placing 15 ml. of blood in tubes containing oxalate in #1; nothing in #2, which should be allowed to precipitate; and #3 containing topical thrombin.

tion, such as that proposed by Baudo et al.,[388] may be considered in these cases.

To reduce the frequency of intraoperative DIC, efforts to diagnose the specific coagulant deficit should be made in order to indicate appropriate replacement therapy.

TRANSFUSION REACTIONS

The dangers of transfusion reactions can never be overstressed; despite the modern methods of blood unit coding, cross matching, and blood bank organization, the possibility of untoward reactions occurring from blood transfusions is a fact of life in busy operating rooms where major surgery is undertaken frequently.

Although accurate available data are lacking, it is apparent that these reactions are distressingly common phenomena. Moreover, constant alertness for them should be maintained, because timely and appropriate treatment may prevent disastrous consequences of iatrogenic errors.

Transfusion reactions have been classi-

fied in two broad categories: immediate reactions, ordinarily observed within 48 hours of administration, and delayed reactions, usually appearing after the fifth day following transfusion; the first type is mediated by isosensitization with antigen transfer, whereas the second is characterized by transmission of diseases, notably serum hepatitis. In this chapter, only the former type of complication will be dealt with.

In order to identify, diagnose, and treat these reactions, procurement of the following information is necessary. In addition to consideration of the patient's clinical history, it is important to evaluate the previous transfusion history, indications for transfusion, physical signs and symptoms occurring during the reaction time, volume, and type of component infused. To investigate further, determinations of plasma and urine hemoglobin and serum bilirubin, the Shumm test for haptoglobin, confirmation of serum compatibility between donor and recipient samples, and aerobic and anaerobic cultures of both bloods should be made.

In an analysis of 2293 reactions from transfusion, Baker, Moinichen, and Nyhus[389] found allergic (45.6 per cent) and febrile (43.5 per cent) instances to be much more common than hemolytic (9.9 per cent) and other forms (1.0 per cent) of transfusion reactions.

ALLERGIC REACTIONS

In the awake patient, itching, erythema, urticaria, chills, and fever are manifestations of hypersensitivity to the transfused blood; occasionally laryngeal edema and bronchospasm are also seen. The onset of symptoms may appear even before the unit has been totally transfused. The cause is rarely identified, but an antigen-antibody reaction is presumably implicated.[390]

In the anesthetized patient, the first warning signs may be the appearance of erythema along the pathway of the vein where the blood is entering the circulation, and the presence of urticaria on the chest, face, and neck may follow. Changes in vital signs are rarely seen.

Patients with a history of transfusion reactions, atopy, hay fever, or multiple drug allergies appear to be more susceptible to this complication. In these instances, the prophylactic administration of antihistaminic drugs appears to curtail the frequency with which these reactions are seen, but should not be used routinely. Whenever one of these reactions is diagnosed during the transfusion of the first unit, it is rarely necessary to interrupt transfusion, because the reaction is transient and responsive to treatment.[391] However, if a reaction occurs during the second unit transfusion, it is impossible to ascertain which unit was the origin of the reaction, and it is justifiable to discontinue the second unit and attempt to identify the precise nature of the reaction. Diphenhydramine HCl, 50 mg given intravenously, is usually enough to treat mild episodes; for more severe bouts, epinephrine, 0.3 to 0.6 mg subcutaneously, and hydrocortisone, 250 mg intravenously, may be resorted to. In every case, close observation is advisable; however, if respiratory distress due to laryngeal edema is present, cold oxygen mist and the intravenous injection of dexamethasone may be indicated, as well as insuring patency of the airway. The in-halation of racemic epinephrine has also been recommended.

FEBRILE REACTIONS

The transfusion of donor blood containing leukocyte antigens to a recipient with leukocyte antibodies is thought to be the mechanism responsible for this untoward response, which is most frequently seen in patients who have received transfusion therapy repeatedly.

At least 300 ml or more of blood is characteristically necessary to elicit a febrile reaction, usually manifested by chills and fever and confirmed by negative blood cultures or other evidence of pyrogens.[390]

Since these types of reactions are most likely to occur in patients with chronic hematologic disorders requiring multiple transfusions, differential centrifugation, partial filtration, and even the use of washed red blood cells have been recommended in these high-risk individuals. The removal of large numbers of non-viable (stored) erythrocytes from the circulation by the reticuloendothelial system may occasionally produce fever.

Treatment is usually supportive, with antipyretics and intravenous fluids; nevertheless it is perhaps best to discontinue the blood until hemolytic reaction is ruled out.[391] Again, the importance of monitoring the patient's body temperature during anesthesia is emphasized, because an upward trend would be an early sign of recognition of this type of complication.

PYROGEN REACTIONS

These complications were seen more frequently before disposable transfusion equipment was used routinely. Then, bacteria, denatured proteins, foreign bodies, and toxins were difficult to remove from rubber and glass items and could affect the recipient when reused.

Currently, the most likely source is external contamination by the personnel who take part in the preparation and administration of blood and its products. Pathogenic and nonpathogenic bacteria have been found to be the cause of these reactions, which are manifested as a rapid rise in temperature with gradual fall. Symptomatic treatment is usually all that is necessary to abort these benign problems of transfusion therapy.[392] More recently, plasticizers and their metabolites have been found in the blood of patients receiving transfusions from plastic bags, indicating that the plastic material of the bag is not necessarily inert, but that some of its products pass into the contained blood and upon entering the recipient's circulation may undergo degradation.[393] The consequences of this chemical contamination are as yet unknown but undoubtedly deserve investigation. The effects of these degraded metabolites on different organ functions will have to be determined in order to resolve this dilemma.

Going against accepted concepts, the fact is that certain bacteria can survive the acidity and low temperatures at which blood is usually stored. This is possible because certain microorganisms such as Pseudomonas, Paracolon and E. coli can metabolize citrate and obtain the nutrients to remain alive in those adverse circumstances. Bacterial growth may be recognized by a dark brown, nearly black color in the plasma when it is allowed to separate from the red cell mass. If infused, hypotension, hyperpyrexia, and bleeding diathesis may supervene.[392] When in doubt, blood bags should be returned to the blood bank, because prophylaxis is more effective than treatment, which in this case would have to consist of the heroic measures used to combat septic shock.

HEMOLYTIC REACTIONS

These undoubtedly were the main cause for the delay in acceptance of blood transfusions as a therapeutic tool before blood groups were identified.

Red cell lysis can take place intravascularly, liberating hemoglobin into the circulating plasma and in extravascular sites such as the reticuloendothelial system characterized by hyperbilirubinemia and little or no hemoglobinemia.

When the amount of free hemoglobin in plasma exceeds 25 mg per 100 ml, hemoglobinuria occurs, eliminating about one third of the free hemoglobin through this pathway. Some of the hemoglobin is reabsorbed in the renal tubules, and most of the iron subsequently released is stored as hemosiderin and the rest as protein-bound ferritin.

Incompatibility due to antibodies is produced by the transfusion of red cells to a subject whose plasma contains an antibody that is readily lytic in vitro, that is, anti-A or anti-B. When small volumes of blood are transfused, up to 50 per cent of the erythrocytes may be lysed; with larger volumes nearly 90 per cent of the cells are lysed. Mild delayed reactions may occur and are manifested only by hyperbilirubinemia.

A frank hemolytic transfusion reaction may occur even with the infusion of very small amounts of whole blood or packed red cells. As a rule, the smaller the amount required to produce signs or symptoms, the greater are the resulting morbidity and mortality. A better prognosis is expected when larger quantities of blood were infused before the reaction was detected.

A feeling of heat along the vein where the blood is being transfused, flushing of the face, as well as chills, fever, and chest and flank pain may herald the onset of hemolysis. Occasionally, the patients themselves have volunteered the information of "knowing that something is wrong" or "I know that I am dying." Tachycardia and dyspnea occur in advanced stages of the reaction. From studies in animals, the pathogenesis of this condition appears to be due to pulmonary vascular obstruction, subsequent fall of cardiac output, and diminished tissue perfusion.[394]

Unexplained oozing in the operating site during blood transfusion may be the first indication of hemolytic reactions during anesthesia. Tachycardia, hypotension, and hemoglobinemia may soon appear. Renal failure sometimes follows incompatible transfusion and is probably caused by deposition of hemoglobin in the renal glomeruli and tubules, decreasing the glomerular filtration rate and altering the pH of the urine.

Early stimulation of diuresis by the administration of mannitol has been thought to be of value in aborting the renal impairment produced by this entity.[397, 398] Blood transfusion can be continued only after rematching with a freshly drawn sample. To maintain cardiac output, dopamine has been tried with rewarding results. The use of sodium infusions to alkalinize the urine and prevent precipitation of hemoglobin in the distal tubules has had controversial results, as has the use of adrenocorticosteroids.[399]

Considerable hemolysis with negative serologic reaction is usually asymptomatic and is manifested by jaundice 24 to 48 hours after transfusion. The mechanism for this derangement is obscure, but it is probably related to a deficiency of glucose-6-phosphate dehydrogenase. It is considered that about 50 per cent of the non-viable red cells are removed from the circulation within a few minutes of their transfusion and little if any hemoglobin produced by this mechanism is found free in plasma, thus confirming their extravascular destruction.

Delayed hemolytic transfusion reaction can occur when the amount of the antibody in the recipient's serum may be too low to produce rapid hemolysis. It is of interest, though, that septic and massively traumatized patients hemolyze serologically compatible transfused blood. This has been explained by the development of an anamnestic immune response with a rapid rise in antibody titer, eventually resulting in hemolysis. In this case, corticosteroid therapy may be of value.[399, 400]

Thrombocytopenia can occur after transfusions if the recipient develops a circulating platelet antibody, resulting in lysis of both the recipient's platelets and the transfused platelets. This has been noted to occur mostly in middle-aged women, and thus far no explanation for its pathophysiology has been found; however, there appears to be an indication that coating of the recipient platelets with donor platelet antigen produces subsequent nonspecific platelet lysis.[401] Large doses of steroids and transfusion of platelet concentrates are used as treatment.

Simulated intravascular hemolysis can occur under the following circumstances:

1. Hemolytic transfusion reactions have been noted when whole blood is passed through a reservoir containing 5 per cent dextrose in water or 25 per cent saline. This is probably due to cell swelling on exposure to hypotonic solutions, followed by rupture. Entry of distilled water into the circulation, such as in transurethral prostatic resection, can produce massive hemolysis. One thousand milliliters of water intravenously can result in hemoglobin plasma levels between 250 and 400 mg per 100 ml.

2. Overheating transfused blood to 44°C can result in hemolysis and denaturation of proteins.

3. Transfusion of frozen blood may result in a relatively benign hemoglobinuria without some of the serious immunological side effects. Frozen blood bags that have been rewarmed with considerable hemolysis present have a purple appearance and should be discarded.

4. External pressure required for rapid transfusions may produce significant hemolysis; even more may occur if the transfusion is through very narrow orifices, creating turbulence.

5. Following cardiopulmonary bypass, various degrees of hemolysis can occur, usually dependent on the duration of the bypass, the flow rate of perfusion, and the type of oxygenator used.

6. Hemolysis, massive enough to produce anemia, has been seen after the insertion of defective heart valves or any other devices within the heart.

OTHER EFFECTS OF TRANSFUSION

Results of Citrate Administration

Citrate intoxication occurring after massive blood transfusion remains a debatable issue. From the work by Bunker et al.,[402] it was found that citrate, if given in large amounts at a fast rate, may result in decreased myocardial contractility, arterial hypotension, Q-T segment abnormalities, and bradycardia. However, it was also shown that adults with adequate liver perfusion and function may tolerate the citrate contained in 1 unit of blood when given every five to seven minutes. Most untoward effects resulting from citrate overdose can be reversed by administration of calcium, and thus calcium has been advocated for treatment and even for prophylaxis of this entity.[403]

Since the metabolism of 1 mm of citrate produces 3 mEq of bicarbonate, it would be expected to lower the level of hydrogen ions; thus transfusion of large volumes does not result in acidosis as long as citrate continues to be metabolized. It does, however, generate citrate as substrate available for aerobic metabolism and eventual formation of bicarbonate.

On the other hand, the infusion of stored blood depleted of 2,3-diphosphoglycerate (2,3-DPG), with high oxygen affinity into acidotic animals has been noted to decrease oxygen delivery up to nine hours later.[404]

Howland and his coworkers,[405, 406] after acquiring extensive data with massive blood transfusions, have shown the warming and neutralization of acidity of these large volumes of cold, acid blood to be of greater benefit than calcium.

This same group[407] noted that the levels of ionized calcium are depressed during massive transfusion but only temporarily, and that this had no hemodynamic effect as long as circulating blood volume was maintained, as determined by central venous and pulmonary capillary wedge pressures. Therefore, calcium salts need not be administered unless hypotension develops. In some instances, levels of total calcium and albumin correlate with each other and establish criteria for adequate distribution of blood and fluid replacement.[408] Patients receiving colloid solutions have higher albumin and oncotic pressure than those receiving crystalloids.[409] Calcium was shown to be not only unnecessary but also possibly detrimental, leading to ventricular fibrillation when administered to patients with low body temperature.[400]

In the author's experience, the latter concept has been applied with satisfactory results; nevertheless, as long as the patient's temperature remains within normal limits, the slow intravenous injection of calcium chloride has resulted in improved cardiovascular function in anhepatic patients or those with severe liver and pancreatic failure. Equally effective has been the intravenous injection of calcium when used to treat hypotensive episodes resulting from inadequate blood replacement.

Other biochemical alterations resulting from massive blood replacement may be deduced from the list of changes occurring in stored blood, as listed in Table 8–9. Bicarbonate is indicated only when evidence of metabolic acidosis is present, as measured in arterial blood samples.

Hyperkalemia

As blood is stored, red cells gradually lyse; thus older bank blood may have plasma potassium concentrations as high as 21 mEq per liter. Although hyperkalemia could potentially develop, in reality this is the exception rather than the rule in rapid blood transfusion. A re-entry of K^+ ions into other erythrocytes occurs when blood is prewarmed and when it enters the circulation. In the postoperative period, metabolic alkalosis actually fosters elimination of K^+ ions through the kidneys, in attempt to retain H^+ ions. If hyperkalemia occurs, it can result in cardiac arrhythmias and hypotension secondary to lowered cardiac contractility. Elevated T waves are seen in the electrocardiogram, and high serum K^+ levels are found in laboratory determinations.

Hyperkalemia can be treated by calcium

Table 8–9   *Biochemical Comparison Between Stored Bank and Circulating Bloods*

Indices	Normal Blood*	Bank Blood
pH	7.40	6.65
Temp. C°	37.5	4–6
Hematocrit	45	41
Protein gm./100 ml.	7–8	7.3
K^+ mEq./L.	4.5	7–30†
Ca^{++} mEq./L.	5	0.5
Na^+ mEq./L.	140	170
O_2 Saturation %	98	35.3
Pco_2	40	191
Lactate mEq./L.	1.3	5.65
Pyruvate mEq./L.	0.07	0.22
Cytric acid mEq./L.	0.15	11.0
Platelets/ml.	230,000	0
Factors V, VIII %	100	50

*Arterial blood.
†Varies with the time of storage.

administration; calcium chloride is preferred, since it contains about four times more ionized Ca^{++} than gluconate. Glucose and insulin can also accelerate the re-entry of plasma K^+ into red blood cells.

Temperature

Since stored blood is usually kept at 4° C, the administration of large volumes would certainly lower the recipient's body temperature. Blood is rewarmed while being administered by passing it through a coil of tubing immersed in a water bath that is kept at a temperature between 37 and 39° C. Electrical warmers have also been used effectively. Microwave ovens for rewarming multiple blood bags are effective, though overheating has been known to occur.

Pulmonary Emboli and Detritus

One need only look at a used blood transfusion filter to be concerned about the ultimate destiny of the clots, fibrin, and other material that are usually included in the contents of most blood transfusion bags. Gervin et al.[410] and Barrett and collaborators[411] have shown the substantial amount of microaggregates contained in stored blood, and their lodging in the pulmonary circulation, and proposed this as one of the mechanisms involved in post-traumatic respiratory insufficiency. These findings have led to the acceptance and requirement of filters that would have smaller mesh than the commonly used blood filters, which have 40 to 80 micron mesh. Instead, micropore filters with 20 micron mesh have been suggested. However, these filters also slow down the flow of the transfused blood. As a solution, a multilayer, graduated density filter composed of nonwoven polyester fiber has been proposed in order to achieve high flow rate, ample volume capacity, and efficient particle removal.[412]

Effects of Anesthetic Agents upon the Hematopoietic System

This subject is of particular interest, not only because it deals with the action of anesthetic agents on a body system seldom given consideration during the daily practice of anesthesia but also because, as has been suggested, it may represent a potential professional hazard for anesthesiologists.[210]

Here, as in other cases, the challenge of a problem encountered in the clinic led to laboratory experimentation, only to be followed by a return to the human species for possible application. In doing so, further reasons for studying this subject were noted, for a remote possible association of anesthesia, radiation, and whatever other pollution dangers we are exposed to in our current working conditions had been revealed.

Among other cellular effects, halothane causes significant depression of neutrophil chemotaxis.[413] In vitro, halothane can suppress lymphocyte transformation in response to phytohemagglutinin.[414] Local anesthetics also alter the membrane characteristic of platelets and reversibly inhibit their aggregation and release.[415]

Interestingly enough, Ames et al.[12] have shown that patients anesthetized for six hours or longer with 50 per cent nitrous oxide may have evidence of megaloblastic bone marrow depression for up to 24 hours. These findings were attributed to interference with vitamin B_{12} or folic acid leading to imposed thymidine synthesis and were partially reversed by the administration of B_{12}. This concept was further supported by the observation that conversion of homocysteine to methionine (a B_{12} dependent reaction) is nearly prevented in rats exposed to 50 per cent nitrous oxide for 6 hours.[9]

Certain physical properties make nitrous oxide a desirable gas for providing analgesia by inhalation outside the operating room.[416] Relying on the then current concept of the "nobility" of nitrous oxide, Bjorneboe,[417] in 1953, advocated curarization and mechanical ventilation with nitrous oxide-containing atmospheres for patients suffering from severe tetanus, and this form for treatment was adopted. In 1955, Gormsen[418] first reported agranulocytosis and thrombocytopenia in one patient who had received a variety of drugs, among them nitrous oxide, curare, and chlorpromazine; however, the latter two were incriminated at the time as the possible cause of the hematologic alterations. The next year, Lassen et al.[419] studied the same phenomenon and experimentally reproduced it in other individuals with tetanus, having correlated the occurrence of leukopenia with the inhalation of nitrous oxide. Furthermore, the need for frequent blood transfusions in order to maintain the hemoglobin level, as well as what was described as "depression of erythropoiesis of the megaloblastic type" and peripheral thrombocytopenia, were manifestations of a certain degree of pancytopenia. All these effects reversed when the inhalation of the anesthetic was discontinued. These initial reports were followed by others equally striking.[420, 421, 422]

The leukopenic effects of nitrous oxide were confirmed and applied to a potential therapeutic use by Lassen and Kristensen[423] when patients with myelogenous leukemia with leukocytosis had a drop of white blood cells to a normal count after breathing nitrous oxide for three to five days.

Although these observations remained valid, Petrovsky and Yefuni[424] failed to observe leukopenia in patients inhaling nitrous oxide-oxygen mixtures for various periods of time to relieve postoperative pain. Nevertheless, Lefemine and Harken[425] and Parbrook[426] have recommended that its inhalation be limited to a maximum of 48 hours.

However, it was not until an animal experimental model was found that dose response and interactions with other drugs and circumstances were elucidated. For this, Green and Eastwood[427] exposed mixed strain albino rats to varied concentrations of nitrous oxide. A concentration of 40 per cent produced a 50 per cent drop in white blood cells in 15 days, whereas 80 per cent nitrous oxide caused leukopenia of 80 per cent in five days. The bone marrow of these rats showed a progressive hypoplasia as exposure to the gas was prolonged. Reproduction of marrow cells was arrested, and mitosis ceased to appear. Similar studies conducted by Parbrook[428] demonstrated the reversibility of such an effect. He also noted that the presence of surgical wounds enhanced the leukopenia, whereas the inhalation of nitrous oxide delayed wound healing. In animal species, rats and mice were found to be satisfactory for studies of protracted nitrous oxide treatment;[429] appetite and weight loss were not as marked as those observed in guinea pigs and rabbits. Among rats, interstrain differences appeared in adult animals. A combination of Sprague/Dawley and wild rat has been noted to be the most sensitive model for these studies.[430]

Certain primates are also suitable for investigation. "Anesthesia-like states" produced in rhesus monkeys by inhalation of helium and nitrogen at high pressures (40 to 60 atm) have resulted in peripheral lymphocytopenia.[431]

Still the question of whether this action was limited to nitrous oxide remained undisclosed. Using a similar experimental model, Aldrete and Virtue[432, 433] carried out a series of observations with other anesthetic gases. The continuous administration of subanesthetic concentrations of ethylene (60 per cent), cyclopropane (6 per cent), acetylene (50 per cent), and xenon (70 per cent) for six days resulted in various degrees of leukopenia with certain reduction in erythrocyte and thrombocyte counts. In addition, there was a fall in the cellularity of bone marrow aspirates, as well as changes in the granulocyte-erythroblast ratio (Table 8–10). In contrast, the inhalation of 80 per cent helium, argon, neon, sulfur hexafluoride and air, under the same experimental conditions, produced no significant effects.[434] The factors of lower food ingestion and decreased activity were also ruled out as being influential in the production of the findings previously described (Table 8–10).[435]

Bruce and Koepke[436] reported a peripheral granulocytopenia and an inhibition of dividing bone marrow granulocytes in rats inhaling halothane for three to five days. Further confirmation of this action could be speculated on, because somewhat similar hematologic alterations have been reported as sequelae of prolonged exposure to benzene,[135, 136] urethane,[437] alcohol, and single injections of barbiturates in dogs.[438] Since all these substances have "narcotizing" qualities, one can only postulate that the studies described suggest that drugs with anesthetic properties not only have depressant effects on the central nervous system but also possess an inhibitory action on hematopoiesis.

Nunn et al[439] studied the effects of halothane and/or nitrous oxide on division of cultured murine bone marrow cells, noting that halothane from 0.5 per cent to 2 per cent caused from gradual depression to almost total inhibition. The effects of 75 per cent nitrous oxide were equivalent to 0.5 per cent halothane. There was adequate recovery from 1 per cent but not from 2 per cent halothane. The mechanisms for this action on cells are complex, varying from depression of incorporation of labeled thy-

Table 8-10 *Effects of Prolonged Inhalation of Gases on the Blood Elements of Rats*

Group	Gas Concentration In Oxygen	Mean Variations of Blood Cell Counts (Per Cent of Initial Value)			Bone Marrow Cellularity Changes	Per Cent of Initial Hematocrit Value
		Leukocytes	Erythrocytes	Thrombocytes		
1	Air	+15.2	+2.8	+3.5	None	+4
2	Air — less food	+10	+1	+1	None	+5
3	Air — reserpine	+4	+3	+1	None	+2
4	100% oxygen	−11	−12	−2	None	−4
5	63% air	+6	+2	+2	None	+2
6	70% nitrous oxide	−69.9*	−13.2	−20.2†	−40%	−2
7	80% sulfur hexafluoride	+10	+11.2	+0.2	None	+2
8	80% helium	−1	−1	−4	None	+2
9	80% neon	−4	−2	−3	None	+2
10	80% argon	−6	−2	−3	None	+1
11	65% xenon	−30*	−18†	−4	−25%	−4
12	60% ethylene	−48.2*	−11.2	−19.3†	−30%	+2
13	6% cyclopropane	−65.6*	−14	−13.5	−30%	+8
14	50% acetylene	−56.6	−18†	−22†	−30%	−8

Alterations of blood cell counts, bone marrow cellularity, and hematocrit in rats exposed to various gases: Except for the group inhaling sulfur hexafluoride (during nine days), all the groups were subjected to six days of exposure. Cyclopropane was mixed with 20 per cent oxygen and 74 per cent air. (From Aldrete and Virtue, with the permission of the publisher.)
  * = $p < .001$.
  † = $p < .05$.

midine into DNA to delay of entry into mitosis resulting in multipolar mitosis and multinucleate cells. On the other hand, fentanyl and droperidol failed to elicit any apparent toxicity on human bone marrow cultures.[440]

An interesting, but at the same time threatening, evidence of relationships between anesthesia and the reticuloendothelial system was insinuated in the statistical scrutiny of the causes of death among anesthesiologists conducted by Bruce and collaborators.[210] In a study that included the junior, active, and retired members of the American Society of Anesthesiologists encompassing the years 1947 to 1966, there were 441 deaths. In correlating the causes of death in this professional group with those occurring in American males generally and in male policyholders of an insurance company, it was observed that anesthesiologists appear to have a low incidence of lung cancer and a slightly lower than average incidence of coronary artery disease; however, high rates of suicide and malignancies of lymphatic and reticuloendothelial tissues were significantly evident. More recently, however, two excellent epidemiological and objective studies[441, 442] provided evidence that average anesthetists not only live longer than surgeons and family doctors but

they do not seem to have any more susceptibility to develop fatal cancer, liver, or kidney diseases than other physicians. Surprisingly enough, suicide accounted for about 19 per cent of the deaths noted in one study.[442]

The chronic exposure of anesthesia personnel to anesthesia gases is certainly not a contribution to health, and preferably should be avoided. In accordance with the recommendation of Hallen et al.[443] and the experience in our practice, serious consideration of reduction of the amount of wasted anesthetic vapors is in order. This can be safely accomplished by the simple expedient of using low inflows[444] and/or disposing of the wasted gases outside the operating room.[445] The final solution to this question remains undiscovered, and it continues to be a challenge to those with intuition and curiosity about their own fate.

Effects of Anesthetic Gases and Vapors on Coagulation

From time to time, one of these compounds has been incriminated as producing an increase in blood loss in the operative field. It was not too long ago that experienced surgeons felt they could identify the anesthetic agent given to their patients by the amount of blood apparent immediately after the skin was incised. This contention was common when ether and cyclopropane were frequently used, and, although pharmacologically the action of the latter upon capillary sphincters has been proved, implying capillary stasis, one can readily distinguish the use of the former by the widely recognizable odor. At any rate, it is not doubted that with hypercarbia, acidosis, and vasodilatation, bleeding in the operating site may seem more apparent than when local anesthetic drugs with added vasoconstrictors are employed.

Specifically, the fluorinated ether methoxyflurane has been incriminated as producing changes in the coagulation process. Thuries[446] observed hypofibrinogenemia and hypofibrinemia in patients anesthetized with methoxyflurane alone; these were ameliorated when induction of anesthesia was attained with a steroid drug. Somewhat similar findings were noted in rat, dog, and man receiving methoxyflurane anesthesia; but in this study, the platelet count was also slightly diminished.[447]

Meda[448] demonstrated decreased ADP-induced platelet aggregation in vitro produced by methoxyflurane, halothane, diethylether, cyclopropane, and nitrous oxide; however, Lichtenfeld and collaborators[449] failed to confirm any significant change in platelet aggregation in patients anesthetized with halothane, nitrous oxide, or enflurane in clinical concentrations.

Although more prolonged exposure would be required in order to make an emphatic statement, it must be taken into consideration that other factors such as other medications (aspirin), renal or hepatic disease, surgical stress, and release of tissue procoagulants may play a role during anesthesia and surgery.

REFERENCES

1. Virchow, R. L. K.: White blood. Neue Notizen a.d. Geb. d. Nat. und Helike, Weimar 36:151, 1845. In Major, R. H.: Classic Decriptions of Disease. 3rd ed., Springfield, III., Charles C Thomas, 1945, p. 510.
2. Herbert, V.: Megaloblastic anemia. N. Engl. J. Med. 272:340, 1963.
3. Herbert, V., Streiff, R. R., and Sullivan, L. W.: Notes on vitamin B₁₂ absorption: Autoimmunity and childhood pernicious anemia. Medicine 43:679, 1964.
4. Reich, P. R.: Hematology: Pathophysiologic Basis for Clinical Practice. Boston: Little, Brown, and Company, 1978, pp. 74–80.
5. Sullivan, L. W.: Differential diagnosis and management of the patient with megaloblastic anemia. Amer. J. Med. 48:609, 1970.
6. Castle, W. B.: Factors involved in the absorption of vitamin B₁₂. Gastroenterology 37:377, 1959.
7. Herbert, V.: Nutritional requirements for vitamin B₁₂ and folic acid. Amer. J. Clin. Nutr. 21:743, 1968.
8. Lichtman, M. A. (Ed.): Hematology for Practitioners. Boston: Little, Brown, and Company, 1978, p. 135.
9. Nunn, J. F., and Chanarin, I.: Editorial. Nitrous oxide and vitamin B₁₂. Brit. J. Anaesth. 50:1089–1090, 1978.
10. Banks, R. G. S., Henderson, R. J., and Pratt, J. M.: Reactions of gases in solution. Part III: Some reactions of nitrous oxide with transition-metal complexes. J. Chem. Soc. (A) 2886, 1968.
11. Lassen, H. C. A., Henriksen, E., Neukirch, F., and Kristensen, H. S.: Treatment of tetanus. Severe bone marrow depression after prolonged nitrous oxide anaesthesia. Lancet 1:527, 1956.
12. Ames, J. A. L., Burman, J. F., Rees, G. M., et al: Megaloblastic haemopoiesis in patients receiving nitrous oxide. Lancet 2:339, 1978.
13. Sullivan, L. W., Lubby, A. L., and Streiff, R. R.: Studies on the daily requirement of folic acid in infants and the etiology of folate deficiency in goat's milk megaloblastic anemia. Amer. J. Clin. Nutr. 18:311, 1966.
14. Herbert, V., Zalusky, R., and Davidson, C. S.: Correlation of folate deficiency with alcoholism and associated macrocytosis, anemia and liver disease. Ann. Intern. Med. 58:977, 1963.
15. Sullivan, L. W., and Herbert, V.: Suppression of hematopoiesis by ethanol. J. Clin. Invest. 43:2048, 1964.
16. Hoffbrand, A. V., and Necheles, T. F.: Mechanisms of folate deficiency in patients receiving phenytoin. Lancet 2/528, 1968.
17. Streiff, R. R.: Malabsorption of polyglutamic folic acid secondary to oral contraceptives. Clin. Res. 17:345, 1969.
18. Rosenberg, I. H., Streiff, R. R., Godwin, H. A., and Castle, W. B.: Impairment of intestinal deconjugation of dietary folate. Lancet 2:530, 1968.
19. Moore, F. D.: The effects of hemorrhage on body composition. N. Engl. J. Med. 273:567, 1965.
20. Gillies, I. D. S.: Anaemia and anaesthesia. Brit. J. Anaesth. 46:589, 1974.
21. Noble, W. H. Early changes in lung water after haemorrhagic shock in pigs and dogs. Canad. Anaesth. Soc. J. 22:39, 1975.
22. Roberts, J. G., Foëx, P., Clarke, T. N. S., et al: Haemodynamic interactions of high-dose propranolol pretreatment and anaesthesia in the dog. III: The effects of haemorrhage during halothane and trichloroethylene anaesthesia. Brit. J. Anaesth. 48:411, 1976.
23. Horan, B. F., Prys-Roberts, C., Hamilton, W. K., and Roberts, J. G.: Haemodynamic responses to enflurane anaesthesia and hypovolemia in the dog, and their modification by propranolol. Brit. J. Anaesth. 49:1189, 1977.

24. Horan, B. F., Prys-Roberts, C., Roberts, J. G., et al.: Haemodynamic responses to isoflurane anaesthesia and hypovolemia in the dog, and their modification by propranolol. Brit. J. Anaesth. 49:1179, 1977.

25. Tanifuji, Y., and Eger, E. I.: Effect of arterial hypotension on anaesthetic requirement in dogs. Brit. J. Anaesth. 48:947, 1976.

26. Cullen, D. J., and Eger, E. I.: The effects of hypoxia and isovolemic anemia on the halothane requirement (MAC) of dogs. III: The effects of acute isovolemic anemia. Anesthesiology 32:46, 1970.

27. Erslev, A. J.: Anemia of chronic renal disease. Arch. Intern. Med. 126:774, 1970.

28. Boddy, L., Lawson, D. H., and Linton, A. L.: Iron metabolism in patients with chronic renal failure, Clin. Sci. 39:115, 1970.

29. Marcus, A. J.: Platelet function. N. Engl. J. Med. 280:1278, 1969.

30. Eschbach, J. W., Funk, D., Adamson, J., Kuhn, L., Scribner, B. H., and Finch, C. A.: Erythropoiesis in patients with renal failure undergoing chronic dialysis. N. Engl. J. Med. 276:653, 1967.

31. Hampers, C. L., Streiff, R. R., Nathan, D. G., et al: Megaloblastic hematopoiesis in uremia and in patients with long-term hemodialysis. N. Engl. J. Med. 276:551, 1967.

32. Aldrete, J. A., Daniel, W., O'Higgins, J. W., Homatas, J., and Starzl, T. E.: Analysis of anesthetic related morbidity in human recipients of renal homografts. Anesth. Analg. 50:321, 1971.

33. Graves, C. L., and Allen, R. M.: Anesthesia in the presence of severe anemia. Rocky Mount. Med. J. 63:35, 1970.

34. Jandl, J. H.: Anemia of liver disease. Observations on its mechanism. J. Clin. Invest. 34:390, 1955.

35. Lieberman, F. L. and Reynolds, T. B.: Plasma volume in cirrhosis of the liver: Its relationship to portal hypertension, ascites and renal failure. J. Clin. Invest. 46:1297, 1967.

36. Aldrete, J. A.: Anesthesia and intraoperative care. In Starzl, T. E.: Experience in Hepatic Transplantation. Philadelphia, W. B. Saunders Co., 1969, pp. 81-111.

37. Ajlouni, K., and Doeblin, T. D.: The syndrome of hepatitis and aplastic anaemia. Brit. J. Haematol. 27:345, 1974.

38. Böttiger, L. E., and Westerhom, B. Aplastic anaemia. III. Aplastic anaemia and infectious hepatitis. Acta Med. Scand. 192:323, 1972.

39. Semi-annual tabulation of Reports Compiled by the Registry on Blood Dyscrasias (March 20, 1963). Chicago: American Medical Association, 1963.

40. Nagao, T., and Mauer, A. M.: Concordance for drug-induced aplastic anemia in identical twins. N. Engl. J. Med. 281:7, 1969.

41. Rubin, D., Weisberger, A. S., Botti, R. E., and Stornasli, J. P.: Changes in iron metabolism in early chloramphenicol toxicity. J. Clin. Invest. 37:1286, 1958.

42. Saidi, P., Wallerstein, R. O., and Aggeler, P. M.: Effect of chloramphenicol on erythropoiesis. J. Lab. Clin. Med. 57:247, 1961.

43. Bowman, W. D.: Abnormal ringed sideroblasts in various hematological disorders. Blood 18:662, 1961.

44. Cotton, H. B., and Harris, J. W.: Familial pyridoxine responsive anemia. J. Clin. Invest. 41:1352, 1967.

45. Moorhouse, J. A., and Mathewson, F. A. L.: Familial hemolytic anemia: Concurrent crises in three members of a family. Canad. Med. Assoc. J. 75:133, 1956.

46. Dacie, J. V.: The Hemolytic Anemias: The Congenital Anemias. New York, Grune and Stratton, 1960, pp. 82-150.

47. Emerson, C. P., Jr., Shen, S. C., Ham, T. H., and Castle, W. B.: The mechanism of blood destruction in congenital hemolytic jaundice. J. Clin. Invest. 26:1180, 1947.

48. Schwartz, S. I., Bernard, R. P., Adams, J. T., and Bauman, A. W.: Splenectomy for hematologic disorders. Arch. Surg. 101:338, 1970.

49. Singer, D. B.: Post-splenectomy sepsis. In Rosenberg, H. S., and Bolande, R. P. (eds.): Perspectives in Pediatric Pathology. Chicago, Year Book, 1973, pp. 285-312.

50. Ducla-Soares, A., and Parreira, F.: Anémie elliptocytique familiale. Etude de 3 cas personnels. Sang 29:33, 1958.

51. Blackburn, E. K., Jordan, A., Lytle, W. J., Swan, H. T., and Tudhope, G. R.: Hereditary elliptocytic haemolytic anaemias. J. Clin. Path. 11:316, 1958.

52. Motulsky, A. G., Singer, K., Crosby, W. H., and Smith, V.: The life span of the elliptocyte. Hereditary elliptocytosis and its relationship to other familial hemolytic diseases. Blood 9:57, 1954.

53. Dacie, J. V.: The congenital haemolytic anaemias. Hereditary non-spherocytic haemolytic anaemia, "atypical" and unclassified types, "erythropoietic porphyria" and congenital Heinz-body anaemia. In The Hemolytic Anaemias. New York, Grune and Stratton, 1960, pp. 171-199.

54. Tanaka, K. S., Valentine, W. N., and Miwa, S.: Pyruvic kinase deficiency in hereditary nonspherocytic hemolytic anemia. Blood 19:267, 1962.

55. White, J. M.: The unstable haemoglobin disorders. Clin. Haematol. 3:333, 1974.

56. Marks, P. A., Banks, J., and Gross, R. T.: Genetic heterogeneity of glucose-6-phosphate dehydrogenase deficiency. Nature 194:454, 1962.

57. Kushavovskii, M. S.: Acute drug-induced hemolytic anemia associated with met- and sulfhemoglobinemia (glucose-6-phosphate dehydrogenase deficiency in the erythrocytes). Probl. Hemat. 11:59, 1966.

58. Siniscalco, M., Bernini, L., and Latte, B.: Linkage data involving G-6-PD deficiency, colour blindness and hemophilia. 2nd Int. Conf. on Human Genetics, Rome, Abst. 120. Amsterdam: Excerpta Medica, 1961.

59. Westing, D. W., and Pisciotta, A. V.: Anemia, cataracts, and seizures in patients with glucose-6-phosphate dehydrogenase deficiency. Arch. Intern. Med. 118:385, 1966.

60. Lehman, H., and Huntsman, R. G.: Man's Hemoglobins. Philadelphia, J. B. Lippincott Co., 1966.

61. Roughton, F. J. W.: Transport of oxygen and carbon dioxide. In Fenn, W. O. and Rahn, H.: Handbook of Physiology, Respiration, Vol. 1. Washington, D. C., Amer. Phys. Soc., 1964, pp. 767-827.

62. Pertuz, M. F., and Lehmann, H.: Molecular pathology of human hemoglobin. Nature 219: 902, 1968.

63. Huehns, E. R., and Bellingham, A. J.: Diseases of function and stability of hemoglobin. Brit. J. Haematol. 17:1, 1969.

64. Heller, P.: Hemoglobinopathic dysfunction of the red cell. Amer. J. Med. 41:799, 1966.

65. Dresbach, M.: Elliptical human red corpuscles. Science 19:469, 1904.

66. Hahn, E. V., and Gillespie, E. B.: Sickle cell anemia. Arch. Intern. Med. 39:233, 1927.

67. Pauling, L., Itano, H. A., Singer, S. J., and Wells, I. C.: Sickle cell anemia, a molecular disease. Science 110:543, 1949.

68. Apthorp, G. H., and Lehmann, H.: Sickle cell anemia. Proc. Roy. Soc. Med. 57:178, 1964.

69. Neel, J. V.: The inheritance of sickle cell anemia. Science 110:64, 1949.

70. McCormick, F.: Abnormal hemoglobins. II: The pathology of sickle cell trait. Am. J. Med. Sci. 92:329, 1961.

71. Dalal, F. Y., Schmidt, G. B., Bennett, E. J., and Ramamurthy, S.: Sickle cell trait: a report of a postoperative neurological complication. Brit. J. Anaesth. 46:387, 1974.

72. Harris, J. W., Brewster, H. H., Ham, T. H., et al: Studies on the destruction of red blood cells: X: The biophysics and biology of sickle cell disease. Arch. Intern. Med. 97:145, 1956.

73. de Laval, M. R., Taswell, H. F., Bowie, E. J. W., and Danielson, G. K.: Open heart surgery in patients with inherited hemoglobinopathies, red cell dyscrasias, and coagulopathies. Arch. Surg. 109:618, 1974.

74. Ahulu-Konotry, F. I. D.: The sickle cell diseases. Arch. Intern. Med. 133:611, 1974.

75. Couley, C. L., and Carache, S.: Mechanisms by which some abnormal hemoglobins produce clinical manifestations. Seminars Hematol. 4:53, 1967.

76. Etteldorf, J. N., Tharp, C. P., and Turner, M. D.: Studies on the cardiovascular dynamics with sickle cell anemia. Amer. J. Dis. Child 90:571, 1955.

77. Femi-Pearse, D., Gaziouglu, K. M., and Yu, P. N.: Pulmonary function studies in sickle cell disease. J. App. Physiol. 28:574, 1970.

78. Shelley, W. M., and Curtis, E. M.: Bone marrow and fat embolism in sickle cell anemia and sickle cell hemoglobin C disease. Bull. Johns Hopkins Hosp. 103:8, 1958.

79. Kennedy, A. C., and Valtis, D. J.: Oxygen dissociation curve in anemia of various types. J. Clin. Invest. 33:1372, 1954.

80. Konotey-Ahulu, F. I. D.: Sicklaemic human hygrometers. Lancet 1:1003, 1965.

81. Anderson, R., Cassell, M., Mullinaux, G., and Chaplin, H., Jr.: Effect of normal cells on viscosity of sickle cell blood. In vitro studies and report of six years' experience with a prophylactic program or "partial exchange transfusion." Arch. Intern. Med. 111:286, 1963.

82. Brody, J. L., Goldsmith, M. H., Park, S. K., and Soltys, H. D.: Symptomatic crisis of sickle cell anemia treated by limited exchange transfusion. Ann. Intern. Med. 72:327, 1970.

83. Elegbeleye, O. O., Akinsete, F. I., Afonja, A. O., and Femi-Pearse, D. Ventilatory response to carbon dioxide in patients with homozygous sickle-cell disease. Brit. J. Anaesth. 48:249,1976.

84. Sickle cell anaemia and anaesthesia. Brit. J. Med. 2:1263, 1965.

85. Gilbertson, A. A.: The management of anaesthesia in sickle cell states. Proc. Roy. Soc. Med. 60:631, 1967.

86. Hilkowitz, G., and Jacobson, A.: Hepatic dysfunction and abnormalities of serum proteins and serum enzymes in sickle-cell anemia. J. Lab. Clin. Med. 57:856, 1961.

87. Gilbertson, A. A.: Anesthesia in West African patients with sickle cell anemia, haemoglobin SC disease and sickle cell trait. Brit. J. Anaesth. 37:614, 1965.

88. Holzmann, L., Finn, H., Lichtman, H. C., and Harmel, M. H.: Anesthesia in patients with sickle cell disease: A review of 112 cases. Anesth. Analg. 48:566, 1969.

89. Ciliberti, B., Mazzia, V., Mark, L., and Marx, G.: Sickle cell disease and anesthesia. (One case report of postoperative mortality.) New York J. Med. 4:548, 1962.

90. Griffin, D. R.: Sickle-cell disease as it relates to anesthesia: Report of two cases. Anesth. Analg. 45:826, 1966.

91. Guinee, W. S., Heaton, J. A., Barreras, L., and Diggs, L. W.: Effects of general anesthesia on sicklemic patients. Anesthesiology 29:193, 1968.

92. Virtue, R. W., Myers, D., and Aldrete, J. A.: Postanesthetic administration of doxapram hydrochloride and/or oxygen at an altitude of 1 mile. Anesth. Analg. 51:1, 1972.

93. Knudsen, J.: Duration of hypoxemia after uncomplicated upper abdominal and thoracoabdominal operations. Anaesthesia 25:372, 1970.

94. Diggs, L. W.: Sickle cell crisis. Amer. J. Clin. Path. 44:1, 1965.

95. Brown, R. A.: Anaesthesia in patients with sickle cell anemia. Brit. J. Anaesth. 37:181, 1965.

96. Anstall, H. B., Huntsman, R. G., Lehmann, H., Hayward G. H., and Weitzman, D.: The effect of magnesium on blood coagulation in human subjects. Lancet 1:814, 1959.

97. Giesecke, A. H., Morris, R. E., Dalton, M. D., et al.: Of magnesium, muscle relaxants, toxemic parturients and cats. Anesth. Analg. 47:689, 1968.

98. Watson-Williams, E. J.: Use of low molecular weight dextran in sickle cell anaemia. Proc. Roy. Soc. Med. 60:636, 1967.

99. Stevens, A. R.: Splenectomy in sickle cell anemia. Arch. Intern. Med. 125:883, 1970.

100. Shotton, D., Crockett, C. L., and Leavell, B. S.: Splenectomy in sickle cell anemia. Blood 6:365, 1951.

101. Jandl, J. H., and Aster, R. H.: Increased splenic pooling and pathogenesis of hypersplenism. Amer. J. Med. Sci. 253:383, 1967.

102. Grace, D. A., and Winter, C. C.: Priapism: An appraisal of management of twenty-three patients. J. Urol. 99:301, 1968.

103. Pietras, J. R., Cromie, W. J., and Duckett, J.:

Ketamine as a detumescence agent during hypospadias repair. J. Urol. *121*:654, 1979.

104. Surana, R. B., Cott, R. B., and Ferguson, A. D.: Studies in sickle-cell anemia. XXXI. Preliminary observations on the use of indomethacin in the treatment of thrombotic crises. Med. Ann. DC *35*:593, 1966.

105. Nalbandian, R. M., Houghton, B. C., Henry, R. L., and Wolf, P. L.: The molecular basis for the oral prophylactic use of urea in the treatment of sickle cell anemia. Fed. Proc. *30*:684, 1971.

106. Nalbandian, R. M., Henry, R. L., Nichols, B. M., Kessler, D. L., Camp, F. R., Jr., and Vining, K. K., Jr.: The molecular basis for the treatment of sickle cell crisis. Ann. Intern. Med. *72*:795, 1970.

107. Shapiro, N. D., and Poe, F.: Sickle cell disease: An anesthesiological problem. Anesthesiology *16*:771, 1955.

108. Fouche, H. H., and Switzer, P. K.: Pregnancy with sickle cell anemia. Review of the literature and report of cases. Amer. J. Obstet. Gynec. *58*:468, 1949.

109. Barreras, L., and Diggs, L. W.: Sodium citrate orally for painful sickle cell crises. J.A.M.A. *215*:762, 1971.

110. Konotey-Ahulu, F. I.: Anaesthetic deaths and the sickle-cell trait. Lancet *1*:267, 1969.

111. Motulsky, A. F., and Stamatoyannopoulos, G.: Drugs, anesthesia and abnormal hemoglobins. Ann. N.Y. Acad. Sci. *151*:807, 1968.

112. Pearson, H. A.: Thalassemia intermedia. Genetic and biochemical considerations. Ann. N.Y. Acad. Sci. *119*:390, 1964.

113. Ingram, V. M.: A molecular model for thalassemia. Ann. N.Y. Acad. Sci. *119*:390, 1964.

114. Kaplan, E., and Zuelzer, W. W.: Erythrocytic survival studies in childhood. II. Studies in Mediterranean anemia. J. Lab. Clin. Med. *36*:517, 1950.

115. Necheles, R. F., Steiner, M., and Baldini, M.: The *in vitro* synthesis of hemoglobin by human bone marrow in thalassemia. Blood *25*:897, 1965.

116. Orr, D.: Difficult intubation: A hazard in thalassemia. A Case Report. Brit. J. Anaesth. *39*:585, 1967.

117. Smith, E. W., and Krevans, J. R.: Clinical manifestations of hemoglobin C disorders. Johns Hopkins Med. J. *104*:17, 1959.

118. Edwards, R.: Anaesthesia for caesarian section in haemoglobin SC disease complicated by eclampsia. A Case Report. Brit. J. Anaesth. *45*:757, 1973.

119. Sawitsky, A., and Ozaeta, P. B., Jr.: Disease-associated autoimmune hemolytic anemia. Bull. N.Y. Acad. Med. *46*:411, 1970.

120. Burnet, M.: Autoimmune disease. Brit. Med. J. *2*:645, 1959.

121. Dacie, J. V., and DeGruchy, G. C.: Autoantibodies in acquired haemolytic anaemias. J. Clin. Pathol. *4*:253, 1951.

122. Coombs, R. R. A., Mourant, A. E., and Race, R. R.: A new test for the detection of weak and "incomplete" Rh agglutinins. Brit. J. Exp. Path. *26*:255, 1945.

123. Evans, R. S., Turner, E., Bingham, M., and Woods, R.: Chronic hemolytic anemia due to cold agglutinins. J. Clin. Invest. *47*:691, 1968.

124. Schubothe, H.: The cold hemagglutinin disease. Seminar Hematol. *3*:27, 1966.

125. Crosby, W. H.: Paroxysmal noctural hemoglobinuria. Blood *6*:270, 1952.

126. Vos, G. H., Petz, L., and Fudenberg, H. H.: Specificity of acquired haemolytic anaemia autoantibodies and their serological characteristics. Brit. J. Haematol. *19*:57, 1970.

127. Rudaev, I. A. A.: On the preparation and administration of intubation anesthesia in patients with hypoplastic and aplastic anemia. Eksp. Khir. Anest. *13*:60, 1968.

128. Lees, M. H.: Case of immune aplastic haemolytic anaemia. Brit. Med. J. *1*:110, 1960.

129. Boyett, J. D., and Butterworth, C. E.: Lead poisoning and hemoglobin synthesis. Amer. J. Med. *32*:844, 1962.

130. Albahary, C.: Lead and hemopoiesis. The mechanism and consequences of the erythropathy of occupational lead poisoning. Amer. J. Med. *52*:367, 1972.

131. Lichtman, H. C., and Feldman, F.: In vitro pyrrole and porphyrin synthesis in lead poisoning and iron deficiency. J. Clin. Invest. *42*:830, 1963.

132. Harris, J. W.: Studies on the mechanism of drug-induced hemolytic anaemia. J. Lab. Clin. Med. *44*:809, 1956.

133. Whitaker, J. A., and Viett, T. J.: Fluorescence of erythrocytes in lead poisoning in children. An aid to rapid diagnosis. Pediatrics *24*:734, 1958.

134. Aldrete, J. A.: Unpublished data.

135. Erf, L. A., and Rhoads, C. P.: The hematological effects of benzene (benzol) poisoning. J. Indust. Hyg. Toxicol. *21*:421, 1939.

136. Das, K. C., Sen, N. N., Chaterjee, J., and Aikat, B. K.: Some observations on benzene-induced hypoplastic marrow in tissue culture. Ind. J. Med. Res. *51*:890, 1963.

137. Ockner, R. K., and Schmid, R.: Acquired porphyria in man and rat due to hexachlorobenzene intoxication. Nature *189*:499, 1961.

138. Schmid, R.: Cutaneous porphyria in turkey. N. Engl. J. Med. *263*:397, 1960.

139. Prankerd, T. A. J.: Haemolytic effects of drugs and chemical agents. Clin. Pharmacol. Ther. *4*:334, 1962.

140. Zieve, L.: Jaundice, hyperlipidemia and hemolytic anemia: Heretofore unrecognized syndrome associated with alcohol fatty liver and cirrhosis. Ann. Intern. Med. *48*:471, 1958.

141. Smith, J. A., Lonergan, E. T., and Sterling, K.: Spur-cell anemia. Hemolytic anemia with red cells resembling acanthocytes in alcoholic cirrhosis. N. Engl. J. Med. *271*:396, 1964.

142. Alpert, L. I., and Benisch, B.: Hemangioendothelioma of the liver associated with microangiohepatic hemolytic anemia. Amer. J. Med. *48*:624, 1970.

143. Brain, M. C.: Microangiopathic hemolytic anemia. Ann. Rev. Med. *21*:133, 1970.

144. Luke, R. G., Talbert, W., Siegel, R. R., and Holland, N.: Heparin treatment for postpartum renal failure with microangiopathic haemolytic anaemia. Lancet *1*:750, 1970.

145. Lynch, E. C.: Microangiopathic hemolytic anemia in carcinoma of the stomach. Gastroenterology *52*:88, 1967.

146. Seligson, U.: Microangiopathic hemolytic anemia

and defibrination syndrome in metastatic carcinoma of the stomach. Israel J. Med. Sci. 4:69, 1968.

147. Kasabach, H. H., and Merritt, K. K.: Capillary hemangiomas with extensive purpura. Amer. J. Dis. Child. 59:1063, 1940.

148. The hemolytic-uremic syndrome. New Eng. J. Med. 281:1072, 1969.

149. Gianantonio, C., Vitacco, M., and Mendilaharzu, F.: The hemolytic-uremic syndrome. J. Pediatr. 64:478, 1964.

150. McClean, N. M., Jones, C. H., and Sutherland, D. A.: Haemolytic uremic syndrome: A report of one outbreak. Arch. Dis. Child. 41:76, 1966.

151. Ham, T. H.: Hemoglobinuria. Amer. J. Med. 18:990, 1955.

152. Buckle, R. M.: Exertional (march) hemoglobinuria: Reduction of haemolytic episodes by use of sorbo-rubber insoles. Lancet 1:1136, 1965.

153. Payne, R. B.: Low plasma haptoglobin in march hemoglobinuria. J. Clin. Path. 19:170, 1966.

154. Pollard, T. D., and Weiss, I. W.: Acute tubular necrosis in a patient with march hemoglobinuria. N. Engl. J. Med. 283:803, 1970.

155. Reich, C., Seife, M., and Kessler, B. J.: Gaucher's disease: A review and discussion of 20 cases. Medicine 30:1, 1951.

156. Medoff, A. S., and Bayrd, E. D.: Gaucher's disease in 29 cases: Hematological complications and effect of splenectomy. Ann. Intern. Med. 40:481, 1954.

157. Felty, A. R.: Chronic arthritis in the adult associated with splenomegaly and leukopenia. Johns Hopkins Med. J. 35:16, 1924.

158. Ruderman, M., Miller, L. M., and Pinals, R. S.: Clinical and serological observations on 27 patients with Felty's syndrome. Arthritis Rheum. 11:377, 1968.

159. Mason, D. T., and Morris, J. J.: The variable features of Felty's syndrome. Amer. J. Med. 36:463, 1964.

160. Finch, C. A., and Finch, S.: Idiopathic hemochromatosis. Medicine 34:381, 1955.

161. James, T. N.: Pathology of the cardiac conduction system in hemochromatosis. N. Engl. J. Med. 271:92, 1964.

162. Ayvazian, J. H.: Xanthinuria and hemochromatosis. N. Engl. J. Med. 270:18, 1964.

163. Reissmann, K. R.: Studies on the mechanism of erythropoietic stimulation in parabiotic rats during hypoxia. Blood 5:372, 1950.

164. Stohlmann, F., Jr.: Erythropoiesis. N. Engl. J. Med. 267:342, 1962.

165. Pearson, H. A.: Recent advances in hematology. Pediatrics 69:466, 1966.

166. Jacobson, L. O., Goldwasser, E., Fried, W., and Plzak, L.: Role of the kidney in erythropoiesis. Nature 179:633, 1957.

167. Erslev, A. J., and Gabuzda, T. G.: Pathophysiology of Blood. 2nd ed., Philadelphia, W. B. Saunders, 1978, pp. 31–34.

168. Nathan, D. G., Schupak, E., Stohlmann, F., Jr., and Merrill, J. P.: Erythropoiesis in anephric man. J. Clin. Invest. 43:2158, 1964.

169. Okumewick, J. P., and Fulton, D.: Comparison of erythropoietin response in mice following polycythemia induced by transfusion or hypoxia. Blood 36:239, 1970.

170. Benesch, R., and Benesch, R. E.: The effect of organic phosphates from the human erythrocyte on the allosteric properties of hemoglobin. Biochem. Biophys. Res. Commn. 26:162, 1967.

171. Valtis, D. J., and Kennedy, A. C.: Defective gas-transport function of stored red blood cells. Lancet 1:119, 1954.

172. Dawson, R. B., and Ellis, T. J.: Hemoglobin function of blood stored at 4° C in ACD and CPD with adenine and inosine. Transfusion 10:113, 1970.

173. Bunn, H. F., May, M. H., Kocholaty, W. F., et al.: Hemoglobin function in stored blood. J. Clin. Invest. 48:311, 1969.

174. Schweizer, O., and Howland, W. S.: 2,3-diphosphoglycerate levels in CPD-preserved bank blood. Anesth. Analg. 53:516, 1974.

175. Beutler, E., and Wood, L.: In vivo regeneration of red cell 2,3-diphosphoglyceric acid (DPG) after transfusion of stored blood. J. Lab. Clin. Med. 74:300, 1969.

176. Valeri, C. R.: Viability and function of preserved red cells. N. Engl. J. Med. 284:81, 1971.

177. Oski, F. A., and Delivoria-Papadopoulos, M.: The red cell 2,3-diphosphoglycerate and tissue oxygen release. Pediatrics 77:941, 1970.

178. Snyder, L. M., and Reddy, W. J.: Thyroid hormone control of erythrocyte 2,3-diphosphoglyceric acid concentration. Science 169:879, 1970.

179. Miller, W. W., Delivoria-Papadopoulos, M., Miller, L., and Oski, F. A.: Oxygen releasing factor in hyperthyroidism. J.A.M.A. 211:1824, 1970.

180. Delivoria-Papadopoulos, M., Oski, F. A., and Gottlieb, A. J.: Oxygen-hemoglobin dissociation curves: Effect of inherited enzyme defects of the red cell. Science 165:601, 1969.

181. Bunn, H. F., and Jandl, J. H.: Control of hemoglobin function within the red cell. N. Engl. J. Med. 282:1414, 1970.

182. Lenfant, C., Torrance, J., English, E., et al.: Effect of altitude on oxygen binding by hemoglobin and on organic phosphate levels. J. Clin. Invest. 47:2652, 1968.

183. Monge, C., and Whittembury, J.: Increased hemoglobin-oxygen affinity at extremely high altitudes. Science 186:843, 1974.

184. Benesch, R., and Benesch, R. E.: Intracellular organic phosphates as regulators of oxygen release by hemoglobin. Nature 221:618, 1969.

185. Chanutin, A., and Curnish, R. R.: Effect of organic and inorganic phosphates on the oxygen equilibrium of human erythrocytes. Arch. Biochem. Biophys. 121:96, 1967.

186. Eaton, J. W., Faulkner, J. A., and Brewer, G. J.: Response of the human red cell to muscular activity. Proc. Soc. Exp. Biol. Med. 132:886, 1969.

187. Kracke, R. R., and Parker, F. P.: The relationship of drug therapy to agranulocytosis. J.A.M.A. 105:960, 1935.

188. Moeschlin, S., and Wagner, K.: Agranulocytosis due to the occurrence of leukocyte-agglutinins (pyramidon and cold agglutinins). Acta Haemat. 8:29, 1952.

189. Alcoba, L. M.: Drug-induced agranulocytosis with medullary plasmacytosis and hyperglobulinemia. Rev. Clin. Exp. 103:316, 1966.

190. Yunis, A. A., and Bloomberg, G. R.: Chloram-

phenicol toxicity: Clinical features and pathogenesis. Prog. Haemat. 4:138, 1964.

191. Scott, J. L., Finegold, S. M., Belkin, G. A., and Lawrence, J. S.: A controlled double blind study of the hematological toxicity of chloramphenicol. N. Engl. J. Med. 272:1137, 1965.

192. Weisberger, A. S., Armentrout, S., and Wolfe, S.: Protein synthesis by reticulocyte ribosomes. I. Inhibition of polyuridylic acid-induced ribosomal protein synthesis by chloramphenicol. Proc. Nat. Acad. Sci. 50:86, 1963.

193. Lawrence, J. S.: Leukopenia: Its mechanism and therapy. J. Chron. Dis. 6:351, 1957.

194. Yunis, A. A., Arimura, G. K., Lutcher, C. L., Blasquez, J., and Halloran, M.: Biochemical lesion in dilantin-induced erythroid aplasia. Blood 30:587, 1967.

195. Kaplan, S. S., and Fink, M. E.: Drug induced agranulocytosis. Conn. Med. 32:32, 1968.

196. Pisciotta, A. V., and Kaldahl, J.: Studies on agranulocytosis. IV. Effects of chlorpromazine on nucleic acid synthesis of bone marrow cells in vitro. Blood 20:364, 1962.

197. Pisciotta, A. V.: Drug induced leucopenia and aplastic anemia. Clin. Pharmacol. Ther. 12:13, 1971.

198. Mowat, A. G.: Haematologic aspects of systemic disease: Connective tissue disease. Clin. Haematol. 1:573, 1972.

199. Wiik, A., and Munthe, E.: Complement-fixing, granulocyte-specific antinuclear factors in neutropenic cases of rheumatoid arthritis. Immunology 26:1127, 1974.

200. Lewis, C. L., and Patterson, E.: Leukopenia after postmastectomy irradiation. J.A.M.A. 235:747, 1976.

201. Irey, H. S.: Adverse drug reactions and death: A review of 827 cases. J.A.M.A. 236:575, 1976.

202. Reizenstein, P., and Edgardk, K.: Mortality in agranulocytosis. Lancet 2:293, 1974.

203. Palva, I. P., Mustala, O. O., and Salokannel, S. J.: Drug-induced agranulocytosis. III. Response to corticosteroids. Acta Med. Scand. 192:51, 1972.

204. Morley, A. A., Carew, J. P., and Baikie, A. G.: Familial cyclical neutropenia. Brit. J. Haematol. 13:719, 1967.

205. Duane, G. W.: Periodic neutropenia. Arch. Intern. Med. 102:462, 1958.

206. Page, A. R., and Good, R. A.: Studies on cyclic neutropenia. Amer. J. Dis. Child. 94:623, 1957.

207. Burger, C. L., Harris, W. W., Anderson, N. G., Bartlett, T. W., and Kniseley, R. M.: Virus-like particles in human leukemia plasma. Proc. Soc. Exp. Biol. Med. 115:151, 1964.

208. March, H. C.: Leukemia in radiologists 10 years later: With review of pertinent evidence for radiation leukemia. Amer. J. Med. Sci. 242:137, 1961.

209. Lange, R. D., Maloney, W. C., and Yamawaki, T.: Leukaemia in atom bomb survivors. Blood 9:574, 1954.

210. Bruce, D. L., Eide, K. A., Linde, H. W., and Eickenhoff, J. E.: Causes of death among anesthesiologists: A 20-year survey. Anesthesiology 29:565, 1968.

211. The connection between tandearil and leukemia. Svensk. Farm. T. 70:211, 1966.

212. Evans, A. E.: Central nervous system involvement in children with acute leukemia: A study of 921 patients. Cancer 17:256, 1964.

213. Berlin, N. I., Lawrence, J. H., and Lee, H. C.: The pathogenesis of the anemia of chronic leukemia. Measurement of the lifespan of the red blood cell with glycine 2-C^{14}. J. Lab. Clin. Med. 44:860, 1954.

214. Block, J. B., Carbone, P. P., Oppenheim, J. J., and Frei, E.: The effect of treatment in patients with chronic myelogenous leukemia. Biochemical studies. Ann. Intern. Med. 59:629, 1963.

215. Galton, D. A. G., and Till, M.: The treatment of chronic leukaemias. Brit. Med. Bull. 15:79, 1959.

216. Rall, D. P.: Conference on obstacles to the control of acute leukemia. Experimental studies of the blood-brain barrier. Cancer Res. 25:1572, 1965.

217. Rowley, J. P.: A new consistent chromosomal abnormality in chronic myelogenous leukaemia identified by quinacrine fluorescence and Giemsa staining. Nature 243:290, 1973.

218. Stenman, U. H., Simons, K., and Grasbeck, R.: Vitamin B$_{12}$-binding proteins in normal and leukemic human leukocytes and sera. Scand. J. Clin. Lab. Invest. 21:202, 1968.

219. Galton, D. A. G.: Chemotherapy of chronic myelogenous leukemia. Semin. Hematol. 6:323, 1969.

220. Kyle, R. A., Kiely, J. M., and Stickney, J. M.: Acquired hemolytic anemia in chronic lymphocytic leukemia and the lymphomas. Arch. Intern. Med. 104:61, 1959.

221. Dacie, J. V.: Secondary or symptomatic haemolytic anemias. In The Haemolytic Anaemias: Congenital and Acquired, Part III. 2nd ed., London, Churchill, 1967, p. 729.

222. Fiddles, P., Penny, R., Wells, T. V., and Rozenberg, M. C.: Clinical correlations with immunoglobulin levels in chronic lymphatic leukemia. Aust. N. Z. J. Med. 4:346, 1972.

223. Bentvelzen, P., Hilgers, J., Yohn, D. S.: Advances in Comparative Leukemia Research. Amsterdam, Elsevier/North Holland Biomedical Press, 1978, pp. 55–105.

224. Haut, A. Wintrobe, M. M., and Cartwright, G.: The clinical management of leukemia. Amer. J. Med. 28:777, 1960.

225. Freymann, J. G., Vender, J. B., Marler, E. A., and Meyer, D. G.: Prolonged corticosteroid therapy of chronic lymphocytic leukemia and the closely allied malignant lymphomas. Brit. J. Haematol. 6:303, 1960.

226. Thomson, A. E., and Robinson, M. A.: Cytocidal action of colchicine in vitro on lymphocytes in chronic lymphocytic leukaemia. Lancet 2:868, 1967.

227. Sinn, C. M., and Dick, F. W.: Monocytic leukemia. Amer. J. Med. 20:588, 1956.

228. Doan, D., and Wiseman, B.: The monocyte, monocytosis, and monocytic leukosis. Ann. Intern. Med. 8:383, 1934.

229. Lynch, M. J.: Monocytic leukemia. Canad. Med. Assoc. J. 70:670, 1954.

230. Plenderleith, I. H.: Hairy cell leukemia. Canad. Med. Assoc. J. 102:1054, 1970.

231. Baldini, M., Fudenberg, H. H., Fukutake, K., and Dameshek, W.: The anemia of the Di Guglielmo syndrome. Blood 14:334, 1959.

232. Di Guglielmo, G.: Acute erythemic disease. In

Proceedings, Sixth Congress of the International Society of Hematologists. New York, Grune and Stratton, 1958, p. 33.

233. Dameshek, W., and Baldini, M.: The Di Guglielmo syndrome. Blood 13:192, 1958.

234. Sheets, R. F., Drevets, C. C., and Hamilton, H. E.: Erytholeukemia (Di Guglielmo syndrome). Arch. Intern. Med. 111:295, 1963.

235. Kotlarek-Haus, S., Halawa, B., and Domanski, I.: Contribution to the acute erythroleukemia. Przegl. Lek. 22:758, 1966.

236. Griffiths, L. L., and Brews, V. A. L.: The electrophoretic pattern in multiple myelomatosis. J. Clin. Path. 6:187, 1953.

237. Hutter, O. R., and Kostial, K.: Effect of magnesium and calcium ions on the release of acetylcholine. J. Physiol. 124:234, 1954.

238. Zimmerman, H. H., and Hall, W. H.: Recurrent pneumonia in multiple myeloma and some observations on immunological response. Arch. Intern. Med. 103:173, 1959.

239. Bloch, K. J., and Maki, D. G.: Hyperviscosity syndromes associated with immunoglobulin abnormalities. Semin. Hematol. 10:113, 1973.

240. Bayrd, E. D.: The bone marrow on sternal aspiration in multiple myeloma. Blood 3:987, 1948.

241. Laget-Corsin, L.: Problems of anesthesia and resuscitation posed by the dysglobulinemias. Anesth. Analg. (Paris) 25:145, 1968.

242. Kyle, R. A., Jowsey, J., Kelly, P. J., and Taves, D. R.: Multiple myeloma bone disease: The comparative effect of sodium fluoride and calcium carbonate or placebo. N. Engl. J. Med. 293:1334, 1975.

243. Gilbert, H. S.: The spectrum of myeloproliferative disorders. Med. Clin. N. Amer. 57:355, 1973.

244. Bowdler, A. J., and Prankerd, T. A.: Primary myeloid metaplasia. Brit. Med. J. 1:1352, 1961.

245. Rosenbaum, D. L., Murphy, G. W., and Swisher, S. N.: Hemodynamic studies of the portal circulation in myeloid metaplasia. Amer. J. Med. 41:360, 1966.

246. Waldenström, J.: Three new cases of purpura hyperglobulinaemia. Acta Med. Scand. Suppl. 1952, p. 226.

247. Forget, B. G., Squires, J. W., and Sheldon, H.: Waldenström macroglobulinemia with generalized amyloidosis. Arch. Intern. Med. 118:363, 1966.

248. Morel-Maroger, L., Basch, A., Danon, F., Weroust, P., and Richet, G.: Pathology of the kidney in Waldenström's macroglobulinemia. N. Engl. J. Med. 283:123, 1970.

249. Zollinger, H. U.: Die pathologische Anatomie der Makroglobulinämie Waldenström. Helv. Med. Acta 25:153, 1958.

250. Dutcher, T. F., and Fahy, J. L.: The histopathology of the macroglobulinemia of Waldenström. J. Nat. Cancer Inst. 22:887, 1959.

251. Mackay, I. R., Eriksen, N., Motulsky, A. G., and Volwiler, W.: Cryo- and macroglobulinemia: Electrophoretic, ultracentrifugal and clinical studies. Am. J. Med. 20:564, 1956.

252. Franklin, E. C., Lowenstein, J., Bigelow, B., and Meltzer, M.: Heavy chain disease. A new disorder of serum γ-globulins. Amer. J. Med. 37:332, 1964.

253. Osserman, E. F., and Takatsuki, K.: Clinical and immunochemical studies of four cases of heavy (Hγ²) chain disease. Amer. J. Med. 37:351, 1964.

254. Burkitt, D.: Sarcoma involving jaws in African children. Brit. J. Surg. 46:218, 1958–59.

255. Clinicopathological Conference: Lymphosarcoma in a St. Louis girl clinically and histologically resembling Burkitt's African lymphoma. Amer. J. Med. 38:96, 1965.

256. Aldrete, J. A.: Nasotracheal intubation. Surg. Clin. N. Amer. 49:1209, 1969.

257. Waters, D. J.: Guided blind endotracheal intubation. Anaesthesia 18:158, 1963.

258. Maizels, M., Prankerd, T. A. J., and Richards, J. D. M.: Haematology in Diagnosis and Treatment. London, Tindall and Cassell, 1968, pp. 199–207.

259. Binder, R. A., and Gilbert, H. A.: Muramidase in polycythemia vera. Blood 36:228, 1970.

260. Berlin, N. I.: Differential diagnosis of the polycythemias. Semin. Hematol. 3:209, 1966.

261. Modan, B., and Lilienfeld, A. M.: Polycythemia vera and leukemia. The role of radiation treatment. Medicine 44:305, 1965.

262. Wassermann, L. R., and Gilbert, H. S.: Complications of polycythemia vera. Semin. Hematol. 3:199, 1966.

263. Coleman, A. J., and Sliom, C. M.: Polycythaemic hypoxaemia and general anesthesia. A case report. Brit. J. Anaesth. 38:653, 1966.

264. Wasserman, L. R., and Gilbert, H. S.: Surgery in polycythemia vera. N. Engl. J. Med. 269:1226, 1963.

265. Gaarder, A., Jonsen, J., Laland, S. Hellem, A., and Owren, P. A.: Adenosine diphosphate in red cells as a factor in the adhesiveness of human blood platelets. Nature 192:531, 1961.

266. Stefanini, M., and Chatterjea, J. B.: Studies on platelets. IV. A thrombocytopenic factor in normal human blood plasma or serum. Proc. Soc. Exp. Biol. Med. 79:623, 1952.

267. Zucker, M. B., and Lundburgh, A.: Platelet transfusions. Anesthesiology 27:385, 1966.

268. Harrington, W. J.: The Purpuras. Disease-a-Month. Chicago: Year Book Publications, July, 1957.

269. Bunting, W. L., Kiely, J. M., and Campbell, D. C.: Idiopathic thrombocytopenic purpura. Arch. Intern. Med. 108:733, 1961.

270. Corn, M., and Upsham, J. D.: Evaluation of platelet antibodies in idiopathic thrombocytopenic purpura. Arch. Intern. Med. 109:157, 1962.

271. Ackroyd, J. F.: The immunological basis of purpura due to drug sensitivity. Proc. Roy. Soc. Med. 55:30, 1962.

272. Hill, J. M., and Loeb, E.: Massive hormonal therapy and splenectomy in acute thrombotic thrombocytopenic purpura. J.A.M.A. 173:778, 1960.

273. Borchgrevink, C. F.: Platelet adhesion in vivo in patients with bleeding disorders. Acta Med Scand. 170:231, 1961.

274. Bonnin, J. A., Cohen, A. K., and Hicks, N. D.: Coagulation defects in a case of systemic lupus erythematosus with thrombocytopenia. Brit. J. Haemat. 2:168, 1956.

275. Terragna, A., and Spirito, L.: Thrombocytopenic

purpura in an infant after administration of ace-tylsalicylic acid to the wet-nurse. Minerva Pediatr. *19*:613, 1967.

276. Quick, A. J.: Acetylsalicylic acid as a diagnostic aid in hemostasis. Amer. J. Med. Sci. *254*:392, 1967.

277. Derham, R. J., and Rogerson, M. M.: The Schönlein-Henoch syndrome and collagen disease. Arch. Dis. Child. *27*:139, 1952.

278. Djerassi, I., Farber, S., and Evans, A. E.: Transfusions of fresh platelets concentrates to patients with secondary thrombocytopenia. N. Engl. J. Med. *268*:221, 1963.

279. Cooper, T., Stickney, J. M., Pease, G. L., and Bennett, W. A.: Thrombotic thrombocytopenic purpura. Amer. J. Med. *13*:374, 1952.

280. Panner, B.: Nephritis of Schönlein-Henoch syndrome. Arch. Path. *74*:230, 1962.

281. Haggerty, R. J., and Eley, R. C.: Varicella and cortisone. Pediatrics 78:160, 1956.

282. Reynolds, R., and Etsten, B.: Anesthesia for splenectomy in patients with blood dyscrasia. J.A.M.A. *164*:137, 1957.

283. Jacoby, J., Hamelberg, W., and Jones, J., Jr.: Hypersplenism as an anesthetic problem. Anesth. Analg. *39*:527, 1962.

284. Touvet, J., Montague, J., Julien, M., and Larrieu. J. M.: Quelques reflexions sur l'anesthesie et la reanimation dans la chirurgie due purpura thrombocytopenique. Anesth. Analg. (Paris) 22:577, 592, 1965.

285. Wilkinson, F., and McKeage, F. J.: Anesthesia for splenectomy. Canad. Med. Assoc. J. *47*:553, 1947.

286. Saunders, W. H.: Hereditary hemorrhagic telangiectasia. Arch. Otolaryng. 76:245, 1962.

287. Merskey, C.: The occurrence of haemophilia in the human female. Quart. J. Med. *20*:299, 1951.

288. Whissell, D. Y., Hoag, M. S., Aggeler, P. M., Kropatkin, M., and Garner, E.: Hemophilia in a woman. Amer. J. Med. 38:119, 1965.

289. Graham, J. B., Barrow, E. M., and Roberts, H. R.: Possible implications of the autosomal and X-linked hemophilia phenotypes. Thromb. et Diath. Haemorrh. Suppl. *17*:151, 1965.

290. Patek, A. J., Jr., and Taylor, F. H. L.: Hemophilia. II. Some properties of a substance obtained from normal human plasma effective in accelerating the coagulation of hemophilic blood. J. Clin. Invest. *16*:113, 1937.

291. Biggs, R., and MacFarlane, R. G.: Hemophilia and related conditions. Brit. J. Haematol. *4*:1, 1958.

292. Fudeta, H., Hashimoto, Y. K., and Mori, K.: Anesthesia in patients with hemophilia A and B. Japan. J. Anesth. 25:718, 1976.

293. Brinkhaus, K. M.: The Hemophilias. Chapel Hill, N. C., University of North Carolina Press, 1964, p. 69.

294. Stites, D. P., Hershgold, E. J., Perlman, J. D., et al.: Factor VIII detection by hemagglutination inhibition: Hemophilia A and von Willebrand's disease. Science *171*:196, 1971.

295. Bloom, A. L.: Immunological detection of blood coagulation factors in hemorrhagic disorders. *In* Haffhrand, A. V., et al.: Recent Advances in Haematology. London, Churchill-Livingston, 1977.

296. Pearson, H. A.: Recent Advances in Hematology. Pediatrics 69:466, 1966.

297. McMillan, C. W., Diamond, L. D., and Surgenor, P. M.: Treatment of classic hemophilia: Use of fibrinogen rich in Factor VIII for hemorrhage and surgery. N. Engl. J. Med. *265*:224, 1961.

298. Kekwick, R. A., and Wolf, P.: A concentrate of human antihaemophilic factor — its use in six cases of haemophilia. Lancet *1*:647, 1957.

299. Wagner, R. H., McLester, W. D., Smith, M., and Brinkhaus, K. M.: Purification of antihemophilic factor (Factor VIII) by amino acid precipitation. Thromb. Diath. Haemorrh. *12*:64, 1964.

300. Pool, J. G., and Shannon, A. E.: Production of high-potency concentrates of antihemophilic globulin in a closed bag system. N. Engl. J. Med. *273*:1443, 1965.

301. Fraenkel, G. J.: Surgery in hemophilia. J. Roy. Coll. Surg., Edinburgh 3:54, 1957.

302. Kasper, C. K., Dietrick, S. L., and Rappaport, S. I.: Hemophilia prophylaxis with Factor VIII concentrates. Arch. Intern. Med. *125*:1004, 1970.

303. Lazerson, J.: Prophylactic infusion therapy in hemophilia. Hosp. Pract. *12*:49, 1979.

304. Aronstein, A.: Prophylaxis in haemophilia: A double blind control trial. Brit. J. Haematol. *33*:81, 1976.

305. Sampson, J. F., Hamstra, R., Aldrete, J. A.: Management of hemophiliac patients undergoing surgical procedures. Anesth. Analg. 58:113, 1979.

306. Dufour, J., D'Auteuil, P., and Dionne, P.: Tooth extraction under hypnosis in a hemophiliac. Rev. Franc. Odontostomat. *15*:955, 1968.

307. Trieger, N., and McGovern, J. J.: Evaluation of corticosteroids in hemophilia. N. Engl. J. Med. *266*:432, 1962.

308. Sinclair, J. H.: Loss of blood following the removal of teeth in normal and hemophiliac patients. Oral Surg. *23*:415, 1967.

309. Lucas, O. N., Finkelman, A., and Tocantins, L. M.: Management of tooth extraction in hemophiliacs by the combined use of hypnotic suggestion, protective splints and packing of socket. J. Oral Surg. *20*:488, 1962.

310. Yonezawa, T.: A case report: Local cooling under tourniquet on hand surgery for a hemophilic patient. Japan. J. Anesth. *14*:141, 1965.

311. Wadwa, S., and Bahl, C. P.: Repeated anaesthesia in a hemophilic patient. J. Indian Med. Assoc. *49*:435, 1967.

312. Simon, E., Roux, C., and Moret, J.: Drug combinations in the treatment of pain in hemophiliacs. Bibl. Haemat. *26*:78, 1966.

313. Neumark E.: What to avoid in the treatment of pain in hemophilia. Bibl. Haemat. *26*:87, 1966.

314. Alagille, D.: Treatment of pain in hemophiliacs. Sem. Ther. *39*:588, 1963.

315. Hrodek, O., and Norakova, M.: The treatment of pain and some psychological problems in the hemophiliac. Bibl. Haemat. *26*:73, 1966.

316. Bithell, T. C., Pizarro, A., and MacDiarmid, W. D.: Variant of Factor IX deficiency in female with 45, X Turner's syndrome. Blood *36*:169, 1970.

317. Brafield, A. J., Madras, M. B., and Case, J.: The stability of Christmas factor. A guide to the management of Christmas disease. Lancet 2:867, 1956.

318. Aggeler, P. M.: Plasma thromboplastin component (PTC) deficiency: A new disease resembling hemophilia. Proc. Soc. Exper. Biol. Med. 79:692, 1952.

319. Bruning, P. F., and Loeliger, E. A.: Prothrombal: A new concentrate of human prothrombin complex for clinical use. Brit. J. Haemat. 21:377, 1971.

320. Hoag, M. S., Johnson, F., and Robinson, J.: Treatment of hemophilia B with a new clotting factor concentrate. N. Engl. J. Med. 280:581, 1969.

321. Kasper, C. K.: Surgical operation in hemophilia B. Use of Factor IX concentrate. Calif. Med. 113:4, 1970.

322. Biggs, R., Bidwell, E., Handley, D. A., MacFarlane, R. G., Trueta, J., Elliot-Smith, A., Dike, G. W. R., and Ash, B. J.: The preparation and assay of a Christmas-factor (Factor IX) concentrate and its use in the treatment of two patients. Brit. J. Haemat. 7:349, 1961.

323. Geratz, J. D., and Graham, J. B.: Plasma thromboplastic component (Christmas factor, Factor IX) levels in stored human blood and plasma. Thromb. Diath. Haemorrh. 4:376, 1960.

324. Graham, J. B.: Stuart clotting defect and Stuart factor. Thromb. Diath. Haemorrh. Suppl. 1:22, 1960.

325. Aballi, A. J., Banus, V. L., de Lamerens, S., and Rosenzweig, S.: Coagulation studies in the newborn period. IV. Deficiency of Stuart-Power factor as a part of the clotting defect of the newborn. Amer. J. Dis. Child. 9:549, 1959.

326. Lewis, J. H., and Ferguson, J. H.: Afibrinogenemia. Report of a case. Amer. J. Dis. Child. 88:711, 1954.

327. Quick, A. J.: Genetic aspects of hemostasis. A review. Thromb. Diath. Haemorrh. 20:209, 1968.

328. Gitlin, D., and Borges, W. H.: Studies on the metabolism of fibrinogen in two patients with congenital afibrinogenemia. Blood 8:679, 1953.

329. McFarlane, R. G.: A boy with no fibrinogen. Lancet 1:309, 1938.

330. Barry, A., and Delage, J. M.: Congenital deficiency of fibrin stabilizing factor: Observation of a new case. N. Engl. J. Med. 272:943, 1965.

331. Hougie, C., Barrow, E. M., and Graham, J. B.: Stuart clotting defect. I. Segregation of a hereditary hemorrhagic state from the heterogeneous group heretofore called "stable factor" (SPCA, proconvertin, Factor VII) deficiency. J. Clin. Invest. 36:485, 1957.

332. Ackroyd, J. F.: Function of Factor VII. Brit. J. Haemat. 2:397, 1956.

333. Dische, F. E.: Blood-clotting substances with "Factor VII" activity: A comparison of some congenital and acquired deficiency. Brit. J. Haemat. 4:201, 1958.

334. Furnival, C. M., McKenzie, R. J., Blumgart, L. H.: The mechanism of impaired coagulation after partial hepatectomy in the dog. Surg. Gynec. Obstet. 143:81, 1976.

335. Beck, E., Duchert, F., Ernst, M.: The influence of fibrin stabilizing factor on the growth of fibroblasts in vitro and wound healing. Thromb. Diath. Haemorrh. 6:485, 1961.

336. Ikkala, E., and Mevonlinna, J. R.: Congenital deficiency of fibrin stabilizing factor. Thromb. Diath. Haemorrh. 7:567, 1962.

337. Hardisty, R. M., and Pinninger, J. L.: Congenital afibrinogenemia: Further observations on the blood coagulation mechanism. Brit. J. Haemat. 2:139, 1956.

338. Graham, J. B.: Biochemical genetic speculations provoked by considering the enigma of von Willebrand's disease. Thromb. Diath. Haemorrh. Suppl. 11:119, 1963.

339. Biggs, R., and Matthews, J. M.: The treatment of hemorrhage in von Willebrand's disease and the blood level of Factor VIII (AGH). Brit. J. Haematol. 9:203, 1963.

340. Cornu, P., Larrieu, M. J., Caen, J., and Bernard, J.: Transfusion studies in von Willebrand's disease. Effect on bleeding time and Factor VIII. Brit. J. Haematol. 9 189, 1963.

341. Blomback, M., Jorpes, J. E., and Nilsson, I. M.: Von Willebrand's disease. Amer. J. Med. 34:263, 1963.

342. Quick, A. J.: Platelets in the Minot-von Willebrand syndrome. Thromb. Diath. Haemorrh. 12:313, 1967.

343. Blackburn, E. K.: Primary capillary haemorrhage (including von Willebrand's disease). Brit. J. Haematol. 7:239, 1961.

344. Zucker, M. B.: In vitro abnormality of the blood in von Willebrand's disease correctable by normal plasma. Nature 197:601, 1963.

345. Caen, J., and Cousin, C.: Le trouble d'adhésivité "in vivo" des plaquettes dans la maladie de Willebrand et les thromboasthénnies de Glanzmann. Nouv. Rev. Franc. Hemat. 2:685, 1962.

346. Quick, A. J.: Salicylates and bleeding: The aspirin tolerance test. Amer. J. Med. Sci. 252:265, 1966.

347. Quick, A. J.: Bleeding time after aspirin ingestion. Lancet 1:50, 1968.

348. Perkins, H.: Correction of the hemostatic defects in von Willebrand's disease. Blood 30:375, 1967.

349. Bowes, J. B.: Anaesthetic management of haemothorax and haemoptysis due to von Willebrand's disease. Brit. J. Anaesth. 41:894, 1969.

350. Larrieu, M. J., Caen, J., Lelong, J. C., and Bernard, J.: Maladie de Glanzmann. Nouv. Rev. Franc. Hemat. 1:662, 1961.

351. Haridsty, R. M., Dormandy, K. M., and Hutton, R. A.: Thromboasthenia. Brit. J. Haemat. 10:371, 1964.

352. Van Creveld, S., Ho, L. K., and Veder, H. A.: Thrombopathia. Acta Haemat. 19:199, 1958.

353. Rodriguez-Erdman, F.: Bleeding due to increased intravascular blood coagulation. Hemorrhagic syndromes caused by consumption of blood-clotting factors (consumption coagulopathies). N. Engl. J. Med. 273:1370, 1965.

354. Cafferata, H. T., Aggeler, P. M., Robinson, A. J., and Blaisdell, F. W.: Intravascular coagulation in the surgical patient. Amer. J. Surg. 118:281, 1969.

355. Verstraete, M., Amery, A., and Vermylen, C.: Diagnostic hints for intravascular coagulation and its treatment with heparin. Acta Clin. Belg. 18:480, 1963.

356. Rapaport, S. I., Tatter, D., Coeur-Barron, N., and Hjort, P. F.: Pseudomonas septicemia with intravascular clotting leading to generalized

Shwartzman reaction. N. Engl. J. Med. 271:80, 1964.

357. Corrigan, J. J., Jr., Ray, W. L., and May, N.: Changes in the blood coagulation system associated with septicemia. N. Engl. J. Med. 279:851, 1968.

358. Starzl, T. E., Boehming, H. J., Amemiya, H., Wilson, C. B., Dixon, F. J., and Giles, G. R., Simpson, K. M., and Halgrimson, C. G.: Clotting changes, including disseminated intravascular coagulation during rapid renal homograft rejection. N. Engl. J. Med. 283:383, 1970.

359. Kasabach, H. H., and Merritt, K. K.: Capillary hemangioma with extensive purpura. Amer. J. Dis. Child. 59:1063, 1970.

360. Pelletier, L. L., Bond, D. M., Romig, D. A., et al.: Disseminated intravascular coagulation and hepatic necrosis. Complications of infectious mononucleosis. J.A.M.A. 235:1144, 1976.

361. Margolis, J.: Activation of Hageman factor by saturated fatty acids. Austr. J. Exper. Biol. Med. Sci. 40:505, 1962.

362. Good, R. A., and Thomas, L.: Inhibition by heparin of local and generalized Shwartzman reactions. J. Lab. Clin. Med. 40:804, 1952.

363. Shapiro, S. S., and McKay, D. G.: Prevention of generalized Shwartzman reaction with sodium warfarin. J. Exp. Med. 107:377, 1958.

364. Albrechtson, O. K., and Skjodt, P.: Complications during fibrinogen therapy in case of abruptio placentae. Acta Obst. Gynec. Scand. 43:129, 1964.

365. McKay, D. G., and Corey, A. E.: Cryofibrinogenemia in toxemia of pregnancy. Obstet. Gynec. 23:508, 1964.

366. Reid, D. E., Weinger, A. E., and Roby, C. C.: Intravascular clotting and afibrinogenemia, presumptive lethal factors in syndrome of amniotic fluid embolism. Amer. J. Obstet. Gynec. 66:465, 1953.

367. Reid, H. A., Chan, K. E., and Thean, K. C.: Prolonged coagulation defect in Malayan viper bite. Lancet 1:621, 1963.

368. Korst, D. R., and Kratochvil, C. H.: "Cryofibrinogen" in case of lung neoplasm associated with thrombophlebitis migrans. Blood 10:945, 1955.

369. McKally, M., and Vasicka, A.: Generalized Shwartzman reaction and hypofibrinogenemia in septic abortion. Obstet. Gynec. 19:359, 1962.

370. Kunzer, W., and Aalam, F.: Treatment of acute haemolytic uraemia syndrome with heparin. Lancet 1:1106, 1964.

371. Botti, R. E., and Ratnoff, O. D.: Clot-promoting effect of soaps on long chain fatty acids. J. Clin. Invest. 42:1569, 1963.

372. Meeks, E. A., Jay, J. B., and Heaton, L. D.: Thrombocytopenic purpura occurring with large hemangioma. Amer. J. Dis. Child. 90:349, 1951.

373. McNamara, J. J., Burran, E. L., Stremple, J. F., et al.: Coagulopathy after major combat injury. Am. Surg. 176:243, 1972.

374. Miller, R. D.: Complications of massive blood transfusions. Anesthesiology 39:82, 1973.

375. Ellison, N.: Diagnosis and management of bleeding disorders. Anesthesiology 47:171, 1977.

376. Attar, S., Boyd, A., Layne, E., McLaughlin, J., and Mansberger, A. R.: Alterations in coagulation and fibrinolytic mechanisms in acute trauma. J. Trauma 9:939, 1969.

377. Clifton, E. E.: Possibilities of development of fibrinolytic activity with new and projected agents. Angiologica (Basel) 5:146, 1968.

378. Maeck, J. V., and Billiaucus, H.: Heparin in treatment of toxemia of pregnancy: Preliminary report. Amer. J. Obstet. Gynec. 55:326, 1948.

379. Von Franken, I., Johnson, L., Olsson, P., and Betterquist, L.: Heparin treatment of bleeding. Lancet 1:70, 1963.

380. Saba, H. I., Herion, J. C., Walker, R. I., et al.: Effect of lysosomal cationic proteins from polymorphonuclear leukocytes upon the fibrinogen and fibrinolysis system. Thromb. Res. 7:543, 1975.

381. Graham, G. A., Emerson, C. P., and Angle, T. J.: Postoperative hypofibrinogenemia: Diffuse intravascular thrombosis after fibrinogen administration. N. Engl. J. Med. 257:101, 1957.

382. Guimbretiere, J., and Lebeaupin, P. R.: Acideepsilon-aminocaproique: Premiers resultats therapeutiques dans certain syndromes hemorragiques. Anesth. Analg. (Paris) 21:339, 1964.

383. Von Kaulla, K. N.: Synthetic activators of fibrinolysis which possess anticoagulant property. Experientia 21:439, 1965.

384. Nilsson, I. M., Bjorkman, S. E., and Anderson, L.: Clinical experiences with ε-aminocaproic acid as antifibrinolytic agent. Acta Med. Scand. 170:487, 1961.

385. Bernstock, L., and Hirson, C.: Thrombotic thrombocytopenic purpura. Remission on treatment with heparin. Lancet 1:28, 1960.

386. Cuocolo, R. Spamrinato, N., and Pica, M.: Behavior of hematic fibrinolytic activity in relation to various types of anesthesia. Rass. Int. Clin. Ter. 45:731, 1965.

387. Kuznetsova, B. A., and Zhilin, I. U. N.: The effect of anesthesia on the blood coagulation system and fibrinolytic activity in patients with pulmonary tuberculosis. Grudn. Khir. 9:66, 1967.

388. Baudo, F., Cipriani, D., and De Cataldo, F.: Coagulation disorders with consumption of coagulation factors, probably due to drug hypersensitivity. Minerva Med. 58:4618, 1967.

389. Baker, R. J., Moinichen, S. L., and Nyhus, L. M.: Blood transfusion reaction: A reappraisal of surgical incidence and significance. Ann. Surg. 169:684, 1969.

390. Perkins, H. A., Payne, R., Ferguson, J., and Wood, M.: Nonhemolytic febrile transfusion reactions. Vox Sang. 11:578, 1966.

391. Merritt, J. A., and Maloney, W. C.: Untoward reactions to blood transfusions. N. Engl. J. Med. 274:1426, 1966.

392. Freisleben, E.: Elucidation of transfusion reactions. Scand. J. Clin. Invest. (Suppl. 100)19:16, 1967.

393. Jaeger, R. J., and Rubin, R. J.: Plasticizers from plastic devices: Extraction, metabolism and accumulation by biological systems. Science 170:460, 1970.

394. Halmagyi, D. F., Stargecki, B., McRae, J., and Homer, G. J.: The lung as the main target organ in the acute phase of transfusion reaction in the sheep. J. Surg. Res. 3:418, 1963.

395. Giesecke, A. H.: Identification of transfusion

reactions during anesthesia. Anesth. Analg. 42:121, 1961.

396. Perkins, H. A.: Postoperative coagulation defects. Anesthesiology 27:456, 1966.

397. Bluemle, L. W.: Hemolytic transfusion reactions causing acute renal failure. Postgrad. Med. 38:484, 1965.

398. Schmidt, P. J., and Holland, P. V.: Pathogenesis of acute renal failure associated with incompatible transfusion. Lancet 2:1169, 1967.

399. Binder, J. C.: Incompatible blood transfusions during operation. Brit. J. Anaesth. 31:271, 1959.

400. Howland, W. S., Jacobs, R. G., and Goulet, A. H.: An evaluation of calcium administration during rapid blood replacement. Anesth. Analg. 39:557, 1960.

401. Spellman, G. C.: Corticosteroid treatment of transfusion reaction from incompatible blood of ABO type. J.A.M.A. 169:1622, 1959.

402. Bunker, J. P., Bendixen, H. H., and Murphy, A. J.: Hemodynamic effects of intravenously administered sodium citrate. N. Engl. J. Med. 266:372, 1962.

403. Nahas, G. C., Manger, W. M., and Ultmann, J. E.: Transfusion acidosis. Bibl. Haemat. 19:610, 1964.

404. Mondzetenowski, J. P., Guy, J. T., Bromberg, P. A., Metz, E. N., and Balcerzak, S. P.: Oxygen delivery following transfusion of stored blood. II. Acidotic rats. J. App. Physiol. 37:64, 1974.

405. Howland, W. S., Schweizer, O., and Boyan, C. P.: The effect of buffering on the mortality of massive blood replacement. Surg. Gynec. Obstet. 121:777, 1965.

406. Howland, W. S., Schweizer, O., and Boyan, C. P.: Massive blood replacement without calcium administration. Surg. Gynec. Obstet. 119:814, 1964.

407. Kahn, R. C., Jascott, D., Carlon, G. C., Schweizer, O., et al.: Massive blood replacement: Correlation of ionized calcium, citrate, and hydrogen ion concentration. Anesth. Analg. 58:274, 1979.

408. Howland, W. S., Schweizer, D., Carlon, G. C., et al.: Cardiovascular effects of low levels of ionized calcium during massive transfusion. Surg. Gynec. Obstet. 145:581, 1977.

409. Carlon, G. C., Kahn, R. C., Bertoni, G., et al.: Rapid volume expansion in patients with interstitial lung disease. Anesth. Analg. 58:13, 1979.

410. Gervin, A. S., Mason, K. G., and Wright, C. B.: Microaggregate volumes in stored human blood. Surg. Gynec. Obstet. 139:519, 1974.

411. Barrett, J., Davidson, I., and Dhurandhar, H. N.: Pulmonary microembolism associated with massive transfusion. II. The basic pathophysiology of its pulmonary effects. Ann. Surg. 182:56, 1975.

412. Marshall, B. E., Wurzel, H. A., Ellison, N., et al.: Microaggregate formation in stored blood. III. Comparison of Bentley, Fenwall, Pall and Swank micropore filtration. Circ. Shock 2:249, 1975.

413. Stanley, T. H., Hill, G. E., Portas, M. R., et al.: Neutrophil chemotaxis during and after general anesthesia and operation. Anesth. Analg. 55:668, 1976.

414. Cullen, B. F., Sample, W. F., and Chretien, P. B.: The effect of halothane on phytohemagglutinin-induced transformation of human lymphocytes in vitro. Anesthesiology 36:206, 1972.

415. Feinstein, M. B., Fiekers, J., and Fraser, C.: An analysis of the mechanism of local anesthetic inhibition of platelet aggregation and secretion. J. Pharmacol. Exp. Ther. 197:215, 1976.

416. Parbrook, G. E.: Therapeutic uses of nitrous oxide: A review. Brit. J. Anaesth. 40:365, 1968.

417. Bjornehoe, M., Ibsen, B., and Johnsen, S.: Case of tetanus treated with curare, tracheotomy and positive pressure ventilation with nitrous oxide and oxygen anesthesia. Ugeskr. Laeg. 115:1535, 1953.

418. Gormsen, J.: Agranulocytosis and thrombocytopenia in a case of tetanus treated with curare and chlorpromazine. Danish Med. Bull. 2:87, 1955.

419. Lassen, H. C. A., Henriksen, E., Neukirch, F., and Kristensen, H. S.: Treatment of tetanus: Severe bone marrow depression after prolonged nitrous oxide anesthesia. Lancet 2:527, 1956.

420. Wilson, P., Martin, F. I. R., and Last, P. M.: Bone marrow depression in tetanus: Report of a fatal case. Lancet 2:527, 1956.

421. Henriksen, E.: Tetanus and nitrous oxide anesthesia. Nordisk. Med. 56:1418, 1956.

422. Sando, M. J. W., and Lawrence, J. R.: Bone marrow depression following treatment of tetanus with protracted nitrous oxide anesthesia. Lancet 1:588, 1958.

423. Lassen, H. C., and Kristensen, H. S.: Remission of chronic myelogenous leukemia following prolonged nitrous oxide inhalation. Dan. Med. Bull. 6:252, 1959.

424. Petrovsky, B. V., and Yefuni, S. N.: Therapeutic inhalation anaesthesia. Brit. J. Anaesth. 37:42, 1965.

425. Lefemine, A. A., and Harken, D. E.: Postoperative care following open-heart operations: Routine use of controlled ventilation. J. Thor. Card. Surg. 52:207, 1966.

426. Parbrook, G. D.: Postoperative pain relief: Comparison of methadone and morphine when used concurrently with nitrous oxide anesthesia. Brit. Med. J. 2:616, 1966.

427. Green, C. D., and Eastwood, D. W.: Effects of nitrous oxide inhalation on hemopoiesis in rats. Anesthesiology 24:341, 1963.

428. Parbrook, G. D.: Exposure of experimental animals to nitrous oxide containing atmospheres. Brit. J. Anaesth. 39:119, 1967.

429. Parbrook, G. C.: Leucopenic effects of prolonged nitrous oxide treatment. Brit. J. Anaesth. 39:114, 1967.

430. Green, C. D.: Effects of nitrous oxide on RMA and DNA synthesis in the hemopoietic system. In Fink, B. R.: Toxicity of Anesthetics. Baltimore, Williams and Wilkins, 1968, pp. 114–122.

431. Brauer, R. W., Way, R. O., and Perry, R. A.: Anesthetic effects of hyperbaric environment. In

Fink, B. R.: Toxicity of Anesthetics. Baltimore, Williams and Wilkins, 1968, pp. 241–258.

432. Aldrete, J. A., and Virtue, R. W.: Effects of prolonged inhalation of hydrocarbon gases. Anesthesiology 28:238, 1967.

433. Aldrete, J. A., and Virtue, R. W.: Prolonged inhalation of inert gases by rats. Anesth. Analg. 46:562, 1967.

434. Aldrete, J. A., and Virtue, R. W.: Effects of prolonged inhalation of anesthetic and other gases on blood and marrow of rats. In Fink, B. R.: Toxicity of Anesthetics. Baltimore, Williams & Wilkins, 1968, pp. 105–113.

435. Aldrete, J. A.: Effects of prolonged inhalation of inhalation anesthetic agents on formed elements of blood and bone marrow of rats. Thesis for partial fulfillment of the requirements for the degree of Master of Sciences, University of Colorado Graduate School, June, 1967.

436. Bruce, D. L., and Koepke, J. A.: Changes in granulopoiesis in the rat associated with prolonged halothane anesthesia. Anesthesiology 27:811, 1966.

437. Paterson, E., Haddow, A., Thomas, I. A., and Watkinson, J. M.: Leukemia treated with urethane. Lancet 1:677, 1946.

438. Usenik, E. A., and Cronkite, E. P.: Effects of barbiturate anesthetics on leukocytes in normal and splenectomized dogs. Anesth. Analg. 44:167, 1965.

439. Nunn, J. F., Sturrock, J. E., and Howell, A.: Effect of inhalation anaesthetics on division of bone marrow cells in vitro. Brit. J. Anaesth. 48:75, 1976.

440. Stamenkovick, L., van Leersum, R. H., Dicke, K. A., et al.: Effects of droperidol and fentanyl on human bone marrow cultures. Anaesthesia 32:328, 1977.

441. Doll, R., Peto, R.: Mortality among doctors in different occupations. Brit. Med. J. 1:1433, 1977.

442. Lew, E. A.: Mortality experience among anesthesiologists, 1954–1976. Anesthesiology 51:195, 1979.

443. Hallen, B., Ehrner-Samuel, H., and Thomason, M.: Measurements of halothane in the atmosphere of an operating theatre and in expired air and blood of the personnel during routine anesthetic work. Acta Anaesth. Scand. 14:17, 1970.

444. Usubiaga, L., Aldrete, J. A., and Fiserova-Bergerova, V.: Influence of gas flows and operating room ventilation on the daily exposure of anesthetists to halothane. Anesth. Analg. 51:968, 1972.

445. McIntyre, J. W. R., and Russel, J. C.: Removal of halothane and methoxyflurane from waste anaesthetic vapours. Canad. Anaesth. Soc. J. 14:333, 1967.

446. Thuries, S.: Methoxyflurane et coagulation. Anesth. Analg. Reanim. 22:593, 1965.

447. Smith, E. B., Petty, W. C., and Carr, J. S.: Effect of methoxyflurane on clotting properties in the rat, dog, and man. American Society of Anesthesiology, Annual Meeting, San Francisco, October 27, 1969.

448. Meda, I.: The effects of volatile general anesthetics on adenosine-diphosphate-induced platelet aggregation. Anesthesiology 34:405, 1971.

449. Lichtenfeld, K. M., Schiffer, C. A., and Helrich, M.: Platelet aggregation during and after general anesthesia and surgery. Anesth. Analg. 58:293, 1979.

9

Gastrointestinal Disorders

By RICHARD P. SAIK, M.D., CLIFF CHADWICK, M.D.,
and JORDAN KATZ, M.D.

Nausea and Vomiting
Fistula
Planned Fistulas
Obstruction
Constipation and Diarrhea
GI Bleeding: Hematemesis, Melena, Rectal
  Bleeding
Malabsorption
Surgical Nutrition
Peritonitis
Liver Disease
Jaundice
Disorders of the Esophagus
  Diverticula
  Achalasia
  Diffuse Esophageal Spasm
  Paraesophageal Hernia
  Esophageal Perforation
  Esophageal Moniliasis
  Corrosive Esophagitis
  Reflux Esophagitis and Stricture
  Barrett's Syndrome
  Benign Neoplasms
  Esophageal Webs
  Mallory-Weiss Syndrome
  Lower Esophageal Ring
  Esophageal Disturbances Associated with
    Systemic Disease
Disorders of the Stomach and Duodenum
  Foreign Bodies
  Corrosive Gastritis
  Association of Gastric and Duodenal
    Ulceration with Other Diseases
  Suppurative Gastritis
  Granulomatous Gastritis
  Neoplasms of the Stomach
  Gastric Volvulus
  Vagotomy Operations with Intraoperative
    Testing
Disorders of the Small Intestine
  Neoplasms of the Small Intestine
  Peutz-Jeghers Syndrome
  Vascular Lesions
  Regional Enteritis (Crohn's Disease)
  Tuberculous Enteritis

Typhoid Enteritis
Diverticula
Radiation Enteritis
Pneumatosis Cystoides Intestinalis
Bypass Operations for Obesity
Disorders of the Large Intestine
  Ulcerative Colitis
  Granulomatous Colitis (Crohn's Disease)
  Pseudomembranous Colitis
  Actinomycosis
  Amebiasis
  Tuberculosis
  Ischemic Colitis
  Schistosomiasis
  Villous Adenomas
  Gardner's Syndrome
  Chagas' Disease
  Volvulus
  Angiodysplasia
Disorders of the Pancreas
  Pancreatitis
  Pancreatic Cysts
  Cystic Fibrosis in Adults
Disorders of the Liver
  Pyogenic Liver Abscess
  Amebic Liver Abscess
  Echinococcosis (Hydatid Disease)
  Primary Carcinoma
  Major Hepatic Resection
  Gilbert's Syndrome
  Dubin-Johnson Syndrome
  Drugs and the Liver
Disorders of the Gallbladder and
  Extrahepatic Biliary System
  Choledochal Cysts
  Gallstone Ileus
  Ascending Cholangitis
  Primary Sclerosing Cholangitis
  Carcinoma of the Biliary Tree
Anesthetic Considerations
  General Considerations
  Vomiting
  Fluid Replacement
  Parenteral Nutrition
  Specific Disorders

Many diseases of the gastrointestinal tract with different causes develop similar alterations of function. The first portion of this chapter is devoted to a discussion of pathophysiologic processes common to many of the disease entities mentioned. After this, selected individual disorders of the gastrointestinal system are briefly described. Finally, anesthetic implications are presented, again covering alterations common to many diseases and, in appropriate instances, suggestions relevant to a particular disorder.

NAUSEA AND VOMITING

Nausea and vomiting may occur separately but are closely allied. Nausea is the sensation of an iminent need to vomit. Nausea usually precedes vomiting, which may be associated with almost any disease of the gastrointestinal tract and can lead to a variety of complications. In spite of its frequency, the act of vomiting is not well understood physiologically. Most neurophysiologists agree that a center controlling vomiting exists in the medulla oblongata through which all reflex arcs pass, whether peripheral or central. Actually two centers exist; one is a chemoreceptor implicated with drug-induced vomiting and the other is an integrating center concerned with the act itself.

Afferent fibers are known to arise in the gastrointestinal tract and run via the vagal and sympathetic pathways, yet neither vagotomy and/or sympathectomy alone abolishes vomiting of peritonitis.

The major etiologic factors in vomiting include stimuli from the gastrointestinal tract, central causes, and blood borne factors. The gastrointestinal causes are varied. Obstruction will mechanically cause vomiting, and the higher the level of obstruction, the more rapid the onset. Inflammatory diseases such as appendicitis induce vomiting via visceral reflexes, as does distention of the bowel.

Vomiting can lead to laceration of the gastroesophageal mucosa with severe bleeding (Mallory-Weiss syndrome) or spontaneous rupture of the esophagus (Boerhaave's syndrome). Aspiration of vomitus can produce severe respiratory problems (Mendelson's syndrome). More frequently, the clinical problems are due to metabolic, fluid, electrolyte, and acid-base alterations resulting from the gastrointestinal fluid loss. The nature and severity of these changes are due to multiple factors (the basic disease, the pathophysiological processes leading to the vomitus, the intensity and duration of vomiting, and the quantity and quality of the vomitus).

Initially, the significant physiologic alteration is loss of extracellular volume caused by the loss of water and electrolytes. With persistent vomiting, acid-base and electrolyte abnormalities become more evident. These changes will vary, depending upon the electrolyte and hydrogen ion lost, because the vomitus may consist of gastric juice primarily or a mixture of gastric juice, intestinal secretion, pancreatic secretion, and bile.

If the loss is primarily gastric juice, metabolic alkalosis results, owing to the rapid loss of hydrogen and chloride ions and the accumulation of bicarbonate ions in the blood. With the accumulation of bicarbonate ions, the rate and depth of respiration may be decreased in an attempt by the body to conserve HCO_3. There may be partial restoration of the blood pH toward normal.

Metabolic alkalosis is often accompanied by hypokalemia. In addition to the potassium being lost in gastric juice, there may be an increase in the renal excretion of potassium. With the reduction of extracellular potassium concentration, there is a shift of hydrogen and sodium into the cells in exchange for potassium, and this may then result in an intracellular acidosis with a coexistent extracellular alkalosis. In addition, despite the extracellular alkalosis, the urine may be found to be acid.

If the vomitus contains intestinal secretion (bile and pancreatic secretion in addition to gastric juice), the shift in acid-base balance may be toward metabolic acidosis, depending upon the electrolyte and hydrogen ion concentrations in the vomitus.

Fluid therapy is based upon the replacement of fluid volume and electrolytes. Replacement of chloride is essential, and this can usually be accomplished with administration of normal saline solutions. With hypokalemia, KCl should also be administered to correct the potassium and chloride deficit once urine output is adequate. If vomiting is due to causes other than gastric outlet obstruction, saline solutions may still be used for the initial fluid therapy, because volume replacement is probably the most important factor. The subsequent solution should be based upon the clinical response and the blood electrolyte concentrations and pH.

FISTULAS

Gastrointestinal fistulas are abnormal communications between the stomach or intestine and another segment of bowel, a hollow viscus (bladder, ureter, gallbladder), blood vessel, or skin. The important clinical problems are related to fluid and electrolyte losses, malnutrition, infection, and skin irritation. The severity of the physiological alterations will be determined in part by the location, the extent of the gastrointestinal tract bypassed by the fistula, the size, and the duration of drainage. The majority of acute fistulas are secondary to surgical procedures and may be due to suture line leaks, anastomotic disruptions, or suturing or injuring the bowel during abdominal closure. Others may arise from inflammatory processes, ischemic necrosis of the bowel, or tumor. Adequate nutritional management is essential for all external gastrointestinal fistulas. Spontaneous closure is more than twice as likely (89 per cent versus 37 per cent) in patients receiving over 1600 calories a day compared with those who did not. Mortality rates range from 6 to 21 per cent but are highest (52 per cent) in those who have had irradiation for malignant disease. The best operative approach is excision of the involved area and anastomosis.

Gastric and Duodenal Fistulas. These fistulas are usually complications of gastric or duodenal surgery, especially gastric resection, and arise from gastrojejunal or duodenal stumps. The fluid loss from these is often great, because they may discharge up to 7 liters per day. The initial major problem is the rapid dehydration that occurs. Electrolyte and acid-base abnormalities are related to the composition of the fistula output; the fluid may be acid or alkaline, because it is a mixture of gastric, duodenal, jejunal, pancreatic, or biliary secretions. Decompression of the stomach, rational antibiotic therapy, and total parenteral nutrition have become essential to the management of these patients.

Gastrojejunocolic Fistula. Stomal ulcer-

ation may be responsible for a direct communication between the stomach and the transverse colon. It is not the bypass of the intestine by gastric contents that causes the diarrhea but the reflux of feces into the small bowel and the resulting irritation and increased bacterial growth. Resulting malabsorption in diarrhea can be corrected by a proximal colostomy, allowing adequate nutrition before definitive and more radical surgery.

Small Bowel Fistulas. Although the output of this fistula may vary, depending on size and other factors such as distal obstruction, the output is usually lower than in duodenal fistula. In general, the higher the fistula is in the small bowel, the more serious is the problem. Not only is the amount of fluid and electrolyte loss greater (3 to 5 liters of fluid lost are not uncommon) but also a larger segment of intestine is functionally lost for absorption and nutrition. It is important to identify the site of the fistula and ascertain if there is distal obstruction as soon as possible. Barium studies and fistulograms are useful for this purpose and may also determine if an abscess cavity exists or if more than one segment of the intestine is involved. Serious infection with septicemia or peritonitis is a prominent feature of small bowel and colonic fistulas, resulting in death in 85 per cent of these patients.

Colonic Fistulas. The fluid and electrolyte losses from these fistulas usually do not produce serious clinical problems, because the losses are similar to those from ileostomies and colostomies. Nutrition is usually also not a problem. However, these fistulas may be associated with intraperitoneal abscesses or infection and with wound infection.

Pancreatic Fistulas. These fistulas may develop as a result of ductal disruption secondary to trauma, surgery, or drainage of pseudocysts. The volume loss rarely exceeds 1.5 liters a day, although it may be as high as 2.5 liters. Volume depends upon the amount of gland drained by the fistula. The fluid loss may be hypertonic with respect to plasma. Fluid and electrolyte depletion is not common unless the fistula drains most of the pancreas. Diagnosis is confirmed by the elevated amylase content. Almost all will close spontaneously but vigorous fluid replacement is indicated. Malnutrition due to loss of enzymes may require enzyme replacement. Pure pancreatic fistulas will not affect the surrounding skin. If autodigestion and irritation of the surrounding skin occur, then either infection is present or the fistula is mixed with small bowel content, thus activating the pancreatic enzymes.

Biliary Fistulas. These fistulas may be external or internal and partial or complete. External biliary fistulas are usually complications of operations on the gallbladder or biliary tract (ligature slipping off the cystic duct or injury to the common duct). The volume output may vary from 250 to 1500 ml per day, which may result in electrolyte depletion with a greater loss of base than acid (low chloride and high concentration of bicarbonate). Internal fistulas may occur with kidney, ureter, and other parts of the gastrointestinal tract, and may lead to acute or chronic cholangitis secondary to the inflammatory mass. Prothrombin deficiency can also occur secondary to malabsorption of vitamin K. These fistulas also lead to steatorrhea and excessive loss of calcium, progressing to osteoporosis. Another complication associated with an internal fistula is bowel obstruction presenting as gallstone ileus.

Gastroileal Fistula. This fistula is caused by anastomosing the stomach to the ileum instead of the jejunum in performing a gastrojejunostomy, resulting in rapid weight loss, diarrhea, and inanition. A marginal ulcer can occur in the ileum near the anastomosis, and severe bleeding may result.

Urinary Enteric Fistulas. Pyeloduodenal fistulas may result secondary to operative trauma, infection, or erosion of a calculus. The major physiological alteration is due to the urine passing into the duodenum with absorption of an excessive amount of chloride, leading to a hyperchloremic acidosis. A rectovesical or colovesical fistula may be associated with rectal neoplasm, diverticulitis, or an endoscopic procedure or operation; it usually results in a chronic urinary tract infection.

Ileostomy. Although recent improvements in techniques and care of ileostomies have reduced some of the problems associated with them, complications may still occur. Some of these are intestinal obstruction, retraction, stenosis, prolapse, ileostomy dysfunction, and stomal fistulas. The usual output of a mature ileostomy is 500 to 700 cc per day. Ileostomy dysfunction, which is probably due to a partial obstruction of the ileostomy, may lead to increased bowel motility and pressure, resulting in fulminating losses of small bowel contents through the opening. Another complication associated with an ileostomy is a high incidence of renal calculi.

Planned Fistulas. Many fistulas are created for therapeutic purposes and must be considered in the same light as the pathological entities described above. Temporary gastrostomies or nasogastric drainage mimics gastric fistula. Esophagostomy, ileostomy, and colostomy may all be performed as a preliminary to bypassing an area of pathology and leak. Long intestinal tubes used in therapy for small bowel obstruction may have been in place for a week or more, similarly creating a functional small bowel fistula.

OBSTRUCTION

Esophagus. Esophageal obstruction may be acute or chronic. The etiology is quite variable and includes foreign body, carcinoma, neuromuscular disorders, stricture, or congenital anomalies. Clinical manifestations depend in part upon the onset, severity, extent, duration, and level of obstruction in addition to the cause.

Acute obstruction usually produces only a slight dilatation of the proximal esophagus with accumulation of secretions. With gradual obstruction there may be marked proximal dilatation. There is no retention of secretion or food initially, because the esophagus is able to compensate for the increased peripheral resistance by increased peristalsis. However, in time there is decompensation of the muscle with marked dilatation and retention of food and secretion. In acute obstruction the accumulation of secretion may produce aspiration pneumonia; chronic obstruction may lead to repeated episodes of aspiration pneumonia. Fortunately, unlike the pneumonia caused by aspiration of acid gastric juice, these attacks are usually mild. With chronic prolonged obstruction, all the consequences of starvation and malnutrition will also become evident.

Pylorus. Pyloric obstruction may be acute or chronic. With acute obstruction, vomiting is the prominent feature. The pathophysiological changes associated with vomiting caused by gastric outlet obstruction have been discussed. Pyloric obstruction may increase the volume of gastric secretion and thereby aggravate the loss of gastric juice by vomiting.

With a more gradual chronic pyloric obstruction, food retention may occur, which then leads to stimulation of gastric secretion via gastrin release; as a result, gastric erosion or ulcer may occur. With prolonged pyloric obstruction all the consequences of malnutrition may develop.

Small Intestine. The three most frequent causes of small intestinal obstruction are adhesions, internal hernia, and neoplasms of the bowel. Other causes include congenital abnormalities, volvulus, intussusception, inflammatory processes, trauma, and iatrogenesis (e.g., potassium-induced stricture, radiation changes). Mortality ranges from 1 to 3 per cent with adhesions and hernias to 41 per cent in those patients with obstruction from a malignancy. The relatively lower mortality rates become generally higher (20–40 per cent) when a strangulated obstruction is present. Eight per cent of mechanical bowel obstructions involve the small bowel, and only 20 per cent involve the colon. The severity of the altered physiological processes caused by the obstruction will depend upon the type of bowel obstruction, the location, the extent, and the duration.

Simple mechanical obstruction of the small intestine is physical obstruction of the bowel lumen without compromise of the bowel blood supply. The obstruction produces distention of the proximal bowel caused by the accumulation of fluid and gas. Fluid accumulates rapidly in the lumen as the result of a negative net flux of fluid across the mucosa. This negative flux is due chiefly to decreased absorption of water and electrolytes, but bowel distention also promotes increased intestinal secretions. Isotope studies have clearly demonstrated that absorption of ingested fluid and of upper gastrointestinal digestive secretions are but a part of a much larger exchange of fluid between the body and lumen of the gastrointestinal tract. A fasting individual ingesting 1000 cc of water will absorb 500 cc of that. In addition, he will have secreted and reabsorbed 5000 cc of fluid via the intestinal lumen. A net negative flux (absorption) of 500 cc thus normally occurs. In obstruction, a positive flux exists with decreased absorption as well as increased secretion; the percentage to which each mechanism participates is unclear. The fluid in the bowel consists of saliva, gastric juice, bile, pancreatic juice, and intestinal secretion (see Figure 9–1).

With continued secretion of intestinal fluid into the lumen and increase in dilatation of the bowel, there is further loss of fluid by accumulation of fluid in the wall of the bowel itself. This process may progress to exudation of the fluid into the peritoneal cavity. The edema of the bowel wall may further increase the loss into the third space by a decrease in absorptive capacity of the mucosa. In addition to these losses, fluid rich in electrolytes may be lost by vomiting and/or intestinal intubation. The intestinal gases are derived principally from swallowed air, and only a little results from bacterial fermentation and diffusion from blood. Normally, most of the gases are absorbed from the intestine, but this is also impaired. Stasis may also lead to bacterial growth in the small intestine. Much of the intestinal distention above a mechanical obstruction can be attributed to swallowed air (70 per cent nitrogen). Nitrogen diffuses poorly, since partial pressure differences between the plasma and the intestine are small. One of the major effects of intestinal intubation is to suck out swallowed air, thereby decreasing the harmful effects of the distention contributed by intestinal gas.

The vomiting and sequestration of fluid into the bowel lumen and wall may lead to hypovolemia, shock, renal insufficiency, and ultimately death. Initially the main disturbance is loss of volume and salt, but without treatment it may lead to acid-base disturbances. Unlike pyloric obstruction, obstruction of the intestine will alter the acid-base imbalance toward acidosis and hypokalemia. In addition to these changes, distention also decreases the effective pulmonary ventilation by elevating the diaphragm, adding a respiratory component to the acidosis.

A closed loop obstruction is obstruction of the bowel at two levels, thereby preventing movement of the gas and fluid within the segment in either an aboral or an adoral direction. This form of obstruction is dangerous, because it may progress rapidly to strangulation obstruction. A rapid transfer of fluid into the gut lumen occurs, along with

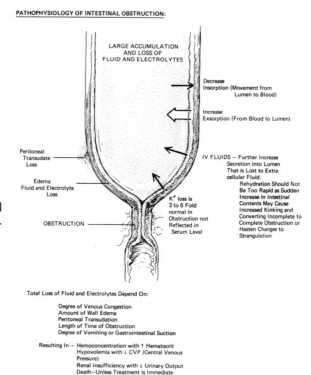

PATHOPHYSIOLOGY OF INTESTINAL OBSTRUCTION:

LARGE ACCUMULATION
AND LOSS OF
FLUID AND ELECTROLYTES

Decrease
Insorption (Movement from
Lumen to Blood)

Increase
Exsorption (From Blood to Lumen)

Peritoneal
Transudate
Loss

Edema
Fluid and Electrolyte
Loss

IV FLUIDS — Further Increase
Secretion into Lumen
That is Lost to Extra-
cellular Fluid.
Rehydration Should Not
Be Too Rapid as Sudden
Increase in Intestinal
Contents May Cause
Increased Kinking and
Converting Incomplete to
Complete Obstruction or
Hasten Changes to
Strangulation

K⁺ loss is
3 to 6 Fold
normal in
Obstruction not
Reflected in
Serum Level

OBSTRUCTION

Total Loss of Fluid and Electrolytes Depend On:

Degree of Venous Congestion
Amount of Wall Edema
Peritoneal Transudation
Length of Time of Obstruction
Degree of Vomiting or Gastrointestinal Suction

Resulting In — Hemoconcentration with ↑ Hematocrit
Hypovolemia with ↓ CVP (Central Venous
Pressure)
Renal Insufficiency with ↓ Urinary Output
Death—Unless Treatment is Immediate.

Figure 9–1. Pathophysiology of intestinal obstruction. (From Nadrowski, L. F.: Rev. Surg. *31*(6):381, 1974.)

rapid increase in the intraluminal pressure, which then leads to interference with the blood and lymph flow. This may then lead to ischemia and subsequent necrosis with all the complications associated with strangulated obstruction. With necrosis, perforation of this segment may occur.

Strangulated obstruction is obstruction of the lumen of the bowel associated with impairment of the bowel vascular supply. This type of obstruction involves the small bowel more frequently than the colon. In addition to the pathophysiological change noted above, other events occur, leading to an acute emergency. The vascular impairment first involves the venous return, producing extravasation of bloody fluid into the bowel wall and lumen, which in turn causes hypovolemia. With edema and further obstruction, the arterial return is compromised, producing necrosis of the bowel. Ischemia promotes an invasion of the bowel wall with bacteria, which may also pass across the bowel into the peritoneal cavity. There is production of both endo- and exotoxins. Absorption of these substances induces toxicity and septic shock.

Management is designed to have the patient in the best possible condition to undergo surgery and anesthesia. The patient with a strangulated obstruction is an immediate emergency, whereas a patient seen within 24 hours of a simple mechanical obstruction can be operated upon after a few hours of preparation including routine work-up, fluid replacement, x-rays, and gastric decompression. If obstruction has been present longer than 24 hours, it may be in the patient's best interest to have a longer period of preoperative preparation. Moderate hypokalemia may require 6 to 12 hours to restore potassium levels, but more severe abnormalities may take upwards of 24 to 36 hours. Colloid replacement may be necessary, and preoperative antibiotics are administered by most surgeons. Fluid replacement is guided by clinical signs, urine output, and central venous pressure. During this period, gastric decompression ("short tubes") removes gas and fluid, reducing the risk of aspiration and slowing the progression of distention. "Long tubes" (Miller-Abbott and Cantor are the most common) are useful to decompress the small bowel, thereby decreasing painful symptoms for the patient while making the operation easier for the surgeon by reducing the risk of enterotomy and increasing visibility during the procedure. Intestinal intubation is often used in definitive therapy for patients with

a) partial small bowel obstruction, b) carcinomatosis, and c) early postoperative obstruction. Long intestinal intubation should not be attempted for definitive treatment of complete obstruction, since the diagnosis of strangulation is often impossible clinically and the recurrence rate of obstruction, if intubation is successful, can be over 30 per cent.

Colon. Although mechanical obstruction of the colon also produces distention caused by accumulation of secretions and gas, it progresses more slowly than small bowel obstruction. The consequences of the progressive distention depend upon the competence of the ileocecal valve. If the valve is incompetent, there is partial decompression of the obstructed colon by reflux of fluid and gas into the ileum, with progressive dilatation of the small bowel and feculent vomiting. If the valve is competent, a closed loop obstruction results. The intraluminal pressure increases in the closed loop and may result in rupture. The cecum, because of its large diameter, is the most common site of rupture. The high intraluminal pressure may also compromise the circulation to the bowel and lead to patches of ischemia, gangrene, and eventually perforation.

Intestinal intubation slows the progression of distention but is not as effective as for small bowel obstruction. A barium enema preoperatively will often help to delineate the pathology and the level of obstruction. After fluid and electrolyte resuscitation, an immediate diverting colostomy is indicated.

Paralytic Ileus. Paralytic ileus implies physiologic obstruction of the intestine without physical obstruction of the lumen. Ileus occurs following all abdominal operations, and recovery is different in the different segments of the gastrointestinal tract. The common causes of non-operative ileus include intra-abdominal sepsis, retroperitoneal pathology such as hematoma, ureteral colic, neurological disease, and systemic causes such as toxemia and electrolyte abnormalities. There is lack of normal propulsion of gas and fluid distally because of diminished or absent peristalsis or uncoordinated propulsive movements. The basic mechanism is not entirely clear, but the sympathetic nervous system appears to play an important role. Usually the small bowel and large bowel are involved, with

marked distention caused by fluid accumulation and swallowed air. The sequestration of fluid in the bowel lumen may be significant and may produce hypovolemia, but this effect is usually not as great as with mechanical bowel obstruction. The intraluminal pressure usually does not rise as high as with mechanical obstruction, but it may be sufficient to produce edema in the gut wall. Marked distention of the bowel may severely impair pulmonary ventilation. Rarely is surgery indicated. Gastric suction or intestinal intubation along with newer pharmacologic agents is helpful. Parasympathomimetic drugs, vasopressin, and A-ganglion blockers have all reportedly been helpful. Metoclopramide has been useful in some cases of gastric atony.

Acute Gastric Dilatation. Acute gastric dilatation may result after surgical procedures, anesthetics, or trauma. The basic mechanism of this complication is not entirely clear, but it usually begins with gastric distention. There is progressive accumulation of gastric secretion and air, and within a few hours the volume in the stomach may approximate 4 to 5 liters. The distention and accumulation of fluid result in dehydration, hypovolemia, and mechanical interference with respiration and cardiac function, and may lead to shock and death. Sudden massive vomiting and aspiration of gastric contents may also lead to death. The treatment consists of decompression with a nasogastric tube and replacement of the fluid loss. Some of the clinical symptoms of shock are probably neurogenic in origin, because decompression may reverse many of the signs very rapidly.

CONSTIPATION AND DIARRHEA

CONSTIPATION

Constipation is a term used to denote abnormal retention of stool, infrequent bowel movements, stools of insufficient quantity, or stool that is abnormally dry and hard.

Psychologic, neurogenic, and mechanical factors (such as tumors, intussusception, or volvulus) and use of drugs can lead to constipation.

Obstipation, which is the absence of passage of both flatus and feces, suggests a mechanical obstruction. This may result in massive abdominal distention and respiratory compromise. Intestinal "toxemia" may occur, with distention from abnormal absorption of bacterial toxins, leading to a septic presentation. Cecal perforation can result from colonic obstruction, but in about 15 per cent of patients the ileocecal valve is incompetent, allowing for back-up into the lower small bowel.

DIARRHEA

Intestinal transit varies with the amount and quantity of food, and frequently with the emotional state of the individual. Generally the healthy stomach completely empties in three to four hours, with chyme then reaching the cecum within four hours. Cecal contents are semiliquid; much of the water absorption takes place in the colon. Diarrhea is the frequent passage of excessively liquid stools. There are numerous causes of diarrhea, including diseases of the gastrointestinal tract, diseases of multiple other organ systems, medication, and therapy such as radiation. Emotional problems are a frequent cause of chronic diarrhea. Organic problems can include inflammatory bowel disease, malignancy, tumor, and infections, including parasites. Many tumors, such as carcinoids and Zollinger-Ellison tumor, secrete hormones inhibiting intestinal absorption and stimulating transit. Metabolic disorders such as uremia may also lead to diarrhea.

It is commonly believed that water absorption occurs primarily in the colon, and that, therefore, diarrhea is due to a defect in the colonic mucosa. The colon is normally presented with only 400 to 500 cc of fluid from the ileum daily, and all but 100 cc of water is absorbed by the colonic mucosa. On the other hand, the small intestine is presented with 7 liters of fluid, which are secreted into the gastrointestinal tract, as well as 1 to 2 liters, which are ingested per day. All but 400 to 500 cc is absorbed by the small intestine. It is obvious that the small intestine is the primary organ in water absorption, and diarrhea may result from either small bowel or large bowel disease.

Diarrhea may result from impaired intestinal absorption of water and electrolytes, abnormal intestinal motility, increased absorption of fluid and electrolytes into the gut lumen, and an increase in osmotically active substances in the lumen. In severe diarrhea, the fluid volume deficit and electrolyte imbalance are primarily caused by the marked increase in lost volume, because diarrheal stools tend to be somewhat less hypotonic than normally formed stools. The volume loss may vary from 1000 to 4000 cc per day. Acid-base balance shifts toward a metabolic acidosis because of several factors. Fecal sodium and chloride concentrations are usually lower than plasma levels, whereas potassium and bicarbonate levels are higher; therefore, there is loss of bicarbonate ions in the stool. Starvation and hypovolemia may increase the endogenous production of acids, and dehydration may compromise renal function. In addition, hypokalemia may result from loss of potassium in the stool. Some entities, such as villous adenoma, may secrete a potassium-rich fluid. These complications may be accentuated if the diarrhea includes an appreciable loss of proteins or blood. The concentration of protein in stool is negligible except in cases of exudative diarrhea.

GASTROINTESTINAL BLEEDING: HEMATEMESIS, MELENA, RECTAL BLEEDING

Bleeding may be the presentimg symptom in more than 30 per cent of patients with a wide variety of gastrointestinal diseases. Hematemesis, the vomiting of blood, may be accompanied by melena, the passage of black, tarry stools. As little as 50 ml of blood can produce melena. The tarry color is attributable to the production of acid hematin by the action of gastric acid on hemoglobin or the production of sulfide from heme.

Rapid bleeding can result in hypotension and shock. It is frequently difficult to estimate the amount of blood loss, since hemoglobin and hematocrit levels are unreliable unless equilibration has occurred. As bleeding progresses, the heart rate increases and cardiac output is decreased. Myocardial ischemia may result as well as reduced renal blood flow, leading to either oliguria or anuria. Azotemia may occur as a result of breakdown of blood by bacterial action in the gastrointestinal tract. This usually does not happen with colonic bleeding. It is of great importance to determine blood clotting factors in these patients. Rapid bleeding and clotting may bring about a consumptive coagulopathy resulting in thrombocytopenia, prolonged prothrombin time, and other clotting defects. Bleeding may stop with the administration of platelets, vitamin K, and fresh frozen plasma, obviating an emergency operation or making its performance less of a risk.

Bleeding may be so rapid that attempts to resuscitate the patient completely are fruitless and immediate anesthesia and operation without diagnostic procedures are necessary. The stomach should be lavaged to decrease the risk of aspiration, using an Ewald tube if necessary. If time permits, upper G.I. endoscopy is of value. Diagnostic angiography can locate arterial bleeding sites in about 90 per cent of cases if bleeding is occurring at a rate of 3 to 5 ml per minute. Arterial catheters can be used for infusion of vasopressin (0.1–0.2 unit/min) to slow the rate of bleeding but are generally not superior to intravenous vasopressin. This method can be used while the patient is being readied for surgery and may be therapeutic in 50 to 80 per cent of cases. Arterial catheters may have an advantage over the intravenous route only for embolizing small arterial bleeders with small clots if vasopressin fails.

Bleeding distal to the ligament of Treitz is usually manifested by melena or red rectal bleeding (hematochezia) and is usually of colonic origin. Bleeding from the distal small bowel is rare and can be due to a Meckel's diverticulum, polyps, intussusception, Crohn's disease, tumors, and/or vascular abnormalities. The most common cause of massive colonic bleeding is diverticulosis, whereas carcinoma represents the most common source of moderate bleeding. Angiodysplasia is becoming more recognized as a cause of massive bleeding from the colon and has a predilection for the ascending colon. Selective angiography is of particular use in localizing and treating bleeding from diverticulosis and angiodysplasia. Many of these patients are elderly and have associated cardiovascular disease, and an emergency operation is not desirable if avoidable.

MALABSORPTION

Although the small intestine is the major site of absorption of water, nutrient materi-al, and electrolytes, malabsorption may result not only from diseases of the small intestine but also from biliary, pancreatic, or gastric diseases. The malabsorption may be limited to only one element or substance, or it may include multiple substances.

In many of the malabsorption states, steatorrhea and diarrhea occur, with progressive weight loss. There may be malabsorption of the fat-soluble vitamins (A, D, K) and calcium. Hypoprothrombinemia may result from faulty absorption of vitamin K. Tetany and osteomalacia can occur from inadequate absorption of calcium caused by vitamin D deficiency and formation of soap with fatty acids. Anemia can result from folic acid or vitamin B_{12} malabsorption or from iron deficiency. With severe or prolonged malabsorption, protein deficiency can result. The clinical manifestations will obviously vary, depending upon the pathophysiological processes, etiology, severity, and duration of the malabsorption.

Gastric Disorders. Total or subtotal gastrectomy may be followed by mild to severe metabolic, digestive, and nutritional disorders. In general, the deficiency syndromes are directly related to the extent of the gastric resection.

After total gastrectomy all patients lose weight, but this problem may be minimal in patients with partial gastrectomy. The weight loss and the difficulty in maintaining weight seem to be related to several factors; however, many mechanisms are not clear. Steatorrhea may be due to bypassing the duodenum (steatorrhea is more frequent in patients with Billroth II than with Billroth I), bacterial growth in the afferent loop, pancreatic disorder, or intestinal mucosal disease. Minimal steatorrhea may not be clinically significant, especially if the patient maintains his weight. However, it is important to be aware of the other defects which may be associated with steatorrhea: calcium deficiency and vitamin A, D, or K deficiency.

Anemia is another common postgastrectomy disorder. Iron deficiency anemia is more commonly seen in females than in males. The exact cause of this deficiency is not clear, but poor iron absorption may be due to surgical bypass of the duodenum. The anemia is usually mild and will respond to oral iron therapy. Megaloblastic anemia caused by vitamin B_{12} deficiency will develop in all patients after total gastrectomy and in some after partial gastrectomy. In the latter group, the deficiency is seen seven to eight years after resection, more frequently in patients who were operated upon for gastric ulcer than for duodenal ulcer, and in those who were reconstructed with a Billroth II rather than a Billroth I. In patients with total gastrectomy, the vitamin B_{12} deficiency is due to intrinsic factor deficiency and not to the absorptive mechanism. After partial gastrectomy the defect may be due to lack of intrinsic factor or to the overgrowth of bacteria in a stagnant loop of bowel competing for vitamin B_{12}. The deficiency or lack of intrinsic factor is corrected with parenteral vitamin B_{12}. The anemia caused by a blind loop may respond to vitamin B_{12} or antibiotics, but surgical correction may be required.

Hepatic and Biliary Causes. Malabsorption may result from hepatocellular disease, bile not reaching the intestine, or interruption of the enterohepatic circulation of bile. Bile salts are important in the emulsification of fat for hydrolysis, formation and transfer of micelles into the intestinal mucosa, and activation of lipase. Interference of these functions leads to malabsorption of fats. Associated with this steatorrhea, there may be malabsorption of fat-soluble vitamins (A, D, K) and calcium.

Small Intestinal Causes. Malabsorption caused by intestinal factors may be related to abnormalities of motility, total absorptive surface area, mucosa, vascular lesions, and bacterial overgrowth. The absorptive surface area of the intestine may be decreased by surgical bowel resection, bypass, or intestinal fistula. The severity of the malabsorption is related in part to the extent, site, and duration of the decreased surface.

Massive resection (two thirds or more) of the small intestine can result in impairment of the absorption of virtually all food constituents, leading to a state closely related to starvation. Malabsorption is due not only to the decrease in absorptive surface area but also to rapid transit time. If the distal bowel is included in the massive resection, the enterohepatic recirculation is interrupted. With prolonged depletion, pancreatic enzyme deficiency may result, aggravating the malabsorption. There is malabsorption of fat and protein but less often of carbohydrates. The protein depletion results from impaired absorption as well as from increased me-

tabolism caused by caloric deficiency. In addition to steatorrhea, patients may develop calcium deficiency, magnesium deficiency, and anemia.

Most adult patients can function relatively well with 50 per cent loss of the small bowel. The section of the bowel that is lost is also important. Steatorrhea appears to be greater if the duodenum and jejunum are excised. Vitamin B_{12} deficiency may result if the distal 6 to 8 feet of ileum is resected. Iron absorption occurs primarily in the duodenum. Calcium is absorbed primarily in the duodenum and jejunum, but more hypocalcemia is seen in patients with lower bowel resections.

Pancreatic Causes. Pancreatic enzymes are important in the digestion of carbohydrate, protein, and fat. However, with pancreatic deficiency, these food components can still be partially digested and absorbed because of the intestinal enzymes. The defect in digestion and absorption varies considerably. A person with no pancreatic proteolytic enzyme may be able to digest and absorb 25 to 75 per cent of protein and 60 to 90 per cent of fat ingested. Pancreatic insufficiency may result from protein malnutrition, mucoviscidosis, congenital defect of enzyme formation, chronic pancreatitis, carcinoma of the pancreas, and pancreatic resection.

Blind Loop Syndrome. This clinical syndrome results from the stasis of gut content sufficient to allow abnormal bacterial overgrowth. The exact pathogenesis is not known, but the malabsorption is associated with bacterial overgrowth. This syndrome may result from surgical blind loop, fistulas, strictures, and diverticula of the small bowel. Vitamin B_{12} absorption is decreased and may lead to macrocytic megaloblastic anemia, peripheral neuropathy and subacute combined degeneration of the spinal cord, glossitis, and weight loss similar to that of pernicious anemia. Steatorrhea may be common, and this may lead to deficiency of vitamins A, D, and K, which may further impair the nutrition of the patient.

Protein-Losing Enteropathy. The loss of serum proteins into the gastrointestinal tract is of minor significance because proteins are digested into their constituent amino acids, which are then reabsorbed and utilized. In patients with certain gastrointestinal diseases, there may be a marked increase in the loss of serum proteins into the gastrointestinal tract. Normal subjects catabolize 5 to 11 per cent of their intravascular pool of albumin or gamma globulins daily, but patients with gastrointestinal loss may catabolize over 60 per cent of the plasma pool daily. The excess over normal is then lost into the gastrointestinal tract. When the rate of protein loss exceeds the body's capacity to synthesize that protein, hypoproteinemia results. Protein loss into the gastrointestinal tract differs from loss caused by an injured kidney, because serum proteins of all molecular sizes diffuse into the gastrointestinal tract, whereas usually only the smaller serum proteins are lost into the urine. With extensive or severe renal damage, macroglobulins are also lost. The reduction in serum protein concentrations is not uniform for all proteins. In general, the concentrations of proteins with longest normal survival (albumin and gamma globulin) are decreased most severely. However, albumin synthesis in the liver can be doubled with albumin loss, but immunoglobulin synthesis appears to be increased only by antigenic stimuli and not with decreased plasma concentrations. The clinical picture varies, depending on the basic gastrointestinal disease. Iron, copper, calcium, lipids, and lymphocytes may also be lost into the gastrointestinal tract.

Hypoproteinemia and edema may be the only major manifestations with minimal gastrointestinal symptoms. Other findings include growth retardation, hypocalcemia, tetany, iron deficiency anemia, eosinophilia, lymphocytopenia, and aminoaciduria. Edema is frequently massive. There may be effusion into the serous cavities, and diarrhea may be present. Over 40 gastrointestinal disorders have been described with excessive gastrointestinal protein loss, e.g., gastric carcinoma, giant hypertrophy of the gastric mucosa, atrophic gastritis, regional enteritis, Whipple's disease, lymphosarcoma of the bowel, ulcerative colitis, and allergic gastroenteropathy.

SURGICAL NUTRITION

The majority of patients undergoing surgery withstand the brief period of catabolism and starvation without difficulty. Many, however, approach surgery in a malnourished state, heightening the risk of morbidity and mortality and often succumbing to starvation rather than their underlying disorder. In some instances, preventing weight loss and replacing depleted energy reserves allows for healing, prolonged chemotherapy, and even remission in the disease process itself. Postoperatively, the catabolic effect on nitrogen balance is often greater than starvation alone. A negative nitrogen balance of 12 gm may be seen after three days of starvation and can be expected to be over 20 gm after three days in a patient with a ruptured appendix and peritonitis.

Baseline. The Nutrition Board of The National Research Council have noted that normal patients require approximately 1 gm of protein and 35 kcal per kg of body weight or 1400 kcal per square meter of body surface area per day. These requirements vary with age, sex, and level of activity. With surgery and injury these needs are higher. Dudrick has noted that a complicated surgical patient requires between 2500 and 4000 kcal/day with 12 to 24 gm of nitrogen. These are in addition to the needs for vitamins and essential trace elements.

Method for Nutritional Support. Partial starvation can be tolerated by a normally nourished patient for at least one week. Adequate fluids with appropriate electrolytes and a minimum of 150 gm of glucose minimizes protein catabolism and prevents acidosis.

Nasogastric Tube, Gastrostomy, Jejunostomy. When possible, the gastrointestinal tract should be chosen as the highest priority means of establishing alimentation. Nasogastric or nasopharyngeal tubes can be used for blended diets administered through the small bore plastic tubes in patients unwilling or unable to swallow. It is inadvisable to use these methods, however, for a patient who is not awake or who is mentally obtunded and/or on a respirator. Aspiration of gastric content is a problem that often occurs even around a snug-fitting tracheostomy or endotracheal tube.

Feeding can be performed distal to the pylorus or even distal to a fistula by using a long intestine tube (Cantor) or a planned jejunostomy. Gastrostomies offer few advantages over nasogastric intubation and alleviate only the nasopharygeal irritation, parotitis, and/or the small amount of esophageal reflux that has been noted with nasogastric tubes. Also, gastrostomies have been associated with an array of their own interesting complications, such as bleeding, skin irritation, leak, and peritonitis.

Elemental Diets. These diets are available for patients who need complete nutritional support or as supplements for patients in whom residue is not desirable or in whom only part of the small bowel is available for absorption of simple sugars and amino acids. The diets are formulated and synthesized out of known chemical nutrients such as purified amino acids and simple carbohydrates. They contain no bulk and thus give no residue. They may be administered via gastrostomies or nasogastric or jejunostomy tubes (see Table 9–1).

Elemental diets have been found to be useful in protein depleted patients with a variety of gastrointestinal diseases, such as ulcerative or granulomatous colitis, malabsorption syndrome, short bowel syndrome, gastric or small bowel fistulas, and multiple trauma or burns. The diets have been used during preoperative bowel preparation in the place of other feeding for their lack of bowel residue properties. An additional benefit of elemental diets has been the demonstration that there is a resultant decrease in the volume of gastric juice output as well as enzyme and exocrine pancreatic secretions, suggesting their use in patients in whom the gastrointestinal tract should be at rest, such as those with inflammatory disease and acute pancreatitis. In as many as 50 per cent of patients enterocutaneous fistulas have reportedly closed when the patients were fed elemental diets distal to their fistula.

The complications are minimal and include nausea, vomiting, and diarrhea and usually secondary to the high osmolality as well as hypertonic nonketotic coma. Hyperglycemia and glycosuria have been reported.

Parenteral Alimentation. When the gastrointestinal tract is not available for feeding or its use is inadvisable, parenteral routes must be used. Infusions of 5 per cent glucose (isotonic) are inadequate to meet the caloric requirements of the patient even if given in large quantities approaching water intoxication. Use of peripheral hypertonic solutions leads to vein thrombosis and a high incidence of thrombophlebitis.

The demonstration by Dudrick and coworkers that complete nutritional needs can be met by use of hypertonic, high caloric solutions with protein hydrolysates infused through an indwelling catheter in a major vein such as the vena cava has revolutionized the field of surgical nutrition. The blood flow in these vessels is rapid enough to ensure rapid mixing of the hypertonic mixture and prevent phlebitis. A ratio of at least 150 kcal per gram of nitrogen must be given and in quantities greater than the basic caloric needs to achieve a positive nitrogen balance and spare protein breakdown. The demonstration that the growth rates of beagle puppies receiving IV alimentation were comparable to those of normal puppies was dramatic and convincing.

Solutions available for total parenteral nutrition vary from hospital to hospital. Most are designed to hold approximately 100 kcal/1000 cc and include a 5 per cent solution of protein hydrolysate or crystalline amino acids in addition to 30 per cent dextrose. A typical order would be as follows: 5 per cent Travamine in D3OW with NaCl 50 mEq, KCl 50 mEq, Mg 8-12 mEq, Ca 10 mEq, HPO_4 30 mEq/L, add 5 ml of multivitamins to each liter. Trace elements can be added by administering a unit of plasma or whole blood on a weekly basis. In addition, vitamins K and B_{12}, folic acid, iron, calcium, and phosphate can be added daily or on a weekly basis. The choice of adding sodium chloride or sodium bicarbonate depends on the acid-base status of the patient. Daily serum elec-

Table 9–1 *Approximate Composition per 1800 cc of Elemental Nutrients*

	Vivonex 100	Vivonex 100 HN	Flexical-1000 cc
Kcal	1800	1800	1000
Carbohydrates, gm	407	379	148
Protein, gm	37	75	22
Nitrogen, gm	59	12	35
Fat, gm	13	0.8	31
Sodium, mEq	104	60	20
Potassium, mEq	54	32	35
Osmolality, mOsm/L	1175	844	845

trolytes should be monitored initially, along with BUN, and frequently thereafter. If casein hydrolysate solutions are used, phosphorus need not be added, since adequate levels will be present. Infusions are started gradually with 1 to 2 liters per day. Vital signs, central venous pressure, urinary output, and urine sugar are checked every six hours, and blood sugars are checked daily. Glucose intolerance is common and may rise initially as high as 400 mg per 100 ml. The rate of infusion usually can be adjusted not to exceed a urine glucose greater than a 3+ reaction. However, occasionally insulin may have to be administered subcutaneously.

Access route for administration of total parenteral nutrition (TPN) is of central importance, since it was initially the development of the concept of high flow admixing with hyperosmotic solution that led to the feasibility of TPN. One of the preferred routes is the subclavian vein cannulated under a strictly sterile technique with catheter placement in the superior vena cava or right atrium. An internal jugular route or "long line" cannulation via a "cut down" on an antecubital vein is also useful but generally has a lower rate of success. For more prolonged use or at-home alimentation, an A-V fistula using a vein graft can be constructed, as for dialysis. Care of the access site is of paramount importance, since this represents the source of a large percentage of the complications attending TPN. Antibiotic ointment is placed around the catheter entrance through the skin. This, and the sterile occlusive dressing, is changed every two to three days. Every four to six days the transfixing suture is removed and the catheter itself is replaced by a new sterile one over a guide wire. The line is used solely for TPN and not for other infusions, medications, or blood sampling. The care is important enough and is often so specialized that many institutions employ a TPN team or specialty nurse whose only job is to care for the TPN access sites.

Any seriously ill patient suffering from malnutrition, sepsis or trauma when the GI tract cannot be used for feeding can benefit from TPN. Specifically:

1. Infants with GI anomalies, tracheoesophageal fistula, gastroschisis, omphalocoele, or intestinal atresia.

2. Infants who fail to thrive secondary to gastrointestinal insufficiency with malabsorption, enzyme deficiencies, meconium ileus, or short bowel syndrome.

3. Adults with short bowel secondary to massive resection or fistula.

4. Malnourished patients with obstructions such as achalasia, stricture, cancer of the esophagus, gastric carcinoma, or pyloric obstruction.

5. Surgical patients with prolonged paralytic ileus, multiple injuries, or abdominal trauma.

6. Malabsorption due to sprue, pancreatic insufficiency, ulceration colitis, and regional enteritis.

7. Patients who cannot eat or who regurgitate following metabolic disorders, intracranial surgery, and central nervous system trauma.

8. Patients with excessive metabolic demands, such as severe trauma, full thickness burns, major fractures, or soft tissue trauma.

9. Patients with major disease of the gastrointestinal tract, as in granulomatous enterocolitis, ulcerative colitis, or tuberculous enteritis.

10. Certain paraplegics and quadriplegics with decubitus ulcers when soilage is a problem.

11. Preoperatively in a patient with prolonged severe malnutrition.

Complications occur frequently enough that serious attention must be given to the above indications for the use of TPN. There are basically three categories: mechanical, infectious, and metabolic. Placement of a catheter can result in pneumothorax, hemothorax, or hydrothorax; subclavian artery injury; cardiac arrhythmias; air embolus, or catheter embolism. Thrombophlebitis or thrombosis of the superior vena cava is fortunately rare. Infectious complications range from skin problems to fatal septicemia. Fewer than 5 per cent of all patients have sepsis but in approximately 20 per cent of those cases this sepsis is fungal in origin. One of the earliest signs of sepsis may be the sudden development of glucose intolerance. With the development of fever in a patient on TPN, catheter sepsis should be considered first, and the catheter should be removed and the tip cultured, along with the blood and TPN fluid. A catheter can be replaced in the opposite subclavian vein. As mentioned above, these problems are common and serious enough to justify specialization of care for these catheters.

Metabolic problems are rare when the patient is closely monitored but are listed in Table 9–2.

Fat Emulsions. Complications with TPN as administered via a central vein catheter and/or the need for essential fat in a given patient may indicate the use of intralipid, either to maintain sufficient nutrition or as a weekly supplement to that patient on central TPN. Intralipid is a 10 per cent emulsion of fat (1.1 cal per ml) derived from soybean oil, phospholipid, and glycerin. The fat particles are about 0.5 micron in diameter and the solution is isotonic, thus making it suitable for peripheral intravenous administration. This may be useful in a patient with sepsis when a central line may be an excessive risk.

The principal advantage of intralipid is its high caloric content and isotonicity, making it possible to provide 2000 to 3000 calories per day through a peripheral vein. However, it is expensive, and limitations in the rate of utilization and biochemical efficiency (as well as the need for some carbohydrate and protein) make it wise not to exceed 60 per cent of the day's caloric intake from this source.

Intralipid cannot be mixed with drugs or electrolytes. A filter must be used. Adverse reactions include nausea, dyspnea, cyanosis, and allergic reactions, among others. Clinical experience thus far is somewhat limited.

Peripheral Amino Acids for Protein Sparing. The goal is to minimize protein loss when there is a condition of negative caloric balance. Although patients are expected to lose weight, the loss is hoped to be principally from fat rather than muscle stores. Two liters of a 3 to 5 per cent amino acid solution provides 10.3 grams of nitrogen and can be administered peripherally with 5 per cent glucose and/or supplemented with 500 ml of intralipid.

This scheme has been used in obese patients undergoing weight reduction, those with fatty infiltrates in their liver following prolonged TPN or small bowel bypass, and for short periods in postoperative patients. There is as yet no clinical evidence that amino acids have any practical advantage over conventional 5 per cent glucose solutions; however, they greatly add to the expense.

PERITONITIS

Peritonitis may be primary (no peritoneal source of infection) or secondary (usually to disease within the abdominal cavity). The severity of clinical manifestations is determined in part by some of the following factors: age of the patient, extent (localized, diffused), virulence of the organism, amount and duration of contamination, and the cause (chemical, infectious).

Early effects of peritonitis are on the respiratory system and are due to pain and high diaphragms as a result of distention. Tachypnea caused by pain may initially produce respiratory alkalosis. Eventually shallow respiration and inhibition of coughing produce an accumulation of secretions, leading to atelectasis and respiratory acidosis.

There is loss of water, electrolytes, and proteins into the peritoneal cavity and extracellular tissue spaces. In addition there is loss of fluid into the tissues of the bowel secondary to adynamic ileus, water retention, and dilutional hyponatremia. Contraction of intravascular volume leads to hypotension, anuria, and shock. In some forms of peritonitis with septicemia there may be peripheral circulatory pooling which aggravates the contracted volume and shock. With diffuse peritonitis there are severe alterations of the cardiovascular and respiratory systems. Hypovolemic shock and septic shock are characterized by low cardiac output. Because of inadequate perfusion of the tissues, metabolic acidosis results. The body attempts to compensate by increased respiratory effect, but this leads to greater oxygen demand by muscles. A vicious cycle is thus begun. In addition pyrexia increases oxygen requirement.

Aggressive treatment of respiratory failure should consist of increasing respiratory efficiency, at the same time decreasing the oxygen requirement. The fluid replacement of patients with peritonitis must be flexible and guided by continuous monitoring of the urine output, blood pressure, hematocrit, and venous pressure.

Acute renal insufficiency may also result from diffuse peritonitis. Not all the mechanisms leading to the renal failure are known, but decreased renal perfusion caused by hypovolemia, hypertension, and vasoconstriction probably play the major roles.

Table 9–2 *Metabolic Complications of Intravenous Hyperalimentation*

Problems	Possible Causes
I. Glucose metabolism:	
A. Hyperglycemia, glycosuria, osmotic diuresis, hyperosmolar non-ketotic dehydration and coma	Excessive total dose or rate of infusion of glucose; inadequate endogenous insulin; glucocorticoids; sepsis
B. Ketoacidosis in diabetes mellitus	Inadequate endogenous insulin response; inadequate exogenous insulin therapy
C. Postinfusion (rebound) hypoglycemia	Persistence of endogenous insulin production secondary to prolonged stimulation of islet cells by high-carbohydrate infusion
II. Amino acid metabolism:	
A. Hyperchloremic metabolic acidosis	Excessive chloride and monohydrochloride content of crystalline amino acid solutions
B. Serum amino acid imbalance	Unphysiologic amino acid profile of the nutrient solution; differential amino acid utilization with various disorders
C. Hyperammonemia	Excessive ammonia in protein hydrolysate solutions; arginine, ornithine, aspartic acid and/or glutamic acid deficiency in amino acid solutions; primary hepatic disorder
D. Prerenal azotemia	Excessive protein hydrolysate or amino acid infusion
III. Calcium and phosphorus metabolism:	
A. Hypophosphatemia	
1. Decreased erythrocyte 2,3-di-phosphoglycerate	Inadequate phosphorus administration, redistribution of serum phosphorus into cells and/or bone
2. Increased affinity of hemoglobin for oxygen	
3. Aberrations of erythrocyte intermediary metabolites	
B. Hypocalcemia	Inadequate calcium administration; reciprocal response to phosphorus repletion without simultaneous calcium infusion; hypoalbuminemia
C. Hypercalcemia	Excessive calcium administration with or without high doses of albumin; excessive vitamin D administration
D. Vitamin D deficiency; hypervitaminosis D	Inadequate or excessive vitamin D administration
IV. Essential fatty acid metabolism:	
Serum deficiencies of phospholipid linoleic and/or arachidonic acids; serum elevations of △-5,8,11-aicosatrienoic acid	Inadequate essential fatty acid administration; inadequate vitamin E administration
V. Miscellaneous:	
A. Hypokalemia	Inadequate potassium intake relative to increased requirements for protein anabolism; diuresis
B. Hyperkalemia	Excessive potassium administration especially in metabolic acidosis; renal decompensation
C. Hypomagnesemia	Inadequate magnesium administration relative to increased requirements for protein anabolism and glucose metabolism
D. Hypermagnesemia	Excessive magnesium administration; renal decomposition
E. Anemia	Iron deficiency; folic acid deficiency; vitamin B-12 deficiency; copper deficiency; other deficiencies
F. Bleeding	Vitamin K deficiency
G. Hypervitaminosis A	Excessive vitamin A administration
H. Elevations in SGOT, SGPT and serum alkaline phosphatase	Enzyme induction secondary to amino acid imbalance, excessive glycogen and/or fat deposition in the liver
I. Cholestatic hepatitis	Decreased water content of bile

(From Dudrick, S.J.: Manual of Surgical Nutrition; American College of Surgeons. Philadelphia, W. B. Saunders Co., 1975.)

LIVER DISEASE

Portal Hypertension. The normal portal pressure is less than 300 mm. of water. Some of the causes of portal hypertension are increased hepatoportal flow without obstruction, postsinusoidal obstruction of the hepatic veins, presinusoidal obstruction of the portal veins (intra- and extrahepatic), and increased central venous pressure.

ETIOLOGY

1. Increased hepatoportal flow
   a. Hepatic arterial-portal vein fistula
   b. Splenic A-V fistula
   c. Intrasplenic origin
2. Extrahepatic outflow obstruction
   a. Budd-Chiari syndrome
   b. Right heart failure
3. Obstruction of extrahepatic portal system
   a. Congenital
   b. Cavernous transformation of portal vein
   c. Infection
   d. Trauma
   e. External compression
4. Intrahepatic obstruction
   a. Nutritional cirrhosis
   b. Postnecrotic cirrhosis
   c. Biliary cirrhosis
   d. Other fibrotic diseases, hemochromatosis, Wilson's disease
   e. Infiltrative disease
   f. Vein occlusion — Schistosomiasis

Over 90 per cent of patients with portal hypertension have nutritional cirrhosis and alcoholism. Portal pressure can be assessed preoperatively by hepatic vein wedge cannulation, much like a wedged pulmonary artery pressure estimating left atrial filling. At the same time, portal vein venography can be obtained to document the status of flow, varices, and patency of the portal vein.

The most serious complication of portal hypertension is bleeding from esophageal varices. The therapeutic regimen is directed at effective control of bleeding and may be nonoperative or operative. About 30 per cent of patients with varices can be anticipated to bleed. Approximately 70 per cent who have bled from varices die within one year and 60 per cent rebleed massively in one year. A prophylactic shunt is not advised, since predicting the 30 per cent of cirrhotics with varices that will bleed is impossible. On the other hand, about 25 per cent of those having portacaval shunt operations will have a neurological disturbance after. Acute hemorrhage in cirrhotics can be assumed to be coming from the varices in upward of 50 per cent of patients, 30 per cent having gastritis and the rest bleeding from ulcer, Mallory-Weiss tears, or other disorder. Esophagoscopy is the single most important diagnostic technique to differentiate variceal bleeding from gastritis or Mallory-Weiss tears and should be performed first in all patients. Upper GI series will verify the presence of varices and possibly the presence of ulcer disease. A note of caution: demonstration of varices in a patient in shock may be difficult during endoscopy and any bleeding from the lower esophagus must be looked on with suspicion.

Rapid control of bleeding is a necessity. Balloon tamponade with the Sengstaken-Blakemore tube requires careful attention to details to avoid complications. The tube should be checked prior to insertion, the placement checked with x-rays, and the maintenance of pressure and traction monitored. Complications include pressure necrosis of the esophagus, aspiration, and asphyxiation when the tube slips out of the stomach into the pharynx. Recurrence of bleeding is not uncommon. Tube compression can be used while preparing a patient for surgery. Intravenous vasopressin (Pitressin) constricts the splanchnic circulation and reduces portal pressure by about 40 per cent. Twenty units infused over 10 to 20 minutes or continuously infused at 0.2 unit/ml/min has provided temporary cessation of bleeding in 70 to 90 per cent of patients. Recurrent bleeding may occur in over 50 per cent of patients. Arfonad has been used to produce generalized hypotension. Many clinicians in Europe have begun using sclerotherapy via the flexible endoscope, but experience in this country is as yet limited.

All of the non-operative methods are thus less than optimal. Surgical therapy includes transesophageal ligation, cannulation of the thoracic duct, esophagogastric devascularization, and transection of the esophagus with re-anastomosis and various portacaval shunt operations. Mortality rates for all procedures approach 75 per cent in emergency situations. Since only portacaval shunting provides a definitive treatment scheme, all other procedures have largely been abandoned. All patients undergoing emergency shunt should have fresh blood available. This provides necessary clotting factors often diminished in hepatic disease, and avoids the increased ammonia content and decreased platelet and prothrombin supply characteristic of banked blood. Intestinal cathartics with enemas and magnesium sulfate should be started immediately to prevent encephalopathy. Sodium salt solutions should be avoided, since these patients conserve sodium, and total body stores are high despite serum dilution. Large amounts of potassium may be required in addition to vitamin K, glucose, and protein. Many of these patients have a significant A-V shunt intrahepatically and have a hyperdynamic state with huge cardiac outputs. Rapid digitalization has been used in these individuals prior to operation to prevent cardiac failure.

Ascites. The pathogenesis of ascites in liver disease is complex and not fully understood. Several factors appear to be important in the formation of ascites: portal hypertension with increased hydrostatic pressure (postsinusoidal obstruction), lowered plasma colloidal osmotic pressure, increased plasma aldosterone concentration with retention of sodium and water, and possible excessive lymph production.

Hepatic Coma. Patients with liver disease may develop a metabolic encephalopathy that is related to the portosystemic shunt; it can occur naturally or it can be due to surgery. The exact relationship between ammonia metabolism and hepatic coma is not fully understood. The patient is characterized by a variable disturbance of consciousness, mental confusion, inappropriate activity, increased muscle activity, hyperventilation, exaggerated reflexes, and hepatic tremor or asterixis. Clinically, hepatic coma is often precipitated by gastrointestinal bleeding, overeating of proteins, and surgery. Other factors that may be important are any tendency to alkalosis (which increases ammonia toxicity), severe infection, sedation, diuretics, and hypokalemia.

Treatment is directed at reducing the ammonia concentration in the blood. Blood in the gastrointestinal tract should be removed by stomach irrigation, enemas, and cathartics. Dietary protein is drastically reduced, and calories are given as carbohydrates. Neomycin is used to decrease the bacterial action. The hypokalemia and alkalosis

should be treated with potassium. Other methods of treatment that have been used include glutamic acid or arginine, wholebody hypothermia, exchange resins, hemodialysis, exchange transfusion, and cross-circulation experiments with living human volunteers or isolated pig livers.

Liver disease produces many other alterations of physiologic functions. The liver is the major site of detoxification of many drugs, and therefore the pharmacologic action of these drugs may be prolonged. Endocrine changes may occur because of altered hepatic metabolism or conjugation and excretion of hormones by the liver. Magnesium deficiency and hypokalemia may aggravate muscle weakness. Hypoglycemia may occur as a result of massive liver necrosis or impairment of hepatic glycogenolysis and gluconeogenesis. Hypoprothrombinemia may result from malabsorption of vitamin K.

Patients with liver disease may develop hematological abnormalities. Anemia may be caused by hemolysis, iron deficiency, folic acid deficiency, or bleeding. Thrombocytopenia and granulocytopenia may be associated with the anemia.

Renal function may be altered in patients with liver disease caused by reduced renal blood flow secondary to a decreased blood volume and cardiac output. There may be kidney damage caused by the agents producing the liver disease or by shock. The hepatorenal syndrome is not fully understood at present. The patient with liver disease who develops hepatorenal syndrome has histologically normal kidneys, oliguria, azotemia, and high urine osmolality with a low sodium content.

JAUNDICE

Jaundice, meaning "yellow," refers to the presence of an excess of bile pigments in the body tissues and serum and may be the presenting sign in a number of hepatic and nonhepatic diseases. Evaluation of the patient is directed toward defining whether the jaundice is due to a surgically correctable lesion. Although elevated serum bilirubin levels in the infant can result in kernicterus and irreversible damage to the central nervous system, in the adult, longer periods of hyperbilirubinemia may be tolerated. Loss of appetite and fever can result in weight loss. Pruritus can lead to rashes and excoriation and may be a disturbing symptom. Extrahepatic obstruction can result in acholic stools and subsequent malabsorption. Liver function chemistries often discern the particular medical disease causing jaundice, but mechanical problems are often more difficult to elucidate, since x-ray examinations depend on the liver's ability to concentrate and excrete dye. More direct examination involves liver biopsy, transhepatic cholangiography, ultrasonography, laparoscopy, endoscopic retrograde cholangiopancreatography, and ultimately and equally important, if not more so, exploratory laparotomy. Laparotomy and correction of extrahepatic obstruction is of some immediate importance because of the risk of biliary cirrhosis, which may be irreversible, and possibly the hepatorenal syndrome, which can accompany liver failure. In addition the gram-negative sepsis and shock that can occur with mechanical extrahepatic obstruction is unpredictable, carrying a mortality of upward of 80 per cent.

DISORDERS OF THE ESOPHAGUS

DIVERTICULA

Esophageal diverticula may be classified by location (pharyngoesophageal, thoracic, supradiaphragmatic) or as traction or pulsion diverticula.

Pharyngoesophageal or Zenker's Diverticula (Pulsion). These diverticula are formed by protrusion of the pharyngeal mucosa posteriorly between the inferior constrictor muscle of the pharynx and the cricopharyngeus muscle resulting from incoordination of the pharyngoesophageal junction. Diverticula usually occur in patients over 50 and are rare under age 30. Symptoms that may result depend partly on the size of the diverticulum and include dysphagia, regurgitation of undigested or partially digested food, gurgling in the throat accompanying swallowing, and swelling of the neck with eating. If the diverticula are large and produce obstruction of the esophagus, they may lead to regurgitation, coughing, choking spells, and aspiration, especially at night. Weight loss, malnutrition, and lung complications may develop. In general, the only available treatment is surgical excision of the diver-

ticulum. The diverticulum should be emptied, prior to surgery, of secretions, food, and barium to prevent aspiration and contamination.

Thoracic Diverticula (Traction). These diverticula are located in the middle one third of the esophagus at about the level of the left main bronchus and are thought to develop by traction on the esophagus secondary to lymph node inflammation. They rarely produce symptoms, because the neck of the diverticulum is broad and there is less tendency for food to collect. Operation is indicated only if complication of the diverticulum occurs, such as a diverticulitis, perforation, hemorrhage, or fistula formation. Complications are rare, however.

Supradiaphragmatic (Epiphrenic Diverticulum, Pulsion). These unusual diverticula, which occur in older patients, are found in the distal esophagus. Symptoms include dysphagia, pain, and occasionally hemorrhage. They are often associated with other esophageal motility disorders. Treatment in general is symptomatic. Surgery is indicated only if symptoms are severe or progressive. The problem of aspiration and suppurative pneumonitis is not as common as in Zenker's diverticulum.

ACHALASIA

Achalasia of the esophagus, or cardiospasm, is a disorder of esophageal motility characterized by absence of peristalsis and failure of vestibular relaxation after deglutition. The exact cause of the disease is not known, but achalasia is generally thought to be a disease with a neurogenic basis. The primary defect is not known, but there is an absence or decrease of ganglion cells of Auerbach's myenteric plexus in many of the patients. Vagus nerve changes and decreased cell counts of the medullary dorsal motor nucleus have also been described.

Achalasia may occur at any age but it is most frequently noticed between the ages of 30 and 50. It occurs in both males and females, with no sex predilection. The clinical onset is insidious, with the earliest and most constant symptom being dysphagia. Initially the dysphagia may be intermittent, but later it becomes persistent. Pain is not a common symptom, but it may occur early in the disease. Regurgitation may occur, especially at night, and may lead to pulmonary complications. With prolonged symptoms, the patient may also lose weight and develop all the problems of malnutrition. Furthermore, gradual dilatation of the esophagus results, with stasis of food and saliva that is difficult to evacuate, resulting in risk of aspiration. Treatment may be medical or surgical until an enlarged, dilated esophagus develops, in which case surgical resection is usually required.

Medical treatment consists of mechanical, pneumatic, or hydrostatic dilatation of the narrowed segment. The major acute complication of this method of treatment is perforation of the esophagus. The surgical treatment most commonly used is esophagomyotomy (modified Heller procedure).

Although most achalasia seen in the United States is idiopathic in nature, similar findings may occur in Chagas' disease (*Trypanosoma cruzi*). (See diseases of the colon.)

Diffuse Esophageal Spasm

Diffuse esophageal spasm usually occurs in the middle-aged and has no sex predilection. The cause of this condition is not known. Histologically the smooth muscle, except for thickening, is normal and ganglion cells are present. The disease may be related to primary involvement of the vagal afferent system. Symptoms are usually intermittent dysphagia or pain or both. Pain is the prominent symptom, presenting as moderate substernal discomfort or, in some cases, mimicking angina. Although symptoms are triggered or aggravated by eating, they may occur spontaneously. Symptoms are not usually incapacitating. Occasionally patients may lose weight, and many of them are high-strung and nervous.

Patients undergoing surgery must be selected very carefully. To be considered as surgical candidates they should have serious disability from their symptoms and no evidence of other gastrointestinal disorder.

Paraesophageal Hernia

This is a relatively uncommon hernia. The esophageal junction remains below the hiatus, but a part or all of the stomach extends alongside the esophagus into the thorax. Unlike sliding hiatus hernia, esophageal reflux is not a problem. Major complications are vascular congestion, ulceration in the herniated part of the stomach, hemorrhage, and obstruction. Occasionally a portion of the stomach can become strangulated, necessitating an emergency operation. Other abdominal organs such as the spleen, colon, or small bowel may be involved in the hernia. Because these severe complications may develop even in asymptomatic paraesophageal hernias, surgical repair is generally indicated.

Esophageal Perforation

Perforation or rupture of the esophagus is a serious complication associated with high mortality and morbidity. It may result from a variety of causes: secondary to esophageal instrumentation, ingestion of foreign body, spontaneous rupture associated with vomiting (Boerhaave's syndrome), external trauma, peptic ulcer, and devascularization of the esophageal wall. Although perforation can occur at any level of the esophagus, the two common sites are at the junction of the pharynx and esophagus and the lower esophagus just above the diaphragm. Perforation causes contamination of the paraesophageal tissue to a variable degree. Contamination with food, air, and bacteria may be more extensive with spontaneous rupture or trauma than with endoscopic perforation, because in the latter case the patient has usually been fasted for a period of time and the problem is generally recognized immediately. The anatomic location of the perforation is important. Perforation of the cervical esophagus produces contamination in the neck but also may extend down into the mediastinum. Perforation of the subphrenic esophagus may produce peritonitis. Thoracic esophageal perforation produces contamination of the mediastinum, and interstitial emphysema frequently extends upward into the neck.

In addition to the mediastinitis, these patients may have pneumothorax and/or pleural effusion. The clinical manifestations resulting from the mediastinitis include sequestration of body fluids, bacterial contamination, hypovolemia, and pleural space involvement. The accumulation of air and fluid may lead to interference with cardiorespiratory dynamics. With cervical perforation, pain, fever, and dysphagia are the common symptoms. Cervical crepitus and tenderness may be present on physical examination. Thoracic esophageal perforation may cause chest pain, fever, dyspnea, cervical crepitus, Hamman's sign, cyanosis, and shock. Subphrenic esophageal perforation produces signs similar to perforation of a duodenal ulcer. In spontaneous rupture (Boerhaave's syndrome) excruciating pain (mimicking a pulmonary embolus or myocardial infarction) and the other clinical manifestations of perforation occur after an episode of vomiting. Treatment consists of parenteral antibiotics and correction of fluid and electrolyte imbalance. Perforations require exploration with closure or repair if possible and, most important, adequate drainage. Complications that may develop are cervical or mediastinal abscesses, empyema, and esophagopleural or cutaneous fistulas.

The results of surgical treatment of cervical esophageal perforation are good (survival, 90 to 95 per cent). Mortality of thoracic and abdominal esophageal perforations varies from 10 to 30 per cent. With spontaneous rupture the mortality is quite high (30 to 50 per cent). A major factor in the high mortality and morbidity appears to be a delay in diagnosis and treatment beyond 24 hours.

ESOPHAGEAL MONILIASIS

Monilial esophagitis is produced by invasion of the esophageal mucosa by Candida in a mycelian phase which leads to destructive changes. The yeast phase is noninvasive. The infection leads to marked mucosal inflammation, erosion, ulceration, and pseudomembrane and pseudotumor formation. These lesions may produce massive hemorrhage, perforation, or fungemia with dissemination to other organs. Although esophageal moniliasis may occur in patients without concurrent diseases, it is most commonly found in those with underlying neoplasia. Frequently the patients are receiving antimicrobials, antimetabolites, adrenal steroids, or radiation therapy. Common symptoms are pyrosis, dysphagia, and odynophagia. Because of these symptoms, the oral intake of fluid and food may be poor. Treatment consists of supportive measures and appropriate antifungal chemotherapy.

Surgical treatment is limited to the treatment of complications.

CORROSIVE ESOPHAGITIS

Intentional or accidental ingestion of strong alkali or acid produces chemical burns of the esophagus and at times the stomach. Commercial lye solution (95 per cent NaOH) is the most common agent ingested. The extent and severity of injury depend upon the agent, amount, concentration, nature (liquid, solid), and duration of contact. If a small amount is ingested, only the mouth and pharynx may be burned. With a greater ingestion, the middle and distal esophagus may be affected. If the stomach is involved, the antral area is most commonly injured. Two of the early complications that can occur are perforation and mediastinitis. The major complication in the chronic phase is stricture. Early treatment consists of ingestion of and irrigation with large volumes of water or saline solutions, neutralization with the appropriate agents (e.g., vinegar, sodium bicarbonate), antibiotics, and steroids. The treatment of the stricture may require dilatation by bougienage, resection of the stricture, or bypass with stomach, colon, or intestine.

REFLUX ESOPHAGITIS AND STRICTURE

The most common cause of esophagitis is reflux of acidic gastric juice into the lower esophagus, which most commonly accompanies a sliding hiatal hernia but exists 15 per cent of the time without an anatomical hernia. Corrosive esophagitis from ingestion of a strong acid or alkali is less common. Since the esophageal mucosa is sensitive also to alkaline secretions, reflux esophagitis may occur after operative procedures that have reduced gastric acid output and/or have disturbed the motility and normal physiologic sphincter mechanisms of the stomach, pylorus, or lower esophagus.

Dysphagia, regurgitation, substernal or epigastric pain, and heartburn are the most common symptoms. Dysphagia is more prominent later in the history of the disease when stricture formation is occurring. Upper gastrointestinal series is most commonly used to demonstrate reflux of barium and hiatal hernia but entails a high degree of inaccuracy, often missing minor changes. Esophagoscopy with biopsy is now essential to objectively confirm the presence and grade of esophagitis. Manometry, acid perfusion studies (Bernstein's test), pH monitoring, and acid clearing studies have all been helpful in confirming the diagnosis.

The essence of treatment is to prevent reflux or minimize its effects. Weight reduction, bland diets, antacids, elimination of heavy meals, elevation of the head of the bed at night, and cimetidine have all been used in treatment. It is important to recognize intractability early and to recommend surgical therapy before allowing fibrosis and stricture to occur.

Three common operative repairs are currently used: 1) Belsey Mark IV operation, a 270° horizontal gastric plication to the diaphragm, sometimes performed intraabdominally but usually transthoracically; 2) Nissen fundoplication, a vertical 360° wrap of the lower esophagus by the fundus; and 3) Hill repair, fixation of the lesser curvature to the median arcuate ligament. All three operations essentially 1) reduce the hiatal hernia and return a segment of the esophagus within the high pressure abdominal area, 2) re-create the angle of His at the cardioesophageal junction, and 3) suture the lower esophagus and stomach to prevent a recurrence of the "sliding" into the mediastinum. All patients facing surgery are at an increased risk of aspiration and many tend to be obese. The approach used for each patient is determined on an individual basis and is dependent upon the skills of the surgeon. Transthoracic approaches are favored when a previous number of abdominal operations have been performed, and abdominal procedures are favored when associated abdominal pathology may exist. Some now advocate parietal cell vagotomy along with operative repair, both for the advantages of surgical exposure and for the acid reduction. Recurrence of reflux can be assessed symptomatically by x-rays, or by physiological testing. In general, all of the above operations are about 80 per cent successful. Some objective evidence would favor the Nissen fundoplication for superior clinical results, but many forms of breakdown have been described. Complications besides recurrence of reflux include postoperative dysphagia, "gas-bloat syndrome," gastric distention, bleeding, abscess, inadvertent splenectomy, esophagogastric fistula, postoperative respiratory problems including pneumonia, and incomplete relief of symptoms.

Stricture. When a patient develops a stricture secondary to reflux, the operative morbidity and mortality are increased. For this reason conservative measures at bougienage are usually attempted first. Many of these individuals are malnourished and should be placed in positive nitrogen balance by total parenteral nutrition, as discussed earlier, or by feeding once bougienage is succesful. Standard operative repair of the hiatal hernia alone may be successful along with bougienage. Occasionally with severe stricture formation, a Thal patch can be used if a short segment is involved, or esophagogastrectomy or esophagectomy with bowel interposition if the stricture is long. Most resections are accompanied by a pyloroplasty to enhance emptying. All these procedures are excessive, carrying risk, and should be attempted only if more conservative techniques fail.

BARRETT'S SYNDROME

Normally a variable length of the distal esophagus (0.75 to 2.0 cm.) is lined by columnar epithelium without parietal cells. In some patients columnar epithelium may line most of the lower esophagus. This change is probably acquired and not congenital and is a sequel of reflux esophagitis. Deep chronic peptic ulcers may develop in this area, which then lead to other complications, such as perforation with mediastinitis, massive hemorrhage, or stricture. Barrett's syndrome consists of an esophagus lined by columnar epithelium, chronic peptic ulcer, and/or esophageal stricture.

BENIGN NEOPLASMS

Benign tumors of the esophagus are rare. Dysphagia is the most frequent symptom, although many are asymptomatic. The most common benign tumors are the leiomyomas. They are usually intramural and extramucosal, but can be pedunculated and multiple. Other benign tumors include cysts and papillomas.

ESOPHAGEAL WEBS

Fibrous webs occur at various levels of the esophagus. Upper esophageal webs may be associated with anemia (Plummer-Vinson syndrome). This syndrome is usually seen in middle-aged, edentulous women with atrophic oral mucosa. Clinical manifestations include dysphagia, glossitis, spooning of nails, and iron deficiency anemia. Treatment consists of dilatation of the stricture and treatment of the anemia.

MALLORY-WEISS SYNDROME

A linear tear of the mucosa of the esophagogastric junction without muscular disruption may occur after retching or vomiting. This tear then may lead to significant bleeding. Conservative management may stop the bleeding; if not, the laceration has to be repaired surgically.

LOWER ESOPHAGEAL RING

This ring is located at the esophagogastric junction and may cause intermittent dysphagia of solid foods if the diameter of the lumen is under 13 mm. The usual treatment is dilatation of the stricture and treatment of the underlying pathology, which in a large number of instances is esophageal reflux.

ESOPHAGEAL DISTURBANCES ASSOCIATED WITH SYSTEMIC DISEASE

Myasthenia Gravis. Patients may complain of mild dysphagia. There are weakness of the pharyngeal musculature and a decrease in the esophageal peristaltic waves which disappear in the lower esophagus. On barium swallow, the barium is retained in the pyriform sinuses and may be aspirated into the trachea. Dysphagia may be associated with other neuromuscular disorders such as myotonia dystrophica, amyotrophic lateral sclerosis, Parkinson's disease, or stroke.

Scleroderma. Symptoms seen commonly with this disorder are dysphagia, regurgitation, heartburn, and other symptoms of esophageal obstruction. Treatment is dilatation of the strictures. If the strictures cannot be dilated, surgical resection may be required. Other collagen diseases may also produce dysphagia and esophageal dysfunction.

DISORDERS OF THE STOMACH AND DUODENUM

FOREIGN BODIES

A variety of individual foreign bodies may be ingested. Most pass into the duodenum and eventually are passed in the stool. Complications associated with foreign bodies if they do not pass into the duodenum are penetration of the gastric wall by sharp objects, ulcerations which may lead to pain and bleeding, or obstruction. These complications require surgical removal of the foreign body.

Bezoars may produce the following symptoms and complications: abdominal pain, nausea, vomiting, weight loss, weakness, obstruction, ulceration, and inanition. Trichobezoars (hairballs), phytobezoars (accumulation of vegetable fibers), trichophytobezoars (a combination of the two), diospyrobezoars (persimmon fibers), and concretions (precipitated or solidified chemicals, e.g., shellac-resin mass) are the more common types found. Trichobezoars are usually found in females under 30, and phytobezoars in males over 30. Surgical removal is indicated because mortality from hemorrhage and ulceration is quite high without surgery.

CORROSIVE GASTRITIS

Intentional or accidental ingestion of strong alkali or acid usually produces chemical burns of the mouth, pharynx, and esophagus, but gastric burns can occur. Strong acids tend to produce more damage than alkali in the stomach, because the latter is partially neutralized by the gastric acid. The treatment consists of evacuation, dilution, lavage and neutralization, antibiotics, sedation, and intravenous fluids. Early complications that may occur are hemorrhage or perforation; a late complication is outlet obstruction secondary to scarring.

ASSOCIATION OF GASTRIC AND DUODENAL ULCERATION WITH OTHER DISEASES

Zollinger-Ellison Syndrome. This syndrome is characterized by fulminating ulcer diathesis, pronounced gastric hypersecretion, and non-beta islet cell tumors of the pancreas. Severe diarrhea may also be associated with this syndrome. The age distribution is from eight to over 80, but the greatest incidence is in the third, fourth, and fifth decades. Some of the characteristic clinical features are 1) intractable ulcer, unusual location of an ulcer, or multiple ulcers; 2) gastric hypersecretion, a 12-hour nocturnal collection of over 1000 cc or over 200 mEq of HC1 under basal condition, with only a relatively slight increase in acid output after maximal stimulation with histamine or Histalog; 3) severe diarrhea; 4) steatorrhea; 5) hypokalemia; 6) recurrence after adequate surgical treatment; and 7) high serum gastrin levels. These findings are not present in all patients, because some may have gastric hypersecretion without ulcer but with severe diarrhea. Sixty per cent of these tumors are malignant and may metastasize. Tumors may be found in the duodenum in addition to the pancreas and are frequently multiple. Twenty to 25 per cent of patients have other functioning endocrine adenomas. The glands that may be affected are the parathyroid, pituitary, thyroid, and adrenal cortex. In the surgical management of these patients, total gastrectomy is used most frequently. The use of long term H_2 receptor blockade with cimetidine has been useful in decreasing gastric acid output and managing the symptomatology. Many are now advocating medical treatment and nutritional support prior to exploratory laparotomy and complete excision of the tumor if possible, total gastrectomy being reserved for complications of medical therapy and if the tumor cannot be removed (e.g., metastatic).

Hyperparathyroidism. There may be a slightly higher incidence of peptic ulcer disease in patients with hyperparathyroidism, but the relationship between the two is not clear. Hypercalcemia does stimulate antral gastrin release. In addition, ectopic gastrin production has been documented in parathyroid tissue. Thirty per cent of patients with ulcerogenic tumors of the duodenum may be hyperparathyroid (Werner-Morrison syndrome).

Adrenal Dysfunction and Steroids. There is an increased incidence of peptic ulceration with Cushing's disease, as well as with exogenous administration of adrenocortical steroids. All the mechanisms that lead to the ulcerations are not known. Increase in acid secretion is probably not a major factor. The decrease and chemical alterations of the gastric mucus may be important. Steroid ulcers are seen more commonly in patients with rheumatoid arthritis than in patients with ulcerative colitis. The ulcers occur more frequently in the stomach than in the duodenum. They may be asymptomatic and only become evident after a severe complication such as hemorrhage or perforation. If these patients require surgical treatment, they are often poor risks because of their primary disease.

Stress Ulcers. Stress ulcers may occur after major operations or severe trauma. A serious complication or sepsis after the initial injury seems to increase their incidence. Very commonly, the combination of these features occur in the surgical intensive care setting in an already seriously ill patient. Mortality from gastric hemorrhage approaches 80 per cent in many reports. An associated but etiologically different type of peptic ulceration is related to major burns (10 to 20 per cent of moderate to severe burns produce Curling's ulcers). Intracranial disease or injury is associated with peptic ulceration (Cushing's ulcer). Stress ulcerations occur more frequently in the stomach than in the duodenum. They are usually multiple and vary from superficial erosions to deep submucosal ulcers. They can present with perforation or hemorrhage, resulting in high morbidity and mortality, but more commonly exist for days without bleeding, as noted by routine fiberoptic endoscopy. Physiologic disruption of the gastric mucosa barrier has been observed in animal models, with hydrogen ion back diffusion in advance of gross mucosal changes, but this is difficult to monitor in man and does not correlate well with the occurrence of clinical gastritis and ulceration. If the underlying disease is reversible, stress ulceration is considered a temporary derangement best treated by prophylaxis. Uncontrollable hemorrhage is treated surgically by vagotomy, suture ligation, gastrectomy if necessary, and occasionally total gastrectomy. Intravenous infusion with vasopressin (Pitressin) has been of limited usefulness and is a temporary measure. The incidence of surgical procedures, however, is dropping because of the increasing expertise in intensive care and the increasing awareness of the problem. Total parenteral nutrition, patient monitoring, cimetidine, and continuous regulation of intragastric pH to 7.0 with antacid has resulted in marked diminution in the occurrence of acute gastric mucosal disease. Prostaglandin is now being investigated as a cytoprotective agent that may be useful in future prophylaxis against gastric mucosal disruption.

Pulmonary Disease. There is an increased incidence of peptic ulcers in patients with chronic pulmonary disease (severe chronic emphysema, cor pulmonale). Duodenal ulcer is seen more commonly than gastric ulcer. The mechanisms that lead to ulcerations are not clear, although chronic hypoxia does result in increased gastric acid output.

Liver Disease. The incidence of peptic ulceration is increased in patients with cirrhosis and those who have undergone portacaval shunts. The pathophysiology of this type of ulcer is not completely understood but it appears to be the result of a jejunal hormone normally degraded in the liver that stimulates acid output.

Pancreatic Exocrine Disease. The incidence of peptic ulcer is increased in patients with chronic pancreatitis. The exact pathophysiological relationship between ulcer disease and pancreatic disease is not clear.

Massive Small Bowel Resection. This procedure is associated with an increased incidence of peptic ulcerations. The ulcers may be due to an increase in gastric secretion on the basis of lack of inhibitory factors. In some cases increases in serum gastrin have been noted.

Drugs. Many drugs may produce gastric mucosal injury or aggravate the ulcer diatheses. The more common offenders include aspirin, phenylbutazone, indomethacin, caffeine, alcohol, nicotine, and steroids.

SUPPURATIVE GASTRITIS (PHLEGMONOUS OR NECROTIZING GASTRITIS)

This is a rare infection of the gastric wall. The infecting organism is usually *hemolytic streptococcus,* but other organisms may be involved. It is most commonly seen in middle-aged male alcoholics with hypochlorhydria. The mode of infection is not clearly known. Some of the symptoms and complications that may occur are acute epigastric pain, vomiting, which may be hemorrhagic, sepsis, spreading cellulitis, abscess formation, and perforation. Progression to death can occur in a few hours. Treatment consists of massive antibiotics and supportive care. Operative treatment may be required for the complications. *Necrotizing gastritis* is usually due to fusiform and spirochetal organisms commonly found in the mouth. They may produce necrosis and gangrene of the gastric wall. Similar complications can result.

GRANULOMATOUS GASTRITIS

Tuberculosis of the stomach is usually secondary to active pulmonary tuberculosis. The lesion may consist of multiple ulcers or diffuse hypertrophic thickening of the stomach wall. Treatment is similar to pulmonary tuberculosis. Operative treatment may be necessary for obstruction or destruction of the stomach wall. *The gastric lesion of tertiary syphilis* may present with epigastric fullness, weight loss, and anemia. The treatment is adequate penicillin therapy, but operation may be required for the late complication of obstruction. *Eosinophilic infiltration* of the stomach is characterized by focal or diffuse eosinophilic infiltrate of the granulomatous variety. The cause is unknown. Symptoms of obstruction, ulceration, or hemorrhage may result. Treatment is similar to the management of benign tumors of the stomach.

NEOPLASMS OF THE STOMACH

Benign Tumors. Benign tumors of the stomach are relatively uncommon. They may be mucosal tumors or intramural tumors. Gastric adenomas may be single or multiple, polypoid or sessile; they tend to occur in the antrum. The majority of patients are over 60, are achlorhydric and have atrophic gastritis. Most of these tumors produce no symptoms, but they may be associated with epigastric distress, anemia (hypochromic or macrocytic pernicious anemia), nausea and vomiting, or intermittent obstruction.

Intramural tumors of the stomach occur in

middle-aged and older patients. They may be leiomyomas, fibromas, fibromyomas, schwannomas, neurofibromas, neuroblastomas, lipomas, hemangiomas, glomus tumors, or ectopic pancreatic tissue. Clinical manifestations that may result from these tumors are hemorrhage, abdominal distress, episodic vomiting, and the symptoms of outlet obstruction. Treatment is local excision or partial gastric resection, depending on the location and size of the tumor.

Carcinoid Tumors. See section on the small intestine.

Lymphomas and Sarcomas. Gastric *lymphomas* may be secondary to disseminated disease or may be primary in the stomach (lymphosarcoma, reticulum cell sarcoma, Hodgkin's disease). Treatment of primary lymphomas consists of gastric resection or total gastrectomy if confined to the stomach, followed by postoperative x-ray therapy. The five-year survival rate is about 35 to 40 per cent.

Leiomyosarcomas often present with abdominal pain, weight loss, chronic bleeding, or severe acute hemorrhage. Surgical treatment is gastric resection if the lesion is confined to the stomach. The five-year survival rate is about 50 per cent.

GASTRIC VOLVULUS

Torsion of the stomach may occur along either the long or the transverse axis of the stomach. Relaxation or loss of the support of the stomach permits this to occur. Volvulus may be associated with hiatal hernia, eventration of the diaphragm, ventral hernia, gastric tumors, gastric ulcer, or chronic dilatation of the stomach. Acute gastric volvulus presents with sudden epigastric pain and vomiting followed by retching. Complete or partial obstruction of both ends of the stomach may result in marked distention, progressing to shock. The symptom triad consists of 1) unproductive retching, 2) localized epigastric pain, and 3) inability to pass a tube into the stomach. Strangulation can occur with volvulus, and this of course increases the urgency of treatment. Treatment consists of reducing the volvulus, correcting the associated abnormalities if the risk is reasonable, and a partial gastrectomy with vagotomy if necessary. A corrective procedure should be performed at a second operation if there is any question of risk.

VAGOTOMY OPERATIONS WITH INTRAOPERATIVE TESTING

Vagotomy is playing a more and more critical role in the surgical management of duodenal ulcer disease, and, while not uncommon, testing for completeness of vagotomy during the operation is being performed at only a few medical centers. As selective vagotomy becomes more accepted, documenting the adequacy of vagotomy will become important. Over 90 per cent of ulcer recurrences following vagotomy are attributed to incomplete vagotomy. A successful intraoperative test that would alert the surgeon to this problem intraoperatively would be of critical importance.

Many methods are currently operable, but all have their limitations. In all cases, cooperation with the anesthesiologist is essential. Administration of medications and assistance with instrumentation may be needed. Furthermore, anticholinergics and antihistamine (H_2-blockers) cannot be used preoperatively.

Electrostimulation of the vagus and monitoring changes of intragastric pressure was first introduced in 1958 but has not been generally used, since it is cumbersome and time consuming, and requires special instrumentation to record motility changes. Staining techniques require exposure of the nerve, and the intraoperative use of other "vagal stimulants," such as insulin and 2-deoxy-D-glucose, is dangerous and not accurate. Currently, most commonly used methods measure the well documented change in fundic mucosal pH that occurs following denervation. pH varies from 1.2 to over 3.0. The use of pH probes requires a gastrotomy and careful contact over the entire mucosal surface. Other methods utilize Congo Red, an azine dye indicator that turns red to black below pH 3.0 and adheres to the gastric mucosa. Congo Red color changes can be noted via a gastrotomy or pyloroplasty incision and via fiberoptic endoscope passed just prior to intubation of the patient. Congo Red has been used before, in the days of gastrectomy, to allow surgeons to determine the margin between the antrum and the fundus and now allows determination of innervated and denervated mucosa in the era of vagotomy. Drawbacks still exist regarding the validity of a negative test, since anesthetics alone depress gastric secretion. Pentagastrin has been used as a stimulant, but ideal doses, time of observation, and long term follow-up have not been determined or corroborated. The test is simple and safe, and if accurate may satisfy the needs of an intraoperative vagotomy test; it has been used in many vagotomy patients thus far.

DISORDERS OF THE SMALL INTESTINE

NEOPLASMS OF THE SMALL INTESTINE

Both benign and malignant neoplasms of the small bowel are relatively rare. They occur most commonly in the fifth to seventh decades with equal sex distribution. The two most common complications of these tumors are bowel obstruction and bleeding. The obstruction may result from intussusception, a constricting lesion, or volvulus. Bleeding is usually occult, slow, and intermittent, producing an iron deficiency anemia. Rarely, these neoplasms may produce bloody stools. Vascular tumors and myomas are most commonly associated with bleeding. Other complications that may occur are perforation with peritonitis, internal fistula, or abscess formation. Some of the common symptoms are nausea, vomiting, pain, diarrhea with mucus, and weight loss.

Malignant Neoplasms. Adenocarcinomas are the most common malignant neoplasms of the small bowel. They are more common in the duodenum than in the ileum. Lesions in the duodenum frequently bleed and may also produce obstructive jaundice. The jejunal and ileal lesions tend to present with small bowel obstruction. Treatment is wide resection, including adjacent lymph nodes; duodenal tumors require pancreatoduodenectomy. The resectability rate is only about 40 per cent, and the overall five-year survival rate is only 20 per cent.

Sarcomas are most commonly found in the ileum. They tend to grow outside the bowel and present as abdominal masses without obstruction.

Lymphomas occur more commonly in the lower segments of the small bowel, may be multiple, and are more common in males than in females. Complications that can occur include perforation, malabsorption, and pneumatosis cystoides intestinalis. The treatment is wide resection and possibly radiation. Long-term survival varies from 10 to 40 per cent.

Leiomyosarcomas are often present as large tumors and frequently produce bleeding. The five-year survival rate is about 40 to 50 per cent.

Carcinoid. Carcinoid tumors can occur at any place in the gastrointestinal tract from the gastric cardia to the anus. They are also found in the bronchus and may occur in teratomas. Approximately 46 per cent are found in the appendix, 28 per cent in the ileum, and 17 per cent in the rectum. These tumors are usually small (less than 1.5 cm) and frequently multiple (29 per cent). They may also be associated with other primary malignant neoplasms. The malignant potential depends on the size and location of the tumor. Very few appendiceal carcinoids metastasize, but about a third of ileal carcinoids do. The larger tumors tend to metastasize. Multiple tumors are found in 30 per cent of small bowel carcinoid. Treatment consists of resection of the primary lesion with the mesentery containing the lymphatic drainage of the area. Even with widespread metastatic disease, all resectable tumors should be removed. The five-year survival rate after curative resection is 70 per cent. Even with metastasis, five-year survival is reported to be 27 per cent.

Malignant carcinoid tumors may produce the so-called carcinoid syndrome, which has the following manifestations: intermittent red or purplish flushing of the trunk and face, diarrhea, asthma, tachycardia, arthralgia, and pellagra-like skin changes. Normally only about 1 per cent of dietary tryptophan is metabolized to form serotonin, most going to form protein and niacin. Malignant carcinoids can divert as much as 60 per cent of tryptophan into the serotonin pathways, leaving a niacin deficiency. Serotonin is broken down by the liver to 5-hydroxyindoleacetic acid (5-HIAA) and is excreted in the urine (normal 2–10 mg/day). By bypassing the liver and entering the systemic circulation directly serotonin accumulates contributing to the carcinoid syndrome. Pulmonary stenosis or tricuspid insufficiency may develop as a result of subendothelial fibrosis of the valves, which may then lead to cardiac failure. The flushing may be precipitated by food, alcohol, or emotional stress. Usually the duration of flushing is brief, but it may last several hours. Diarrhea is usually sudden in onset and is watery. Recent studies suggest that, in addition to production of serotonin, carcinoid tumors secrete several biologically active peptides that may be responsible for some aspects of the syndrome. Carcinoids at different levels of the gastrointestinal tract have slightly different characteristics. Upper GI tract carcinoids tend to elaborate kallikrein, which in turn gives rise to kinins. In addition, histamine and ACTH may be produced by these functioning carcinoids. Mid-gut carcinoids secrete serotonin, and lower gastrointestinal tract lesions (such as rectal carcinoids) may not secrete any substance and tend not to take up silver staining. Treatment of patients with this syndrome is not entirely satisfactory, because in most patients not all the neoplastic tissue can be removed. However, an attempt should be made to remove as much of the primary and metastatic tumor as possible for relief from some of the undesirable symptoms. In considering surgical treatment, it is important to remember that approximately 40 per cent of the patients live only one to four years.

Benign Neoplasms. Benign tumors of the small bowel include leiomyomas, lipomas, adenomas, polyps, hemangiomas, neurogenic tumors, and fibromas. The signs and symptoms of these tumors are related to obstruction and hemorrhage: nausea, vomiting, abdominal pain, and melena. Other complications that can occur are peritonitis and fistula formation. In general, these tumors should be excised.

Peutz-Jeghers Syndrome. This syndrome is characterized by multiple polyps of the gastrointestinal tract, especially the small bowel, and melanin spots of the oral mucosa, lips, palms of the hands, and soles of the feet. The condition is familial, and inheritance is as a simple mendelian dominant. The polyps are thought to be hamartomas without malignant potential. Complications that can occur are hemorrhage and obstruction caused by intussusception. Surgical therapy is indicated only for the complications, because usually not all the polyps can be removed without making the patient a short-gut cripple.

VASCULAR LESIONS

Osler-Weber-Rendu Syndrome (Hereditary Hemorrhagic Telangiectasia). This syndrome is characterized by telangiectasia of the mucous membrane of the nasal or oral cavities, viscera, or skin, a familial occurrence, and repeated hemorrhages. Associated pulmonary arteriovenous fistulas may be present. The major complication is gastrointestinal hemorrhage, which usually does not become evident until after the fourth decade. Because of the extensive involvement, surgical treatment is not entirely satisfactory.

Hemangiomas. Hemangiomas may be capillary, cavernous, or mixed. The complications are due to local destruction, hemorrhage, obstruction, perforation, and sepsis. Surgical treatment is indicated only for the complications.

REGIONAL ENTERITIS (CROHN'S DISEASE)

Regional enteritis is an inflammatory disease of unknown cause that may involve the stomach, duodenum, jejunum, ileum, colon, and anus. Clinically the disease most frequently involves the terminal ileum. It is primarily a disease of young adults, although it may develop in older patients and in the very young. Diseased small bowel demonstrates thickening of the bowel wall and involvement with granulomas through all layers, with the submucosa showing the greatest increase. There is marked narrowing of the lumen (string sign on x-ray), mucosal modularity (cobblestone appearance), ulceration, and thickening of the mesentery with enlargement of the lymph nodes. Mesenteric fat tends to grow and encroach around the bowel wall, and several loops may become matted together. Early or acute enteritis will demonstrate hyperemia, dullness of the serosa, edema of the mesentery, and a "soft" thickening of the bowel wall as opposed to the chronic changes noted above. Only a minority of the patients with acute disease progress to chronic regional enteritis, and most can be treated conservatively.

The cause of Crohn's disease is at yet unknown but a chronic infectious process has been hypothesized based on findings of virus-like inclusion bodies within cells from surgical specimens. Allergic or autoimmune as well as hereditary factors have also been implicated.

The disease may involve any segment of the gastrointestinal tract from esophagus to rectum. One of the clinical hallmarks of regional enteritis is the involvement of separate "skip-areas" with normal bowel in between. In about one third of patients, both small and large bowel are involved. Another group of patients classicially have the disease limited to the ileum. Uncommonly the disease can be limited to the colon with a predilection for the right colon.

Clinical manifestations depend upon the extent of the disease process, site of involvement, and complications. Common findings are abdominal pain, diarrhea, low grade fever, leukocytosis, and tenderness in the right lower quadrant. Patients may also have weight loss, weakness, and fatigue. The complications that may occur include obstruction, internal fistulas, abscess formation, perforation, enterocutaneous fistulas, and hemorrhage. While bleeding is rare, infectious complications such as abscess, fistulas, etc., occur in upward of 50 per cent. Emergency surgery is rarely needed but is not infrequent. Most patients have diarrhea, steatorrhea, and frank malnutrition. Total parenteral nutrition is now an accepted mainstay for medical treatment. Approximately one third of fistulas can be healed on bowel rest and adequate intravenous nutrition. Remission of the disease is common on this regimen, as described above, along with other measures such as vitamin supplements, sulfonamide therapy, symptomatic treatment of diarrhea, and steroids. Low doses of Imuran have been used with some success but more often have been ineffective and quite toxic. Systemic antibiotics are used for secondary infectious complications.

Indications for surgery are failure of medical therapy, complications as noted previously, and a continued downhill course despite adequate medical treatment. Surgical treatment may be resection of the diseased segment, with primary anastomosis or bypass of the diseased area. Operative mortality is about 2 to 5 per cent (8-10 per cent for reoperations) and the recurrence rate is reported at 35 to 50 per cent. The morbidity is higher in patients who have been on large doses of steroids for prolonged periods. Because of high recurrence rates, surgical therapy is now used conservatively. To remove all diseased bowel is no longer the goal, rather, the attempt is to preserve as much intestine for as long as possible, with recurrent disease expected. Increasing numbers of malignancies have been reported of late

in association with this disease, adding to the concern. In addition, a minority of patients (less than 50 per cent) get no recurrence following surgery and can be rehabilitated completely. In some cases, a mild recurrence can be managed on proper medical therapy.

TYPHOID ENTERITIS

Typhoid fever is an acute systemic infection caused by *Salmonella typhi*. Malaise, headache, and fever are noted during the incubation period. Diarrhea and high fever start about the third week. The serious complications which can occur are hemorrhage, perforation, and acute cholecystitis. Complications are due to ulceration and erosion of blood vessels in Peyer's patches. Gross bleeding is present in 10 to 20 per cent of all cases, but perforation occurs in only about 2 per cent. Treatment consists of chloramphenicol, steroids to reduce toxicity, and intravenous fluids and blood if necessary. Mortality should be less than 5 per cent. Operative treatment is indicated only when absolutely necessary for correction of complications.

TUBERCULOUS ENTERITIS

Tuberculosis of the intestine is caused most commonly by the human strain of the organism. The ileocecal area is involved in 85 per cent of the patients with tuberculous enteritis. Most of the patients have no signs or symptoms; but when they occur, pain, weight loss, nausea, and diarrhea are noted. Complications that can occur include obstruction, free perforation into the peritoneal cavity, abscess, fistulas, and hemorrhage. Systemic complications include malnutrition and amyloidosis. The primary treatment is antitubercular chemotherapy. Surgical management is limited to treatment of complications.

DIVERTICULA

False diverticula of the small bowel are most commonly found in the jejunum, although they may occur in the duodenum and ileum. Jejunal diverticula are usually found in patients over 50, with no sex preponderance. A variety of clinical manifestations may result from these diverticula. Patients may develop intermittent periumbilical or epigastric pain, profuse watery diarrhea, weight loss, and nausea and vomiting. In these patients there may be hypertrophy and dilatation of the jejunal segment with the diverticula as well as hypermotility of the segment. Diverticula may also be associated with malabsorption, steatorrhea, and anemia. The anemia is most commonly megaloblastic. The mechanisms of the malabsorption are not fully known, but abnormal growth of bacteria may interfere with absorption. The medical treatment consists of replacement of vitamin B_{12}, folic acid, oral iron, and calciferol as indicated. Oral antibiotics have been used with good results in some of these patients. Surgical resection has also been followed by improvement in malabsorption in a few patients. Jejunal diverticula can also present as an acute diverticulitis. Complications which can occur are perforation, peritonitis, abscess formation, adhesions, and intestinal obstruction. These complications may require surgical treatment with resection of the involved segment.

RADIATION ENTERITIS

Damage to small bowel from irradiation is now diminishing as a result of better radiotherapy techniques. Patients receiving abdominal radiotherapy frequently develop anorexia, nausea, and diarrhea during and after treatment. These symptoms can usually be controlled with medication and usually subside with completion of therapy. However, symptoms may persist in some patients for several months after therapy or may recur after several months. Some of the clinical manifestations of established actinic enteritis are cramping abdominal pain, alternating constipation and diarrhea, and vomiting. A mass may be palpable in the abdomen. There may be malabsorption of fat, vitamin B_{12}, and calcium, and loss of protein and blood into the intestine with resulting anemia and low serum albumin. Some patients have improved with steroid therapy. Indications for operative treatment are progression of the clinical signs and symptoms on adequate medical therapy and complications such as perforation, obstruction, abscess, or fistulas (enterovesical, en-

terovaginal). The treatment of choice is resection of the diseased bowel segment. The immediate operative mortality is approximately 17 per cent.

PNEUMATOSIS CYSTOIDES INTESTINALIS

This rare condition is manifested by gas-filled cysts in the wall and mesentery of the gastrointestinal tract. Eighty-five per cent of the cases are associated with other lesions of the gastrointestinal tract such as peptic ulcer and diverticulitis, and 15 per cent are primary. These cysts may be submucosal or subserosal, and the common sites are the jejunum, ileocecal area, and colon. Complications are rare, but the following may occur: hemorrhage, obstruction (caused by volvulus, intussusception, or external compression), malabsorption, and tension pneumoperitoneum. No treatment is needed except for the associated disease and rare complications. The cysts may disappear spontaneously.

BYPASS OPERATIONS FOR OBESITY

The term morbid obesity usually is applied to the individual who has reached two to three times his or her ideal weight as defined on insurance tables and who has maintained this weight for five or more years despite efforts by the patient, family, and physicians to determine an endocrinological cause and/or to sustain reduction. Mortality rates of men weighing more than 254 pounds at ages 15 to 39 are 200 per cent of expected levels. Obese individuals are at risk from cardiovascular disease, liver and biliary disease, and multiple disorders such as social, physiological, and economic problems that disturb the quality of their life. Psychiatrists are only successful in 1 per cent of patients.

To deal with this problem, a variety of small intestinal bypass procedures have been developed to decrease absorption resulting in diarrhea. All patients considered should meet the criteria of morbid obesity and have had all organic causes ruled out, be free of psychiatric disease, be motivated and informed, be less than 50 years of age, and be available for follow-up.

Thorough preoperative workup includes

lipid, cortisol, thyroid, liver, renal, and pulmonary studies. Most operative complications are related to the obesity and not to the operation per se. Oxygen saturation is affected by the obesity, by positioning, and by the packs and retraction necessary during surgery. Forty per cent oxygen does not usually result in adequate arterial oxygenation during these operations. Ventilation and blood pressure determinations can be physically difficult. Veins are not as accessible, and decreased vital capacity, tidal volume, and expiratory reserve are usual.

Many different operative techniques are used. Most use a transverse incision which best allows extension and adequate visualization. In addition, postoperative wound complications may be lessened. In the obese, visualization and mobilization of the bowel may be difficult. Panniculectomy is added to the procedure by some surgeons. In addition, cholecystectomy is advocated when stones are present to eliminate postoperative cholecystitis, a potential problem. One of the first operations used involved anastomosing 14 inches of proximal jejunum to the distal 4 inches of the ileum, end to side, with the proximal part of the distal jejunum closed. Other variants include an end to end jejunal-ileal anastomosis with the bypassed segments drained into the cecum or colon to obviate reflux of chyme, which may prevent the desired amount of weight loss. Various regimens have been used, such as the proximal 10 inches to the distal 10 inches of ileum and 40 cm of proximal jejunum to the distal 4 cm of ileum. The attempt is to preserve the preferential absorptive capacity of the upper small bowel along with the fat and enterohepatic recirculation capacity of the distal ileum. The proximal portion of the bypass segment is anchored to the abdominal wall to prevent intussusception.

The results and complications have been variable. Operative mortalities range from 4 to 6 per cent. The rate of complications is high, averaging about 30 per cent, with thrombophlebitis, pulmonary embolism, coronary occlusion, and peritonitis not infrequent. By far the most common complication relates to the wound and ranges from subcutaneous collections of liquefied fat and serum to frank wound dehiscence. The rehospitalization rate is 50 per cent. Weight loss initially can be precipitous until three months postoperatively, reaching a plateau at anywhere from one to three years after the operation, when compensatory hypertrophy and elongation of the bowel occurs. Patients can expect to lose an average of one third of their preoperative weight.

Complications are usual. About 1 per cent lose excessive amounts of weight, and 5 to 20 per cent have inadequate weight loss, all requiring revision. Diarrhea of up to 20 stools per day is usual but, hopefully, can be controlled to 10 per day by the use of Lomotil or paregoric, by restricting fat, and by adding medium chain triglycerides to the diet. The most troublesome complication is the hepatic changes that occur. From 60 to 90 per cent have fatty infiltration preoperatively, which increases after bypass. Most improve when the weight loss plateaus but must be followed by serial liver biopsy. Most obese patients preoperatively are chronically protein malnourished. This must be corrected prior to bypass. Five per cent of patients go on to have liver failure requiring reversal of the bypass. Jaundice, hypoprothrombinemia, fluid retention, hypoalbuminemia, elevation of liver enzymes, anorexia, and nausea accompany liver failure. Essential amino acid alimentation has been helpful. Other problems noted include deficiencies in potassium, calcium, magnesium, and vitamin B_{12}. Generally there is a decrease in blood pressure and an amelioration in the severity of diabetes, if present. Excess gastric secretion may increase the risk of peptic ulceration. Alopecia is noted in about 4 to 33 per cent and about 7 per cent develop renal stones of calcium oxalate. Problems with the intestine itself include internal herniation, volvulus, intussuception, and bypass enteritis, which may be due to changes in pH allowing for enhanced bacterial growth.

Gastric Bypass. Many surgeons have abandoned the intestinal bypass procedures mentioned above and are utilizing gastric bypass or gastric partition. The proximal 10 per cent of the stomach is anastomosed to a loop or Roux-en-Y limb of jejunum with no more than a 1.2 cm opening. Others have used stapling across the proximal gastric pouch, removing two or three staples, thus avoiding an anastomosis. It is too early to judge the effectiveness and results of these procedures; however, all the complications dependent on obesity per se would be expected to be the same as with the intestinal bypass procedures. Nausea and vomiting are more frequent but diarrhea is much less. Patients undergoing gastric bypass have not yet demonstrated significant liver deterioration, and this plus the lack of diarrhea combined with acceptable weight loss bodes well for the future.

Ileal Bypass for Hyperlipidemia. Whereas massive small bowel bypass for obesity is now abandoned or utilized with caution, bypass of the distal one third of the small bowel has been a benefit for the non-obese hyperlipidemic patients with atherosclerosis. Bypass of the ileum increases fecal loss of normally absorbed cholesterol, both endogenous and exogenous, as well as resulting in a reduced bile salt pool. Those who have not responded to medication, cholesterol-lowering drugs, or anion exchange resins, can be considered for ileal bypass. Serum cholesterol and lipid reduction of up to 40 per cent has been maintained for three to five years. Operative mortality is usually related to atherosclerotic cardiovascular disease and is about 2 per cent. Patients with types III and IV hyperlipoproteinemia and a positive family history and symptoms have been considered candidates for the procedure. Amelioration in occurrence of angina and claudication, and exercise tolerance has been reported. Regression of xanthelasma and stabilization of coronary arteriographic findings can be expected.

DISORDERS OF THE LARGE INTESTINE

ULCERATIVE COLITIS

Idiopathic ulcerative colitis is an acute and chronic ulcerative inflammatory disease of the colon and rectum of unknown etiology. The possibility that autoimmune mechanisms may be involved has received considerable attention. The condition occurs more frequently in females than in males. It affects whites more often than blacks, and the incidence in Jews is about three times that in non-Jews. The highest disease incidence occurs in the third and fourth decades, although it may occur in the young. Ulcerative colitis may vary clinically from mild with minimal symptoms to acute fulminant cases. It has a tendency to remissions and exacerbations. The disease is often indistinguishable from granulomatous colitis. However, in ulcerative colitis, the left side or the entire colon is usually involved and the disease is most often limited to the mucosa and submucosa.

Some of the clinical manifestations that may occur are severe diarrhea with blood, pus, and mucus, rectal tenesmus, cramping lower abdominal pain, anorexia, malaise, weakness, and weight loss. Recurrence may be precipitated by emotional stress, dietary indiscretion, pregnancy, and upper respiratory infection. Complications of ulcerative colitis are perforation, toxic megacolon, hemorrhage, carcinoma, perirectal or rectovaginal fistulas, abscesses, and malabsorption. Systemic complications include iron deficiency anemia, electrolyte and fluid imbalances, vitamin B_{12} and folate deficiency, hyponatremia, and retarded growth and sexual development. Extracolonic manifestations that may occur include iritis, arthritis, erythema nodosum, arthralgia, pyoderma gangrenosum, spondylitis, pericholangitis, hepatitis, cirrhosis, interstitial pancreatitis, acute psychosis, and thrombophlebitis.

Treatment consists of steroids, Azulfidine, antidiarrheal agents, diet, and vitamin and mineral supplements. Steroids may be given parenterally, orally, or in retention enemas. More recently, small doses of Imuran have been used with improvement in some of the patients. Most patients experience a prolonged period of weight loss, malnutrition, and electrolyte imbalance. It is unusual to see a patient who is intractable to medical therapy who will not benefit from a period of total parenteral nutrition prior to surgery. During this time, vitamins and electrolyte replacement should be given. Surgical intervention may be necessary for hemorrhage, perforation, obstruction, toxic megacolon, carcinoma, failure of medical management, and severe extracolonic complications. Total proctocolectomy with ileostomy is the treatment of choice. Some have advocated rectal sparing operations when the rectum appears normal. Recurrence of the disease in the rectal stump, however, is quite high (>60%). In those patients free of ileitis and in whom the diagnosis is secure, a continent ileal pouch (KOCH) can be constructed that offers distinct advantages over the usual ileostomy. Complication rates remain high in the hands of surgeons not experienced with the technique. The mortality rate for elective operations is about 3 to 5 per cent.

A late complication of ulcerative colitis is carcinoma. The risk of carcinoma during the first ten years after the onset of the disease is not high, but then the risk increases 2 per cent per year. The risk is greater in patients with total colonic involvement and in patients whose symptoms began before age 25. The average age of patients with ulcerative colitis who develop carcinoma is 37. The five-year survival rate of ulcerative colitis patients with carcinoma is 20 per cent, compared to 40 per cent in idiopathic carcinoma of the colon.

The incidence of toxic megacolon is about 1.6 to 2 per cent of cases with colitis; it is a dreadful complication. The cause of the toxic dilatation is not known, but certain temporal relationships have been noted: administration of opiates, barium enema during an acute attack, and administration of anticholinergics. Clinical manifestations of toxic megacolon include marked dilatation of part or all of the colon, abdominal pain, fever, tachycardia, anemia, prostration with shock, and severe toxicity. Medical management consists of gastrointestinal decompression, parenteral fluids and electrolytes, blood, antibiotics, and steroids. If the patient is taking opiates or anticholinergics, they are discontinued. Operative treatment is indicated if there is perforation or no improvement with adequate intensive medical care. The operative treatment of choice is total proctocolectomy with ileostomy, but subtotal colectomy with ileostomy without removal of the rectum may be performed if the patient's condition is poor. The mortality rate for emergency operation for ulcerative colitis is about 20 per cent.

GRANULOMATOUS COLITIS (CROHN'S DISEASE)

Crohn's disease most commonly affects the terminal ileum but may involve the colon alone or in association with small bowel disease and is a variant of the disease discussed above. The cause of the disease is unknown. Some of the typical clinical manifestations include intermittent or continuous diarrhea (usually not grossly bloody), weight loss, abdominal cramping pain, low grade fever, anemia, abdominal mass in the right lower quadrant, and weakness. Perianal lesions and fistulas (rectovesical, rectovaginal) are common. As compared with ulcerative colitis, diarrhea and bleeding are less pronounced, while strictures and fistulas are more common. Acute hemorrhage and toxic megacolon are not usually seen. In general, while the risk of cancer is lower than in ulcerative colitis, the mortality from colectomy is similar; recurrences are greater, leading to a decreased percentage of complete rehabilitation. Medical treatment is basically similar to that of ulcerative colitis. Indications for operative treatment are failure of medical therapy to control the disease, fistulas, extensive perianal pathology, obstruction, and hemorrhage. The surgical treatment depends on the extent of the disease and varies from segmental resection and anastomosis to total protocolectomy with ileostomy. Emergency operations are less frequently required than with ulcerative colitis. With segmental resection, the recurrence rate may be as high as 40 per cent. Recurrence of the disease in the small bowel after total proctocolectomy has been reported to be as low as 3 per cent. The incidence of complications is increased in patients who have been on large doses of steroids for prolonged periods.

PSEUDOMEMBRANOUS COLITIS

This is a severe, acute, necrotizing inflammatory disease of the gastrointestinal tract. The cause is not completely understood, but it has been associated with antimicrobial therapy. Lincomycin and clindamycin have been implicated with diarrhea in 21 per cent and frank colitis in 10 per cent of patients receiving a course of therapy. A variety of antibiotics including ampicillin, tetracycline, Chloromycetin, and cephalosporins have also been involved. Suppression of intestinal bacteria by antibiotics may be an important factor, and recent isolation of clostridial toxin in stools of patients with the disease and subsequent inoculation in rabbits followed by production of the disease are suggestive. Symptoms may develop after abdominal operations, in the second to eighth postoperative day. Clinical manifestations include severe voluminous diarrhea, fever, tachycardia, hypotension, shock dehydration, oliguria, electrolyte and protein loss, abdominal distention, weakness, and disorientation. Diarrhea is profuse, watery, and often green but may be bloody. Volume of the stool may exceed 10 liters per day. Treatment consists of discontinuing unnecessary antibiotics, aggressive electrolyte and fluid replacement, albumin and blood as needed, ACTH, and specific antimicrobials based on stool cultures. Vancomycin therapy has been suggested. A few patients, refractory to cessation of antibiotics and medical therapy, have required emergency colectomy. This is a severe process, with the mortality rate varying between 30 and 80 per cent.

ACTINOMYCOSIS

This infection, produced by the fungus *Actinomyces israelii*, involves primarily the cecum and appendix and may present as an appendicitis with perforation. Some of the clinical manifestations that may be present are abdominal pain in the right lower quadrant, spiking fever, chills, vomiting, weight loss, and a palpable abdominal mass. Sulfur granules in the drainage suggest the diagnosis. Complications that can occur include abscess formation, sinus tract, and fistulas. Treatment consists of penicillin or tetracycline with surgical drainage and excision as indicated.

AMEBIASIS

This infectious disease, caused by the protozoa *Entamoeba histolytica*, involves the cecum, ascending colon, and rectum with ulcerations. Asymptomatic infections are relatively common. Acute amebic dysentery usually presents with increasingly severe diarrhea over a period of several days associated with abdominal cramps. The stools are semifluid with flecks of blood-stained mucus, but in severe cases the stools may be grossly bloody. The acute attack usually subsides, followed by periods of recurrences and remission. Some of the clinical manifestations in the chronic form of the disease are weight loss, intermittent diarrhea (two to four stools per day with blood and mucus), abdominal cramping pain, and low grade fever. Amebic titers should be obtained to confirm the diagnosis. Complications that can occur include liver abscesses, perforation, and amebomas. Amebomas occur most commonly in the cecum or sigmoid colon and may produce bleeding and symptoms of obstruction. Sur-

gical resection of the bowel in a patient with untreated amebomas or amebiasis can lead to peritonitis and fistula formation. Treatment consists of drugs and, rarely, surgical treatment of the complications.

TUBERCULOSIS

Tuberculosis of the colon is usually secondary to pulmonary tuberculosis. The cecum and ascending colon are most frequently involved. Patients may be asymptomatic or have diarrhea, abdominal pain, and anemia. Complications include hemorrhage, perforation, obstruction, and fistula formation. The treatment is essentially similar to the treatment of pulmonary tuberculosis, and surgical treatment is limited to the treatment of complications. If tuberculosis is suspected preoperatively, the patient should be placed on antituberculosis chemotherapy.

ISCHEMIC COLITIS

Ischemic colitis may present as a transient ischemic episode with rapid healing or stricture formation, or as a fulminant, catastrophic disease with gangrene of the bowel. Ischemia of the colon can result from thrombosis of the inferior mesenteric artery, embolization of the inferior mesenteric artery (uncommon), inferior mesenteric vein thrombosis, surgical ligation of the inferior mesenteric artery, abdominal aortic angiography, or low flow states (nonocclusive ischemia). Clinical manifestations depend on the cause of the ischemia, collateral circulation, and extent and rapidity of the ischemia. The incidence of spontaneous ischemic colitis is greatest in the sixth to eighth decades. Patients may complain only of mild diarrhea and abdominal pain. However, with acute occlusion of the artery, they can have the following clinical manifestations: cramping lower abdominal pain, diarrhea that may become bloody, fever, and tenderness in the left lower quadrant of the abdomen. These may regress completely, progress to perforation and peritonitis, or later present with symptoms of stricture. Mild episodes are usually transient and may be treated medically with antibiotics, oral restriction, and intravenous fluids. Barium enemas may reveal "thumbprinting" or ulceration which reverts back to normal within a few days. Anticoagulation is not advisable. Emergency operation is indicated for gangrene of the bowel, perforation, and peritonitis, and elective operation may be required for strictures producing obstruction.

SCHISTOSOMIASIS

This is a parasitic disease caused by the blood flukes *Schistosoma mansoni, S. haematobium,* and *S. japonicum.* The freshwater snails that serve as intermediate host for *Schistosoma mansoni* are found in South America and Puerto Rico. Some of the clinical manifestations that may be seen early are pruritic dermatitis, fever, abdominal pain, cough, hemoptysis, urticarial rash, headache, tenesmus, and hepatosplenomegaly. With chronic infection the patients may present with hematemesis, melena, ascites, weight loss, alternating diarrhea and constipation, and fever. Complications include liver damage, colonic polyps, and bowel strictures. Treatment is chemotherapy, with surgery indicated for some of the complications.

VILLOUS ADENOMAS

Although these adenomas occur in both the colon and rectum, the majority (60 to 70 per cent) are found in the rectum. They occur in either sex, with the highest incidence in the sixth and seventh decades. Some of the common clinical manifestations are rectal discharge of blood and mucus, constipation or diarrhea, and weight loss. In a few of these patients there may be considerable loss of mucus (up to 3 liters per day) from the tumor surface, producing serious electrolyte depletion. Severe hypokalemia, hypochloremia, hyponatremia, dehydration, azotemia, and even shock may result from the loss. Aggressive replacement therapy is indicated. Several factors influence treatment. Invasive adenocarcinoma is present in over one third of the lesions. The incidence of malignancy is increased in large tumors (>6 cm). The entire tumor, including its base, must be excised. If malignancy is present, the operation is the standard cancer-type resection. Both benign and malignant lesions may recur locally.

GARDNER'S SYNDROME

This is an inherited disease (autosomal dominant), characterized by multiple colonic polyps, soft-tissue tumors, and osseous neoplasms. The benign osteomas or exostoses are frequently found in the mandible or skull. The soft tissue tumors may be epidermoid or sebaceous cysts, desmoid tumors, lipomas, or neurofibromas. Excessive fibrous reaction may occur after operations. Colonic polyps may not develop until age 30 or 40, after the appearance of the osseous and soft-tissue tumors. The malignant potential of these polyps is similar to that of familial polyposis, and therefore they require surgical treatment.

CHAGAS' DISEASE

This is a disease caused by a protozoan parasite, *Trypanosoma cruzi.* The acute infection usually occurs in the first decade of life, and only a small minority of infected cases are recognized. Many patients are asymptomatic. Clinical manifestations may include malaise, anorexia, intermittent or continuous fever, unilateral palpebral edema, hepatomegaly, tachycardia, and cardiac failure. No effective drug therapy is available. In the chronic form of the disease, the patient may remain asymptomatic for ten to 30 years. However, chronicity can include progressive diffuse chronic myocarditis, megacolon, and megaesophagus. The latter conditions are due to damage to the nerve plexuses in the walls of the colon and esophagus. The megacolon may produce fecal impaction, severe chronic constipation, and volvulus, and surgical treatment may be required.

VOLVULUS

Volvulus, rotation of a segment of bowel about its mesenteric axis sufficient to produce obstruction, occurs in areas of colon freely movable and elongated or where points of fixation are close together. About 80 per cent of cases occur in the sigmoid, 15 per cent in the cecum, and the rest involve transverse colon. Volvulus is the third most common cause of colonic obstruction in the United States.

Most patients have a history of chronic constipation with dilatation and elongation of the colon. Two groups of patients are susceptible: 1) those with severe psychiatric or neurologic disease such as parkinsonism, often in an institution and on sedatives and muscle relaxants, and 2) the elderly with serious cardiovascular and pulmonary disease who tend to be inactive.

Symptoms include cramping abdominal pain, progressively marked abdominal distention, obstipation, and absence of flatus. Nausea and vomiting leads to dehydration after several hours. Respiratory embarrassment can ensue because of the distention and pressure on the diaphragms. The presence of severe shock and toxicity may indicate that strangulation has occurred. Plain films of the abdomen are often diagnostic, showing a "bent-inner tube" sign, and barium enema is confirmatory, demonstrating a "bird's beak" appearance at the area of torsion.

Treatment of this problem is complicated by the advanced age of this group of patients who often have severe associated disease. Fluid and electrolyte replacement and monitoring of urinary output are essential. In 80 to 90 per cent, detorsion of the volvulus can be done by proctoscopic examinations or with a rectal tube. Occasionally detorsion by barium enema is possible. The fiberoptic colonoscope may be of help in reduction and has recently been used in cases of sigmoid volvulus. Tube deflation alone carries a mortality of 2 per cent. Emergency resection or operative derotation is necessary if tube detorsion is unsuccessful. Detorsion alone is followed by a recurrence of volvulus in a majority of patients (>50%). Elective resection with a mortality of 10 per cent after tube detorsion is the treatment of choice for better risk patients. Emergency resection carries a mortality of as high as 20 to 30 per cent, and if the bowel is strangulated the operative mortality may be as high as 50 per cent.

Cecal volvulus is quite different. The diagnosis by abdominal x-ray is less clear and the presentation may be like that of a small bowel obstruction. Tube derotation is not possible, and strangulation is common and tends to occur early in the course of the process. Some surgeons prefer cecopexy to right hemicolectomy for the initial episode. The mortality rate is about 10 per cent.

ANGIODYSPLASIA

Although diverticulosis is commonly regarded as the most common cause of profuse lower gastrointestinal bleeding, vascular ectasias are being recognized with increasing frequency as a cause of bleeding from the colon in the elderly. These lesions are also called angiomas, angiodysplasias, and arteriovenous malformations. They characteristically occur in older patients, are not associated with other skin angiomas, are primarily in the cecum and ascending colon, and tend to be small and multiple. They are hypothesized as degenerative lesions associated with aging and occurring as a result of partial, intermittent low grade obstruction of submucosal veins by years of muscular contraction of the colon.

Many of the patients have diverticula which, in the past, have been confused with angiodysplasia as the source of bleeding. The bleeding can vary from occult to massive hemorrhage. Fully one third of patients have had previous admissions and operations for prior lower gastrointestinal bleeding. All patients should have clotting studies, upper and lower gastrointestinal x-rays, and sigmoidoscopy. Colonoscopy has had limited usefulness when bleeding is active. Selective angiography has been the most useful single diagnostic modality and often is therapeutic when the source of bleeding can be identified. In the majority of patients bleeding stops spontaneously, but recurrence of bleeding is high. If bleeding persists, infusion of vasoconstrictive agents or small preformed clot emboli through a selectively placed angiographic catheter has been successful in almost 75 per cent of patients. If angiographic techniques fail, an emergency segmental colectomy or right hemicolectomy is performed. The number of patients undergoing such emergency colectomies thus far is too small to calculate as accurate mortality.

DISORDERS OF THE PANCREAS

ACUTE PANCREATITIS

The basic cause of acute pancreatitis is not known, but some of the etiologic factors have been well documented. These include gallstones, alcoholism, operative trauma, external trauma, peptic ulcers, hyperparathyroidism, mumps, and hereditary pancreatitis. Other etiologic factors that have been implicated are hyperlipemia, hemochromatosis, toxins, autoimmune mechanisms, and vascular factors. The clinical manifestations vary considerably, because acute pancreatitis ranges from edematous pancreatitis to hemorrhagic pancreatitis. The pain is often in the epigastrium, radiating directly to the back; it is relieved by sitting up and leaning forward. Vomiting is common and may aggravate the pain. Other manifestations that may occur are fever, tachycardia, mild jaundice, and cyanosis. Shock may be present, owing to loss of fluid and blood into the peritoneal cavity. There may be pleural effusions. Serum calcium can be depressed, producing carpopedal spasm. Treatment consists of intravenous fluids and electrolytes, colloid and blood as required, nasogastric suction, narcotics for pain, anticholinergics, antibiotics, insulin and calcium as needed, and occasionally magnesium sulfate or parathyroid extract for tetany. No objective evidence exists that the use of either anticholinergics or antibiotics shortens the course of an attack of acute pancreatitis. Cimetidine has not been of benefit in early studies, yet the primary goal of therapy is to decrease stimuli to the gland while replacing fluid and electrolytes, and providing nutrition. Parenteral nutrition has been useful in patients with persistent and lingering cases.

Complications that may result from acute pancreatitis are pseudocyst, abscess, necrosis or thrombosis of vessels, and perforation of the stomach or duodenum. With repeated attacks of acute pancreatitis, the patient may develop diabetes mellitus and pancreatic insufficiency. Exploratory laparotomy is indicated in acute pancreatitis for some of the complications mentioned previously (abscess, pseudocysts) if there is uncertainty of diagnosis, if there is increasing jaundice, and if the patient continues to deteriorate. Retroperitoneal hemorrhage from acute hemorrhagic pancreatitis is a dreaded complication carrying a mortality of from 80 to 100 per cent. Peritoneal lavage has been suggested to benefit the course, but laparotomy is usually performed to stem the bleeding and adequately drain the retrogastric space or to perform a total pancreatectomy.

Pancreatitis affects multiple systems including the kidneys, liver, brain, and cardiopulmonary system. Acute respiratory disease or "wet lung" leading to ultimate pulmonary failure is not an uncommon mode of death in these patients.

CHRONIC PANCREATITIS

Chronic pancreatitis is a progressive, sclerotic inflammation of the pancreas of variable causation. Clinical manifestations may include persistent epigastric pain that radiates to the back and is aggravated by eating, anorexia, weight loss, diabetes mellitus, steatorrhea, malnutrition, and frequently narcotic addiction. Treatment consists of a well-balanced diet, vitamin supplements, no alcohol, replacement of pancreatic enzymes, mild sedation, and management of diabetes mellitus. Indications for surgical intervention are correctable coexistent biliary tract disease, pseudocysts or abscesses, increasing frequency of acute attacks, and failure of medical treatment. The operative procedures, including sphincterotomy, pancreatojejunostomy, and 95 per cent pancreatectomy, must be strictly individualized after adequate exploration and pancreatography at the time of operation. Almost all procedures have a low likelihood of succeeding in pain prevention if alcohol, the most common causative agent, is not avoided.

PANCREATIC CYSTS

True cysts (lined with epithelium) of the pancreas may be congenital, parasitic, neoplastic, or retention cysts. These benign tumors of the pancreas most commonly occur in the sixth and seventh decades and occur more frequently in females than in males. They may be asymptomatic or may present with the clinical manifestations of an abdominal mass, abdominal discomfort, or occasional jaundice. The treatment of choice is surgical excision of the cyst.

Pseudocysts (no epithelial lining) usually result from pancreatitis or trauma, but neoplasms and parasites are rare causes. Over 80 per cent of cystic lesions of the pancreas are pseudocysts. Some of the clinical manifestations of pseudocysts are abdominal pain, fever, abdominal mass, nausea, vomiting, anorexia, occasional pleural effusion, and jaundice. Complications include obstructive jaundice, secondary infection of the cyst, hemorrhage into the cyst, or rupture of the cyst into the peritoneal cavity or an adjacent viscus. Diagnosis by ultrasonography has become more common and has uncovered small cysts that can be followed and may disappear. Larger cysts (greater than 2 cm) accompanied by symptoms are operated upon 1) because of the high incidence of infection and hemorrhage, and 2) because after six weeks, a thick fibrous capsule develops, which lessens the chance for spontaneous resolution and allows the surgeon to achieve internal drainage. Various operative procedures have been described that must be individualized, depending on the findings at the time of surgery. These include simple external drainage, marsupialization, extirpation, and internal drainages such as cystogastrostomy, cystoduodenostomy, Roux-en-Y cystojejunostomy, and transduodenal sphincterotomy. With marsupialization or external drainage, pancreatic cutaneous fistulas may develop.

CYSTIC FIBROSIS IN ADULTS

Cystic fibrosis of the pancreas in adults is uncommon. This is a genetic disease inherited as an autosomal recessive characteristic. Approximately 5 per cent of patients with cystic fibrosis live past the age of 17. Two thirds of adult patients are males. The clinical manifestations vary, depending on the severity of the disease, but the major cause of mortality and morbidity is the chronic pulmonary disease caused by airway obstruction. These patients may develop bronchiectasis, atelectasis, hemoptysis, pneumothorax, and cor pulmonale. Other clinical features that may develop are due to pancreatic insufficiency, and rarely cirrhosis of the liver and diabetes mellitus may be present. Intestinal complications in adults may include fecal impaction, intestinal obstruction, and ileocolic and colocolic intussusception.

DISORDERS OF THE LIVER

PYOGENIC LIVER ABSCESS

Pyogenic liver abscesses are relatively rare and have decreased even more since the widespread use of antibiotics. They are most commonly seen in patients in the sixth or seventh decade of life. The liver can be invaded by bacteria from ascending cholangitis (secondary to obstruction of the common bile duct), by way of the portal vein (intraperitoneal sepsis) or hepatic artery (bacteremia), by implantation of microorganisms from trauma, and by direct extension of infection. The most commonly offending organisms are E. coli and S. aureus. Other gram-negative organisms such as P. vulgaris and A. aerogenes have also been cultured from abscesses. Bacteroides is increasingly more prevalent, which emphasizes the need to perform anaerobic cultures. In many cases, no organism is cultured. Liver abscesses may be single or, more commonly, multiple. Clinical manifestations include malaise, high spiking fever, right upper quadrant or epigastric abdominal pain, anorexia, and weight loss. There may be mild jaundice, an enlarged tender liver, an elevated right diaphragm, limitation of diaphragmatic excursion, and pleural effusion. Complications that occur are perforation into the peritoneal cavity or subphrenic space and extension into the pleural cavity and sepsis. Diagnosis is made by ultrasonography, isotope scans, and angiography. Treatment consists of appropriate antibiotics and surgical drainage if the abscess is amenable to drainage. The reported mortality rate has varied from 20 to 90 per cent. More recently the mortality has decreased with earlier diagnosis.

AMEBIC LIVER ABSCESS

Approximately 3 to 5 per cent of patients with intestinal amebiasis will develop the complication of hepatic amebiasis. Hepatic amebiasis is most commonly found in young adult males. A high proportion of these patients with liver involvement will have no amebae in their stool. The hepatic abscesses are usually solitary and are located most frequently in the upper part of the right lobe. Typically the appearance of the pus has been described as chocolate sauce or anchovy paste. Clinical manifestations include right upper quadrant abdominal pain, tenderness over the liver, fever, chills, weight loss, weakness, jaundice, and an elevated diaphragm. Complications that may result are secondary infection by pyogenic organisms, rupture of the abscess into the subhepatic or subphrenic space, pleural pulmonary complications (empyema, pulmonary abscess, bronchohepatic fistula), rupture into the peritoneal cavity producing generalized peritonitis, or bloodstream invasion. Treatment consists of proper drug therapy, most commonly metronidazole. Surgery may be indicated for the secondary complications and to resect residual abscess cavities that cannot be drained. Needle aspiration or extraserous external drainage can be attempted for persistent abscesses after a course of drug therapy.

ECHINOCOCCOSIS (HYDATID DISEASE)

Human echinococcosis is a disease caused by infestation with the small tapeworm, *Echinococcus granulosus* or *Echinococcus multilocularis.* The natural carriers are domestic dogs, wolves, and foxes and the most common natural intermediate host is the sheep, although cattle, deer, and hogs may also be infected. Man is infected by ingestion of the eggs. The larvae erupt into cysts, most frequently in the liver. Some may reach the lungs and rarely the brain, heart, kidney, or spleen. A liver cyst may not produce any symptoms for many years. If the cyst ruptures or leaks, the following clinical manifestations may occur: pruritus, urticaria, asthma, jaundice, biliary colic, and anaphylactic shock if the cyst ruptures suddenly. Sudden death may occur. The liver cyst may become infected with pyogenic bacteria or rupture into the peritoneal cavity, leading to seeding of daughter cysts. Pulmonary cysts may be asymptomatic or may obstruct the bronchi or rupture into the bronchus. In addition to pulmonary symptoms, cysts in the brain may produce signs and symptoms of increased intracranial pressure, and cysts of the kidney may produce renal damage. The treatment is surgical removal of the intact cysts. The cyst should be aspirated and hydrogen peroxide, Lugol's iodine, formalin, or absolute alcohol instilled to prevent seeding. In some patients, the allergic symptoms or anaphylactic shock will require treatment. The reported mortality varies from less than 5 per cent to 15 per cent.

PRIMARY CARCINOMA

Primary carcinoma of the liver is uncommon in the United States but not unusual in Japan, China, and some of the African countries where it may represent 17 to 53 per cent of all cancers. It is most commonly found in the fourth to sixth decades of life, although there is also a peak incidence in infancy and childhood. Males are affected more frequently than females. Although the cause of hepatic cancer is unknown, it is related to cirrhosis (postnecrotic more often than Laennec's), malnutrition, parasitic infection of the liver (liver flukes), toxins, and fungal contamination of food. Cirrhosis is present in 60 per cent of patients with hepatocellular carcinoma, which occurs in 4.5 per cent of all cirrhotic patients. Three types of carcinomas are recognized: hepatoma, cholangioma, and mixed type. The initial clinical manifestation of primary carcinoma of the liver may be rapid deterioration of a patient with cirrhosis for no obvious reason. The patient may develop weakness, cachexia, weight loss, ascites, epigastric or right upper quadrant abdominal pain, gastrointestinal bleeding (bleeding into the peritoneal cavity or bleeding varices), edema, jaundice, fever, and an enlarged, tender, irregular liver. The treatment is hepatic resection if the lesion is solitary, if there are no metastases, and if it appears that there will be adequate functioning liver parenchyma after resection. Direct arterial perfusion with 5-fluorouracil has achieved a 25 per cent temporary response rate. Hepatic artery ligation has been attempted as an adjunctive measure with minimal success. The prognosis is grim, with five year survivals of about 14 per cent overall and 36 per cent following "curative" resections.

MAJOR HEPATIC RESECTION

Since the liver has so many important metabolic and physiological functions normally, it is not surprising that significant biochemical, physiological, and metabolic changes occur after major hepatic resections. The understanding and treatment of these alterations are important. Major hepatic resections are usually performed for traumatic injury of the liver or for tumor. Mortality appears to be related to the percentage of liver resected, but the most important factor is the amount of functioning liver tissue that remains. It has been estimated that upward of 80 per cent of the liver can be removed with little or no alteration in hepatic function. In patients with hepatic carcinoma who have cirrhosis, the preoperative preparation with albumin, vitamins A, D, and K, and a high calorie, high carbohydrate diet is important. During surgery, excessive hemorrhage is usually due to mechanical loss and not to alterations of the coagulation mechanism. However, the patient may require blood or other colloid in excess of the estimated blood loss caused by splanchnic bed sequestration. Continuous intravenous fructose or 10 per cent glucose should be given to prevent hypoglycemia (depletion of liver glycogen) until the patient is capable of an adequate oral intake. Total parenteral alimentation is of value pre- and postoperatively. Protein synthesis is depressed, and intravenous albumin (25 to 100 gm) should be given daily to maintain the serum albumin and serum oncotic pressure. There is a decrease in serum triglyceride for about one week, and there is lipid accumulation in the liver remnant. There is usually a transient rise in the serum bilirubin, with the level returning to below 1 mg per 100 ml in one to three weeks. Prothrombin time and partial thromboplastin time may be prolonged. The deficiency should be corrected by administration of vitamin K_1 and fresh frozen plasma. Low serum potassium or inorganic phosphorus may occur. Antibiotics are indicated. Drugs that are metabolized by the liver must be used cautiously. The normal liver has a tremendous capacity for regeneration. The rate of regeneration of human liver after resection is not definitely known, but in dogs there is regeneration of 80 to 90 per cent of the original liver weight in three weeks after two thirds hepatic resection. The capacity of liver regeneration of the cirrhotic liver is very limited, and therefore the mortality is much greater in these patients.

GILBERT'S SYNDROME (IDIOPATHIC UNCONJUGATED HYPERBILIRUBINEMIA)

This syndrome is characterized by mild unconjugated hyperbilirubinemia, usually less than 4 mg per 100 ml, without demonstrable hepatic disorder, hemolysis, or excessive bilirubin production. The serum bilirubin may fluctuate with elevation during stress. There is no significant abnormality of liver function or histology. Gilbert's disease is inherited as an autosomal dominant. No treatment is required for this condition.

DUBIN-JOHNSON SYNDROME

This syndrome is characterized by an elevated serum level of conjugated bilirubin. The conjugated bilirubin is not excreted normally by the liver cells. Although the defect is inborn, jaundice may not be recognized until adulthood. Jaundice may fluctuate, and exacerbation may be associated with mild right upper quadrant abdominal pain and anorexia. In addition to the elevated unconjugated bilirubin, there may be moderate BSP retention. The other liver function tests are normal. Oral cholecystography may show faint or no visualization. No therapy is required.

DRUGS AND THE LIVER

Many new therapeutic agents introduced into clinical medicine have effects on the liver. Some of the effects have little clinical significance, but others may lead to death. Many drugs are metabolized by the liver, which converts them to more water-soluble compounds. The enzymes for oxidation, reduction, conjugation, and hydrolysis are located in the hepatic microsomes, part of the smooth endoplasmic reticulum of the liver cell. Certain drugs, agents, or factors may stimulate or increase the rate of drug metabolism by the liver caused by enzyme induction. Examples include phenobarbital, stress, alcohol, cigarette smoking, and polycyclic aromatic hydrocarbons. This enzyme induction is nonspecific. With enzyme induction, if the original compound is active, the drug becomes less effective and less toxic, whereas if the metabolite is more active than the original compound, effectiveness and toxicity may increase with time.

Drugs may interfere with bilirubin metabolism at the various steps. They may displace bilirubin from its binding with serum albumin, compete with uptake by the cell, interfere with transport through the hepatic cell, increase the load of unconjugated bilirubin on the liver cell, inhibit the conjugation of bilirubin, and compete with bile salts and micelle formation. The response of the liver to a drug may alter the metabolism of a second drug. Two drugs may compete for the same metabolic pathway in the liver.

Direct Hepatic Toxicity. Certain substances of drugs are direct hepatotoxins producing hepatic necrosis. Many of these drugs are also toxic to the kidneys. The effects on the liver may vary from mild elevations of transaminase activity to severe necrosis. Toxic effects may become manifest several years after exposure.

Hepatitis-Like Reactions. The incidence of hepatitic reaction to drugs is low (one in 1000 to one in 10,000 of persons exposed). These reactions are quite similar to ordinary acute viral hepatitis and are usually unrelated to dose or duration of exposure, but occur more frequently after multiple exposures. Hepatitis can develop one to 10 weeks after onset of therapy but usually occurs within the first month. Reported mortality has varied from 20 to 40 per cent. Clinical manifestations include fever, anorexia, malaise, confusion, and jaundice. The liver may be enlarged and tender unless there is massive necrosis. In patients who survive, recovery is complete and cirrhosis or relapses are rare.

Cholestasis. Many drugs may produce cholestasis. A large number of unrelated drugs produce this reaction, which is not related to dosage or duration of therapy. The sulfonylurea derivatives form the largest group of drugs that produce this complication. A sensitized person may develop jaundice after ingestion of only one tablet. Clinical manifestations usually become apparent one to three weeks after use of the drug and may include fever, right upper quadrant pain, rash, eosinophilia, agranulocytosis, and obstructive jaundice. Usually the jaundice is mild and lasts a few days, but cholestasis may be present up to three years even though the inflammatory reaction disappears within six to 12 weeks. However, complete recovery is the general rule.

Granulomas. Several drugs may produce sarcoid-like granulomas in the liver. Patients may be asymptomatic but may develop mild jaundice, hepatomegaly, eosinophilia and elevated alkaline phosphatase.

Tetracycline Steatosis. Large doses of intravenous tetracycline may produce injury to the liver and should be avoided, especially in pregnant women and patients with malnutrition. Hepatic failure has developed in pregnant women receiving large doses of intravenous tetracycline. The mechanism of this reaction is unknown.

The Use of Drugs in Patients with Liver Disease. Liver disease may alter the dose requirement of some drugs. In patients with liver disease some drugs may be metabolized more slowly than normal; others are metabolized normally. In addition, hepatic dysfunction may alter the response of a target organ, and the toxicity of drugs for organs other than the liver may be enhanced because of the change in metabolism.

Some of the drugs or compounds which may have effects on the liver as described here are listed in Table 9–3.

DISORDERS OF THE GALLBLADDER AND EXTRAHEPATIC BILIARY SYSTEM

CHOLEDOCHAL CYST

Congenital cystic abnormalities of the biliary system can occur anywhere along the biliary ducts. The most common form of extrahepatic cyst occurs more frequently in females, and over 30 per cent are diagnosed in the first decade of life. Cystic dilatations can occur along the entire common hepatic common duct, localized to the distal common duct, or as a diffuse fusiform dilatation of the common duct. They present with pain and jaundice that may be intermittent but can progress to complete obstruction, cholangitis, biliary cirrhosis, or spontaneous rupture. Surgical alternatives include a cystojejunostomy with or without a Roux-en-Y limb, cystoduodenostomy, or excision with hepatodochojejunostomy. Cholecystectomy is also advised. Congenital diverticula can be resected.

GALLSTONE ILEUS

Obstruction of the small bowel by an impacted gallstone is an infrequent occurrence. Gallstone ileus causes 1 to 2 per cent of all small bowel obstructions but may be associated with a mortality as high as 10 per cent. Largely this is a disease of the aged, with an average age of 64, over half of whom have associated diabetes and/or major cardiovascular problems.

The gallstone usually erodes into the gastrointestinal tract followed by a cholecystoenteric fistula caused by pressure and

Table 9–3   *Drugs Having Effects on the Liver*

Direct hepatic toxicity:
 Actinomycin D
 Alcohol
 Carbon tetrachloride
 Chloroform
 Dinitrophenol
 Heavy metals
 Methotrexate
 Mithramycin
 Mitomycin C
 Phosphorus
 Poisonous mushrooms
 Stilbamidine
 Tannic acid
 Tetracyclines
 Tromethamine (Tham)

Hepatitis-like reactions:
 Acetohexamide (Dymelor)
 Alpha-methyldopa (Aldomet)
 Chloramphenicol (Chloromycetin)
 Chlortetracycline (Aureomycin)
 Cinchophen (Atophan)
 Diphenylhydantoin (Dilantin)
 Ethionamide (Trecator)
 Halothane (Fluothane)
 Indomethacin (Indocin)
 Iproniazid (Marsilid)
 Isoniazid
 6-Mercaptopurine
 Nialamide (Niamid)
 Novobiocin (Albamycin, Panalba)
 Para-aminosalicylic acid
 Penicillin
 Phenelzine (Nardil)
 Phenylacetylurea (Phenurone)
 Phenylbutazone (Butazolidin)
 Pyrazinamide (PZA)
 Streptomycin

 Sulfamethoxypyridazine (Kynex)
 Tranylcypromine (Parnate)
 Trimethobenzamide (Tigan)
 Triptyline derivatives
 Zoxazolamine (Flexin)

Cholestasis:
 Aminosalicylic acid (PAS)
 Amitriptyline (Elavil, Triavil)
 Arsphenamine
 Carbamazepine (Tegretol)
 Carbarsone
 Chlordiazepoxide (Librium, Protensin)
 Chlorpromazine (Thorazine)
 Chlorpropamide (Diabinese)
 Chlorthiazide (Diuril)
 Ectylurea (Nostyn)
 Erythromycin estolate (Ilosone)
 Mepazine (Pacatal)
 Methimazole (Tapazole)
 Methyltestosterone (Metandren)
 Nitrofurantoin (Furadantin)
 Norethandrolone (Nilevar)
 Para-aminobenzyl caffeine
 Phenindione (Hedulin)
 Prochlorperazine (Compazine)
 Promazine (Sparine, Prozine)
 Propylthiouracil
 Sulfadiazine
 Thioridazine (Mellaril)
 Thiouracil
 Tolbutamide (Orinase)
 Triacetyloleandomycin (TAO, Cyclamycin)

Granulomas:
 Diphenylhydantoin (Dilantin)
 Phenylbutazone (Butazolidin)
 Sulfonylurea derivatives

inflammation. Fistula tracts to all parts of the gastrointestinal tract and even into the pleural cavity have been reported. The duodenum is most commonly involved because of its proximity and likelihood to be involved with inflammatory adhesions to the gallbladder. The site of obstruction is usually at the narrowest portion of the gastrointestinal tract, the distal ileum. Obstruction has been reported at all levels, however, including the colon.

Most patients have a past history of cholelithiasis but recent symptoms are uncommon. Jaundice occurs in about 10 per cent. Nausea, cramping, and vomiting occur as with other small bowel obstructions and there may be extremely large losses of fluid into the intestine, with edema, ulceration, or necrosis of the bowel, and ultimately perforation may result. Fluids and electrolyte replacement similar to that required for small bowel obstruction, as discussed

above, is required. After fluid replacement and nasogastric tube decompression, an operation for localization and removal of the stone is necessary. Either concomitantly or at a planned interval cholecystectomy with closure of the fistula (usually closed by the time of surgery) is performed with the decision based on the status of the patient. Without cholecystectomy, recurrent symptoms and complications occur in upward of one third of patients. Many are extremely ill and depleted and a prolonged operation, which may involve a common duct exploration, is not advisable in the emergency situation.

ASCENDING CHOLANGITIS

Acute cholangitis is a well known but vague and uncommonly diagnosed clinical complex. Since its description by Charcot in 1877, only sporadic references have appeared, the most complete of these describing only 36 patients. The difficulty lies in distinguishing cholangitis from severe cholecystitis. The initially described triad of chills and spiking fever, jaundice, and right upper quadrant pain must be expanded to include bacteremia and sepsis. When, accompanied by lethargy and hypotension, it has been termed suppurative cholangitis. The distinction is important since, in cholangitis, infection has involved the biliary ductal system, often under increased pressure, with resultant cholangiovenous reflux of organisms and sepsis. Gram-negative sepsis and shock may be imminent and when present carries a mortality of 60 per cent.

The overwhelming majority of patients have calculous disease of the biliary tract, some having cholangitis secondary to stricture, trauma, and rarely carcinoma. An interesting group is made up of those who demonstrate transitory cholangitis following manipulation of the common duct, that is, during T-tube cholangiography and mechanical extraction of retained stones. They may develop sepsis and even shock but require no immediate surgery, since continued obstruction does not exist.

The great majority of patients are elderly, two thirds being over 80 years of age. In general, the incidence of both infection and biliary calculi increases with age. Over 90 per cent of patients have positive biliary cultures, most commonly *E. coli* and Klebsiella, but often Streptococcus, Pseudomonas, and Bacteroides, and a combination of more than one organism complicating antibiotic coverage is noted. Most of these patients have associated disease, in particular cardiovascular problems. Despite the obvious hesitancy to operate, if the diagnosis can be made, immediate laparotomy is indicated within a 24 hour period. Appropriate blood cultures should be obtained and broad spectrum antibiotics started. Correction of shock and fluid deficits together with mannitol and colloid replacement to maintain urinary output are essential. Correction of hypoglycemia by infusion of hypertonic glucose has been helpful in reversing the lethargy. Many of these patients have an increased fibrinolysis and thrombocytopenia perhaps secondary to endotoxemia, and clotting studies should be obtained. Operative intervention should be planned when the patient is most stable and should include cholecystectomy and drainage of the common duct. Operative mortality with an aggressive surgical approach can be as low as 15 to 20 per cent. If the disease exacerbates and shock occurs before surgery, 60 per cent of patients can be expected to die. Likewise, nearly 100 per cent of patients "conservatively" treated with cholecystostomy will not survive, since the common duct has not been decompressed. Nowhere is an orderly stepwise approach to the patient with early diagnosis as essential as in this emergent group of patients.

PRIMARY SCLEROSING CHOLANGITIS

Primary sclerosing cholangitis is an uncommon disease involving all parts of the extrahepatic biliary duct system and occasionally the intrahepatic radicles. There is a progressive thickening of the bile duct walls encroaching upon the lumen. A number of cases have been associated with ulcerative colitis, Riedel's trauma and retroperitoneal fibrosis. It is difficult to exclude sclerosing carcinoma as a diagnosis, and this is often possible only after a long follow-up period. The exact cause is unknown. Infection, allergy, autoimmunity, and disseminated collagen disease have all been implicated. The mucosa is intact and normal but the duct walls may be as much as eight times normal thickness.

The disease usually occurs in middle age with jaundice, pain, nausea and vomiting, and sometimes fever. In longstanding cases portal hypertension from biliary cirrhosis may occur, with bleeding varices and ascites. Treatment usually consists of antibiotics to prevent cholangitis and bile salts to increase fluidity of the bile. Steroid therapy, because of its anti-inflammatory component, has been useful. Surgery in an attempt to drain the common duct with a T-tube may be necessary to maintain liver function. Internal shunts have been used but often occlude. The gallbladder is usually not removed, since it may be of use for subsequent drainage of bile.

CARCINOMA OF THE EXTRAHEPATIC BILE DUCT

This lesion is uncommon and is much less frequent than pancreatic and ampullary carcinoma. It is often indistinguishable from sclerosing cholangitis and occurs most frequently in males in the sixth and seventh decades. The tumor is often firm and involves the entire thickness of the duct but may become polypoid, projecting into the lumen. All are adenocarcinomas, and over 75 per cent are metastatic at the time of surgery, with a high incidence of multiplicity noted up and down the ducts, suggesting intraluminal spread. Characteristically there is a rapid onset of jaundice and pruritus with abdominal pain and weight loss. Transhepatic cholangiography is very helpful in diagnosis and a planned preoperative rational surgical approach. Depending on the location of the tumor, surgery may be curative or palliative, with each being more difficult the closer to the liver and the more intrahepatic the location of the tumor. Resection of the tumor is possible on occasion along with hepatojejunostomy. Prolonged palliation with decompression of the intrahepatic ductal system can be done using a U-shaped tube passing through the liver substance, through the obstruction, and out the common duct. Either operation is extensive, and most patients require a postoperative period of alimentation to restore positive nitrogen balance. Clotting factors must be restored, since liver dysfunction is so common. The average postoperative survival is only four months.

ANESTHETIC CONSIDERATIONS

As stated at the beginning of this chapter, anesthetic considerations will be divided into two areas: 1) those that are common to all gastrointestinal diseases and 2) those that relate to specific disease entities.

GENERAL CONSIDERATIONS

It is the responsibility of every anesthesiologist to be cognizant of those factors involving the gastrointestinal system that may influence the well being of the patient. This includes traditional questions about the patient's recent oral intake. The anesthesiologist should also ascertain whether the patient may have any pathologic condition that might influence the induction or conduct of the anesthetic. For example, a history of dysphagia or abnormal regurgitation

might influence the way in which the induction is managed. Specific gastrointestinal disorders may drastically alter the patient's homeostatic state and may have profound physiologic implications. Elective surgery for uncomplicated gallbladder disease may pose no particular pathophysiologic stress. However, the patient requiring emergency surgery for bowel obstruction or correction of high output enterocutaneous fistula will require careful assessment of the physiologic state of multiple organ systems.

Gastrointestinal disorders may have wide-ranging influences on other organ systems. For example, abnormal fluid losses due to vomiting or fistula can result in electrolyte disturbances that might affect the function of many organ systems.

Using hypokalemia caused by vomiting as an illustration, effects on cardiac rhythm, neuromuscular transmission, and central nervous system function can be noted. Similarly, the dehydration associated with vomiting, fistula drainage, or diarrhea would obviously affect the patient's blood volume, cardiac function, renal function, and even cerebral function. The patient with a gastrointestinal bleed or bowel obstruction is at particular risk for regurgitation or vomiting during induction, with the possibility of severe pulmonary sequelae. These examples serve to illustrate the wide-ranging effects that the gastrointestinal system may have on multiple organ systems.

In preparing a patient for anesthesia and surgery, the physician attempts to restore the patient as closely as possible to a normal physiologic state. A word of caution is in order regarding the time frame in which this is accomplished. As a rule, the slow and deliberate correction of the patient's volume status, electrolytes, and blood gases is to be recommended. Attempts at rapid intervention often lead to further deterioration in the patient's status. For example, the rapid administration of fluids to a dehydrated patient may bring about heart failure and pulmonary edema even if the volume of fluid replaced is less than that lost secondary to the pathologic process. As a general rule, the farther from normal that a patient's physiologic parameter is and the longer the patient has been in this condition, the slower should be the return of that parameter to normal.

In summary, the pathophysiologic changes that disorders of the gastrointestinal system cause have multiple effects on many organ systems. A slow and controlled return to normal homeostasis before anesthetic and surgical intervention is in the patient's best interest. Multiple re-evaluations during the course of this return to normal is ideal. Only when acute intervention for a life threatening condition is required should the therapeutic pretreatment be abandoned or hurried.

VOMITING

Vomiting represents a normal reflex mechanism by which the body rids itself of upper gastrointestinal contents. The reflex may be stimulated by numerous factors, such as emotional via cortical afferents or unaccustomed motion through vestibular afferents. Some metabolic products and drugs as well as factors causing irritation to the GI tract may also trigger this reflex. Vomiting is particularly likely to be associated with disorders of the GI tract.

Vomiting represents a complex and multifaceted reflex arc. Stimulation of the GI tract, especially the stomach, by distention or chemical irritation, results in impulses to the medulla via vagal and sympathetic afferents. The vomiting center is located in the medulla near the tractus solitarius at the level of the dorsal motor nucleus of the vagus. From here, the efferent arc is completed via the fifth, seventh, ninth, tenth, and twelfth cranial nerves as well as through the spinal nerves to the diaphragm and abdominal muscles. The act of vomiting involves the orchestration of numerous neuromuscular signals. The results are 1) taking a deep breath; 2) raising the hyoid bone to open the cricoesophageal sphincter; 3) closure of the glottis; 4) lifting of the soft palate; 5) simultaneous contraction of the diaphragm and abdominal muscles, which increases intra-abdominal pressure; and finally 6) relaxation of the gastroesophageal junction, allowing expulsion of gastric contents. Simultaneous reflex peristalsis helps empty the stomach as well as move upper intestinal contents into the stomach.

Chemical afferents to the medulla may also trigger vomiting. The chemoreceptor trigger zone is located bilaterally in the floor of the fourth ventricle above the area postrema. Drugs such as apomorphine, narcotics, copper sulfate, and digitalis derivatives, as well as various toxins, may stimulate this area, which can cause vomiting via interneural connections to the vomiting center.

In the alert, healthy patient the act of vomiting per se usually does not cause any unwanted sequelae. However, this is not the case in the perioperative period. The anesthesiologist is primarily concerned with two complications of vomiting. The most feared is aspiration and its resultant pulmonary complications. The other concerns the metabolic and physiologic implications of protracted vomiting.

Every practicing anesthesiologist knows that the potential for vomiting and aspiration exists in all patients regardless of how the anesthetic is being delivered. Under usual conditions the possibility of vomiting in the healthy patient who has had nothing by mouth for a period of six to eight hours is quite small, because the usual emptying time of the stomach is approximately four hours. However, as in all biological systems, there is marked individual variation. Certain conditions delay gastric emptying time, including pregnancy, apprehension, pain, drugs, and the presence of various diseases. It is especially wise, then, to consider any patient coming to surgery with an underlying gastrointestinal problem as one who has the potential for vomiting and aspiration.

Certain anesthetic precautions will help to minimize the chance of vomiting and aspiration in all patients. An important initial step is to reduce the preoperative anxiety level of the patient by carefully and thoughtfully explaining the procedures that will be followed during induction and emergence. Since many procedures are done while the patient is responsive, it is beneficial to have the full cooperation and understanding of the patient. All adult patients for elective surgery should have nothing by mouth at least eight hours prior to induction. A smooth, controlled induction with careful administration of drugs that may have emetic potential, and avoidance of hypotension and cerebral hypoxia from any cause, will greatly reduce the chances of vomiting. In managing a difficult airway, specific care should be taken not to distend the stomach with positive pressure ventilation. In addition, distention of any hollow viscus, the bladder or rectum for example, can stimulate the vomiting reflex. Perhaps most importantly the pharynx should not be instrumented while the patient is only lightly or partially anesthetized.

The risks of vomiting and aspiration may be further reduced in some patients by pharmacologic pretreatment. Patients coming to surgery for reasons other than acute gastrointestinal emergencies may be benefited by premedication with antiemetics, anticholinergics, and antihistaminics. Some clinicians like to include an antiemetic of the phenothiazine or butyrophenone type with the preoperative medications. Drugs in these groups, such as chlorpromazine or droperidol, are thought to act by inhibiting the effects of emetic substances on the chemotactic trigger zone. In addition to this action, promethazine has antihistaminic properties that may help in blocking the contribution of the vestibular inputs to the vomiting center. These drugs find their main usefulness in decreasing the incidence of postoperative nausea and vomiting.

Centrally acting anticholinergics such as scopolamine are effective in blocking emesis associated with vestibular stimulation such as motion sickness, but do not help with other causes of nausea and vomiting.

Anticholinergics and antihistamines are used to decrease gastric secretion and acidity. Since it has been well established that pulmonary injury from aspiration is directly correlated with the volume and acidity of the aspirate, controlling these factors can help reduce the sequelae of aspiration. Atropine seems to be of no help in this respect. Glycopyrrolate has been found to be effective in increasing gastric pH but only if given in amounts equal to or greater than 0.4 mg. The most effective drug for gastric drying and for increasing gastric pH is cimetidine. This drug is a specific H_2 blocking antihistamine that has become a valuable drug in the anesthetic armamentarium.

Any condition in which food or intestinal fluids are collected in areas that are not physiologically emptied adds to the potential of vomiting. In the esophagus the various diverticula can collect food. It has been noted that Zenker's or pulsion type diverticula in the upper esophagus are usually filled with food contents. Although attempts at suction and inducing vomiting have been tried in these patients, it would be fair to say that there is no guarantee that the contents of a diverticulum can be adequately emptied prior to the actual surgical excision or manipulation of the diverticulum during surgical correction. In these cases, the induction must be managed so as to minimize the chances of regurgitation of diverticular contents.

Farther down the gastrointestinal tract, stasis or obstruction can produce the potential for vomiting, either by distention of bowel or by toxic products produced which might directly stimulate the vomiting and/or chemotactic centers in the medulla. Although acute bleeding or food retention in a patient who has partially or totally obstructed viscera is an obvious reason for vomiting, it must be remembered that the intestinal secretions themselves are produced at a greater rate than they are absorbed. Therefore, all patients with gastrointestinal semiobstruction or total obstruction should be considered to have a high potential for vomiting and hence aspiration.

The pre-induction management of such patients should include prehydration, correction of any electrolyte abnormality, and optimizing of blood gases. The gut should be decompressed and drained as much as possible, usually via various suctioning devices. A large-bore nasogastric tube should be continued until the actual time of anesthetic induction. Unless there is a specific contraindication, suction tubes should be removed prior to the start of anesthesia in order to prevent the chance of reflux around the tube. The tube may then be replaced after the airway has been secured.

The particular anesthetic plan decided on will depend on the patient's condition, planned procedure, surgical requirements and patient preference. In those instances when vomiting and aspiration are particularly likely, one usually considers regional anesthesia or a general anesthetic with an awake intubation or perhaps a general anesthetic with a rapid sequence of intubation.

The use of regional anesthesia where feasible should be considered. There is no guarantee, however, that vomiting will not occur. An anesthetic mishap or unforeseen surgical problems may force a rapid change of anesthetic plan.

Hypotension associated with regional technique may cause vomiting and should be avoided if possible. Surgical traction on peritoneal structures can cause vomiting during what otherwise may be an adequate level of anesthesia. The patient under regional anesthesia should be able to protect his airway; however, this may have been compromised by intravenous sedation or by a high level of anesthesia impairing the ability to cough. Despite these problems, regional anesthesia may be the technique of choice in some instances.

The use of awake endotracheal intubation is perhaps the safest way to secure an airway in an appropriate patient. This is usually done with direct visualization or blindly via the nasotracheal route. Awake laryngoscopy and intubation requires good topical anesthesia to the pharynx and larynx and/or blocks of the superior laryngeal and glossopharyngeal nerves. The use of a styleted tube makes it easier to place the tube into the glottis without stimulating other pharyngeal structures. Blind nasotracheal intubation is usually more comfortable for the patient, since it avoids laryngoscopy with resultant pressure on the back of the tongue. It is best accomplished with a small, soft, well lubricated tube passed through a well topicalized nares. Despite the safety of awake intubation, aspiration may still occur because of the necessary anesthesia to the upper airway.

The technique of rapid sequence intubation as outlined here has proved to be of great safety for the patient at significant risk of aspiration. Before this technique is chosen, however, the anesthesiologist must assure himself that the patient's airway is conducive to a rapid and uncomplicated intubation. The problems that have arisen with this technique are almost invariably due to an inability to intubate the patient after the commitment has been made to proceed. While the patient is spontaneously breathing oxygen by mask, 3 to 6 mg of *d*-tubocurarine or 1 mg of pancuronium bromide (Pavulon) is administered to the patient. This will act to prevent fasciculations and the associated increase in intragastric pressure following relaxation with succinylcholine. Three to five minutes will allow adequate time for the "precurarization" to become effective as well as for the lungs to be denitrogenated. At this point, anesthesia is induced with an intravenous hypnotic, and is immediately followed by a large dose of depolarizing muscle relaxant, for example, 1 mg of succinyl-

choline per pound. At this time a trained assistant should apply firm circoid pressure to occlude the esophagus. This technique, as demonstrated by Selick, is quite effective in stopping gastric regurgitation. However, as was pointed out by Selick, in the face of active vomiting, esophagus pressures may become high enough to pose the threat of esophageal rupture. While the intravenous medications are taking effect, the anesthetist should refrain from positive pressure ventilation, as this may force gas into the stomach and increase the chance of vomiting and regurgitation. As soon as the patient becomes relaxed (approximately one minute), laryngoscopy and intubation with rapid inflation of the cuff on the tube should follow in a smooth controlled manner.

Despite the best precautions, aspiration may occasionally occur, as a result of frank vomiting or, more commonly, from silent regurgitation. The severity of aspiration pneumonitis depends on the material aspirated as well as on the volume. Gastric contents with a pH of less than 2.5 produce the most severe pathology, an immediate chemical burn. The volume necessary to produce injury varies from study to study. Most authors agree that a volume greater than 25 ml is sufficient to cause significant injury in the adult. The patient may become acutely ill immediately or may not show signs for up to 12 hours after the event. The usual signs are wheezing, cyanosis, tachycardia, and tachypnea. As pulmonary edema develops, plasma volume decreases and hypotension may develop. The blood gases show hypoxemia secondary to pulmonary ventilation perfusion mismatch. The PA_{CO_2} can be variable, although a combined respiratory and metabolic acidosis is common.

As soon as aspiration has been detected, the patient should be put on his right side, head down about 25 degrees, and the airway suctioned as expeditiously as possible. A cuffed endotracheal tube should be passed quickly to secure the airway, facilitate oxygenation, and allow for suctioning of the tracheobronchial tree. Bronchoscopy may be necessary to remove large food particles. It should be done by someone experienced in bronchoscopy, with careful attention given to maintaining adequate oxygenation and ventilation. Determining the pH of the aspirated material may give valuable prognostic information. Pulmonary lavage to clear the airway of aspirated material has been advocated by some; however, this only succeeds in further spreading the offending material and removing surface active material. Since pulmonary injury is almost immediate, it is ineffectual to attempt to neutralize the aspirate.

X-rays should be taken to see if any obvious large areas of atelectasis exist that might indicate the presence of an unsuspected foreign body. It is well known that the x-rays immediately after aspiration may appear relatively benign, the extent of damage secondary to aspiration being seen radiographically only hours later. The clinician should not be lulled into a sense of well being because of a benign chest film.

Further therapy of aspiration pneumonitis may require mechanical ventilation with PEEP in order to maintain acceptable blood gases. Bronchodilators such as aminophylline may be of use in combating the bronchospasm that often accompanies aspiration. Administration of antibiotics as a prophylactic measure is controversial, although it is indicated in the face of secondary infection or if evidence exists that pathologic organisms were aspirated. The use of steroids in aspiration is also controversial. There seems to be no harm in a short course of steroid therapy, which may be beneficial during the first 72 hours.

Prolonged vomiting can also cause problems of which the anesthesiologist must be aware. Among the most important of these are dehydration and electrolyte and acid base disturbances. Prolonged vomiting of gastric contents will result in a metabolic alkalosis. If, however, vomiting includes mixtures of pancreatic and biliary secretions, the exact metabolic disturbance cannot be predicted. The patient's condition may vary from that of metabolic alkalosis to that of metabolic acidosis. Usually the kidneys are able to compensate for such disturbances of homeostasis. However, renal function may have been compromised by diuretic drugs, abnormal hormone states, or decreased perfusion secondary to hypovolemia and hypotension. Inadequate dietary replacement of Na^+, K^+, and Cl^- will also make it impossible for renal compensation to occur.

In the usual case of vomiting the prime loss is that of hydrogen and chloride ions. With the loss of hydrogen ions there is an accumulation of bicarbonate in the plasma. This would normally be cleared by the kidneys; however, because of the need to conserve sodium and a relative lack of chloride ion, a potassium deficit develops. This tends to sustain an extracellular alkalosis and intracellular acidosis as potassium moves out of cells and hydrogen ions move into cells. The renal bicarbonate threshold is raised and a "paradoxical aciduria" will develop in the face of extracellular metabolic alkalosis. Adequate replacement of potassium, chloride, and sodium ions will correct this condition.

If significant amounts of pancreatic juice and bile are lost during protracted vomiting, the acid-base changes may be quite different. Pancreatic juice, an iso-osmotic solution with a pH between 8.0 and 8.3 (approx. 115 mEq/L bicarbonate), is produced at over a liter per day. Bile also is usually alkaline, although pH ranges from 5.7 to 8.0 have been reported. From 50 to 1000 ml per day is made. Significant loss of these fluids will result in metabolic acidosis. Hydrogen ions will move into cells in exchange for potassium, resulting in increased plasma potassium levels. Increasing amounts of potassium will be lost into the urine, leading to total body hypokalemia associated with metabolic acidosis.

The implications of protracted vomiting are many and must be considered by the anesthesiologist. It is impossible to list all the consequences of such altered homeostasis, but a few examples will illustrate the point. Metabolic acidosis can impair myocardial function, increase peripheral vasoconstriction, and lead to cardiovascular collapse. Metabolic alkalosis will cause the oxyhemoglobin dissociation curve to be shifted to the left, with resultant decreased oxygen delivery to the tissues. Hypokalemia can have profound effects on all excitable cells. Disturbances in myocardial conduction and rhythmicity can lead to sudden death, especially in the face of digitalis therapy. Muscle weakness is a common sign of hypokalemia, leading to respiratory insufficiency in severe cases. Smooth muscle function is also impaired, contributing to gastric distention and paralytic ileus.

The acid-base status of a patient can significantly influence the actions of many drugs used during anesthetic management. Although the anesthetic MAC of inhalation agents is not altered between pH 6.9 and 7.6, the influence of blood pH on the effects of fixed anesthetic agents can be clinically important. Blood pH will determine the ratio of un-ionized to ionized forms for many drugs; it should be recalled that it is the un-ionized form of a drug that more readily crosses biologic membranes. For many drugs, acid-base status will also influence the proportion of drug that is free as apposed to bound to plasma proteins. It is the free form that is available to reach the site of action. Another method by which pH can influence drug action is by altering the ionic milieu in which the drug's action takes place.

Thiopental is a weak acid with a pKa of 7.6. Therefore, using the Henderson-Hasselbalch equation, at a pH of 7.4 we find that 61 per cent of the drug will be in the un-ionized form. Lower pH values will increase the proportion of un-ionized (membrane diffusible) drug. Protein binding is also influenced by pH, with a maximum of thiopental bound to plasma proteins at a pH of 8.0. Consequently, an acidotic patient will have more drug available to enter the central nervous system. This will be even more important in the patient who is hypoproteinemic or who has been given drugs that will compete for binding sites. Acid-base gradients between CSF and blood are also important in determining drug distribution. For example, if plasma is made relatively alkalotic compared to CSF by bicarbonate injection, it will favor the diffusion of thiopental out of the CNS.

Narcotics are weak bases and, as such, their ionization characteristics are opposite to those of barbiturates. Fentanyl, for example, has a pKa of 7.5, and consequently will be 44 per cent un-ionized at physiologic pH. Increasing blood pH will increase the proportion of un-ionized drug. It has been shown in dogs that respiratory alkalosis will result in higher and prolonged brain levels of this drug. Predictions can be difficult, however, since ventilatory and pH changes can alter protein binding and cerebral flow in a differential manner.

Neuromuscular blocking agents are also influenced by the acid-base status of a patient. It is known that respiratory acidosis will potentiate the effects of nondepolarizing neuromuscular blocking agents. Surprisingly, acute metabolic alkalosis may have a similar effect, although this probably is secondary to decreased calcium and potassium levels. As might be expected, hypokalemia will augment a pancuronium-induced block and will necessitate larger than usual doses of neostigmine for reversal. These examples illustrate the consequences that altered acid-base metabolism may have on anesthetic agents, and serve to emphasize that, to whatever degree possible, the physiologic alterations of protracted vomiting should be corrected prior to anesthetic and surgical intervention.

FLUID REPLACEMENT

Derangement of fluid balance in gastrointestinal disorders is one of the major sequelae in this group of diseases. Sources of obvious loss include vomiting, suctioning, diarrhea, and fistula drainage. Less obvious losses include sequestration of fluid within bowel and peritoneal cavity and tissue edema. Whenever possible, fluid replacement therapy should be based on measurements of volume and composition of fluid losses. Where this is not possible, losses must be estimated and results of therapy carefully monitored.

If one considers that total secretion of fluid into the intestinal tract under normal conditions approximates 10 liters per day, it is obvious that volume and electrolyte disturbances that occur secondary to pathologic conditions may vary considerably. No fixed formula or amount of fluid replacement could be established as a routine until the amount and composition of the particular fluid lost is known. In addition, since the pathologic processes are in a dynamic state, variations may occur from one day to another. In the patient with intestinal obstruction or paralytic ileus, most of the loss is not obvious and body weight may remain stable. This does not mean that a state of dehydration does not exist, since intravascular fluid volume may be markedly decreased. It has been estimated that at the earliest time any degree of intestinal obstruction can be noted radiographically, there is approximately 1500 ml of fluid within the lumen of the bowel. As the obstruction becomes more established, deficits can approximate 6000 ml; with severe intestinal obstruction, losses of fluid within the lumen can exceed 7 liters.

Once any element of dilatation exists within the lumen of the gut, the ability of the mucosal surface to absorb fluid in the normal manner is inhibited. This inhibition roughly correlates to the degree of distention present. In addition, any distention may produce an increase in intestinal secretions. Rising intraluminal pressure eventually compromises the blood supply to the bowel, resulting in ischemia and the threat of perforation.

If loss of fluid into nonphysiologic spaces is combined with decreased oral intake and increased losses due to hyperpyrexia, the picture of severe dehydration and debility results. In the case of acute dehydration it has been estimated that a fluid loss of 1500 to 2000 ml produces oliguria and thirst; a loss of 3000 ml causes increasing oliguria, tachycardia, and postural hypotension. An acute loss of 6 per cent of body weight or 4 to 5 liters of extracellular fluid represents a potentially catastrophic situation. In the more chronic states, extracellular losses of as much as 10 per cent of body weight (7 to 8 liters) can be tolerated.

Fluid replacement therapy should consist of 1) administration of normal daily requirements, 2) matching of abnormal daily losses, and 3) replacement of estimated deficits. Normal adult fluid requirements are estimated to be about 2500 ml of water, 50 mEq sodium, 90 mEq chloride, and 40 mEq potassium. This estimate allows for 1500 ml urine output (enough to allow for renal compensation of minor imbalances) as well as 1000 ml per day for insensible losses (i.e., loss through the lungs and skin). These requirements are approximated by infusing 30 to 35 ml per kg per day of 0.2 normal saline with 20 mEq per liter of potassium. In addition to this, abnormal losses such as nasogastric suction output or fistula drainage should be replaced on a ml per ml basis with appropriate electrolyte solution.

Finally, estimated deficits in volume, sodium, chloride, potassium, and bicarbonate should be calculated. When these determinations are made at regular intervals it is possible to formulate an appropriate solution to be infused.

In actual practice, the first goal of fluid therapy for the patient who has had an acute loss of fluids is return to a normal volume status. Initially, a solution of isotonic saline should be started, with enough given to achieve positive responses from the patient. These include return of pulse, blood pressure, and pulse pressure toward normal, improvement in skin color and temperature,

restoration of urinary output, rise in central venous pressure, and reversal of other signs of dehydration. While the emergent condition is being taken care of, investigation as to the make up of fluid losses and the nature of blood electrolytes and acid-base status can be better evaluated. Additional replacement therapy with appropriate solutions can then be started.

The most common fluid and electrolyte abnormalities associated with gastrointestinal disease are hypovolemia, metabolic alkalosis, metabolic acidosis, and hypokalemia. As stated above, treatment of hypovolemia should be the first priority. Metabolic alkalosis is best treated by administration of sodium chloride and potassium chloride solutions. This will allow the kidneys to lower the bicarbonate threshold and correct the alkalosis. In case of metabolic acidosis, judicious replacement of bicarbonate will be effective. A useful formula for bicarbonate replacement is milliequivalents of sodium bicarbonate needed to return standard bicarbonate normal = 0.3 × weight in kilograms × base deficit. One half to two thirds of this amount can be given rapidly, with additional therapy depending upon blood gas analysis. Potassium deficits can be estimated with the aid of a potassium content capacity vs. serum potassium graph (Fig. 9–2). Extracellular alkalosis should always raise the question of hypokalemia, as discussed above. Similarly hypokalemia should be expected with metabolic acidosis, especially if serum potassium is normal or below normal. Therapy consists of adequate potassium replacement. However, potassium should not be administered until adequate urine output has been established and then only at rates of less than 20 mEq per hour unless constant physician monitoring is available. Concentrations greater than 40 mEq per liter should not be infused via peripheral veins, since this will cause pain and sclerosing of the vein.

PARENTERAL NUTRITION

Malnutrition is a common consequence of diseases of the gastrointestinal tract. In recent years physicians have become more aware of this problem and are becoming more aggressive in its prevention and correction. The science of parenteral nutrition has become well established in medicine

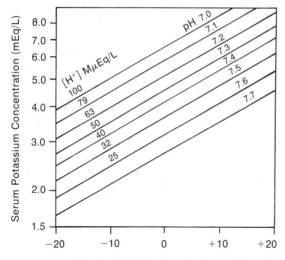

x-axis: Potassium Per Cent Depletion or Excess

Figure 9–2. The relationship between serum potassium concentration, blood pH, and per cent change in content capacity. (From Scribner, P. H. [ed.]: University of Washington Teaching Syllabus for the Course on Fluid and Electrolyte Balance. 7th revision, 1969, pp. 73–76.)

and has greatly altered the management and prognosis of patients with gastrointestinal as well as other diseases. The anesthesiologist as a member of the health care team must also be aware of the physiologic consequences of malnutrition as well as the special problems associated with parenteral nutrition that may affect anesthetic management.

Malnutrition can occur especially rapidly in the patient with gastrointestinal disease. Such patients lose their appetite and decrease oral intake; also, many conditions are associated with protein loss into the gut or via fistula drainage. Malabsorption may be a part of the picture, with deficiencies of B_{12}, folate, and iron commonly occurring. If such a patient is febrile, suffering from an inflammatory process, or septic, the added increase in metabolic expenditure can result in severe malnutrition within days.

Many of the pathogenic consequences of malnutrition are now well recognized and can involve all organ systems. Hypoalbuminemia directly reflects protein malnutrition. Other serum proteins such as transferrin and immunoglobulins are also reduced. Lymphocytes become significantly reduced, further compromising immunocompetence. Not surprisingly, most starved patients die from infection. Impaired wound healing has been long recognized as a consequence of protein-calorie malnutrition. Other changes include decrease in total blood volume, with red cell mass diminished relatively more than plasma volume. As starvation progresses, intracellular structural proteins are lost, and there is a concomitant loss of intracellular ions, especially potassium. It has been estimated that an otherwise healthy average man can survive about 70 days of starvation; this would be associated with an approximate 50 per cent weight loss.

Energy is stored as fat, protein, and glycogen. Of these, liver glycogen represents the only readily available source of glucose for metabolism by brain, red blood cells, and other organs. If an otherwise healthy 70 kg person is fasted, liver glycogen stores will be depleted within 24 hours. After this time period, glucose is provided by gluconeogenesis from protein breakdown. Urinary nitrogen excretion will consequently increase to 10 to 15 grams per day. This represents about 75 grams of protein loss. If fasting continues, nitrogen loss will decrease to less than 2 gm/day by the end of two weeks. The reason for this is a switch to predominantly fat metabolism, as the brain, heart, and other organs utilize keto acids, which are derived from free fatty acid oxidation, as fuel. It is well known that infusion of 100 to 150 gm of glucose per day will cut the initial protein loss by over 50 per cent; however, this will also prevent conversion to primarily fatty acid metabolism. If this is allowed to continue, the long-term result may be more protein wasting than would have been the case with total starvation. This illustrates the need for an early decision regarding adequate parenteral nutrition rather than waiting until weight loss and protein depletion are well advanced.

The indications for parenteral nutrition are quite broad. It may be used as an adjunct to oral or gastric tube feeding in cases where these more traditional modes are inadequate to provide the necessary nutrient load. An example of this would be the patient who has a constrictive lesion of the esophagus and has become chronically malnourished secondary to inadequate oral intake. A weight loss of 10 per cent or greater is a general indication for parenteral nutrition. The nutritionally debilitated patient being prepared for surgery will be benefited by correction of his nutritional status. Improved immunologic competence and wound healing should reduce the incidence of postoperative complications. Continuation of parenteral nutritional support into the postoperative period has similar benefits. This is especially true in those conditions such as perforated viscus or acute pancreatitis, where peritonitis would be expected to result in a protracted paralytic ileus. Parenteral nutrition may be the prime mode of therapy in conditions such as inflammatory bowel disease and enterocutaneous fistula. For example, it is well established that surgery should be avoided if at all possible in many instances of chronic relapsing regional enteritis. The advent of peripheral venous alimentation has served to broaden the indications for intravenous nutritional support because of its decreased risk of complications. The decision to start parenteral nutrition must be individualized, taking into account the nutritional status, the metabolic demands, and the feasibility or lack thereof of meeting those demands by oral or gastric alimentation.

A rational approach to parenteral nutrition must include an understanding of the energy and nutritive requirements of patients with various pathologic conditions. It has been shown that patients undergoing uncomplicated elective surgery have postoperative energy expenditures that do not differ significantly from preoperative values. A patient with multiple fractures, however, may have a 20 per cent increase in resting metabolic expenditure, and a patient with a major infection such as peritonitis may have up to a 30 to 50 per cent increase in resting metabolic expenditure (RME). In order to ensure positive nitrogen balance and weight gain, it is recommended that 50 per cent more calories be provided than the estimated RME. For example, a 70 kg patient with peritonitis would have a normal basal metabolic rate of 1800 calories and a resting metabolic expenditure of about 2520 calories, and should be given about 3780 calories of nutritional support. The optimum calorie-to-nitrogen ratio has been estimated to be 120 to 180 calories per gram of nitrogen, and, as such, the above patient would receive about 25 grams of nitrogen as protein. In addition to adequate calories and protein, total parenteral nutrition must include necessary electrolytes, vitamins, trace elements, and essential fatty acids.

Standard solutions for parenteral nutrition deliver calories as a 25 per cent dextrose solution. The hypertonicity of such solutions led to the coining of the term hyperalimentation. Such solutions must be delivered via a central venous route to minimize the incidence of thrombosis. Protein is delivered with this solution as either protein hydrolysates or as solutions of crystalline amino acids. The improved efficacy in uptake of crystalline amino acid solutions is responsible for the widespread use of this formulation. Solutions include both essential and nonessential amino acids and are delivered as a 4.25 per cent amino acid and 25 per cent dextrose solution. Once formulated, the solution must be used reasonably rapidly, since a spontaneous browning reaction will occur. This is not a problem with sorbitol solutions, as sometimes used in Europe. Fructose may be used as the calorie source and has the advantage of not requiring insulin to enter cells. This may be of advantage in the diabetic patient.

Adequate amounts of electrolytes and minerals must be supplied with the infusion. This is especially true of intracellular ions such as potassium, phosphate, magnesium, and calcium, which are rapidly utilized during metabolism. Large amounts of vitamins C and B complex should be given on a daily basis, as these are rapidly utilized during stress. The fat soluble vitamins A, E, and D may be given at weekly intervals to help prevent hypervitaminosis. Additionally, vitamin B_{12}, folate, and vitamin K may be required. Requirements for trace elements have not been established but these must be supplied in prolonged total parenteral nutrition. They may be supplied with blood products or given via injection.

When dealing with patients receiving hyperalimentation one should be especially aware of the possible complications associated with this mode of therapy. Hyperalimentation catheters are usually placed via the subclavian route. Catheter placement is associated with about a 5 per cent complication rate, including pneumothorax, brachial plexus injury, and hemothorax. Subclavian thrombosis secondary to prolonged hyperalimentation has been found to be a more common complication than was once thought. The anesthesiologist should be alert to the possibility of an unrecognized mechanical complication.

Sepsis is the most serious complication of

hyperalimentation. The incidence has declined with scrupulous attention to detail, regular dressing changes, and assurance that the infusion route is not violated for drug administration or CVP measurement. One multi-institution study reported a 7 per cent septicemia incidence, half due to Candida and half due to other bacteria. Institutions with special "hyperal teams" have reported lower incidences. For those conditions in which prolonged hyperalimentation is required, the Broviack catheter, which is tunneled subcutaneously prior to entry into a large vein, is becoming popular.

The metabolic implications of hyperalimentation are the most important to the anesthesiologist. Normal man has a glucose tolerance of about 0.5 gm/kg/day. However, in cases of severe stress such as sepsis, malnutrition, or surgery, decreased insulin secretion as well as peripheral insulin resistance can lead to glucose intolerance. For these reasons hyperalimentation should be started slowly and gradually increased. If hyperglycemia develops, insulin may be added to the infusion. Similarly, to prevent rebound hypoglycemia, hyperalimentation solutions should be tapered prior to discontinuation. During anesthesia and surgery the infusion rate should be slowed and blood glucose monitored. When it is impossible to monitor intraoperative blood glucose, it is perhaps best to discontinue hyperalimentation prior to surgery.

As mentioned previously, significant amounts of potassium and phosphate may be utilized with hyperalimentation. It may be necessary to add additional amounts of these substances to prevent deficiencies. Hypophosphatemia may cause neurologic dysfunction as well as decreasing levels of 2,3-DPG and a shift of the oxyhemoglobin dissociation curve to the left. Hyperchloremic metabolic acidosis has been a problem with some hyperalimentation solutions because of excessive chloride loads. The current practice of formulating solutions with acetate salts has largely resolved this problem. These examples illustrate the importance of preoperative assessment of electrolyte, mineral, and acid-base status in patients on parenteral alimentation regimens.

The physician dealing with the hyperalimentation patient should also be aware of the fact that CO_2 production will be increased. This may present a problem in weaning the patient from mechanical ventilation. If this becomes a problem, decreasing the infusion rate or switching to a lipid calorie source with a lower respiratory quotient may be helpful. Lipids per unit kilocalorie produce less CO_2 than comparable protein solutions.

The advent of fat emulsions for parenteral nutrition has added significant flexibility to the management of patients requiring parenteral alimentation. Fat emulsions have the advantage of being concentrated sources of energy; that is, it is possible to supply more calories in a similar volume of infused solution. They are a readily available source of essential fatty acids. Essential fatty acids are required for prostaglandin synthesis, normal wound healing, and red cell membrane integrity. Fat emulsions are not hypertonic and so can be infused in peripheral veins, thereby reducing the risks of sepsis. Further, fat infusions are not wasted by the kidneys.

The most commonly used fat emulsion is made up of soybean oil emulsified in water with egg phosphates. The solution is made isotonic by the addition of 2.5 per cent glycerol. Particle sizes are comparable to natural chylomicrons. Blood clearance studies have shown that the kinetics is also similar to that of natural chylomicrons. Animal studies have indicated that positive nitrogen balance and weight gain are more efficiently achieved when fat is included as a calorie source in total parenteral nutrition. The optimal proportion of calories supplied by fat is not known but it is usually given to supply approximately one half of total calorie requirements.

As with standard hyperalimentation solutions, lipid infusions should be started slowly (0.5 gm/kg/day) and gradually increased to 2 to 5 gm per kg per day. A number of adverse reactions have been reported, including febrile responses, anemias, and abnormalities of coagulation. Decreased pulmonary diffusion capacity has been observed that may last for four hours. The addition of small amounts of heparin (e.g., $2500\mu/500$ ml) reportedly prevents this by increasing the rate of blood clearance. Blood gases and pulmonary mechanics were found to be unaltered. Lipid infusions should be used cautiously in case of abnormal fat metabolism, adult onset diabetes mellitus, severe liver disease, coagulopathies, and severe pulmonary disease.

SPECIFIC DISORDERS

Introduction. Common pathophysiologies of gastrointestinal disorders and their anesthesiologic implications have been mentioned in the prior sections. Similarly, many of the disorders discussed in the first part of this chapter do not have unique anesthetic considerations beyond those mentioned in the general discussion and will not be individually presented here.

Disorders of the Esophagus. Of extreme importance to the anesthesiologist is the patient who presents with esophageal obstruction secondary to tumor or radiation, or both. The chronic malnutrition that may result from such a lesion has already been mentioned. Other complications, such as weakening of the esophageal wall and leakage of its contents into the mediastinum and pleural cavities, present a more immediate problem. Another complication, in the carcinoma patient, could be direct extension of tumor into major bronchi. The formation of tracheoesophageal fistulas is a well-known clinical entity. It is therefore important before anesthetizing a patient for excision of the esophageal lesion to know the exact extent to which the tumor has invaded other tissues. In cases in which extension to the trachea or bronchial tree is a possibility, preanesthetic bronchoscopy should be performed, not only to delineate the extent of resection from a surgeon's point of view but also to inform the anesthesiologist as to what he might be facing at the time of intubation. It is quite possible that endotracheal intubation could start bleeding because of friable tumor tissue, perforate the trachea, or acutely obstruct the airway by traumatically freeing the tumor into the lumen of the airway.

Mediastinitis, if it occurs, is a serious problem, causing emphysema, pneumonitis, pericarditis, and subcutaneous emphysema. Both tension pneumomediastinum and tension pnemothorax may result, with severe compromise of circulation and respiration. Correction of these complications preoperatively by judicious drainage, antibiotics, and pulmonary physiotherapy is essential for optimal anesthetic management.

Esophageal perforations can occur from other factors as well, including foreign bodies, severe vomiting, external trauma, ulcer, and ingestion of liquid or solid toxins.

Disorders of the Stomach. Peptic ulcer, one of the most common gastric disorders, offers no unusual problems other than those secondary to its complications, namely bleeding and risk of aspiration and perforation. However, those ulcers associated with hyperparathyroidism and steroid treatment are of particular importance because of the basic effects of these underlying causes on other systems of the body.

Macrocytic anemia secondary to atrophic gastritis from any cause should be corrected prior to surgery. It must be remembered that many times these patients are normovolemic. Blood component therapy, packed cells in this instance, might be better treatment than whole blood.

Disorders of the Bowel. A number of bowel disorders and their anesthetic considerations have already been mentioned. Of particular concern to the anesthesiologist is the presence of obstruction, since this is such a frequent feature of diseases of the bowel and has numerous implications regarding anesthetic management. Aside from those factors that have already been mentioned, special attention must be given to the possibilities of respiratory embarrassment secondary to elevation of the diaphragm by massively distended bowel. The added work of breathing that this represents to a patient who may already be debilitated by malnutrition and electrolyte abnormalities can rapidly lead to respiratory failure.

The mass of an obstructed bowel can also have dramatic hemodynamic effects that may not be predictable. Sudden decompression of distended bowel may result in rapid dilatation of splanchnic venous beds. This dilatation of capacitance vessels with loss of effective circulating blood volume may lead to profound hypotension and shock. Conversely, the bowel obstruction may have compressed the inferior vena cava and impeded blood return to the heart. Sudden decompression may in this case result in a hyperdynamic state or possibly even cardiac failure. Decompression, therefore, should be done gradually, allowing time for hemodynamic compensation.

When considering the anesthetic approach to the patient with bowel obstruction, a number of factors must be reviewed. Vomiting, fluid status, acid-base balance, and nutritional factors have already been discussed. The question of regional versus general anesthesia is an interesting one.

It is well known that the elimination of sympathetic tone by spinal or epidural anesthesia causes an increase in motor activity of the bowel. Whether or not this occurs in distended bowel is not clear. However, the possibility of perforation by increased intraluminal pressures secondary to unchecked vagal activity has been mentioned. The incidence of this complication is unknown. Regional anesthesia should not be considered to be absolutely contraindicated in the patient with bowel obstruction but rather should be considered in relation to the patient and the surgical situation. If general anesthesia is chosen, particular attention must be given to the choice of inspired gases. Nitrous oxide presents a particular problem because of its greater blood solubility compared with nitrogen, which accounts for approximately 70 per cent of trapped intraluminal gas. Since nitrous oxide has 34 times the blood solubility of nitrogen, it will diffuse into the intraluminal gas at a much faster rate than nitrogen can diffuse out. The resulting increased intraluminal volume can be dramatic. It has been shown in dogs that 70 to 80 per cent inspired N_2O concentration can cause a 75 to 100 per cent increase in intraluminal volume within two hours. Therefore, anesthetic mixtures high in nitrous oxide should not be used in closed bowel obstruction. This makes a nitrous oxide–narcotic-relaxant technique unsuitable. Potent inhalation agents are also not ideal, since they decrease splanchnic circulation, which may be critical in cases of already marginal visceral circulation.

The anesthesiologist should also be alert to less common disorders of the bowel. The Peutz-Jeghers syndrome can occasionally be diagnosed by an alert anesthesiologist who notices rather distinctive pigmented spots on the lips. However, in this disorder bleeding is usually limited to the gastrointestinal tract itself. In contrast to this, the vascular lesions of Osler-Weber-Rendu disease indeed present as telangiectasias on the mucous membranes of the oral cavities. Airway insertion and endotracheal intubation could stir up significant bleeding. The association of arteriovenous fistula with this disorder should be noted, because high output cardiac failure is a possible sequela.

Infectious disorders of the large bowel are usually not seen at surgery; however, complications can require correction. It is important for the anesthesiologist to realize that diseases such as amebiasis, actinomycosis, and tuberculosis are just intestinal forms of systemic infections. It is quite probable that patients with intestinal amebiasis also have invasion of the liver. Only 10 per cent of these present with clinical signs of liver infection or abscess. The pus from a liver abscess can gain access to any structure in the vicinity. Rupture through the diaphragm into the lungs is not unknown, and bronchial-hepatic fistulas can be formed. Similarly, amebae can invade the central nervous system and lungs. It is unnecessary to go over the effects of such diffuse involvement in this chapter. What is important from the anesthesiologist's point of view is to realize that a patient being operated on for sequelae of an infectious process within the gastrointestinal tract may be afflicted with various systemic complications. The diffuseness of the infection and its overall effects on body homeostasis must be evaluated.

Carcinoid Tumors. Carcinoid tumors are relatively rare and are usually associated with the gastrointestinal tract. Many are secreting in nature and provide serious challenges to anesthetic management. Less than 25 per cent of patients with carcinoid tumors have the carcinoid syndrome, and most of these patients have liver metastases. The syndrome is marked by vasomotor symptoms of flushing and cyanosis, bronchospasm, hypo- or hypertension, diarrhea, and right sided valvular disease of the heart. The syndrome can be quite variable and its expression depends on the proportion of various vasoactive substances secreted. Of the many substances known to be secreted, bradykinin and serotonin seem to be the most important from an anesthetic point of view. Bradykinin appears to be the chief cutaneous flush mediator. Histamine secretion is now believed to occur mainly in patients with gastric carcinoids. Bradykinins are potent vasodilators and are thought to cause the severe hypotension sometimes seen during anesthesia. The effects on extravascular smooth muscle contraction give rise to bronchoconstriction, which is seen to accompany hypotension and flushing. Serotonin has positive inotropic and chronotropic effects on the myocardium and variable effects on peripheral circulation. It is thought to be responsible for the hypertension sometimes seen during anesthesia. It also is the cause of increased gut motility and diarrhea in carcinoid patients.

The preoperative management of these patients should include careful assessment of their primary symptomatology, as this may give an indication of possible intraoperative problems. Clinical evidence of valvular heart lesions should be sought and cardiac failure treated if necessary. Large doses of corticosteroids prior to anesthesia appear to be helpful in inhibiting the formation of kinins. Aprotinin is a kallikrein trypsin inhibitor that has been claimed to be effective in the treatment of bradykinin crisis and has been recommended for prophylactic use in patients whose symptoms are suggestive of bradykinin secretion. Those patients with mainly serotoninergic dysfunction should be given antiserotonin drugs preoperatively. Methotrimeprazine has been recommended as the drug of choice. It should be remembered that this drug is a phenothiazine derivative with potent analgesic properties and may reduce anesthetic requirements.

The anesthetic management of patients with carcinoid tumors should include careful and extensive monitoring. Volume loading prior to induction will insure adequate intravascular reserves in case of hypotensive crisis on induction. A careful, smooth induction must be stressed and may be facilitated by topical anesthetic spray of the larynx after muscle relaxation. The use of succinylcholine has been discouraged because of the possibility of increasing intraabdominal pressure, as a result of muscle fasciculation, which may stimulate the release of hormones from the tumor. Anesthetic agents with significant hypotensive properties such as halothane or ethrane should be avoided. Drugs that are known to release histamine, for example, morphine and d-tubocurarine, are contraindicated, since they may trigger hypotension and bronchospasm. The anesthetics of choice would seem to be a thiopental, fentanyl, nitrous oxide, and pancuronium technique.

Regional anesthesia offers no benefit and is in fact contraindicated because the associated hypotension may precipitate a bradykininergic crisis that is often refractory to the usual modes of therapy. Vasopressors of the catecholamine type, or those that act by releasing catecholamines, should be avoided as they are known to activate tumor kallikrein. Angiotensin and methoxamine are recommended for the treatment of such hypotension.

Disorders of the Pancreas. Of importance to the anesthesiologist are the operations done on patients with pancreatic insufficiency. In addition to those factors mentioned previously having to do with malabsorption disorders, it must be remembered that chronic pancreatitis may lead to diabetes mellitus and all its sequelae. In its early stages acute derangements in fluid and electrolyte balance occur. Decrease in calcium is fairly frequent; this should be replaced by calcium gluconate or calcium chloride preoperatively, bringing calcium levels as close to normal as possible. Similarly, hypokalemia, which is part of the process of pancreatitis, should be corrected by intravenous potassium replacement, using blood electrolyte and ECG monitoring in order to prevent potassium overload.

Cystic fibrosis of the pancreas is the expression in that organ of mucoviscidosis, a generalized congenital defect of exocrine glands, resulting in excessive loss of electrolytes in sweat, saliva, and tears and overproduction of abnormally thick mucus. The pancreas is progressively replaced with fibrous tissue, and there is an insufficiency of exocrine secretion by the gland, leading to malabsorption and steatorrhea. The disease may manifest itself in the newborn as meconium ileus, accounting for approximately 20 per cent of the intestinal obstruction of the newborn. Bronchial obstruction may progress to chronic pulmonary disease with bronchiectasis, retained secretions, pneumonitis, and lung abscess. In addition to the usual problems encountered with the malabsorption disorders, patients with cystic fibrosis of the pancreas present with the problem of a severely compromised pulmonary tree. Emphasis on preoperative clearing of the secretions by postural drainage, liquefaction and suctioning, antibiotic therapy, and pulmonary physiotherapy is mandatory. Hyponatremia caused by an abnormally active sodium pump must be looked for and sodium replaced prior to anesthesia.

Insulinomas are rare tumors of the pancreas that arise from the beta cells of the islets of Langerhans. They may be benign or malignant. The primary symptoms of these tumors are paroxysms of severe hypoglycemia caused by excessive secretions of insulin. It is suggested that prior to surgery these patients receive an intravenous infusion containing glucose to forestall the possibility of a hypoglycemic crisis during preoperative fasting. Pretreatment with corticosteroids will also help to maintain an adequate blood sugar level. It has been suggested that the anesthetic of choice would be an inhalation agent such as halothane, which is known to produce a relative, although mild, hyperglycemia during the operative period. Others have suggested a narcotic-nitrous oxide-relaxant technique, which has minimal effect on carbohydrate metabolism. Using this technique combined with blood glucose determinations every 5 to 10 minutes (using Dextrostix), it should be possible to determine the completeness of tumor removal. Incomplete tumor removal would be indicated by falling glucose levels, while complete removal would be marked by rising glucose levels within 10 or 15 minutes.

Disorders of the Liver. Hepatic disease has many anesthetic implications because of the wide range of pathophysiologic conditions it may cause. Defects in blood coagulation result from an interaction of multiple factors. Simple obstructive jaundice will lead to decreased vitamin K absorption and a resultant decrease in prothrombin and factors VII, IX, and X. Severe liver disease will lead to a reduction in all liver synthesized clotting factors (i.e., I, II, V, VII, X). Hypersplenism and thrombocytopenia may be found in 50 per cent of patients with severe cirrhotic liver disease.

A complex anemia is frequently seen in these patients. Contributing factors include occult or frank blood loss into the gastrointestinal system as well as decreased red cell formation in the marrow. There is increased hemolysis as well as sequestration of red blood cells in the spleen. Inadequate vitamin intake and absorption add a vitamin deficiency component to the anemia.

Jaundice may result from excessive bilirubin in the blood secondary to hemolysis or from reduced hepatic uptake, conjugation, or excretion of bile. Elevated levels of protein bound or indirect bilirubin can interact with some anesthetic drugs by displacing them from protein binding states.

Alcohol abuse is a frequent cause of liver disease. The common clinical impression that alcoholic patients have a higher tolerance for anesthetics has been substantiated for thiopental-Demerol-N_2O anesthesia.

This is explained on the pharmacokinetic basis of increased drug metabolism secondary to hepatic enzyme induction, although pharmacodynamic actions at the level of the central nervous system may also be important. Once such a patient's liver disease becomes advanced, however, the patient may become extremely sensitive to such drugs, as there is insufficient functioning hepatic tissue to metabolize them.

Long-standing liver disease often results in progressive hepatic fibrosis. As portal flow decreases, collateral canals form to return the blood to the systemic circulation, resulting in esophageal varices. The clinician must be alert to the possibility of inducing variceal bleeding when passing a nasogastric tube or instrumenting the lower esophagus. Ascites is frequently also a problem in these patients. It is formed by elevated portal pressures as well as decreased plasma oncotic pressure secondary to hypoalbuminemia. Severe ascites causes massive abdominal distention and raised diaphragms, leading to ventilatory insufficiency. Ascitic fluid has even been known to enter the pleural cavities, causing hydrothorax.

Hepatic encephalopathy may develop in cases of extensive portal to systemic shunting due to naturally developing collaterals or surgical portacaval anastomosis. This complex syndrome is characterized by disturbances of consciousness, fluctuating neurologic signs, and asterixis. The cause of this syndrome is unknown, although it is usually associated with high levels of abnormal nitrogenous substances, such as ammonia, within the systemic circulation. Many fixed anesthetic agents must be given with great care in such patients, since the effects may be profound and long lasting. Recent work with specially formulated hyperalimentation solutions promises to be of help in the nutritional support of patients with liver disease as well as in the treatment of hepatic encephalopathy.

Progressive renal failure is a serious complication of advanced hepatic disease. Often the basic pathophysiology causing the hepatic disease (e.g., the deposition of copper in Wilson's disease) is common to both organs. However, more often the changes in renal function are secondary to hyperaldosteronism with sodium retention and potassium excretion, abnormal antidiuretic hormone function, and decreased renal blood flow.

When one considers the many pathophysiologic implications of hepatic disease it becomes clear that the anesthetic plan must be carefully thought out and well understood. This is especially true with regard to the administration of fixed anesthetic agents. It is well known that the effects of succinylcholine may be prolonged in patients with liver disease because of decreased levels of plasma pseudocholinesterase, which is produced in the liver. Pancuronium may be required in greater than the usual amounts to reach a given end point. This has been explained on the basis that a large amount of the drug is bound to gamma globulin, which is often increased in patients with liver disease. However, the duration of neuromuscular block may be prolonged, since at least a proportion of the drug is cleared by the hepatic metabolism. The examples serve to illustrate the importance of understanding the altered pharmacology of many drugs in the patient with hepatic disease.

Many drugs used in the practice of anesthesia have the potential for causing hepatic injury. This has been an especially confusing issue in regard to the potent inhalation agents. The particulars of this controversy will not be dealt with here. It is sufficient to say that potent inhalation agents have advantages and disadvantages of which one should be fully aware. Volatile anesthetics have the advantage of providing a complete anesthetic that can be readily eliminated without depending on hepatic or renal function. The potent inhalation agents, however, have been shown to reduce hepatic blood flow to a greater extent than some other anesthetic techniques. Since anesthetic induced hepatic necrosis has been produced in animal models given a mildly hypoxic anesthetic mixture in the presence of induced enzyme systems, the concern becomes obvious. If a general anesthetic must be given to a patient with hepatic disease, it is best to maintain a light level of anesthesia, maintain normocapnea, and insure adequate oxygen in the inspired mixture.

REFERENCES

General

Artz, C. P., and Hardy, J. D. (eds.): Management of Surgical Complications. 3rd ed. Philadelphia, W. B. Saunders Company, 1975.

Condon, R. E., and Nyhus, L. M. (eds.): Manual of Surgical Therapeutics. Boston, Little, Brown and Company, 1969.

Davenport, H. W.: Physiology of the Digestive Tract. 2nd ed. Chicago, Year Book Medical Publishers, 1966.

Preston, F. W., and Beal, J. M. (eds.): Basic Surgical Physiology. Chicago, Year Book Medical Publishers, 1969.

Schwartz, S. I., Hume, D. M., Lillehei, R. C., Shires, G. T., Spencer, F. C., and Storer, E. H. (eds.): Principles of Surgery. New York, McGraw-Hill Book Company, 1969.

Welch, C. E.: Medical progress: Abdominal surgery. N. Engl. J. Med. *284*:424, 471, 534, 1971.

Vomiting

Bruno, M. S., Grier, W. R. N., and Ober, W. B.: Spontaneous laceration and rupture of esophagus and stomach. Mallory-Weiss syndrome, Boerhaave syndrome and their variants. Arch. Intern. Med. *112*:574, 1963.

Cummins, A. J.: The physiology of symptoms. III. Nausea and vomiting. Amer. J. Dig. Dis. 3:710, 1958.

Davenport, H. W.: Physiology of the Digestive Tract. 2nd ed. Chicago, Year Book Medical Publishers, 1966.

Dobbins, W. O., III: Mallory-Weiss syndrome: A commonly overlooked cause of upper gastrointestinal bleeding. Report of three cases and review of the literature. Gastroenterology *44*:689, 1963.

Drucker, W. R., and Wright, H. K.: Physiology and pathophysiology of gastrointestinal fluids. Curr. Prob. Surg., May, 1964.

Richman, H., and Abramson, S. F.: Mendelson's syndrome: Diagnosis, therapy, and prevention. Amer. J. Surg. *120*:531, 1970.

Fistulas

Anderson, M. C., and Schiller, W. R.: The exocrine pancreas. *In*: Preston, F. W., and Beal, J. M. (eds.): Basic Surgical Physiology. Chicago, Year Book Medical Publishers, 1969.

Baker, R. J., Bass, R. T., Zajtchuk, R., and Strohl, E. L.: External pancreatic fistula following abdominal injury. Arch Surg. 95:556, 1967.

Beal, J. M., and Moody, F. G.: Postoperative complications of duodenal surgery. Surg. Clin. N. Amer. *44*:379, 1964.

Beal, J. M.: The stomach. *In* Preston, F. W., and Beal, J. M. (eds.): Basic Surgical Physiology. Chicago, Year Book Medical Publishers, 1969.

Davenport, H. W.: Physiology of the Digestive Tract. 2nd ed. Chicago, Year Book Medical Publishers, 1966.

Drucker, W. R., and Wright, H. K.: Physiology and pathophysiology of gastrointestinal fluids. Curr. Prob. Surg., May, 1964.

Edmunds, L. H., Jr., Williams, G. N., and Welch, C. E.: External fistulas arising from the gastrointestinal tract. Ann. Surg. *152*:445, 1960.

Hardy, J. D.: Small bowel fistulas and ileostomy. *In* Randall, H. R., Hardy, J. D., and Moore, F. D. (eds.): Manual of Preoperative and Postoperative Care. Philadelphia, W. B. Saunders Company, 1967.

Hardy, J. D.: High-output gastrointestinal fistula. *In* Hardy, J. D. (ed.): Critical Surgical Illness. Philadelphia, W. B. Saunders Company, 1971.

Jesseph, J. E., and Bachulis, B. L.: Surgical accidents and errors. *In* Harkins, H. N., and Nyhus, L. M. (eds.): Surgery of the Stomach and Duodenum. 2nd ed. Boston, Little, Brown and Company, 1969.

Jordan, G. L., Jr.: Pancreatic fistula. Amer. J. Surg. *119*:200, 1970.

Marshall, S. F., and Knud-Hansen, J.: Gastrojejunocolic and gastrocolic fistulas. Ann. Surg. *145*:770, 1957.

Moore, H. G., Jr.: Complications of gastric surgery. *In* Harkins, H. N., and Nyhus, L. M. (eds.): Surgery of the Stomach and Duodenum. 2nd ed. Boston, Little, Brown, and Company, 1969.

Moretz, W. H.: Inadvertent gastro-ileostomy. Ann. Surg. *130*:124, 1949.

O'Brien, P. H.: Fluid and electrolyte balance. *In* Preston, F. W., and Beal, J. M. (eds.): Basic Surgical Physiology. Chicago, Year Book Medical Publishers, 1969.

Pearlstein, L., Jones, C., and Polk, A.: Gastrocutaneous fistula: Etiology and treatment. Ann. Surg. *187*:223, 1978.

Preston, F. W.: The intestine and rectum. *In* Preston, F. W., and Beal, J. M. (eds.): Basic Surgical Physiology. Chicago, Year Book Medical Publishers, 1969.

Preston, F. W., and Beal, J. M.: The liver and biliary tract. *In* Preston, F. W., and Beal, J. M. (eds.): Basic Surgical Physiology. Chicago, Year Book Medical Publishers, 1969.

Reber, H. A., Roberts, C., Way, L., and Dumpley, J.: Management of external gastrointestinal fistulas. Ann. Surg. *188*:460, 1978.

Rousselot, L. M., and Slattery, J. R.: Immediate complications of surgery of the large intestine. Surg. Clin. N. Amer. *44*:397, 1964.

Schwartz, S. I.: Complications. *In* Schwartz, S. I., et al. (eds.): Principles of Surgery. New York, McGraw-Hill Book Company, 1969.

State, D.: Immediate complications of gastric surgery. Surg. Clin. N. Amer., *44*:371, 1964.

Obstruction

Barnett, W. O.: Strangulation obstruction. *In* Hardy, J. D. (ed.): Critical Surgical Illness. Philadelphia, W. B. Saunders Company, 1971.

Byrne, J. J., and Cahill, J. M.: Acute gastric dilatation. Amer. J. Surg. *101*:301, 1961.

Catchpole, B. N.: Ileus: Use of sympathetic blocking agents in its treatment. Surgery *66*:811, 1969.

Condon, R. E., and Zacheis, H. G.: Intestinal obstruction. *In*: Condon, R. E., and Nyhus, L. M. (eds.): Manual of Surgical Therapeutics. Boston, Little, Brown and Company, 1969.

Drucker, W. R., and Wright, H. K.: Physiology and pathophysiology of gastrointestinal fluids. Curr. Prob. Surg., May 1964.

Hammond, J. B., and Scanlon, E. F.: The esophagus. *In* Preston, F. W., and Beal, J. M. (eds.): Basic Surgical Physiology. Chicago, Year Book Medical Publishers, 1969.

Harkins, H. N., and Nyhus, L. M. (eds.): Surgery of the Stomach and Duodenum, 2nd ed. Boston, Little, Brown and Company, 1969.

Heimbach, D. M., and Crout, J. R.: Treatment of paralytic ileus with adrenergic neuronal blocking drugs. Surgery *69*:582, 1971.

Nadronski, L.: Pathophysiology and current treatment of intestinal obstruction. Rev. Surg. *31*:381, 1974.

Schwartz, S. I., and Storer, E. H.: Manifestations of gastrointestinal disease. *In* Schwartz, S. I., et al. (eds.): Principles of Surgery. New York, McGraw-Hill Book Company, 1969.

Stewardson, R., Bombeck, C. T., and Nyhus, L. M.: Critical operative management of small bowel obstruction. Ann Surg. *187*:189, 1978.

Wangenstein, O.: Understanding the bowel obstruction problem. Amer. J. Surg. *135*:131, 1978.

Warren, W. D.: Small intestinal obstruction. *In* Randall, H. R., Hardy, J. D., and Moore, F. D. (eds.): Manual of Preoperative and Postoperative Care. Philadelphia, W. B. Saunders Company, 1967.

Wilson, B. J.: Postoperative ileus. *In* Randall, H. R., Hardy, J. D., and Moore, F. D. (eds.): Manual of Preoperative and Postoperative Care. Philadelphia, W. B. Saunders Company, 1967.

Woodward, E. R.: Stomach and duodenum. *In* Randall, H. T., Hardy, J. D., and Moore, F. D. (eds.): Manual of Preoperative and Postoperative Care. Philadelphia, W. B. Saunders Company, 1967.

Diarrhea

Davenport, H. W.: Physiology of the Digestive Tract. 2nd ed. Chicago, Year Book Medical Publishers, 1966.

Drucker, W. R., and Wright, H. K.: Physiology and pathophysiology of gastrointestinal fluids. Curr. Prob. Surg., May 1964.

Low-Beer, T. S., and Read, A. E.: Progress report. Diarrhoea: Mechanisms and treatment. Gut *12*:1021, 1971.

Schwartz, S. I., and Storer, E. H.: Manifestations of gastrointestinal disease. *In* Schwartz, S. I., et al. (eds.): Principles of Surgery. New York, McGraw-Hill Book Company, 1969.

Malabsorption

Borgström, B., Dahlqvist, A., Lindberg, T., and Thaysen, E. H.: The basis of malabsorption. *In* Bittar, E. E., and Bittar, N. (eds.): The Biological Basis of Medicine, Vol. 5. London, Academic Press, 1969.

Floch, M. H.: Recent contributions in intestinal absorption and malabsorption (a review). Amer. J. Clin. Nutr, *22*:327, 1969.

Jeffries, G. H., Weser, E., and Sleisenger, M. H.: Progress in gastroenterology: Malabsorption. Gastroenterology *56*:777, 1969.

Kirsner, J. B.: Clinical observations on malabsorption. Med. Clin. N. Amer. *53*:1169, 1969.

Sheehy, T. W., and Floch, M. H.: The Small Intestine: Its Function and Diseases. New York, Harper & Row, 1964.

Wright, H. K., and Tilson, M. D.: The short gut syndrome: Pathophysiology and treatment. Curr. Prob. Surg., June 1971.

Surgical Nutrition and Elemental Diets

Aguirre, A., Fischer, J. E., and Welch, C. E.: The role of surgery and hyperalimentation in therapy of gastrocutaneous fistulae. Amer. Surg. *180*:393, 1974.

Blackburn, G. L., Flatt, J. P., Clove, G. A., and

O'Donnel, T. E.: Peripheral intravenous feeding with isotonic amino acid solution. Am. J. Surg. 125:447, 1973.

Bruegyman, J. L.: Infection control in parenteral nutrition. J.A.M.A. 224:1429, 1973.

Burk, S., Hobar, I., Hakansson, I., and Wretlind, A.: Nitrogen sparing effect of fat emulsion compared with glucose in the post-operative period. Acta Chir. Scand. 142:423, 1976.

Dillon, J., Jr., Schaffner, W., Van Way, C., III, and Meng, H.: Septicemia and total parenteral nutrition. J.A.M.A. 223, 1341, 1973.

Dudrick, S., Long, J., Steiger, E., and Rhoads, J.: Intravenous hyperalimentation. Surgery 68:726, 1970.

Dudrick, S., MacFadyen, B., Van Buren, C., Ruberg, R., and Maiymart, A.: Parenteral hyperalimentation: Metabolic problems and solutions. Ann. Surg. 176:259, 1972.

Greenberg, G. R., Marliss, E., Anderson, G., et al.: Protein sparing therapy in post-operative patients. Effects of adding hypocaloric glucose or lipid. N. Engl. J. Med. 294:1411, 1974.

Mullen, J., Hargrove, C., Dudrick, S., Fitts, L., and Rosatio, E.: Ten years' experience with intravenous hyperalimentation and inflammatory bowel disease. Ann. Surg. 187:523, 1978.

Siberman, H., Freehau, M., Fong, G., and Rosenblatt, N.: Parenteral nutrition with lipids. J.A.M.A. 238:1380, 1977.

Voitk, A., Brown, R., Echave, V., McArdle, A. H., Curd, F., and Thompson, I.: Use of an elemental diet in the treatment of complicated pancreatitis. Amer. J. Surg. 125:223, 1973.

Voitk, A. J., Echave, V., Brown, R. A., McArdle, A. A., and Gurd, F.: Elemental diet in the treatment of fistulas of the alimentary tract. Surg. Gynecol. Obstet. 137:68, 1973.

Protein-Losing Enteropathy

French, A. B.: Protein-losing gastroenteropathies. Amer. J. Dig. Dis. 16:661, 1971.

Waldmann, T. A.: Protein-losing enteropathy. Gastroenterology 50:422, 1966.

Peritonitis

Altemeier, W. A., Culbertson, W. R., and Fullen, W. D.: Intra-abdominal sepsis. Adv. Surg. 5:281, 1971.

Hedberg, S. E., and Welch, C. E.: Suppurative peritonitis with major abscesses. In Hardy, J. D. (ed.): Critical Surgical Illness. Philadelphia, W. B. Saunders Company, 1971.

Skillman, J. J., Bushnell, L. S., and Hedley-Whyte, J.: Peritonitis and respiratory failure after abdominal operations. Ann. Surg. 170:122, 1969.

Storer, E. H.: Peritonitis and intraabdominal abscesses. In Schwartz, S. I., et al. (eds.): Principles of Surgery. New York, McGraw-Hill Book Company, 1969.

Liver Disease

Berci, G., Morgenstein, L., Shore, J., and Shapire, S.: A direct approach to the differential diagnosis of jaundice. Amer. J. Surg. 126:372, 1973.

Conn, H. O.: A rational program for the management of hepatic coma. Gastroenterology 57:715, 1969.

Elias, E., Hamlyn, A. N., Jarn, S., Long, R. G., Summerfield, J., Dick, R., and Sherlock, S.: A randomized trial of percutaneous transhepatic cholangiography with the Chiba needle versus endoscopic retrograde cholangiography for bile duct visualization in jaundice. Gastroenterology 71:439, 1976.

Goldstein, L., Sample, W., Kodell, B., and Werner, M.: Gray-scale ultrasonography and thin needle cholangiography. J.A.M.A. 238:1041, 1977.

Henley, K. S.: Ascites and renal failure in liver disease: Principles of management. Amer. J. Dig. Dis. 16:363, 1971.

Kaplan, M., Juler, G., Stanton, W., and Eisenman, J.: Rapid and accurate preoperative diagnosis of obstructive jaundice. Arch. Surg. 188:828, 1974.

McDermott, W. V., Jr.: Liver and portal vein. In Randall, H. R., Hardy, J. D., and Moore, F. D. (eds.): Manual of Preoperative and Postoperative Care. Philadelphia, W. B. Saunders Company, 1967.

Schwartz, S. I.: Liver. In Schwartz, S. I., et al. (eds.): Principles of Surgery. New York, McGraw-Hill Book Company, 1969.

Walls, W. D., and Losowsky, M. S.: The hemostatic defect of liver disease. Gastroenterology 60:108, 1971.

Witte, M. H., Witte, C. L., and Dumont, A. E.: Progress in liver disease: Physiological factors involved in the causation of cirrhotic ascites. Gastroenterology 61:742, 1971.

Esophagus

General

Kramer, P.: Progress in gastroenterology: Esophagus. Gastroenterology 54:1171, 1968.

Pope, C. E., II: Progress in gastroenterology: The esophagus: 1967 to 1969. Gastroenterology 59:460, 615, 1970.

Wilkins, E. W., Jr., and Skinner, D. B.: Surgery of the esophagus. N. Engl. J. Med. 278:824, 887, 1968.

Zboralske, F. F., and Friedland, G. W.: Medical progress: Diseases of the esophagus. Present concepts. Calif. Med. 112:33, 1970.

Diverticula

Dorsey, J. M., and Randolph, D. A.: Long-term evaluation of pharyngoesophageal diverticulectomy. Ann. Surg. 173:680, 1971.

Ellis, F. H., Jr.: Pharyngo-esophageal diverticula and cricopharyngeal incoordination. Mod. Treat. 7:1098, 1970.

Localio, S. A., and Stahl, W. M.: Diverticular disease of the alimentary tract, Part II: The esophagus, stomach, duodenum and small intestine. Curr. Prob. Surg., Jan. 1968.

Payne, W. S., and Claggett, O. T.: Pharyngeal and esophageal diverticula. Curr. Prob. Surg., April 1965.

Achalasia

Cassella, R. R., Brown, A. L., Jr., Sayre, G. P., and Ellis, F. H., Jr.: Achalasia of the esophagus: Pathologic and etiologic considerations. Ann. Surg. 160:474, 1964.

Ellis, F. G.: The aetiology and treatment of achalasia of the cardia. Ann. Roy. Coll. Surg. Eng. 30:155, 1962.

Nemir, P., Jr., Fallahnejad, M., Bose, B., Jacobwitz, D., Frobese, A. S., and Hawthorne, H. R.: A study of the cause of failure of esophagocardiomyotomy for achalasia. Amer. J. Surg. 121:143, 1971.

Diffuse Esophageal Spasm

Bennett, J. R., and Hendrix, T. R.: Diffuse esophageal spasm; a disorder with more than one cause. Gastroenterology 59:273, 1970.

Gillies, M., Nicks, R., and Skyring, A.: Clinical manometric and pathological studies in diffuse oesophageal spasm. Brit. Med. J. 2:527, 1967.

Kramer, P.: Diffuse esophageal spasm. Mod. Treat. 7:1151, 1970.

Paraesophageal Hernia

Culver, G. J., Pirson, H. S., and Bean, B. C.: Mechanism of obstruction in para-esophageal diaphragmatic hernias. J.A.M.A. 181:933, 1962.

Hill, L. D., and Tobias, J. A.: Paraesophageal hernia. Arch. Surg. 96:735, 1968.

Esophageal Perforation

Bruno, M. S., Grier, W. R. N., and Ober, W. B.: Spontaneous laceration and rupture of esophagus and stomach. Mallory-Weiss syndrome, Boerhaave syndrome and their variants. Arch. Intern. Med. 112:574, 1963.

Burford, T. H., and Ferguson, T. B.: Esophageal perforations and mediastinal sepsis. In Hardy, J. D. (ed.): Critical Surgical Illness. Philadelphia, W. B. Saunders Company, 1971.

Foster, J. H.: Esophageal perforation. Mod. Treat. 7:1284, 1970.

Esophageal Moniliasis

Holt, J. M.: Candida infection of the oesophagus. Gut 9:227, 1968.

Sherlock, P., Goldstein, M. J., and Eras, P.: Esophageal moniliasis. Mod. Treat. 7:1250, 1970.

Smith, J. M. B.: Mycoses of the alimentary tract. Gut 10:1035, 1969.

Corrosive Esophagitis

Haller, J. A., Jr., and Andrews, H. G.: Pathophysiology and management of acute corrosive burns of the esophagus. Mod. Treat. 7:1182, 1970.

Hollinger, P. H.: Management of esophageal lesions caused by chemical burns. Ann. Otol. 77:819, 1968.

Marchand, P.: Caustic strictures of the oesophagus. Thorax 10:171, 1955.

Moody, F. G., and Garrett, J. M.: Esophageal achalasia following lye ingestion. Ann. Surg. 170:755, 1969.

Reflux Esophagitis and Stricture

Boesly, S.: The acid perfusion test. Scand. J. Gastroent. 12:241, 1977.

Boesly, S.: Continuous esophageal pH recording and acid clearing test. Scand. J. Gastroent. 12:245, 1977.

Demeester, T., Johnson, L., and Kent, A.: Evaluation of current operations for the prevention of gastroesophageal reflux. Ann. Surg. 180:511, 1974.

Hiebert, C.: The recognition and management of gastroesophageal reflux without hiatal hernia. World J. Surg. 1:445, 1977.

Hill, L., Ives, R., Stevenson, J., and Pearson, J.: Reoperation for disruption and recurrence after Nissen fundoplication. Arch. Surg. 114:542, 1979.

Polk, H.: Fundoplication for reflux esophagitis: Misadventures with this operation of choice. Ann. Surg. 183:645, 1976.

Saik, R., Greenburg, A. G., and Peskin G.: A study of fundoplication disruption and deformity. Amer. J. Surg. 134:19, 1977.

Skinner, D.: Complications of surgery for gastroesophageal reflux. World J. Surg. 1:485, 1977.

Barrett's Syndrome

Burgess, J. N., Payne, W. S., Andersen, H. A., Weiland, L. H., and Carlson, H. C.: Barrett esophagus: The columnar–epithelial-lined lower esophagus. Mayo Clin. Proc. 46:728, 1971.

Heitmann, P., Csendes, A., and Strauszer, T.: Esophageal strictures and lower esophagus lined with columnar epithelium: Functional and morphologic studies. Amer. J. Dig. Dis. 16:307, 1971.

Johnston, J. H., Jr.: Gastric lined esophagus associated with rings and stenoses. Ann. Surg. 173:641, 1971.

Jordan, P. H., Jr., and Longhi, E. H.: Diagnosis and treatment of an esophageal stricture (ring) in a patient with Barrett's epithelium. Ann. Surg. 169:355, 1969.

Other Diseases

Bruno, M. S., Grier, W. R. N., and Ober, W. B.: Spontaneous laceration and rupture of esophagus and stomach. Mallory-Weiss syndrome, Boerhaave syndrome and their variants. Arch. Intern. Med. 112:574, 1963.

Dobbins, W. O., III: Mallory-Weiss syndrome: A commonly overlooked cause of upper gastrointestinal bleeding. Report of three cases and review of the literature. Gastroenterology 44:689, 1963.

Fischer, R. A., Ellison, G. W., Thayer, W. R., Spiro, H. M., and Glaser, G. H.: Esophageal motility in neuromuscular disorders. Ann. Intern. Med. 63:229, 1965.

Goyal, R. K., Glancy, J. J., and Spiro, H. M.: Lower esophageal ring. N. Engl. J. Med. 282:1298, 1355, 1970.

Postlethwait, R. W., and Sealy, W. C.: Experiences with the treatment of 59 patients with lower esophageal web. Ann. Surg. 165:786, 1967.

Rinaldo, J. A., Jr., and Gahagan, T.: The narrow lower esophageal ring: Pathogenesis and physiology. Amer. J. Dig. Dis. 11:257, 1966.

Schmidt, A., and Lockwood, K.: Benign neoplasms of the esophagus. Acta Chir. Scand. 133:640, 1967.

Watson, R. R., O'Connor, T. M., and Weisel, W.: Solid benign tumors of the esophagus. Ann. Thorac. Surg. 4:81, 1967.

Winship, D. H.: Management of esophageal problems in patients with collagen vascular disease. Mod. Treat. 7:1241, 1970.

Stomach

General

Harkins, H. N., and Nyhus, L. M. (eds.): Surgery of the Stomach and Duodenum. 2nd ed. Boston, Little, Brown and Company, 1960.

Kirsner, J. B.: Peptic ulcer: A review of the recent literature on various clinical aspects. Gastroenterology 54:611, 945, 1968.

Menguy, R. B.: Stomach. In Schwartz, S. I., et al. (eds.): Principles of Surgery. New York, McGraw-Hill Book Company, 1969.

Foreign Bodies

Condon, R. E., and DeVito, R. V.: Other surgical diseases of the stomach and duodenum. In Harkins, H. N., and Nyhus, L. M. (eds.): Surgery of the Stomach and Duodenum. 2nd ed. Boston, Little, Brown and Company, 1969.

DeBakey, M., and Ochsner, A.: Recent advances in surgery. Bezoars and concretions. A comprehensive review of the literature with an analysis of 303 collected cases and a presentation of eight additional cases. Surgery 4:934, 1938; 5:132, 1939.

Holmes, T. W., Jr.: Polybezoar and gastrointestinal foreign bodies. Amer. J. Surg. 103:487, 1962.

Association of Gastric and Duodenal Ulceration with Other Diseases

Friesen, S. R.: Zollinger-Ellison Syndrome. Curr. Prob. Surg., April 1972.

Hinchey, E. J., Hreno, A., Benoit, P. R., Hewson, J. R., and Gurd, F. N.: The stress ulcer syndrome. Adv. Surg. 4:325, 1970.

Menguy, R., and Eiseman, B.: Extragastric factors associated with peptic ulcer. Curr. Prob. Surg., August 1964.

Nagel, C. D.: The nature and treatment of stress ulcers: A review. Calif. Med. 112:19, 1970.

Oberhelman, H. A., Jr.: Physiological Principles of Gastric Surgery. Springfield, Ill., Charles C Thomas, Publisher, 1968.

Ptak, T., and Kirsner, J. B.: Zollinger-Ellison syndrome, polyendocrine adenomatosis and other endocrine associations with peptic ulcer. Adv. Intern. Med. 16:213, 1970.

Saik, R. P., Greenburg, A. G., Farris, J. M., and Peskin, G. W.: The practicality of the Congo red test or is your vagotomy complete? Amer. J. Surg. 132:144, 1976.

Schmitz, E. J.: The Zollinger-Ellison syndrome. In Harkins, H. N., and Nyhus, L. M.: Surgery of the Stomach and Duodenum, 2nd ed. Boston, Little, Brown and Company, 1969.

Gastritis

Booher, R. J., and Grant, R. N.: Eosinophilic granuloma of the stomach and small intestine. Surgery 30:388, 1951.

Chazan, B. I., and Aichison, J. D.: Gastric tuberculosis. Brit. Med. J. 2:1288, 1960.

Cooley, R. N., and Childers, J. H.: Acquired syphilis of the stomach. Gastroenterology 39:201, 1960.

Gonzalez-Crussi, F., and Hackett, R. L.: Phlegmonous gastritis. Arch. Surg. 93:990, 1966.

Higgins, G. A., Lamm, E. R., and Yutzy, C. V.: Eosinophilic gastroenteritis. Arch. Surg. 92:476, 1966.

Marks, I. N., Banks, S., Werbeloff, L., Farman, J., and Louw, J. H.: The natural history of corrosive gastritis: Report of five cases. Amer. J. Dig. Dis. 8:509, 1963.

Sayer, R. B., Waddel, M. C., Sawyer, K. C., and Greer, J. C.: Emphysematous gastritis. Gastroenterology 53:452, 1967.

Thompson, C. R., Ashurst, P. M., and Butler, T. J.: Survey of haemorrhagic erosive gastritis. Brit. Med. J. 3:283, 1968.

Neoplasms of the Stomach

Beard, R. J., Gruebel Lee, E. C., Haysom, A. H., and Melcher, D. H.: Noncarcinomatous tumors of the stomach. Brit. J. Surg. 55:535, 1968.

Ellis, H. A., and Lannigan, R.: Primary lymphoid neoplasms of the stomach. Gut 4:145, 1963.

Naqvi, M. S., Burrows, L., and Kark, A. E.: Lymphoma of the gastrointestinal tract: Prognostic guides based on 162 cases. Ann. Surg. 170:221, 1969.

Pack, G. T.: Unusual tumors of the stomach. Ann. N.Y. Acad. Sci. 114:985, 1964.

ReMine, W. H.: Gastric sarcomas. Amer. J. Surg. 120:320, 1970.

Gastric Volvulus

Figiel, L. S., and Figiel, S. J.: Acute organo-axial gastric volvulus. Amer. J. Roent. 90:761, 1963.

Gosin, S., and Ballinger, W. F., II: Recurrent volvulus of the stomach. Amer. J. Surg. 109:642, 1965.

Small Intestine

General

Colcock, B. P., and Braasch, J. W.: Surgery of the Small Intestine in the Adult. Philadelphia, W. B. Saunders Company, 1968.

Storer, E. H.: Small intestine. In Schwartz, S. I., et al. (eds.): Principles of Surgery. New York, McGraw-Hill Book Company, 1969.

Tumors

Beck, A. R., and Jewett, T. C.: Surgical implications of the Peutz-Jeghers syndrome. Ann. Surg. 165:299, 1967.

Brooks, B. S., Waterhouse, J. A. H., and Powell, D. J.: Malignant lesions of the small intestine. Brit. J. Surg. 55:405, 1968.

Colcock, B. P., and Braasch, J. W.: Surgery of the Small Intestine in the Adult. Philadelphia, W. B. Saunders Company, 1968.

Dorman, J. E., Floyd, C. E., and Cohn, I., Jr.: Malignant neoplasms of the small bowel. Amer. J. Surg. 113:131, 1967.

Grahame-Smith, D. G.: Progress report: The carcinoid syndrome. Gut 11:189, 1970.

Halpern, M., Turner, A. F., and Citron, B. F.: Hereditary hemorrhagic telangiectasia. Radiology 90:1143, 1968.

Jeghers, H., McKusick, V. A., and Katz, K. H.: Generalized intestinal polyposis and melanin spots of the oral mucosa, lips, and digits. N. Engl. J. Med. 241:993, 1031, 1949.

Naqvi, M. S., Burrows, L., and Kark, A. E.: Lymphoma of the gastrointestinal tract: Prognostic guides based on 162 cases. Ann. Surg. 170:221, 1969.

Oates, J. A., and Butler, T. C.: Pharmacologic and endocrine aspects of carcinoid syndrome. Adv. Pharmacol. 5:109, 1967.

Ostermiller, W., Joergenson, E. J., and Weibel, L.: A clinical review of tumors of the small bowel. Amer. J. Surg. 111:403, 1966.

Wilson, H., Cheek, R. C., Sherman, R. T., and Storer, E. H.: Carcinoid tumors. Curr. Prob. Surg., Nov. 1970.

Regional Enteritis

Colcock, B. P.: Regional enteritis. Curr. Prob. Surg., June 1965.

Gitnick, G. L., Arthur, M., and Shibata, I.: Cultivation of viral agents from Crohn's disease. Lancet 2:215, 1976.

Law, D. H.: Regional enteritis. Gastroenterology 56:1086, 1969.

Lennard-Jones, J. E., and Morson, B. C.: Changing concepts in Crohn's disease. Disease-a-Month, August 1969.

Parent, K., and Mitchell, P.: Bacterial variants: Etiologic agents in Crohn's disease? Gastroenterology 71:365, 1976.

Tyer, F., Steiger, E., and Dudrick, S.: Adenocarcinoma of the small intestine and other malignant tumors complicating regional enteritis. Ann. Surg. 169:510, 1969.

Weedom, D., Shoite, R., Ilstrip, D., Huizenga, K., and Taylor, W.: Crohn's disease and cancer. N. Engl. J. Med. 289:1099, 1973.

Other Inflammatory Diseases

Abrams, J. S., and Holden, W. D.: Tuberculosis of the gastrointestinal tract. Arch. Surg. 89:282, 1964.

Bentley, G., and Webster, J. H. H.: Gastrointestinal tuberculosis: A 10 year review. Brit. J. Surg. 54:90, 1967.

Colcock, B. P., and Braasch, J. W.: Surgery of the Small Intestine in the Adult. Philadelphia, W. B. Saunders Company, 1968.

Huckstep, R. L.: Recent advances in the surgery of typhoid fever. Ann. Roy. Coll. Surg. Eng. 26:207, 1960.

Woodward, T. E., and Smadel, J. E.: Management of typhoid fever and its complications. Ann. Intern. Med. 60:144, 1964.

Other Diseases

DeCosse, J. J., Rhodes, R. S., Wentz, W. B., Reagan, J. W., Dworken, H. J., and Holden, W. D.: The natural history and management of radiation-induced injury of the gastrointestinal tract. Ann. Surg. 170:369, 1969.

Kushlan, S. D.: Pneumatosis cystoides intestinalis. J.A.M.A. 179:699, 1962.

Localio, S. A., and Stahl, W. M.: Diverticular disease of the alimentary tract. Part II: The esophagus, stomach, duodenum and small intestine. Curr. Prob. Surg., January 1968.

Mason, G. R., Guernsey, J. M., Hanks, G. E., and Nelson, T. S.: Surgical therapy for radiation enteritis. Oncology 22:241, 1968.

Mujahed, Z., and Evans, J. A.: Gas cysts of the intestine (pneumatosis intestinalis). Surg. Gynec. Obstet. 107:151, 1958.

Ileal Bypass for Hyperlipidemia

Buchwald, H., and Varco, R.: A bypass operation for obese hyperlipidemic patients. Surgery 70:62, 1971.

Griffen, W., Young, V., and Stevenson, C.: A prospective comparison of gastric and jejunoileal bypass procedures for morbid obesity. Ann. Surg., 186:500, 1977.

Payne, I. H., and DeWind, L.: Surgical treatment of obesity. Amer. J. Surg. 118:141, 1969.

Phillips, R.: Small intestinal bypass for the treatment of morbid obesity. Surg. Gynecol. Obstet. 145:455, 1978.

Scott, H. W.: Metabolic surgery for hyperlipidemia and atherosclerosis. Amer. J. Surg. 23:3, 1972.

Scott, H. W., Dean, R., Shull, H., and Gluck, F.: Results of jejunoileal bypass in two hundred patients with morbid obesity. Surg. Gynecol. Obstet. 145:661, 1977.

Strauss, R., and Wise, L.: Operative risks of obesity. Surg. Gynecol. Obstet. 146:286, 1978.

Large Intestine

General

Turell, R. (ed.): Diseases of the Colon and Anorectum. 2nd ed. Philadelphia, W.B. Saunders Company, 1969.

Ulcerative Colitis and Granulomatous Colitis

Barker, W. F.: Fulminant ulcerative colitis: Toxic megacolon, perforation, and hemorrhage. *In* Hardy, J. D. (ed.): Critical Surgical Illness. Philadelphia, W. B. Saunders Company, 1971.

Glotzer, D. J., Gardner, R. C., Goldman, H., Hinrichs, H. R., Rosen, H., and Zetzel, L.: Comparative features and course of ulcerative and granulomatous colitis. N. Engl. J. Med. 282:588, 1970.

Goligher, J.: The outcome of excisional operations for primary and recurrent Crohn's disease of the large intestine. Surg. Gynecol. Obstet. 148:1, 1979.

Judd, E. S.: Current surgical aspects of toxic megacolon. Surgery 65:401, 1969.

Morson, B. C., and Bussey, H. J. R.: Predisposing causes of intestinal cancer. Curr. Prob. Surg., February 1970.

Nugent, F. W.: Medical management of inflammatory disease of the colon. Surg. Clin. N. Amer. 51:807, 1971.

Nugent, F. W., Veidenheimer, M., Meissner, W., and Haggitt, R.: Prognosis after colonic resection for Crohn's disease of the colon. Gastroenterology 65:398, 1973.

Prohaska, J. V.: The inflammatory diseases of the large and small bowel. Curr. Prob. Surg., March 1969.

Steinberg, D., Allan, R. N., Brooke, B., Cooke, W. T., and Alexander-Williams, J.: Sequelae of colectomy and ileostomy: Comparison between Crohn's colitis and ulcerative colitis. Gastroenterology 68:33, 1978.

Thomford, N. R., Rybak, J. J., and Pace, W. G.: Toxic megacolon. Surg. Gynecol. Obstet. 128:21, 1969.

Turnbull, R. B., Schofield, P. F., and Hawk, W. A.: Nonspecific ulcerative colitis. Adv. Surg. 3:161, 1968.

Wright, R.: Progress in gastroenterology: Ulcerative colitis. Gastroenterology 58:875, 1970.

Zetzel, L.: Medical progress: Granulomatous (ileo) colitis. N. Engl. J. Med. 282:600, 1970.

Other Colitis

Abrams, J. S., and Holden, W. D.: Tuberculosis of the gastrointestinal tract. Arch. Surg. 89:282, 1964.

Bartlett, J., Onderdonk, A., and Cisners, R.: Clindamycin associated colitis in hamsters: Protection with vancomycin. Gastroenterology 73:772, 1977.

Bentley, G., and Webster, J. H. H.: Gastrointestinal tuberculosis: A 10 year review. Brit. J. Surg. 54:90, 1967.

Earlam, R. J.: Gastrointestinal aspects of Chagas' disease. Amer. J. Dig. Dis. 17:559, 1972.

Fagin, R. R., and Kirsner, J. B.: Ischemic diseases of the colon. Adv. Intern. Med. 17:343, 1971.

Gelfand, M. D., and Krone, D. L.: Non-staphylococcal pseudomembranous colitis. Amer. J. Dig. Dis. 14:278, 1969.

Hummel, R. P., Altemeier, W., and Hill, E. O.: Iatrogenic staphylococcal enterocolitis. Ann. Surg. 160:551, 1964.

Laranja, F. S., Dias, E., Nobrega, G., and Miranda, A.: Chagas' disease. A clinical, epidemiologic, and pathologic study. Circulation 14:1035, 1956.

Levine, B., Peskin, G., and Saik, R. P.: Drug induced colitis as a surgical disease. Arch. Surg. 111:987, 1976.

McMahon, J. E.: A study of some clinico-pathological manifestations in Schistosoma mansoni infections in Tanzania. Ann. Trop. Med. 61:302, 1967.

Rowland, A. K.: Progress report: Intestinal schistosomiasis. Gut 12:663, 1971.

Tedesco, R.: Antibiotic associated pseudomembranous colitis with negative proctosigmoidoscopy examination. Gastroenterology 77:295, 1979.

Williams, L. F., Jr., Bosniak, M. A., Wittenberg, J., Manuel, B., Grimes, E. T., and Byrne, J. J.: Ischemic colitis. Amer. J. Surg. 117:254, 1969.

Villous Adenoma and Gardner's Syndrome

Babior, B. M.: Villous adenoma of the colon. Study of a patient with severe fluid and electrolyte disturbances. Amer. J. Med. 41:615, 1966.

Morson, B. C., and Bussey, H. J. R.: Predisposing causes of intestinal cancer. Curr. Prob. Surg., February 1970.

Nicoloff, D. M., Ellis, C. M., and Humphrey, E. W.: Management of villous adenomas of the colon and rectum. Arch. Surg. 97:254, 1968.

Thomas, K. E., Watne, A. L., Johnson, J. G., Roth, E., and Zimmermann, B.: Natural history of Gardner's syndrome. Amer. J. Surg. 115:218, 1968.

Volvulus

Anderson, A., Bergdohl, L., and Van Der Linden, W.: Volvulus of the cecum. Ann. Surg. 181:876, 1975.

Arnold, G., and Nance, F.: Volvulus of the sigmoid colon. Ann. Surg. 177:527, 1973.

Shoospow, D., and Berardi, R.: Volvulus of the sigmoid colon. Dis. Col. Rect. 19:535, 1976.

Angiodysplasia

Boley, S., Sammartano, R., Brandt, L., and Sprayregen, S.: Vascular ectasias of the colon. Surg. Gynecol. Obstet. 149:353, 1979.

Talman, E., Dixon, D., and Gutierrez, F.: Role of arteriography in rectal hemorrhage due to arteriovenous malformation and diverticulosis. Ann. Surg. 190:203, 1979.

Pancreas

General

Anderson, M. C.: Review of pancreatic disease. Surgery 66:434, 1969.

Acute Pancreatitis

Gleidman, M. L., Bolooki, H., and Rosen, R. G.: Acute pancreatitis. Curr. Prob. Surg., August 1970.

Paloyan, E.: The forms of pancreatitis. Curr. Prob. Surg., June 1967.

Williams, R. D.: Acute necrotizing pancreatitis. In Hardy, J. D. (ed.): Critical Surgical Illness. Philadelphia, W. B. Saunders Company, 1971.

Chronic Pancreatitis

Child, C. G., III, Frey, C. F., and Fry, W. J.: A reappraisal of removal of ninety-five per cent of the distal portion of the pancreas. Surg. Gynecol. Obstet. 129:49, 1969.

Gillesby, W. J., and Puestow, C. B.: Pancreaticojejunostomy for chronic relapsing pancreatitis. An evaluation. Surgery 50:859, 1961.

Warren, K. W.: Surgical management of chronic relapsing pancreatitis. Amer. J. Surg. 117:24, 1969.

Pancreatic Cysts and Pseudocysts

Balfour, J. F.: Pancreatic pseudocysts: Complications and their relation to the timing of treatment. Surg. Clin. N. Amer. 50:395, 1970.

Becker, W. F., Pratt, H. S., and Ganji, H.: Pseudocysts of the pancreas. Surg. Gynecol. Obstet. 127:744, 1968.

Piper, C. E., ReMine, W. H., and Priestley, J. T.: Pancreatic cystadenomata. Report of 20 cases. J.A.M.A. 180:648, 1962.

Rosenberg, I. K., Kahn, J. A., and Walt, A. J.: Surgical experience with pancreatic pseudocysts. Amer. J. Surg. 117:11, 1969.

Cystic Fibrosis in Adults

Brusilow, S. W.: Cystic fibrosis in adults. Ann. Rev. Med. 21:99, 1970.

di Sant'Agnese, P. A., and Talamo, R. C.: Pathogenesis and physiopathology of cystic fibrosis of the pancreas. Fibrocystic disease of the pancreas (mucoviscidosis). N. Engl. J. Med. 277:1287, 1344, 1399, 1967.

Liver

General

Schwartz, S. I.: Surgical Diseases of the Liver. New York, McGraw-Hill Book Company, 1964.

Sherlock, S.: Diseases of the Liver and Biliary System. 4th ed. Oxford, Blackwell Scientific Publications, 1968.

Pyogenic Liver Abscess

Altemeier, W. A., Schowengerdt, C. G., and Whiteley, D. H.: Abscesses of the liver: Surgical considerations. Arch. Surg. 101:258, 1970.

Butler, T. J., and McCarthy, C. F.: Pyogenic liver abscess. Gut 10:389, 1969.

Gaisford, W. D., and Mark, J. B. D.: Surgical management of hepatic abscess. Amer. J. Surg. 118:317, 1969.

Amebic Abscesses

Abbruzzese, A. A.: Hepatic amebiasis. Amer. J. Gastroent. *54*:464, 1970.
Grigsby, W. P.: Surgical treatment of amebiasis. Surg. Gynecol. Obstet. *128*:609, 1969.

Echinococcosis

Hankins, J. R.: Management of complicated hepatic hydatid cysts. Ann. Surg. *158*:1020, 1963.
Katz, A. M., and Pan, C.: Echinococcus disease in the United States. Amer. J. Med. *25*:759, 1958.
Taiana, J. A.: Thoracic hydatid echinococcosis: Diagnosis and treatment. Dis. Chest *49*:8, 1966.

Primary Carcinoma and Major Hepatic Resection

Curutchet, H. P., Terzy, J. J., Kay, S., and Lawrence, W., Jr.: Primary liver cancer. Surgery *70*:467, 1971.
El-Domeiri, A. A., Huvos, A. G., Goldsmith, H. S., and Foote, F. W.: Primary malignant tumors of the liver. Cancer *27*:7, 1971.
Fortner, J. G., Beattie, E. J., Shiu, M. H., Howland, W. S., Watson, R. C., Gaston, J. P., and Benua, R. S.: Surgery in liver tumors. Curr. Prob. Surg., June 1972.
Stone, H. H., Long, W. D., Smith, R. B., and Haynes, C. D.: Physiologic considerations in major hepatic resections. Amer. J. Surg. *117*:78, 1969.

Congenital Hyperbilirubinemias

Arias, I. M.: Chronic familial nonhemolytic jaundice with conjugated bilirubin in the serum. Gastroenterology *43*:588, 1962.
Mandema, E., de Fraiture, W. H., Nieweg, H. O., and Arends, A.: Familial chronic idiopathic jaundice (Dubin-Sprinz disease) with a note on Bromsulphalein metabolism in this disease. Amer. J. Med. *28*:42, 1960.
Powell, L. W., Hemingway, E., Billing, B. H., and Sherlock, S.: Idiopathic unconjugated hyperbilirubinemia (Gilbert's syndrome). A study of 42 families. N. Engl. J. Med. *227*:1108, 1967.

Drugs and the Liver

Conney, A. H.: Drug metabolism and therapeutics. N. Engl. J. Med. *280*:653, 1969.
Schaffner, F., and Raisfeld, I. H.: Drugs and the liver: A review of metabolism and adverse reactions. Adv. Intern. Med. *15*:221, 1969.
Sherlock, S.: Drugs and the liver. Brit. Med. J. *1*:227, 1968.
Zimmerman, H. J.: The spectrum of hepatotoxicity. Perspect. Biol. Med. *12*:135, 1968.

Disorders of the Gallbladder and Extrahepatic Biliary System

Alonse-Lej, F., Rever, W. B., and Pessagno, D. J.: Congenital choledochal cyst, with a report of 2, and an analysis of 94 cases. Surg. Gynecol. Obstet. *108*:1, 1958.
Balmer, S. D., and Burson, L. C.: One-step repair for cholecystoduodenal fistula and gallstone ileus. Arch. Surg. *90*:313, 1965.

Charcot, J. M.: Lesons sur les maladies du foie de voires filiaires et de Reins. Paris, Faculté de Medecine de Paris, 1877.
Dow, R. W., and Lindenauer, S. M.: Acute obstructive suppurative cholangitis. Ann. Surg. *169*:272, 1969.
Saik, R. P., Greenburg, A. G., Farris, J., and Peskin, G. W.: Spectrum of cholangitis. Amer. J. Surg. *130*:143, 1975.
Saik, R. P., Greenburg, A. G., and Peskin, G. W.: Cholecystostomy hazard in acute cholangitis. J.A.M.A. *235*:2412, 1976.
Sakso, K., Seitzinger, G. L., and Garside, E.: Carcinoma of the extrahepatic bile duct: Review of the literature and report of 6 cases. Surgery *41*:416, 1957.
Terblanche, J., Saunders, S. J., and Louew, J. H.: Prolonged palliation in carcinoma of the main hepatic duct junction. Surgery *71*:728, 1972.
Thorbjarnarson, B.: Carcinoma of the bile ducts. Cancer *12*:708, 1959.
Warren, K., Athanassiades, S., and Monge, J.: Primary sclerosing cholangitis: A study of 42 cases. Amer. J. Surg. *111*:23, 1966.
Warshaw, A. L., and Bartlett, M. K.: Choice of operation for gallstone intestinal obstruction. Ann. Surg. *164*:1051, 1966.

Anesthetic Considerations

Ainslie, S. G., Eisele, J. H., and Corkill, G.: Fentanyl concentrations in brain and serum during respiratory acid-base changes in the dog. Anesthesiology *51*:293, 1979.
Barnett, W. O.: Experimental strangulated intestinal obstruction — a review. Gastroenterology *39*:34, 1960.
Beeson, P. B., and McDermott, W.: Textbook of Medicine. 13th ed. Philadelphia, W.B. Saunders Company, 1971, pp. 1618–1639.
Belinkoff, S., and Hall, O. W., Jr.: Anesthesia in intestinal obstruction. Anesth. Analg. *30*:96, 1951.
Berry, R. E. L.: Obstruction of the small and large intestine. Surg. Clin. N. Amer. *39*:1267, 1959.
Best, C. H., and Taylor, N. B.: The Physiologic Basis of Medical Practice. 7th ed. Baltimore, Williams and Wilkins Company, 1961, Chapter 50.
Biebuyck, J. F.: Effects of anaesthetic agents on metabolic pathways: Fuel utilisation and supply during anaesthesia. Brit. J. Anaesth. *45*:263, 1973.
Borison, H. L., and Wang, S. C.: Physiology and pharmacology of vomiting. Pharmacol. Rev. *5*:193, 1953.
Bruce, D. L.: Anesthetic implications of fasting. Anesth. Analg. *50*:612, 1971.
Brunner, E. A.: Normal nutrition in man: Anesthesiologic implications. Anesth. Analg. *50*:620, 1971.
Cahill, G. F., Jr.: Control of body fuel utilization during starvation. *In* Conference on Energy Metabolism and Body Fuel Utilization. Cambridge, Harvard University Press, 1966.
Cahill, G. F., Jr.: Starvation in man. N. Engl. J. Med. *282*:668, 1970.
Cohn, I., Jr., and Atik, M.: Strangulation obstruction — closed loop studies. Ann. Surg. *153*:94, 1961.
Davenport, H. W.: Physiology of the Digestive Tract. 2nd ed. Chicago, Year Book Medical Publishers, 1966.
Dodd, R. B.: Problems in anesthesia for intestinal obstruction. South. Med. J. *45*:805, 1952.
Dudrick, S. J., Wilmore, D. W., and Vars, H. M.: Long-

term total parenteral nutrition with growth in puppies and positive nitrogen balance in patients. Surg. Forum *18*:356, 1967.

Dundee, J. W.: Anesthesia for acute intestinal obstruction. Brit. J. Anaesth. *22*:131, 1950.

Fine, J.: The cause of death in acute intestinal obstruction. Anesth. Analg. *40*:150, 1961.

Fischer, J. E.: Total Parenteral Nutrition. Boston, Little, Brown and Company, 1976, pp. 3–55, 187–230, 305–336.

Goodman, L. S., and Gilman, A.: The Pharmacological Basis of Therapeutics. 4th ed., New York, Macmillan Company, 1970, pp. 169–645.

Guyton, A. C.: Textbook of Medical Physiology. 4th ed., Philadelphia, W. B. Saunders Company, 1971, pp. 780–782.

Hood, J. H.: Clinical considerations of intestinal gas. Ann. Surg. *163*:359, 1966.

McClelland, R. N., Shires, G. T., Baxter, C. R., Coln, G. D., and Carrico, J.: Balanced salt solutions in the treatment of hemorrhagic shock. J.A.M.A. *199*:166, 1967.

Merin, R. G., Samuelson, P. N., and Schalch, C. S.: Major inhalation anesthetics and carbohydrate metabolism. Anesth. Analg. *50*:625, 1971.

Millar, R. D., and Way, W. L.: Inhibition of succinylcholine-induced increased intragastric pressure by non-depolarizing muscle relaxants and lidocaine. *34*:185, 1971.

Moore, F. D.: Metabolic Care of the Surgical Patient. Philadelphia, W. B. Saunders Company, 1959, Chapters 24, 25, and 26.

Moore, F. D., and Brennan, M. F.: Intravenous feeding. N. Engl. J. Med. *287*:862, 1972.

Moore, F. D., and Shires, G. T.: Moderation. Ann. Surg. *166*:300, 1967.

Neill, L. W., Shires, T., and Jenkins, M. T.: Problems caused by intestinal obstruction. *In* Greene, M. (ed.): Anesthesia for Emergency Surgery. Philadelphia, F. A. Davis Company, 1963, Chapter 7.

Randall, H. T.: Fluid and electrolyte therapy in surgery. *In* Schwartz, S. I., et al. (eds.): Principles of Surgery. New York, McGraw-Hill Book Company, 1969, pp. 46–83.

Ruggera, G., and Taylor, G.: Pulmonary aspiration in anesthesia. West. J. Med. *125*:411, 1976.

Saidman, L. J.: Uptake, distribution and elimination of barbiturates. *In* Eger, E. I. (ed.): Anesthetic Uptake and Action. Baltimore, Williams & Wilkins Co., 1974, pp. 264–284.

Schwartz, S. I., and Storer, E. H.: Manifestations of gastrointestinal disease. *In* Schwartz, S. I., et al. (eds.): Principles of Surgery. New York, McGraw-Hill Book Company, 1969, pp. 830–867.

Sellick, B. A.: Cricoid pressure to control regurgitation of stomach contents during induction of anaesthesia. Lancet 2:404, 1961.

Sheldon, G.: Hyperalimentation: Its rationale and effect on anesthetic management. *In* 1979 Annual Refresher Course Lectures. American Society of Anaesthesiologists, 1979, Lecture 120.

Sheldon, G. F., Plzak, L. F., Jr., Watkins, G. M., et al.: Inorganic phosphate and the oxyhemoglobin dissociation curve. Surg. Forum *22*:81, 1971.

Shields, R.: The absorption and secretion of fluid and electrolytes by the obstructed bowel. Brit. J. Surg. *52*:774, 1965.

Shires, G. T.: What's new in surgery, shock and metabolism. Surg. Gynecol. Obstet. *124*:284, 1967.

Shires, G. T., Coln, D., Carrico, J., and Lightfoot, S.: Fluid therapy in hemorrhagic shock. Arch. Surg. *88*:688, 1964.

Shires, T., and Adwan, K. O.: A review of the advances in management of mechanical obstruction of the small intestine. Amer. Surg. *24*:431, 1958.

Shires, T., Williams, J., and Brown, F.: Acute change in extracellular fluids associated with major surgical procedures. Ann. Surg. *154*:803, 1961.

Stoelting, R. K.: Responses to atropine, glycopyrrolate, and Riopan of gastric fluid pH and volume in adult patients. Anesthesiology *48*:367, 1978.

Stoelting, R. K.: Gastric fluid pH in patients receiving cimetidine. Anesth. Analg. *57*:675, 1978.

Wilmore, D. W., Moylan, J. A., Helmkamp, G. M., and Pruitt, B. A: Clinical evaluation of 10% intravenous fat emulsion for parenteral nutrition in thermally injured patients. Ann. Surg. *178*:503, 1973.

Winning, T. J., Brock-Utne, J. G., and Downing, J. W.: Nausea and vomiting after anesthesia and minor surgery. Anesth. Analg. *56*:674, 1977.

Specific Disorders

Bolooki, H., and Gliedman, M. L.: Peritoneal dialysis in treatment of acute pancreatitis. Surgery *64*:466, 1968.

Brown, B. R.: Anesthetic hepatic toxicity: A scientific problem? *In* 1979 Annual Refresher Course Lectures. American Society of Anesthesiologists, 1979. Lecture 106.

Chalmers, T. C.: Pathogenesis and treatment of hepatic failure. N. Engl. J. Med. *263*:23, 77, 1960.

Chalmers, T. C., Eckhardt, R. D., Reynolds, W. E., Cigarroa, J. G., Jr., Deane, N., Reifenstein, R. W., Smith, C. W., and Davidson, C. S.: The treatment of acute infectious hepatitis. Controlled studies of the effect of diet, rest, and physical reconditioning on the acute course of the disease and of the incidence of relapses and residual abnormalities. J. Clin. Invest. *34*:1136, 1955.

Churchill-Davidson, H. C. (ed.): A Practice of Anaesthesia. 4th ed., Philadelphia, W. B. Saunders Company, 1978, pp. 1193–1228.

Conrad, M. E., Schwartz, F. D., and Young, A. A.: Infectious hepatitis — a generalized disease. A study of renal gastrointestinal and hematologic abnormalities. Amer. J. Med. *37*:789, 1964.

Cooperman, L. H.: Effects of anaesthetics on the splanchnic circulation. Brit. J. Anaesth. *44*:976, 1972.

Di Sant'Agnese, T. A., and Talamo, R. C.: Medical progress. Pathogenesis and physiopathology of cystic fibrosis of the pancreas. N. Engl. J. Med. *277*:1287, 1344, 1399, 1967.

Dormandy, T. L.: Gastrointestinal polyposis with mucocutaneous pigmentation (Peutz-Jeghers syndrome). N. Engl. J. Med. *256*:1093, 1141, 1186, 1957.

Dreiling, D. A., Janowitz, H. D., and Perrier, C. Z.: Pancreatic Inflammatory Disease: A Physiologic Approach. New York, Harper and Row, 1964.

Dykes, M. H. M.: Anesthesia and the Liver. Boston, Little, Brown and Company, 1970.

Eger, E. I., II, and Saidman, L. J.: Hazard of nitrous oxide anesthesia in bowel obstruction and pneumothorax. Anesthesiology *26*:61, 1965.

Engel, G. L.: Biologic and physiologic features of ulcerative colitis. Gastroenterology *40*:313, 1961.

Garceau, A. J., Chalmers, T. C., and the Boston Inter-Hospital Liver Group: The natural history of cirrhosis. N. Engl. J. Med. 267:469, 1963; 271:1173, 1964.

Grace, N. D., Muench, H., and Chalmers, T. C.: Present status of shunts for portal hypertension in cirrhosis. Gastroenterology 50:684, 1966.

Gross, J. B., and Comfort, M. W.: Chronic pancreatitis. Amer. J. Med. 21:596, 1956.

Ham, J.: Factors affecting administration of neuromuscular blocking agents. In 1979 Annual Refresher Course Lectures. American Society of Anesthesiologists, 1979. Lecture 121.

Handbook of Physiology, Section 6: Alimentary Canal. Vol. II: Absorption. American Physiological Society, 1967.

Howat, D. D. C.: Anaesthesia for biliary and pancreatic surgery. Proc. Roy. Soc. Med. 70:152, 1977.

Jeffries, G. H., Weser, E., and Sleisenger, M. H.: Malabsorption. Gastroenterology 56:777, 1969.

Kleine, J. W., Khouw, Y. H., and Heeres, M.: Management of anesthesia during surgery for patients with carcinoid syndrome. Acta Anaesth. Belg. 28:165, 1977.

Lamont, A. S. M., and Jones, D.: Anaesthetic management of insulinoma. Anaesth. Intens. Care 6:261, 1978.

Law, D. H.: Regional enteritis. Gastroenterology 56:1086, 1969.

Lennard-Jones, J. E., Lockhardt-Mummery, H. E., and Morson, B. C.: Clinical and pathological differentiation of Crohn's disease and proctocolitis. Gastroenterology 54:1162, 1968.

Lieber, C. S.: Metabolic derangement induced by alcohol. Ann. Rev. Med. 18:35, 1967.

Lieber, C. S., Jones, D. P., and Decarli, L. N.: Effects of prolonged ethanol intake: Production of fatty liver despite adequate diets. J. Clin. Invest. 44:1009, 1965.

Littman, A., and Hanscom, C. H.: Current concepts: Pancreatic extracts. N. Engl. J. Med. 281:201, 1969.

Marston, A.: Mesenteric arterial disease. The present position. Gut 8:203, 1967.

Mason, R. A., and Steane, P. A.: Carcinoid syndrome: Its relevance to the anesthetist. Anesthesia 31:228, 1976.

Miller, R., Patel, A. U., Warner, R. R. P., and Parnes, J. H.: Anaesthesia for the carcinoid syndrome: A report of nine cases. Canad. Anesth. Soc. J. 25:240, 1978.

Mixter, C. G., Jr., Keynes, W. M., and Cope, O.: Further experience with pancreatitis as a diagnostic clue to hyperparathyroidism. N. Engl. J. Med. 266:265, 1962.

National Halothane Study: Report of the National Institutes of Health. Bethesda, Md., 1969.

Prince, A. M., Hargrove, R. L., Szmuness, W., Cherubin, C. E., Fontana, B. J., and Jeffries, G. H.: Immunologic distinction between serum and infectious hepatitis. N. Engl. J. Med. 282:987, 1970.

Sawyer, C. C., Eger, E. I., Fink, B. R. (eds.): Bahlman, S. H., et al.: Metabolism of inhalation anesthetics. In Cellular Biology and Toxicity of Anesthetics. Baltimore, Williams and Wilkins Company, 1972, pp. 238–244.

Schenker, S., McCandless, C. W., Brophy, E., and Lewis, M. S.: Studies on the intracerebral toxicity of ammonia. J. Clin. Invest. 46:838, 1967.

Schiff, L.: Disease of the Liver. 3rd ed. Philadelphia, J.B. Lippincott Company, 1969.

Schwachman, H., Kulczycki, L. L., and Khaw, K. T.: Studies in cystic fibrosis: A report on sixty-five patients over 17 years of age. Pediatrics 36:689, 1965.

Schwartz, S. I.: Principles of Surgery. New York, McGraw-Hill Book Company, 1969, pp. 536–539, 887–891.

Senior, J. R.: Post-transfusion hepatitis. Gastroenterology 49:315, 1965.

Sherlock, S.: Diseases of the Liver. 4th ed. Oxford, Blackwell Scientific Publications, 1968.

Sherlock, S.: Hepatic coma. Gastroenterology 41:1, 1961.

Sleisenger, M. H.: Malabsorption syndrome. N. Engl. J. Med. 281:111, 1969.

Spock, A., Heick, H. M. C., Criss, H., and Logan, W. S.: Abnormal serum factor in patients with cystic fibrosis of the pancreas. Pediat. Res. J. 1:173, 1967

Stone, H. H., and Donnelly, C. C.: The anesthetic significance of serotonin secreting carcinoid tumors. Anesthesiology 21:203, 1960.

Tammisto, T., and Takki, S.: Nitrous oxide–oxygen–relaxant anaesthesia in alcoholics: A retrospective study. Acta Anaesth. Scand. (Suppl.) 53:68, 1973.

Trey, C., Lipworth, L., Chalmers, T. C., Davidson, C. S., Gottlieb, L. S., Popper, H., and Saunders, S. J.: Fulminant hepatic failure. Presumable contribution of halothane. N. Engl. J. Med. 279:798, 1968.

Truelove, C. S., and Edwards, F. C.: The course and prognosis in ulcerative colitis. Gut 4:229, 1963.

Wilcox, R. G., and Isselbacher, K. J.: Chronic liver disease in young people. Amer. J. Med. 30:185, 1961.

Zetzel, L.: Granulomatous ileocolitis. N. Engl. J. Med. 282:600, 1970.

10

Morbid Obesity and Other Nutritional Disorders

By NORMAN H. BLASS, M.D.

Morbid Obesity
Protein-Calorie Malnutrition States
  Thermal Injury
  Anorexia Nervosa

Cachexia of Malignancy
Kwashiorkor and Marasmus
Parenteral Hyperalimentation
Vitamin Deficiency States

Although nutrition has been a recognized science for many years, it was not until the recent advent of surgery for the treatment of morbid obesity that it engendered widespread interest. It was in the process of attempting drastic weight reduction by surgical means that the critical role played by nutrition was properly assessed. From there, it was a logical step to extend the knowledge gained in such procedures to all surgery performed on patients who suffer from diseases or conditions marked by improper nutrition.

Improper nutrition can be manifested by dietary deficiencies or excesses, depending usually upon the economic status of the country in which the individual lives. Economically advanced nations face the ever present problem of obesity, whereas the underprivileged areas have their share of hunger and starvation.

MORBID OBESITY

Despite widespread publicity concerning its various adverse affects on health, obesity still remains the most common nutritional disorder in the United States. Studies suggest that a weight of 20 per cent over the ideal is associated with a mortality that is increased as high as 50 per cent above the norm.

Although we lack a precise and accurate definition of obesity, the term "morbid obesity" may be used to describe anyone weighing twice the predicted weight for age, sex, body build, and height according to the Metropolitan Life Insurance Company tables.

The most important physiologic disorders associated with obesity are of the cardiovascular and pulmonary systems.

Many early investigators reported patients whose symptoms were characterized by obesity, hypoxemia, and alveolar hypoventilation, the so-called "pickwickian syndrome." However, the pickwickian syndrome is seen in only 8 per cent of morbidly obese people. The majority of this class of patients have hypoxemia without hypercarbia.

Obese patients may have alterations in respiratory muscle function, chest wall compliance, and intra-abdominal and intrathoracic pressures. According to Tucker and

Sieker (1960), postural changes particularly alter lung function in obese persons. Functional residual capacity becomes progressively smaller as the subject changes from the erect to the seated and finally to the Trendelenburg position. This effect is secondary to the progressive elevation of the diaphragm by the abdominal viscera. The characteristic changes found in pulmonary function tests are hypoxemia, marked reduction in expiratory reserve volume, maximum volume ventilation, and functional residual capacity, but only a slight reduction in vital capacity. Chest compliance is definitely reduced, but unless an additional burden is placed upon the pulmonary system, lung compliance is only minimally reduced.

These deleterious functional alterations are associated with a constant increase in the work of breathing. To counteract this phenomenon, the obese person regulates his or her breathing by decreasing tidal volume and increasing respiratory rate. This worsens ventilation to the already poorly ventilated dependent portions of the lung, which become more atelectatic, thus increasing shunting. There is a lowering of the Pa_{O_2} without evidence of diffusion defect; but an increased alveolar-arterial oxygen tension difference occurs. It has also been emphasized that airway closure within tidal volume ranges may contribute to regional hypoventilation and to hypoxemia. There may be regional differences in lung compliance and gas mixing, producing uneven gas distribution. This is made worse by the early airway closure.

There is a curvilinear relationship between pulmonary function tests and degree of obesity. This apparently confirms the fact that as weight increases, there is a progressive reduction in certain lung functions. However, the Pa_{O_2}, while lower than for normal subjects, does not correlate with the degree of obesity.

Insofar as circulatory function is concerned, massive obesity imposes an additional work load on the heart, concomitant with an increased basal metabolism and exercise intolerance. The demands of the excess body tissue mass lead to an increase in cardiac output. Studies have shown that there can be a doubling of the cardiac output when there is an excess of 100 kg in weight. Since heart rate remains essentially unchanged, this increase in cardiac output must be produced by an increase in the stroke volume.

While there is no precise correlation between excess weight and systemic hypertension, there is a significant incidence of both pulmonary and peripheral arterial hypertension. This hypertension, plus the increase in stroke volume, leads to an increase in the work of the heart, mainly left ventricular work. The ECG frequently reveals left axis deviation and left ventricular hypertrophy. Heart weight increase and heart diameter enlargement occur frequently in obese patients, and this is in proportion to the excess poundage. This increase is due to the hypertrophy of the ventricles, particularly the left ventricle.

There is an increase in blood and plasma volume, but the predicted volume and flow per unit weight of body mass is less than in normal-sized subjects. Studies have shown that there is no significant change in organ blood flow. The cerebral and renal blood flows are essentially unchanged. Splanchnic blood flow is increased. (Apparently the fat tissue depots are the major recipients of this increase in cardiac output.)

Heart failure is much more common in the morbidly obese person, as is pulmonary hypertension. There is an increase in pulmonary capillary wedge pressure during exercise, and hypoxia is not uncommon.

Diabetes mellitus and generalized arteriosclerosis occur more commonly in the markedly obese patient than in the normal population but there is no linear relationship to the degree of obesity.

Bedell (1958) differentiated between simple obesity and the pickwickian syndrome by classifying obese patients into three groups according to pulmonary function. In the first group, he placed those who had normal arterial oxygen saturation with reduced expiratory volume, reduced breathing capacities, and reduced maximal flow rate. In the second group, he placed those who did not have lung disease but did have arterial hypoxemia without hypercapnia. The third group included those who had alveolar hypoventilation, intrinsic lung disease, or central nervous system lesions. According to Bedell, obese people with normal lungs and a normal respiratory center do not exhibit alveolar hypoventilation.

It is pertinent to note that because of the

sheer size of these patients, they have been neglected as a group in regard to their special needs and problems. To delineate conditions peculiar to the morbidly obese, it is helpful to divide their problems into three categories: mechanical, psychological, and physiological.

Mechanical. The following types of problems are common. Hospital gurneys available for transporting patients may be of insufficient width and sturdiness for some of these grossly overweight individuals. Furthermore, nurses and orderlies assigned to these patients may be loath to lift them in order to avoid any potential injury to themselves.

The possible inadequacy of the operating table must also be recognized. The standard operating table is approximately 20 inches (50 cm) wide, and it is not unknown for these extremely large patients to require two standard tables in order to be maintained in a successful surgical position.

Another problem occurs when attempting to obtain an accurate blood pressure reading. Even when using a large cuff (such as that used on the thigh), it has been shown that there can be as much as a 20 torr error on the elevated side when using a cuff, compared with direct arterial measurement.

Starting an intravenous line can also impose difficulties, owing to excess adipose tissue preventing the palpation of a suitable vein. Furthermore, it is not unknown for an artery to be entered mistakenly. It is frequently less hazardous to do a cut-down in order to start a satisfactory intravenous line, and one often finds it expeditious to percutaneously approach the external or internal jugular vein in order to obtain a secure, intravenous route.

Positioning the patient provides an additional challenge. It may be difficult to identify the usual anatomic landmarks if one plans to use regional anesthesia. Furthermore, when the patient lies supine, the diaphragm cannot move freely against the weight of the abdominal wall and its contents, and there is increased effort in breathing. The lithotomy and Trendelenburg positions further contribute to this increased effort. The supine position can lead to obstruction of the circulation because of aortocaval compression, produced by the sheer mass of the abdomen. If the patient is placed in the prone position, ventilation

becomes extremely difficult. It is recommended that when an extremely obese patient must assume the prone position, techniques using endotracheal anesthesia with controlled ventilation should be utilized.

The size of the needles chosen to perform regional block can constitute yet another area in which the anesthetist must be alert to the special needs of this class of patient. The needles must be selected carefully as to length, and it is probably wise to choose a needle with a larger diameter and therefore less flexibility than usual.

Psychological. Within the psychological realm, obese patients tend to be misunderstood, resulting in a situation wherein their very cooperation may be lost. Contrary to popular opinion, most obese individuals are depressed, guilty about their eating habits, and upset about their physical condition. Moreover, they have a distorted body image. It is imperative that while the patient is awake, all personnel, including nurses, orderlies, surgeons, and anesthetists be extremely careful not to make disparaging remarks about the patient's size, body configuration, or general appearance. Furthermore, it has been shown that some patients, even under general anesthesia have recall of what is said in the operating room. Therefore, it is important to make no untoward remarks about the patient's body build while he or she is apparently asleep. The individual may smile and laugh with you, but inwardly, he or she may become depressed, leading to a defensive state that may preclude satisfactory cooperation during perioperative care.

Thus, psychological preparation of the patient is probably one of the most important parts of the preoperative visit, since a cooperative patient is an essential element for successful recovery. To achieve this cooperation, it is necessary for the anesthesiologist to explain the preparation involved prior to surgery, the procedure that will occur in the surgical suite, and the possible events in the recovery room. It will be necessary to describe the planned procedure, to discuss the possibility of an awake nasal or oral intubation, and to explain that a ventilator may be used postoperatively.

As an aid to psychological preparation, one must be careful in utilizing such drugs as diazepam or barbiturates, since they can produce respiratory depression as well as the benefit of their calming effect. It cannot be overemphasized that while these patients may appear clinically stable, they may very well be on the brink of respiratory disaster.

Obese people, like infants, tend to utilize food as a means to relieve apprehension, which is a prominent feature of their psychological makeup. When we bring these patients to surgery, we prevent oral intake, thus removing one of their psychological crutches.

To summarize, it is important to understand that patients who are markedly obese manifest low self-esteem and exhibit passive aggressiveness along with vulnerability to depression, which may be hidden by an outward show of joviality. They also have a distortion of body image, are self-conscious, and have a veritable sense of helplessness and ineffectiveness.

Physiological. A tendency toward thoracolumbar lordosis and thoracic curvature is produced by the large and protruding abdomen. There is limitation of rib movement and of the ability to raise the lower portion of the sternum. The excess layers of fat on the chest wall and abdomen splint both the chest wall and the diaphragm, limiting excursion. This leads to increased effort in breathing, and ventilation deteriorates with certain changes in position. Interestingly, there is no direct linear relationship between the effort required in breathing and the degree of obesity. Although hypoxemia is relatively frequent, hypoventilation characterized by a rise in Pco_2 is of low incidence because those portions of the lung that remain perfused and ventilated can clear increased amounts of CO_2, as a result of the CO_2 diffusion capacity and the characteristics of its dissociation curve. However, this is in delicate balance and can be disturbed with such maneuvers as the Trendelenburg position or the use of a general anesthetic.

As a baseline preoperative measurement of the patient's status, a detailed history (particularly with reference to exercise capabilities), an electrocardiogram, arterial blood gas, pulmonary function tests, and a chest x-ray are appropriate parameters to assess prior to subjecting the patient to anesthesia and the stress of surgery. If the patient is to undergo abdominal surgery directed at reducing his or her obesity, or

has had intestinal bypass surgery in the past, it would be advisable to evaluate the status of the liver.

During examination of the patient preoperatively, the mobility of the patient's neck, its range and motion, and the amount of adipose tissue should be carefully noted and any potential difficulty in intubation anticipated. One should never compromise the patient's ability to maintain his or her own airway until assured that ventilation can be satisfactorily maintained. If one anticipates a problem, an awake nasal or oral intubation under topical anesthesia should be considered. The use of the fiberoptic laryngoscope or bronchoscope sometimes avoids a problem situation.

As to the surgical procedure itself, Vaughn and others have demonstrated that during intra-abdominal surgery, an FI_{O_2} greater than 0.4 is frequently necessary in order to produce satisfactory oxygen tension in an otherwise normal but morbidly obese patient. In other words, during abdominal procedures, one can anticipate that pulmonary gas exchange already compromised will further deteriorate. It has been shown that the placement of packing beneath the diaphragm may result in a fall of the Pa_{O_2} to as low as 65 torr even with an FI_{O_2} of 0.4. The Trendelenburg position also may cause a decrease in the oxygen tension of the blood. Salem et al. (1978) have shown that PEEP, when used in the morbidly obese patient, can produce a significant decrease in the oxygen tension and that PEEP and CPAP should probably be avoided in such cases.

One particular group of patients deserves special mention. These are individuals who have been morbidly obese and have already undergone some type of intestinal short-circuiting surgery for the treatment of their obesity. They manifest certain metabolic and physical changes that will influence the anesthesiologist and affect the choice of anesthetic technique.

All patients who have had an ileojejunostomy for obesity have diarrhea, and any electrolyte imbalance resulting from this can significantly alter the patient's cardiac and anesthetic status.

Since the original surgery was designed to prevent absorption of various nutrients, malnutrition may be one price exacted for the weight loss. As caloric intake together with weight is reduced, proteins are used as an energy source. It is not surprising therefore, that hypoproteinemia can occur which is further worsened because absorption of amino acids from the intestinal tract is impaired. In fact, the pattern observed in the early postoperative period is similar to that seen in malnourished children with kwashiorkor.

Protein deficiency that occurs during pregnancy may have some deleterious effects on the fetus. Intrauterine growth retardation as a result of the mother's low protein levels is not unusual.

Other manifestations of malnutrition are produced by inadequate absorption of fecal fat and the reduced absorption of fat soluble vitamins. This leads to reduced intestinal absorption of fatty acids and an increased production of bile salts from cholesterol, with a consequent drop in plasma cholesterol. (This may be considered a beneficial result for the patient.) There is vitamin deficiency, with the absorption of vitamin B_{12} being uniformly impaired. This is accompanied by a loss of electrolytes in the stools, and the serum potassium is frequently reduced, necessitating potassium supplementation for most patients. There have been reports of low magnesium and low calcium, and the occurrence of hypocalcemic tetany in some cases.

An interesting phenomenon that occurs in a number of patients is a polyarthritis with migratory arthralgia that can involve all joints. Some of these patients may have to be placed on corticosteroids and may be taking this medication when seen by the anesthesiologist.

Liver disease is one of the more common and perplexing problems facing both surgeon and anesthesiologist planning surgery upon a patient who has had previous intestinal bypass surgery. Liver biopsy often reveals fatty infiltration, and liver function tests may show a wide range of abnormal results. There are several theories as to the causation of the liver disease. These include protein deficiency, deficiency of vitamins and bile acids, and absorption of toxic products. The latter may arise within the bypassed small bowel segment and is probably due to bacterial infestation of the excluded segment.

Other types of surgery to correct morbid obesity are the gastric stapling and gastric bypass operations. When gastric bypass is performed, 90 per cent of the stomach is left in continuity with the duodenum. The remaining 10 per cent is anastomosed to the jejunum. The most encouraging aspect of either the bypass or the stapling procedure is that the numerous metabolic problems that have been so troublesome for patients who have had an ileojejunal bypass are usually not observed. The severe electrolyte disturbances and hepatic failure common to the former type of procedure have not generally been seen. However, nausea and vomiting when the patient overeats are not unusual and must be recognized as potential problems in fluid and electrolyte management.

PROTEIN-CALORIE MALNUTRITION STATES

Nutritional deficiency is an important major health problem in underdeveloped nations of the world and is not unknown in the more economically fortunate countries. While conditions of malnutrition in the poorer nations are usually manifested as kwashiorkor and marasmus, the more developed countries see their share of the protein-calorie deficiency syndromes in patients who suffer from major thermal injury, anorexia nervosa, the cachexia of malignancy, or other chronic, debilitating diseases.

THERMAL INJURY

Burns encompassing large areas of the body produce a hypercatabolic state; the patient's resting metabolic needs may double the normal requirements. It is also not unusual for as much as 30 grams of nitrogen per 24 hours to be excreted via the urine, and this, of course, places extremely heavy demands on lean body mass. Body energy stores and muscle protein are used preferentially. Loss will occur despite continual parenteral and enteral administration. The major problems in extensively burned patients are increased nutritional requirements, impaired intake, loss of the skin barrier to heat, and water loss. There is a combination of increased evaporative loss, radiation heat loss, and increased metabolic rate, making daily fluid requirements frequently three to five times greater than normal. There are also internal derangement of cellular metabolism and alterations in intracellular electrolytes.

This catabolic state also leads to impaired wound healing, altered immune response, with greatly increased risks of sepsis, and increased respiratory work. The hypermetabolic response is not related to caloric expenditure but is secondary to obligatory evaporative water loss from the burn area and an increased catecholamine release following hypothalamic stimulation. It is suspected that the effect of prostaglandins on the neurohypophyseal arch is the etiology for the excess catecholamine release.

In patients with major burns, the pharmacokinetics of drugs with predominantly urinary excretion pathways, such as aminoglycosides, may be altered by changes in renal function. In some cases, the glomerular filtration rate may decrease, particularly in the early period after the burn or in the following weeks when sepsis becomes a major problem. At other times, it may increase greatly over normal values. These changes can be assessed by creatinine clearance, which should be monitored routinely, especially in younger burn patients. When creatinine clearance is increased, the excretion of drugs may be more rapid and their plasma half-life decreased. Plasma levels should then be checked and the dosage modified as indicated. Since peak levels of a given dose to a patient remain unchanged, a decreased interval between doses would be preferred to an increase in the size of the dose. Drugs used in anesthesia that rely mainly or entirely on urinary excretion for cessation of action, such as gallamine, should have their dosage adjusted accordingly.

ANOREXIA NERVOSA

Anorexia nervosa involves a myriad of physical, emotional, and behavioral changes occurring in people who starve themselves because of an aversion to food or fear of weight gain. There is a dearth of research into this disease process. The sine qua non symptom for the diagnosis of the disease is substantial loss of body weight due to intensive caloric restriction. However, it is pertinent to know that the syndrome frequently may be associated with uncontrolled and excessive eating without satiation or awareness of hunger. Whatever the psychologic makeup of the patient, the symptoms of the disease entity are identical with those of externally produced starvation. The disease is accompanied, however, by so serious a psychologic and metabolic derangement that one third of these unfortunate people remain chronically ill or succumb to the disorder. Although there are frequent endocrinologic abnormalities, the disease entity is primarily a disturbance of the psyche. Anorexia nervosa is not that unusual a condition. Crisp (1974) found an incidence of 1 per 200 among young females.

While apparently obesity and anorexia nervosa are at opposite ends of the nutritional scale, they may well be external manifestations of the same emotional problem. Both involve disturbances in body image, perception of effective and visceral sensations, and an overall sense of ineffectiveness.

The anorectic, however, may manifest only selective alimentary inhibition. Protein deficiency may or may not be significant. Nevertheless, the patient usually manifests hypotension, bradycardia, hypothermia, and diminished endocrine function suggestive of a functional anterior hypothalamic deficiency. The patient also manifests dehydration, hypokalemia and leukopenia. The neutropenia, when severe, may predispose to infection. Anemia and loss of cell mass are usually found, and the ECG may reveal cardiomyopathy.

CACHEXIA OF MALIGNANCY

Cachexia of malignancy should be defined to include anorectic effects as well as other metabolic changes produced in the tumor-bearing host. Decreased food intake or absorption leads to cachexia. The spectrum of cachexia ranges from the patient with mild weight loss and no apparent symptoms referable to a malignant process to a patient with severe wasting disease, marked weakness, and grossly evident metastatic malignancy. Anorexia, a frequent problem in cancer patients, is a major cause of the cachexia; decreased absorption also contributes. However, the pathophysiology of the anorexia is not well understood, and probably many factors are involved. There are variables pertaining to the tumor, its size, the presence or absence of metastases, and the host variables, such as the presickness nutritional status of the patient and the patient's emotional response to the illness itself.

Cachexia manifests itself by weakness, pale, taut skin, edema, and ulcerations. There is no simple correlation between the type of tumor, the anatomic site of involvement, the caloric intake, and the degree of cachexia. (A patient might have widespread metastases and little or no evidence of cachexia.)

Chemical mediators produced by the tumor may lead to the cachectic syndrome. Anemia may occur in cancer patients without hemolysis or bleeding. There are also profound alterations of host lipid metabolism and protein depletion with hypoalbuminemia.

KWASHIORKOR

Kwashiorkor is a life-threatening disease characterized by a severe form of malnutrition that usually occurs in children in underdeveloped nations. Characteristically, the disease surfaces when infants are weaned after a long period of breast feeding and placed on a diet relatively high in carbohydrates but extremely low in protein.

The children are found to be small in stature with a failure to grow in a manner commensurate with their age. There is peripheral edema dependent upon the degree of protein deficiency. Protein synthesis is impaired. A deficiency in lipoproteins, which prevents free fatty acids from being metabolized properly and results in their accumulation, leads in turn to a fatty liver. The excess carbohydrate produces a secondary hyperinsulinism that further inhibits gluconeogenesis, particularly in the liver, and, more important, contributes to a hypoglycemic state, especially during stressful periods. There is a diminution in total body stores of potassium, calcium, and magnesium. A gross electrolyte disturbance is common to all organ systems. Electrocardiographic abnormalities, such as reduced voltage and S-T segment changes, are frequent

and may persist in spite of what appears to be adequate treatment, attesting to the severe damage to the myocardium itself. There is an inability of the body to maintain temperature along with a tendency toward anemia with iron deficiency, normocytic or macrocytic anemia being frequently seen. Death is usually due to infection, abnormalities of electrolytes, or liver failure.

MARASMUS

Marasmus is a protein-calorie abnormality of young children. It is manifested by a severe diminution of the intake of calories, but the protein-calorie balance apparently is reasonably well maintained. As in kwashiorkor, there is an associated loss of potassium, the major biochemical deficit. Furthermore, the administering of carbohydrates may shift the available potassium back into the cell, causing a further diminution of the serum potassium level.

Anesthetic Management in Protein-Calorie Deficiencies. It would obviously be advantageous to have the patient brought to a state of near normal nutrition prior to surgery. Before the advent of parenteral hyperalimentation this was frequently impossible. While there are no available statistics as to intraoperative mortality from anesthesia and surgery in patients who are starved, the intraoperative risk is probably increased.

The hyperkeratosis, dermatosis, and ulcerations that occur in the skin of patients with malnutrition warrants careful placement of the patient on the operating table and protection of these areas, as well as the eyes.

Dehydration is a common symptom, but one must be careful that the rapid administration of blood, fluid, or albumin does not precipitate pulmonary edema. Hypothermia is frequently observed. The temperature drop may be so severe that the anesthetics administered, such as halothane and ethrane, may have their biodegradation and excretion mechanisms altered. Overdosage may occur because of reduced need.

The lowered body temperature affects the neuromuscular junction and the acetylcholine released, with prolongation of neuromuscular blockade. Apparently moderate hypothermia antagonizes the nondepolarizing muscle relaxant and potentiates the depolarizing agents. At very low temperatures, the production of acetylcholine is reduced and the nondepolarizing agents are markedly potentiated. It is entirely possible that it may be unnecessary to use muscle relaxants in a severely debilitated individual.

Regional anesthesia, such as field or nerve blocks, causes little if any adverse systemic reactions and should be utilized whenever applicable.

Hypoproteinemia, a major manifestation of protein-calorie deficiency disease states, is of significance during anesthetic management because albumin is largely responsible for the protein binding of many drugs. Its reduced concentration can increase the effect of a given dose of drug, since it is the unbound portion of the drug that is physiologically active. Consideration of this effect should lead to reduced dosage of drugs during anesthesia, particularly barbiturates and muscle relaxants.

PARENTERAL HYPERALIMENTATION

Total parenteral nutrition is the continuous infusion of nutrients via a central line in order to achieve a positive nitrogen balance and to prevent catabolism. Its use can be lifesaving in some protein-calorie malnutrition states. However, there are characteristic problems associated with the procedure that the anesthesiologist should know. These problems may be mechanical or metabolic, or both.

Mechanically, the anesthesiologist should understand the proper care of the catheter. The catheter must not be used for administration of drugs or fluids except those used for parenteral nutrition. The dressing, which probably will be changed every four hours, should be occlusive and antibacterial. Aseptic technique cannot be overemphasized, because it has been shown that catheter sepsis generally results from skin contamination. Hematogenous spread, while possible, is of secondary importance.

Metabolic complications may be classified as follows:

1. Fluid overload — leading to hypertonicity and vascular congestion if an excess of hydrolysate is administered.

2. Electrolyte imbalance — leading to hypernatremia and hyperchloremia, indicative of hypertonicity. This requires solute-free water load for correction. Hyponatremia and hypochloremia may occur, since a prescribed amount of sodium is necessary in order to excrete any given water load. If sodium is lacking in sufficient quantity, there may be an inappropriate excretion of antidiuretic hormone with resulting hyponatremia and a consequent inability to excrete the water load.

3. Hypo/hyperkalemia and other element imbalances — hypokalemia usually is the result of an inadequate intake of potassium, since 3 mEq of potassium are required for every gram of nitrogen retained. Hypokalemia is manifested by progressive weakness and a tendency to edema formation. The kidneys may lose their ability to concentrate urine, and permanent renal damage may occur from the changes in the tubular cells. Mental symptoms may also appear, in addition to which the heart muscle is adversely affected. Glucose intolerance may result.

Hyperkalemia, while less of a problem, usually results from administration of excess potassium. In the presence of metabolic acidosis, even the administration of otherwise average daily requirements of potassium may lead to hyperkalemia and the development of ventricular fibrillation.

Hypocalcemia develops when inadequate amounts of calcium are administered to the patient or when attempting to increase the phosphate ion without concomitant calcium.

Hypophosphatemia may occur if the intake of phosphate ion is inadequate, especially when total parenteral nutrition lasts more than seven to 10 days. There may also be redistribution of the phosphate ion into muscle cells and into red blood cells, leading to a decrease in 2,3-DPG and a shift of the oxygen dissociation curve to the left with an increased affinity of hemoglobin for oxygen. With a decrease in phosphate ion, there is a decrease in muscle strength and a possibility of respiratory arrest.

Magnesium balance is rarely a clinical problem because the skeleton provides a large reservoir of magnesium that even long-term parenteral nutrition does not deplete significantly.

Hyperglycemia leading, in turn, to hyperosmolar nonketotic coma is a potential danger during glucose administration if too

Table 10–1   *Metabolic Complications of Intravenous Hyperalimentation*

Problems	Possible Etiologies
I. Glucose metabolism:	
A. Hyperglycemia, glycosuria, osmotic diuresis, hyperosmolar non-ketotic dehydration and coma	Excessive total dose or rate of infusion of glucose; inadequate endogenous insulin; glucocorticoids; sepsis
B. Ketoacidosis in diabetes mellitus	Inadequate endogenous insulin response; inadequate exogenous insulin therapy
C. Postinfusion (rebound) hypoglycemia	Persistence of endogenous insulin production secondary to prolonged stimulation of islet cells by high-carbohydrate infusion
II. Amino acid metabolism:	
A. Hyperchloremic metabolic acidosis	Excessive chloride and monohydrochloride content of crystalline amino acid solutions
B. Serum amino acid imbalance	Unphysiologic amino acid profile of the nutrient solution; differential amino acid utilization with various disorders
C. Hyperammonemia	Excessive ammonia in protein hydrolysate solutions; arginine, ornithine, aspartic acid and/or glutamic acid deficiency in amino acid solutions; primary hepatic disorder
D. Prerenal azotemia	Excessive protein hydrolysate or amino acid infusion
III. Calcium and phosphorus metabolism:	
A. Hypophosphatemia 1. Decreased erythrocyte 2,3-diphosphoglycerate 2. Increased affinity of hemoglobin for oxygen 3. Aberrations of erythrocyte intermediary metabolites	Inadequate phosphorus administration, redistribution of serum phosphorus into cells and/or bone
B. Hypocalcemia	Inadequate calcium administration; reciprocal response to phosphorus repletion without simultaneous calcium infusion; hypoalbuminemia
C. Hypercalcemia	Excessive calcium administration with or without high doses of albumin; excessive vitamin D administration
D. Vitamin D deficiency; hypervitaminosis D	Inadequate or excessive vitamin D administration
IV. Essential fatty acid metabolism: Serum deficiencies of phospholipid linoleic and/or arachidonic acids, serum elevations of Δ-5,8,11-eicosatrienoic acid	Inadequate essential fatty acid administration; inadequate vitamin E administration
V. Miscellaneous:	
A. Hypokalemia	Inadequate potassium intake relative to increased requirements for protein anabolism; diuresis
B. Hyperkalemia	Excessive potassium administration especially in metabolic acidosis; renal decompensation
C. Hypomagnesemia	Inadequate magnesium administration relative to increased requirements for protein anabolism and glucose metabolism
D. Hypermagnesemia	Excessive magnesium administration; renal decompensation
E. Anemia	Iron deficiency; folic acid deficiency; vitamin B_{12} deficiency; copper deficiency; other deficiencies
F. Bleeding	Vitamin K deficiency
G. Hypervitaminosis A	Excessive vitamin A administration
H. Elevations in SGOT, SGPT, and serum alkaline phosphatase	Enzyme induction secondary to amino acid imbalance; excessive glycogen and/or fat deposition in the liver
I. Cholestatic hepatitis	Decreased water content of bile

much or too rapid infusion is given. Therefore, adequate insulin coverage must be maintained.

Metabolic acidosis may occur because of the development of hyperchloremic acidosis from the synthetic amino acids being administered.

Miscellaneous aberrations that may occur include anemia, resulting from a deficiency of iron, folic acid, vitamin B_{12}, copper, and zinc. There may also be associated phospholipid alterations in the membrane of red cells when a deficiency of essential fatty acids causes diminished ability of the red blood cells to deliver oxygen. There may be increased platelet adhesiveness, which can lead to hypercoagulation. In addition, a deficiency of vitamin B_{12} may result in bleeding, subsequently leading to anemia, and there may be a rise in liver enzymes from excess glycogen or fat deposition in the liver.

VITAMIN DEFICIENCIES

A severely restricted diet often leads to one or more vitamin deficiencies. Even when the diet is apparently adequate, there may be an inherent inability of the body to absorb or utilize the particular vitamin. This is especially true in periods of extra utilization such as during pregnancy.

Vitamin B Group. It is generally true that a deficiency of one member of the vitamin B group leads to or is associated with a deficiency in the rest of the B group. Vitamin B_1 deficiency, beriberi, is most commonly found in such areas as the southern part of the United States and eastern Asia and is often associated with the ingestion of polished rice. This disease process is often precipitated by hard work, pregnancy, and lactation.

The disease itself may have predominately cardiovascular or neurological symptoms, although most patients manifest a mixed syndrome. Cardiovascular manifestations of the disease consist of palpitations, weakness, shortness of breath, a dilated peripheral vascular bed, and a cardiac output increased in proportion to decreases in peripheral resistance. There is an accumulation of lactic and pyruvic acids in tissue and body fluids; there is also shunting of blood across capillary beds and renal retention of sodium and water. High output cardiac failure, with increased oxygen consumption, may occur.

When neurological manifestations predominate (dry beriberi), mental aberrations and peripheral neuropathy are noted. Recent memory and abstract thought processes are impaired. There is muscle wasting, diminution of vibratory sense, loss of reflexes, and possible cranial nerve involvement.

This disease entity is also characteristic of the chronic alcoholic, and this state of confusion in its chronic form is known as Korsakoff's psychosis.

During treatment with intravenous vitamin B_1, it is important to remember that increasing cardiac failure may result even while the peripheral vascular abnormality is being quickly corrected because of the rapid increase in total resistance. Cardiac glycosides alone do not cure the congestive heart failure produced by this disease but, when administered concomitantly with vitamin B_1, they are usually efficacious.

Owing to the high output failure that is present and the increased oxygen consumption, high oxygen concentrations are mandatory during anesthesia. Halothane may reduce cardiac work load and lower blood pressure, reducing the metabolic requirement of oxygen to some extent. Theoretically, during regional anesthesia, the maximally functioning heart might not be able to compensate for the decrease in peripheral vascular resistance. However, clinically, this has not been documented. Furthermore, because of the peripheral neuropathy, there may be abnormal sympathetic responses during anesthesia, with resulting hypotension.

Vitamin B_{12} (riboflavin), a member of the flavoprotein group of specific proteins, has an important function in cell respiration, but changes brought about by its deficiency are of little clinical importance and thus do not concern anesthetic management.

Vitamin B_6 (pyridoxine) deficiency is a relatively rare situation. Since this vitamin is not stored in the body, deficiency may occur as a result of malabsorption or other defective intestinal function. It is of interest, however, that patients who are on drugs such as Apresoline and Isoniazid, may manifest a deficiency of vitamin B_6, while patients with hypochromic anemia, who are occasionally refractory to routine therapy, may respond to vitamin B_6 even if there is no response to iron therapy.

Vitamin K. This vitamin is not stored in the body. A constant supply is required for synthesis of the coagulation factors II, VII, IX, and X. Any pathologic process that affects fat absorption, GI motility, or bacterial flora can affect the production of vitamin K. This deficiency can be rapidly alleviated however, when the vitamin is administered parenterally. Symptoms will abate in about 1 to $1\frac{1}{2}$ hours, and both the prothrombin time and the partial thromboplastin time will revert to normal in 4 to 12 hours. Vitamin K should be given intramuscularly or subcutaneously whenever possible because there have been cases of anaphylaxis reported during intravenous administration of this drug.

Vitamin D Deficiency (Rickets). Rickets occurs because of impaired bone mineralization. It is now known that vitamin D is a precursor of a hormonal system. Vitamin D is stored in great abundance in skin and can be converted by sunlight into vitamin D_3. Hence, in sunlight, vitamin D is not a dietary requirement at all. Whether it is ingested or formed by ultraviolet radiation in man, vitamin D is metabolically inert and must undergo transference within the body to the active metabolites. This is accomplished by the liver and kidney. In view of the above, vitamin D can be considered a hormone because there are large supplies of precursors available. It is synthesized in the liver and kidney, and its active products are secreted into the general circulation to be taken up by tissues elsewhere in the body.

Rickets usually occurs as a result of poverty, ignorance, or participation in fad diets. It is most often found in premature infants and children fed nonenriched cow's milk. Rickets also occurs in various malabsorption states, when calciferol absorption is impaired. Insofar as anesthesia is concerned, careful management of possible cardiac dysrhythmias and the recognition of a reduced requirement for neuromuscular blocking agents is indicated in view of the hypocalcemia. Monitoring with a peripheral nerve stimulator is also indicated.

Vitamin C Deficiency (Scurvy). Scurvy, a disease of ancient vintage, was a problem for many years, especially among sailors deprived of fresh fruit for long periods. This was controlled in the British Navy by stocking limes for long journeys. (The British are still occasionally referred to as "Limeys.") Today, interestingly, scurvy is manifesting itself again with a relatively new modification. A certain percentage of the population, particularly in the United States, has the habit of taking vitamin C in megavitamin doses compared with the dose necessary for adequate body nutrition. Doses greater than 1 gm a day may induce increased catabolism of the vitamin, a condition that continues after the dosage has been reduced. Increased catabolism may produce a "rebound scurvy" if doses of 1 gm daily are stopped abruptly rather than tapered off. Sometimes this may happen when a patient is admitted to the hospital. The physician in charge of the case may not know about the patient's penchant for extremely high doses of vitamin C, and fail to prescribe it. This leads to rebound scurvy with appearance of the classic symptoms, including capillary fragility, hemorrhage, bony changes and irritability. There is gingivitis with loosened teeth giving rise to possible difficulties in intubation. Defective synthesis of norepinephrine and serotonin with vasomotor instability can occur. Macrocytic anemia may ensue, since vitamin C is necessary for folic acid metabolism. All of the symptoms will respond to increased amounts of vitamin C.

REFERENCES

Morbid Obesity

Alexander, J. K.: Obesity and cardiac performance. Am. J. Cardiol. *14*:860, 1964.

Alexander, J. K., Amad, K. H., and Cole, V. W.: Observations on some clinical features of extreme obesity, with particular reference to cardiorespiratory effects. Am. J. Med. *32*:517, 1962.

Alexander, J. K., Horton, R. W., Miller, W., et al.: The effect of upper abdominal surgery on the relationship of airway closing point to end-tidal position. Clin. Sci. *43*:137, 1972.

Ames, F. C., et al.: Liver dysfunction following small-bowel bypass for obesity: Nonoperative treatment of fatty metamorphoses with parenteral hyperalimentation. J.A.M.A. *235*:1249, 1976.

Anderson, J., et al.: Pulmonary function in obese patients scheduled for jejuno-ileostomy. Acta Anaesth. Scand. *21*:346, 1977.

Backman, L., Freyschuss, U., Hallberg, D., et al.: Cardiovascular function in extreme obesity. Acta Med. Scand. *193*:432, 1973.

Barrera, F., Reidenberg, M. M., Winters, W. L., et al.: Ventilation-perfusion relationships in the obese patient. J. Appl. Physiol. *26*:420, 1969.

Bedell, G. N., et al.: Pulmonary function in obese patients. J. Clin. Invest. 37:1049, 1958.

Bendezo, J. E., et al.: Certain metabolic consequences of jejuno-ileo bypass. Am. J. Clin. Nutr. 29:366, 1976.

Bendixen, H. H.: Morbid Obesity. ASA Refresher Courses, 6:1, 1978.

Berlines, K., Fujy, H., Lee, D. H., et al.: Blood pressure measurements in obese persons. Comparison of intraarterial and auscultatory measurements. Am. J. Cardiol. 8:10, 1961.

Brown, R. G., et al.: Hepatic effects of jejunoileal bypass for morbid obesity. Am. J. Surg. 127:53, 1974.

Catenacci, A. J., Anderson, J. O., and Boersma, D.: Anesthetic hazards of obesity. J.A.M.A. 175:657, 1961.

Chernick, R. M.: Respiratory effects of obesity. Canad. Med. Assoc. J. 80:613, 1959.

Drenick, E. D., et al.: Bypass enteropathy: Intestinal and systemic manifestations following small-bowel bypass. J.A.M.A. 236:269, 1976.

Fisher, A., Waterhouse, T. D., and Adams, A. P.: Obesity: Its relation to anaesthesia. Anaesthesia 30:633, 1975.

Fox, G. S.: Anaesthesia for intestinal short circuiting in the morbidly obese with reference to the pathophysiology of gross obesity. Canad. Anaesth. Soc. J. 22:307, 1975.

Hollenbeck, J. I., et al.: An etiologic basis for fatty liver after jejunoileal bypass. J. Surg. Res. 18:83, 1975.

King, G. E.: Errors in clinical measurement of blood pressure in obesity. Clin. Sci. 32:223, 1967.

Kisk, G. P., et al.: Intestinal bypass in marked obesity: Long-term metabolic sequelae. Ann. Surg. 41:786, 1975.

McIntyre, J. W. R.: Problems for the anesthetists in the care of the obese patient. Canad. Anaesth. J. 15:317, 1968.

McKenzie, R., et al.: Anesthesia for jejunoileal shunt: A review of 88 cases. Anesth. Analg. 54:65, 1975.

Phillips, R. B.: Small intestinal bypass for the treatment of morbid obesity. Surg. Gynecol. Obstet. 146:455, 1978.

Putnam, L., Jenicek, J. A., and Allen, C. A.: Anesthesia in the morbidly obese patient. South. Med. J. 67:(12) 1411, 1974.

Salem, M. R., Dalal, F. Y., Zygmunt, M. P., et al.: Does PEEP improve intraoperative arterial oxygenation in grossly obese patients? Anesthesiology 48:280, 1978.

Sharp, J. T., Henry, J. P., Sweeny, S. K., et al.: The total work of breathing in normal and obese man. J. Clin. Invest. 43:728, 1964.

Sixt, R., Baker, B., and Kral, J.: Closing volume and gas exchange in obese patients before and after intestinal bypass operation. Scand. J. Resp. Dis. (Suppl.) 95:65, 1976.

Soderberg, M., Thomson, D., and White, T.: Respiration, circulation and anesthetic management in obesity. Investigation before and after jejunoileal bypass. Acta Anaesth. Scand. 21:55, 1977.

Tucker, D. H., and Sieker, H. O.: The effect of change in body position on lung volumes and intrapulmonary gas mixing in patients with obesity. Am. Rev. Resp. Dis. 82:787, 1960.

Vaughn, R. W., et al.: Anesthetic considerations in jejunoileal small bowel bypass for morbid obesity. Anesth. Analg. 53:421, 1974.

Vaughn, R. W., Engelberdt, R. D., and Wise, L.: Postoperative hypoxemia in obese patients. Ann. Surg. 53:877, 1974.

Vaughn, R. W., and Wise, L.: Intraoperative arterial oxygenation in obese patients. Ann. Surg. 184:35, 1976.

Vaughn, R. W., et al.: Postoperative alveolar arterial oxygen tension difference: Its relation to the operative incision in obese patients. Anesth. Analg. 54:433, 1975.

Vaughn, R. W., et al.: Effect of position (semirecumbent versus supine) in postoperative oxygenation in markedly obese subjects. Anesth. Analg. 55:37, 1976.

Woods, J. R., et al.: The jejunoileal bypass and pregnancy. Obstet. Gynecol. Surg. 33:(11) 697, 1978.

Protein Calorie Malnutrition States

Bemis, K. M.: Current approaches to the etiology and treatment of anorexia nervosa. Psychological Bull. 85:(3) 593, 1978.

Border, J. R.: Metabolic response to short-term starvation, sepsis and trauma. In Cooper, P. (ed.): Surgery Annual 1970. New York, Appleton-Century Crofts, 1970, Vol 2.

Brenton, D. P., et al.: Hypothermia in kwashiorkor. Lancet 1:410, 1967.

Campbell, P. S., Rosen, E. N., Fanaroff, A., et al.: The continuing high mortality of protein-calorie undernutrition in children. S. African Med. J. 43:605, 1969.

Costa, G.: Cachexia, the metabolic component of neoplastic disease. Cancer Res. 37:2327, 1977.

Crisp, A. H.: Primary anorexia nervosa or adolescent weight phobia. Practitioner 212:525, 1974.

Currere, P. W.: Metabolic and nutritional aspects of thermal injury. Burns 2:16, 1976.

DeWhip, W.: Working conference on anorexia and cachexia of neoplastic disease. Cancer Res. 30:2816, 1970.

DeWys, W. D.: Anorexia in cancer patients. Cancer Res. 37:2354, 1977.

Dippe, S. E.: Anorexia nervosa: A self imposed disease. Arizona Med. 36:(3) 171, 1978.

Dunlap, W. M., et al.: Anemia and neutropenia caused by copper deficiency. Ann. Intern. Med. 80:470, 1974.

Gaines, D. M., et al.: Perceptual experiences in anorexia nervosa and obesity. Canad. Psychiat. Assoc. J. 23:249, 1978.

Henden, D. N., et al.: Humoral mediators of nontemperature dependent hypermetabolism in 50% burns in adult rats. Surg. Forum 28:37, 1977.

Hughes, W. T., et al.: Protein-calorie malnutrition. Am. J. Dis. Child. 128:44, 1974.

Mukherjee, K. L.: Classification of protein-calorie undernutrition in children. Arch. Dis. Child. 42:647, 1967.

Schussler, I., et al.: Anorexia nervosa: Current theory and clinical application. J. Florida Med. Assoc. 65:(5) 345, 1978.

Scrimshaw, N. J., and Belar, M.: Malnutrition in underdeveloped countries. N. Engl. J. Med. 272:137, 1965.

Vis, H. L.: Protein deficiency disorders. Postgrad. Med. J. 45:107, 1969.

Wilmore, D. W.: The Metabolic Management of the Critically Ill. New York, Plenum Publishing Co., 1977.

Wilmore, D. W., et al.: Catecholamines: Mediators of the hypermetabolic response to thermal injury. Ann. Surg. *180*:(4) 653, 1974.

Woik, T. H., et al.: Tropical problems in nutrition. Ann. Intern. Med. *79*:901, 1973.

Yarborough, M. F., et al.: Nutritional management of the severely injured patient. Contemp. Surg. *13*:15, 1978.

Parenteral Hyperalimentation

Abbott, W. M.: Indications for parenteral nutrition. *In* Fischer, J. E. (ed.): Total Parenteral Nutrition. Boston, Little, Brown & Co., 1976.

Dudrick, S. J., and Long, J. M.: Applications and hazards of intravenous hyperalimentation. Ann. Rev. Med. 28:517, 1977.

Dudrick, S. J., et al.: Parenteral hyperalimentation: Metabolic problems and solutions. Ann. Surg. *176*:259, 1972.

Kay, R. G., et al.: A syndrome of acute zinc deficiency during total parenteral alimentation in man. Ann. Surg. *183*:331, 1976.

Lindor, K. D., et al.: Liver function values in adults receiving total parenteral nutrition. J.A.M.A. *241*: (22) 2398, 1979.

Ryan, J. A., et al.: Catheter complications in total parenteral nutrition: A prospective study of 200 consecutive patients. N. Engl. J. Med. *290*:757, 1974.

Scheflan, M., et al.: Intestinal adaptation after extensive resection of the small intestine and prolonged administration of parenteral nutrition. Surg. Gynecol. Obstet. *143*:757, 1976.

Wilmore, R. W., et al.: Parenteral nutrition in burn patients. *In* Fischer, J. E. (ed.): Total Parenteral Nutrition. Boston, Little, Brown, & Co., 1976.

Winters, R. W., et al.: Intravenous nutrition in the high risk infant. New York, John Wiley and Sons Inc., 1975.

Vitamin Deficiencies

Akbarian, M., Yankopoulos, N. A., and Abelmann, W. H.: Hemodynamic studies in beri beri heart disease. Am. J. Med. *41*:197, 1966.

Ansell, J. E., Kumer, R., and Deyben, D.: The spectrum of vitamin K deficiency. J.A.M.A. *238*:40, 1977.

Arnstein, A. R., and Frame, B.: Primary hypophosphatemic rickets and osteomalacia. A review. Clin. Orthop. *49*:109, 1966.

Barrett-Connor, E.: The etiology of pellagra and its significance for modern medicine. Am. J. Med. *42*:859, 1967.

Clinical nutrition. Vitamin C toxicity. Nutr. Rev. *34*:236, 1976.

Daly, W. J., McNutt, K., and Todhunter, E. W.: Niacin. Nutr. Rev. 33:289, 1975.

Gravallese, M.: Circulatory studies in Wernicke's encephalopathy. Circulation 25:836, 1957.

Hankes, L. V.: Tryptophan: Abnormal metabolism in pellagra patients. Metabolism 19:465, 1970.

Hodges, R. E., et al.: Clinical manifestation of ascorbic acid deficiency in man. Am. J. Clin. Nutr. 24:432, 1971.

Johnson, J. E.: Hypocalcemia and cardiac arrhythmias. Am. J. Dis. Child. *115*:373, 1968.

Martz, D. M.: Acute brain syndrome secondary to niacin deficiency. Am. J. Psychiat. *122*:215, 1965.

Potts, J. T., and Deftos, L. J.: Parathyroid hormone thyrocalcitonin, vitamin D, bone and bone mineral metabolism. *In* Bondy, P. (ed.): Diseases of Metabolism. 6th ed., Philadelphia, W. B. Saunders Co., 1969.

Rivlin, R. S.: Riboflavin metabolism. N. Engl. J. Med. *283*:463, 1970.

Sauderbech, E. H., et al.: Thiamine requirements of the adult human. Am. J. Clin. Nutr. 23:67, 1970.

Sebrell, W. H.: A clinical evaluation of thiamine deficiency. Ann. N. Y. Acad. Sci. 98:563, 1962.

Slaywitz, B. A., Siegel, N. J., and Pearson, H. H.: Megavitamins for minimal brain dysfunction. A potentially dangerous therapy. J.A.M.A. *238*:1749, 1977.

Suttie, J. W.: Vitamin K and prothrombin synthesis. Nutr. Rev. *31*:105, 1973.

Tampaichits, V., et al.: Clinical and biochemical studies on adult beri-beri. Am. J. Clin. Nutr. 23:1017, 1970.

Vilter, R. W.: Effects of ascorbic acid deficiency in man. *In* Sebrell, W. H., Jr., and Harris, R. S. (eds.): The Vitamins. New York, Academic Press, 1967, Vol. 1, p. 457.

11

Renal Diseases

By R. I. MAZZE, M.D., and M. J. COUSINS, M.B.

Effect of Anesthetic Agents in Patients
  with Normal Renal Function
  Circulatory Effects
  Sympathetic Nervous System
  Endocrine System
Diagnosis of Renal Impairment and
  Interpretation of Renal Function Studies
Effects of Drugs in Patients with
  Reduced Renal Function
  Premedicant Agents
  Anesthetic Agents and Adjuvant Drugs
Renal Diseases
  Acute Glomerulonephritis
  Pyelonephritis
  Renal Papillary Necrosis

Nephrotic Syndrome
Diabetes Mellitus
Rheumatoid Arthritis
Gout
Systemic Lupus Erythematosus (SLE)
Periarteritis Nodosa
Other Systemic Diseases
Nephrotoxins
Acute Renal Failure
  Acute Renal Failure Due to Prerenal
    Causes
Dialysis and Renal Transplantation
  Dialysis
  Renal Transplantation

EFFECT OF ANESTHETIC AGENTS IN PATIENTS WITH NORMAL RENAL FUNCTION

Before considering the renal effects of anesthesia and operation in patients with kidney disease, it is important to assess these effects in surgical patients without renal disease. All general anesthetic agents depress renal function: urinary flow, glomerular filtration rate (GFR), renal blood flow (RBF), and electrolyte excretion are reduced.[1-7] This consistent and generalized depression of renal function can be attributed to many factors, including the type and duration of surgical procedure; the physical status of the patient, especially that of the cardiovascular and renal systems;[8-10] preoperative and intraoperative blood volume and fluid and electrolyte balance;[11-13] and the choice of anesthetic agent.[6] Changes in renal function following spinal and epidural anesthesia tend to parallel the degree of sympathetic blockade and therefore the amount of hypotension that is produced.[14]

In most cases the changes in renal function associated with anesthesia and surgery are completely reversible at the end of the operative procedure.

The depression in renal function caused by anesthetic agents is due to their direct and indirect effects. The indirect effects on the circulatory, sympathetic nervous, and endocrine systems are, by far, the most important. In animals, ether, cyclopropane, and halothane have direct effects on sodium transport,[15] whereas in man methoxyflurane causes direct depression of renal tubular function.[16, 17]

CIRCULATORY EFFECTS

During general anesthesia RBF may be depressed as a consequence of renal vasoconstriction, systemic hypotension, or both. Drugs that evoke the greatest increase in catecholamine excretion, such as cyclopropane and diethyl ether,[18] tend to support systemic blood pressure but in so doing cause a marked increase in renal vascular resistance, a decrease in RBF, and a marked depression in renal function.[7] Halothane and thiopental, though not evoking a catecholamine response, are associated with a moderate increase in renal vascular resistance as blood is shunted away from the kidney to compensate for hypotension induced by myocardial depression and peripheral vasodilatation.[5] Renal blood flow and GFR fall with these agents but not as much as with anesthetic agents that stimulate catecholamine release. Finally, anesthetic drugs with alpha-adrenergic blocking activity,[19] such as droperidol, the tranquilizer component of Innovar, appear to cause the smallest changes in renal hemodynamics and function.[6]

SYMPATHETIC NERVOUS SYSTEM

The blood vessels of the kidney are supplied with sympathetic constrictor fibers derived from the T4-L1 spinal cord segments via the celiac and renal plexuses. There is no sympathetic dilator or parasympathetic innervation of the kidney. Under a wide variety of physiologic conditions, normal and abnormal, RBF is regulated to maintain stability of GFR. The best evidence for the role of the sympathetic nervous system in the renal effects of anesthesia is provided by Berne's experiments in dogs with one normal and one denervated kidney.[20] Prior to induction of anesthesia, the RBF and GFR of a denervated and normally innervated kidney are the same. However, following induction of anesthesia, RBF and GFR decrease on the normally innervated side, whereas no changes are seen on the denervated side. These changes must be due to an anesthetic induced increase in vasoconstrictor tone of the innervated kidney.

Autoregulation of RBF and GFR occurs in unanesthetized animals and may also be present during general anesthesia. In animals anesthetized with the intravenous agents pentobarbital and chloralose, and with halothane, RBF and GFR vary only slightly over an arterial pressure range of 80 to 180 mm Hg.[21, 22] By contrast, autoregulation does not appear to be present in surgical patients undergoing general anesthesia with the inhalation agents. Decreases in

RBF and GFR of 50 per cent or more have been reported with ether, cyclopropane, and halothane anesthesia, although blood pressure has been stable and above 80 mm Hg.[2, 4-7] Studies in humans are more difficult to control than those in animals and, at the moment, the evidence is conflicting.

ENDOCRINE SYSTEM

Endocrine effects on renal function during anesthesia are also of importance and are closely tied to the circulatory effects discussed above. Most important in regulating urine volume is the antidiuretic hormone (ADH).

Release of ADH is controlled by osmoreceptors in the carotid body and the pituitary that are sensitive to osmolality changes of approximately 2 per cent.[23] An increase in the osmolality of blood causes reflex release of ADH, which is carried by the blood to the kidneys and is taken up by the distal tubules and collecting ducts. This causes an increase in tubular reabsorption of water; since solute excretion is essentially unchanged, urine volume falls and concentration is increased. When sufficient water is absorbed, the osmolality of plasma is lowered and ADH release is suppressed. In like fashion, a decrease in plasma osmolality causes suppression of ADH release with resulting formation of dilute urine. Decreased intravascular volume also stimulates ADH release, probably through reflex baroreceptor mechanisms.[24] Until recently, it had been assumed that general anesthetic agents and narcotics caused release of ADH. However, development of radioimmunoassay techniques for ADH measurement have permitted precise measurements of this hormone in surgical patients. It is now clear that neither morphine nor light halothane anesthesia stimulates high levels of ADH secretion. The increase in ADH levels that accompanies operation with these anesthetics is most likely due to a stress response that can be attenuated with deeper anesthesia.[25]

Epinephrine, norepinephrine, and the renin-angiotensin system are involved in control of RBF, in that elaboration of these substances produces a marked increase in renal vascular resistance with a decrease in RBF.[26] Norepinephrine, the primary adrenergic transmitter substance, is known to increase in concentration during cyclopropane and ether anesthesia, with little change occurring during halothane or thiopental administration.

Renin secretion ultimately results in the formation of the pressor and renal vascular constricting substance angiotensin II. Variation of plasma renin activity has been shown to occur during anesthesia but its significance remains obscure.[27] Recent development of a specific angiotensin II antagonist, saralasin, has allowed delineation of the role of the renin-angiotensin system in blood pressure control during anesthesia.[28] Although anesthesia with halothane, enflurane, ketamine, and fluroxene did not result in significant increases in plasma renin activity, the renin-angiotensin system played a significant role in the maintenance of blood pressure during halothane and enflurane administration.

Aldosterone is responsible for moment-to-moment regulation of sodium excretion by the kidney. Its release is primarily dependent on volume depletion as mediated by baroreceptors in the carotid sinus. Secondary pathways for aldosterone release involve circulating angiotensin level, ADH concentration, and renin-angiotensin formation. Anesthetics are known to affect these systems and may influence the primary volume-sensitive mechanisms as well as alter the circulatory pressures that activate the carotid baroreceptors.[29, 30]

Table 11–1 summarizes published reports of changes in renal function observed during general anesthesia in man. Detailed reviews of the effects of anesthesia on the kidney have recently been published by Cousins and Mazze,[35] Bastron and Deutsch,[36] and Larson et al.[37]

DIAGNOSIS OF RENAL IMPAIRMENT AND INTERPRETATION OF RENAL FUNCTION STUDIES

The patient's past medical history is the single most important piece of information in establishing the presence of renal disease. Physical findings, aside from those associated with hypertension, are minimal until renal disease is far advanced. In patients without history of renal or systemic disease, urinalysis is sufficient preoperative laboratory screening for identification of kidney disease. If disease is present, more precise methods of assessing renal function are necessary.

Laboratory tests useful in determining the presence and extent of kidney disease are noted below.

Urinalysis. Urinalysis, consisting of urinary appearance, pH, specific gravity, protein content, sugar content, and microscopic examination, is one of the most readily available, inexpensive, and informative laboratory tests.

1. Appearance of the urine indicates whether there is bleeding in the genitourinary tract, infection, or systemic disease.

2. pH: Although the kidneys share regulation of acid-base balance with the lungs, they are the sole pathway of excretion for the 60 mEq of hydrogen ion, or nonvolatile acid, that each day is produced by normal metabolism. The three main processes by which the kidney excretes an acid urine are the reabsorption of bicarbonate from glomerular filtrate, the acidification of buffers in the tubular urine, and the production of ammonia in tubular cells with its subsequent excretion as ammonium ion. Therefore, the ability to acidify urine is a measure of renal competence.[38]

3. Urinary specific gravity is a measure of concentrating ability and therefore of tubular function. A similar but more specific test is determination of urinary osmolality, which is a measure of the number of particles per unit volume of solvent. Tubular fluid is isotonic as it passes through the proximal tubule, but it rapidly becomes hypertonic as it descends deep into the medulla through the narrow segment of the loop of Henle. As chloride is reabsorbed from the ascending limb of the loop of Henle, tubular fluid becomes hypotonic. In the distal tubules and collecting ducts, ADH acts, facilitating the passage of sodium-free fluid into the interstitium of the renal medulla, resulting in the formation of small amounts of concentrated urine. In the absence of ADH, sodium reabsorption continues in the distal tubules, but there is no reabsorption of water so that large volumes of dilute urine are produced.[39] The elaboration of concentrated urine (specific gravity, 1.030; 1050 milliosmoles per kilogram [mOsm per kg]) is indicative of excellent

Table 11-1 Renal Function Studies During General Anesthesia

Author	Agent	Depth	Premedication	RBF	GFR	Filtration Fraction	Urine Volume	Na Excretion	K Excretion	Remarks
						% of Control				
Burnett[1] (1949)	Ether	1st–2nd plane	None	62	78	131	55	—	—	No fluid information
Habif[2] (1951)	Ether	2nd plane	Atropine, meperidine	48	61	132	42	37	48	250 ml./hr. of 5% dextrose or normal saline (NS)
Miles[3] (1952)	Ether	Light / Deep	Atropine / Atropine	65 / 42	78 / 57	124 / 142	— / —	— / —	— / —	No fluid information
Burnett[1] (1949)	Cyclopropane	1st–2nd plane	None	46	69	148	56	—	—	No fluid information
Habif[2] (1951)	Cyclopropane	2nd plane	Meperidine, atropine	31	45	156	32	16	32	250 ml./hr. of 5% dextrose or normal saline
Miles[3] (1952)	Cyclopropane	Light / Deep	Atropine / Atropine	72 / 34	74 / 45	109 / 150	—	— / —	—	No fluid information
Deutsch[7] (1967)	Cyclopropane	2nd plane	None	58	61	114	35	33	122	Hydrated $\bar{c}$ 1 L. of 4% fructose; nonoperated
Mazze[4] (1963)	Halothane	0.5–1.0% / 1.2–3.0%	Morphine, scopolamine / Morphine, scopolamine	39 / 31	52 / 42	134 / 126	43 / 36	43 / 36	117 / 108	No fluids during surgery
Barry[9] (1964)	Halothane	0.5–1.0% / 1.2–3.0%	Morphine, scopolamine / Morphine, scopolamine	88 / 53	92 / 60	104 / 110	— / —	— / —	— / —	Hydrated before and during surgery $\bar{c}$ 15 ml./hr. of 1/3 NS
Deutsch[5] (1966)	Halothane	2nd plane	None	62	81	139	37	36	—	Hydrated $\bar{c}$ 1 L. of 4% fructose; nonoperated
Cousins[31] (1976)	Enflurane	0.8–1.4%	Morphine, scopolamine	77	79	103	67	—	—	Hydrated before and during surgery $\bar{c}$ 15 ml./hr. of 1/3 NS
Mazze[32] (1974)	Isoflurane	1.2%	Morphine, scopolamine	51	63	119	34	—	—	Hydrated before and during surgery $\bar{c}$ 15 ml./hr. of 1/3 NS
Auberger[34] (1965)	Methoxyflurane	0.6–0.8%	Atropine	70	79	111	46	—	—	No fluid information
Habif[2] (1951)	Thiopental	2nd plane	Meperidine, atropine	70	68	97	48	30	57	250 ml./hr. of 5% dextrose or normal saline
Deutsch[23] (1969)	Thiopental, nitrous oxide	Light	Morphine, atropine	64	73	122	41	39	104	Hydrated $\bar{c}$ 1 L. of 4% fructose; nonoperated
Gorman[6] (1966)	Neuroleptanalgesia	2nd plane	None	97	97	100	58	66	80	No fluids during surgery

tubular function, whereas urinary toxicity fixed at that of plasma (specific gravity 1.010; 300 mOsm per kg) may be indicative of renal disease. The ability to dilute urine persists long after concentration defects are present, so urinary osmolality of 50 to 100 mOsm per kg may be found in the presence of advanced renal disease.[40]

4. Protein in the urine is usually a sign of renal disease. The most common cause of proteinuria is the escape of normal plasma protein through a defective glomerular membrane. However, proteinuria may also be due to failure of normal tubular reabsorption of protein, abnormally increased concentrations in the plasma of normal plasma proteins, or the presence in the plasma of abnormal protein, which is then passed in the urine. Patients without renal disease may have proteinuria after strenuous exercise or after standing for several hours. Massive proteinuria is always abnormal and is usually indicative of severe glomerular damage.[41]

5. Glucose is freely filtered and reabsorbed by the proximal tubule. Glycosuria is usually indicative of diabetes mellitus, but may mean that the patient's ability to reabsorb glucose has been exceeded by an abnormally heavy load presented to the tubules. This occurs frequently in the hospitalized patient who is receiving intravenous glucose infusions.

6. Microscopic examination of the urine may reveal the presence of casts, bacteria, and various cell forms, thereby supplying diagnostic information in the patient with renal disease. It can also be of importance in determining whether abdominal complaints are renal or intestinal in origin.

Complete Blood Count. Hemoglobin or hematocrit determinations are of value in determining the extent of anemia associated with renal disease. Cell and platelet counts are of particular importance in patients receiving immunosuppressive therapy or with coagulation abnormalities.

Blood Urea Nitrogen (BUN). BUN concentration is a valuable index of general kidney function. Urea is freely filtered at the glomerulus, with about one third of the filtered amount reabsorbed when urine flow is more than 2 ml per minute. BUN concentrations remain normal despite reductions in glomerular and tubular function of 50 per cent or more. Therefore, a normal BUN concentration in a patient with a history of renal disease indicates only that the disease is not far advanced. Excretion of drugs eliminated by the kidney may be quite abnormal despite BUN concentrations in the normal (10 to 20 mg per cent) or slightly elevated (24 to 35 mg per cent) range. A high protein diet tends to raise BUN concentration slightly, whereas serum creatinine concentration is unaffected.

Serum Electrolytes. Sodium, potassium, and chloride concentrations should be determined if impairment of renal function is suspected. These tests will remain normal until renal function is markedly impaired, at which time hyperkalemia, with or without hyperchloremic acidosis, may be present.

pH and Blood Gases. If the patient has significant renal disease, metabolic acidosis may be present. Arterial blood pH, standard bicarbonate, and PCO_2 should be determined to measure the extent of acid-base balance.

Chest X-Ray. This may help to determine the presence of hypertensive cardiovascular disease, pericardial effusion, or uremic pneumonitis.

Electrocardiogram (ECG). The ECG reflects the toxic effect of potassium excess more closely than does determination of serum potassium concentration. Tall peaked T waves, depression of the ST segment, widening of the QRS complex, and ventricular arrhythmias occur as hyperkalemia progresses. Digitalis toxicity caused by decreased renal digitalis excretion may be present and can best be detected by examination of the ECG. Therapeutic doses of digitalis shorten the QT interval, depress the ST segment, and lower or invert the T wave. Toxic doses exaggerate these changes and, in addition, frequently cause ventricular premature contractions that may be coupled or tripled, producing bigeminal or trigeminal rhythms. The ECG may also reveal hypocalcemia, which together with hyperkalemia and digitalis excess is potentially the most likely cause of arrhythmias during anesthesia in uremic patients. Finally, the ECG may be of value in diagnosing hypertensive and ischemic heart disease.

EFFECTS OF DRUGS IN PATIENTS WITH REDUCED RENAL FUNCTION

When severe renal disease is present the action of drugs may be altered owing to anemia, serum protein and electrolyte abnormalities, body fluid relocation, and abnormal cell membrane activity.[42] Drugs eliminated in unchanged form by the kidney alone (e.g., gallamine) are contraindicated because therapeutic levels are sustained for prolonged periods of time.[43] Drugs that are metabolized and then excreted (e.g., morphine) are presumed to be more suitable for administration in the patient with impaired renal function. The products of drug metabolism are usually more polar forms of the parent compound[44] and hence are more readily excreted in the urine. Little is known about the toxicity of these compounds when they cannot be eliminated in normal fashion, but they can be quite harmful. Inorganic fluoride, derived from biotransformation of methoxyflurane, is an example of a metabolite that is more toxic than the parent compound.[45] A review of drug action in patients with renal disease is presented in the monograph by Reidenberg.[46]

Since patients with severe renal disease are debilitated, they could have impaired mechanisms of biotransformation in addition to markedly decreased renal excretion of drugs. Uremia also may be accompanied by CNS depression, so drugs with CNS depressant activity should be administered with caution. Dosage reductions of 25 to 50 per cent are appropriate in most cases, depending on the severity of renal impairment.

PREMEDICANT AGENTS

Barbiturates. The long-acting barbiturates barbital and phenobarbital should be avoided because they are primarily excreted unchanged in urine.[47] Short-acting agents such as thiopental, pentobarbital, and secobarbital are more satisfactory because they are inactivated by hepatic metabolism or depend upon redistribution for termination of action.

Belladonna Alkaloids. As much as 50 per cent of belladonna alkaloids such as atropine and hyoscyamine are excreted unchanged by the kidney, so dosage should be modified in patients with severe renal disease.[48] Scopolamine is almost completely metabolized prior to excretion and is preferable if the use of a drying agent is indicated. However, the anuric patient often has dry, friable mucous membranes, so antisialagogues may not be necessary.

Phenothiazine and Benzodiazepine Compounds. Both phenothiazine and benzodiazepine (Valium) are metabolized in the liver, so impairment of renal function probably does not affect their duration or intensity[49, 50] of action. In addition to tranquilizing properties, these compounds have antiemetic effects, a desirable action in patients with renal failure. Phenothiazine derivatives are known to produce alpha-adrenergic blockade, which may accentuate cardiovascular instability in uremic patients. Diazepam has a half-life in excess of 24 hours, so it may not be the best choice in patients with pre-existing CNS depression. CNS depressants with short half-lives appear more appropriate.

Narcotics. The action of narcotics is intensified and prolonged in proportion to the severity of renal disease, but this is probably related to the patient's debilitated state rather than to the lack of metabolism or excretion. Both morphine and meperidine are almost completely metabolized before excretion;[55] however, little is known about the toxicity of their metabolic products.

ANESTHETIC AGENTS AND ADJUVANT DRUGS

Inhalation Agents. Although most inhalation anesthetic agents are biotransformed to some extent, and the products of metabolism are often eliminated by the kidney, these drugs do not rely on renal excretion for reversal of their therapeutic effects. Therefore, in patients with mild or moderate impairment of renal function, all inhalation agents except methoxyflurane and perhaps enflurane are suitable for administration in usual clinical doses.[17] Enflurane is metabolized to inorganic fluoride[31, 51] and, thus, is a potential nephrotoxin. Clinical and animal studies have not borne out this concern.[31, 51-54] Therefore, when indicated, enflurane may be administered to patients with renal disease with due regard for its theoretical potential for nephrotoxicity.

In the uremic patient hyperkalemia, hypocalcemia, and acidosis may cause increased myocardial irritability. Therefore, agents that sensitize the heart to catecholamines, such as cyclopropane or halothane, should be administered with great caution. Hypercarbia may be particularly dangerous in patients predisposed to cardiac irregularities, so hypoventilation must be avoided.

Nitrous oxide concentration should not exceed 50 per cent because of the decreased oxygen-carrying capacity associated with the anemia of uremia and the increased intrapulmonary shunting that occurs during general anesthesia.

Intravenous Agents. Metabolic degradation and excretion play a negligible part in emergence from anesthesia produced by a single dose of thiopental. However, sleeping time is increased in proportion to the degree of uremia.[57] Sixty-five to 75 per cent of thiopental is bound in the ionized form to albumin. Since albumin concentration is markedly reduced in uremia, binding is decreased and a greater proportion of thiopental is available to reach receptor sites. In addition, the pK of thiopental is in the physiologic range, so that the acidosis of uremia reduces the ionized or readily bound form of the drug. Although the latter changes are less important than those that are due to decreased serum albumin concentration, in combination they reduce the quantity of thiopental necessary to produce anesthesia. An additional explanation for the decreased drug requirement in uremic patients may be the alteration in the blood-brain barrier that is said to occur with this condition.[58] The same considerations are true for methohexital, although metabolism plays a slightly greater part in termination of its therapeutic effect.

Propanidid, a phenoxyacetic amine, and althesin, a steroid anesthetic not available in the United States, are rapidly metabolized in the liver. They appear to be suitable for use in patients with severe renal impairment, although experience with them is less than with intravenous barbiturates.[59]

Neuroleptanalgesia, when employed with concentrations of nitrous oxide up to 50 per cent, is a satisfactory anesthetic technique for the uremic patient. Both droperidol and fentanyl are metabolized prior to excretion.[19] When used in combination with N_2O, neuroleptanalgesia has been reported to produce less intraoperative depression of RBF and GFR than occurs with inhalation agents.[6] This is probably due to alpha-adrenergic blockade produced by the butyrophenone component, droperidol.

Muscle Relaxants. Succinylcholine has been used without difficulty in patients with decreased and absent renal function. Its metabolic products, succinic acid and choline, are nontoxic; however, a metabolic precursor of these two compounds, succin-

ylmonocholine, can produce a nondepolarizing block if large amounts accumulate.[60] Since succinylmonocholine is excreted by the kidney, care must be exercised that only minimal doses of succinylcholine are administered. Pseudocholinesterase levels may be reduced[61, 62] following hemodialysis, so use of a test dose of 5 to 10 mg of succinylcholine and a nerve stimulator will be of value in avoiding prolonged apnea. Succinylcholine administration produces a rapid but transient rise in serum potassium concentration of 0.5 mEq/L in normal patients, whereas in traumatized, burned, or neurologically injured patients the increase may be as great as 3 to 4 mEq/L. The latter rise, combined with the usually occurring sympathomimetic response to succinylcholine administration, may be particularly dangerous in the uremic patient in whom pre-existing hyperkalemia, hypocalcemia, acidosis, and diminished ability to excrete potassium tend toward production of ventricular arrhythmias. In the recently dialyzed patient with renal failure, the risk of hyperkalemia following succinylcholine administration appears to be no greater than in patients without renal disease.[63]

Curare has been used with success in patients with limited or absent renal function. In patients with normal renal function, curare-induced paralysis is terminated by redistribution, with approximately 38 per cent of the drug excreted unchanged by the kidney.[64] The patient with renal impairment and the anephric patient with a transplanted kidney excrete less curare, so the duration of neuromuscular blockade will be prolonged if dosage is not reduced by 25 to 50 per cent.

Gallamine[43] and decamethonium[65] rely almost entirely on urinary excretion for termination of their action. Therefore, their use in patients with decreased renal function should be avoided.

Pancuronium is the most commonly used muscle relaxant in poor risk patients, including those with renal disease. Its pharmacokinetics in patients with renal disease are similar to those of curare.[64, 66] Termination of action depends predominantly upon redistribution, with hepatic metabolism and renal excretion playing lesser roles. Dosage reductions of 25 to 50 per cent are necessary if prolonged block is to be avoided.

Ganglionic Blockers. Pentolinium and hexamethonium are quaternary ammonium compounds and are excreted unchanged solely by the kidneys. Their use should be avoided when production of hypotension is a therapeutic aim.[67] Occasionally, some patients with poorly controlled renal hypertension will develop hypertensive crises during stimulation associated with intubation or surgical incision. The action of trimethaphan (Arfonad) is terminated enzymatically by cholinesterase[68] rather than by renal excretion, so it should be used to control blood pressure in these situations.

Digitalis. Digoxin and lanatoside C, digitalis preparations with relatively rapid onset and short duration, are excreted in the urine in unchanged form.[69] Digitalis leaf and digitoxin are metabolized and then excreted in the urine, but little is known about the cardiovascular activity of their metabolic products. The administration of digitalis to the patient with reduced renal function is always hazardous; the addition of an anesthetic in this situation compounds the risk. Initial digitalization or changes in digitalis dosage should be avoided prior to surgery.[70] Blood levels should be obtained to assist in avoiding toxicity.

Vasopressors and Antihypertensive Agents. Patients with severe renal disease are frequently taking antihypertensive medication, most commonly thiazide diuretics, methyldopa, and beta adrenergic blocking agents. These patients may be hypovolemic, so anesthesia must be induced slowly and with smaller dosages of anesthetic agents; otherwise, profound hypotension may ensue. If a vasopressor is necessary, then direct alpha-adrenergic stimulators (e.g., phenylephrine) are most effective. Unfortunately, this type of vasopressor causes the greatest interference with renal circulation.[71] Although the beta stimulator isoproterenol maintains heart and brain perfusion without renal vasoconstriction, it also increases myocardial irritability. The best solution to this therapeutic dilemma is to substitute measures such as elevation of the legs and blood volume expansion, thereby avoiding the use of these drugs.

Methyldopa reduces both central and peripheral norepinephrine levels and is known to interact with anesthetic agents in a dose-related fashion, lowering the minimum alveolar concentration (MAC) of anesthetic required for analgesia.[72] Depression of MAC may be enhanced by the debility of uremia. In contrast, prior administration of the monoamine oxidase (MAO) inhibitor iproniazid elevates central norepinephrine levels and causes an increase in MAC.

Monoamine oxidase inhibitors are occasionally used in patients with renal disease to control mental depression. Interaction of MAO inhibitors with analgesics and vasopressors occurs in anesthetized patients[73] and may be accentuated in uremia.

RENAL DISEASES

Many renal diseases, such as glomerulonephritis, although of moderately high incidence, are not frequently encountered by the anesthesiologist. Others, such as chronic pyelonephritis, are seen more often but are recognized as not requiring specific anesthetic management. In this section, pathophysiologic and functional changes encountered in renal disease are discussed as the diseases present in their acute form. However, most of the conditions are progressive, with functional impairment directly proportional to the amount of nephron damage. When far advanced, the pathophysiology and metabolic changes are similar to those seen in acute renal failure but often are better tolerated because of their slower onset. The end stage of functional impairment is referred to as chronic renal failure, although this is not a specific pathologic diagnosis. References for diseases described from here through page 474 are not included in this section unless they have specific relevance to anesthetic management. Complete discussions are found in Renal Disease,[74] edited by D.A.K. Black, and Diseases of the Kidney,[75] edited by Maurice Strauss.

ACUTE GLOMERULONEPHRITIS

Acute glomerulonephritis (type I nephritis, acute hemorrhagic nephritis, acute diffuse nephritis) usually has an abrupt onset and is characterized by albuminuria, hematuria, hypertension, and edema. It is most common in children and in young adults, but can occur in the elderly. Acute glomerulonephritis is frequently preceded by an upper respiratory infection, hemolytic streptococcus, group A type 12 being the most common pathogen; however, the preceding infection may be a common cold, pneumococcal pneumonia, or a variety of other antigens. All glomeruli are usually involved, with epithelial crescent formation, periglomerular inflammation, and fibrinoid necrosis of glomeruli and their arterioles seen in the most severe cases.

The two most serious complications of acute glomerulonephritis are hypertensive encephalopathy and acute heart failure. There is usually no evidence of increased intracranial pressure in patients with hypertensive encephalopathy. The condition is readily reversed when blood pressure is lowered, suggesting that excessive cerebral vasoconstriction rather than cerebral edema is the cause. Heart failure associated with glomerulonephritis occurs as a result of increased demand on the heart secondary to hypervolemia and hypertension. Left ventricular failure can be life threatening, so immediate venesection and antihypertensive therapy are indicated.

Renal function tests provide an accurate guide to the severity of the lesion in glomerulonephritis, but the contribution of extrarenal factors that compromise renal function, such as vomiting and heart failure, must be taken into account. BUN is slightly elevated, but tubular function is normal and renal concentrating ability is unaffected. Twenty-four-hour urine volume is usually normal, but in severe cases oliguria may occur. In these cases hyperkalemia, acidosis, refractory anemia, or intercurrent infection may also be present. In addition to antihypertensive drugs, patients with severe glomerulonephritis may be taking digitalis, diuretics, large doses of corticosteroids, and antibiotics.

More than 90 per cent of patients with acute glomerulonephritis recover completely in three or four weeks. Two to 3 per cent of patients die in the acute phase, secondary to heart failure, cerebrovascular accident, renal failure, or infection. Seven or 8 per cent of patients develop chronic glomerulonephritis, the disease progressing either rapidly (2 to 10 years) or slowly (10 to 40 years), with death occurring from renal failure or the complications of hypertension. In patients with a slowly progressive clinical course, it is often difficult to obtain a history of a previous acute attack. Albuminuria and hypertension are the presenting signs, with the differential diagnosis including chronic pyelonephritis, ischemic renal disease, the residual lesion of toxemia of pregnancy, amyloid disease, renal artery stenosis, and diabetic nephrosclerosis.

Membranous glomerulonephritis (type II nephritis, glomerulocapillary nephritis, subacute parenchymatous nephritis, lipoid nephrosis) is an irreversible form of diffuse glomerulonephritis in which the glomerular lesion develops slowly throughout the course of the disease. Edema is the most prominent clinical feature, although proteinuria may be present for months or years before edema becomes obvious. The nephrotic syndrome (proteinuria, hypoproteinemia, and edema) is often present, although its duration and intensity are not related to the severity of the renal lesion. The onset of hypertension is gradual, with the severity comparable to the extent of the structural lesion.

There is no documented anesthetic experience in patients with glomerulonephritis. If proteinuria and hypertension are noted as incidental findings in a patient scheduled for elective surgery, the procedure should be deferred until an adequate renal workup can be performed. If acute glomerulonephritis is diagnosed, elective surgery should be postponed for approximately 30 days. Ninety per cent of patients will completely recover during that period of time. There is no advantage to postponing necessary elective surgery in patients with an established diagnosis of progressive acute glomerulonephritis or with membranous glomerulonephritis, because in these cases the lesion gradually worsens and complete recovery is rare. When emergency procedures are indicated in patients with acute glomerulonephritis, a careful evaluation of the cardiovascular system is indicated. Heart failure may be present but can be greatly improved by venesection. Removal of 500 to 1000 ml of blood may help to reduce blood pressure to normotensive levels.[76] Patients probably will be receiving antihypertensive medication, and possibly digitalis and corticosteroids as well, so the anesthesiologist should be aware of the interaction of anesthetic agents with these drugs. If impairment of renal function is minimal, then all anesthetic agents and techniques, with the exception of methoxyflurane, are acceptable. Spinal or epidural anesthesia may be particularly useful because of the sympathetic blockade and resulting internal phlebotomy that are produced by these techniques. If there is extensive renal damage, then particular care must be exercised in the choice and administration of anesthetic agents and adjunctive drugs (see section on Effect of Drugs in Patients with Reduced Renal Function).

PYELONEPHRITIS

Acute and chronic pyelonephritis are two of the most commonly diagnosed renal conditions in contemporary medicine. Acute pyelonephritis is characterized by the sudden onset of chills, a rise in body temperature to 102 to 105° F, dull pain in the kidney region, and symptoms of cystitis. The greatest significance of acute pyelonephritis to the anesthesiologist is that it may simulate surgical diseases of the gastrointestinal tract, most frequently appendicitis. Anesthetic management of patients with acute pyelonephritis requiring emergency surgery is aimed at reduction of body temperature and correction of dehydration, if present. Significant impairment of renal function is rarely present with the initial attack or early in the course of chronic pyelonephritis.

The term chronic pyelonephritis describes the late stage of recurrent bacterial infection of the kidney. However, many different disease processes may cause similar signs and symptoms, with renal functional and histological changes almost indistinguishable from those of chronic pyelonephritis. Some of these disease processes are 1) renal ischemia secondary to arteriosclerosis, renal artery stenosis, or renal infarction; 2) chronic interstitial nephritis secondary to analgesic (phenacetin) abuse or to hypersensitivity to compounds such as sulfanilamides or phenytoin (Dilantin); 3) radiation injury; and 4) obstruction. Histologically, the kidney of chronic pyelonephritis shows disproportionately greater changes in the tubules and interstitium than in the glomeruli. Tubules may show very severe changes, appearing damaged either directly by the acute inflammatory process or by ischemia subsequent to vascular narrowing.

Changes in renal function are directly related to the extent of renal involvement. There is disproportionate injury to medullary structures with early impairment of ability to concentrate urine. Excessive sodium and potassium loss, reduced ability to secrete a strongly acid urine, and inability to increase ammonia production in response to acidosis also have been described.

The most serious anesthetic problem in patients with long-standing chronic pyelonephritis is that of deranged fluid balance with dehydration and hypovolemia.[10] Because they are unable to concentrate urine effectively, patients with chronic pyelonephritis often have a daily urine output of 3 or more liters. If operated upon late in the day, they will have been without fluid intake for 14 or more hours, during which time urine and insensible water loss may exceed 2 liters. Replenishment of intravascular volume prior to induction of anesthesia with a solution such as Ringer's lactate is essential; otherwise, vasodilatation produced by induction of anesthesia will result in profound hypotension. Patients with chronic pyelonephritis present no other specific difficulties. Hypertension is not usually part of the syndrome, and renal insufficiency is a late complication.

RENAL PAPILLARY NECROSIS

Occasionally, in acute or chronic pyelonephritis a portion of medullary tissue, usually the tip of the papilla, becomes ischemic and sloughs away from the remainder of the kidney parenchyma. Formerly, this was thought to occur only rarely, accompanied by high fever, uncontrolled infection, and rapid deterioration in the clinical state. It was recognized in association with diabetes mellitus or urinary tract obstruction and was often a terminal event in patients with extensive chronic pyelonephritis and superimposed acute pyelonephritis. A more subtle form of renal papillary necrosis, recognizable by pyelography but not accompanied by manifestations of severe infection or clinical deterioration, is now known to occur most frequently in association with chronic abuse of phenacetin-containing analgesics. Renal papillary necrosis should not be considered as a disease entity in itself but rather as a manifestation of other disease processes.

NEPHROTIC SYNDROME

The nephrotic syndrome is also not a specific disease entity. The term signifies a stage in a variety of renal disorders in which proteinuria is severe enough to lead to hypoproteinemia and to cause metabolic responses that result in excessive retention of water and salt. Hence the triad of proteinuria, hypoproteinemia, and edema. Approximately 80 per cent of the cases of nephrotic syndrome are secondary to glomerulonephritis, with the remaining 20 per cent caused by metabolic, infectious, genetic, and autoimmune diseases, toxic agents, or obstructive vascular phenomena.

The formation of edema in the nephrotic syndrome is secondary to an increase in glomerular permeability. Serum proteins, primarily albumin, are lost in tubular fluid, ultimately appearing in the urine. As hypoalbuminemia progresses, there is diminished intravascular colloid osmotic pressure, resulting in sequestration of edema fluid into the interstitial space. Hypovolemia occurs and with it decreased RBF and GFR. These changes in renal hemodynamics and blood volume lead to increased aldosterone secretion with increased reabsorption of sodium and water and formation of additional edema fluid. As the disease progresses, hypertension also occurs.

Patients with the nephrotic syndrome occasionally present for emergency surgery. They may be receiving diuretics, steroids, and antihypertensive medications. Assessment of the circulatory status is critical. Measurement of central venous pressure will be helpful in determining whether hypovolemia is present. If so, albumin infusion, 25 to 50 gm, will help restore blood volume and probably lead to diuresis of edema fluid and reduction in BUN concentration. Preoperative measurement of renal function is valuable as a guide to the extent of the renal lesion. Potassium supplementation prior to surgery may be necessary owing to deficiencies secondary to the disease process itself or induced by administration of diuretics or corticosteroids. Low serum protein levels result in reduced protein binding of drugs such as thiopental; thus more drug is available to act at receptor sites.

DIABETES MELLITUS

Renal involvement in diabetes mellitus is common, with approximately 11 per cent of deaths in diabetics caused by renal failure. Lesions are most commonly found in the glomeruli but may also be seen in the tubules and arterioles. In addition, acute pyelonephritis is at least twice as common in diabetics as in nondiabetics. In the juvenile diabetic, evidence of renal involvement, manifested by proteinuria, appears 10 to 15 years after diabetes is diagnosed. Proteinuria, at first intermittent, becomes constant and massive, leading to the nephrotic syndrome. Azotemia and hypertension are late manifestations of diabetic nephropathy. Death occurs approximately three years after the nephrotic syndrome develops. In adult onset diabetes mellitus, the course of renal disease is not so rapid, but death from renal failure may occur. Necrotizing papillitis may be present in either juvenile or adult onset diabetes. This is a severe type of pyelonephritis in which the vascular supply of the papilla is compromised by thrombosis secondary to infection or vascular lesions in the renal medulla. Preoperative renal function studies should be obtained in diabetic patients to determine whether renal disease is present and, if so, the extent to which it has progressed.

RHEUMATOID ARTHRITIS

Uremia is the cause of death in approximately 25 per cent of patients with rheumatoid arthritis. Several different primary renal lesions have been noted. Focal glomerulonephritis is the most common, with renal amyloidosis the next most frequent. Chronic interstitial nephritis and renal papillary necrosis related to analgesic abuse were found in 22 per cent of a series of 80 patients with rheumatoid arthritis. Specific rheumatoid vascular lesions and gold-induced renal lesions also have been noted in the kidneys of patients with rheumatoid arthritis. As with other collagen diseases, hypertension is frequent, so patients may be receiving antihypertensive medication in addition to corticosteroids and salicylates. The latter drug may interfere with coagulation by causing inhibition of platelet agglutination. Since tubular disease is common in rheumatoid arthritis, patients tend to lose large quantities of salt and water. Vigorous hydration prior to induction of anesthesia may be necessary. Renal function studies should be obtained in patients with rheumatoid arthritis to determine whether renal involvement is present.

GOUT

Renal failure is the cause of death in approximately 25 per cent of patients with primary gout. Several types of lesions are seen: interstitial nephritis, advanced arteriosclerosis, and nephrosclerosis associated with hypertension; tubular hydronephrosis secondary to tophus formation; and glomerulosclerosis.

About 40 per cent of patients with gout have some form of renal involvement as manifested by albuminuria, cylindruria, low GFR, or elevated BUN concentration. Renal involvement is progressive, and all stages may be seen. Preoperative evaluation of renal function in all patients with gout is essential. Following surgery, there may be an exacerbation of the symptoms of gout, especially in patients with decreased renal function, because they are unable to excrete the increased load of uric acid resulting from surgical catabolism.

Methoxyflurane administration results in an increase in serum uric acid.[17] This may lead to an exacerbation of gout, so methoxyflurane administration to patients with this disease is contraindicated.

SYSTEMIC LUPUS ERYTHEMATOSUS (SLE)

Approximately two thirds of patients with SLE have renal involvement, most commonly demonstrating glomerular lesions. Some patients show only mild focal changes in the glomerular tuft and may recover completely with steroid therapy. Others have more severe, proliferative, membranous processes of glomeruli with necrosis, interstitial infiltration, edema, fibrosis, and tubu-

lar damage. These patients tend to have a poor prognosis. Patients with advanced SLE are invariably receiving antihypertensive medication and corticosteroids. Because the natural history of the disease is one of periods of activity and remission, careful assessment must be made to ensure that elective surgery is done during a quiescent period.

PERIARTERITIS NODOSA

Renal involvement in periarteritis nodosa is frequent, with glomerular lesions predominating. Functional impairment may range from mild to total renal failure. Hypertension is usually a feature of this disease. Patients may be taking antihypertensive medications as well as large doses of corticosteroids. Prognosis in patients with periarteritis nodosa is variable, so nonemergency surgery is best deferred until the progress of the disease is determined.

OTHER SYSTEMIC DISEASES

Renal involvement is common in many systemic diseases, such as subacute bacterial endocarditis, amyloidosis, myelomatosis, hepatic cirrhosis, leukemia, sickle cell disease, macroglobulinemia, sarcoidosis, Henoch-Schönlein purpura, and Marfan's syndrome. Glomerular lesions are seen in most of these diseases, but tubular and vascular lesions can occur. Assessment of renal status is important in the preanesthetic evaluation of the patient. Urinalysis and blood urea nitrogen or serum creatinine determination are the most valuable laboratory tests.

NEPHROTOXINS

The kidney is particularly susceptible to damage from drugs or poisons because of its rich blood supply, increased concentration of excreted compounds in renal tubular cells during reabsorption or secretion, and concentration of fluids in the renal medulla. The amount of damage produced by nephrotoxins depends on many factors, such as the duration and intensity of exposure, the degree of toxin binding to plasma protein and tissues other than kidney, the degree and duration of binding to renal tissue, and the rapidity of renal or extrarenal elimination. Toxic damage to the kidney may be either acute or chronic, may predominantly affect glomerular or tubular function or cause generalized renal damage, and can be manifested by anuria, oliguria, or polyuria. An extensive review on the subject of toxic nephropathy has been written by Schreiner and Maher.[77]

Methoxyflurane Nephrotoxicity. In 1966, Crandell et al. reported 16 cases of toxic nephropathy among 94 patients receiving methoxyflurane anesthesia.[16] The condition was characterized by polyuria, hypernatremia, increased serum osmolality, elevated BUN concentration, and excessive weight loss. Patients were unable to elaborate a concentrated urine following water deprivation or pitressin administration. In a later randomized, prospective evaluation of methoxyflurane administration in patients without renal disease, Mazze et al. confirmed Crandell's findings.[17] In six of 12 patients receiving methoxyflurane-oxygen anesthesia, a syndrome characterized by polyuria, lack of responsiveness to pitressin infusion, marked weight loss, and delayed return to preoperative concentrating ability was observed. Also noted were hypernatremia, serum hyperosmolality, elevated BUN, increased serum creatinine, increased serum uric acid, and a decrease in uric acid clearance. Subsequent studies related nephrotoxicity to the degree of methoxyflurane metabolism.[45] Two toxic metabolites, inorganic fluoride and oxalic acid, were identified, with the former most likely causing renal dysfunction associated with methoxyflurane anesthesia. Development of an animal model in Fischer 344 rats confirmed the role of inorganic fluoride as the primary nephrotoxin and further showed the lesion to be dose related.[78] Fluoride acts as a nephrotoxin probably by interfering with the development of a hypertonic interstitial renal medulla, abolishing the environment necessary for the functioning of the countercurrent system of urinary concentration and dilution. High concentrations of fluoride may bring about these changes by inhibiting Na^+ and K^+ ATPase, the activity of which is essential for the function of the ion pump in the ascending limb of the loop of Henle. Also, fluoride is a potent vasodilator, so it may interfere with function of the countercurrent system

by causing an increase in medullary blood flow; this would result in a washout of sodium from the medullary interstitium and would abolish its hypertonicity. It is unlikely that lack of ADH is a factor in the concentrating defect, as polyuria after either methoxyflurane anesthesia or fluoride injection is resistant to vasopressin administration.[78] The lesion is not due to molecular, that is, unbiotransformed methoxyflurane, and treatment with barbiturates prior to methoxyflurane administration increases the extent of renal damage.[79] The lesion in man also appears to be dose-related.[80] However, toxic interaction with antibiotics such as tetracycline and gentamicin and other potentially nephrotoxic drugs may cause renal damage even when methoxyflurane dosage is low.[81-83]

Because of its potential for adverse renal effects there should be clear indications for the use of methoxyflurane whenever it is selected for administration. Generally speaking, methoxyflurane should not be administered for procedures lasting more than two hours as the sole agent for producing muscle relaxation in patients with kidney disease, in patients receiving enzyme-inducing drugs, or in patients having operative procedures that might normally be expected to compromise renal function.

Enflurane is also metabolized to inorganic fluoride but to a much lesser extent than methoxyflurane.[31, 51, 52] Its administration is accompanied by a clinically insignificant urinary concentrating defect.[52] At the present time, enflurane is not considered a nephrotoxin. When indicated, it may be administered to patients with mild to moderately advanced renal disease.[53]

Approximately 50 per cent of toxic nephropathies are due to poisoning with heavy metals or organic solvents. Mercury, carbon tetrachloride, ethylene glycol, and radiologic contrast media are the most common offenders. The type of damage varies with the nephrotoxin; carbon tetrachloride causes acute proximal tubular necrosis with rapid development of oliguric renal failure; ethylene glycol is metabolized to oxalic acid, which is then deposited within the renal parenchyma as calcium oxalate crystals, producing marked proximal tubular dilation and obstruction; sulfonamides form insoluble crystals that are deposited within the renal tubules, pelvis, and ureters; radiologic contrast media have caused acute tubular necrosis following oral administration for visualization of the gallbladder and after intravenous injection for pyelography or arteriography; streptomycin, vancomycin, kanamycin, and neomycin share the common property of eighth cranial nerve damage and nephrotoxicity. Bacitracin, polymyxin, colistin, gentamicin, amphotericin B, and tetracycline produce tubular damage that in its severest form may result in acute tubular necrosis. Tetracycline nephrotoxicity is due to its deterioration with formation of anhydrotetracycline and epianhydrotetracycline. However, renal lesions have been reported even following the administration of fresh tetracycline.

Kidney damage in acute metal nephropathies usually affects the proximal convoluted tubule, with glycosuria, aminoaciduria, and excessive urinary loss of phosphate and urate occurring in the majority of patients. There is also impaired acidification of the urine, excessive urinary loss of potassium, and impaired urinary concentrating ability. Glomerular changes are rarely seen in acute metal nephropathies, but they may be seen in chronic metal nephropathies. The nephrotic syndrome may occur following mercury, gold, or thallium poisoning. Heavy metal poisoning is treated by the administration of ethylenediaminetetra-acetate (EDTA).

Nephropathies secondary to drugs, poisons, and heavy metal may interest the anesthesiologist in several ways. He may be called upon to anesthetize patients who have been receiving large doses of antibiotics or who have had frequent doses of radiographic contrast media for diagnostic purposes. These drugs are particularly hazardous in patients with renal impairment, as their excretion may be reduced and toxic levels may develop rapidly. Patients with toxic nephropathies may also require emergency surgery. They should be treated as outlined in the section on Effects of Drugs in Patients with Reduced Renal Function.

ACUTE RENAL FAILURE

Acute renal failure (acute tubular necrosis, ATN, lower nephron nephrosis) is defined as the sudden inability of the kidneys to vary urine volume and content appropriately in response to homeostatic needs.[84]

The causes of acute renal failure may be divided into three broad categories, based on the predominant antecedent factor, viz., circulatory problems impairing renal perfusion (prerenal), primary renal disease (renal), and obstruction of the urinary tract (postrenal). Inevitably there is some overlapping between these three groups.

The diagnosis of acute renal failure is made when urinary flow remains below 20 ml per hour in a patient who is adequately hydrated, has stable blood pressure, and has a patent urinary outflow tract. The urine that is formed has increased sodium content, a characteristic sediment when examined microscopically, and very little urea when compared with the rising blood urea content.[84]

The most obvious problem arising from acute renal failure is the inability to maintain the dynamic balance between dietary intake of food and water and production of waste products. The abnormalities that occur are summarized as follows:[85]

1. There is a progressive rise in serum urea, creatinine, uric acid, some amino and organic acids, polypeptides, sulfate, and phosphate.

2. Serum potassium rises 0.3 to 3 mEq per liter per day except when there is concomitant loss from diarrhea or vomiting.

3. Serum sodium and calcium usually fall.

4. Hypermagnesemia is frequent.

5. Serum proteins are decreased.

6. Total reducing substance in the serum is consistently elevated and true hyperglycemia is common. This may be either sensitive or resistant to insulin.

7. Elevation of total lipids, cholesterol, phosphorus, and neutral fats occurs.

8. Elevation of hydrogen ion concentration is consistently present.

The kidney is an endocrine as well as an excretory organ. Disorders of renin-angiotensin and aldosterone secretion occur and are in part responsible for the hypertension that ensues. Reduced erythropoietin production results in anemia, low platelet count, and clotting abnormalities.

Heart failure and abnormalities in liver function are often present in patients with renal shutdown. Infection is common and difficult to treat because of altered excretion of antibiotics, with rapid development of toxic levels of these drugs.

Oliguria may persist for as long as a

month (usually 10 to 18 days) before diuresis occurs, signifying the beginning of the recovery phase. During the diuretic phase, urine volume gradually increases until as much as 5 or 6 liters of urine are produced daily. Management of the patient is directed at maintaining fluid and electrolyte balance in the face of these large losses. Finally, concentrating ability gradually returns toward normal.

In many patients this sequence of events does not occur and death ultimately ensues from arrhythmias, bleeding, or infection. The mortality rate from acute renal failure has been reduced in recent years, in part because of earlier and more frequent dialysis, but it is still greater than 25 per cent. The most significant feature determining survival is the condition of the patient prior to the onset of acute renal failure, probably explaining the 85 per cent survival associated with renal failure in pregnancy.

A variation of the aforementioned syndrome is nonoliguric acute renal failure.[86] In this condition the antecedent causes may be the same as in classic oliguric renal failure but an oliguric or anuric phase is never identifiable. Polyuria occurs, accompanied by an increase in BUN and serum creatinine concentrations as well as decreases in other indices of renal function. Prognosis is better in nonoliguric renal failure, as the therapeutic difficulties of the oliguric phase are not encountered. This condition is similar to the syndrome seen in patients suffering renal dysfunction following methoxyflurane anesthesia.[16, 17]

ACUTE RENAL FAILURE DUE TO PRERENAL CAUSES

It is in this group of patients that the anesthesiologist has a unique opportunity to reduce the incidence of renal failure and to favorably influence the outcome of incipient renal failure. Although the pathophysiology of renal failure is not completely understood, several points seem clear. The renal circulation is one of the first to be compromised when circulatory homeostasis is threatened. There is diminution of total renal blood flow with a significant shift of distribution from the rapid flow compartment, thought to represent superficial cortical flow, to the deeper regions of the kidney.[37, 87] This sustained preglomerular vasoconstriction causes a reduction in renal cortical perfusion sufficient to markedly reduce glomerular perfusion. The small quantity of filtered fluid is quickly and almost completely reabsorbed in the proximal tubule. Consequently, there is a loss of intratubular volume and pressure and a tendency for the tubules to collapse. In some cases, interstitial edema and precipitation of solute in the tubules further compromise excretory function. This sequence leads to additional ischemia and finally to necrosis of the tubular epithelium.[88]

If renal vasoconstriction and ischemia can be reversed early in their course, or prevented by prophylactic measures in high risk patients, then the classic picture of acute renal failure may not develop.[10, 89-91] Situations accompanied by a definable incidence of renal failure are as follows:

1. Cardiopulmonary bypass or surgery of the aorta.[92-94]
2. Major biliary tree surgery.[95]
3. Procedures in which large volumes of blood may be transfused.[73]
4. Hypovolemic hypotension.[97]
5. Lengthy or extensive surgical procedures in older patients.[98]
6. Surgery in patients with pre-existing renal disease.[10, 99]
7. Obstetric complications such as abruptio placentae.[88]
8. Major trauma.[96, 100]
9. Transfusion of mismatched blood.[100]

In some patients with these conditions, vigorous preoperative and intraoperative hydration will prevent renal complications.[89, 93] In others, hydration and administration of diuretics may be of value in reversing oliguria and preventing development of acute renal failure.[97]

In patients in whom the risk of renal failure is high, the importance of urine output as a vital sign is equal to that of pulse rate, respiratory rate, and blood pressure. An indwelling urethral catheter should be inserted prior to surgery, and hourly urinary volume should be measured. Correction of fluid volume losses should be carried out with appropriate crystalloid and colloid solutions, including blood. Prior to induction of anesthesia, a fluid load of Ringer's lactate or a similar solution equal to 10 ml per kg of body weight should be infused. This should be followed each hour by intraoperative infusion of maintenance fluids equal to urinary output plus 5 ml per kg of body weight.

If urinary output is less than 75 to 100 ml per hour with this regimen, then provided that signs of circulatory overload are not present, intravenous mannitol, 12.5 to 20 gm, should be administered within a five minute period. If the initial response to this therapy is positive but urine output decreases again, then a 20 per cent mannitol drip should be started and infused at a rate necessary to maintain urine flow at 75 to 100 ml per hour.[13] Alternatively, furosemide, 20 to 40 mg, administered intravenously, may be of value. Recently, dopamine in low doses, 1 to 5 μg per kg per minute, has been recommended for the treatment of oliguria.[101] Even in the absence of heart failure this drug may increase RBF. However, in doses higher than 10 to 20 μg per kg per minute the alpha adrenergic stimulating effect of dopamine may predominate and RBF may decrease. If there is no response or only a partial response to fluid, diuretic, and dopamine therapy, then the clinical situation must be reevaluated. Acute renal failure may have occurred and a restrictive fluid regimen may be necessary.

Emergency or urgent surgery is occasionally indicated in patients with acute renal failure. Whenever possible, dialysis should be carried out the day before operation. Spinal and epidural anesthesia should not be administered if clotting abnormalities are present, but other regional techniques may be useful. Endotracheal intubation should be avoided when possible because of the danger of producing hemorrhage in the airway of patients with bleeding tendencies. Drugs should be administered, based on considerations outlined in the section on Effects of Drugs in Patients with Reduced Renal Function.

For additional information pertaining to the problems of anesthesia in patients with acute renal failure, the reviews of Vandam et al., Jacobson et al., and Mazze should be consulted.[71, 102, 103] General considerations pertaining to treatment of renal failure can be found in the monograph by Merrill.[85]

DIALYSIS AND RENAL TRANSPLANTATION

The steady improvement in techniques of hemodialysis, from the first artificial kidney developed in 1944 by Kolff and Bert[104] to the current practice of home dialysis,[105] has resulted in additional years of productive life for patients with chronic renal failure. It has also increased the frequency with which the anesthesiologist meets patients on dialysis programs, not only for renal transplantation but also for surgery unrelated to renal disease.

DIALYSIS

Only two techniques are presently used, peritoneal dialysis and hemodialysis. The dialysis principle involves equilibration of waste products in the patient's blood across a semipermeable membrane to the dialysis bath. The dialysis fluid may be hypertonic or hypotonic to plasma, resulting in removal or addition of fluid to the patient's extracellular fluid volume. In peritoneal dialysis the patient's peritoneum is used as the exchange membrane, avoiding the need for vascular cannulas and expensive equipment. Peritonitis is a constant danger, and pain during dialysis may be severe. Future refinement may make this a cheap and acceptable form of chronic dialysis.

Hemodialysis is by far the most common dialysis technique used today. Short Teflon or silicone rubber-shunted cannulas are permanently inserted in the forearm or lower leg, employing local infiltration anesthesia. Several anesthetic precautions are appropriate. Uremic patients may be debilitated, in which case smaller doses of all drugs, including local anesthetics, should be administered. Hyperkalemia, acidosis, and overhydration can combine to cause myocardial irritability; therefore, local anesthetic solutions containing epinephrine should be used with caution. In addition, epinephrine-induced vasoconstriction may make cannula insertion more difficult. Brachial plexus block may greatly facilitate introduction of the cannula by producing excellent analgesia and peripheral vasodilatation; however, caution must be exercised not to exceed safe dosage limitations.

In the interval between treatments, clotting does not occur because the shunted circuit is short and blood flow is rapid (150 to 300 ml per minute). During hemodialysis, which is performed two or three times weekly and may require 10 to 14 hours, both the patient and the external circuit are heparinized to prevent clotting. Serial serum electrolyte and hematocrit determinations should be carried out and abnormalities corrected by altering the dialysis bath fluid.

RENAL TRANSPLANTATION

Dialysis and transplantation are complementary to the treatment of chronic renal failure, because dialysis is needed to restore the patient to the best possible condition prior to surgery.

Selection, Preparation, and Anesthetic Management of the Donor. The ideal donor is a monozygotic twin, because no immunologic problems arise following transplantation. However, five year survival rates of greater than 70 per cent can also be expected with genetically related donors and immunosuppressive drug therapy.[106] It is important to remember that donors are subjected to an operation that they do not require for their own physical well-being; therefore, they must be in optimal condition prior to surgery. The greatest risk is from surgical hemorrhage, so blood and appropriate intravenous channels must be available should transfusion be necessary. It is the responsibility of all physicians involved in donor care to be sure that their patients understand the risks involved and that they have given legal authorization for the operation.

Choice of anesthetic agent for the donor does not appear to be critical; however, deep anesthesia with hypotension should be avoided, as it will cause greater depression of renal function, particularly urinary flow, than light anesthesia in the transplanted kidney.[13] Muscle relaxants may be administered as for any other operative procedure. An adequate amount of balanced salt solution should be administered to ensure brisk urinary flow from the donor kidney. It may be advisable not to administer drugs solely dependent upon the kidneys for excretion, because donors will acutely lose 50 per cent of their renal tissue. Although the remaining kidney can usually maintain normal function, excretory reserve is diminished. This could become significant if homeostasis is threatened, e.g., by spasm of renal vessels caused by aortic manipulation or by sudden hemorrhage.

Preoperative Treatment of the Recipient. Bilateral nephrectomy is usually performed prior to kidney transplantation to help control hypertension and infection. If possible, both nephrectomy and transplantation should be accomplished before the patient develops complications of advanced renal disease such as infection, pericarditis, and peripheral neuropathy. Hemodialysis in the 24 hours prior to transplantation will result in the patient being in the best possible condition at the time of operation. Patients have a normochromic, normocytic anemia that should be corrected during dialysis by transfusion of packed red blood cells.[108] However, hemoglobin levels of more than 9 to 10 gm per cent are difficult to attain and should not be a therapeutic aim because of the danger of producing circulatory overload. Normal bleeding time, serum creatinine concentration below 10 mg per cent, and BUN less than 60 mg per cent can be expected following hemodialysis. Serum potassium concentration should be reduced to 4.0 to 5.0 mEq per liter. Metabolic acidosis is infrequent following adequate dialysis. Prior to dialysis, hypertension may be present, and heart failure, pericardial effusion, pleural effusion, and pulmonary congestion may also be in evidence. Digitalis administration is extremely hazardous because of the danger of digitalis toxicity caused by diminished excretion and by alterations in electrolyte balance associated with hemodialysis.[70]

When the donor kidney is from a cadaver, there is less time for adequate preoperative preparation of the recipient.[61, 109] Nephrectomy and transplantation may have to be done as a combined procedure. Increased intraoperative morbidity and mortality can be anticipated owing to the greater magnitude of preoperative biochemical derangement and the prolonged anesthesia and surgery times.[110] Intravenous infusion of glucose-insulin solution or rectal instillation of sodium-loaded cation exchange resins will help to reduce elevated serum potassium concentration. Mild acidosis is usually well tolerated; however, bicarbonate levels should not be allowed to fall below 20 mEq per liter. Sodium bicarbonate rather than lactate is preferable for correcting deficits, because lactate is not well metabolized in uremia.[42] In spite of these therapeutic measures, the patient's general condition will not improve as much as after full preoperative hemodialysis; this should be strived for in all cases. In recent years, methods of extracorporeal perfusion and preservation have been developed that have extended viability of cadaver kidneys beyond 48 hours, so renal transplantation in less than optimally prepared patients should occur with diminishing frequency.[111]

Anesthetic Management of the Recipient. A number of reviews have been written on this subject, and they should be read for a more detailed discussion.[70, 97, 109, 112] Premedication for nephrectomy or transplantation should be with reduced doses of the usual agents. Ideally, the patient will have been dialyzed the day prior to surgery, so the dialysis record should be examined to note changes in body weight and vital signs and to determine whether blood has been administered. A reduction in body weight of several pounds, accompanied by an increase in hematocrit out of proportion to the number of blood transfusions administered, should alert the anesthesiologist to the possibility that the patient may be hypovolemic.

General anesthesia is usually employed for nephrectomy, whereas both general and regional anesthesia have been administered with good results for transplantation.[61, 70, 109, 110, 112] The denervated kidney may be more responsive to circulating catecholamines than if normally innervated,[113] so agents that cause catecholamine release — cyclopropane and ether[18] — should be administered with caution. Muscle relaxants excreted completely by the kidney — gallamine and decamethonium—should not be administered to the recipient. Succinylcholine administration may result in prolonged neuromuscular block because reductions in pseudocholinesterase levels have been reported to occur following hemodialysis.[61, 62, 115] However, it has been safely administered both for intubation and intraoperative relaxation in patients with absent renal function. Hyperkalemia following succinylcholine administration does not appear to be a problem in uremic patients on dialysis, because the rise in serum potassium concentration is no greater than in patients without renal disease.[63, 116] However, it is not known if even small rises in serum potassium concentration in nondia-

lyzed, hyperkalemic patients will cause arrhythmias. Curare and pancuronium are primarily excreted by the kidney, and cases of prolonged paralysis have been reported with both, usually after administration of usual or even larger than usual doses. Recurarization has been reported in both drugs, probably because the duration of action of neostigmine is less than that of the muscle relaxants in patients with renal failure.[117] It should be emphasized, however, that succinylcholine, curare, and pancuronium have all been administered safely to patients with renal failure when dosages are reduced and a neuromuscular function monitor is used to assess the extent of blockade. Based on considerations of renal function and drug excretion, a satisfactory anesthetic technique would include thiopental for induction of anesthesia, succinylcholine for endotracheal intubation, halothane, 50 per cent N_2O and oxygen for maintenance of anesthesia, and pancuronium for intraoperative relaxation. As noted in the introductory section, a technique including droperidol may have a beneficial effect on renal perfusion, but experience with this drug in patients with impaired renal function is not well documented.

There is a theoretical advantage in using regional techniques; because muscle relaxants are not required, endotracheal intubation and the attendant possibility of respiratory infection are avoided, and fewer depressant drugs are required. In addition, the block may be kept low, because the procedure is entirely extraperitoneal and in the lower half of the abdomen. However, the technique of continuous intra- and postoperative local heparinization of the transplanted kidney may contraindicate the use of continuous regional techniques.[106, 107] Hypotension is not reported to occur with regional anesthesia if adequate hydration has been carried out prior to administration of the block.[118] However, if hypotension does occur, direct-acting pressor agents (norepinephrine, methoxamine, phenylephrine) should be avoided, as they reduce renal perfusion. Of the centrally acting pressors, dopamine and methylamphetamine have been shown to increase RBF,[71, 101] although isoproterenol may also be beneficial owing to its positive inotropic and chronotropic effects on the heart and relaxing effect on peripheral blood vessels. Atropine alone may be sufficient to restore blood pressure if hypotension is accompanied by bradycardia.

Fluid administration must be carried out with the knowledge that anephric patients frequently have either increased or decreased blood volume. Systemic arterial and central venous pressure (CVP), pulse rate, and auscultation of the chest should be used as guide lines for fluid replacement. Hypovolemia should be suspected if examination of the previous day's dialysis record shows an increase in hematocrit out of proportion to the amount of transfused blood; it is confirmed by a greater than expected acute fall in central venous and arterial pressure following induction of anesthesia. Hypervolemia is recognized by a rise in CVP and signs of pulmonary congestion. Adequate hydration should ensure a copious diuresis when the arterial anastomosis is completed if ischemia time of the transplanted kidney has been brief.

The recipient and donor are frequently anesthetized in the same or adjacent operating rooms to ensure maximal coordination of the two surgical teams. The donor kidney is placed extraperitoneally in the recipient's contralateral iliac fossa.[119] The renal artery is anastomosed to the internal iliac artery, the renal vein to either the external or common iliac vein, and the ureter to the bladder. When ischemia time is short, approximately 30 minutes, diuresis ensues, with initial urinary output occasionally greater than 1 liter per hour. If ischemia time is two or more hours, as in cadaver kidney transplantation, a variable period of oliguria or anuria may occur. The use of mannitol or furosemide is indicated in these patients. Immunosuppressive therapy is commenced at the time of operation, employing large doses of drugs such as azathioprine (Imuran) and prednisone. The former may cause leukopenia, in addition to suppressing antibody formation, thereby rendering the patient more susceptible to infection.

Renal function after successful transplantation follows one of several patterns. There may be a brisk diuresis with adequate excretion of waste products, the only major postoperative problem being to avoid dehydration and electrolyte imbalance. In other cases, despite a high rate of urine flow, metabolic products accumulate, with renal function resembling that seen in the early diuretic phase of acute tubular necrosis. Hemodialysis is not necessary, because a recovery phase soon follows. A third general pattern is one of variable periods of anuria or oliguria, followed by a diuretic phase and then recovery of renal function. Postoperative management is aimed at avoiding fluid and electrolyte imbalance, employing hemodialysis whenever necessary to assist the patient in excreting toxic products of metabolism.

REFERENCES

1. Burnett, C. H., Bloomberg, E. L., Shortz, G., Compton, D. W., and Beecher, H. K.: A comparison of the effects of ether and cyclopropane anesthesia on renal function of man. J. Pharmacol. Exp. Ther. 96:380, 1949.
2. Habif, D. V., Papper, E. M., Fitzpatrick, H. F., Lowrance, P. M., Smythe, C., and Bradley, S. E.: The renal and hepatic blood flow, glomerular filtration rate, and urinary output of electrolytes during cyclopropane, ether, and thiopental anesthesia, operation, and the immediate postoperative period. Surgery 30:341, 1951.
3. Miles, B. E., De Wardener, H. E., Churchill-Davidson, H. C., and Wylie, W. D.: The effect on the renal circulation of pentamethonium bromide during anesthesia. Clin. Sci. 11:73, 1952.
4. Mazze, R. I., Schwartz, F. D., Slocum, H. C., and Barry, K. G.: Renal function during anesthesia and surgery. I. The effects of halothane anesthesia. Anesthesiology 24:279, 1963.
5. Deutsch, S., Goldberg, M., Stephen, G. W., and Wu, W.: Effects of halothane anesthesia on renal function in normal man. Anesthesiology 26:793, 1966.
6. Gorman, H. M., and Craythorne, N. W. B.: The effects of a new neuroleptanalgesic agent (Innovar) on renal function in man. Acta Anaesth. Scand. (Suppl) 24:111, 1966.
7. Deutsch, S., Pierce, E. C., Jr, and Vandam, L. D.: Cyclopropane effects on renal function in normal man. Anesthesiology 28:547, 1967.
8. Hayes, M. A., and Goldenberg, I. S.: Renal effects of anesthesia and operation mediated by endocrines. Anesthesiology 24:487, 1963.
9. Barry, K. G., Mazze, R. I., and Schwartz, F. D.: Prevention of surgical oliguria and renal-hemodynamic suppression by sustained hydration. N. Engl. J. Med. 270:1371, 1964.
10. Seitzman, D. M., Mazze, R. I., Schwartz, F. D., and Barry, K. G.: Mannitol diuresis: A method of renal protection during surgery. J. Urol. 90:139, 1963.
11. Boba, A., and Landmesser, C. M.: Renal complications after anesthesia and operation. Anesthesiology 22:781, 1961.
12. Hutchin, P., McLaughlin, J. S., and Hayes, M. A.: Renal response to acidosis during anesthesia

and operation. Ann. Surg. *154*:9, 145, 161, 1962.

13. Mazze, R. I., and Barry, K. G.: Prevention of functional renal failure during anesthesia and surgery by sustained hydration and mannitol infusion. Anesth. Analg. *46*:61, 1967.

14. Papper, E. M., and Ngai, S. H.: Kidney function during anesthesia. Ann. Rev. Med. *7*:213, 1956.

15. Andersen, N. B.: Effect of general anesthetics on sodium transport in the isolated toad bladder. Anesthesiology *27*:304, 1966.

16. Crandell, W. B., Pappas, S. G., and Macdonald, A.: Nephrotoxicity associated with methoxyflurane anesthesia. Anesthesiology *27*:591, 1966.

17. Mazze, R. I., Shue, G. L., and Jackson, S. H.: Renal dysfunction associated with methoxyflurane anesthesia: A randomized prospective clinical evaluation. J.A.M.A. *216*:278, 1971.

18. Price, H. L., Linde, H. W., Jones, R. E., Black, G. W., and Price, M. L.: Sympathoadrenal responses to general anesthesia in man and their relation to hemodynamics. Anesthesiology *20*:563, 1959.

19. Janssen, P. A. J., Niemegeers, J. E., Schellekens, K. H. L., Verbruggen, F. J., and van Neuten, J. M.: The pharmacology of dehydrobenzperidol, a new potent and short acting neuroleptic agent chemically related to haloperidol. Arzneimittel-Forsch *13*:205, 1963.

20. Berne, R. M.: Hemodynamics and sodium excretion of denervated kidney in anesthetized and unanesthetized dog. Am. J. Physiol. *171*:148, 1952.

21. Shipley, R. E., and Study, R. S.: Changes in renal blood flow, extraction of inulin, glomerular filtration rate, tissue pressure and urine flow with acute alterations of renal artery blood pressure. Am. J. Physiol. *167*:676, 1951.

22. Bastron, R. D., Perkins, F. M., and Pyne, J. L.: Autoregulation of renal blood flow during halothane anesthesia. Anesthesiology *46*:142, 1977.

23. Robertson, G. L.: Vasopressin in osmotic regulation in man. Ann. Rev. Med. *25*:315, 1974.

24. Moran, W. H., and Zimmerman, B.: Mechanism of antidiuretic hormone control of importance to the surgical patient. Surgery *62*:639, 1967.

25. Philbin, D. M., and Coggins, C. H.: Plasma antidiuretic hormone levels in cardiac surgical patients during morphine and halothane anesthesia. Anesthesiology *49*:95, 1978.

26. Jacobson, W. E., Hammarsten, J. F., Heller, B. I.: The effects of adrenaline upon renal function and electrolyte excretion. J. Clin. Invest. *30*:1503, 1951.

27. Pettinger, W., Tanaka, K., Keeton, K., et al.: Renin release, an artifact of anesthesia and its implications in rats. Proc. Soc. Exp. Biol. Med. *148*:625, 1975.

28. Miller, E. D., Jr, Longnecker, D. E., and Peach, M. J.: The regulatory function of the renin-angiotensin system during general anesthesia. Anesthesiology *48*:399, 1978.

29. Robertson, J. D., Swan, A. A. B., and Whitteridge, D.: Effect of anesthetics on systemic baroreceptors. J. Physiol. Lond. *131*:463, 1956.

30. Price, H. L., and Widdicombe, J.: Actions of cyclopropane on carotid sinus baroreceptors and carotid body chemoreceptors. J. Pharmacol. Exp. Ther. *135*:233, 1962.

31. Cousins, M. J., Greenstein, L. R., Hitt, B. A., and Mazze, R. I.: Metabolism and renal effects of enflurane in man. Anesthesiology *44*:44, 1976.

32. Mazze, R. I., Cousins, M. J., and Barr, G. A.: Renal effects and metabolism of isoflurane in man. Anesthesiology *40*:536, 1974.

33. Deutsch, S., Bastron, R. D., Pierce, E. C., Jr., and Vandam, L. D.: The effects of anaesthesia with thiopentone, nitrous oxide, narcotics and neuromuscular blocking drugs on renal function in normal man. Br. J. Anaesth. *41*:807, 1969.

34. Auberger, V. H., and Heinrich, J.: Methoxyflurane und Nierenfunktion. Der Anaesthesist *14*:202, 1965.

35. Cousins, M. J., and Mazze, R. I.: Anaesthesia, surgery and renal function. Anaesth. Intensive Care *1*:355, 1973.

36. Bastron, R. D., and Deutsch, S.: Anesthesia and the Kidney. New York, Grune and Stratton, 1976.

37. Larson, C. P., Jr., Mazze, R. I., Cooperman, L. H., and Wollman, H.: Effects of anesthetics on cerebral, renal and splanchnic circulation. Anesthesiology *41*:169, 1974.

38. Elkinton, J. R., McCurdy, D. K., Buckalew, V. M., Jr.: Hydrogen ion and the kidney. *In* Black, D. A. K. (ed.): Renal Disease. 2nd ed., Philadelphia, F. A. Davis Co., 1967, pp. 110–133.

39. Wirz, V. H., Hargitay, B., and Kuhn, W.: Lokalisation des Konzentrierungsprozesses in der Niere durch direkte Kryoskopie. Helv. Physiol. Acta *9*:196, 1951.

40. Kleeman, C. R., Adams, D., and Maxwell, M. H.: The defect in urinary dilution associated with chronic renal disease. Clin. Res. *7*:77, 1959.

41. Hardwicke, J., and Soothill, J. F.: Proteinuria. *In* Black, D. A. K. (ed.): Renal Disease. 2nd ed., Philadelphia, F. A. Davis Co., 1967, pp. 252–274.

42. Schreiner, G. E., and Maher, J. F.: Uremia: Biochemistry and Pathogenesis; Treatment. Springfield, Ill., Charles C Thomas, 1961.

43. Feldman, S. A., Cohen, E. N., and Golling, R. C.: The excretion of gallamine in the dog. Anesthesiology *30*:593, 1969.

44. Fingl, E., and Woodbury, D. M.: General principles. *In* Goodman, L. S., and Gilman, A. (eds.): The Pharmacological Basis of Therapeutics. 4th ed. New York, Macmillan Co., 1970, pp. 1–35.

45. Mazze, R. I., Trudell, J. R., and Cousins, M. J.: Methoxyflurane metabolism and renal dysfunction: Clinical correlation in man. Anesthesiology *35*:247, 1971.

46. Reidenberg, M. M.: Renal Function and Drug Action. 1st ed., Philadelphia, W. B. Saunders Co., 1971.

47. Foster, C. A.: Sedative and hypnotic drugs. *In* Wylie, W. D., and Churchill-Davidson, H. C. (eds.): A Practice of Anesthesia. Chicago, Year Book Publishers, 1961, pp. 634–650.

48. Gosselin, R. E., Gabourel, J. D., and Willis, J. H.: The fate of atropine in man. Clin. Pharmacol. Ther. *1*:597, 1960.

49. Williams, R. T., and Parke, D. V.: The metabolic fate of drugs. Ann. Rev. Pharmacol. *4*:85, 1964.

50. Randall, L. O., Heise, G. A., Schallek, W., Bag-

don, R. E., Banziger, R., Boris, A., Moe, R. A., and Abrams, W. B.: Pharmacological and clinical studies of Valium, a new psychotherapeutic agent of the benzodiazepine class. Curr. Ther. Res. 3:405, 1961.

51. Hitt, B. A., Mazze, R. I., Beppu, W. J., Stevens, W. C., and Eger, E. I. II: Enflurane metabolism in rats and man. J. Pharmcol. Exp. Ther. 203:193, 1977.

52. Mazze, R. I., Calverley, R. K., and Smith, N. T.: Inorganic fluoride nephrotoxicity: Prolonged enflurane and halothane anesthesia in volunteers. Anesthesiology 46:265, 1977.

53. Carter, R., Heerdt, M., and Acchiardo, S.: Fluoride kinetics after enflurane anesthesia in healthy and anephric patients and in patients with poor renal function. Clin. Pharmacol. Ther. 20:565, 1976.

54. Sievenpiper, T. S., Rice, S. A., McClendon, F., Kosek, J. C., and Mazze, R. I.: Renal effects of enflurane anesthesia in Fischer 344 rats with pre-existing renal insufficiency. J. Pharmacol. Exp. Ther. 211:36, 1979.

55. Way, W. L., and Trevor, A. J.: Sedative-hypnotics. Anesthesiology 34:170, 1971.

56. Sharpless, S. K.: Hypnotics and sedatives. In Goodman, L. S., and Gilman, A. (eds.): The Pharmacological Basis of Therapeutics. 4th ed., New York, Macmillan Co., 1970, pp. 121–134.

57. Dundee, J. W., and Richards, R. K.: Effect of azotemia upon the action of intravenous barbiturate anesthesia. Anesthesiology 15:33, 1954.

58. Freeman, R. B., Sheff, M. G., Maher, J. F., and Schreiner, G. E.: The blood-cerebrospinal fluid barrier in uremia. Ann. Intern. Med. 56:233, 1962.

59. Clarke, R. J. S., and Dundee, J. W.: Clinical studies of induction agents. XV: A comparison of the cumulative effects of thiopentone, methohexitone and propanidid. Br. J. Anaesth. 38:401, 1966.

60. Foldes, F. F., McNall, P. G., and Birch, J. H.: The neuromuscular activity of succinylmonocholine iodide in anaesthetized man. Br. Med. J. 1:967, 1954.

61. Wyant, G. M.: The anaesthetist looks at tissue transplantation: Three years' experience with kidney transplants. Canad. Anaesth. Soc. J. 14:255, 1967.

62. LeVine, D. S., and Virtue, R. W.: Anaesthetic agents and techniques for renal homotransplants. Canad. Anaesth. Soc. J. 11:425,1964.

63. Miller, R. D., Way, W. L., Hamilton, W. K., and Layzer, R. B.: Succinylcholine induced hyperkalemia in patients with renal failure? Anesthesiology 36:138, 1972.

64. Miller, R. D., Matteo, R. S., Benet, L. Z., Sohn, Y. J.: The pharmacokinetics of d-tubocurarine in man with and without renal failure. J. Pharmacol. Exp. Ther. 202:1, 1977.

65. Paton, W. D. M., and Zaimis, E. J.: Methonium compounds. Pharmacol. Rev. 4:219, 1952.

66. McLeod, K., Watson, M. J., and Rawlines, M. D.: Pharmacokinetics of pancuronium in patients with normal and impaired renal function. Br. J. Anaesth. 48:341, 1976.

67. Peters, L.: Renal tubular excretion of organic bases. Pharmacol. Rev. 12:1, 1960.

68. Bodman, R. I.: Controlled hypotension. In Hewer, C. L. (ed.): Recent Advances in Anaesthesia and Analgesia. 10th ed., London, J. & A. Churchill, Ltd., 1967, pp. 90–117.

69. Ashley, J. J., Brown, B. T., Okita, G. T., and Wright, S. E.: The metabolites of cardiac glycosides in human urine. J. Biol. Chem. 232:315, 1958.

70. Vandam, L. D., Harrison, J. H., Murray, J. E., and Merrill, J. P.: Anesthetic aspects of renal homotransplantation in man. Anesthesiology 23:783, 1962.

71. Churchill-Davidson, H. C., Wylie, W. D., Miles, B. E., and de Wardner, H. E.: The effects of adrenaline, nonadrenaline and methedrine on renal circulation during anesthesia. Lancet 2:803, 1951.

72. Miller, R. D., Way, W. L., and Eger, E. I. II: The effects of alpha-methyldopa, reserpine, guanethidine and iproniazid on minimum alveolar anesthetic requirement (MAC). Anesthesiology 29:1153, 1968.

73. Schmidt, K. F., and Roth, R. H.: Interaction of psychotropic drugs with agents employed in clinical anesthesia. Clin. Anaesth. 3:60, 1967.

74. Black, D. A. K.: Renal Disease. 2nd ed. Philadelphia, F. A. Davis Co., 1967.

75. Strauss, M. D.: Diseases of the Kidney. Boston, Little, Brown and Co., 1963.

76. Wilson, C.: The natural history of nephritis. In Black, D. A. K. (ed.): Renal Disease. 2nd ed., Philadelphia, F. A. Davis Co., 1967, pp. 225–251.

77. Schreiner, G. E., and Maher, J. F.: Toxic nephropathy. Am. J. Med. 38:409, 1965.

78. Mazze, R. I., Cousins, M. J., and Kosek, J. C.: Dose-related methoxyflurane nephrotoxicity in rats: A biochemical and pathological correlation. Anesthesiology 36:571, 1972.

79. Cousins, M. J., Mazze, R. I., Kosek, J. C., Hitt, B. A., and Love, F. V.: The etiology of methoxyflurane nephrotoxicity. J. Pharmacol. Exp. Ther. 190:530, 1974.

80. Cousins, M. J., and Mazze, R. I.: Methoxyflurane nephrotoxicity: A study of dose-response in man. J.A.M.A. 225:1611, 1973.

81. Mazze, R. I., and Cousins, M. J.: Combined nephrotoxicity of gentamicin and methoxyflurane anesthesia in man. Br. J. Anaesth. 45:394, 1973.

82. Barr, G. A., Mazze, R. I., Cousins, M. J., and Kosek, J. C.: An animal model for combined methoxyflurane and gentamicin nephrotoxicity. Br. J. Anaesth. 45:306, 1973.

83. Kuzucu, E. Y.: Methoxyflurane, tetracycline, and renal failure. J.A.M.A. 211:1162, 1970.

84. Barry, K. G., and Mally, J. P.: Oliguric renal failure: Evaluation and therapy by intravenous infusion of mannitol. J.A.M.A. 179:510, 1962.

85. Merrill, J. P.: The Treatment of Renal Failure. 2nd ed., New York, Grune and Stratton, 1965, pp. 96–118.

86. Vertel, R. M., and Knochel, J. P.: Nonoliguric acute renal failure. J.A.M.A. 200:118, 1967.

87. Hollenberg, N. K., Epstein, M., Rosen, S. M., et al.: Acute oliguric renal failure in man: Evidence for preferential renal cortical ischemia. Medicine 47:455, 1968.

88. Schreiner, G. E.: Acute renal failure. *In* Black, D. A. K. (ed.): Renal Disease. 2nd ed., Philadelphia, F. A. Davis Co., 1967, pp. 309–326.

89. Barry, K. G., Mazze, R. I., and Schwartz, F. D.: Prevention of surgical oliguria and renal hemodynamic suppression by sustained hydration. N. Engl. J. Med. *207*:1371, 1964.

90. Luke, R. G., Linton, A. L., Briggs, J. D., and Kennedy, A. C.: Mannitol therapy in acute renal failure. Lancet *1*:980, 1965.

91. Cantarovich, F., Galli, C., Benedetti, L., et al.: High dose furosemide in established acute renal failure. Br. Med. J. *2*:449, 1973.

92. Norman, J. C.: Renal complications of cardiopulmonary bypass. Dis. Chest. *54*:50, 1968.

93. Thompson, J. E., Vollman, R. W., Austin, D. J., and Kartchner, M. M.: Prevention of hypotensive and renal complications of aortic surgery using balanced salt solution: Thirteen year experience with 670 cases. Ann. Surg. *167*:767, 1968.

94. Lundberg, S.: Renal function during anesthesia and open-heart surgery in man. Acta Anaesth. Scand. (Suppl.) *27*:1, 1967.

95. Dawson, J. L.: Postoperative renal function in obstructive jaundice: Effect of a mannitol diuresis. Br. Med. J. *1*:82, 1965.

96. Teschan, P. E., Post, R. S., Smith, L. H., Abernathy, R. S., Davis, J. H., Gray, D. M., Howard, J. M., Johnson, K. E., Klopp, E., Mundy, R. L., O'Meara, M. P., and Rush, B. F., Jr.: Posttraumatic renal insufficiency in military casualties. Am. J. Med. *18*:172, 1955.

97. Barry, K. G., Cohen, A. C., Knochel, J. P., Whelan, T. J., Jr., Beisel, W. R., Vargas, C. A., and LeBlanc, P. C., Jr.: Mannitol infusion. II. The prevention of acute renal failure during resection of an aneurysm of the abdominal aorta. N. Engl. J. Med. *264*:967, 1961.

98. Rush, B. F., Fishbein, R., and Wilder, R. J.: Effect of operative trauma upon renal function in older patients. Ann. Surg. *162*:863, 1965.

99. Sawyer, K. C., Sawyer, R. B., and Robb, W. C.: Postoperative renal failure. Am. J. Surg. *106*:668, 1963.

100. Baxter, C. R., and Maynard, D. R.: Prevention and recognition of surgical renal complications. Clin. Anesth. *3*:322, 1968.

101. Reid, P. R., and Thompson, W. L.: The clinical use of dopamine in the treatment of shock. Johns Hopkins Med. J. *137*:276, 1975.

102. Jacobsen, E., Christiansen, A. H., and Lunding, M.: The role of the anesthetist in the management of acute renal failure. Br. J. Anaesth. *40*:442, 1968.

103. Mazze, R. I.: Critical care of the patient with acute renal failure. Anesthesiology *47*:138, 1977.

104. Kolff, W. J., and Berk, H. T. J.: Artificial kidney, dialyzer with great area. Acta Med. Scand. *117*:121, 1944.

105. Merrill, J. P., Schupak, E., Cameron, E., and Hampers, C. L.: Hemodialysis in the home. J.A.M.A. *190*:468, 1964.

106. Lucas, Z. J., Palmer, J. M., Payne, R., Kountz, S. L., and Cohn, R. B.: Renal allotransplantation in humans. I. Systemic immunosuppressive therapy. Arch. Surg. *100*:113, 1970.

107. Cousins, M. J.: Hematoma following epidural block. Anesthesiology *37*:263, 1972.

108. Eschbach, J. W., Jr., Funk, D. D., Schribner, B. H., and Finch, C. A.: A study of the anemia of chronic renal failure. Clin. Res. *14*:167, 1966.

109. Strunin, L.: Some aspects of anaesthesia for renal homotransplantation. Br. J. Anaesth. *38*:812, 1966.

110. Clinical Anesthesia Conference: Anesthetic problems in patients of maintenance dialysis. N.Y. State J. Med. 583–585, Feb. 1969.

111. Belzer, F. O., and Kountz, S. L.: Preservation and transplantation of human cadaver kidney: A two year experience. Ann. Surg. *172*:394, 1970.

112. Katz, J., Kountz, S. L., and Cohn, R.: Anesthetic considerations for renal transplant. Anesth. Analg. *46*:609, 1967.

113. Bromage, P. R.: Comparison of vasoactive drugs in man. Br. Med. J. *2*:72, 1952.

114. Flacke, W., and Alper, M. H.: Actions of halothane and norepinephrine on the isolated mammalian heart. Anesthesiology *23*:793, 1962.

115. Holmes, J. H., Nakamoto, S., Sawyer, K. C., Jr.: Changes in blood composition before and after dialysis with the Kloff twin coil kidney. Trans. Am. Soc. Artif. Intern. Organs *4*:16, 1958.

116. Koide, M., and Waud, B. E.: Serum potassium concentrations after succinylcholine in patients with renal failure. Anesthesiology *36*:142, 1972.

117. Miller, R. D., and Cullen, D. J.: Renal failure and postoperative respiratory failure: Recurarization? Br. J. Anaesth. *48*:253, 1976.

118. Cousins, M. J., and Wright, C. J.: Graft, muscle and skin blood flow changes after epidural block in vascular surgery. Surg. Gynecol. Obstet. *133*:59, 1971.

119. Merrill, J. P., Murray, J. E., Harrison, J. H., and Guild, W. R.: Successful homotransplantation of human kidney between identical twins. J.A.M.A. *160*:277, 1956.

12

Neurological Disorders

By LESLIE B. KADIS, M.D.

Basal Ganglia Degeneration
(Movement Disorders)
  General Discussion
  Neuroanatomic and Neurophysiologic
    Consideration
  Primary Symptoms and
    Clinicopathological Correlations
  Specific Disease Entities
Motor Neuron Degeneration
Other Forms of Motor Degeneration
  Chronic Polyneuropathies
  Spinocerebellar Degeneration
  Syringomyelia
  Spinal Cord Trauma

Demyelinating Diseases
The Mucopolysaccharidoses
The Gangliosidoses
Other Inherited Diseases
  Mongolism (Down's Syndrome)
  Klippel-Feil Syndrome
  Arnold-Chiari Malformation
  Familial Dysautonomia (Riley-Day
    Syndrome) and Orthostatic
    Hypotension Syndrome of Shy-Drager
Neuroectodermal Disorders

BASAL GANGLIA DEGENERATION (MOVEMENT DISORDERS)

GENERAL DISCUSSION

The group of diseases that have in common disorganization in motion can be best understood in terms of their similar pathophysiology. The entities considered include Parkinson's disease, Huntington's chorea, Sydenham's chorea, torsion dystonia, and spasmodic torticollis. All have in common symptoms that are labeled chorea, athetosis, and dystonia, although these symptoms occur for other reasons as well. They may also occur after cerebrovascular insufficiency, as a consequence of drug administration (most notably phenothiazines and butyrophenones), or after trauma or cerebral hypoxia. Since the function that is deficient in all these entities is in the basal ganglia, it is not surprising that the medical, surgical, and anesthetic considerations are similar.

NEUROANATOMIC AND NEUROPHYSIOLOGIC CONSIDERATION

The corpus striatum consists of three well-defined areas, the caudate nucleus, putamen, and globus pallidus. These structures lie on the lateral side of the anterior horn of the lateral ventricle and are separated by the internal capsule. The corpus striatum, the red nucleus in the tegmentum of the mid-brain, the substantia nigra in the mid-brain at the level of the superior colliculus, and the subthalamic nuclei on the dorsal aspect of the cerebrum compose the basal ganglia. These nuclei, together with the afferent fibers that pass from the corpus to the red nucleus via the thalamopallidalrubral system and connect with the pontine reticular system, and hence with the main spinal connections, are collectively known as the extrapyramidal system.

Based on anatomic considerations, it seems that the extrapyramidal system should function as a motor system, but in fact much of the present literature suggests that it serves as a modulator of sensory communication from the fusiform muscle receptors via the gamma afferent fibers to the anterior horn cell and motor system. The muscle and the fusiform fibers are part of a servomechanism that reflexly sets the length of the muscle fiber. The control mechanism is actuated by loading and unloading the muscle.[1] In the presence of a lesion in the extrapyramidal system, the efferent limb of the sensory arc is lost and the fusiform fibers are no longer able to initiate activity. It is not surprising that delayed initiation of motor behavior (akinesia) and disorders of muscle tone are primary symptoms of lesions in the basal ganglia.

More recent developments stress the role of dopaminergic fibers in the basal ganglia as inhibitors of the extrapyramidal system[2] and that much of the symptomatology of Parkinson's disease, for example, is caused by deficiency in the enzyme dopamine beta hydroxylase which converts dopamine to norepinephrine.[3] This mechanism similarly explains the exaggerated response that some parkinsonian patients have to exogenously administered norepinephrine. It also explains the chorea that is found in patients with thyroid disease, since tyrosine is a precursor of both thyroxine and dopamine. Further interactional elements occur as a result of the ability of thyroxine to sensitize striatal receptors to dopamine.[4]

PRIMARY SYMPTOMS AND CLINICOPATHOLOGICAL CORRELATIONS

Clinically, the symptoms that result from lesions in the basal ganglia can be seen as part of a continuum. Athetosis represents an intermediate state between chorea on one hand and dystonia on the other.[1] Most often one symptom blends into the next, and frequently the primary disease process is progressive with an evolving clinical picture.

Athetosis is defined as an instability of posture. During voluntary movement, the instability results in alternation between flexion and extension, most exaggerated in the upper extremities. The net result is a severe limitation of motor ability. Facial muscles may be involved, with grimacing and dysarthria. Lesions in the putamen are responsible for this symptom. In chorea, rapid "pseudopurposive" involuntary movements are seen and voluntary movement is interrupted, leading to hypotonia. Disorganization of associated movements contributes to the pronounced lack of coordination. Hemiballismus is a related symptom, but it is usually unilateral. Although a lesion of the caudate nucleus produces choreoid movements, hemiballismus occurs when the contralateral subthalamic nucleus is involved. This is explained on the basis of an interruption in the efferent pathways from the corpus striatum passing through the subthalamic nuclei on their way to their spinal connection.

Dystonia, an exaggeration of muscle tone, results when (as in the case of athetosis) the putamen is involved, but with dystonia the process is often more diffuse. Lesions in both the thalamus and cortex are frequently implicated. The symptoms of hypertonicity may be limited as in spasmodic torticollis or diffuse as in torsion dystonia.

Finally, we come to the rigidity and tremor that characterize Parkinson's syndrome and that often occur together when the globus pallidus is involved. The rigidity results from an exaggerated stretch reflex, so that each increase in tension reflexly produces a further increase in tension, and there is no stretch relaxation at high load factors. When this rigidity occurs in the face of rhythmic alternating contractions of opposing muscle groups (tremor), the "cogwheel rigidity" of Parkinson's syndrome is seen.[2]

SPECIFIC DISEASE ENTITIES

Sydenham's Chorea. Sydenham's chorea occurs primarily in children. It is seen most frequently in females, usually as a consequence of beta hemolytic streptococcal infection; it is rarely fatal, but recurs within a year in as many as 30 to 35 per cent of children. Of particular importance is the association of chorea with endocarditis (20 per cent) and the high incidence of electrocardiographic abnormalities in asymptomatic siblings.[1] Frequently irritability and emotional lability are seen, although more severe mental symptoms do occur infrequently. The electroencephalograph is consistent with a diffuse process, in that a generalized cerebral dysrhythmia with slow waves, 4 to 6 cps, is seen. At autopsy, scattered areas of cell degeneration are found in the cortex, basal ganglia, substantia nigra, and cerebellum, as is arteritis with hyalinization of small vessels.

The onset of symptoms is often insidious, but the diagnosis is not difficult when one is faced with choreiform movements in a child. Often these involuntary movements are most prevalent in the upper extremities and stop during sleep. They may also be diminished by phenothiazines and barbiturates, and these two drugs form the primary basis for symptomatic treatment.[2] Some patients, however, may be treated with cortical steroids, L-dopa, and a dopa decarboxylase inhibitor which may complicate anesthetic management.[3, 4]

Although there is no literature specifically related to the anesthetic management of Sydenham's chorea, a plan could be readily developed. Careful evaluation of cardiac status with particular reference to ECG is essential. Treatment with antibiotics as in rheumatic heart disease may be indicated. Premedication with barbiturates will reduce involuntary movements and apprehension and facilitate induction. During awakening, choreiform movements may be exaggerated, and careful attention to fixation of intravenous and other important equipment is required. The choice of anesthetic technique for maintenance of anesthesia can be made independently from considerations of the neurologic components of the disease.

Huntington's Chorea (Chronic Progressive Chorea, Adult Chorea). Huntington's chorea is a heredofamilial disease transmitted as a mendelian dominant, with an incidence of seven per 100,000.[5] The late onset (35 to 40 years), familial association, and mental deterioration all contribute to its perpetuation in spite of our knowledge of the genetics and the predictability of its occurrence. At autopsy, degeneration is widespread, with shrinkage of the caudate nucleus particularly apparent. The diagnosis is evident when chorea, ataxia, dysarthria, defective mentation and judgment, and mood lability are present and there is a positive family history. The course is progressive, but phenothiazines, particularly fluphenazine (Prolixin), may control the chorea and emotional lability. Davies[6] reported an abnormal response to thiopental, with delayed awakening, generalized tonic spasms, and tight jaws in one patient on two separate occasions. On the third occasion, nitrous oxide supplemented with diethyl ether was used without complications.

More recent anesthetic experience in two patients with Huntington's chorea focused on the alleged barbiturate hyposensitivity and abnormal pseudocholinesterase activity and successfully managed a patient using atropine, droperidol, and fetanyl as premedicants, 100 mg thiopental and 4 mg pancuronium for endotracheal intubation, and maintained these patients with a mixture of 1 per cent halothane in nitrous oxide–oxygen.[7] These items contain the essential elements of a sound anesthetic regimen for management of patients with Huntington's chorea: premedication with phenothiazine or diazepam, a narcotic induction with a small dose of a barbiturate, and maintenance with nitrous oxide supplemented by halothane.

Torticollis. Torticollis, or "wry neck," has received a good deal of attention in the surgical literature, because it lends itself to surgical treatment. It also represents a limited form of torsion dystonia. However, torticollis may also be seen as a sequel of encephalitis lethargica, as a symptom of extrapyramidal disease, after trauma to the cervical spine, in Klippel-Feil syndrome, and with amyotrophic lateral sclerosis. The most frequent mode of presentation is insidious onset in a male in the fourth decade.[8] Spasmodic contractions are seen in the sternocleidomastoid, trapezius, and splenius muscles, and the resultant posture depends on which muscles are predominantly involved. Although emotionally charged situations aggravate the condition and the diagnosis of hysteria is frequently considered, an organic basis is often found. In spite of this, surgical approaches have had variable long-term effects and the overall prognosis is poor.[9] The management of these patients is currently in a state of flux and includes pharmacotherapy, surgery, and electromyographic biofeedback. When surgery is used, the operation currently favored is an anterior rhizotomy at C1 and C3 bilaterally, with subarachnoid section of the spinal accessory nerve. This procedure requires that the patient be sitting, and a wire-wound (armored) endotracheal tube may be required. Furthermore, it is often difficult to locate the first cervical nerve, and C2 through C4 rather than C1 through C3 may inadvertently be sectioned. When this occurs, postoperative respiratory distress may follow because of involvement of the phrenic nerve.[10] Also, residual spasm in the trapezius muscle may present difficulties postoperatively, and additional surgery may be required. Swallowing may also be difficult if the patient cannot reflexly lift his chin. Careful observation during the first postoperative feeding is indicated. Cerebral ischemia has been reported as a consequence of laminectomy at this level because of mechanical interference with flow in the vertebral arteries. There are no reports of anesthetic difficulty during induction. The airway is not usually impeded with either rotation or extension of the neck, and the response to muscle relaxants would be normal. Sedation will often ameliorate the condition, and there are no reports of adverse response to barbiturates. These agents should be included in the preoperative medication and to facilitate induction.

Torsion Dystonia. Torsion dystonia (dystonia musculorum deformans, Oppenheim's disease) is a more severe form of spasmodic torticollis that occurs in children 5 to 15 years of age. It is a rare, slowly progressive disease that occurs predominantly in families of Russian Jews. The onset is gradual, but in the full-blown picture involuntary writhing movements and torsion spasms are characteristic. The spasm commonly involves the vertebral column, and lordosis and scoliosis are seen when the disease is of long duration. Oxygen and carbon dioxide transport may be impaired. Since the symptoms are relieved during sleep, barbiturate premedication and induction are indicated. Steen[11] reported on the use of rectal sedation, administered in the hospital room to children, followed by intravenous induction with barbiturates and maintenace with nitrous oxide-oxygen, and supplemented with a relaxant and meperidine. No complications were noted. Bony changes in the cervical spine were not seen in children, and awake endotracheal intubation was not required. Adults, on the other hand, may have a fixed cervical spine, and it may be impossible to maintain the airway once anesthesia is induced. Awake intubation of the trachea may be required. Davis and Daves[12] more recently reported the successful management of one patient utilizing diazepam for premedication, thiopental for induction, pancuronium for intubation, and enflurane with its special muscle relaxing properties for maintenance of anesthesia.

Parkinson's Syndrome. Parkinson's syndrome (paralysis agitans) may follow central nervous system trauma or carbon monoxide or manganese poisoning, or may occur as a consequence of various psychoactive drugs. It may also be seen following encephalitis lethargica, but most commonly the cause is unknown. The incidence in the population is 187 per 100,000, and patients with Parkinson's syndrome are seen regularly in the operating suite. Although the pathophysiology is unclear, except in a general sense, the substantia nigra is usually involved at autopsy. Clinically, onset occurs in the sixth to eighth decade, with gradual onset of a fine tremor, dysarthria, mask-like facies, and decreased movement. Pain in the muscles is a frequent accompaniment, and patients with Parkinson's syndrome may be referred to a pain clinic.

Continued research on the metabolism of biogenic amines in the brain has led to the concept that the Parkinson's syndrome results from an abnormality in the conversion of dopa (1,3,4-dihydroxyphenylalanine) to dopamine and epinephrine and thence to the use of L-dopa in the treatment of patients with Parkinson's disease. Thus it is not surprising that chlorpromazine and haloperidol, which interfere with catecholamine metabolism at the receptor site, should produce Parkinson's syndrome.[13] Treatment is with either or both of the synthetic antispasmodics — trihexylphenidyl HCL (Artane) and benztropine (Cogentin). When akinesia is the major presenting symptom, L-dopa may be useful. When tremor is the primary complaint, surgical treatment (pallidectomy or ventrolateral thalamotomy) may provide relief. The latter two procedures are not used in the face of hypertension or akinesia, because both symptoms may be exaggerated by the surgical intervention.[14]

The anesthetic and surgical requirements for chemopallidectomy have been well documented. A responsive, well-sedated state is desired, because the stereotactic procedure requires communication with the surgeon. Under light barbiturate anesthesia[15] or following droperidol and phenoperidine,[16] a pneumoencephalogram is performed to identify the lateral ventricles. Under local anesthesia a cryogenic probe is inserted through burr holes with the aid of a stereotactic device, and the lesion is produced. During light sleep the tremor disappears but returns as soon as the patient is aroused, thus providing the surgeon with an indication of the accuracy of the lesion. When movements are sufficiently great, as in torsion dystonia or cerebellar ataxia, general anesthesia may be required. In the latter case, barbiturate sedation and induction can be used and anesthesia maintained with nitrous oxide-oxygen, as in the case of torsion dystonia.

Patients with Parkinson's disease have a high incidence of associated problems and may require surgery for different reasons, and these patients may be receiving L-dopa, with its known ability to sensitize the cardiovascular system. However, the short half-life of L-dopa and the availability of peripheral decarboxylase inhibitors, which mitigate most of the peripheral effects of L-dopa, suggest that these patients can continue to receive that medication up to and including the day before surgery and that the medication can be reinstituted immediately following surgery.

Other rare syndromes that affect the basal ganglia and present similarly to the aforementioned diseases include status marmoratus (double athetosis), which appears during the first year of life, and Hallervorden-Spatz disease (pigmentary degeneration of the globus pallidus). The latter is similar to Wilson's disease with the exception of liver pathology. Creutzfeldt-Jacob disease (spastic pseudosclerosis), a rare progressive disease of middle life with a rapid course, often presents as a disease of the basal ganglia, but soon pyramidal and cerebellar signs become apparent, as do signs of deterioration of mental function. There is no documentation of anesthetic experience, although brain biopsy has been performed and presumably an anesthetic administered.

MOTOR NEURON DEGENERATION

Amyotrophic lateral sclerosis (motor system disease, motor neuron disease) is a degenerative disease of motor cells throughout the central nervous system. Males are more commonly affected than females. When the degenerative process is limited to the motor cortex and the efferent pathways, the syndrome of primary lateral sclerosis occurs; when the disease involves brainstem nuclei, it goes by the name of pseudobulbar palsy; and when it is limited to the spinal cord anterior horn cells, it is called progressive muscular atrophy.[1]

The disorder has its peak incidence in the ages between 40 and 60; it has been described at all ages but is quite uncommon in childhood and early adult life. Werdnig-Hoffmann disease (q.v.) bears a marked similarity to amyotrophic lateral sclerosis, with certain specific exceptions, and ordinarily occurs in the first three years of life. In most series of patients with amyotrophic lateral sclerosis males are affected more commonly than females. Although uncommon, well-documented instances of familial genetically patterned disease occur, and family histories have been traced for both a dominant and a recessive pattern of inheritance. In Guam and the Mariana Islands the disease is endemic, having an incidence perhaps 100 times that of its occurrence in other documented countries. The Chamorro Indians of that area are subject to the disease. There are a high familial incidence and frequent association with another disorder, the Parkinson-dementia complex, which has no clear analogue in this country. Whether the disease in this area is genetically determined or related to environmental factors has thus far not been established, despite intensive epidemiological and clinical surveys. However, because of the pattern of the disease, the possibility of a "slow virus" has been suggested, and attempts are being made, so far unsuccessfully, to transmit the disease to higher primates and other animals. No satisfactory etiologic factors have been determined.

The clinical course of the disease is marked by signs affecting both upper and lower motor neuron processes. Although signs of both systems are almost invariably identifiable when the disease is well established, one or the other may predominate for some time in the early evolution. A common mode of onset is with atrophy, weakness, and fasciculations, very often involving the intrinsic hand muscles; but most muscles are involved within one to two years. Occasionally, the first symptoms may be those related to spasticity and associated spastic weakness, especially in the lower extremities. As the disease progresses, both spasticity and atrophy may be evident in many muscles despite the apparent paradox of a muscle overcontracting at a time when it is wasting. Since the atrophic process is not uniform in a muscle group, those muscle fibers still persisting are often quite adequate to demonstrate the increased resting tone and increased response to passive movement which are the hallmarks of spasticity. Similarly, the deep tendon reflexes are often hyperactive (upper motor neuron lesion symptoms), but this phenomenon is variable, and it is not uncommon to find patients typical in all other respects whose reflexes are hyperactive. It is typical to emphasize that rapidly advancing dysfunction of the upper motor neuron is associated with decreased superficial abdominal reflexes, extensor plantar responses, and, when bilateral, urinary urgency and eventual incontinence; but these signs are often tardy or even quite late in development, although spasticity may be prominent.

In some individuals the early signs and, in fact, the principal early progression of the disease may be most prominent in bulbar innervated striated muscle. Again, the predominant affection may start as atrophy or as spasticity of function, although again both components become well established in the later stages of the disorder. Early bulbar symptoms are commonly those that affect the precision of speech and result in poor enunciation of lingual, labial, and dental sounds. Disorders of swallowing are particularly troublesome, with nasal regurgitation and tracheal aspiration being both disabling and dangerous aspects of the muscle dysfunction. For reasons that are quite unclear, the ocular muscles are uniformly spared. When the bulbar musculature suffers predominantly from lower motor neuron involvement, atrophy of the tongue and flaccid posture of the palate are noted, whereas when upper motor neuron signs are most evident the tongue may appear small from spastic contraction and the gag reflex may be spastically hyperactive. In addition, a curious inability to control emotional responses is present. It appears from interviewing patients closely that affect and feel-

ing tone may be quite normal, and yet when confronted with some stimulus that evokes a small degree of sadness in its thought or implications the patient may burst into uncontrollable spasms of facial emotional response, including tears, gagging, and spastic respiratory sobs, requiring many seconds or sometimes minutes to subside. Similar outbursts of choking, gasping laughter may be provoked by a mildly humorous stimulus, the end appearance of the patient being very hard to distinguish from that occasioned by a depression-evoking stimulus.

Early symptomatology may include the complaint of troublesome, although rarely severe, cramping and aching sensations, especially in the lower extremities. These are probably not related to the fascicular twitchings that are a characteristic sign in this disease. The fasciculations consist of simultaneous contraction of bundles of contiguous muscle fibers which, when close to the surface, are often visible through the skin. They are more evident with fatigue and are increased with exercise. Although patients may notice and comment upon them, they very often are unaware of these muscular twitchings until they are pointed out. In amyotrophic lateral sclerosis the muscular twitching is almost always evident in a variety of areas, as opposed to the very common benign fasciculations that commonly persist for hours or days in one specific bundle of fibers and have no pathologic significance. The usual course of the disease is inexorable progression, without periods of arrest of evolution, to death within three years, although an occasional individual survives past ten years from first symptoms. When bulbar involvement is early, the span of time to profound disability, medical complications, or suicide is apt to be shorter.

Examination of the cellular, protein, and chemical contents of blood and spinal fluid reveals no abnormalities of a specific nature. In advanced and bedridden individuals, serum enzyme changes associated with nonspecific muscle wasting may be identified, but they are no more specific than those that may occur in the disabled or bedridden patient from other causes. Electromyography is helpful in demonstrating signs of muscle denervation and fibrillation potentials in muscles not yet demonstrating clinical signs. Although this finding is not pathognomonic of this disease, the demonstration of a wide distribution of motor atrophy may be important in excluding other disorders. Muscle biopsy demonstrates again only a pattern of muscle fiber loss appropriate for denervation.

Although the prognosis is hopeless, symptomatic benefit is occasionally achieved by directing drug therapy to the complaints of leg cramps and toward the reduction of spasticity.

Recently attention has been called to the occurrence of this disease syndrome process in association with an underlying carcinoma. Most commonly this has been in association with carcinoma of the lung, but it also has been reported in association with a wide variety of other primary carcinomas. Like the other so-called remote effects of carcinoma on the nervous system, the neurologic signs are believed to be due to an abnormal factor elaborated by the neoplasm or by the body in response to some effect of the neoplasm. In this case, position and vibratory sensation are diminished as a result of involvement of the posterior columns.

Werdnig-Hoffmann disease begins within the first year of life, and is considered when the child fails to progress in the landmarks of motor development. By one year of age the pattern of muscular weakness is often clearly developed and usually involves the muscles of the back and pelvic and shoulder girdles, progressing later to the distal limb musculature. On occasion, the diaphragm may be involved early on in the course of the disease, with obvious implications for anesthesia and post-anesthetic recovery.[2] The children are often quite healthy looking in the early stages. The deep tendon reflexes are usually lost, response to sensory stimuli appears quite normal, and examination by muscle biopsy and electromyography demonstrates signs of motor denervation. Early on it may be quite difficult, in the absence of specific testing, to separate the hypotonia and weakness from a considerable variety of other disorders, particularly ones affecting muscle function, from this disorder. Frequently the term "the floppy infant" is used to describe the hypotonic child.

This genetically determined disorder affects the sexes equally and is transmitted as an autosomal recessive gene. The parents are healthy, and the detection of the carrier state has so far not been successful.

The process ordinarily progresses inexorably to death, often in a few months from observed onset, but temporary remissions have been reported and longer survivals noted.

No specific therapy is known, but because of the occasional relatively benign outcome and the possibility of arrest of the process, careful nursing care and attention to the physical problems posed by muscle weakness may sometimes be rewarding.

OTHER FORMS OF MOTOR DEGENERATION

These diseases usually follow the well-defined courses of the typical pictures described in textbooks. Their progress is variable but inexorable, with the exception of Guillain-Barré disease, and there is at present no curative therapy.

The cause is unknown, although speculation has implicated slow virus infective, metabolic, and autoimmune etiologies among others. The diseases are commonly inherited on either an autosomal or a sex-linked basis.

Guillain-Barré, although well documented in the anesthesia literature, may require some special consideration because this is one of the few disorders in which surgery may in fact alter the course of the disease. While the disease is often preceded by respiratory or gastrointestinal infection, both immunizations and surgery have been implicated.[1] The acute weakness that begins in the legs and spreads rostrally to the arms and trunks, and in 50 per cent of cases to the bulbar musculature, may produce a severe respiratory emergency requiring intensive care. Of significant import is the autonomic disturbance that results from chromatolysis of the anteromediolateral cell column and the autonomic ganglia, producing severe cardiovascular instability.[2] Inappropriate secretion of antidiuretic hormone has also been noted. The mortality rate may be as high as 20 per cent, although a more common figure is 5 per cent. Anesthetic considerations are particularly challenging, especially when onset occurs during the last stage of pregnancy, at which time the risk to both mother and fetus is high. This increased risk results from exacerbation of a disease,[3] cardiovascular instability, and sensitivity to positive pressure ventilation or tracheal suction.[4] Whenever possible, it seems prudent to use local anesthesia. If this is not possible, then agents that either activate the sympathetic nervous system or at least are not sympatholytic should be used. Techniques using agents such as nitrous oxide–oxygen supplemented by ketamine or narcotics are indicated. Particular attention should be directed toward maintenance of blood volume and the potential for fluid shifts that result from positional changes and to the frequent cardiac dysrhythmias that occur. It also seems wise to avoid barbiturates and phenothiazines, both of which may produce profound cardiovascular depression.

CHRONIC POLYNEUROPATHIES

These hereditary diseases are often found in conjunction with other degenerative disorders. They are primarily lesions of the peripheral nerves, with secondary anterior horn cell and posterior column loss: The peripheral nerves may be felt to have smooth, firm enlargement. Therefore, mixed lower motor neuron and sensory loss and pain are common.

Charcot-Marie-Tooth disease is of varying severity, ranging from chronic moderate involvement in the dominant form to the much more severe recessive form in which the patient may be a bedridden cripple by the age of 20. It produces lower motor neuron disease, primarily in the legs, together with vasomotor and secondary impairment. Déjérine-Sottas disease is much more widespread, with involvement of the whole of the peripheral nervous system from the cranial nerves downward.

One important consideration is the presence of a high creatine phosphokinase, which, although most often present in the myopathic disorders, may be seen in the neuropathic disorders as well. Most specifically, this has been reported in Charcot-Marie-Tooth disease[5] and occasionally in amyotrophic lateral sclerosis.

SPINOCEREBELLAR DEGENERATION

Friedreich's ataxia causes a degeneration of the spinocerebellar and pyramidal tracts,

together with dorsal root ganglion atrophy. There is therefore mixed upper and lower motor neuron disease, with the cerebellar signs featured predominantly. These are typically ataxia, dysarthria, and nystagmus, combined with weakness, spasticity, and atrophy. Both position and vibration sense are lost. These patients frequently suffer from coexisting diseases of other systems, in particular cardiac disease, murmurs, myocarditis, and ECG changes.

Right ventricular hypertrophy may result in a 10 per cent decrease in blood oxygenation, while the dysfunction in calcium regulation often produces an increase in the resting heart rate. As many as 30 per cent of patients may have an elevated cardiac output related to the increase in resting heart rate. It may be helpful to consider a beta-blocking agent to combat the disturbed myocardial oxygen transport.[1] Sudden death is common.

Anesthetic Considerations. Recently several reports of anesthesia in patients with varying forms of amyotrophic lateral sclerosis have appeared in the literature.[2–6] Mostly these workers have been concerned with the hypersensitivity to depolarizing muscle relaxants and the potential for cardiovascular collapse that follow succinylcholine-induced hyperkalemia. In addition, patients with amyotrophic lateral sclerosis may show signs of a myasthenic syndrome,[6] with degradation in the muscle response to supramaximal tetanic stimulation. Rosenbaum and his colleagues[3] found, as would be expected, a prolonged recovery time following the administration of 20 mg of gallamine, with full recovery requiring neostigmine. These workers recommend a test dose of *d*-tubocurarine in 3.0 mg increments to avoid this problem.

Additional anesthetic hazards may be anticipated, but these have not been adequately documented. Patients with progressive bulbar palsy may have loss of the pharyngeal muscles and present an increased danger of aspiration. This danger period may extend from the preoperative period through the operative period and into the postoperative phase, when neurologic signs may be enhanced.[7] Spasticity, for example, may become sustained tetanus,[1] or the deficit in other muscle groups (pharyngeal or respiratory) may be exaggerated with the developed subsequent complications.

Premedication with morphine, secobarbital, and atropine has been tolerated quite well. The ECG should be monitored to warn of impending cardiac arrhythmias. Induction with thiopental has been used without difficulty. Nondepolarizing muscle relaxants should be used when muscle relaxation is required, using incremental doses; observing the muscle response to tetanic stimulation may be important, although the unequal involvement of the different muscle groups may make this procedure unreliable. Maintenance of anesthesia with nitrous oxide–oxygen, supplemented with a more potent agent such as halothane, will allow excellent control over muscle tone. However, patients with amyotrophic lateral sclerosis may be chronically ill and blood volume may be severely depleted.

The anesthetic considerations in infants with Werdnig-Hoffmann disease are similar to those of amyotrophic lateral sclerosis but are tailored to the special needs of the infant. More than likely these children will require postoperative ventilation, and passage of a nasotracheal tube during anesthesia may be indicated.

SYRINGOMYELIA[1-8]

Syringomyelia is defined as a chronic, slowly progressive degeneration of the spinal cord and medulla, with cavitation and gliosis within the substance of the cord. Frequently, syringomyelia develops in association with other anomalies, such as spina bifida, Arnold-Chiari malformation, basilar impression, cervical rib, and platybasia.[1] It may have its embryologic origin in imperfect closure of the neural tube with persistence of embryonic cell rests and gliosis, which precedes cyst (syrinx) formation.[2] Frequently there is a communication between the syrinx and the fourth ventricle in conjunction with either partial or total obstruction of cerebral spinal fluid outflow tracts. The intracranial pulsation extends downward, with gradual distention of the syrinx and subsequent impingement on neural structures.[3] This gradual process probably accounts for the late onset of the congenital anomaly, usually in the second decade.

The clinical picture is variable and depends on the level at which the syrinx develops, but the onset is usually gradual and associated with muscle weakness and wasting. Since the syrinx is located in the central region of the spinal cord, pain and temperature sensation are diminished as the fibers cross the ventral commissure, whereas the fibers that carry touch go to the posterior tract and may not be involved. Occasionally the reverse situation does occur, in that touch, rather than pain and temperature, is involved, but the mechanism for this is not clear.[4] The site of the syrinx may be determined clinically or by myelography, but this may not be adequate and laminectomy or suboccipital craniotomy may be required for precise localization. The mortality rate is fairly high, with some series approaching 15 per cent,[5] and although numerous surgical procedures have been tried, the results are variable. Difficulties result from postoperative complications when syringobulbia and a large cervical enlargement are present. Arachnoiditis of the fourth ventricle is not insignificant and is a usually fatal problem.

The anesthetic management of patients with syringomyelia obviously depends on many factors. The occurrence of associated anomalies, as mentioned above, is one. Also, these patients are chronically ill and may have depleted blood volume and reduced total body water and electrolytes, and contemplated operation may require difficult surgical positions. A few points are generally applicable: 1) Increased intracranial pressure initiated by strong coughing may be transmitted to the cord and may result in severe permanent damage.[6] 2) Scoliosis, which occurred in 63 per cent of patients in one series, may produce abnormalities of the ventilation-perfusion ratio and predispose to pulmonary complications. 3) If an orthopedic procedure is planned, such as insertion of Harrington rods to correct the scoliosis, the cyst may be adherent and a fluid leak may develop and introduce cord damage. Each of these suggests the particular need for detailed attention to pulmonary function. A smooth induction with an intravenous agent following adequate premedication is required. Endotracheal intubation may have to be performed while the patient is in the awake state when vocal cord paralysis (particularly with syringobulbia) is present, but more than likely that individual will already have a tracheostomy tube in place.

The choice of muscle relaxants may be important, because patients with muscle-wasting disease may have a hyperkalemic response to depolarizing muscle relaxants on the one hand or increased sensitivity to non-depolarizing agents on the other. Using a muscle twitch monitor as a guide should be considered. The electrocardiogram should be monitored to warn of impending cardiac arrhythmias. Temperature should also be monitored in view of the autonomic (sweating) disturbance and poor thermal regulation. The choice of a particular anesthetic agent for maintenance does not seem to be as important as skill in administering and maintaining a smooth anesthetic course.

SPINAL CORD TRAUMA

The problems of spinal cord trauma with resultant spinal cord shock and paraplegia represent a major additional threat to the patient, should he require surgery, and a special challenge to the anesthesiologist. Jousse and colleagues (1968) reviewed the literature in 1968 and found reports of 546 surgical and anesthetic deaths in 2600 patients. Thirty-five of these (6.4 per cent) occurred postoperatively, with cardiac arrest occurring in 15. Although these arrests were not fatal when they occurred during anesthesia, they nonetheless underscore the dimension of the problem for the anesthesiologist.

There are several reports and reviews of anesthetic literature on patients with spinal cord trauma and paraplegia.[10-14] From these reports it seems reasonable to subdivide the paraplegic syndrome into phases: acute (less than three weeks), intermediate (three days to three months), and chronic (greater than three months). This division may be useful, because it defines a group of patients in the intermediate state (note the overlap between intermediate and acute) who may have an elevated serum potassium and an abnormal response to depolarizing blocking agents.[15-16] It may also be useful to think in terms of the level of the lesion. Those patients with transections above the level of the splanchnic outflow (above T7) demonstrate significant vascular instability, with both hypertensive and hypotensive responses reflexly initiated by changes in the vasculature below the level of the lesion. A brief outline follows of the problems that may be encountered:

1. Autonomic hyperreflexia occurs when the lesion is above T7 and may be complicated by the hypovolemia that is common in chronically ill patients. This hyperreflexia can be controlled by general anesthesia with halothane, which can be deepened by administration of the anesthetic as needed. Heart block, a frequent occurrence, may also be a complicating factor, and monitoring the ECG is essential. The heart block may be reflexly induced as a baroreceptor response to vasoconstriction above the lesion, and it may be necessary to stop the surgery until the anesthetic is deepened. Although spinal anesthesia has been reported to eliminate these hazards, the blood volume problem and technical difficulties (distorted skeletal structure) may make this technique too hazardous. Often the autonomic reaction is initiated following bladder (or bowel) distention and is seen most frequently during transurethral surgery. A mass reflex with visceral and motor response may be seen. This reflex can also be controlled by deepening the anesthesia and removing the stimulus.

2. Temperature regulation is dependent to a large extent on control of circulation to the skin, and this is impaired in patients with cord transections. In fact, the patient may be poikilothermic below the level of the lesion. Temperature monitoring and appropriate thermal controls are essential.

3. The respiratory system is frequently involved when muscles of respiration are involved. Most important, the decreased vital capacity and expiratory reserve volume predispose to postoperative pulmonary complications. As would be expected, pneumonia is a frequent cause of death. Kyphoscoliosis with ventilation-perfusion abnormalities follows long-standing muscle imbalance, and monitoring arterial blood gases while using high oxygen techniques may be required. Adequate attention to chest physiotherapy pre- and postoperatively is essential.

4. With each year that passes in paraplegics there is an increased likelihood of renal complications, and 60 per cent have impaired renal function after ten years. Amyloidosis is seen frequently, with protein loss and reduction in total body sodium and potassium. These abnormalities may account in part for the reports of abnormal responses to anesthetics, but this has not been thoroughly documented.

5. Mechanical problems are common causes of decubitus ulcer formation in paraplegics whose cutaneous circulation is impaired. These ulcers may form on all exposed surfaces, even with protection of the skin during short surgical procedures. Particular care in moving and turning the anesthetized paraplegic is essential.

6. Finally, patients in the intermediate stage often have elevated serum potassium and respond to depolarizing muscle relaxants, with further increases in potassium (as high as 11 mEq per liter), and ventricular fibrillation has been reported in several instances.[16] There is some question as to whether or not prior administration of a nondepolarizing agent protects against this event. Since the complication of postrelaxant hyperkalemia has been reported to occur from the third to the eighty-third post-trauma day, the recommendation has been made that only non-depolarizing muscle relaxants be used.

A summary of the recommendations in patients with spinal cord lesions includes the use of anticholinergics to minimize unwanted baroreceptor responses, high levels of oxygen in the inspired air to minimize hypoxia following tracheal stimulation, assisted rather than controlled respirations to limit unwanted Valsalva responses, and moderate levels of general anesthesia with halothane anesthesia to minimize blood pressure rises. Hypertensive responses can successfully be treated with sodium nitroprusside as well.

DEMYELINATING DISEASES

The demyelinating diseases represent a large group of diseases whose pathologies merge into one another but which may be separated on clinicopathologic grounds.[1] The group includes acute disseminated encephalomyelitis after acute infections such as measles, chickenpox, or smallpox, or after smallpox or rabies vaccination; acute hemorrhagic leukoencephalitis; disseminated myelitis with optic neuritis (neuromyelitis optica, Devic's disease); diffuse sclerosis (Schilder's disease, leukodystrophy, Baló's disease, Krabbe's disease, Schanz's disease, Merzbacher's disease); central pontine myelosclerosis; and the clinically most important member of the group, multiple sclerosis (disseminated sclerosis).

Multiple sclerosis is a relatively common disease that affects 500,000 Americans and has an overall incidence of 60 to 70 per 100,000, with marked regional variations. The incidence ranges from 128 per 100,000 in the Shetland Islands of Scotland to a low of 2 per 100,000 in South Africa.[2]

The pathologic lesions include an ingrowth in oligodendroglia, with increased oxidative enzymes in the distribution of the myelin sheath, and the development of sclerotic plaques that represent microglial overgrowth in other areas of the central nervous system. The diffuse symptomatology of the disease relates to the location of these plaques. Perivascular cuffing and edema, with subsequent demyelination and conduction block, account for much of the acute symptomatology. This is particularly evident in the optic nerve. A prolonged latency period in the visual-evoked response can often be demonstrated. The presence of glycoprotein antigens, and particularly the HLA-DW2 determinant, suggest a genetic factor, while the increase in immunoglobulin G in the cerebrospinal fluids, which are specific for myelin, point to the role of autoimmune factors. Evidence of viralleading allergy has also been noted in the high incidence of viral antibodies in affected individuals.[3] Usually the disease develops in young adults with rapid onset of symptoms, including motor weakness, visual symptoms, numbness, and paresthesias; but later, other symptoms, including euphoria, loss of bladder control, nystagmus, and long tract signs, develop. Although the acute course may be rapid, more frequently there are remissions with the development of new symptoms every two to three years. This recurrence may be associated with trauma, infection, or an increase in body temperature (see below). There is some evidence that ACTH offers some help with the acute disease, but this probably does not change the overall prognosis, which is grave. When the onset occurs in the older age group (45 years), prognosis is worse and there is less likelihood of remission.[4] In addition to the usual surgical problems, these patients may present for anterior rhizotomy to relieve spasticity or ventrolateral thalamotomy to relieve the intention tremor; the anesthetic management of these particular situations will be discussed below.

In diffuse sclerosis the onset occurs in

younger people (usually below age 14). with visual impairment progressing to spastic paralysis and mental deterioration, suggesting the diffuse nature of the process. The diffuse nature is confirmed by the finding of generalized slowing of the EEG and cerebral atrophy. Some of the leukodystrophies have been thought to be due to enzymatic defects in myelin formation.

There are over 100 anesthetics reported in the literature. Baskett and Armstrong[5] reported four cases and noted several complications. Two of their patients received thiopental for induction and had significant new symptoms on awakening, including paresis, numbness, and loss of bowel and bladder function. These symptoms responded to ACTH. The second patient did not receive thiopental for a second procedure. He had no problems on awakening. The third patient had four separate anesthetics and developed new symptoms on two occasions, but the onset of new symptoms was not related to the administration of thiopental. Four patients similarly developed postanesthetic problems that may or may not have been related to the administration of thiobarbiturate. Siemkowicz, on the other hand,[6] used thiopental in eleven cases without difficulty and noted that the deterioration that appeared in five cases was clearly related to the occurrence of surgical pyrexia. He used combinations of atropine, thiopental, Valium, fentanyl, and nitrous oxide-oxygen, supplemented with halothane. Bamford and his colleagues[7] evaluated the relationship between anesthesia, surgery, and relapses in patients with multiple sclerosis. He reported on 88 procedures in 42 patients and noted a relapse rate of 0.26 per patient year as compared with the accepted 0.44 per patient year. The outstanding conclusion of these findings suggests again that anesthesia, with the possible exception of subarachnoid block, poses no additional hazards to the patient. What does seem to be important is that in all cases new symptoms resolved, usually within 10 days. Particular attention, however, must be paid to the prevention of pyrexia, since small elevations in body temperature (as little as 1° C) may produce new symptoms. Small temperature elevation induces changes that occur at the site of the demyelinating lesions. One test for multiple sclerosis has been induced rises in temperature. These findings relating temperature and the onset of symptoms have been summarized by Davis (1970).[8]

Other considerations include the presence of a myotonic-like syndrome that may confuse the picture in the event of an abnormal response to muscle relaxants. With the myotonic-like syndrome seen in multiple sclerosis, the EMG is normal and thus can be readily differentiated from drug-induced myotonia.[9] Also, patients with multiple sclerosis have an abnormality in the blood-brain barrier, as would be expected with the perivascular involvement.[10] Although we may predict an abnormal response to all anesthetic agents, this has not been documented.

With the aforementioned considerations in mind, the following anesthetic plan will be outlined. Premedication with diazapam has been used effectively and without problems in the treatment of spasticity in patients with multiple sclerosis, and may be used for premedication. Similarly, induction of anesthesia can be accomplished with diazepam or thiopental, an anesthesia maintained with nitrous oxide-oxygen supplemented with halothane or enflurane when myotonic features are present. Incremental doses of nondepolarizing muscle relaxants minimize the dangers of hyperpyrexia, sometimes seen with depolarizing agents. Careful attention to body temperature during the procedure may prevent postanesthetic problems, but if new symptoms develop after anesthesia they are usually self-limited or respond to the ACTH. Finally, these patients may already be treated with steroids and may require prophylactic preoperative or intraoperative steroids. There is no information regarding administration of anesthesia in any of the other demyelinating diseases.

THE MUCOPOLYSACCHARIDOSES[1-3]

The mucopolysaccharidoses are hereditary disorders characterized by an abnormal metabolism of the polysaccharides chondroitin sulfuric acid B and heparitin monosulfate. These substances accumulate in abnormal amounts in the cells of practically every organ and system in the body, with the brain, heart, liver, and spleen most severely affected. The exact mechanism for the abnormal metabolism of the polysaccharides is not known. It has been suggested that the disorders may result from a defective binding to protein of the mucopolysaccharides. This would result in a free diffusibility of the polysaccharides and subsequent overproduction in the tissues of origin.

Over the past few years, increasing knowledge about the enzymatic deficiencies in this group of disorders has led to the introduction of experimental therapies, characterized by the infusion of plasma protein fractions rich in the deficient enzyme.[4, 5, 6] The interaction of these enzyme fractions with various anesthetic agents is not known. However, given the consideration that they are administered in the form of plasma protein fractions, it is entirely possible that the uptake and distributions of water and fat soluble agents would possibly be affected.

Seven distinct varieties of the mucopolysaccharidoses have been differentiated by combined clinical, genetic, and biochemical study. They are more or less arbitrarily designated mucopolysaccharidoses I through VII.

Hurler's syndrome (gargoylism, mucopolysaccharidosis I) is probably the best known. The condition is inherited as an autosomal recessive with a prevalence of one in 40,000 and is characterized by an increased production of both chondroitin sulfuric acid B and heparitin monosulfate.

The clinical manifestations of Hurler's syndrome include dwarfism, frontal bossing, hypertelorism, thick lips, large tongue, and hepatosplenomegaly. The neck is exceedingly short, and the thorax, on which the head appears to rest directly, is deformed. Nasal congestion, noisy mouth breathing, and frequent upper respiratory infections occur in essentially all patients with Hurler's syndrome. The malformation of the facial and nasal bones is probably, in large part, responsible. Abnormality of the tracheobronchial cartilages, together with that of the upper airway, may be responsible for the susceptibility to respiratory infection in these patients. Bronchopneumonia is a frequent cause of death.

The cardiovascular changes include valvular lesions and coronary artery disease. The involvement of the valves follows the same frequency of distribution as in rheumatic heart disease (mitral more than aortic, more than tricuspid, more than pulmonary). Endocardial, pericardial, and myocardial diseases also occur. Congestive heart failure is common, and death is frequently due to cardiac disease. Angina may be present with involvement of the coronary arteries. The anatomic basis of this is the deposition of mucopolysaccharides in the intima of the coronary arteries and in the heart valves with extensive occlusive disease of the coronary arteries.

There is marked gross and histologic involvement of the liver, but surprisingly the impression given is that little functional impairment occurs. Mental deterioration is severe. Of the mucopolysaccharidoses, Hurler's syndrome produces death at the earliest age on the average. There is no specific therapy. Most patients die before the age of 10 from pulmonary infection or cardiac failure. Inguinal hernia is frequent, and diastasis recti and umbilical hernia are almost invariable. These defects are most often what brings such patients to the operating room.

Hunter's syndrome (mucopolysaccharidosis II) is similar to, but clinically less severe than, Hurler's syndrome. It is inherited in an X-linked recessive way. The incidence appears to be one in 60,000. These patients excrete excessive amounts of chondroitin sulfuric acid B and heparitin sulfate in the urine. These patients often survive to their thirties; the oldest known patient with mucopolysaccharidosis II died at the age of 60.

Sanfilippo's syndrome (mucopolysaccharidosis III) is characterized by severe, progressive mental retardation, with less severe somatic changes. These patients only excrete large amounts of heparitin monosulfate. No cardiac abnormalities have been described. These patients can probably survive to the age of 40.

Morquio's syndrome (mucopolysaccharidosis IV) is characterized by severe skeletal changes that may lead to symptoms of spinal cord and medullary compression with unimpaired intelligence. Such patients are strikingly dwarfed, and inguinal hernias are frequently seen. Aortic regurgitation is an almost constant feature, and the urinary excretion of keratosulfate is increased. The incidence of this syndrome is one in 40,000.

Most of these patients die before the age of 20.

Scheie's syndrome (mucopolysaccharidosis V) presents with nearly normal intelligence and selective excretion of chondroitin sulfuric acid B. Aortic regurgitation and the carpal tunnel syndrome are commonly seen in these patients. Skeletal abnormalities are not severe. The frequency of the syndrome is unknown. The life span of these patients has not been determined accurately, but one patient has reached the age of 47.

The Maroteaux-Lamy syndrome (mucopolysaccharidosis VI) is characterized by normal intelligence, severe skeletal abnormalities, increased excretion of chondroitin sulfuric acid B, and absence of cardiac disease. This condition is quite rare.

I cell disease (mucopolysaccharidosis VII) presents with an abnormal increase in intracellular lipid, even more so than mucopolysaccharides.

Published anesthetic experience with this condition is very brief. It consists of a series of 14 cases reported by Wooley, Morgan, and Hays[7] from the Children's Hospital of Los Angeles, and 10 patients reported by Coran and Eraklis[8] from the Children's Hospital and Medical Center and Harvard Medical School. Unfortunately, in neither of the two series were patients classified as to the type of mucopolysaccharidosis; instead, they were classified as Hunter-Hurler syndrome. Birkinshaw[9] reported on one specific case of an anesthetic administered to a patient with Morquio's syndrome.

The 24 patients underwent a total of 31 operations, 20 of which were inguinal or umbilical herniorrhaphies. Tonsillectomy and adenoidectomy or adenoidectomy alone was the second most frequent operation, with a total of five. The age at operation ranged from seven days to 13 years, but 26 of the 31 operations (84 per cent) were done under the age of four years. In Wooley's series, complications included excessive secretions, difficult or impossible intubation, postoperative tracheostomy for respiratory obstruction, excessive bleeding from the surgical site, and one case of cardiac arrest under open drop ether anesthesia. Seventy per cent of the complications in this series were related to maintenance of airway during operation.

In Coran's series, the anesthetic difficulties were again related to obstruction of the upper airway. Profuse thick secretions occasionally led to severe intraoperative laryngospasm. Preoperative barbiturates and opiates were avoided, and secretions were minimized by larger than usual doses of atropine. Postoperatively, patients were placed in oxygen tents with high humidity. The patients were well hydrated with intravenous fluids, to avoid formation of thick secretions. Serious upper airway obstruction was reported in two patients, but they were managed without tracheostomy.

What was most important in Birkinshaw's report was the danger of subluxation of the atlantoaxial joint with relaxation and subsequent spinal cord transection. (This is also a possible danger in Hurler's syndrome, as spastic quadriplegia may follow C1–C2 subluxation.)[10] Birkinshaw also reiterated the well-known problems with intubation of the trachea that result from distortions in facial structures, as well as the cardiovascular problems.

The deposition of mucopolysaccharides is a function of time; consequently, systemic involvement (namely, heart and lungs) will increase with age. Since most of the patients found in the literature were children or adolescents at the time of surgery, the following ideas concerning anesthetic management refer to this age group in particular.

The difficulties faced by the anesthesiologist taking care of these patients will depend on the type of mucopolysaccharidosis, the degree of systemic involvement, the age of the patient, and the operation planned. Thus it is anticipated that mucopolysaccharidoses I, II, IV, and VI will be the most difficult to manage. The importance of having a definite diagnosis prior to surgery should be stressed. Unfortunately, some operations are performed before a diagnosis is made. The general term "heritable disorder of connective tissue" should be avoided. This term also includes patients with Marfan's syndrome, Ehlers-Danlos syndrome, osteogenesis imperfecta, and fibrodysplasia ossificans progressiva — entities easily differentiated from the mucopolysaccharidoses and presenting altogether different problems for the anesthetist.

The preoperative preparation of these patients is critical. Respiratory infections should be cleared by treatment with antibiotics, after sensitivity studies. Age permitting, all available means to improve respiratory function should be used (e.g., IPPB, postural drainage, chest physiotherapy). The cardiac status should be assessed and, if advisable, treatment with digitalis preparation and/or diuretics instituted. Liver function studies should be done. When subluxation is a potential hazard, it may be possible to sit the patient in a rigid plaster-of-paris brace to maintain the anatomic relationships at the atlantoaxial joint. Intubation can then be carried out while the patient is awake and should relaxation occur the normal anatomic relationships will be maintained.

Premedication with barbiturates, tranquilizers, and opiates is best avoided, so as to prevent respiratory depression and airway obstruction preoperatively and postoperatively. The use of large doses of belladonna alkaloids to minimize secretions is debatable. Thin, watery secretions can be controlled in this way, but thick secretions will get thicker and more difficult to handle. If a belladonna drug is used, scopolamine is the drug of choice, not atropine. It is a better drying agent and its cardiac effects are less.

The vast majority of patients suffering from the mucopolysaccharidoses will require a general anesthetic because of their age, mental status, and skeletal deformities. In adults with mucopolysaccharidosis V, regional anesthesia might be suitable. Of the inhalation agents, diethyl ether is contraindicated, because of its known capacity to increase secretions. Keeping in mind that airway obstruction is the most frequent complication, the anesthetic technique chosen should minimize this possibility in the intra- as well as in the postoperative period. For this reason, most intravenous agents and relaxants are better avoided. The use of ketamine for certain procedures warrants investigation.

A smooth induction with an inhalation agent, followed by endotracheal intubation after a good topical anesthesia, with the patient breathing spontaneously, is the ideal. It should be remembered that many of these children will be difficult to intubate because of anatomic deformities. The anesthetic gases should be humidified during the procedure and intravenous fluids given to prevent drying up of mucosae and inspissation of secretions.

Postoperatively, these patients should be placed in an oxygen tent with high humidity and monitored closely until completely awake. The danger of airway obstruction is as great in the postoperative as in the intraoperative period.

THE GANGLIOSIDOSES[1-4]

The group of diseases that go under the name of gangliosidoses are also known as neurolipidoses and glycogen storage diseases. There are also several eponyms for these diseases that reflect different aspects of the chemical syndromes. These include Tay-Sachs disease, Niemann-Pick disease, and Gaucher's disease. The complex glycolipids, gangliosides, and globosides that are normally turned over by the cell require that the carbohydrate portion be hydrolyzed. Deficiency in the specific enzymes allows the accumulation and storage of different substances in the cell. For example, the accumulation of ganglioside monosialate $(G_{M2})^2$ produces the progressive neuromuscular disorder of Tay-Sachs disease and of Sanderhoff's disease, a variant of Tay-Sachs. Experimental enzyme replacement shows some signs of hope in treating these otherwise progressively unrelenting disorders.[5]

The diseases are characterized as familial neurodegeneration, with evidence of onset in late infancy as early dementia. Cerebellar and pyramidal tract signs may be evident when ganglioside G_{M1} is isolated and the generalized form is diagnosed. With ganglioside G_{M2} (Tay-Sachs disease, amaurotic familial idiocy, Batten's disease) a visceral lesion is seen in Auerbach's plexus, as well as hepatic siderosis, and microglia and giant cell foci are found in the brain. The storage disorder is also present in the reticuloendothelial system. G_{M3} storage results in a neurovisceral form of the disease, whereas in Niemann-Pick disease diffuse neuronal storage of a different material with different histochemical properties is noted. Interestingly enough, many cases with significant variance are appearing in the literature. For example, endocardial fibroelastosis, with its consequent cardiac problems, has been reported in Niemann-Pick disease,[6] some pulmonary involvement[7] and thromboplastin antecedent (Factor XI) deficiency[8] in Gaucher's disease.

Regardless of the defect, the course of the disease is inexorable, although there are different clinical forms with different rates of progression. In spite of the marked metabolic derangement, as evidenced by increased hexosamine and decreased protein synthesis, the anesthetic management has been uncomplicated. The author has been involved in anesthesia for brain biopsy in three affected infants with no untoward consequences. Nitrous oxide-oxygen-halothane anesthesia was used. Muscle relaxants and narcotics were also used without difficulty.

The problem in Gaucher's disease is considerably different, as combined portal and venacaval hypertension has been noted, and splenic[9] and renal[10] transplantations have been required. The anesthetic management of these problems appears to be more related to the surgical procedure and the cardiodynamic problems than to the metabolic-enzymatic difficulties.

OTHER INHERITED DISEASES

DOWN'S SYNDROME (MONGOLISM)

Mongolism occurs in one in 600 births and accounts for 10 per cent of institutionalized mental retardates.[1] The entity is characterized by mental deficiency and multiple musculoskeletal and other congenital abnormalities of varying significance. The multiple congenital abnormalities result when, during cell division, the Down-21 chromosome (Denver numbering system) divides abnormally, producing a trisomic zygote that may or may not be lethal. The abnormality occurs most frequently in mothers over 35 years old, but the cause is not clear. (For an excellent review of autosomal abnormalities the reader is referred to the article by Smith.[2]) Usually the diagnosis can be made in an infant with hypotonia and the classic stigmata. The stigmata include abnormal nostril direction, abnormal toe, short fifth digit, curved fifth digit, squared head, epicanthal fold, and simian crease. But although any one of these may be seen in normal infants (15 per cent), the presence of three or more usually indicates mongolism. When these infants die in infancy, as they do in 60 per cent of the cases, death is usually a result of complications of their cardiac abnormality, which occurs in 66 per cent. There is, however, no good correlation between the frequency of occurrence of stigmata and the presence of congenital heart disease, perhaps suggesting that individuals with many more positive indices die in utero.[3]

Also associated with the skeletal and cardiac anomalies are abnormalities in serotonin and catecholamine metabolism. The significance of the low excretion of free and conjugated epinephrine is not clear, but it may be related to the poor stress response seen in these infants.[4] On the other hand, enzymatic defects occur at many levels, including the conversion of tryptophan to serotonin, tyrosine to epinephrine, and amino acids to taurine.[5] These biochemical abnormalities may result more frequently when the muscular defects are associated with translocation rather than trisomy of the gene,[6] and may represent a variant of the usual Down's syndrome. Abnormalities of serotonin metabolism may have great clinical significance for infants with mongolism; 97.7 per cent of those infants have hypotonia, as evidenced by an inability to maintain posture when held in a prone position (Landau reflex). This hypotonia may be corrected entirely by the administration of 5-hydroxytryptamine (precursor of serotonin), 0.06 to 2.1 mg per kilogram per day over four to six weeks.[7] Unfortunately the side effects of motor restlessness, vomiting, diarrhea, opisthotonos, hypertension, and cutaneous flush may be severe, but they usually respond to reduction of the dosage. There is no correlation of hypotonia with the abnormal response to muscle relaxant or respiratory distress, and the importance of the finding of hypotonia is not clear as regards anesthesia.

There are very few specific reports of anesthesia given to children with mongolism, although they have come to surgery for cardiac abnormalities, umbilical hernias, and undescended testes as well as the usual unrelated surgical illnesses. Preoperative preparation may safely include a drying agent, because the inability to lacrimate is not associated with other secretory problems. Preoperative evaluation must be thorough to evaluate the likelihood of congenital cardiac abnormalities, and the management of children with these particular anomalies depends on the pathophysiology demonstrated. Lassen and colleagues[7] studied cerebral oxygen consumption in unpremedicated children with Down's syndrome. These children were usually placid and cooperative, and accepted a mask induction with 3 per cent halothane and oxygen quite well. The trachea was intubated after 30 mg of gallamine, and anesthesia was maintained for 30 minutes without sequelae; this technique could be generally recommended. It was found that children with Down's syndrome had normal oxygen consumption, as compared with children with other neurologic mental deficiencies. There is an increased rate of respiratory infections that may be related to the high level of the enzyme superoxide dismutase. This enzyme inactivates the superoxide radicals that are normally active in the body's defense against infection.

Of particular importance is the changing attitude toward children with Down's syndrome. Early intelligence testing (IQ) in children with Down's syndrome was most usually performed on institutionalized children. As more and more children are managed at home, a greater potential for leading a productive life has been recognized, and a concerted effort is being made to help parents work effectively with these children. There is a "movement" to protect the rights of children with Down's syndrome, and as this movement gathers force we will not be surprised to see more and more of these children come to surgery for correction of their anatomic lesions. An awareness of the improved life outlook for children with Down's syndrome will help anesthesiologists to relate more effectively to the children and their families.

KLIPPEL-FEIL SYNDROME

Klippel-Feil syndrome refers to congenital fusion of the cervical vertebrae and represents an embryologic failure of differentiation of these structures. Most frequently, the C2 and C3 vertebrae are involved (Type II), although en bloc fusion of all cervical vertebrae, including C1 and the base of the skull, may be seen (Type I).[9] In patients with Type I, the bull neck, with limited range of motion of the neck, and other congenital malformations may be present. Patients with Klippel-Feil syndrome may present with neck pain and cervical radiculitis, basilar artery insufficiency, or quadriparesis. In its most severe form thoracic vertebrae are involved as well, and kyphoscoliosis with a significant pulmonary disability has been reported.[10] Occasionally,

basilar impression (platybasia), in which the base of the skull is flattened in the cervical spine, occurs. Compression of the pons and medulla and stretching of the cranial nerves may all be symptomatic.

The problems encountered in the anesthetic management depend almost entirely on the degree of neck fixation, jaw protrusion, and bull neck. It is quite likely that awake intubation of the trachea will be required,[11] because it may be virtually impossible to ventilate these patients during general anesthesia with or without muscle relaxant supplements. Furthermore, it may be necessary to keep the endotracheal tube in place after the anesthetic until the patient is fully responsive. The presence of cleft palate may further complicate the problem, increasing the potential for aspiration of secretions. Maintenance of anesthesia should not present problems, although basilar artery insufficiency and pulmonary disability will have to be considered. Again the association of other major anomalies with Klippel-Feil syndrome may create as much of a challenge for the anesthesiologists as the primary disorder itself. To name a few of the most important from the standpoint of management of the anesthesiologist would be only to begin the list and increase the awareness of the anesthesiologist for these potential hazards. These include: renal agenesis, aortic coarctation, cervical facial deformity, aplasia of one lung, and multiple internal organ pathology.

ARNOLD-CHIARI MALFORMATION

The Arnold-Chiari malformation comprises a group of congenital hindbrain anomalies in which there is downward displacement of the vermis of the cerebellum into the cervical canal, with caudal displacement of the lower pons and medulla.[12] Most patients present with a high cervical cord lesion and present to surgery for cervical laminectomy and release of increased intraspinal pressure. Usually the symptoms appear in the first four months of life, with hydrocephalus that results from narrowing of the aqueduct. Hydromyelia and later syringomyelia occur frequently. A meningomyelocele is also commonly present.

Surgery is hazardous, because respiratory arrest and loss of consciousness may follow flexion of the neck, and this complication may be missed when the patient is unconscious during general anesthesia. It may be useful to sit the patient up and flex the neck preoperatively to assess the likelihood of respiratory problems caused by anatomic deficiencies.[13] The loss of consciousness may be averted if ventricular puncture is performed prophylactically to relieve pressure.[14]

Children with the Arnold-Chiari malformation may have laryngeal stridor, but pulmonary function is nonetheless normal and the stridor is thought to be due to increased intracranial pressure.[15]

Whenever possible, awake endotracheal intubation to avoid undue positional changes of the neck, light anesthesia, and spontaneous respiration are recommended.[16] When bony or dural decompression is accomplished, immediate results are good. Posterior fossa exploration may have a high morbidity.

FAMILIAL DYSAUTONOMIA (RILEY-DAY SYNDROME) AND ORTHOSTATIC HYPOTENSION SYNDROME OF SHY-DRAGER

These two entities have several features in common. They both have their onset in infancy, are progressive, and begin with symptoms of autonomic lability, such as hypertension in the Riley-Day syndrome and orthostatic hypotension in the Shy-Drager syndrome. Such patients develop symptoms consistent with diffuse central nervous system involvement. In the Riley-Day syndrome hyperpyrexia, emotional lability, and insensitivity to pain predominate.[17] In the Shy-Drager syndrome manifestations of degeneration in the basal ganglia and cerebellum may result in Parkinson's syndrome.[18] In both conditions there is increased sensitivity to catecholamines; indeed, a defect in the conversion from L-dopa to norepinephrine has been postulated in patients with the Riley-Day syndrome.

The anesthetic management of both syndromes has been documented. We were able to find reports of 56 anesthetics administered to patients with the Riley-Day syndrome,[19-21] but only one report of anesthesia in a patient with the Shy-Drager syndrome.[22] Several features dictate the anesthetic management: 1) apprehension may be exaggerated; premedication with chlorpromazine, 1 mg per kilogram, and meperidine, 1 mg per kilogram, has been used successfully. 2) The response to blood volume changes may be marked, and a saline load results in increased left ventricular end-diastolic pressure. Thus the preoperative evaluation of the blood volume as well as continued accurate intraoperative measurement of blood loss is required. 3) There is usually a significant fall in blood pressure without a compensatory tachycardia following thiopental induction. This exaggerated fall in blood pressure has also been noted with potent anesthetics such as halothane, methoxyflurane, and diethyl ether. Moreover, since these patients do not sweat or increase their pulse rates, and blood pressure changes are excessive, the common indicators of depth of anesthesia are not valid. Nitrous oxide-oxygen supplemented with succinylcholine and a dilute phenylephrine drip to maintain blood pressure is an anesthetic technqiue that has been well tolerated. 4) Although there are no reports of abnormal response to depolarizing muscle relaxants, it would appear that these may represent a potential danger, because other patients with lower motor neuron disease have had abnormal response to these agents.[23] Similarly, the potential for hyperpyrexia must be considered, and temperature monitoring is required.

Recently, the association of sleep apnea has been quoted in patients with Shy-Drager syndrome.[24] The significance of anesthesia in this case is not clear, but disturbances in sleep are often treated with tricyclic antidepressants on the one hand, and the apneic syndrome may be enhanced by the central nervous system depressants that linger on in the postoperative period on the other hand.

NEUROECTODERMAL DISORDERS

The group of neuroectodermal disorders that include *Sturge-Weber disease, von Hippel-Lindau disease, von Recklinghausen's disease,* and *tuberous sclerosis* are all of particular import to the anesthesiologist because of their association with other biochemical disorder, tumors, and the unusual location of the neuroanatomic deformities.

Usually the onset is in infancy and childhood, and all, with the exception of Sturge-Weber disease, are associated with intracranial neoplasm.[1, 3]

Sturge-Weber disease manifests as unilateral angiomatous lesions to the leptomeninges and upper face, with linear cerebral calcifications in the underlying brain tissue. The port wine stain in an infant with contralateral hemiparesis, seizure disorders, and mental retardation is diagnostic. Occasionally neurologic manifestations may be mild, and a diagnosis of subdural hematoma may be considered. Cisternography with radioactive albumin demonstrates rapid clearance, as would be expected in the presence of this vascular tumor,[2] and the rapid transport of cerebrospinal fluid may modify the uptake and transfer of anesthetic drugs across the blood-brain barrier. This has not been reported to be clinically significant. Unusual locations for the lesion in Sturge-Weber disease, such as one of the vasomotor centers of the brain, may present special problems.[5]

Patients with von Hippel-Lindau disease present with angioblastic lesions in the retina and often the cerebellum and spinal cord. The disease appears to begin in young adults, but because of the slow progression it may not be noted for some time. The specific progressive neurologic sequelae referable to the site of the lesion may be the presenting complaint. Polycystic kidneys, pancreatic cysts, hypernephroma, erythrocytosis, and pheochromocytoma may also be associated.[1, 4] The anesthetic considerations depend on these entities more than on the primary disease. Perhaps the most important specific factor is the surgical requirements for meticulous dissection, because recurrence of the tumor is rare when completely resected. Thus the anesthetic may be exceedingly long.

Neurofibromatosis, or von Recklinghausen's disease, has been appropriately labeled a "bizarre disease."[6] Although its appearance as a heredofamilial disease in one in 3000 births, with café au lait spots, vascular nevi, moles, and other neurocutaneous lesions,[7] seems straightforward, the multiple hollow organ, peripheral nerve, and neuroendocrine involvement and propensity for malignant degeneration create clinical havoc. It may be possible to understand the disease if we consider the primary embryologic neural crest dysfunction on the one hand and the peripheral nerve sheath tumor on the other. Schimke et al.[8] pointed out that medullary thyroid tumor, pheochromocytoma, and neurofibromatosis have developed from a similar embryologic defect that is genetically determined, and thus the simultaneous (6 to 25 per cent) appearance of the entities can be readily appreciated. Moreover, medullary thyroid tumors may produce a calcium-lowering factor (calcitonin), and secondary hyperparathyroidism with hypercalcemia and nephrocalcinosis may be evident. When the tumors appear in the sheath of periosteal nerves, significant bone changes occur; severe kyphoscoliosis has been reported in as many as 50 per cent of the patients.[9] Many other seemingly unrelated defects, such as honeycomb cystic lung changes with uncompensated respiratory alkalosis[10] and renal artery dysplasia with hypertension,[11] are not so readily explained. Numerous unusual locations for the tumor mass have also been reported. Those in the right ventricular outflow tract with production of right ventricular hypertension and in the larynx have the most obvious anesthetic implications. The anesthetist must be prepared for almost any eventuality in a patient with von Recklinghausen's disease. Unrecognized pheochromocytoma may be the most lethal; it has been reported during anesthesia for cesarean section,[12] but abnormal responses to muscle relaxants have also been noted,[13-14] although these latter relationships are not certain. Because of the multiple nature of the tumor, surgical extirpation is usually not considered unless major organ structures are involved. However, if these patients should require surgery, radiologic examination of the lung for cystic lesions and of the spine for kyphoscoliosis, as well as a careful search for previous unrecognized pheochromocytoma, is required. Since the latter search may not reveal evidence of the tumor even when present, the anesthetic may properly be conducted as if the patient did have pheochromocytoma, with the appropriate monitoring and the availability of vasoactive drugs. One additional report[15] noted the use of 20 various general anesthetics and one experience with subarachnoid block in 16 patients with reported difficulty. One patient had a fleshy tumor of the larynx that presented as respiratory stridor but proceeded without untoward anesthetic sequelae. Again, anesthesia seems not to be a problem provided the anesthesiologist is alert to the myriad associated problems with which these patients present. Thiobarbiturates and halothane have been used. Muscle relaxants may be used with particular care in the event of prolonged block.

Tuberous sclerosis (Bourneville's disease) is present in one in 30,000 births. Patients present with a classic triad of epilepsy, mental deficiency, and adenoma sebaceum. The adenomatous lesions are most commonly seen on the skin but may occur in the heart, lungs, or kidneys. Neurologic symptoms, when they occur, are usually minor, such as central facial paralysis.[16] When infiltration of the heart occurs, ectopic beats may be evident.[17] The natural history of patients with tuberous sclerosis is such that 70 per cent are dead before the age of 25, although surgical resection of the epileptogenic foci may modify this figure.[18] Anesthetic experience is limited, although presumably the patients tolerated the anesthesia for craniotomy.

REFERENCES

BASAL GANGLIA DEGENERATION

Neuroanatomic and Neurophysiologic Considerations

1. Cooper, I. D.: Clinical and physiological implications of thalamic surgery for disorders of sensory communication. J. Neurol. Sci. 2:520, 1965.
2. Ngai, S. H., Parkinsonism, levodopa and anesthesia, Anesthesiology 37:344, 1972.
3. Ziegler, M. G., Lake, C. R., Kopin, I. J. Deficient sympathetic nervous response in familial dysautonomia. N. Engl. J. Med. 290:630, 1976.
4. Murphy, G. T., Rosen, A. D., and Babu, M.: Thyrotoxicosis with Huntington's chorea. N.Y. State J. Med. 77:1322–4, 1977.

Primary Symptoms and Clinicopathological Correlations

1. Brain, W. B., and Waltin, J.: Brain's Diseases of the Nervous System. London, Oxford University Press, 1969, pp. 513–1962.
2. Denny-Brown, D.: The Basal Ganglia and Their Relation to Disorders of Movement. London, Oxford University Press, 1962.

Specific Disease Entities

1. Aaron, A. M., Freeman, J. M., and Carter, S.: The natural history of Sydenham's chorea. Amer. J. Med. 38:83, 1965.
2. Aaron, A. M.: Treatment of Sydenham's chorea. Mod. Treatm. 5:351, 1968.
3. Chase, T. W.: Rational approaches to the pharmacotherapy of chorea. Res. Publ. Assn. Res. New Ment. Dis. 55:33, 1976.
4. Green, L. N.: Corticosteroids in the treatment of Sydenham's chorea. Arch. Neurol. 35:53, 1978.
5. Whittier, J. R.: Treatment of Huntington's disease. Mod. Treatm. 5:332, 1968.
6. Davies, D. D.: Abnormal response to anaesthesia in a case of Huntington's chorea. Brit. J. Anaesth. 38:490, 1966.
7. Fareria, J., et al.: Anesthesia and Huntington's chorea. A report of two cases. Br. J. Anaesth. 49:1167, 1977.
8. Sorensen, B. F., and Hamby, W. B.: Spasmodic torticollis. Neurology 16:867, 1966.
9. Mathews, W. B., Beasly, P., Parry-Jones, W., and Garlan, G.: Spasmodic torticollis a combined clinical study. J. Neurol. Neurosurg. Psychiat. 41:485, 1978.
10. Hamby, W. B., and Schiffer, S.: Spasmodic torticollis: Result of cervical rhizotomy in 50 cases. J. Neurol. Surg. 31:323, 1969.
11. Steen, S. N.: Anesthetic management for basal ganglia surgery in patients with Parkinson's syndrome. New York J. Med. 60:3230, 1960.
12. Davis, U. T., and Daves, R. Anesthetic management in a patient with dystonia musculorum deformans, Anesthesiology 5:630, 1975.
13. Klawans, H. L., Jr., and Cohen, M. M.: Diseases of the extrapyramidal system. Disease-a-Month 1–52, 1970.
14. Coleman, D. J., and De Viller, J. C.: Anaesthesia and stereotactic surgery. Anaesthesia 19:60, 1964.
15. Steen, S. N.: Anesthetic management for basal ganglia surgery in patients with movement disorders. Anesth. Analg. 44:66, 1965.
16. Brown, A.: Neuroleptanalgesia for surgical treatment of parkinsonism. Anaesthesia 19:70, 1964.

MOTOR NEURON DEGENERATION

1. Merritt, H. H.: A Textbook of Neurology. Philadelphia, Lea and Febiger, 1967, p. 508.
2. Mullens, R. B., Hayes, A. P., Gold, A. P., Berdon, W. E., and Bowden, J. D.: Respiratory distress as the initial manifestation of Werdnig-Hoffmann disease. Pediatrics 53:33, 1974.

OTHER FORMS OF MOTOR DEGENERATION AND CHRONIC POLYNEUROPATHIES

1. Perel, A., et al: Anesthesia in the Guillain-Barré syndrome. 32:257, 1977.
2. Lichtenfeld, P.: Autonomic dysfunction in Guillain-Barré syndrome. Amer. J. Med. 50:72, 1971.
3. Newberry, A.: Paraplegia, Vol. 32, p. 78, 1977.
4. Sudo, N., Weingold, A.: Obstetric aspects of Guillain-Barré syndrome. Obstet. Gynecol. 45:39, 1975.
5. Richards, W. C.: Anaesthesia and serum creatine phosphokinase levels in patients with Duchenne's pseudohypertrophic muscular dystrophy. Anaesth. Intens. Care 1:150, 1972.

Spinocerebellar Degeneration

1. Huxtable, R.: Cardiac pharmacology and cardio-myopathy in Friedreich's ataxia. J. Canad. Sci. Neurol. 5:83, 1978.
2. Rosenbaum, K. J., Neigh, J. T., and Strobel, G. E.: Sensitivity to nondepolarizing muscle relaxants in amyotrophic lateral sclerosis: Report of two cases. Anesthesiology 35:638, 1971.
3. Cooperman, L. H.: Succinylcholine-induced hyperkalemia in neuromuscular disease. J.A.M.A. 213:1867, 1970.
4. Beach, T. P., Stone, W. A., and Hamelberg, W.: Circulatory collapse following succinylcholine: Report of a patient with diffuse lower motor neuron disease. Anesth. Analg. 50:431, 1971.
5. Moulder, D. W., Lambert, E. H., and Eaton, E. M.: Myasthenic syndrome in a patient with amyotrophic lateral sclerosis. Neurology 9:627, 1951.
6. Wise, R. P.: Muscle disorders and the relaxants. Brit. J. Anaesth. 35:558, 1963.
7. Edwards, A. E., and Bras, J. F.: The enhancement of neurologic signs under anesthesia. Brit. J. Anaesth. 42:337, 1970.

Syringomyelia and Spinal Cord Trauma

1. Huebert, H. T., and MacKinnon, W. B.: Syringomyelia and scoliosis. J. Bone Joint Surg. 51:338, 1969.
2. Willis, W. H., and Weaver, D. F.: Syringomyelia with bilateral vocal cord paralysis. Arch. Otolaryngol. 87:468, 1968.
3. Williams, B.: Syringomyelia. Brit. Med. J. 1:434, 1970.
4. Magee, K., and Schneider, R. C.: Syringomyelia: Loss of deep pain sensation with otherwise normal sensory perception. J.A.M.A. 200:795, 1967.
5. Williams, B.: Critical appraisal of posterior fossa surgery for communicating syringomyelia. Brain 101:223, 1979.
6. Lind, A. R., McNicol, G. W., Bruce, N. A., MacDonald, H. R., and Donald, K. W.: The cardiovascular response to sustained contractions of a patient with unilateral syringomyelia. Clin. Sci. 35:45, 1968.
7. Love, J., and Grofton, R. A.: Syringomyelia: A look at surgical therapy. J. Neurosurg. 24:714, 1966.
8. Groff, R. A., and Pitts, F. W.: Syringomyelia: Current status of surgical treatment. Surgery 56:806, 1964.
9. Jousse, A. T., Wynne-Jones, M., and Breithaupt, D. J.: A follow-up study of life expectancy and mortality in traumatic transverse myelitis. Canad. Med. Assoc. J. 98:770, 1968.
10. Smith, R. B., and Grenvik, A.: Cardiac arrest following succinylcholine in patients with central nervous system injuries. Anesthesiology 33:558, 1970.
11. Desmond, J.: Paraplegia. Problems confronting the anesthesiologist. Canad. Anaesth. Soc. J. 17:435, 1970.
12. Gode, G. R.: Paraplegia and cardiac arrest: Case reports. Canad. Anesth. Soc. J. 17:452, 1970.
13. Ciliberti, B. J., Goldfine, J., and Rovenstine, E. A.: Hypertension during anesthesia in patient with spinal cord injuries. Anesthesiology. 15:273, 1954.

14. Drinker, A. S., and Helrich, M.: Halothane anesthesia in the paraplegic patient. Anesthesiology 24:399, 1963.
15. Tobey, R. E.: Paraplegia, succinylcholine and cardiac arrest. Anesthesiology 32:359, 1970.
16. Stone, W. A., Beach, T. P., and Hamilberg, W.: Succinylcholine — danger in the spinal-cord-injured patient. Anesthesiology 32:168, 1970.

DEMYELINATING DISEASES

1. Brain, T., and Walton, J.: Brain's diseases of the nervous system. London, Oxford University Press, 1969, pp. 476–478.
2. Silberberg, D. H.: Recent concepts of etiology implications for treatment. Mod. Treatm. 7:879, 1970.
3. Abramsky, O., Lisak, R. P., Silberg, D. H., et al: Antibodies to oligodendroglia in patients with multiple sclerosis. N. Engl. J. Med., 297:1207, 1977.
4. Liebowitz, N., Kahana, E., and Alter, M.: Survival and death in multiple sclerosis. Brain 92:115, 1969.
5. Baskett, P. J., and Armstrong, R.: Anaesthetic problems in multiple sclerosis. Are certain agents contraindicated? Anaesthesia 25:397, 1970.
6. Siemkowicz, E.: Multiple sclerosis and surgery. Anaesthesia, 31:1211–16, 1976.
7. Bamford, C., et al.: Anesthesia in Multiple Sclerosis. Can. J. Neurol. Sci. 5:41–4, 1978.
8. Davis, F.: Pathophysiology of multiple sclerosis and related clinical implications. Mod. Treatm. 7:890, 1970.
9. Weintrault, M. I., Megahed, M. S., and Smith, B. H.: Myotonic-like syndrome in multiple sclerosis. New York J. Med. 70:677, 1970.
10. Leins, P. A., Adams, A. H., Wanyik, G., et al.: Disturbance of blood brain barrier in a case of encephalomyelopathy. Bull. L. A. Neurol. Soc. 35:74, 1970.

THE MUCOPOLYSACCHARIDOSES

1. McKusick, V. A.: Heritable Disorders of Connective Tissue. 3rd ed., St. Louis, C. V. Mosby Co., 1966, pp. 325–399.
2. Dorman, A.: *In* Stanbury, J. B., Wyngaarden, J. B., and Frederickson, D. S. (eds.): The Metabolic Basis of Inherited Disease. 2nd ed., New York, McGraw-Hill, 1966, pp. 963–994.
3. Bearn, A. G.: The mucopolysaccharidoses. *In* Beeson, P. B., and McDermott, W. (eds.): Textbook of Medicine, 13th ed. Philadelphia, W. B. Saunders Co., 1971, pp. 1709–1711.
4. Dorfman, A., et al.: The enzymatic defects in Morquio and Maroteaux-Lamy syndrome. Adv. Exp. Med. Biol. 68:261, 1976.
5. Danes, B. S.: Progress report. The influence of plasma infusion on a child with the Hurler syndrome during the first 18 months of life. Birth defects 10:230, 1974.
6. Yatziu, S., et al.: A therapeutic trial of fresh plasma protein infusion over a period of 22 months in two siblings with Hunter's syndrome: Ass. J. Med. Sci. 11:802, 1975.
7. Wooley, M. M., Morgan, S., and Hays, D. M.: Heritable disorders of connective tissue: Surgi-

cal and anesthetic problems. J. Pediat. Surg. 2:325, 1967.

8. Coran, A. G., and Eraklis, A. J.: Inguinal hernia in the Hurler-Hunter syndrome. Surgery, 61:302, 1967.

9. Birkinshaw, K. J.: Anaesthesia in a patient with an unstable neck. Morquio's syndrome. Anaesthesia 30:46, 1975.

10. Brill, C. B., et al.: Spastic quadriparesis due to C1-C2 subluxation in Hurler syndrome. J. Pediatr. 92:441, 1978.

THE GANGLIOSIDOSES

1. Phillipart, M., Martin, J., Warfin, J. J., and Mences, J. H.: Neimann-Pick disease. Arch. Neurol. 20:227, 1966.

2. Cummings, J. M., Dayan, A. D., Aitken, J. N., and Lewis, G. M.: Unusual forms of gangliosidoses involving the brain and viscera. J. Neurol. Sci. 13:137, 1971.

3. Korey, S., Gomez, C. J., Stein, A., Gonaras, J., Suzuki, K., Terry, R., and Weiss, M.: Studies in Tay-Sachs disease. Neuropath. Exp. Neurol. 22:2, 1963.

4. Aronson, S. M., and Aronson, B. B.: Clinical neuropathological conference. Dis. Nerv. Syst. 31:208, 1970.

5. Beutler, E.: Newer aspects of some interesting lipid storage diseases; Tay-Sach and Gaucher's disease. Anesth. J. Med. 126:46, 1977.

6. Westwood, M.: Endocardial fibroelastosis and Niemann-Pick disease. Brit. Heart J. 39:1394, 1977.

7. Scheider, E. L., et al.: Severe pulmonary involvement in adult Gaucher's disease: Am. J. Med. 63:475, 1977.

8. Seligshorn, U., et al.: Coexistence of factor XI (plasma thromboplastin antecedent) deficiency and Gaucher's disease: Iss. J. Med. Sci. 12:1448, 1976.

9. Grath, C. G., et al.: Splenic transplantation in Gaucher's disease. Birth Defects 9:102, 1973.

10. Desnich, S. J., et al.: Renal transplantation in Type II Gaucher's disease. Birth Defects 9:109, 1973.

OTHER INHERITED DISEASES

1. McIntire, M. S., and Dutch, S. J.: Mongolism and generalized hypotonia. Amer. J. Ment. Defic. 68:669, 1964.

2. Smith, D.: Autosomal abnormalities. Amer. J. Obstet. Gynec. 90(Supp.) 1055, 1964.

3. Gibson, D., Pozsonyi, J., and Zarlos, D.: Dimensions of mongolism: II. The interaction of clinical indices. Amer. J. Ment. Defic. 68:503, 1964.

4. Keele, D., Richards, C., Brown, J., and Marshall, J.: Catecholamine metabolism in Down's syndrome, Amer. J. Ment. Defic. 714:125, 1969.

5. Coleman, M. C.: Down's syndrome. Pediatr. Ann. 7:9, 1975.

6. Rosner, F., Ong, B. H., Pain, R. S., and Mahanand, D.: Biochemical differentiation of trisomic Down's syndrome. N. Engl. J. Med. 273:1356, 1965.

7. Bazelon, M., Pain, R., Cavie, V., Hunt, P., Novick, J., and Mahanand, D.: Reversal of hypotonia in infants with Down's syndrome by adminstration of hydroxytryptophan. Lancet 1:1130, 1967.

8. Lassen, N. A., Christensen, S., Hoedt-Rasmussen, K., and Stewart, B. M.: Cerebral oxygen consumption in Down's syndrome. Arch. Neurol. 15:595, 1966.

9. Gunderson, C., Greenspan, R. H., Glaser, G. H., and Lubs, H. A.: the Klippel-Feil syndrome: Genetics and clinical reevaluation of cervical fusion. Medicine 46:491, 1967.

10. Mather, J. S.: Impossible direct laryngoscopy in achondroplasia. Anesthesia 21:245, 1966.

11. Baga, N., Chusid, E. I., and Miller, A.: Pulmonary disability in the Klippel-Feil syndrome. Clin. Orthop. 67:105, 1967.

12. Appleby, A., Foster, J. D., Harkinson, J., and Hudgson, P.: Diagnosis and management of the Chiari malformation in adult life. Brain 91:131, 1968.

13. Rhotron, A. L.: Microsurgery of Arnold-Chiari malformation in adults with and without hydromyelia. J. Neurosurg. 45:473, 1976.

14. Mullen, S., and Raimondes, A.: Respiratory hazards of surgical treatment of the Arnold-Chiari malformation. J. Neurosurg. 19:675, 1962.

15. Kreiger, A. J.: Detwiller, J. S., and Troosicin, S. Z.: Respiratory function in infants with Arnold-Chiari malformation. Laryngoscope 86:818, 1976.

16. Di Piero, A.: Anesthesiologic problems in surgical correction of Arnold-Chiari malformations. Min. Anesth. 35:228, 1969.

17. McCaughey, T. J.: Familial dysautonomia as an anesthetic hazard. Canad. Anasth. Soc. J. 12:558, 1965.

18. Schwarz, G.: Orthostatic hypotension syndrome of Shy-Drager. Arch. Neurol. 16:123, 1967.

19. Mondy, H. W., and Creighton, R. E.: General anesthesia in eight patients with familial dysautonomia. Canad. Anaesth. Soc. J. 18:563, 1971.

20. Bortels, J. M.: Familial dysautonomia. J.A.M.A. 212:318, 1970.

21. Kritcheman, M. M., Schwartz, H., and Papper, E. M.: Experiences with general anesthesia in patients with familial dysautonomia. J.A.M.A. 170:529, 1971.

22. Cohen, C.: Anesthetic management of a patient with the Shy-Drager syndrome. Anesthesiology 35:95, 1971.

23. Cooperman, I. H.: Succinylcholine-induced hyperkalemia in neuromuscular disease. J.A.M.A. 213:1867, 1970.

24. Briskin J. G., et al.: Shy-Drager syndrome and sleep apnea. In Guilleminault, C., and Dement, W. C.: Sleep Apnea. New York, A. R. Liss, 1978.

NEUROECTODERMAL DISORDERS

1. Hoff, J. T., and Bronson, S. A.: Cerebral hemangioblastoma occurring in a patient with von Hippel-Lindau disease. J. Neurosurg. 28:365, 1968.

2. Chang, J. C., Jackson, G. L., and Blatz, N.: Isotopic cisternography in Sturge-Weber syndrome. J. Nucl. Med. 11:551, 1970.

3. Illingworth, R. D.: Pheochromocytoma and cerebellar hemangioblastoma. J. Neurol. Neurosurg. Psychiat. *30*:443, 1967.

4. Rho, Y. M.: von Hippel-Lindau's disease: A report of five cases. Canad. Med. Assoc. J. *101*:135, 1969.

5. Sturge, A.: A case of partial epilepsy apparently due to a lesion of one of the vasomotor centers of the brain. Trans. Clin. Soc. Lon. *12*:162, 1879.

6. Russell, J. Y. W.: Neurofibromatosis: A bizarre disease. Brit. J. Surg. *52*:251, 1965.

7. Pruzanski, W., and Adler, H.: Myotonic dystrophy, acute intermittent porphyria and neurofibromatosis in one patient. Acta Genet. *16*:102, 1966.

8. Schimke, R. N., Hartmann, W. H., Prout, T. E., and Rimon, D. C.: Syndrome of bilateral pheochromocytoma, medullary thyroid carcinoma and multiple neuromas. N. Engl. J. Med. *279*:1, 1968.

9. Singleton, A. O., Jr.: The surgical aspects of multiple neurofibromatosis. Amer. Surg. *36*:451, 1970.

10. Massaro, D., Katz, S., Mathews, M. J., and Higgins, G.: Von Recklinghausen's neurofibromatosis associated with cystic lung disease. Amer. J. Med. *38*:233, 1965.

11. Bourke, E., and Gatenby, P. B. B.: Renal artery dysplasia with hypertension in neurofibromatosis. Brit. Med. J. *3*:681, 1971.

12. Humble, R. M. Phaeochromocytoma, neurofibromatosis and pregnancy. Anaesthesia *22*:296, 1967.

13. Magbagbeola, J. A.: Abnormal responses to muscle relaxants in a patient with von Recklinghausen's disease. Brit. J. Anaesth, *42*:710, 1971.

14. Manser, J.: Abnormal responses in von Recklinghausen's disease. Brit. J. Anaesth. *42*:183, 1970.

15. Fisher, M. D.: Anesthetic difficulties in neurofibromatosis. Anesthesia *30*:648, 1975.

16. Zaremba, J.: Tuberous sclerosis: A clinical and genetical investigation. J. Ment. Defic. Res. *12*:63, 1968.

17. Cosnett, J.: Tuberous sclerosis and cardiac arrhythmia in three Zulu patients. Brit. Med. J. *2*:672, 1969.

18. Perto, P., Weir, B., and Rasmussen, T.: Tuberous sclerosis: Surgical therapy for seizures. Arch. Neurol. *15*:498, 1960.

13

Connective Tissue Diseases

By JOHN H. EISELE, JR., M.D.

Introduction
  Anesthetic Considerations
  Anesthetic Management
Rheumatoid Arthritis
  Other Diseases with Pathology Similar to
    Rheumatoid Arthritis
  Anesthetic Management of Rheumatoid
    Arthritis and Associated Diseases
Collagen Diseases
  Systemic Lupus Erythematosus
  Scleroderma
  Scleredema (Scleredema Adultorum of
    Buschke)
  Anesthetic Management of Scleroderma
    and Scleredema
  Polyarteritis Nodosa (Periarteritis,
    Necrotizing Angiitis)

Cranial (Temporal) Arteritis
Anesthetic Management of Polyarteritis
  Nodosa and Cranial Arteritis
Dermatomyositis (Neuromyositis,
  Polymyositis)
Granulomatous Diseases
  Wegener's Granulomatosis
  Lethal Midline Granuloma
  Anesthetic Management of Wegener's
    Granulomatosis and Lethal Midline
    Granuloma
  Sarcoidosis (Besnier's, Boeck's,
    Schaumann's, or Uveoparotid Fever)
Summary

INTRODUCTION

The supporting system or connective tissue system is the extracellular framework of the body, composed of structural elements, the fibers, set in a nonstructural matrix, the ground substance. Classification of diseases involving the fibers and their ground substance is not an easy division, because many variations of disturbances have to be considered. This chapter treats three groups of diseases primarily involving connective tissue: 1) rheumatoid arthritis and associated or rheumatoid disorders; 2) the so-called collagen diseases, which include systemic lupus erythematosus, scleroderma, periarteritis nodosa, and associated disorders featuring vasculitis, and dermatomyositis; and 3) granulomatous diseases, namely Wegener's granulomatosis, lethal midline granuloma, and sarcoidosis. In reviewing the various pathologic manifestations, emphasis will be placed on the cardiopulmonary system and other areas of special concern to the anesthetist and surgeon.

ANESTHETIC CONSIDERATIONS

There is no known cause for any of these diseases, and with the exception of rheumatoid arthritis the connective tissue disorders are rare. As a consequence, there is very little reported experience on the anesthetic management of patients with these diseases, except rheumatoid arthritis. Likewise, there is no information regarding the effects, if any, of anesthetic drugs on connective tissue disorders. There are, however, at least two important considerations

508

regarding the influence of these diseases on anesthetic management. First, patients with connective tissue diseases have multisystem involvement and are often chronically ill. This means that anemia, hypovolemia, hypoproteinemia, reduced ability to handle stress, and altered responses to drugs are common. Many of these patients have pulmonary manifestations of their disease that present an added risk for anesthesia and surgery. To a lesser extent there may be cardiac, vasomotor, renal, or gastrointestinal involvement. Secondly, and perhaps more important to the anesthetist, is the preoperative drug and treatment history. Most of the connective tissue diseases in the acute form are treated with corticosteroids; thus, a history of some steroid medication is almost inevitable.

It is important, therefore, to clarify some of the physiologic considerations of adrenal function, because there are clinical reports dating back to 1952 of collapse during and after operation in patients who had previously taken steroids.[1] That corticotropin (ACTH) — as well as the hormones of the adrenal gland (cortisol, corticosterone, aldosterone) — could be suppressed by exogenous cortisone was put on firm scientific ground in a study by Graber et al.[2] in 1965, after it became possible to measure plasma corticotropin. In patients receiving supraphysiologic* doses of cortisone for at least a year, the following events occur:

Steroid	Daily Production	Plasma Concentration
Cortisol	25 mg	10 μg/100 ml
Corticosterone	5 mg	2 μg/100 ml
Aldosterone	0.25 mg	0.01 μg/100 ml

1. During the first month after withdrawal, there is a tendency for depression of both corticotropin and 17-OHCS (hydroxycorticosterone) levels, evidence of both hypopituitary and hypoadrenal function. Nevertheless, the diurnal variation that is part of normal physiology is present.

2. Through the second to fifth months corticotropin levels rise to what would be considered an above normal range, whereas 17-OHCS levels tend to remain low (evidence of hyperpituitarism and hypoadrenocorticism).

3. From five to nine months 17-OHCS is

in the normal range, but only by virtue of continued high corticotropin levels.

4. After nine months no differences from untreated patients are detectable.

Roberts[3] referred to the difficulties in interpreting the many reports of postoperative adrenocortical failure. He pointed out that it was often difficult to discern whether the crisis resulted from inadequate corticotropin output, insufficient adrenal response because of glandular atrophy, or some other unrelated problem. There is a wide range of normal values for plasma 17-OHCS in healthy people at any time of day, plus a diurnal variation wherein early morning values are double those at evening. In regard to surgery, Helmreich et al.[4] found only one in 12 normal patients not on steroids who did not have a significant rise in plasma 17-OHCS levels by the middle of the operation. Virtue et al.[5] observed elevations in plasma 17-OHCS owing to anesthesia alone in a group receiving diethyl ether, but the effect was by no means uniform. In studies by Oyama et al.,[6] surgical patients premedicated with atropine and receiving pentobarbital and morphine only showed plasma 17-OHCS below control levels. Halothane-nitrous oxide anesthesia for 40 minutes prior to surgery was associated with an elevation in plasma 17-OHCS (14 to 18 μg per 100 ml), which continued to rise 30 minutes after the start of the operation. This rise did not occur, however, if anesthesia was induced with thiopental. It is of interest that spinal anesthesia prevents this preoperative and intraoperative rise in 17-OHCS.[7] Oyama and Takiguchi[8] also studied plasma corticotropin, which showed a large but transient increase during the first 20 minutes of halothane-nitrous oxide anesthesia and a second peak some 30 minutes after starting the operation. Unfortunately in most of these studies with halothane we do not know the depth of anesthesia.

ANESTHETIC MANAGEMENT

Every patient receiving long-term corticosteroids should be considered abnormal. The question is whether he is sufficiently abnormal to require steroid support to withstand the stress of surgery. A clinical test to separate normal from abnormal responses as well as to determine the degree of abnormality would be useful.

*Normal values for adrenal steroids (after Goodman and Gilman):

Thorn's diagnostic test[9] of giving corticotropin and measuring plasma 17-OHCS over the next hour is worthwhile, but it does not test the corticotropin release mechanism. There are other tests for pituitary-adrenal function, but they are too complex and expensive for routine use. A more practical test for adrenal competency is to measure serum cortisol levels before and one half hour after an injection of 250 μg ACTH intramuscularly.[10] This test seems to be reliable in detecting impaired hypothalamic-pituitary-adrenocortical responses and is preferable to an insulin produced hypoglycemic stress.

In clinical practice, then, we must realize that despite the fact some patients on maintenance levels of steroids are still capable of activating their pituitary-adrenal axis in response to stress, we cannot easily predict who they might be. We are left then with an obligation to provide steroid coverage for these patients when undergoing surgical stress regardless of the magnitude of the procedure, as adrenal insufficiency has been reported following a simple bunionectomy.[11] It would be useful to recall the signs and symptoms of acute adrenal insufficiency: hypotension, restlessness, weakness, anorexia with nausea and abdominal pain, and frequently hyperpyrexia which may be extreme. The treatment, of course, is hydrocortisone intravenously.

There are numerous protocols and regimens put forth to provide coverage for patients who are currently being treated with steroids (either for replacement or other) and for patients who have taken steroids in the past 6 to 12 months. Moore[12] recommends hydrocortisone, 100 mg intravenously every eight hours, starting three hours prior to anesthesia and continued for one to three days. Plumpton and associates[13] carefully studied plasma cortisol levels following several steroid administration techniques on patients known to have inadequate adrenocortical response to stress. The technique listed in Table 13–1 produced plasma cortisol values comparable to the levels seen in normal patients undergoing surgery.

In patients with an established intravenous drip, hydrocortisone sodium succinate (Solu-Cortef) 100 mg is more useful, and following intravenous injection, demonstrable effects are evident within one hour and persist four to six hours, a response similar

Table 13–1

Operation	Drugs	Duration
Major surgery	Hydrocortisone hemisuccinate 100 mg IM 6-hourly	3 Days
Minor surgery	Same	24 Hours
Short procedures	Hydrocortisone hemisuccinate 100 mg IM	Single dose given with premedications

to that following intramuscular administration.

RHEUMATOID ARTHRITIS

General. Rheumatoid arthritis is a systemic disease primarily affecting connective tissue. Although lesions may be widespread, joint inflammation is the dominant clinical manifestation. The course is variable, but tends to be chronic and progressive, leading to characteristic deformities and disabilities.

In contrast to the collagen diseases, rheumatoid arthritis is far from uncommon. Its prevalence may be as high as 2 per cent of the population, and in socioeconomic terms arthritis and rheumatism are second only to heart disease as causes for chronic limitation of activity.[14] Women are affected three times as frequently as men. The disease may begin at any age, but the most common age of onset is in the fourth decade. By contrast, juvenile rheumatoid arthritis (JRA), also referred to as Still's disease, has its onset between ages two and 12, and may be associated with fevers, adenopathy, splenomegaly, and a morbilliform rash, but its pathology is indistinguishable from that of adult rheumatoid arthritis. In terms of epidemiology, there are no clear-cut genetic, familial, racial, or occupational factors involved in either juvenile or adult rheumatoid arthritis.

Etiologically, attention has been focused on autoimmune phenomena, but the exact role of each of the many features of immunity remains in doubt. Serological abnormalities, such as the presence of macroglobulins in the plasma cells of diseased synovial membrane, suggest an antigenetic stimulus in the articular area. Antibodies to tissue components are often found (antinuclear and antithyroid); however, transfusion of these antibodies fails to cause the illness in normal volunteers.

Pathology.   Proliferative inflammation is the outstanding feature of rheumatoid arthritis. The synovial membrane is at first thickened by edema and cell infiltration and later is thrown into folds with hypertrophied villi. As the disease progresses, the synovial tissue grows from the margins onto the joint surface of the articular cartilage or invades between it and the bone. The development of granulation tissue, which eventually is converted into a dense fibrous scar, dominates the later stages of the disease. Erosion of both cartilage and bone can progress to total destruction of the joint with resultant subluxations, deformities, and contractures of periarticular tissue, such as tendons and ligaments (Fig. 13–1).

Clinical Picture.   The typical patient usually appears chronically ill, undernourished, and anemic. It is characteristic that these symptoms are at first intermittent and may disappear for months or years. In most cases, the disease returns and each time assumes a more chronic form. Most adult cases are polyarticular, affecting the small joints of the hands and feet, usually in a symmetric fashion, producing swelling, pain, and limitation of motion. Unlike the collagen diseases or other rheumatic disorders, the disease process tends to persist in any given joint or joints.

Extra-articular manifestations are probably more common than was previously thought. The extent and frequency of visceral involvement with rheumatoid arthritis is difficult to determine because it is often noted only on necropsy. It has been suggested that nonarticular problems in rheumatoid arthritis, in particular vasculitis, are related in some way to steroid therapy. Regardless of their origin, awareness of cardiac, pulmonary, and hematopoietic changes is essential to the care of these patients.

According to Cathcart and Spodick,[15] the incidence of heart disease in 254 patients with rheumatoid arthritis is 35 per cent, compared with 15 per cent in a control group. The most frequent cardiac signs and symptoms are enlargement of the left ventricle, congestive heart failure, and angina pectoris.

"Rheumatoid lung" or specific lung lesions found in rheumatoid arthritis have been extensively described. Lung involvement is usually a diffuse infiltrate. This produces restriction and, hence, loss of compliance. What has not been well appreciated is the loss of chest wall compliance, which accompanies arthritis in the costovertebral and intervertebral joints. When diffuse interstitial fibrosis is present, there may be an associated oxygen diffusion problem in addition to the loss of compliance, and as a result the arterial Po_2 may be lower than normal.

The severity of the lung involvement is usually in keeping with the degree of joint inflammation. In most cases the pulmonary manifestations are preceded by the joint symptoms, but sometimes they appear at the time of recrudescence of joint symptoms, and on rare occasions acute joint and pulmonary involvement appear simultaneously at the onset of the disease.[16] Pulmonary manifestations generally fall into three patterns:

1. Granulomatous lesions such as subcutaneous nodules, which may be hard to distinguish from infectious granulomata, may occur. They may be multiple or coalescent, producing a honeycombed x-ray picture.

2. Diffuse, large silicotic nodules seen in

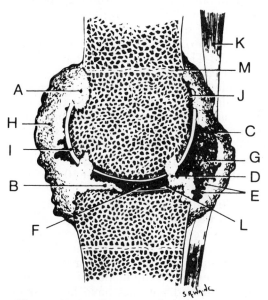

Figure 13–1.   Diagram of changes in a synovial joint in rheumatoid arthritis. A, invasion of subchondral bone; B, erosion of articular cartilage (pannus); C, fibrotic area; D, fibrous adhesions; E, multiple villi. Joint space: F, narrowing; G, loculated effusion; H, laxity of thickened capsule and ligaments; I, articular cartilage; J, subchondral bone; K, muscle; L, fibrocartilage; M, old epiphyseal plate.

the lungs of coal miners with rheumatoid arthritis have been described by Caplan.[17] The nodules may represent an altered tissue reactivity to silica particles.

3. Diffuse interstitial fibrosis may occur without any apparent explanation or related condition. This is perhaps the most common pulmonary lesion associated with rheumatoid arthritis.[18]

Subcutaneous nodules may occur in 5 per cent of rheumatoid arthritics. They are usually found over the elbow or extensor aspect of finger joints, but they have also been occasionally noted in striated muscle, peripheral nerve, heart, lung, uveal tract, and sclera. Lesions resembling subcutaneous nodules have been observed in cardiac valve leaflets and rings, myocardium, and endocardium, although their frequency is hard to estimate.

The most common renal problem with rheumatoid arthritis is amyloidosis, which has been found in up to 20 per cent of autopsies. If severe, this complication can, of course, reduce the excretion of any drugs administered.

Contrary to the visceral involvement, the anemia of rheumatoid arthritis is a more constant clinical finding. About 25 per cent of patients with rheumatoid arthritis have a normocytic hypochromic anemia that has the characteristics of the anemias of chronic infection. This anemia is resistant to treatment with oral iron, and despite the rise in serum levels intravenous iron increases the hemoglobin only slightly. Blood transfusions have been correlated with some clinical improvement and decrease in sedimentation rate.[19] The anemia seen in rheumatoid arthritis is not usually severe, and if the hemoglobin is under 10 gm, other causes should be sought.

Treatment. Basic principles in the treatment of this disease include rest, relief of pain, maintenance of joint function, prevention and correction of deformities by orthopedic principles, and correction of any factors deleterious to the health of the patient. All rheumatoid patients have been or are taking medication. Drugs most frequently used are analgesics and anti-inflammatory agents. The analgesics, acetylsalicylate, phenylbutazone, indomethacin, and many new non-steroidal anti-inflammatory drugs have been extensively used. Gastric disturbance and occult gastrointestinal bleeding are always to be looked for in patients taking the first two drugs.

It is important to remember the effect of salicylates on platelet function. A disturbance of platelet aggregation and release is produced by aspirin, and this can cause unexpected and excessive bleeding even when minimal aspirin is used. Restoration of normal platelet function requires four to seven days, which corresponds to the platelet life span.[20] The best test to evaluate this problem is the bleeding time, which can be done at the bedside.

Sodium salicylate has a direct stimulant effect on metabolism and respiration. In normal man, prolonged salicylate administration increases the sensitivity of the respiratory center to carbon dioxide.[21]

Phenylbutazone has produced occasional bone marrow depression with leukopenia and agranulocytosis. Retention of sodium and water often occurs during the first 10 days of using this drug.

Gold salts have been extensively used in the treatment of rheumatoid arthritis, and there is evidence that these compounds can induce a remission of the disease, especially if treated early. However, dermatitis, stomatitis, renal damage, and bone marrow depression have limited the wide usage of gold.

Systemic use of corticosteroids is effective in suppressing the disease, but there is nearly always a relapse when the drug is stopped. The dangers of inducing a hypoadrenocortical state are well known today, and consequently this drug is employed only after failure of other methods to control the disease. In current practice, however, a large number of patients with rheumatoid arthritis are taking maintenance levels of steroids, and one must be continually on guard for peptic ulceration, aggravation of infection, fracture of long bones, and psychic disturbances.

OTHER DISEASES WITH PATHOLOGY SIMILAR TO RHEUMATOID ARTHRITIS

Ankylosing Spondylitis. Pathologically indistinguishable from rheumatoid arthritis, this is a chronic progressive disease of the sacroiliac and the synovial (apophyseal) joints of the spine, including the surrounding soft tissues. Bony bridges develop along the vertebrae, giving rise to ankylosis and the classic "bamboo spine" x-ray appearance. It differs from rheumatoid arthritis in that the disease is generally confined to the spine and hips, and, unlike rheumatoid arthritis, almost 90 per cent of the patients are males, with onset usually in the late teens. The vertebral and sacroiliac changes give characteristic x-ray pictures that are diagnostic. The impairment of rotating motion and limitation of bending the spine can produce significant restriction of chest expansion. Also noteworthy is the associated occurrence (1 to 4 per cent) of aortitis and aortic insufficiency.

Reiter's Syndrome. This triad of nongonococcal urethritis, conjunctivitis, and subacute or chronic polyarthritis occurs mainly in young adult males. Mucocutaneous lesions are common. The arthritis dominates the clinical picture; it usually lasts three to four weeks, and then undergoes spontaneous remission with recurrences common. Most patients recover completely, but residual joint damage and chronic arthritis do occur.

Sjögren's Syndrome. This disease entity is a combination of keratoconjunctivitis sicca, xerostomia, and rheumatoid arthritis. The joint involvement has no distinguishing characteristics. These patients often exhibit features of collagen diseases, scleroderma, and lupus, and have elevated gamma globulins. The lack of lacrimal and salivary secretions is due to inflammation and fibrosis of these glands. Oral, tracheobronchial, gastric, and vaginal mucosa can also be involved. Enlargement of the submandibular and parotid glands may produce a serious problem in maintaining an airway as well as in visualizing the glottic opening (Fig. 13–2).

Agammaglobulinemia. Approximately 25 per cent of patients with congenital or acquired agammaglobulinemia develop a nonsuppurative form of arthritis with many features of rheumatoid arthritis. The joint involvement, usually asymmetric, either is transient without damage or persists for years with synovial changes indistinguishable from those of rheumatoid arthritis. The incidence of this condition, which responds to salicylates and corticosteroids, is rare; however, it is of considerable interest because of its implication regarding the etiology of rheumatoid arthritis.

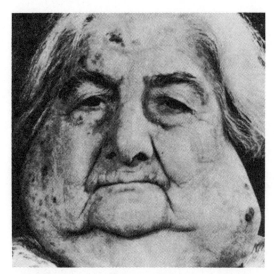

Figure 13–2. Massive enlargement of the parotids in an 82-year-old woman with Sjögren's syndrome. Swelling of the glands was first noted seven years before this photograph was obtained.

ANESTHETIC MANAGEMENT OF RHEUMATOID ARTHRITIS AND ASSOCIATED DISEASES

Because of the frequent occurrence of rheumatoid arthritis and associated diseases, the anesthetist will see many patients requiring surgery for corrective orthopedic procedures and for complications of corticosteroid therapy, as well as for the usual surgical cases. In 1961 Gardner and Holmes[22] reported five cases of rheumatoid arthritis with serious complications related to anesthesia and surgery. In two of these cases, airway or respiratory crisis was caused by rheumatoid arthritis of the small joints of the larynx and by ankylosis of the costovertebral joints.

Involvement of the cricoarytenoid joint may occur in as many as 26 per cent of patients with rheumatoid arthritis.[23] It also may be seen in patients with Reiter's syndrome and systemic lupus erythematosus. The symptoms of cricoarytenoid arthritis in order of their occurrence are a fullness or tightness in the throat, a sensation of a foreign body in the throat, hoarseness or stridor, dysphagia, pain on swallowing, dyspnea, and pain radiating to the ears.[24] Preoperative diagnosis can be made by direct laryngoscopy, whereupon the arytenoid mucosa may appear red and edematous

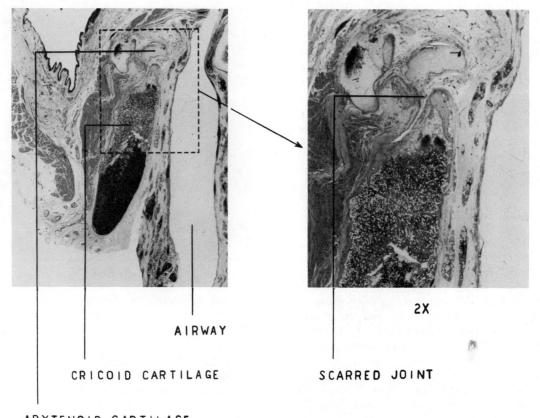

AIRWAY

CRICOID CARTILAGE

SCARRED JOINT

2X

ARYTENOID CARTILAGE

Figure 13–3. Coronal (frontal) section, right half of the larynx from a 61-year-old Caucasian female with severe, generalized rheumatoid arthritis, revealing eburnation of the cartilages, marked fibrosis, and almost complete loss of the right cricoarytenoid joint. (Reprinted with permission of J. A. Phelps, M.D., and the editors of Anesthesiology.)

or thick, rough, and irregular. The glottic opening may be narrowed, and the vocal cords, though normal in appearance, will bow in the middle during inspiration. The degree of cricoarytenoid involvement is apparently related to the activity of the disease. An excellent pathologic presentation of cricoarytenoid arthritis and its problems related to anesthesia is given by Phelps (Fig. 13–3).[25]

Many clinicians believe that for these patients regional anesthesia offers greater safety than general anesthesia. Such an approach is certainly indicated or to be strongly considered for extremity as well as hip surgery. When the operative site precludes a block, preoperative tracheostomy may have to be considered. Edelist in his 1966 review[26] states that the most common airway problem with rheumatoid arthritic patients is a flexion deformity of the cervical spine. He warns that the head and neck

should be manipulated with great care during positioning or intubation, because cervical vertebral erosion and subluxation may occur, especially at the atlantoaxial joint (Fig. 13–4).

Temporomandibular joint arthritis and ankylosis may be the only airway problem in many rheumatoid arthritic patients. If the mouth cannot be opened, nasal intubation or tracheostomy must be performed for insurance of the airway during anesthesia. Temporomandibular joint changes are frequent in JRA,[27] and occasionally these patients have developed ankylosis of the jaw. It is of interest that patients who have only partial limitation, tenderness, or crepitus of the temporomandibular joint do not have an increase in their symptoms after extubation.[28]

A most unusual case of severe cervical spondylosis in a man unable to lift his head off his chest — precluding tracheostomy —

Figure 13-4. *A*, Advanced RA of the cervical spine consisting of resorption of the dens (odontoid) and spinous processes (black arrows), ankylosis of the C2-C3 apophyseal joints, erosions at the joints of Luschka and adjacent end-plates (white arrows), moderate disc narrowing, anterior subluxation of C6-C7 and, finally, generalized demineralization. *B*, Typical "step ladder" subluxations and disc narrowing in advanced RA.

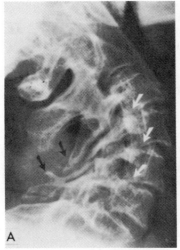
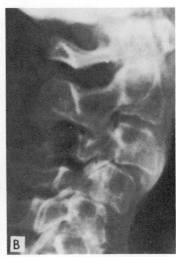

and unable to open his mouth was described by Munson and Cullen.[29] Awake intubation was skillfully performed without moving the patient by using a nasal endotracheal catheter and an oral wire hook to direct the tip of the catheter into the larynx (Figs. 13-5 and 13-6). A cervical osteotomy was then performed so that the head could be extended enough to permit the patient to open his mouth and to heal the ulcers that had formed over the chin and sternum.

It is necessary to assist ventilation during

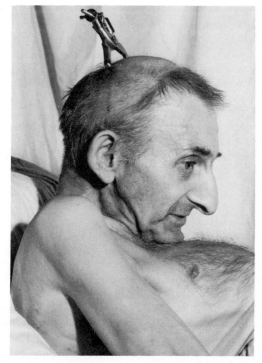

Figure 13-5. A 55-year-old man with a severe, fixed deformity of the cervical spine. Skin ulcerations developed over both mandible and sternum, and he could take nourishment only through a straw. A cervical osteotomy was performed to permit some neck extension.

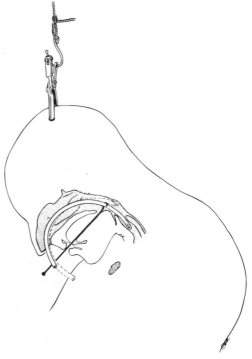

Figure 13-6. Drawing showing position of endotracheal catheter after anterior placement by wire "hook." (Reprinted with permission of Drs. E. S. Munson and S. C. Cullen and the editors of Anesthesiology.)

general anesthesia in patients who have rheumatoid lung changes and possibly costochondral involvement, limiting chest wall expansion. Jenkins[30] states that chronic diffuse interstitial pulmonary fibrosis is the most serious pulmonary lesion in rheumatoid arthritis, and he advises that in western Canada unrecognized tuberculous lung is not uncommon in patients with rheumatoid arthritis. Gardner and Holmes[22] report on two patients with rheumatoid arthritis who died shortly after surgery and apparent satisfactory recovery from anesthesia. One expired two hours after receiving 20 mg of Omnopon for pain, and the other was found dead on the ward some 15 minutes after foot surgery. The authors indicate that rheumatoid arthritics have extreme sensitivity to agents that depress respiratory function, and they question the efficiency with which these patients can mobilize drugs. There is general agreement that rheumatoid arthritic patients should not be left alone postoperatively and that it is best to watch them carefully and even to assist respiratory function.

Anemia in rheumatoid arthritics can be a serious problem, and preoperative evaluation is imperative. Causes for anemia must be investigated, especially in those patients taking drugs with a known tendency to produce gastrointestinal bleeding. The presence of anemia may indicate that hypovolemia and hypoproteinemia also exist. If the hemoglobin is below 9 gm, blood transfusion should be considered prior to elective major surgery.

There is universal agreement that supplemental steroids should be given to the patient who is currently on corticosteroids, or who has been on prolonged therapy within one year of surgery or on prolonged steroid therapy for up to two years prior to surgery when evidence of hypocortisonism existed. For a detailed discussion of this aspect of management, the reader is referred to a discussion earlier in the chapter.

In order to evaluate the operative risk and to determine the hazards attending the management of rheumatoid arthritic patients preoperatively, the following checklist is recommended:

Examination of neck and jaw mobility

Indirect laryngoscopy (if arytenoid arthritis is suspected)

Pulmonary function tests

Chest x-ray

Skeletal x-ray (if there is limitation of the spine)

Blood gas analysis

ECG

Hemoglobin and sedimentation rate

White blood cell and platelet count

Occult blood in stools (if anemic)

Bleeding time (if taking aspirin)

Urinalysis

Creatinine clearance

Liver function tests

Drug therapy history

Previous recent general anesthetics

The same general considerations should govern the management of the associated or rheumatoid diseases. In ankylosing spondylitis it is extremely important to determine the range of motion of the head and neck as well as the spine preoperatively. Spinal or peridural anesthesia may be difficult if not impossible if the intervertebral ligaments are calcified.

In Sjögren's syndrome it would seem appropriate to omit the use of drying agents, because the secretory glands are fibrosed. It would be helpful to employ an anesthesia rebreathing system in order to avoid excessive drying in the airway during endotracheal anesthesia.

COLLAGEN DISEASES

The concept of collagen diseases was advanced in 1942 by Klemperer. It implied pathologic similarities in diseases of unknown etiology which had common alterations in interfibrillary ground substance, proliferation of fibroblasts, a predominant mononuclear inflammatory reaction, and necrosis associated with production of fibrinoid material.

There are many theories regarding the etiology of collagen diseases, including trauma to mast cells, which release substances producing edema and cell infiltration, leading to fibril formation. This was held reasonable because mast cells are most commonly located around blood vessels in the skin, synovial membrane, gastrointestinal tract, cardiovascular system, pleura, pericardium, and lungs. More popular has been the autoimmune hypothesis with the discovery of rheumatoid and LE factors — antibodies directed toward specific host constituents. Antinuclear and anticytoplasmic antibodies, however, are found inconsistently in collagen diseases, and people who are defective in producing antibodies (agammaglobulinemic patients) have a high incidence of connective tissue disorders. It has been repeatedly observed that there is considerable overlap between the various antibodies described in the different connective tissue diseases. Furthermore, some of the lesions, including those seen in rheumatoid arthritis and Hashimoto's thyroiditis, are similar to those produced experimentally by immunologic methods. The higher incidence of these diseases in relation to the increasing use of certain drugs, such as hydralazine, penicillin, and sulfonamides, has led to the suggestion that hypersensitivity may play an important etiologic role, although this consideration is more theoretical than factual.

The following disorders are generally considered collagen diseases: systemic lupus erythematosus, scleroderma, polyarteritis nodosa, and dermatomyositis. Their prevalence in the United States is in the order listed.[31] Also considered by some to be in the classification of collagen diseases are thrombotic thrombocytopenic purpura, temporal or cranial arteritis, Wegener's granulomatosis, and scleredema, all of which are rare.

SYSTEMIC LUPUS ERYTHEMATOSUS (SLE)

General. This disease has numerous manifestations associated with lesions of connective tissue in the vascular system, the dermis, and the serous and synovial membranes. The multitude of visceral manifestations, often present in a complex pattern, make the diagnosis difficult. Lupus is predominantly a disease of women in the child-bearing age. It appears to be more common than previously thought and has no notable racial or geographical distribution.

There are many serum protein alterations, including abnormal serum gamma globulins and factors producing the LE cell, giving rise to the concept that lupus is an autoimmune disorder. The finding of abnormal serum antibodies may be helpful in the diagnosis, because lupus can imitate almost any other clinical entity.

Clinical Picture. The initial clinical picture is variable, although skin and joints are common sites of onset. A characteristic malar facial erythematous rash of butterfly shape is helpful, but it is present in less than half the cases (Fig. 13-7). Changes in pigmentation, telangiectasia, and ulcerations may develop. Joint pain and swelling may resemble that of rheumatoid arthritis and obscure the diagnosis. Renal involvement occurs in 75 per cent of the cases. SLE is associated with a glomerulonephritis that is often progressive and fatal. Over half the patients have involvement of the pericardium, endocardium, or myocardium. When fever and a pericardial friction rub are present, the disease resembles rheumatic fever.

Pleurisy accompanied by a small effusion is a common feature of lupus. There may be

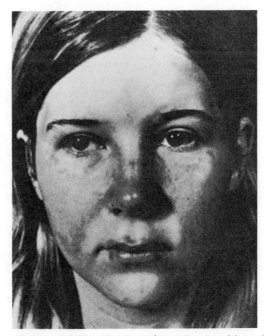

Figure 13-7. Facies of a 19-year-old girl with acute systemic lupus erythematosus. There is a classic butterfly eruption over the bridge of the nose and malar regions.

progressive dyspnea and cyanosis, but fine basilar rales may be the only finding. Pulmonary infiltrates, which appear in many cases, are frequently migratory, and on x-ray suggest basal pneumonitis with focal atelectasis.[32] Sometimes there is a micronodular pattern resembling ground glass. Histologic changes of focal necrosis of alveolar walls may be similar to lesions seen in polyarteritis nodosa and rheumatoid arthritis.

Neurologic signs may be diverse mental reactions, dysphasia, nystagmus, hemiplegia, and polyneuritis. The gastrointestinal tract, liver (lupoid hepatitis), spleen, and lymph nodes may all be involved at some stage of the disease.

The clinical course may be prolonged and is characterized by exacerbations and spontaneous remissions that commonly last months or even years. It is interesting that drugs such as hydralazine, isoniazid, para-aminosalicylic acid, and procainamide over long-term administration can induce the clinical lupus syndrome, including the serum antibodies. This suggests that there may be a host abnormality predisposing to abnormal immunologic reactivity. Judicious use of steroids in the majority of cases results in prolongation of life and a near normal existence.

Anesthetic Management of SLE. The cutaneous lesions (discoid lupus) may present severe nasal and malar eruptions that will make the fit of a face mask difficult. Intubation may be necessary for a good airway; although this should not be a problem, there are rare reports of cricoarytenoid arthritis with a narrowed airway in SLE.[33]

The preparation of lupus patients for surgery may not be easy, because they are generally very sick with fever, often pneumonitis, and renal involvement. It is important that the anesthetist be aware of any and all related problems. In particular, one should check the chest x-ray, serum electrolytes, and blood count. Anemia is very common, and occasionally a hemorrhagic disorder similar to thrombocytopenic purpura may develop. Cryoglobulins have been noted, as well as circulating anticoagulants associated with a prolongation of clotting times. Thus a platelet count and bleeding and clotting time determinations should be made prior to surgery. Platelets and fresh plasma may be indicated at the time of surgery.

In the presence of advanced renal disease the anesthetist must carefully consider the need to give drugs primarily excreted by the kidneys. This includes particularly gallamine and, to a certain extent, curare. Evidence indicates that methoxyflurane would be contraindicated in the presence of existing renal impairment,[34] and that enflurane should be avoided if possible.

Treatment with corticosteroids in this disease is invariably attempted at some time; therefore, adequate preoperative and operative coverage cannot be neglected.

SCLERODERMA (PROGRESSIVE SYSTEMIC SCLEROSIS)

General. This disease causes widespread symmetrical, leathery induration of the skin, followed by atrophy and pigmentation. The skin lesions are the external manifestation of a systemic disease involving muscles, bones, mucous membranes, heart, lungs, intestinal tract, and other internal organs. Scleroderma occurs more often in females, with onset usually between 30 and 50 years of age. There is a local form of this disease, morphea, as well as the generalized form. Histologic diagnosis depends on an increase in otherwise normal collagen fibers. Later there is atrophy of the epidermis, and in some cases calcification develops.

Vasospastic phenomena are seen so commonly in this disease that it has led some investigators to propose a hypersensitivity of autonomic nerves as an important etiologic factor. They have shown a greater increase in peripheral blood flow following intravenous procaine in these patients compared to people without scleroderma.[35] Other investigators believe that monoamine oxidase inhibition may occur in scleroderma, leading to a decrease in catecholamine metabolism.[36] It is proposed that the alpha adrenergic receptors may be abnormally stimulated, since the norepinephrine is broken down at a slower rate.

Clinical Picture. In the classic form the cutaneous changes pass through two stages. Initially there is a brawny, non-pitting edema, giving the hands, feet, and face a puffy white appearance with smoothing of the normal folds. In the second stage the skin becomes waxy, smooth, and tight, so as to be fixed to the deeper structures. This may be more prominent on the fingers, backs of the hands, and ankles. The face becomes masklike (Fig. 13–8). Inability to open the mouth may result from temporomandibular dysfunction, but probably is secondary to changes in perioral soft tissues. A characteristic "fish mouth" appearance is caused by contractions of the mouth and has been noted in varying degrees in 28 per cent of these patients.[37] Weakness and loss of weight are common, and fever and joint pains may also occur sometimes as prodromata.

Raynaud's phenomenon and sclerodactyly, often associated with esophageal involvement, may be present years before skin changes. Dysphagia is one of the most common early symptoms. As the disease advances to the atrophic stage, the skin becomes thinner and adherent to the shrunken muscles. Joint movement may be progressively restricted until the patient resembles a living mummy. Scleroderma of the gastrointestinal tract is common, producing loss of motility, characteristic x-ray changes, and all the complications of inadequate alimentation.

Pulmonary complications occur in almost all cases of scleroderma. Ritchie[38] noted that 21 of 22 scleroderma patients had abnormal lung function. Vital capacity is often reduced, as are the lung volumes, owing to replacement of lung by fibrous tissue and alterations in the elastic properties of the alveoli. Lung compliance is commonly reduced and out of proportion to the lung volume reduction. There is an increase in dead space from widening of the airway, which also reduces resistance, and the result is that these patients breathe at a faster rate to preserve normal alveolar ventilation.

Impaired pulmonary diffusing capacity is common in scleroderma, and, as with sarcoidosis, a lowered diffusing capacity may be present with minimal symptoms or x-ray alterations. Pulmonary hypertension was seen in half of the scleroderma patients studied by Sackner.[31] The degree of restrictive lung disease and diffusion abnormalities correlated poorly with pulmonary artery pressures, suggesting that this hypertension may be another manifestation of widespread vasomotor disturbances.

Cardiac involvement or "scleroderma heart disease" can result from myocardial fibrosis and lead to heart failure. Focal myocardial lesions in scleroderma are seen in the absence of coronary artery disease and appear to be independent of pulmonary, renal, or hypertensive vascular disease. Clinical cardiac dysfunction attributable in whole or in part to primary scleroderma heart disease has been found in 19 per cent of patients with this disease in a study of 52 cases.[39] Most cases of congestive failure are secondary to pulmonary hypertension. Left ventricular hypertrophy may occur as a result of scleroderma of the kidney with severe hypertension. Renal complication is uniformly fatal, because the disease can affect the renal arteries, producing a pathologic picture indistinguishable from malignant nephrosclerosis.

Therapy in scleroderma has not had much effect in changing the clinical course, which finds almost 50 per cent of the patients dead in two years. In many, the disease is chronic and prolonged. Steroids have been extensively used with varying but not encouraging results.

Figure 13–8. Typical facies of scleroderma; smoothness and loss of lines of expression are apparent. Oral aperture is markedly decreased.

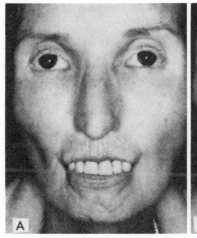
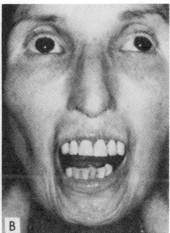

SCLEREDEMA (SCLEREDEMA ADULTORUM OF BUSCHKE)

This is a rare condition which has a benign course. It is characterized by brawny, nonpitting edema of the skin that may resemble scleroderma. It is a diffuse disease of collagen, usually developing a few weeks after infection, most frequently of streptococcal origin. There is sometimes a prodromal period with fever, malaise, and myalgia. Most cases occur in young females; the neck is first involved, with subsequent spread to the face, chest, abdomen, and extremities. Involvement of the tongue and pharynx results in dysphagia, whereas chest wall changes may produce dyspnea. There is usually resolution of the edema in six to 18 months; however, the disease may remain for years.

Scleredema is differentiated from scleroderma because the induration is more prominent in the superficial layers of the skin, and neither atrophy nor pigmentation develops. Hands and feet are rarely involved. Other conditions such as trichinosis, myxedema, and edema of cardiac or renal origin are distinguished by the associated manifestations.

ANESTHETIC MANAGEMENT OF SCLERODERMA AND SCLEREDEMA

Mainly because of the gastrointestinal complications and, to some extent, the consequence of cutaneous calcification, scleroderma patients undergoing surgery are not rare. Occasionally sympathectomies have been done to improve circulation. Anesthetic management of scleroderma has been reported employing conventional agents. Success was assured by careful preparation in anticipation of a difficult intubation.

Tightening of the skin around the mouth may produce severe jaw limitation, and it may thus be important to determine how wide these patients can open their mouths, because intubation may require a nasal approach. A case has been reported of severe oral laceration due to a mouth gag during dental surgery.[40] Pulmonary problems are the rule with these patients; therefore, lung function studies should be performed preoperatively to determine the degree of restrictive disease, the diffusing capacity, and the blood gas values. Evidence of pulmonary hypertension should be looked for on x-ray, ECG, and clinical auscultation for an accentuated pulmonic sound. Ventilation may be difficult in scleroderma patients as a result of altered compliance; consequently, it would seem wise to control breathing, particularly if the preoperative blood gas values were abnormal. It is also important that these patients be observed with great care in the immediate postoperative period, as they may need ventilatory assistance, especially if narcotics were used.

Vasospastic phenomena in scleroderma are so common that one should consider the possible hemodynamic consequences following induction of anesthesia with concomitant vasodilation. The sclerodermic patient may in effect have a reduced circulating plasma volume similar to that of most hypertensive patients (e.g., pheochromocytoma) and thus as the peripheral vascular bed dilates profound hypertension may develop.[41] This occurrence can be anticipated and treated with a plasma expander or if necessary whole blood.

Regional anesthesia in scleroderma may be considered preferable, especially in view of the frequent pulmonary problems. In this regard the author warns against the effect of local anesthetics with epinephrine in cases in which Raynaud's phenomenon exists. An axillary block with 1.5 per cent lidocaine with epinephrine 1:100,000 produced sensory deficits in the fingers for 24 hours in a scleroderma patient.[42] This same patient was then tested with small (2 cc) subcutaneous injections on each side of the umbilicus. One side was made anesthetic with 1 per cent lidocaine for 6 to 7 hours, whereas the other side was anesthetized with 1 per cent lidocaine and 1:100,000 epinephrine for over 10 hours! This surprising result on the anterior abdominal wall suggests that vasomotor instability was widespread and leads one to advise against using local anesthesia with epinephrine in scleroderma.

It should be commented that measurements of blood pressure may be difficult and have been misleading in scleroderma patients with Raynaud's phenomenon. Forearm blood flow is markedly reduced in these patients lying supine at rest, as are skin temperatures. Intramuscular temperature has been recorded at 1.5° C lower than core temperature in this disease.[43] Arterial cannulation may be very difficult in scleroderma patients and should only be attempted in the most critical situations wherein the risk of inadequate pressure recording outweighs the high risk of arterial thrombosis.

POLYARTERITIS NODOSA (PERIARTERITIS, NECROTIZING ANGIITIS)

General. This disease is characterized by widespread vascular lesions reflected in variable signs and symptoms from any organ. The idea that it might be a hyperallergenic reaction to toxic or infectious agents has been popular because the lesions have been produced experimentally, but in most cases there is no allergic history. There are a number of syndromes characterized by arterial inflammatory lesions, and classification at this stage of the disease is difficult. Unlike other collagen diseases, polyarteritis affects males three times more often than females. The lesions involve arteries of medium and small caliber with necrosis, fibrinoid change, and infiltration with leukocytes. Weakening and dilation of the vessel wall may lead to hemorrhage. The vessels are typically involved in a segmental fashion. The lesions are common in the kidneys, heart, gastrointestinal tract, liver, lungs, adrenals, testes, brain, and peripheral nerves.

Clinical Picture. Many patients who acquire polyarteritis already suffer from a chronic or acute respiratory infection. Early symptoms are fever and tenderness of the extremities. Involvement of the alimentary tract, skin, joints, and peripheral nerves are other common early signs. Renal lesions are frequent. They produce a glomerulitis that leads to renal failure in some, whereas in surviving patients renal hypertension results. Abdominal pain, resulting from arteritis of abdominal viscera, and painful peripheral neuritis are common symptoms. There may be involvement of the central nervous system, including subarachnoid hemorrhage, facial palsy, hemiplegia, and convulsions. The coronary vessels may be affected, producing myocardial infarction. Heart failure associated with severe hypertension is often present.

Pulmonary lesions are of interest because they usually precede polyarteritis in other areas, and can mimic asthma, pneumonia, or bronchitis. Focal lesions scattered through the lungs may suggest tuberculosis, sarcoidosis, or carcinomatosis. Unlike other polyarteritis lesions, eosinophilia and sometimes nasal granulomas are present, making it difficult to differentiate this disorder from Wegener's granulomatosis. Rose and Spencer[44] found that lung lesions could precede generalized polyarteritis by years and that treatment with corticosteroids could lead to permanent control.

Other common manifestations of this disease are joint involvement, usually migratory in nature and resembling rheumatic fever. Sometimes chronic deformation of joints occurs, resembling rheumatoid arthritis. Skin lesions are found in 25 per cent of the cases in the form of nodules that vary in size and are frequently tender.

The course of this disease is variable but it is usually fatal when the kidneys, lungs, or heart are involved. Long remissions have occurred and are probably related to steroid therapy. Biopsies have shown suppression of arterial inflammation within weeks after steroid treatment.

CRANIAL (TEMPORAL) ARTERITIS

The relationship between this form of arteritis and polyarteritis is not established. Cranial arteritis is part of a generalized vascular disorder wherein the carotid arterial system is so often involved that it is designated a separate clinical entity. The larger arteries are affected, particularly the temporal and occipital. The disease is a panarteritis, with inflammation starting in the adventitia and spreading into the media. It primarily affects older people of both sexes equally. In most cases the disease subsides in one to two years. The clinical stages may be divided into 1) headache, 2) ocular complications, and 3) systemic complications. The eye manifestations may result from ophthalmoplegic or vascular lesions affecting the optic nerve and retina. Complete blindness is the most common result. Systemic arteritis with skin and visceral lesions, polyneuropathy, and muscle and joint involvement may occur. All patients should be treated with steroids as soon as the diagnosis is made to prevent blindness, although vision cannot be restored to prior levels.

ANESTHETIC MANAGEMENT OF POLYARTERITIS NODOSA AND CRANIAL ARTERITIS

Apparently these patients come to surgery often, with a report from one hospital stating that 10 out of 12 patients with polyarteritis nodosa had abdominal operations.[45] The diagnosed patients either are very sick and hospitalized or are in remission on large doses of steroids. It is of interest to the anesthetist that cases of polyarteritis nodosa and temporal arteritis have been observed with acute pharyngeal edema wherein the uvula and parapharyngeal areas were severely swollen.[46]

Hypertension is invariable with renal involvement and leads to certain anesthetic considerations. It should be important to try to maintain normal blood pressure, because the critical closing pressure in organs affected by arteritis can be altered. This would mean that coronary and cerebral thrombosis are of major concern when hypotension occurs. There are no data available to confirm or refute this precaution.

During active temporal arteritis McGowan[47] reported a case of blindness occurring during general anesthesia in a man 76 years old. The patient had lost his vision in one eye just prior to admission and had signs of laryngeal carcinoma. Temporal artery biopsy confirmed the diagnosis of the associated ocular lesion, and steroid treatment was started. A transient blindness in the good eye occurred two days prior to surgery for laryngectomy. During the operation the blood pressure fell from 160/90 to 120/70 for 20 minutes. The subsequent blindness after anesthesia may or may not have been related to this; nonetheless it has been proposed by the author that elective surgery be postponed during acute temporal arteritis.

The frequent involvement of the lungs and the almost invariable renal complication should alert the anesthetist to the problem of evaluating these patients before surgery. If there is a suggestion of pulmonary involvement, then the degree of lung dysfunction, if any, should be determined by the appropriate tests. Likewise, any degree of renal failure should be known preoperatively.

DERMATOMYOSITIS (NEUROMYOSITIS, POLYMYOSITIS)

General. The hallmarks of this disease are a violaceous skin rash over the face and extremities, nonsuppurative inflammation of striated muscles, and creatinuria. The microscopic appearance of muscle and skin, however, is not pathognomic. The skin, affected in 50 per cent of cases, shows atrophy of the epidermis, whereas the dermis is edematous and mucoid, and the connective tissue is condensed, fibrotic, and infiltrated with cells. The appearance resembles scleroderma, but systemic involvements are quite rare. The muscle fibers become vacuolated and degenerated. Calcinosis may eventually develop in the subcutaneous tissues, muscles, and fascia. The disease is rare, affecting females more than males. Its usual onset is in the 40-to-50-year range; however, it is the most common collagen disease seen in children.

Clinical Picture. The onset is often heralded by a facial rash with edema and vague malaise. The rash spreads in a butterfly distribution as in lupus erythematosus, but it is more bluish. The eyelids may be swollen and show a heliotrope coloration caused by telangiectasis (see Fig. 13–9). The dermal and muscle manifestations do not run parallel. In 50 per cent of the cases rheumatic signs appear in conjunction with the muscle weakness. Muscular involvement is usually bilateral and symmetric, affecting the neck, shoulders, and pelvic muscles. Eventually, there is muscle wasting and stiffness, and fixation of the joints may occur. Diplopia, dyspnea, and impaired sphincter control may be seen. Isolated lung disease is very rare in this disorder; however, Hepper et al.[48] reported three types of pulmonary involvement: 1) aspiration pneumonia that is related to weakness of the muscles involved in swallowing, 2) respiratory insufficiency resulting from progressive weakening of the intercostal and diaphragmatic muscles, and 3) lung involvement from the connective tissue disease itself, described as a patchy infiltrative process throughout both lungs.

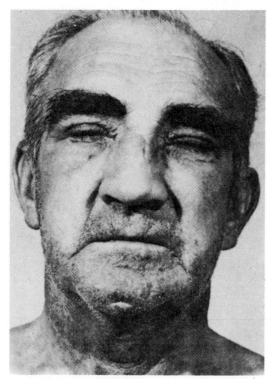

Figure 13–9. Classic skin rash in dermatomyositis. There is marked periorbital edema and erythema with facial edema, especially of the cheeks. There is also dusky erythema of the neck, the sides of the forehead, and the "V" of the neck.

Pathologic specimens show interstitial pneumonitis of a hypersensitive and desquamative type as well as interstitial fibrosis.[49] Intermittent fever, malaise, and anorexia are common, and the course is progressive to death in about half the cases. Those surviving one year may go into a long remission. In the early phase of lung involvement, corticosteroids appear to be effective when used in high dosages.

Anesthetic Management of Dermatomyositis. Since dermatomyositis is a systemic disease, the anesthetist should be concerned with anemia as well as intercurrent infection, which may be frequent in patients who have lost their ability to swallow. These patients do not have the tight skin and hence the problems in opening the mouth encountered in patients with scleroderma.

It seems reasonable that dermatomyositis patients should require less neuromuscular drug because of their diminished muscle mass. There is some evidence to indicate that they may have an altered sensitivity to the muscle relaxants.[50] In examining 10 patients with dermatomyositis, Wylie and Churchill-Davidson found two patients who demonstrated a myasthenic response using a decamethonium test. This means that electromyographically recorded fasciculations were not blocked by decamethonium, which is the finding in myasthenia gravis. One of the two patients, however, had bronchogenic carcinoma and it was not stated whether or not he had a neuropathy. Carcinomas of breast, ovary, lung, and stomach occur in more than 15 per cent of patients with dermatomyositis, and carcinomatous neuropathies are more frequent in these tumors. This is significant in that patients with dermatomyositis may have an occult malignancy associated with neuromuscular weakness and myasthenic responses. Although this complication of dermatomyositis may not be common, it should put the anesthetist on guard so that small test doses of muscle relaxants should always be used if relaxation is required. Furthermore, if at all possible, the muscle twitch response should be monitored.

The high incidence of swallowing and vocal cord dysfunction in this disease requires special anesthetic care to prevent secretions from accumulating.[51] Saliva or sometimes barium may pool in the valleculae and pharynx and fall down the trachea during anesthesia. Endotracheal intubation is strongly indicated in these patients for most operations as well as for postoperative care.

In view of reports of respiratory impairment caused by either aspiration pneumonia or weakness of inspiratory muscles, it is imperative to determine the ventilatory adequacy preoperatively. A vital capacity measurement, blood gas analysis, and chest x-ray, coupled with a good clinical evaluation, will dictate how these patients can best be managed during anesthesia and surgery. If the patient's ventilatory status prior to surgery is marginal with a reduced vital capacity, he should not be permitted spontaneous breathing during surgery and in the immediate postoperative period. The importance of airway protection and adequate ventilation in these patients leads one to choose general rather than regional anesthesia.

GRANULOMATOUS DISEASES

WEGENER'S GRANULOMATOSIS

This is one of a group of clinical and pathologic syndromes forming a spectrum at one end of which there are pure necrotizing and granulomatous lesions without arteritis, and at the other there is pure arteritis without granulomatous reaction. Each disease has certain distinguishing features: population affected, distribution of vascular lesions, size of involved vessels, and histologic details. Wegener's granulomatosis has a constant triad of necrotizing giant cell granulomatosis of the upper respiratory tract and lungs, widespread necrotizing vasculitis of the small arteries and veins, and focal glomerulonephritis. It affects both sexes, mostly those between 20 and 40 years of age. Its onset is insidious, with purulent rhinorrhea, epistaxis, nasal pain, or cough. As the process spreads, it leads to mucosal ulceration and destruction of cartilage and bone in the nose, palate, and orbit, and to pulmonary congestion. It has been reported to cause laryngeal obstruction, suggesting neoplasm and, in another case, tracheoesophageal fistula, both conditions having major anesthetic importance.[52]

Later there is systemic involvement of skin, muscles, bone, peripheral nerves, and kidneys. It is distinguished from lethal midline granuloma by the histologic features of the latter. It must also be distinguished from tuberculosis, sarcoidosis, and mycotic infection. The appearance of chest x-ray in this disease is extremely varied, from increased vascular markings (vasculitis of pulmonary vessels), patchy pneumonia, or diffuse miliary nodularity. One interesting manifestation is the development of asymptomatic and clinically unrecognizable circumscribed neoplasms.[53] These appear suddenly and may undergo central necrosis and cavitation. Diagnosis may be difficult, as neither x-ray nor bronchoscopy has been more than occasionally positive. However, few other procedures have proved more helpful short of thoracotomy.[54] One feature that can differentiate the pulmonary lesions of this disease from neoplasia is the occurrence of progression in one lung while regression is evident in the other lung.[55]

The clinical course is downhill and fatal. Although symptomatic control can be achieved with steroids, the fatal outcome is merely delayed.

LETHAL MIDLINE GRANULOMA

This is a rare, invariably fatal disease resulting in destruction of the midface. It affects men more than women and is most common between 30 and 50 years of age. Ulceration begins in the nose and progressively destroys bone cartilage and skin. The granuloma may replace the midface, nasopharynx, and oropharynx. Nasal congestion, rhinorrhea, or sinusitis may be present for years before other evidence of the disease. Later there may be interference with sight and speech, and, eventually, airway problems. The average course is about one year, death usually resulting from cachexia. The diagnosis must exclude neoplasms and the many infectious processes that produce ulcerations of the nose and upper respiratory tract. The absence of vasculitis distinguishes it from Wegener's granulomatosis. Corticosteroid and radiation therapy occasionally impede the destructive process, and a favorable report has followed the use of methotrexate.

ANESTHETIC MANAGEMENT OF WEGENER'S GRANULOMATOSIS AND LETHAL MIDLINE GRANULOMA

The role of the anesthesiologist in this condition may be very important, because the establishment of a good airway may require careful advance planning owing to the possible structural abnormalities. One should not use the "crash induction" technique without knowing the exact involvement of the lesions, which may be hard to determine preoperatively. A preoperative tracheostomy may often be the wisest course. An often neglected role of the anesthesiologist may be his ability to spot or diagnose abnormalities in such cases when an ulceration or hole in the palate or pharynx may be the first sign of one of these diseases.

The pulmonary infection in Wegener's granulomatosis may progress to widespread consolidation and present a formidable anesthetic risk, especially if arterial oxygen desaturation exists. Regional anesthesia and supplemental oxygen may be preferable in these cases, since there are likely to be infected granulomatous lesions throughout the upper airway.

SARCOIDOSIS (BESNIER'S, BOECK'S, SCHAUMANN'S, OR UVEOPAROTID FEVER)

General. Sarcoidosis is a systemic granulomatous disease characterized by spontaneous and complete remissions in the early stages, and by a slowly progressive course if the disease persists. Lymph nodes, lungs, liver, spleen, eyes, and skin are most often involved, but any tissue or organ may be affected, including the central nervous system and cranial nerves.

The epidemiology and etiology of this disease have evoked a large number of interesting international studies. It occurs in almost all races and all regions of the world. The highest prevalence rate is in Sweden, but neighboring Finland has about the lowest. In the United States there is a preponderance in Negroes and in those born in rural areas, especially in the Southeast. Sarcoid occurs at all ages, the greatest incidence occurring between 20 and 40 years, with a slightly higher rate among females. The production of sarcoid granuloma by a variety of stimuli such as beryllium, zirconium, silica, quartz, and talc has led some to consider sarcoidosis a host reaction pattern involving immunologic mechanisms. *Mycobacterium tuberculosis* and pine pollen have received extensive consideration as etiologic agents, but without general acceptance.

Pathology. The epithelioid cell granuloma or tubercle is the cardinal feature of the tissue reaction in sarcoidosis. Unlike tuberculosis, caseation and necrosis are rare and healing takes place by fibrosis with dense scar formation, which later contracts and becomes hyalinized. All organs and tissues may show evidence of the disease, and the constitutional symptoms are produced almost entirely by the granulomas or scars. The extent of these functional impairments determines the seriousness of the disease.

Clinical Picture. One outstanding and important clinical feature of sarcoidosis is the disparity between the extensive involvement of organs and the mildness or absence of symptoms. Asymptomatic onset occurs most often in North America, whereas acute illness with fever, rash (erythema nodosum), arthralgia, and bilateral hilar adenopathy may be seen at the onset more commonly in Europe. In most cases the symptoms subside in a few months, and complete clearing of the pulmonary changes occurs within two years without specific therapy. If the disease persists, progressive involvement of lung or other organs may occur for years wherein functional impairment of an organ is not rare. Death occurs in only a small proportion of cases.

Pulmonary lesions are characterized by infiltration of the alveolar walls by granuloma, which is replaced by fibrous scar tissue. This reduces effective diffusing surface and, when extensive, can lead to dyspnea and oxygen desaturation. Nickerson[56] describes three distinct areas of pulmonary lesions: pleural, often forming subpleural fibrous masses; peribronchial, occurring as solitary lesions encircling small bronchioles; and septal, occurring as solitary lesions in alveolar septa.

The most clearly recognizable sign of pulmonary sarcoid is the enlarged symmetrical hilar adenopathy whose outer border casts smooth contoured shadows on x-ray. This may lead to extrinsic bronchial obstruction and distal atelectasis, or to infiltration of the bronchial mucosa, which causes asthmatic symptoms[57] and progresses to produce bronchial stenosis.

In a study of the mechanics of ventilation in sarcoidosis, Snider and Doctor[58] showed that 17 of 21 patients had compliance values below normal or at the low end of the normal range. Some of the low compliance values were observed in patients without x-ray evidence of parenchymal disease. Other studies on patients with chronic sarcoidosis and pulmonary fibrosis indicate a reduction in air flow that exceeds the reduction in lung volume, which is consistent with airway obstruction.[59, 60]

In general, the lung volumes are diminished with pulmonary sarcoid infiltration, and the gas transfer factor (diffusing capacity) tends to fall early. Johnson et al.[61] found that the major change was in transfer of gas from alveoli to capillaries, whereas the alveolar capillary volume was less affected.

The upper airway may be involved,

with mucosal infiltrations of the nose, nasopharynx, tonsils, palate, and larynx.[62] All parts of the larynx have been involved, nearly always in association with other parts of the respiratory tract. Women seem to be afflicted in this area more than men. There are numerous cases reported with lobulated swellings of the vocal cords, epiglottis, arytenoids, and aryepiglottic folds, necessitating tracheostomy.[63]

Although the incidence of granulomatous cardiac lesions in autopsied cases of sarcoidosis is 20 per cent,[64] this does not reflect the clinical picture. The most common cardiovascular compliction of sarcoid is right ventricular enlargement. Svanborg[65] observed that seven out of 11 cases with moderate pulmonary fibrosis had an elevated pulmonary artery pressure. Right ventricular failure, however, is no more common than it is with other pulmonary disease.

Sarcoid lesions have been found occasionally in the valves, but more often in the myocardium, sometimes resulting in arrhythmias or heart block (see Fig. 13–10). Ventricular tachycardia is the most frequently reported abnormal rhythm.[66] Cases of sudden death have been recorded with autopsy findings of sarcoid lesions destroying the conducting system. Most patients with cardiac sarcoidosis causing dysfunction present entirely with cardiac problems and have little or no evidence of other organ dysfunction.[67]

Sarcoid lesions have been seen upon occasion in every organ of the body, including the skin, but they are of particular interest when they affect the eyes. According to Scadding,[62] 14 per cent of his cases had symptomatic uveitis at some stage of this disease. It affects primarily the anterior uveal tract, producing iridocyclitis, which is an indication for corticosteroid treatment.

The diagnosis of sarcoidosis is usually based on the clinical findings and a tissue biopsy showing characteristic granulomas. Increased sedimentation rate and hypergammaglobulinemia are common, whereas hypercalcemia and hypercalciuria are present in about 25 per cent of cases. The differential diagnosis includes berylliosis, lymphomas, and tuberculosis. Corticosteroids are indicated for ocular, cardiac, central nervous system, and progressive pulmonary parenchymal involvement, as well as for persistent hypercalcemia.

Anesthetic Management of Sarcoidosis. The pulmonary pathology and, though not as frequent, the cardiac involvement, are the major concerns for anesthetists. One important feature of pulmonary sarcoidosis is the discrepancy between the patient's symptoms and the pathologic changes that may be present. A case from the author's hospital can serve to demonstrate the problem: A 35-year-old man who came to the clinic with blurring of vision caused by a detached retina was scheduled for immediate corrective eye surgery. He had a history of sarcoidosis diagnosed one year previously by chest x-ray (Fig. 13–11) and characteristic skin lesions. He had no pulmonary symptoms, and physical examination revealed slight tachypnea, bronchovesicular breath sounds with minimal dry rales at the lung bases, cervical and axillary adenopathy, and a palpable spleen tip. Preoperative blood gas analysis showed an O_2 saturation of 90 per cent, Pa_{CO_2} 38 mm Hg, pH 7.37, and HCO_3 22 mEq/liter. Endotracheal anesthesia was maintained with halothane-nitrous oxide and oxygen 40 per cent. Shortly after the start of surgery, cyanosis of the fingers and nailbeds was noted, at which time the O_2 was increased to 60 per cent and respiration was vigorously assisted. After 10 minutes an arterial blood gas analysis indicated an O_2 saturation of only 91 per cent, whereupon the nitrous oxide was discontinued. In this case the magnitude of pulmona-

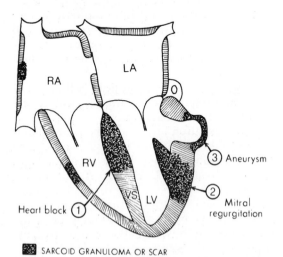

■ SARCOID GRANULOMA OR SCAR

Figure 13–10. Diagram showing the most common sites of sarcoid granulomas or scars in the heart and the most frequent functional consequences of these lesions.

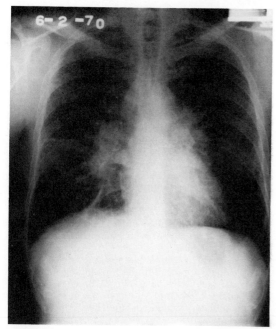

Figure 13–11. Chest x-ray of a 36-year-old man, showing characteristic hilar shadows and parenchymal infiltration of sarcoidosis. When seen preoperatively, he appeared asymptomatic.

ry venous admixture can be easily appreciated. However, the cause, whether from poor O_2 diffusion or ventilation-perfusion discrepancy, was obscure. The point is that a patient with asymptomatic lung disease whose oxygenation on air was marginal became worse during halothane anesthesia inspiring 40 per cent oxygen.

It is important to define pulmonary function status in patients with evidence of pulmonary sarcoidosis prior to operation. In particular, the diffusing capacity should, if possible, be determined. Diffusing capacity under halothane anesthesia was not significantly altered in 12 patients with normal awake diffusion capacities studies by Bergman.[68] However, it is not known what might happen to the diffusing capacity under anesthesia in a patient with a diffusion impairment. A decrease in lung compliance is common in pulmonary sarcoidosis and should be borne in mind prior to anesthesia. In addition to routine pulmonary function studies, diffusing capacity, and blood gas analysis, there should be a cardiac evaluation. In particular, evidence of pulmonary hypertension, right ventricular hypertrophy, and any arrhythmias should be

ascertained. During anesthesia and surgery, ECG monitoring is essential, for if there is sarcoid heart disease, the most common abnormalities are ventricular tachycardia and sudden arrest!

Often sarcoid patients have been on long-term treatment with corticosteroids, in which case preoperative and operative coverage with additional steroids is essential, as discussed earlier in this chapter.

SUMMARY

Patients with connective tissue disorders require surgical operations more frequently than realized. They are a definite challenge and present the anesthetist with many potential problems. Such patients are chronically ill and sometimes are seen during an acute flare-up of their disease, whereupon systemic visceral involvement may be common. The anesthetist must be aware of the patient's general state of health and must search for evidence of pulmonary, cardiac, or hematologic disturbances. Airway problems should be anticipated in many cases, especially in rheumatoid arthritis. A few minutes of careful questioning and examining preoperatively may prevent an unexpected disaster. The history of drug therapy is essential preoperative information, particularly because many of these patients will need augmentation or coverage with steroid drugs.

Lastly, it is important not to forget that more often than not these patients are psychologically affected by their disease, which calls for a greater than normal amount of understanding and sympathy on the part of the anesthetist. The risk of anesthesia in these patients is obviously high and this concern should be shared with the patient and his family as well as with the surgeon. The extra care required for preoperative assessment and preparation, and for intraoperative as well as postoperative vigilance, will assure the patient of the best anesthesia care.

REFERENCES

Connective Tissue Diseases — General

Beeson, P. B., and McDermott, W. (eds.): Cecil-Loeb Textbook of Medicine. 15th ed., Philadelphia, W. B. Saunders Co., 1979.

Hollander, J. L.: Arthritis and Allied Conditions: A textbook of Rheumatology, E. W. Boland et al., section eds., 9th ed., Philadelphia, Lea and Febiger, 1979.

Primer on the rheumatoid diseases. American Rheumatism Association. 7th ed., New York, Arthritis Foundation, 1973.

Sackner, M. A.: Scleroderma. New York, Grune and Stratton, 1966.

Scadding, J. G.: Sarcoidosis. London, Eyre and Spottiswoode, 1967, Chapter 13.

Steroid Therapy

1. Fraser, C. G., Preuss, F. S., and Bigford, W. D.: Adrenal atrophy and irreversible shock associated with cortisone therapy. J.A.M.A. *149*:1542, 1952.
2. Graber, A. L., Ney, R. L., Nicholson, W. E., Island, D. P., and Liddle, G. W.: Natural history of pituitary-adrenal recovery following long-term suppression with corticosteroids. J. Clin. Endocrinol. 25:11, 1965.
3. Roberts, J. C.: Operative collapse after corticosteroid therapy — a survey. Surg. Clin. N. Amer. *50*:363, 1970.
4. Helmreich, M. L., Jenkins, D., and Swan, H.: The adrenal cortical response to surgery. II. Change in plasma and urinary corticosteroid levels in man. Surgery *41*:895, 1957.
5. Virtue, R. W., Helmreich, M. L., and Gainza, E.: The adrenal cortical response to surgery. I. The effect of anesthesia on plasma 17-hydroxycorticosteroid levels. Surgery *41*:549, 1957.
6. Oyama, T., Shibata, S., Matsumoto, F., Takiguchi, M., and Kudo, T.: Effects of halothane anesthesia and surgery on adrenocortical function in man. Canad. Anesth. Soc. J. *15*:258, 1968.
7. Hume, D. M., and Wittenstein, G. J.: The relationship of the hypothalamus to pituitary-adrenocortical function. Proceedings, First Clinical ACTH Conference. Philadelphia, The Blakiston Co., 1950, p. 134.
8. Oyama, T., and Takiguchi, M.: Plasma levels of ACTH and cortisol in man during halothane anesthesia and surgery. Anesth. Analg. 49:363, 1970.
9. Thorn, G. W.: Clinical considerations in the use of corticosteroids. N. Engl. J. Med. *274*:775, 1966.
10. Kehlet, H., Blichert-Toft, M., Lindholm, J., and Rasmussen, P.: Short ACTH test in assessing hypothalamic-pituitary-adrenocortical function. Brit. Med. J. *1*:249, 1976.
11. Salassa, R. M., Bennet, W. A., Keating, F. R., and Sprague, R. G.: Postoperative adrenal cortical insufficiency. Occurrence in patients previously treated with cortisone. J.A.M.A. *152*:1509, 1953.
12. Moore, F. D.: Metabolic Care of the Surgical Patient. Philadelphia, W. B. Saunders Co., 1966, p. 765.
13. Plumpton, F. S., Besser, G. M., and Cole, P. V.: Corticosteroid treatment and surgery. 2. The management of steroid cover. Anaesthesia *24*:12, 1969.

Rheumatoid Arthritis

14. Primer in rheumatic diseases. Special contribution, Part I. Committee of the American Rheumatism Association. J.A.M.A. *190*:127, 1964.
15. Cathcart, E. S., and Spodick, D. H.: Rheumatoid heart disease: A study of the incidence and nature of cardiac lesions in rheumatoid arthritis. N. Engl. J. Med. *266*:959, 1962.
16. Rubin, E. H.: Pulmonary lesions in rheumatoid disease with remarks on diffuse interstitial pulmonary fibrosis. Amer. J. Med. *19*:569, 1955.
17. Caplan, A.: Certain unusual radiological appearances in chests of coal miners suffering from rheumatoid arthritis. Thorax 8:29, 1953.
18. Lee, F. I., and Brain, A. T.: Chronic diffuse interstitial pulmonary fibrosis and rheumatoid arthritis. Lancet 2:693, 1962.
19. Syndas, D. A.: The anemia of rheumatoid arthritis and its treatment with blood transfusions. Acta Rheum. Scand. 7:95, 1961.
20. Weiss, H. J.: Antiplatelet drugs — A new pharmacologic approach to the prevention of thrombosis. Amer. Heart J. *92*:86, 1976.
21. Tenney, S. M., and Miller, R. M.: Respiratory and circulatory actions of salicylate. Amer. J. Med. *19*:498, 1955.
22. Gardner, D. L., and Holmes, F.: Anaesthetic and postoperative hazards in rheumatoid arthritis. Brit. J. Anaesth. *33*:258, 1961.
23. Lofgren, R. H., and Montgomery, W. W.: Incidence of laryngeal involvement in rheumatoid arthritics. N. Engl. J. Med. *267*:193, 1962.
24. Funk, D., and Raymom, F.: Rheumatoid arthritis of the cricoarytenoid joints: An airway hazard. Anesth. Analg. *54*:742, 1975.
25. Phelps, J. A.: Laryngeal obstruction due to cricoarytenoid arthritis. Anesthesiology *27*:518, 1966.
26. Edelist, G.: Principles of anesthetic management in rheumatoid arthritic patients. Anesth. Analg. *43*:227, 1964.
27. Grosfeld, O., Czarnecka, B., Drecka-Kuzan, K., Szymanska-Jagiello, W., and Zyszko, A.: Clinical investigations of the temporomandibular joint in children and adolescents with rheumatoid arthritis. Scand. J. Rheum. 2:145, 1973.
28. Taylor, R. C., Way, W. L., and Hendrixson, R.: Temporomandibular joint problems in relation to the administration of general anesthesia. J. Oral Surg. 26:327, 1968.
29. Munson, E. S., and Cullen, S. C.: Endotracheal intubation in a patient with ankylosing spondylitis of the cervical spine. Anesthesiology *26*:365, 1965.
30. Jenkins, L. C., and McGraw, R. W.: Anesthetic management of the patient with rheumatoid arthritis. Canad. Anaesth. Soc. J. *16*:4, 1969.

Lupus Erythematosus

31. Sackner, M. A.: Scleroderma. New York, Grune and Stratton, 1966.
32. Divertie, M. B.: Lung involvement in the connective tissue disorders. Med. Clin. N. Amer. *48*: 1015, 1964.

33. Sourander, L. B., and Pulkkinen, K.: Simultaneous occurrence of ankylosis of the cricoarytenoid joints with dyspnea and L-E syndrome in rheumatoid arthritis. Acta Rheum. Scand. 8:255, 1962.

34. Cousins, M. J., and Mazzi, R. I.: Methoxyflurane nephrotoxicity. J.A.M.A. 225:1611, 1973.

Scleroderma

35. Wiskemann, A., and Korff, F.: The influence of procaine, griseofulvin, and chloroquine on the circulation of the skin in cases of progressive scleroderma. Derm. Wschr. 37:1033, 1967.

36. Brunjes, S., Arterberry, J. D., Shankel, S., and Johns, V. J., Jr.: Decreased oxidative deamination of catecholamines associated with clinical scleroderma. Arthritis Rheum. 7:138, 1964.

37. Weisman, R. A., and Calcaterra, T. C.: Head and neck manifestations of scleroderma. Ann. Otol. 87:332, 1978.

38. Ritchie, B.: Pulmonary function in scleroderma. Thorax 19:28, 1964.

39. Bulkley, B. H., Klaesmann, P. G., and Hutchins, G. M.: Angina pectoris, myocardial infarction and sudden cardiac death with normal coronary arteries: A clinicopathologic study of 9 patients with progressive systemic sclerosis. Amer. Heart J. 95:563, 1978.

40. Davidson-Lamb, R. W., and Finlayson, M. C. K.: Scleroderma. Complications encountered during dental anesthesia. Anaesthesia 32:893, 1977.

41. Mathews, W. A.: Pheochromocytoma. Clin. Anesth. 3:91, 1963.

42. Eisele, J. H., and Reitan, J. A.: Scleroderma, Raynaud's phenomenon, and local anesthetics. Anesthesiology 34:386, 1971.

43. Brown, G. E., O'Leary, P. A., and Adson, A. W.: Diagnostic and physiologic studies in certain forms of scleroderma. Ann. Intern. Med. 4:531, 1930.

Periarteritis

44. Rose, G. A., and Spencer, H.: Polyarteritis nodosa. Quart. J. Med. 26:43, 1957.

45. Colton, C. L., and Butler, T. J.: The surgical problems of polyarteritis nodosa. Brit. J. Surg. 54:393, 1967.

46. Martin, T.H.: Pharyngeal edema associated with arteritis: A report of two cases. Canad. Med. Assoc. J. 101:229, 1969.

47. McGowan, B. L.: Active temporal arteritis. Amer. J. Ophthal. 64:455, 1967.

Dermatomyositis

48. Hepper, N. G., Ferguson, R. H., and Howard, F. M., Jr.: Three types of pulmonary involvement in polymyositis. Med. Clin. N. Amer. 48:1031, 1964.

49. Olsen, G. N., Swenson, E. W.: Polymyositis and interstitial lung disease. Am. Rev. Resp. Dis. 105:611, 1972.

50. Wylie, W. D., and Churchill-Davidson, H. C.: A Practice of Anesthesia. Chicago, Year Book Medical Publishers, 1962, Chapter 32.

51. Metheney, J. A.: Dermatomyositis: A vocal and swallowing disease entity. Laryngoscope 88:147, 1978.

52. Kulis, J. C., and Nequin, N. D.: Tracheo-esophageal fistula due to Wegener's granulomatosis. J.A.M.A. 191:148, 1965.

53. Blatt, I. M., Seltzer, H. S., Rubin, P., Furstenberg, A. C., Maxwell, J. H., and Schull, W. J.: Fatal granulomatosis of the respiratory tract. Arch. Otolaryn. 70:707, 1959.

54. Landman, S., and Burgener, F.: Pulmonary manifestations in Wegener's granulomatosis. Am. J. Roent. Rad. Nucl. Med. 122:750, 1974.

55. Israel, H. L., and Patchefksy, A. S.: Wegener's granulomatosis of lung: Diagnosis and treatment. Experience with 12 cases. Ann. Intern. Med. 74:881, 1971.

Sarcoidosis

56. Nickerson, D. A.: Boeck's sarcoid: A report of 6 cases in which autopsies were made. Arch. Path. 24:19, 1937.

57. Benedict, E. B., and Castleman, B.: Sarcoidosis with bronchial involvement: Report of a case with bronchoscopic and pathological observations. N. Engl. J. Med. 224:186, 1941.

58. Snider, G. L., and Doctor, L. R.: The mechanics of ventilation in sarcoidosis. Amer. Rev. Resp. Dis. 89:897, 1964.

59. Miller, A., Teirstein, A. S., Jackler, I., Chuang, M., and Siltzbach, L. E.: Airway function in chronic pulmonary sarcoidosis with fibrosis. Am. Rev. Resp. Dis. 109:179, 1974.

60. Levinson, R. S., Metzger, L. F., Stanley, N. N., Kelsen, S. G., Altose, M. D., Cherniack, N. S., and Brody, J. S.: Airway function in sarcoidosis. Am. J. Med. 62:51, 1977.

61. Johnson, R. L., Jr., Lawson, W. H., and Wilcox, W. C. N.: Alveolar capillary block in sarcoidosis. Clin. Res. 9:196, 1961.

62. Scadding, J. G.: Sarcoidosis. London, Eyre and Spottiswoode, 1967, Chapter 13.

63. Miglets, A. W., Viall, J. H., and Kataria, Y. P.: Sarcoidosis of the head and neck. Laryngoscope 87:2038, 1977.

64. Porter, G. H.: Sarcoid heart disease. N. Engl. J. Med. 263:1350, 1960.

65. Svanborg, N.: Studies on cardiopulmonary function in sarcoidosis. Acta Med. Scand. (Suppl.) 366:1, 1961.

66. Chamovitz, D. L., Culley, A. W., and Carlson, K. E.: Cardiac sarcoidosis: Report of a case with paroxysmal ventricular tachycardia. J.A.M.A. 182:574, 1962.

67. Roberts, W. C., McAllister, H. A., Jr., and Ferrans, V. J.: Sarcoidosis of the heart. Am. J. Med. 63:86, 1977.

68. Bergman, N. A.: Pulmonary diffusing capacity and gas exchange during halothane anesthesia. Anesthesiology 32:317, 1970.

14

Muscle Diseases

By JORDAN MILLER, M.D., and CHINGMUH LEE, M.D.

Muscular Dystrophies
Glycogen Storage Diseases
Lipid Storage Myopathies
Myositis Ossificans
Mitochondrial Myopathies
Sarcoplasmic Myopathies

Malignant Hyperthermia
Myasthenias
  Myasthenia Gravis
  Myasthenic Syndrome
Familial Periodic Paralysis

The muscular diseases are all intrinsic disorders of the skeletal muscle cell. Although the causes of these diverse diseases are frequently unknown, it has been possible in most cases to place the defect at or beyond the neuromuscular junction. Although most anesthesiologists have only limited experience with these diseases, the existing literature enables us to modify our anesthetic technique in such a way as to decrease the risk to these patients.

At the start, some general rules that apply to all patients with muscular diseases should be mentioned. Even patients who are capable of fairly normal activities may have decreased muscle reserves to compensate for the stresses of anesthesia and operation. Thus, they are analogous to a partially curarized patient who seems normal but to whom any added stress may be catastrophic. Respiratory failure after upper abdominal surgery is more likely to occur in these patients and the prognosis is graver.

The anesthetic requirements are similar to those of any patient, but the margin of safety is reduced. One should use the smallest amounts of agents that provide satisfactory operating conditions. Fixed dosage schedules should be avoided and continuous adjustments made according to the demands of the situation. Careful monitoring, both of objective and subjective parameters, must continue well into the postoperative period. It should be remembered that narcotics are as much a potential source for respiratory difficulty as the general anesthetic or the muscle relaxants. The patient must demonstrate adequate respiratory reserve and ability to handle secretions before leaving the recovery room. If either of these criteria is not met, mechanical ventilation and the use of an endotracheal tube should be offered. If prolonged ventilatory assistance is required, tracheostomy should be considered.

The preoperative use and teaching of chest physiotherapy and IPPB may avoid many problems in the postoperative period. This is valuable even in those patients in whom respiratory problems are not anticipated. Preventive measures can be lifesaving.

Preoperative baseline measurements of respiratory reserve with at least simple tests of lung function such as vital capacity and maximum inspiratory force, and of blood gases will allow better assessment of these parameters postoperatively. We have been frequently surprised by the poor reserves shown by patients with muscular diseases.

MUSCULAR DYSTROPHIES

These are a group of primary muscular atrophies of unknown cause. They are best characterized by degeneration of the muscle fibers and an increase in the content of fat and fibrous tissue in the muscle[66] in the absence of any evidence of denervation.[45]

The most common and at the same time most severe form is the childhood or Duchenne type. This is characterized by the onset, between the ages of two and six, of weakness in the pelvic girdle, followed rapidly by atrophy in the other proximal muscles.[20] The earlier the onset, the more rapid the downhill course. Frequently the atrophy is preceded by "pseudohypertrophy," which occurs in the calf muscles. This is not true hypertrophy, because the affected muscle is actually weaker than normal. A biopsy shows that the enlargement is due to an increase in fat and fibrous tissue. The muscle, however, does not show the rapid loss of function seen in muscles that just atrophy. Its level of function remains stable, though diminished, while other muscles become functionally useless.

Because the inheritance is sex linked recessive[9], almost all of the reported patients are male. However, there have been some well-documented cases in females. These, it is now thought, are explained by the Lyon hypothesis, which states that in any one cell only one X chromosome is active. The other X in females is inactivated early in the growth of the embryo, and is a chance occurrence. Therefore, it would be expected that in some female heterozygotes the vast majority of cells could have the abnormal X chromosome as the only active one, thus explaining the occasional female with the disease.[73] In addition, female carriers show elevated serum enzymes. Those with the highest enzyme levels would be the ones with the largest proportion of abnormal cells.

Elevated serum enzymes are derived from enzymes released by muscle injury. Aldolase, creatine phosphokinase (CPK), serum glutamic oxaloacetic transaminase (SGOT), lactic dehydrogenase (LDH), and serum glutamic pyruvic transaminase (SGPT) are the most commonly measured. At present this increase in enzymes is thought to result from an increased permeability of the cell membrane to the enzymes located in the sarcoplasm. The enzyme levels are highest early in the disease and decrease as the atrophy progresses. In addition to the loss of enzymes, muscles lose their myoglobin, turning pale early in the disease before fat and fibrous tissue accumulate.[66] The fat that does increase during atrophy is quite resistant to mobilization, even in the presence of inanition. The reason for this is unknown.

Clinically, patients exhibit Gowers' sign, using their hands to climb up their legs in order to arise from the floor. This is necessary because of the early weakness of the pelvic girdle and the relative strength of the arms and shoulders. They cannot walk with heels flat on the ground; they have a waddling gait and a lordotic stance, legs apart and shoulders back. The downhill course of the disease, although variable, is progressive, leading to a wheelchair existence after three to 10 years, and death after five to 20 years.[20] There is a sub-group of about 15 per cent who have a much slower course, and seem to stabilize at about the time of puberty. In those with a slow course, contractures play a major role in the disability.[27] If patients are bedridden for any length of time, they may not recover to their preoperative level of function. This is a major limitation to any surgery and emphasizes the need for physical therapy to prevent contractures.

Cardiac abnormalities occur in a high proportion of these patients, from 50 to 70 per cent,[19, 28, 51, 63, 72] though they are clinically significant in only 10 per cent and in most of these only in the terminal phase of the disease. Arrhythmias occur frequently, even after minor emotional trauma. Atrial tachycardia was reported by Griggs in 65 per cent of his patients. One or more of the following EKG abnormalities have been noted in over 90 per cent of the patients: 1) an increased net R-S in V_1; 2) deep narrow Q in the left precordial leads; 3) RSR' in V_1; 4) polyphasic R in V_1. Mitral valve prolapse demonstrated by echocardiogram[28] is present in 25 per cent. Patients whose cardiac status was fully compensated have died suddenly and unexpectedly. Of the 292 cases reported since 1922, only 140 reports mentioned the cardiac status, and of these 94 were abnormal.[72] The usual picture at autopsy is cardiac dilation with or without hypertrophy. There is frequently a picture of increased connective tissue and fat, as in the skeletal muscle. Fibrosis of the myocardium is limited to the free wall of the left ventricle in Duchenne muscular dystrophy, unlike the fibrosis associated with other forms of muscular dystrophy. There are also respiratory problems, usually the result of pulmonary infections. In a series of 19 autopsies between 1922 and 1951, 12 patients died after acute respiratory infections.[72]

There have been two large series of anesthetic experience published, one by Richards and the other by Cobham, one reporting 43 patients with 61 anesthetics[57] and the other describing anesthetics in 70 patients.[11] Virtually all anesthetic agents have been used. No temperature rise or cardiac arrest was reported in the series. In Richard's study halothane was used 37 times and succinylcholine 12. All were used without subsequent problems. The anesthetic difficulties seemed to parallel the severity of the illness, those with pre-existing respiratory difficulty being most prone to postoperative problems.[44] However, there have been several cardiac arrests reported in patients with Duchenne muscular dystrophy during or immediately after anesthesia.[4, 22, 39, 48, 61] The most frightening aspect seems to be that in most cases the patients had minimal weakness at the time of operation. In several, the arrest first called attention to the Duchenne dystrophy. The reports do not give enough information to allow an explanation. However, elevated CPK and myoglobinuria occurred, in the patients who survived. Acidosis was also common. There were no episodes of hyperpyrexia in any of these patients. The possibility that the inherent membrane defect in Duchenne's muscular dystrophy might make the muscle more susceptible to injury induced by anesthesia cannot be ruled out.

Since most operations are done early in the disease, the incidence of serious anesthetic problems would be expected to be relatively low. The major *predictable* problem would be respiratory depression in patients with minimal reserves. Thus the lightest anesthetic levels should be aimed for. Minimal premedication should be used, with the understanding, however, that many of these children are hostile and withdrawn. Preoperative introduction to chest physiotherapy, IPPB, and its use early in the postoperative periods should keep respiratory complications to a minimum. Except for one patient who showed prolonged apnea after 300 mg of succinylcholine, there was no adverse effect from normal doses of muscle relaxants.[11] There is no report of the use of regional anesthesia in these patients. Field block anesthesia for muscle biopsy has been recommended.[26]

Several unusual complications have occurred postoperatively. Gastric dilatation,[57, 71] heralded by tachycardia and unobtainable blood pressure, occurred in three patients. The combined effects of primary abnormalities in smooth muscle, inactivity, and anesthesia are all thought to lead to the dilatation. The prophylactic use of a nasogastric tube is recommended.

Tachycardia can be minimized by using scopolamine or glycopyrrolate instead of atropine, if the belladonna drugs cannot be avoided entirely.[71] If pentothal is used, it should be given in small incremental doses; with this regimen no problems have been encountered.[71] Another problem noted was difficulty in swallowing, which led to aspiration, respiratory failure, and the death of two patients within 48 hours after minor operations.[7]

Becker dystrophy, a variant of Duchenne dystrophy, is an X-linked muscular dystrophy which is distinguishable from Duchenne dystrophy by its later onset and a much more benign course; most patients are not wheelchair bound before the age of 15 years.[46]

The second type of muscular dystrophy is the fascioscapulohumeral (FSH) form, also known as the benign or Landouzy-Dejerine form. The disease begins in adolescence and has an insidious progression. Patients have weak pectoral and facial muscles; however, the pelvic muscles are much less affected than in the Duchenne type.[20] Occasional patients have signs of the disease as early as six years, but most have recognizable symptoms by the age of 12.[66] Many, however, reach middle age without realizing that they have any abnormality. The mode of inheritance is autosomal dominant, and thus males and females are equally affected. There has been no clear-cut differentiation made between the heterozygous and homozygous forms of the disease, although it is assumed that the homozygous form is worse.

Just as the skeletal muscle weakness is less severe than that in the Duchenne form, the frequency of cardiac involvement is also lower. However, patients have been reported with atrial paralysis.[1] These patients have no atrial electrical activity and cannot be paced electrically from the atrium. Severe bradycardia may be present and life threatening. Ventricular pacing is required in these patients. The most abnormal respiratory finding is a decrease in the vital capacity, owing to the involvement of the accessory muscles of respiration. An average of 15 years after the onset, when two of eight patients were already in wheelchairs, the PCO_2 and the PO_2 remained normal. The carbon dioxide response curve was also normal. However, many patients had recurrent bouts of upper respiratory tract infections.[40] If anesthesia and operation are required, one should aim to prevent respiratory complications.

The third type of dystrophy is called the limb girdle type, a wastebasket classification. There are two subdivisions: Erb's type, in which the shoulder girdle is primarily involved, and the Leyden-Mobius type, with primarily pelvic girdle[20] involvement. The onset occurs at any time from the first to the third decade. The severity is midway between the Duchenne and FSH types. The involvement of the heart varies. In one series three of 26 patients had congestive heart failure.[69] In another series there was none in 18 patients.[73] The most common EKG abnormalities are sinus tachycardia and right bundle branch block. Respiratory problems are similar to those of patients with the FSH form.

There are several less common varieties of muscular dystrophy. One is the distal form. This occurs in Sweden but not elsewhere. The weakness, as the name implies, is primarily distal. The onset is after the age of 30 and the pattern of inheritance is autosomal dominant. It is only slowly progressive.[73] Waters reported another muscular dystrophy,[67] an X-linked humeroperoneal dystrophy with a very slow progression that produced mild disability secondary to weakness and contractures. The patient's predominant findings were cardiac rather than skeletal muscle. Atrial arrhythmias occurred early in the disease and later progressed to atrial paralysis. Sudden death was common between the ages of 30 and 60. The severity of the skeletal muscle disease did not correlate with the cardiac manifestations. Cardiomyopathy may have been present, since fibrosis of the entire ventricle has been reported by others.[28]

One of the most difficult problems in the classification of the muscular dystrophies is the exact position of ocular muscular dystrophy. This type presents before the age of 30, with weakness of the extraocular muscles and ptosis, but rarely diplopia. Symptoms are similar to those of ocular myasthenia gravis.[37, 58, 59] Confusion in classification occurs because biopsies resemble those of muscular dystrophy but progression is very slow without episodes of severe weakness. Fatigue does not make the symptoms worse. If there is extension of weakness, it is limited to the proximal limb muscles, but unlike myasthenia gravis, dysarthria, dysphagia or dyspnea are absent. Despite these dissimilarities, many of the ocular muscular dystrophy patients fit into the myasthenia group[59] because of their exquisite sensitivity to curare. However, more of them are sensitive to curare than are helped by anticholinesterases. In fact, several have been completely paralyzed by 5 to 10 per cent of the usual curarizing dose and then could not have the paralysis reversed by edrophonium. Obviously curariform drugs must be used with extreme caution in these patients, and preparation must be made to ventilate them over many hours. This is particularly true when there is involvement of muscles other than those around the eye.

The one muscular dystrophy that shows the widespread nature of the disease most clearly is myotonic muscular dystrophy, also known as Steinert's disease, Batten-Curschmann's disease, or myotonia atrophica. This form of muscular dystrophy has myotonic symptoms that generally precede the atrophy and weakness. The onset is between the second and fourth decades, and is slowly progressive. Death does not usually occur before the fifth or sixth decade. In spite of the myotonia, the major complaint is weakness, usually of the facial, sternocleidomastoid, and distal muscles. There is pharyngeal weakness with nasal speech.

The myotonic phenomenon consists of a persistent contraction after either voluntary use or mechanical stimulation of a muscle.[60] This prolonged contraction is really a contracture,[42] that is, a contraction with electrical silence. It is sustained without further stimulation by the motor nerve. In addition to the agonist muscles going into contracture, the antagonists also go into a contracture as the patient tries to relax.[16] This has been referred to as afterspasm. Measurements of membrane potential in vivo show values of smaller magnitude than noted in normals or in other forms of myotonia.[52]

Many of the properties of myotonic musculature have been elucidated by the use of various anesthetic techniques. Thus it was shown that the abnormality was not neural in origin because both spinal and regional blocks[16, 43] failed to either prevent or terminate the contractures. Total neuromuscular block with curare[6] also showed the independence of the myotonia from the neuromuscular transmission. Instead, the local infiltration of procaine decreased the myotonia. This observation led to the use of quinine[43] and then procainamide to decrease the myotonia. These drugs are effective both subjectively and objectively in all forms of myotonia, resulting in improvement in the EMG with a more stable resting potential and less spontaneous muscle activity. The anticholinesterases have been said to make the myotonia worse, but in one study there was no change in EMG, except for some twitching in one patient.[43] The use of intra-arterial acetylcholine or choline in these patients gives a response at much lower doses than in normal patients. The response looks like the response in denervated muscle.[45, 53] The use of depolarizing muscle relaxants leads to contracture. In nerve injury of short duration (less than 20 weeks) a similar response is seen in muscles distal to the point of injury. It is of interest that detailed studies of the motor end plate in myotonic muscle show many end plates with profuse subterminal ramifications of the nerves. The same picture is noted in bird and frog muscle, which also responds to succinylcholine with contracture.[53]

The truly systemic nature of myotonic dystrophy[14] can be seen from the wide variety of systems involved. The most common associated abnormality is presenile cataract, which is characteristic for the disease. In many relatives of affected patients this may be the only evidence of the disease. It was once said that cataract occurred in the first generation, muscular abnormality in the second generation, and the full systemic manifestations in the third. This is probably just an artifact resulting from case selection. Frontal baldness in males, testicular atrophy, and intellectual and emotional changes are all common. The testicular changes are primary, rather than due to pituitary abnormalities. The glucose tolerance test is ab-normal, with delayed utilization of glucose and a slow return to normal serum glucoses after the glucose load. Tolbutamide causes an abnormally high increase in insulin (by radioimmunoassay), but the decrease in glucose is only 65 per cent of normal. This would mean that these patients are resistant to insulin of endogenous origin, whereas exogenous insulin produces a normal response.[34] The control mechanisms for insulin release and inhibition are normal in these patients.[35]

The cardiorespiratory abnormalities are of particular concern to anesthesiologists. Cardiac arrhythmias were mentioned as early as 1911 by Griffith, who reported a myotonic dystrophy patient with a heart rate of 36.[10] The most common EKG abnormality is an increased PR interval which is unresponsive to both atropine and nitroglycerin. The P wave has a decreased height, and ST elevations are common. Atrial flutter, which responds to quinidine, has been observed. Digitalis has also been used to control the heart rate associated with flutter. Blood pressure is usually low. Nine of 37 patients who expired in one series died primarily as a result of cardiac failure. One patient had documented cardiomyopathy with lesions similar to those in skeletal muscle.[8] Some patients had Stokes-Adams attacks, as would be expected from the frequent increase in the PR interval. Caution in the use of quinidine must be observed as with any patient liable to Stokes-Adams attacks. The severity of the cardiac disease does not parallel that of the skeletal muscle disease.[69] Cardiac catheterization has shown an increased pulmonary wedge pressure and low cardiac index in several patients.[40] The value of Swan-Ganz catheters for the intraoperative management of these patients is exemplified by the report of Meyers.[47]

Respiratory problems can be discussed in three categories: 1) abnormalities in pulmonary function tests; 2) central nervous system disease, leading to respiratory failure; and 3) problems of the oropharynx.

Pulmonary function abnormalities include a vital capacity that is frequently reduced. In 50 per cent of patients it is decreased by more than 10 per cent. In one patient (a 31-year-old, slightly obese male) it was only half of normal. A major loss is in the expiratory reserve volume. The maximal breathing capacity is also decreased usually to 50 to 70 per cent of normal.[3, 25, 41, 69] The most impressive loss, however, is the reduction in the maximal expiratory pressure. Of 10 patients measured, it averaged 25 per cent of normal.[25] The lungs themselves seem normal. Although this is a picture similar to that seen in restrictive chest wall disease, the mechanism is different. The primary (diaphragm and intercostals) as well as the accessory muscles of respiration have been shown to be abnormal in many of these patients.[3, 40] The diaphragm has been seen to move abnormally on fluoroscopy, and the intercostals are myotonic. The use of quinine to decrease the myotonia has improved the respiratory status.[40]

There are many patients with somnolence, and the question arose as to whether this was a direct or secondary CNS manifestation of the disease. Of the patients studied, several did have mild elevations of the PCO_2 and a low oxygen saturation on room air. There was a shift in the CO_2 response curve to the right (lower sensitivity to CO_2).[41] There was an associated increase in the PCO_2 when patients breathed 100 per cent oxygen. However, with abnormal chest mechanics one cannot be certain that these findings indicate abnormalities in the central control of respiration. The somnolence, however, would not be expected merely on the basis of these relatively mild changes in the blood gases.[8] In addition, one patient showed no change in somnolence with improved respiratory function and restoration of PCO_2 to normal. However, sleep caused an increase in PCO_2, which produced pulmonary hypertension in the patient evaluated. A second patient with somnolence described by Tsueda could not be weaned from a respirator for five days postoperatively.[65] In short, somnolence, personality changes, and occasional CNS atrophy are thought to be primary CNS manifestations of the disease.

The frequent occurrence of pneumonia[44] has led to investigation of the swallowing mechanism in some of these patients. Of four patients who died of pneumonia, two had pulmonary abscesses and one had evidence of aspiration.[15, 69] Of 44 patients studied, all but one showed abnormal swallowing in cineradiography. Of these, 12 had aspiration of radiopaque material without any cough.[55] Many patients without pulmonary symptoms had severe abnormalities

demonstrated on cineradiography. Only males showed the aspiration, although there were many females in the study. Twenty-two patients had chronic cough, four bronchiectasis, three tuberculosis, and three severe emphysema. The difficulty in swallowing was not improved by quinine, procainamide, or steroids. This is consistent with the observation that the swallowing abnormality parallels the atrophy rather than the myotonia. In addition to the esophagus, the stomach shows poor motility. Smooth muscle involvement is thought to be responsible for this. Poor gastric motility may decrease the absorption of oral medication as well as increase the danger of aspiration.[31]

Therapy is aimed at the myotonia and not the atrophy, for which there is no effective treatment. Quinine was the first drug used, and although useful in many patients, it requires mild toxicity before it is effective. Procainamide,[23] on the other hand, works without many of the toxic symptoms. Orally it is given in a dosage of 1 gm four times a day. It is effective in blocking the myotonia after spontaneous effort but not after percussion, and thus may not help relaxation during surgery. It can be administered intravenously in doses to 1000 mg at the rate of 100 mg per minute.

As would be expected, this disease poses a very difficult problem to the anesthesiologist. The patients have many serious problems related to the systemic manifestations of their disease. Thus one must be aware of the serious cardiac problems, and EKG monitoring is mandatory. The arguments for and against prophylactic digitalization are the same as in any other case of mild cardiac disease. Digitalization probably is indicated only when there is manifest congestive failure. Respiratory problems combined with swallowing difficulties require careful attention.[15] Because of the shift in the CO_2 response curve, patients require controlled ventilation during the anesthesia, and may well require postoperative ventilation even after relatively minor surgery. Preoperative blood gases should be obtained as a baseline. Respiratory function tests should include a one-second forced expiratory volume, and if possible, minute ventilation, maximum breathing capacity, and total lung volume. Endocrine abnormalities should not cause any serious problems. If there is an episode of unexplained hypotension with poor response to vasopressors, steroids should be used. The psychological problems require a careful and involved preoperative visit to produce patient cooperation.

It was reported as early as 1915[17] that the myotonic did poorly after anesthesia. After an uneventful ether anesthetic a patient had cyanosis for the next 24 hours. Then in the early 1950's, Dundee[18] reported that thiopentone in these patients produced severe apnea, and was contraindicated. Careful studies have shown that this is not unique to thiopentone but that these patients are particularly sensitive to any respiratory depressant.[5, 21, 24, 32, 68] The depression is not the result of a direct effect on muscle, as was once thought, but a nonspecific effect of depressant medication in a patient with little respiratory reserve. The seriousness of the respiratory problem is well documented by the deaths of four of five patients with respiratory depression in Kaufman's series.[38] In a comment on Kaufman's paper, Hunter described a patient who had pentothal and curare for a hysterectomy, and then required ventilation for four days and had difficulties handling secretions for four weeks.[36] More recently Ravin reported a patient with severe respiratory problems four hours postoperatively because of respiratory obstruction. This patient had appeared to do well in the immediate postoperative period.[56] This is obviously not just the result of a single anesthetic, but rather represents the ease with which these patients can decompensate. As little as 100 mg of pentothal after the usual narcotic premedication has caused apnea. If apnea occurs, the best therapy is ventilation rather than counteracting drugs such as neostigmine, naloxone, or doxapram.[30]

The production of muscle relaxation in a myotonic is one of the most difficult problems facing the anesthesiologist. Nerve blocks cannot guarantee relaxation because the muscles are still subject to the equivalent of percussion myotonia, the stimulus of the surgeon, and electrocautery but provide an ideal anesthetic if relaxation is not needed.[29, 33, 70] Muscle relaxants of the nondepolarizing type have much the same problem in that they only block the motor nerve impulses. They may or may not produce relaxation. The experience with muscle relaxants is best documented by Mitchell.[49] He showed that myotonic patients have normal sensitivity to curare.[2, 49] Use of neostigmine following the use of muscle relaxants has not provoked problems. Though neostigmine has been noted to increase myotonia, this and other reports of its use to reverse nondepolarizing blocks have been uneventful.[13, 14, 49, 56] Deep general anesthesia may also be used to produce relaxation. However, if the general anesthetic is deep, respiration is likely to be depressed for a prolonged period and cardiac function may be unacceptably depressed. The depolarizing muscle relaxants have the same limitations as those of the nondepolarizing type, and in addition there have been many reports of widespread myotonia following their use. Involvement of the muscles of respiration as well as the larynx[54, 64] has made it difficult or impossible to ventilate these patients. The myotonia seems to last as long as or longer than the duration of effect of succinylcholine. Whether the use of procainamide or dantrolene would reduce the occurrence of this reaction is not known. Limitation of the dose of succinylcholine to less than 30 mg at a time has been recommended and would seem to be logical.[53] Since succinylmonocholine also seems to cause myotonia, there may be a limit to the usefulness of repeated small doses. Certainly before the use of a depolarizing relaxant, patients should inhale 100 per cent oxygen. However, not all patients with this disease will exhibit myotonia after depolarizing muscle relaxants, and in fact over half have responded in the normal manner to these agents.[64]

The use of intravenous Lidocaine distal to a tourniquet (Bier block) may be the ideal mode for extremity surgery where relaxation is necessary, because the direct effect of local anesthetics on the muscle might prevent myotonia. There are no reports in the literature of this being used. Althesin (not available in the United States) has been reported to prevent percussion and surgical myotonia without affecting the EMG. Several patients have had successful operations following use of this anesthetic agent either alone or with nitrous oxide.[50, 62]

The postoperative shivering that is so frequently seen with halothane may also produce myotonia. It would seem that balanced anesthesia would be a reasonable choice. Good temperature control would also lessen shivering even with halothane or enflurane.

Pregnancies may prove a hazard. However, pregnancy is rare in these patients because of ovarian atrophy. In patients who do become pregnant, regional anesthesia would seem ideal. Most of these patients have a normal first stage of labor but should not push in the second stage to prevent skeletal muscle contracture and respiratory distress. Uterine atony has been reported to occur after delivery and may require oxytocics and/or massive blood transfusions.[21, 29, 31, 33]

Myotonia congenita was first described by Thomsen in himself and several relatives.[10] It is a rather benign disease in that there is no atrophy, and no known systemic symptoms occur other than those related to muscle. The myotonia is much more widespread than in myotonic dystrophy, and the muscles are frequently increased in size. This disease is much less common than myotonic dystrophy. It is inherited as an autosomal dominant. Though in some families there have been cataracts, cataract is not commonly associated with this disease. There is also good evidence that myotonia congenita is not a variant of myotonic dystrophy, although there are some families in which both diseases have appeared. Drug therapy and methods to produce relaxation in these patients are the same as for myotonic dystrophy patients.

Paramyotonia congenita is characterized by myotonia followed by paresis, usually induced by exposure to cold. There is a resemblance both to hyperkalemic periodic paralysis and to myotonia congenita. The exact placement of this disease in the classification is unclear, but it is probably a subgroup of one or both of the above.

GLYCOGEN STORAGE DISEASES

This group of diseases is particularly interesting from both the clinical and biochemical points of view. Every enzyme deficiency that theoretically could lead to accumulation of glycogen has been found to occur. The theory that glycogen synthesis uses a different enzymatic pathway from glycogen breakdown was actually based on a case of abnormal glycogen storage. Glycogen is a very high molecular weight polysaccharide with many branches. It has two types of glucose-to-glucose bonds, thus permitting this branching (Fig. 14–1). The classification presented of the glycogenoses is that of Cori.[3]

Cori Type I (von Gierke's Disease, Hepatorenal Glycogenosis). The enzyme defect is absence of glucose-6-phosphatase. The mode of inheritance is autosomal recessive. This enzyme functions primarily in the liver to convert glucose-6-phosphate into glucose, which can then be mobilized and transported via the blood stream to the periphery. In this disorder enzymatic conversion is the rate-limiting step and glycogen is stored in excess in the liver. As the synthesis of glycogen continues, the liver increases in size and a large protuberant abdomen appears.

Fasting produces profound hypoglycemia, as the liver cannot release glucose after stimulation with glucagon or epinephrine. The symptoms in the first year of life are secondary to the hypoglycemia. Blood sugars between 15 and 36 mg per 100 ml are not uncommon. Thus one may see convulsions, failure to thrive, and severe acidosis. There is a massive hyperlipemia that must be taken into consideration when interpreting serum values such as sodium, since the lipid fraction contains no sodium (a 20% decrease in serum sodium values is normal in the presence of a 20% lipemia). Renal involvement presents as hyperuricemia and episodes of gout.

The diagnosis is made by infusing glucagon and observing a smaller than expected rise in blood glucose. The small rise that does occur is due to the debrancher enzyme, which frees glucose instead of glucose-6-phosphate. A more accurate test is to give fructose. In normal patients this produces a rise in blood glucose as fructose is rapidly transformed first into fructose-6-phosphate, then glucose-6-phosphate, and finally glucose. Since glucose-6-phosphatase is necessary for this conversion, there is no rise in glucose after the infusion of fructose in these patients.

The best therapy presently available is frequent small carbohydrate feedings. Several people have used thyroxin and glucagon to limit the amount of glycogen synthesis, permitting the glucose to pass through the liver without being taken up and converted to glycogen. The glucose can then supply the brain and other organs.[9] Similarly, portacaval bypass has recently

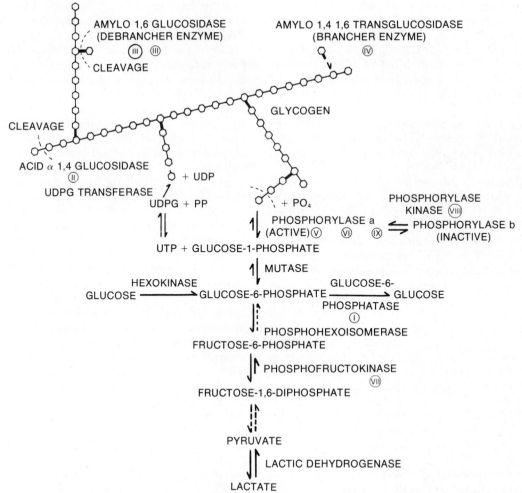

Figure 14–1. Schema of glycogen metabolism. The Roman numerals indicate where defects give rise to the individual types of glycogen storage disease. (Modified from Cornblath, M., and Schwartz, R.: Disorders of Carbohydrate Metabolism. Philadelphia, W. B. Saunders Co., 1966.)

been advocated to improve growth and decrease episodes of hypoglycemia. The mechanism is, again, based on allowing glucose to bypass the liver and thus reach the periphery.[1]

Cox[2] recently reported his experience with 11 surgical procedures performed in the past 10 years. One patient had a cardiac arrest after a one-hour tonsillectomy and could not be resuscitated. Although the remaining 10 patients survived, a single detailed case report emphasizes the serious anesthetic problems. The patient was a 17-year-old boy weighing 32 kg who was kept on nothing per mouth for seven hours prior to operation. On arrival in the operating room he had a pH of 7.24 and a lactic

acidosis. The acidosis progressively worsened in spite of 5 per cent dextrose given intravenously. A total of 90 mEq of $NaHCO_3$ was given to restore his pH from 7.08 to the preoperative value of 7.24. This slowly returned to normal by the next day. Cox feels that large blood loss (18 per cent of predicted blood volume) associated with the surgery contributed to the acidosis. It would seem wise to buffer the blood that has to be given, but it would be even more important to use overnight intravenous dextrose infusion to prevent acidosis prior to the start of surgery. In a series of four patients, Casson has used hyperalimentation for at least one week preoperatively both to improve the patient's general state and to decrease liver size prior to major surgery. Hyperalimentation is then continued postoperatively to allow optimum healing.

The careful frequent measuring of the acid-base status is highly recommended and is essential prior to and during any surgical procedure. Patients have been reported to go into severe acidosis without ketone bodies in the urine,[9] so monitoring of ketones is not adequate. The type of anesthetic seems to make little difference; cyclopropane, ether and halothane have all been used successfully.

Cori Type II (Pompe's Disease, Generalized Glycogenosis, Lysosomal Acid Maltase Deficiency). Lysosomal acid maltase deficiency (alpha-1-4 and 1-6 glucosidase)[3] shows striking clinical heterogeneity. In infantile form there is a deficiency of this enzyme in all tissues. Storage of glycogen occurs in membrane limited sacs and is seen in heart and skeletal muscle and in the nervous system. The onset of symptoms occurs from two to six months, with vomiting, anorexia, weakness, drooling, cyanosis, and dyspnea. The patient looks like a cretin. The primary symptoms are those of failure of the heart and neuromuscular system. Infants are hypotonic, but muscle bulk is good. The electrocardiogram shows 1) short PR interval, 2) high QRS, and 3) depressed ST segments and inverted or peaked T waves. Blood sugar and glucose tolerance tests are normal. Death ensues usually in the first year but may not occur until the third year and is secondary to congestive heart failure or aspiration pneumonia. The presence of increased ventriculoseptal wall thickness and outflow tract obstruction to both right and left sides has been reported and may be contributory to congestive heart failure in these patients.[11, 12] It is not clear how acid maltase deficiency causes muscle damage. One hypothesis is that the lysosomes may be destroyed by the accumulation of glycogen, thus releasing their contents and causing muscle destruction.[13] Kaplan has recently reported anesthetic experience in two patients with this disease. Both patients seemed to tolerate anesthesia using ether, ketamine, halothane, and nitrous oxide and succinylcholine on different occasions.[12] However, only minimal monitoring was reported in these patients and no statement as to intraoperative changes in acid-base status, blood pressure, evidence of myocardial ischemia, or temperature changes were reported.

The late onset forms of the disease do not occur in the same families as the infantile form,[5] and so are thought to be an unrelated genetic abnormality.[3] They are very variable in onset, from childhood to adult patients. The patients do not have cardiac and nervous system involvement. The presence of small amounts of normal enzyme activity in muscle, approximately 7 per cent, may play a role in the later onset of the disease in these patients. There are no data to indicate what the levels of enzymes are in the heart and central nervous system and whether the presence of enzyme in these tissues is, in fact, protective. Adults have weakness of skeletal muscles and present with many of the symptoms of a slowly progressive muscular dystrophy. Ventilatory insufficiency can be life-threatening in these patients, but otherwise they do fairly well. There is no anesthesia experience in adults with this disease.

Cori Type III (Forbes' Disease, Limit Dextrinosis, Debrancher Deficiency). This disease looks like a milder form of Type I; however, there is involvement of cardiac and skeletal muscle. Signs and symptoms disappear after puberty for an unknown reason.[3] Fasting blood sugar is depressed (35 to 50 mg per 100 ml), though not as low as in Type I. There is decreased response to epinephrine, and acetonuria is common. Glucose can be mobilized only if it occurs after a branching point. As a result the glycogen noted is much more branched than usual. Once a branch occurs, that portion of the molecule can no longer be used. Unlike Type I disease, infusion of fructose causes a rise in the blood glucose because the missing enzyme is not involved in the conversion of fructose to glucose. Since gluconeogenesis is possible, the use of a high protein diet is helpful.[14] The electrocardiogram is not a good indicator of the severity of the heart disease. Evidence of congestive failure might not occur even with significant cardiac involvement.

Of the three patients reported in the literature, one had two general anesthetics, both uneventful except for an episode of laryngospasm. The first operation was an open liver biopsy by open drop ether; the second was open heart surgery with the use of bypass to correct subvalvular aortic stenosis. In neither case were blood acid-base values reported. Severe acidosis was present in two patients in spite of preoperative hyperalimentation and the intraoperative use of a 15% dextrose and bicarbonate solution. The acidosis, however, was not progressive. Pancuronium and halothane nitrous oxide were well tolerated. The postoperative course in the patients undergoing portacaval shunts was benign.[1]

Cori Type IV (Andersen's Disease, Brancher Deficiency). This is the rarest of the glycogenoses, with only two reported cases in the literature. Here the glycogen is made abnormally, without branches. All the enzymes needed for the degradation are present; thus the presence of excess "glycogen" is thought to be due to the precipitation of the unbranched polysaccharide, with tissue reaction and loss of availability of glycogen to the tissues. The disease is characterized by cirrhosis and an early death.

There is no reported anesthetic experience with this disease. The severe liver involvement would limit the use of drugs that depend on this organ for metabolism. Bleeding may be a problem and can be treated with fresh frozen plasma to restore clotting factors.

Cori Type V (McArdle's Disease, Myophosphorylase Deficiency).[7] There are at least two distinct immunological types of phosphorylase. The first is found in liver and leukocytes, the second in skeletal muscle. If one is absent, it is absent in all the tissues in which it is normally found; however, the other type will still be found in its usual locations. Characteristically the onset is in childhood, with symptoms of diminished activity and cramping with exercise, followed by weakness.[8] If exercise is continued, muscle contracture (contraction but with EMG silence) and myoglobinuria occur. In one family the onset was in middle age.[6] There is no muscle atrophy until the fifth decade. The classic test for this disease is to determine venous lactate and pyruvate levels after ischemic exercise. In the normal there is a two- to five-fold increase. Here, there is a decrease, as the muscle cannot break down its glycogen and must use lactate and pyruvate for metabolism. Ischemic exercise tolerance is only 10 to 20 per cent of normal, in spite of normal initial muscle strength. Blood sugar rises normally after glucagon or epinephrine, and the exercise tolerance can be increased by treatment with glucagon, dextrose, fructose, or lactate. In the one autopsy in this disease the cardiac muscle was normal. There is a question whether in another patient the uterine musculature was abnormal. One patient was known to have done heavy work until the age of 49, at which time she experienced the classic symptoms and had biopsy proved lack of myophosphorylase. The evidence, however, is strongly in favor of an autosomal recessive inheritance and not of an acquired disease.

Since it is thought that repeated episodes of ischemia lead to eventual atrophy,[10] it would seem unwise to use prolonged tourniquets in these patients, either to reduce blood loss or to permit the use of intravenous local anesthesia. The use of an infusion of dextrose or the use of glucagon to increase the blood sugar would seem wise. Myoglobinuria has been seen after prolonged ischemia and should be watched for; good hydration and mannitol may be necessary to prevent renal damage. There is no experience with use of muscle relaxants in this disease; however, recent reports of myoglobinemia after succinylcholine and halothane[15] should make one wary of using this combination in these patients. Muscle weakness is not very common and will not occur if perfusion is adequate and blood sugar levels are maintained.

Cori Type VI (Hepatophosphorylase Deficiency, Hers' Disease). Mild to moderate degrees of hypoglycemia are caused by the small amounts of phosphorylase in the liver. There is usually a poor response to glucagon and epinephrine. The muscle phosphorylase (being a different enzyme immunologically) and cardiac phosphorylase are both normal, but the leukocyte phosphorylase levels follow those of the liver. One patient was seen to have a bleeding diathesis. Whether it was related to this disease is not known. Liver function is usually not impaired. Except for the prevention of hypoglycemia there is no specific therapy.

Type VII (Tauri, Muscle Phosphofructokinase Deficiency).[17] Symptoms are similar to those in myophosphorylase deficiency. Ischemic exercise leads to the same lack of elevation of lactate. Muscle weakness on strenuous exercise and cramping of muscle and myoglobinuria can occur. Phosphofructokinase, the enzyme that converts either fructose-6-phosphate or fructose-1-phosphate to fructose-1,6-diphosphate, is missing. Since this is necessary for the metabolism of glycogen, glucose, or fructose, none of these compounds would be expected to improve the picture.[17]

Type VIII (Low Hepatic Phosphorylase Activity). Patients show progressive central nervous system degeneration with death in childhood.

Type IX (Deficient Hepatic Phosphorylasekinase activity with predominant hepatomegaly). One patient with two anesthetics, the first with halothane and succinylcholine, produced no reported problems. During the second anesthetic with enflurane after succinylcholine plus ketamine for induction, temperature increased 2° C in two hours and there was evidence of a hypermetabolic state with an increase in arterial PCO_2 and a base excess of -12. The acidosis was at least partially due to ketosis, although adequate serum glucose was documented and extra glucose was given intravenously. No other finding of malignant hyperpyrexia was found in this patient and only minimal changes in CPK occurred postoperatively. The child did well postoperatively.

Type X (Deficient Cyclic, 3,5 AMP Dependent Kinase). Excess glycogen is found in both skeletal muscle and liver. Hepatomegaly is a major sign.

Phosphohexoisomerase deficiency is the lack of the enzyme needed to convert glucose-6-phosphate to fructose-6-phosphate. As expected, fructose relieves the symptoms and permits the production of lactate.[16]

In Types V, VII, and phosphohexoisomerase deficiency high levels of glycolysis, without ischemia, would be expected to produce symptoms. Thus anything that would produce a hypermetabolic state in muscle, such as shivering or hyperthemia, might lead to problems and even myoglobinuria. Careful avoidance of heat loss during the operation with continuous temperature monitoring is indicated. In the patient with proved phosphohexoisomerase deficiency the use of intravenous fructose is warranted.

LIPID STORAGE MYOPATHIES

Another group of myopathies has been found in which there is abnormal metabolism of lipids.[4] A picture of myopathy that is usually slowly progressive is described. So far, two major types have been demonstrated.

Type I (Carnitine Deficiency). Carnitine facilitates the transport of long-chain fatty acids into mitochondria. Its absence in muscle causes weakness. Lipid granules are seen in the muscle. Since fatty acids are not prime substrate but only account for approximately 50 per cent of the energy utilization of muscle, the muscle can be exercised but not to the same extent as normal muscle. Medium-chain fatty acids, which do not require carnitine to get into mitochondria, and dietary carnitine will help most patients. In addition, the use of steroids is also efficacious. It is thought that steroids allow access of long-chain fatty acids into the mitochondria without carnitine. A few patients have been reported with respiratory insufficiency and one with cardiac involvement. A more serious variety of this deficiency has been reported in three patients from the same town. They showed a rapidly progressive myopathy that was lethal.[3] Storage of lipid in muscle, liver, kidney, and myocardium was seen. Though carnitine deficiency was present, a trial of carnitine was without success in one case. An acute metabolic disorder was responsible for the deaths of all of these patients. It was probably related to a hepatic encephalopathy. All patients showed signs of nausea, vomiting, and weakness with the acute episodes.

Type II (Carnitine Palmityl Transferase Deficiency.)[1, 4] Myoglobinuria and muscle cramps are associated with increased plasma triglycerides. Weakness is usually not present, and on ischemic exercise normal lactate production is encountered. On prolonged fasting, however, increased serum levels of muscle CPK and myoglobinuria occur. The onset of muscle cramps, later than with glycogen storage disease, is characteristic. Prolonged fasting leads to myoglobinuria. Exercise enhances the fasting myoglobinuria, and this may be severe enough to cause renal failure.[2] No anesthetic experience has been reported. Glucose would seem to be mandatory to prevent glycogen depletion followed by muscle dependence on long-chain fatty acids. Excessive muscle activity, such as shivering, should be prevented, if possible. Temperature must be rigidly controlled.

MYOSITIS OSSIFICANS

This familial disease usually starts in early childhood and is transmitted as an autosomal recessive. After a minor trauma, a cystlike nodule is first felt under the skin. This is followed by the appearance of true bone in that area. The heart, diaphragm, sphincters, and larynx are spared in this otherwise widespread progressive disease. The major problems are those of fixation of muscles of mastication and the neck. In addition, three fourths of affected individuals have other associated anomalies, such as microdactyly, curved or ankylosed digits and other digital anomalies, absent teeth, and spina bifida, and many of these require surgical correction. Biopsies and other surgical intervention, however, can cause the local formation of bone. Death is usually due to limitation of motion over the trunk, leading to secondary respiratory or cardiac failure. Although death usually occurs in the second to fourth decade, survival to the seventh has been reported.

Anesthetic problems are primarily related to the inability to open the mouth or bend the neck. This cannot be overcome by muscle relaxants once ossification has occurred. Tracheostomy may be of value when direct vision or blind nasal intubation is impossible; however, ossification may occur at the tracheostomy site. Limitation of the chest wall can become a problem as the disease progresses. Steroids have been used for treatment, although their efficacy remains in question.

MITOCHONDRIAL MYOPATHIES

Five types of myopathy have been described in which abnormalities of the mitochondria are seen on muscle biopsy. The most common feature in each of these is long-term myopathy, frequently manifest at birth or in childhood.[10]

The first type to be described in 1959 was named after Luft, who subsequently, in 1962, provided a more detailed account of the metabolic abnormality.[5] The patient was noted to have symptoms from at least age seven but was studied at the age of 35. At that time she was noted to have many of the symptoms of hyperthyroidism, including hyperhidrosis, polydipsia, polyphagia, asthenia, and decreased weight. However, her growth and development were normal by history. She was first treated for hyperthyroidism medically, with an initial decrease in her basal metabolic rate (BMR). Later, after a thyroidectomy, unmistakable signs of myxedema developed, despite a BMR of +100 per cent. Although this was considerably less than her maximum of +270 per cent, she required thyroid replacement therapy. She had not only the expected increased minute ventilation but also an increased functional residual capacity and residual volume: total lung capacity ratio.

The pathologic picture was that of mitochondria of variable size with increased numbers of cristae, which is normal in mitochondria from liver, heart, and diaphragm but not skeletal muscle. The nuclei were surrounded by a clear myofibril-free area. Her uterine and skin mitochondria were normal. A similar picture was seen in a second case reported and described in detail by Haydar and Afifi.[1, 4]

The clinical picture could be explained by biochemical studies that demonstrated loose coupling of oxidative phosphorylation. Loose coupling of oxidative phosphorylation is a situation in which the stepwise oxidation of hydrogen by the cytochrome system does not produce adenosine triphosphate (ATP) from adenosine diphosphate (ADP) in a stoichiometric relationship. Since ADP is produced from ATP during muscle contraction, its concentration is related to the amount of work done by the cell, and thus the metabolic rate normally increases as the available ADP increases. This patient's mitochondria, unlike normal ones, did not decrease the rate of oxidation when ADP was absent from the medium. Thus, the fixed relationship no longer held. Her rate of oxidation of hydrogen was not dependent on availability of ADP. However, her oxidative phosphorylation was not uncoupled, because ATP could be produced if ADP was present. This is mandatory for life, because energy, as high energy phosphate, must be stored for the body to do useful work.

This patient had one anesthetic, for thyroidectomy, which consisted of intravenous Narkotal (5,2 bromoallyl-N-methyl-5-isopropyl barbituric acid) and ether by endotracheal tube. There were no complications during or after the surgery.[6]

Undoubtedly this patient with such a high metabolic rate would benefit from the use of high concentrations of oxygen and a larger than usual minute ventilation. High output respiratory failure might be expected, especially after major surgery, and postoperative ventilation should be considered. Blood gas measurements would also be valuable both before and during surgery, because normal amounts of shunt might produce arterial desaturation owing to the increased A-V O_2 gradient. Short periods of apnea, or decreased perfusion, would be expected to be hazardous. Since this patient's blood volume was almost twice the predicted normal, blood volume measurements would be of value in this disease. Hyperthermia, not seen in the single anesthetic experience, would be a concern, and the use of a temperature monitor would be indicated.

In 1967, van Wijngaarden[9] reported on a patient with the onset of myopathy at the age of four years. At 11 she had slight deltoid weakness and a waddling gait; her BMR was normal. At 15 the disease showed a slow progression, and the BMR was slightly elevated to +24 per cent. The muscle mitochondria were seen to be elongated and annular, with tightly packed cristae. They also demonstrated loosely coupled oxidative phosphorylation but used a normal amount of glucose-6-phosphate per oxygen consumed. How this disease is related to Luft's disease is not known, since the marked weakness relative to the metabolic abnormality certainly produced a quite different clinical picture. No anesthetic experience is reported.

Megaconical myopathy was first described by Shy and Gonatas[8] in an eight-year-old female with mitochondrial abnormality (large and with inclusion bodies) but a normal BMR. The weakness was primarily proximal (pelvic and shoulder girdles, proximal limb muscles, sternocleidomastoids) as in the previous case. There were increased lipid stores, and Engel questions whether this was really a lipidosis.[3]

Pleoconical myopathy was first reported by Gonatas and Shy[3] in an eight-year-old male who had been noted to be a "floppy" baby. He had acute exacerbations of the disease with quadriparesis lasting 10 to 14 days. Here the mitochondria were slightly increased in size but with normal internal architecture. The BMR was, again, normal and there is no anesthetic experience reported.

Coleman et al.[2] reported on two patients with proximal weakness and muscle fatigability noted since ages seven and eight. Both had subsarcolemmal vacuoles and mitochondria with high levels of oxidative enzymes. These patients' biopsies looked like those of Shy and Gonatas but were present only in type I fibers, whereas Shy's patient had these findings in both the type I and type II cells. Type I cells are small and are identified histochemically by their high content of mitochondria and mitochondrial oxidative enzymes. Type II cells are larger but with fewer mitochondria and higher phosphorylase activity.[7] The ultrastructure had not yet been done when the article was published; but there was no evidence of hypermetabolism.

As pointed out in the introduction, careful concerned management is essential for successful anesthesia. This includes minimal required dosage, careful monitoring throughout the procedure and into the postoperative period, and awareness of the potential problems associated with minimal muscle reserve.

SARCOPLASMIC MYOPATHIES

There are three types of histologic abnormalities of skeletal muscle sarcoplasm. These are somewhat more common than the myopathies of mitochondrial origin but are still extremely rare, with only a handful of reported cases in the world literature.

Nemaline Myopathy. Nemaline myopathy was first described in 1963 by Shy et al.[7] By 1967, 11 cases had been reported.[9] The clinical picture has been one of a relatively nonprogressive symmetrical muscle weakness without marked wasting affecting primarily the proximal muscles. Hypotonia is severe in infancy, with resultant late acquisition of motor skills; only one in eight walked by 18 months. In one case the newborn was noted to be weak, and in two of four cyanosis was noted perinatally. In older patients with this disease severe kyphosis is seen that may lead to cord compression and further diminution in muscular power. One patient was reported to have a vital capacity of only 40 per cent of that predicted but with normal flow rates, and her mother, who also had the disease, died of respiratory failure at 63 after an upper respiratory infection.[5] In the one reported autopsy there was no involvement of cardiac or smooth muscle.[6] Cineradiography revealed an asymptomatic abnormality in swallowing. However, two patients have shown rapid progression; one died of cardiac failure at 12 years of age,[3] the other died at 10 months. Diaphragm and intercostal muscles were involved.

Histologically there are 0.5 to 3.0 micron rods found between the normal myofibrils in from 2 to 40 per cent of the muscle fibers. Their origin is from the Z band of the muscle cell. Because the lowest percentage of abnormal cells was in the oldest patient, it is felt that the number of affected cells does not increase with time. There have been no biochemical abnormalities demonstrated to date, although the number of mitochondria in the affected areas was less than in the normal. It seems from the limited data that this is an autosomal dominant disease with incomplete penetrance.[8]

There is no reported anesthetic experience. All biopsies, even in children, have been obtained under local anesthesia.

Myotubular Myopathy. This disorder shows bilateral facial paralysis and internal strabismus, the Mobius syndrome. In addition, there is cranial nerve functional loss. The muscle fibers are round and large, with a clear area devoid of myofibrils around the centrally placed nuclei.[9]

Central core disease was first described by Shy et al. in 1956. A second family was described in 1961 and several more in the following years. Hypotonia and proximal muscle weakness appear in the first year of life, and, as in nemaline myopathy, there is a delay in physical development.[7] This weakness remains without progression throughout life. Lower extremity weakness is more pronounced than upper, and these patients have difficulty walking up stairs and rising from a sitting position. An increased lumbar lordosis is also present. Wasting of muscles has not been prominent in most patients.

Histologically nearly every muscle cell has a densely staining core of altered myofibrils. This core is a region without mitochondria and sarcoplasmic reticulum in an otherwise normal fiber. There is no increase in the connective tissue of the endomysium, nor is there evidence of regenerating fibers. Biochemically, muscle cells of the propositus showed an absence of muscle phosphorylase until activated with AMP (adenosine monophosphate), after which they had 10 per cent of normal. The histologically unaffected father showed the same absence of phosphorylase but on activation had 50 per cent of normal levels. The mother had normal levels of phosphorylase. This differs from McArdle's disease (absence of myophosphorylase), in which patients have no phosphorylase and AMP has no effect. Also serum levels of pyruvate and lactate rise normally in central core disease but not in McArdle's disease. Histochemically the phosphorylase is absent only in the core regions.[2] Serum glutamic oxaloacetic transaminase (SGOT) has been normal in these diseases.[7] It is believed that there is an autosomal dominant mode of inheritance, but the absence of histologic abnormality in the father of the patient described leaves the possibility that this is either a forme fruste (a variable incomplete form of the disease) or recessive inheritance.

Denborough reported a patient from a family with malignant hyperpyrexia who was diagnosed as having central core disease. A muscle biopsy responded abnormally in vitro to halothane.[1] Whether this is a chance association is not now clear. Harrison reported two patients with central core disease who had no problem with halothane anesthesia.[4] One of our patients with this disease had an uneventful open reduction of the hip at another hospital. All other operations have been biopsies done under local anesthesia.

In each of the aforementioned diseases the weakness is relatively nonprogressive and the expected life span is close to normal. However, as in the reported case of a nemaline myopathy death caused by upper respiratory tract infection,[5] musculoskeletal abnormalities and weakness make these patients poor risks. Any operation in which there is splinting of the diaphragm or chest or decreased motion secondary to pain may lead to respiratory failure. Preoperative evaluation of respiratory function would be helpful. Because these patients have been shown by cineradiography to have abnormalities in swallowing, they must be carefully watched to prevent aspiration even after the normal recovery from anesthesia. Muscle relaxants may be necessary in these patients, as their weakness may be only slight. If relaxants are required, a nerve stimulator should first be placed to evaluate what is normal for each patient. Following oxygenation, a small initial dose should be used (succinylcholine, 0.3 mg per kg, or d-tubocurarine, 0.1 mg per kg). Additional doses should be based upon the response to the test dose and be given sparingly. However, because of the nonuniform degree of weakness, the degree of relaxation in the muscles of the hand may not give an accurate picture of the relaxation in the abdominal muscles.

MALIGNANT HYPERTHERMIA

Human malignant hyperthermia (MH) appears to be a pharmacogenetic disorder transmitted by a dominant autosomal gene, although there exists considerable variability in expressivity and possibly also in penetrance of the trait. The possibility of multifactorial or two-gene inheritance has not been ruled out. The seriousness of the problem is underscored by two facts: 1) the mortality rate, until recently, has ranked highest among complications of modern anesthesia; 2) the incidence is not very low, about 1 in 3000 to 15,000 pediatric patients and 1 in 50,000 to less than 1 in 100,000 in the general population.[1, 2, 3, 4] Obviously, the incidence and mortality depend on the criteria of diagnosis.

Clinical Features. In view of the variability of symptoms of the reported cases of MH and the necessity of early diagnosis, it is essential for the anesthesiologist to familiarize himself with the typical features first. The patient is probably in the early teens and has a normal history and physical examination. Some family members may have had an adverse anesthetic experience, though the patient may have had uneventful anesthesia in the past. The patient might have some relatively mild congenital musculoskeletal abnormality, such as strabismus, ptosis, kyphoscoliosis, hernia, club foot, or joint dislocations.[1, 4] Most likely, the patient has received atropine as premedication and succinylcholine to facilitate endotracheal intubation. Retrospectively, the anesthetist might recall that the patient responded to succinylcholine with exaggerated fasciculation and that the relaxation, especially that of the jaw, seemed poor. A potent anesthetic, usually halothane, was subsequently used to maintain anesthesia. Frequently, the concentration of halothane was increased at some point during the operation because the patient "appeared to be light," having tachycardia, hypertension, and poor relaxation. Respiratory movement might increase or appear in spite of "adequate" controlled ventilation. Subsequently, the patient was noted to be hot. The temperature then continued to climb rapidly. An increase from a normal temperature to 40°C in five minutes has been observed. An increase from normal to 44°C within one to two hours of induction of anesthesia is not unusual.[1] Once this happens, the patient would die unless treated immediately and vigorously.

In addition to high temperature, tachycardia and hypertension are almost always observed. As a matter of fact, tachycardia (not fever or rigidity) is the most consistent and earliest clinical sign of MH. Though fever is a relatively late sign, thermogenesis increases early and the resultant progressive venous hypoxemia and lactic acidemia are among the earliest laboratory findings.[5] Many patients become rigid and difficult to ventilate. Cardiac arrhythmias (ventricular premature beat, bigeminy, ventricular tachycardia, and fibrillation) are common and may occur early. Cardiovascular collapse may ensue. Numerous metabolic changes are observed.[1, 3, 5, 6] Metabolic acidosis is manifested as, but not totally explained by, severe lactic acidemia. The severe hypermetabolic state produces severe respiratory acidosis despite attempts at hyperventilation by the anesthetist. Cyanosis and possibly mottling of the skin may occur. Myoglobinemia, myoglobinuria, hyperkalemia, hypocalcemia, elevated serum creatine phosphokinase (CPK) and other muscle enzymes, hemoconcentration, and reduced platelet count are also common observations. If the patient survives the acute fulminant episode, delayed sequelae may soon follow. These include acute renal shutdown, disseminated intravascular coagulopathy, bleeding tendency, cerebral hypoxia

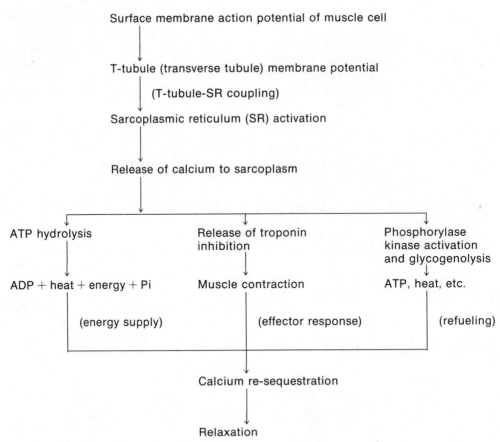

Figure 14–2. Excitation-contraction coupling, contraction, and relaxation of skeletal muscle (simplified scheme of main events.)

and edema, pulmonary edema, and secondarily also myocardial infarction and cerebral vascular accident. Hyperglycemia, increased blood concentration of catecholamines, increased inorganic phosphates, and elevated concentrations of thyroid hormones are also observed.

Variation in the syndrome occurs in almost every aspect of the above described "typical" picture. Babies as young as two months old and geriatric patients as old as 78 years have suffered from MH,[1] although the highest incidence is in the first three decades. With succinylcholine, an unyielding muscle rigidity may ensue immediately, but, instead of a generalized rigidity, an isolated spasm of the jaw muscle making it difficult to intubate the trachea is a common occurrence.[7] With inhalational anesthetics, fever and muscle rigidity tend to be delayed and one third of human MH cases have occurred without rigidity. The onset of temperature elevation can occur during the induction of anesthesia, during operation, after the patient arrives in the recovery room, or even later. Fever may recur in the postoperative day. As an extreme variation from the so-called "typical" case, some of the reported incidents are obviously benign and normothermic. These so-called variations include non-fatal normothermic localized muscle rigidity, elevated CPK without muscle rigidity, and even myoglobinuria without CPK elevation, and may reflect variations in criteria of clinical diagnosis.

Pathogenesis. Figure 14–2 is a simplified scheme of muscle response to the action potential of its cell membrane. Normally, the sarcolemma, the sarcoplasmic reticulum, and the mitochondria actively sequester and store calcium away from the sarcoplasm. When these biological membranes are activated, free calcium is released into the sarcoplasm. Muscle contraction and intracellular catabolic processes ensue. Return of the muscle to the relaxed state requires re-sequestration and clearance of the released calcium from the sarcoplasm. These functions consume energy.

The pathogenesis of MH has been intensely investigated. The syndrome is commonly considered an idiosyncratic self-perpetuating hypercatabolic response precipitated by a variety of causes, particularly halothane, succinylcholine, and other drugs used in the practice of anesthesia. The main defect seems to be the stress- or drug-induced loss by the sarcoplasmic reticulum of its ability to re-sequester calcium.[1, 8, 9] The resultant excess calcium in myoplasm, in turn, causes 1) persistent contracture of the myofibril, 2) excessive activation of ATPase and hydrolysis of ATP with resultant depletion of ATP and creatine phosphate (CP), and 3) activation of ATP regenerating mechanisms (with glycogenolysis), and may secondarily also cause 4) uncoupling of oxidative phosphorylation. This would explain most of the clinical features of "typical" cases of MH. Alpha-adrenergic stimulation seems to play an important etiological factor in initiating or perpetuating the catabolic process, especially the heat production.[10]

The above mechanism of MH, plausible as it is, is not universally accepted but only represents a popular view. As a matter of fact, almost every aspect of it has controversies. Sarcoplasmic reticulum may not be the sole or main site of the defect. Alternative hypotheses attribute the defect to mitochondria or sarcolemma. MH without rigidity is more difficult to explain than MH with rigidity. The question is why the myofibril remains relaxed in the presence of supposedly excessive concentration of free calcium in the sarcoplasm. Also, the membrane defect in MH may not be limited only to the skeletal muscle. Evidence suggests that cells from organs other than skeletal muscle may also be primarily involved. These include the brain, the platelets, the lungs, the heart, and the endocrine organs. The primary involvement of these organs would explain the early occurrence of coma, bleeding tendency, pulmonary edema, cardiac arrhythmia and sudden arrest, and abnormal glucose levels.

Morphological studies of human and porcine MH muscle has revealed a variety of abnormal features. Some of these suggest myopathic, others neuropathic, origin of the pathology. None of these, however, are pathognomonic. Sporadic reports have suggested a relationship between MH and central-core disease, other primary myopathies, and viral myopathy.

Investigations of porcine MH[5, 10, 11, 12, 13] play a major role in our understanding of human MH. Besides the pig model, MH-like syndrome has been observed more recently in dogs,[14] cats,[15] and horses.[16]

Diagnosis. Tentative diagnosis of a "typical" fulminant case of MH can be made on clinical observations alone. Supportive laboratory diagnostic tests can be found on page 549. Suggestive anesthetic experience, muscle cramps and weakness, suspicious family history and unexplained myoglobinuria, elevated CPK, especially if it is anesthesia-induced, abnormal muscular and skeletal build, and a history of difficulty in temperature control should be taken as warning clues to the susceptibility. However, while a working diagnosis of MH should be made without delay and the patient should be treated immediately, a definite diagnosis of MH should be confirmed by more definitive tests. Labeling a patient as being MH susceptible has grave medical and socioeconomic implications. Conditions such as sepsis, pyrogen reaction, thyrotoxicosis, pheochromocytoma, and drug reactions should be ruled out first. In addition, the relation between MH and other muscle diseases described in this chapter is unclear. Some of these, such as myotonic muscular dystrophy for example, may share with MH the common feature that succinylcholine causes rigidity and may precipitate or aggravate muscle damage, and may become a problem in differential diagnosis.

Muscle biopsy may allow positive identification of susceptible subjects and should be performed before definitely labeling a patient as MH susceptible. In vitro, MH susceptible muscle can be made to go into contracture (increased resting tension, not necessarily augmented twitch response to electric stimulation) by exposure to halothane, caffeine, succinylcholine, or potassium.[17, 18] These tests are now available only at major medical centers. Since prophylaxis against MH relies primarily on prediction of susceptibility, predictive tests should be prescribed for high-risk families. In addition to the definitive tests mentioned above, elevated serum CPK has been widely used to predict susceptibility, to diagnose MH, and to follow up an attack. However, it is nonspecific and absence of it does not rule out MH, nor does an increased CPK diagnose MH.

Intraoperative Management. Controversies exist at the present time in aspects of therapy of MH as they do in many other aspects of the disease, with the exception that dantrolene sodium appears generally favored as the drug of choice (see below). For the treatment of a fulminant case of MH, see below. The proper response to a less fulminant or less clear-cut case of MH obviously depends on the certainty of diagnosis and the severity of the case.

Guidelines are not available for definite diagnosis of less fulminant cases of MH, and none of the early signs are pathognomonic. As a result, it is up to each anesthesiologist to decide on the course of action when faced with such cases. We suggest that otherwise *unexplainable* central venous hypoxemia (especially in the absence of arterial hypoxemia), progressive or marked metabolic and/or respiratory acidosis, generalized rigidity, sudden high fever, and other signs of marked hypermetabolism such as high CO_2 production constitute "major signs" for a tentative diagnosis of MH. Other signs, being less specific, should be regarded as "minor signs." They serve to alert the anesthesiologist to search for major signs and to measure pertinent baseline data. Obviously, each major sign should be considered a possible indication for initiation of aggressive treatment and termination of anesthesia as soon as possible, especially if the anesthesiologist believes that a fulminant attack is imminent. The minor signs may serve to suggest changing anesthesia technique. If there is a family history of MH, even minor signs may become indications for more aggressive treatment.

Preplanned Therapeutic Regimen. Recognizing the fulminant time course and the high mortality of improperly treated MH, it is logical to have a preplanned regimen in each operating area for emergent treatment. A local expert should update the regimen and, if possible, personally direct the operation. A suggested plan for fulminant MH is described below. As stated above, modification can be made for less fulminant cases.

PREPLANNED THERAPEUTIC REGIMEN FOR FULMINANT MH

I. The pharmacy should keep a sufficient supply of the intravenous preparation of dantrolene sodium. Oral preparation should also be available.

II. Have readily available some IV fluid in the refrigerator for immediate use. Locate a source of large quantity of crushed ice, sufficient to cover the whole body of an adult. Have canvas, plastic, or cloth sheet, or an inflatable raft as a container to cool the patient in.

III. On working diagnosis of malignant hyperthermia:

(A) Treatment:

1) Terminate any anesthetic that may be triggering the attack. Ventilate patient with 100% oxygen. Sedate, if appropriate, with neuroleptanalgesic, barbiturate, diazepam, or narcotic. Terminate anesthesia and surgery as soon as possible. Change anesthetic technique if anesthesia cannot be terminated. Change soda lime canister, rebreathing hoses, and mask to get rid of incriminated inhalational anesthetics. (Treatment of shivering with chlorpromazine or nondepolarizing muscle relaxants and use of inhalational anesthetics to facilitate cooling are controversial.)

2) Cool the patient. If necessary, submerge the whole body in ice-water mixture. Hydrate with iced intravenous fluids. Use cold gastric lavage, high flow fresh gas input, large minute ventilation, fans, and cooling blanket. Cool the head if possible. Use all available body cavities. Use extracorporeal bypass, or hemodialysis if patient happens to be on one. Avoid unintentional overcooling.

3) Inject, IV, sodium bicarbonate, 1–2 mEq/kg. Repeat as needed, using arterial blood analysis as guide. Increase initial dose if MH is diagnosed late.

4) Monitor constantly the vital signs (axillary and core temperatures, BP, pulse rate, cardiac rhythm, pupil size and reactivity, cyanosis). Arterial catheterization and bladder catheterization are indicated. Central venous line and Swan-Ganz catheter should be considered, but do not delay treatment for these. Monitor urinary output and appearance.

5) Inject, IV, dantrolene*. Add procainamide†, if necessary, under EKG control. Glucocorticosteroids may be considered.

6) Secure high urinary output. Hydrate with iced lactated Ringer's or 5% dextrose solution. Give furosemide (1 mg/kg) and/or mannitol (1 gm/kg), IV.

7) Injection of insulin (10 units) has been advocated to ensure glucose

It is essential to avoid injection of calcium, despite hypocalcemia and despite cardiac depression (observed usually after initial tachycardia and hypertension). Hypocalcemia is a sign of calcium influx into the muscle cell, and the pathogenesis of MH is thought to result from intracellular calcium excess. Supplying calcium will only add fuel to the pathologic process. Also avoid α-adrenergic stimulants.[10]

During convalescence, patients may require significant amounts of potassium because large quantities of potassium are lost as a result of potassium efflux from the cell. However, with intra- and extracellular potassium poorly stabilized, and with possible renal shutdown, administration of potassium has to be carried out with extreme caution.

Elective Anesthesia. Anesthesia may be required for patients suspected to be, or even diagnosed as, MH susceptible. Use local, spinal, or epidural anesthesia, if possible. Use ester but avoid amide local anesthetics. Sedation, neuroleptanalgesia, and general anesthesia with Innovar, diazepam, althesin, barbiturates, narcotics, and nitrous oxide have been used successfully, although nitrous oxide was implicated in one case of MH. Avoid trimeprazine. Glucocorticoids appear harmless or even beneficial. Enflurane and *d*-tubocurarine may precipitate MH but appear less noxious than halothane and succinylcholine. Pancuronium appears safe. Studies in MHS pigs suggest that total spinal or epidural block will prevent the sympathetic response, attenuate the attack, or even prevent the occurrence of MH as a stress reaction, but may not be completely protective if the triggering agent acts heavily and directly on the muscle. The portion of the body not covered by the block is not protected. Lidocaine, *d*-tubocurarine, and chlorpromazine are controversial, and probably should be avoided if possible.

In short, no anesthetic technique should be considered completely safe. Prophylactic use of dantrolene should be considered for patients susceptible to MH. During anesthesia, one should always watch for the

utilization and to reduce hyperkalemia. This should be covered by injection of sufficient glucose, in spite of the frequent finding of hyperglycemia.

(B) Tests:

1) Determine arterial (and central venous) blood gases, acid-base balance, electrolytes (Ca^{++}, K^+, Na^+, Cl^-, phosphate), glucose, and osmolarity; repeat as indicated. Determine Hct (as guide to fluid loss).

2) Test for evidence of muscle damage (elevated serum CPK, LDH, SGOT, myoglobinemia, myoglobinuria), abnormal blood picture (thrombocytopenia, hemolysis, abnormal platelet aggregation), and coagulopathy.

3) The following tests may also be considered: serum catecholamines, thyroid hormone, alkaline phosphatase, and magnesium. Consider 12-lead EKG and EEG after the emergent treatment. Consider culturing of the intravenous fluids to rule out iatrogenic septicemia as the cause of fever.

IV. Continue intensive care:

1) Continue close monitoring and intensive care.

2) Treat recurrent fever, control rapidly fluctuating serum electrolyte and glucose concentrations with great care, avoid administration of calcium.

3) Guard against heart failure, acute pulmonary edema, cerebral edema, coma, hypoxic brain damage, acute renal shutdown, cerebral vascular accident, coagulopathy, and muscle edema, necrosis, and paralysis. Dialyze, if necessary.

V. Follow-up:

1) Consult or refer to medical center with better facilities.

2) Consider confirmative and predictive tests (follow-up on CPK, do muscle biopsy for provocative tests).

3) Consider epidemiological survey of family and relatives. Register with Medic-Alert Foundation.

4) Arrange for socioeconomic assistance, and marital counseling, if necessary.

---

*Dantrolene sodium: dose in human MH remains to be determined. We suggest 1 mg/kg IV slow push with rapid infusion of IV diluent. Repeat as needed (up to a total of 10 mg/kg), provided muscle twitch remains elicitable by nerve stimulation and provided cardiovascular functions remain undepressed, or until satisfactory control of MH is obtained, usually at 2.5 mg/kg. Avoid extravascular infiltration, as the solution has a pH of 9.5.

†Procainamide: 1 gm in 500 ml, IV over a 10-minute period, or 200 mg diluted in 200 ml, IV in 5 minutes; repeat as necessary.

early clues to an impending attack, such as poorly relaxed jaw, tachycardia, hypertension, reduced arterial and venous PO_2 and, obviously, hot skin. Since emotional excitement, high environmental temperature, sympathetic response to a cold environment, fever caused by mild infection, exercise, and muscle injury may be contributory to the triggering and perpetuating process, they should be avoided. Cardiac drugs such as amide local anesthetics (lidocaine), belladonna alkaloids (atropine), cardiac glycosides, calcium, catecholamines, and possibly quinidine should be avoided or used with caution because MH may involve the cardiac muscle. As a matter of fact, patients with cardiomyopathy are thought to be at high risk for MH.

Pharmacology of Dantrolene. Dantrolene sodium is a hydantoin compound used orally in the treatment of chronic skeletal muscle spasticity associated with upper motor neuron diseases such as stroke, cerebral palsy, and spinal cord injury, which may be painful, disabling, or interfering with nursing care.[19] Availability of an intravenous preparation of dantrolen (which was approved for use by the FDA in October 1979) may revolutionize the prophylaxis and treatment of MH.[11, 12, 13] Dose requirement of dantrolene is empirical, and depends, among other factors, upon the severity of the individual episode of MH, a factor that may never be known in the case of successful prophylaxis. Titrate to effect, starting with 1 mg/kg (see p. 548). The muscle relaxant effect of dantrolene has an immediate onset following intravenous injection. One should always be ready to deal with excessive muscle depression when administering dantrolene in large doses. Although the muscle relaxant effect of dantrolene may be accomplished in a few minutes, clinical resolution of the syndrome of MH may require some time. Combined use of procainamide and dantrolene may be desirable because procainamide is more effective for the heart, as dantrolene is for the skeletal muscle. Since dantrolene acts by direct depression of the contractile mechanism of skeletal muscle,[20, 21] its paralytic effect is independent of (and probably additive to) the paralytic effect of neuromuscular blocking agents.[22] Our preliminary observations in the cat have suggested that the paralyzing effect of dantrolene is most readily reversed by germine monoacetate.[22]

While 4-aminopyridine is partially effective, neostigmine is too short-acting and calcium is ineffective. At the present time, respiratory support, not drug therapy, is indicated in patients with a relative dantrolene overdose.

The therapeutic effect of dantrolene in the other muscle diseases outlined in this chapter is unclear at the present time. Perioperatively, it probably should be considered in the anesthetic management of myotonic dystrophy, to provide relaxation and to control contracture and shivering. However, dantrolene may add to the underlying weakness, and patients with muscle diseases might be exceptionally sensitive to the paralyzing effect of dantrolene.

MYASTHENIAS

MYASTHENIA GRAVIS

Myasthenia gravis is characterized by fluctuating weakness that varies throughout the day. The weakness is the primary complaint of the patient, not fatigue, and although weakness is worsened by exercise, patients may not make this correlation. The ocular muscles are the most commonly affected and are involved initially in 40 per cent of patients (eventually in 85%), causing both ptosis and diplopia. Cranial nerve problems are noted, causing limitation of facial movement and orophayrngeal weakness with dysarthria and dysphagia. Limb and neck paresis is common but only when cranial nerve muscles are already involved. Respiratory weakness is less common and is seen almost exclusively during myasthenic crisis.[14]

Myasthenic patients have been classified by Osserman[13] as follows: Group 1, ocular; Group 2-A, mild generalized symptoms; Group 2-B, moderate generalized symptoms with some bulbar symptoms; Group 3, acute severe, presenting in weeks to months with severe bulbar symptoms; Group 4, late severe, marked bulbar symptoms and severe generalized weakness.

The incidence is about 3 per 100,000. It occurs in three times as many females as males between the ages of 10 and 40, though the incidence is equal thereafter. Patients under 16 years of age account for 10 per cent of all cases. Pediatric cases can be divided as follows:[4] 1) Neonatal transient. Approximately 20 per cent of neonates born to myasthenic mothers will have transient neonatal myasthenic symptoms. They require therapy for one to two months. 2) Neonatal persistent — have an onset usually at two to three months of age. 3) Juvenile — are similar to the adult and can be divided as the adult patients are.

Though the causal event is unknown, the vast majority of patients have antibodies to muscle acetylcholine receptors.[5, 7, 12] The antibody is not bound directly to the site that binds acetylcholine but close it. This reduces binding of acetylcholine to the receptor. Previously held theories including excessive hydrolysis of acetylcholine and packets of acetylcholine containing subnormal quantities of acetylcholine at the nerve terminal are less attractive at the present time.

The thymus gland seems intimately involved in the disease process. This observation has led to the use of thymectomy as a therapeutic mode. Approximately two thirds of patients who do not have a thymoma are improved after thymectomy.[14] The improvement may occur rapidly but patients may require several years before significant improvement occurs.[8] Complete remission occurs in about 25 per cent of thymectomy patients. Patients with a thymoma have a lower response to thymectomy, with improvement in only 25 per cent.

The diagnosis of myasthenia can be made both on the clinical symptoms and the characteristic EMG.[16] Clinically, improvement follows the use of an anticholinesterase agent such as edrophonium or neostigmine, though the response may be difficult to evaluate in patients with pure ocular weakness. A small percentage of patients who do not show the characteristic improvement with anticholinesterases may require a curare test for diagnosis.[4] One tenth of the normal curarizing dose (i.e., .03 mg/kg of d-tubocurarine) is drawn into a syringe and given IV in increments to the patient. As soon as exaggeration of symptoms occurs, the test is stopped. Aggravation of symptoms and onset of weakness appearing before one tenth of the normal curarizing dose is given are diagnostic of myasthenia.

Therapy of the disease consists of giving anticholinesterase agents; the most commonly utilized are oral pyridostigmine or neostigmine. Patients seem to prefer pyridostigmine, as its duration of action is longer and it does not cause as many side effects.[14] Ephedrine may also be used to increase the patient's sense of well-being and to potentiate the effects of the anticholinesterase, though the mechanism of action is not understood.[14] More recently, large doses of steroids have been given in the hope of suppressing the antibody to the receptor. Other immunosuppressive agents are not used widely at the present time because their efficacy and long-term side effects have not been as well documented.

Myasthenic crisis is defined as an exacerbation of symptoms that are so severe that they involve the respiratory muscles. It may result directly from increased muscle weakness or be secondary to infection. Oropharyngeal weakness predisposes to respiratory infection. Increased secretion, respiratory infection, and muscle weakness produce a vicious cycle. These symptoms may not satisfactorily respond to anticholinesterase therapy and the patient may well need respirator support.

Cholinergic crisis, which is sometimes difficult to distinguish from myasthenic crisis, is the result of overtreatment of the patient with anticholinesterase agents, causing increased muscle weakness and secretions. It has been recommended that these two crises be distinguished by the injection of edrophonium to a dose of 10 mg in an average 70 kg patient. If improvement in muscle strength occurs, then the patient is undertreated with anticholinesterase therapy. If no increase in muscle strength occurs or if respiratory distress becomes worse, then the patient is probably in a cholinergic crisis. Respiratory support, if needed, should not await the anticholinesterase test. It is possible that some muscles are overtreated, while others are undertreated.

The published anesthetic experience is quite large. However, the vast majority of reports are of patients having thymectomy.[4, 8, 11, 13, 18] The procedure requires no muscle relaxation, and the use of ventilatory assistance is common. However, because myasthenics may have exacerbations of symptoms and may well develop myasthenic crises after any operative intervention, postoperative ventilatory assistance may be required even for peripheral surgery and even without the use of muscle relaxants. Experience with regional and local anesthesia[2, 15] has indicated that, if possible, these techniques should be preferred. However, ester local anesthetics may prove more toxic in these patients. The anticholinesterase agents inhibit pseudocholinesterase and reduce the hydrolysis of ester local anesthetic agents. Small doses, such as tetracaine in spinal anesthesia, would not be contraindicated.

The greatest controversy seems to be about whether the myasthenic patient should be maintained on anticholinesterase therapy preoperatively, intraoperatively, and postoperatively.[2, 3, 4, 13, 18] Patients who are dependent on anticholinesterase therapy for well-being and have more than just ocular symptoms would seem best treated with little break in their usual anticholinesterase therapy regimen. Thus, a patient who describes severe weakness on arising in the morning, who can barely swallow the anticholinesterase pills, and who has trouble with respiration before the first dose of anticholinesterase should continue the drug, particularly if the operation is going to take place late in the morning or in the afternoon. On the other hand, patients who have only mild symptoms can clearly do without their medication, especially if the operative procedure is to take place early in the day. Anticholinesterases do complicate the anesthetic management, as they potentiate vagal responses and, as mentioned, decrease the metabolism of ester local anesthetics. Relaxation may also be more difficult to produce. With an understanding of the drug action, preoperative anticholinesterase therapy should produce little problem for the anesthesiologist.

As mentioned earlier in this chapter, patients with little respiratory reserve tolerate any sedative premedication poorly. Therefore, myasthenics should be given a small premedication, if any, and when premedication is given, the patients must be observed carefully to make sure that the premedication is not excessive. Suggestions that patients be intentionally tired so that muscle relaxation secondary to tiring will aid in intubation seem unnecessary.[3] Patients with an empty stomach may be given intravenous barbiturate for induction, deepened with an inhalational anesthetic and intubated without the use of muscle relaxants. The use of muscle relaxants is controversial. If the patient is to be ventilated postoperatively, the use of very small doses of curare or other nondepolorizing muscle relaxants for an operation requiring muscle relaxation does not seem to be a bad recommendation.[9] However, if the procedure can be performed under inhalation anesthesia alone, the use of muscle relaxants does not seem warranted.[18]

The use of succinylcholine for intubation has both advantages and disadvantages. It is said that myasthenics are less responsive to succinylcholine than normal patients. In our experience, the usual intubating dose of succinylcholine produces adequate relaxation and apparent rapid recovery. However, careful study of their neuromuscular transmission by EMG has shown disturbing results in a number of patients. Phase II block occurs early and is very slow in recovery. We have seen patients who recover to less than 50 per cent of their normal and then maintain this degree of blockade for several hours after a single dose of succinylcholine. The use of anticholinesterase further complicates the response to succinylcholine, since succinylcholine will be poorly metabolized in these patients. The presence of varying levels of anticholinesterase activity will confuse the matter further. However, succinylcholine is not contraindicated in these patients as long as the possibility of prolonged neuromuscular block is understood. Anticholinesterases have also been seen to increase the duration and efficacy of narcotics.

Several groups of investigators have attempted to predict which myasthenic patients will require postoperative ventilation.[11, 13] Adult patients with a vital capacity of less than 2 liters, a duration of disease of greater than six years, and any intercurrent respiratory problems tend to become dependent on postoperative ventilatory support. Bulbar symptoms may[13] or may not[11] contribute to the need for postoperative ventilatory support. Clearly, a larger percentage of patients undergoing major upper abdominal or thoracic surgery will require respiratory support. There is some question as to whether chronic use of anticholinesterases in patients who undergo bowel anastomoses may have a higher incidence of bowel anastomotic leaks.[1] Because of this, it is suggested that patients who have bowel surgery not be given continuous anticholinesterase therapy during the postoperative period, but rather be ventilated if necessary.

Continuous *anticholinergic* therapy may be an alternative.

In spite of major improvement in their clinical symptoms, patients on large dose steroid therapy may still have increased sensitivity to nondepolarizing muscle relaxants. One patient reported by Griggs showed an eight-fold decrease in sensitivity to curare after ACTH therapy. On the other hand, Lake has reported one patient undergoing two successive operations, one two months and the other four months after the start of steroid therapy (with good symptomatic improvement in myasthenic symptoms) who remained exquisitely sensitive to small doses of *d*-tubocurarine. On one occasion, the patient required reversal two hours after 6 mg of curare. Regardless of the preoperative management, postoperative anticholinesterase therapy should be based on the edrophonium test, since the requirements for anticholinesterases change in the postoperative period.[2, 4]

Early extubation, if possible, seems warranted by the published case reports. Our personal practice is to allow a trial of spontaneous ventilation when the patient has an inspiratory force greater than -30 cm of water and a vital capacity of at least 15 cc/kg body weight. The patient is then allowed to maintain ventilation for one to two hours, during which time arterial blood gases are checked to ensure absence of fatigue. In addition, vital capacity measurements and clinical assessment are continued. Under these conditions, anticholinesterase therapy may be reinstituted and the patient may be extubated. Even then it is mandatory that respiratory support be immediately available. We manage these patients in an intensive care unit. Occasionally patients will maintain adequate vital capacity and adequate blood gases with an endotracheal tube in place only to rapidly decompensate on extubation. We feel that these patients are predominantly those who have oropharyngeal weakness and are incapable of taking care of their own secretions and maintaining a patent airway. They are difficult to predict. Only careful evaluation and constant vigilance allows one to extubate them safely.

Pregnancy is a stress to the myasthenic patient. The symptoms respond unpredictably to pregnancy but return to the prepregnant state of weakness immediately post partum.[15, 17] As mentioned earlier, 20 per cent of the newborns of myasthenic mothers will be myasthenic in the neonatal period. These infants require careful evaluation and respiratory support as well as anticholinesterase therapy when indicated.

In summary, the perioperative treatment of the myasthenic must be individualized to the severity of the disease. The use of regional or local anesthesia seems warranted wherever possible. General anesthesia can be performed safely. Postoperatively, patients must be carefully monitored and frequently evaluated, as unpredicted changes in ventilatory status may occur. Use of anticholinesterase agents is still controversial in the immediate preoperative and postoperative periods.

MYASTHENIC SYNDROME (EATON-LAMBERT SYNDROME)

Patients characteristically have weakness, usually in the proximal limb muscles, with the lower more involved than the upper. Rarely are bulbar or ocular muscles involved. Unlike myasthenia gravis, there is an increase in strength on activity. This syndrome has been associated with a carcinoma, most commonly carcinoma of the bronchus, but patients have been observed with thoracic extensions of carcinoma of the prostate, breast, stomach, and rectum.[10] The degree of muscle weakness is not related to the severity of other systemic effects of the tumor such as weight loss and muscle wasting. The carcinoma itself may not be obvious on examination and may take as long as two years after the symptoms of muscle weakness develop before it is discovered. The removal of the tumor does not affect the weakness.[10]

There is reduced muscle response to single nerve stimulus. However, using tetanic stimulation, there is a progressive increase in muscle strength as the frequency and duration of the stimulation are increased.[16] This is the reverse picture from that seen in myasthenia gravis. Post-tetanic potentiation is marked. At the present time, the best evidence is that the number of quanta of acetylcholine released per nerve impulse is decreased but the end-plate sensitivity is normal, again, unlike myasthenia gravis.[6]

Patients are extremely sensitive to both non-depolarizing and depolarizing muscle relaxants, and the weakness after these agents may last for many days.[10] The response to anticholinesterase drugs is poor, but guanidine hydrochloride will produce marked improvement.[6]

Since many of these patients require anesthesia for biopsy and/or treatment of their primary malignancy, anesthesiologists are confronted with a patient who may need general anesthesia and muscle relaxation but in whom muscle relaxants will produce prolonged weakness. The use of an inhalational anesthetic would seem the wisest course. However, if adequate muscle relaxation cannot be provided by the inhalational anesthestic, muscle relaxants may be used with the understanding that prolonged ventilatory assistance may be required. At the end of the procedure, the usual means for evaluating muscle relaxation can be used and anticholinesterase agents given to reverse curariform block. The patient should then be tested for ventilatory adequacy. This should include a trial of spontaneous ventilation to see if the patient requires ventilatory assistance. The usual means and criteria for extubation should be applied to these patients.

FAMILIAL PERIODIC PARALYSIS

There are three distinct types of disorders in this group, hypo-, hyper-, and normokalemic. Although they have many clinical similarities, the mechanisms are very different. The first case in the literature, reported by Shakhnovitch in 1882,[3] describes many of the symptoms of hypokalemic periodic paralysis. The attacks are precipitated by large carbohydrate-containing meals, characteristically a large evening meal, which lead to paralysis on awakening the next morning. Cold, mental stress, infections, surgical or accidental trauma, and menstruation have all been implicated in the onset of paralytic attacks. The paralysis is variable and usually asymmetric, involving primarily the lower and upper extremities, trunk, and neck, but only rarely the cranial nerve distribution or the diaphragm. It is thought that after repeated attacks atrophy ensues, but this is only a late occurrence, and most patients are quite muscular. The deep tendon reflexes may remain intact.[13] Transient bradycardia, cardiac dilatation, and the onset of an apical systolic murmur have been observed. Blood pressure rises, and arrhythmias can occur during attacks. The electrocardiogram shows evidence of hypokalemia. Usually the electrocardiographic abnormalities are more severe than one would predict from the serum potassium. During the attack the basal metabolic rate goes up. Whether this is solely due to the anxiety of the patient is not known. The electromyogram (EMG) shows abnormal lengthening of the action potential as the patient goes into the paralysis, until finally there is electric silence. Improvement is preceded by diaphoresis and diuresis, with a total loss of fluid of from 1 to 3 kg.[13] During recovery the serum potassium returns to normal before the EMG does.[5]

The actions of many drugs have been studied in these patients in an attempt to understand the mechanism of the paralysis. Potassium was found to be therapeutic before the mechanism was understood. If it is given and the uptake is measured, there is first uptake into the muscles and then a paradoxical loss of potassium from the muscles, and recovery ensues.[13] At present it is thought that, for some reason not readily apparent, potassium moves into cells, thus causing the decrease in serum potassium. It is known that the potassium is not lost into the urine or the stool. In vivo intracellular recordings during attacks have shown a reduction in the resting membrane potential.[6, 7] The most attractive theory[6] is that chronic hypokalemia leads to increased intracellular sodium, decreased intracellular potassium, and decreased sodium conductance, making the muscle unresponsive to stimulation. Insulin, under these conditions, will lead to further hypokalemia, as does stimulation of beta receptors (thyrotoxic patients) and rest. Increasing potassium externally will restore excitability. However, an excessive increase in external potassium will make the muscle inexcitable. Large amounts of licorice, which causes hypokalemia by its mineralocorticoid-like activity, can induce attacks. Insulin and glucose are used to induce attacks for diagnosis.[10] The only synthetic glucocorticoid that does not cause crises is triamcinolone, which increases the Na:K excretion ratio in the urine. Extreme limitation in sodium intake and the use of diuretics, plus potassium replacement, has prophylactic value. More recently, the use of 250 to 1000 mg. per day of acetazolamide has been found to prevent attacks. The probable mechanism of action is its ability to produce a metabolic acidosis. Other agents producing metabolic acidosis are similarly protective.[10, 14, 15] $NaHCO_3$ will induce attacks. The effects of respiratory acidosis and alkalosis have not been reported.

Of the cases reported in the literature, approximately 10 per cent died during paralysis.[2] The most common cause is respiratory failure resulting from aspiration pneumonia or infection. Cardiac failure and shock have also been reported.

Autopsies have shown no specific lesion except for vacuoles in the sarcoplasmic reticulum of skeletal muscles, which increase during attacks. The contents of the vacuoles have not been identified.

The disease, as the name implies, is familial. It is usually an autosomal dominant, with high penetrance in males. There are also many sporadic cases, usually occurring in males. These are more difficult to evaluate because affected individuals may have only one attack in a lifetime and the symptoms, particularly in females, may be minimal.

The thyrotoxic variety of periodic paralysis is similar to that found in the hypokalemic type, except that during an attack the fall in serum potassium is usually greater. The incidence is much higher in males than in females, and is highest in Orientals. The paralytic episodes end when the patient is made euthyroid.[4, 7]

There are three reports in the anesthetic literature of anesthesia for patients with hypokalemic periodic paralysis.[1, 8, 12] Each of two patients had three anesthetics and one patient had two anesthetics. In addition, one paper reviewed the experience in a family of eight members with 21 anesthetics between them.[8] All forms of anesthesia were used. One patient developed respiratory failure six hours after an appendectomy and required ventilatory assistance for 36 hours. The patient had a second episode of weakness after a second operation, this time 18 hours postoperatively. In both cases, the patient's potassium was below 3.0 and responded to KCl therapy. All reports were of uneventful intraoperative anesthesia. A retrospective review of 21 anesthetics in eight patients showed six episodes of weakness. In all episodes, the weakness was no greater than what was usually experienced by the patient. Four out of six patients who were

given cyclopropane anesthesia, one out of two patients given halothane, and one out of three patients given Innovar had episodes of weakness. The etiological factors responsible for postoperative weakness cannot be determined from this report. Succinylcholine has been used with no apparent problem. One patient given curare, but with other unrelated problems, seemed to have had a mildly prolonged recovery. The majority of patients who experienced difficulties did so in the first day postoperatively, although they did well immediately on awakening from anesthesia.

The guidelines for anesthetic management of these patients should include warning the patient not to overeat on the night before surgery, and an attempt should be made to decrease the patient's mental stress.

Since there is usually a decrease in the frequency and severity of the attacks in middle age, the patients to be most careful with are those in the younger age groups. Care must also be used to recognize a patient who is undergoing atrophy. Since this runs in certain families, a history of atrophy should be sought. If the patient is on spironolactone, acetazolamide, or other diuretics, the serum electrolytes should be obtained, but should not provoke hasty therapy. However, oral potassium therapy is indicated for those on diuretics and having even the slightest degree of hypokalemia. Care must be used in giving potassium to patients receiving spironolactone, because this agent blocks the action of aldosterone and thus limits the ability of the kidney to excrete excess potassium. The use of dextrose should be limited, and supplementary potassium should be given in order to prevent hypokalemia, because it is well known that when dextrose enters the cell potassium also does. A large salt load can also precipitate paralysis. This is especially true if the sodium is in the form of bicarbonate. Cold is a major cause of paralysis and should be guarded against.

The best form of monitor in the operating room is an electrocardiogram, since changes in the T wave signifying hypokalemia can be constantly watched for. Central venous pressure or Swan-Ganz catheter may be helpful, as cardiac failure is also a concomitant of paralysis in some patients. The effects of muscle relaxants are not well documented and, unless absolutely necessary, should be avoided. Since the muscles are insensitive to even direct electrical stimulation during an attack, the nerve stimulator may not be helpful at that time. However, since respiratory muscles and face muscles are only rarely affected by the disease, the facial nerve can be used in the differential diagnosis of a prolonged paralysis.[13] The use of a nerve stimulator has been reported in one patient.[8] Though the patient appeared normal at the time, the muscle response to electrical stimulation of the ulnar nerve was weak and showed marked post-tetanic potentiation. However, no fade was observed. Thus, a baseline measurement must be obtained before the use of muscle relaxants. The possibility of respiratory failure encourages the use of respiratory assistance, chest physiotherapy, and IPPB.

Patients with spontaneous attacks of paralysis rarely need ventilatory support or an endotracheal tube to prevent aspiration. The cough reflex is usually intact, and in addition gastric acid secretion is markedly diminished. The use of potassium chloride restores function within a few hours in most cases. However, the respiratory status should be checked and the adequacy of the cough evaluated.

It has been suggested that those with particularly severe symptoms have adrenalectomy. If steroids are necessary, triamcinolone would seem the best choice. If paralysis is found to have occurred, the use of from 5 to 15 gm of KCl p.o. will abort the attack. Intravenously, a smaller dose is used (60 meq K^+) over several hours. Frequent monitoring of serum K^+ is mandatory to prevent hyperkalemia. It may take two hours or more for the symptoms to completely disappear.

The hyperkalemic form of periodic paralysis was separated from the hypokalemic form in 1957. The attacks occur after exercise, but sooner than they do in the hypokalemic form. They are unrelated to high carbohydrate meals, and tend to occur when the person is hungry. The attacks are shorter, many lasting only one hour or less, instead of the hours or days of the hypokalemic type. Cold also precipitates attacks, but stress is a less common factor. The attacks start, as do those of the hypokalemic type, in the lower extremities, upper extremities, and trunk, but then go on to include the facial muscles, including the tongue. The age of onset is earlier, with

symptoms seen in infancy.[13] With age, the attacks become less frequent but more severe. Lid lag was at one time thought to be the clinically distinguishing feature between this and hypokalemic periodic paralysis, but this sign is now known to be nonspecific. Respiratory muscles are spared. Pregnancy, especially during the last two trimesters, is associated with an increase in severity of the disease, which slowly remits post partum.[3]

The potassium rises an average of 20 per cent during an attack, but may still be within normal limits. In spite of this, the membrane potential does change with attacks.[11] Membrane potential is reduced, and there is increased sensitivity to acetylcholine injected intra-arterially. The hyperkalemia has been shown to result from an outpouring of potassium from muscles, associated with an increased permeability to sodium and an increase in the intracellular chloride. The administration of potassium provokes the attacks and is used in confirming the diagnosis.

Along with the paralytic episodes many patients exhibit myotonia, most marked on percussion of the tongue and hypothenar muscles.[9] In this respect the disease is quite similar to paramyotonia congenita.[17] Neostigmine has been reported to increase the myotonia, and so care should be used in its administration in these patients. EMG during an attack shows increased spontaneous activity, with marked myotonic discharges. However, with effort, the motor unit discharges are reduced in amplitude but of normal duration.[5] Unlike the hypokalemic paralysis, there is normal propagation of the action potential along the muscle.

The ECG shows peaking of the T waves before and during evidence of paresis. If one gives glucagon or epinephrine, paresis may be aborted, and the ECG shows signs of hypokalemia (U waves and small T wave), although the serum K^+ remains normal.

Insulin and glucose therapy seems at present to be the best way to abort an attack. The use of calcium, epinephrine, thiazide, and glucagon has not been as successful.[9] Prophylatic use of a high sodium, low potassium diet with frequent high carbohydrate feedings decreases the severity of attacks. Acetazolamide decreased the number and severity of attacks in one family, Thiazide was also useful.[9] Both work by kaluresis.[6]

The onset of atrophy is more dependent on the nature of the disease in a particular family than on any other factors now known.

The only report of anesthesia in this disease appeared in 1969, when three anesthetic experiences were described.[3] After pentothal alone for a dental extraction, a patient was paralyzed for several hours. A second patient received general anesthesia for a vaginal delivery (the agent used was not reported) and was paralyzed for several hours. The third case was an uneventful use of spinal anesthesia for a vaginal delivery. Fasting prior to the extraction may have provoked the episode in the first case; we cannot indict the pentothal. The incidence of episodes of paralysis rises in the third trimester of pregnancy, and the occurrence here in one case cannot be shown to be due to the general anesthesia. In view of the limited experience, firm conclusions cannot be drawn. Caution is indicated.

The most important measure in preparation for anesthesia is to prevent carbohydrate depletion by starting dextrose the night before the operation and by using potassium-free and dextrose-rich fluids intraoperatively. Again, the use of an ECG monitor intraoperatively would be of great assistance. Muscle relaxants should be avoided if possible,[16] and if a nerve stimulator is used, it must be remembered that even facial muscles can be paralyzed by hyperkalemia. The ECG should give a clue to the differential diagnosis.

The third and most difficult form of this disease to manage is normokalemic periodic paralysis. The onset is in early childhood, with the attacks often severe and associated with loss of cough reflex. An episode may last for two to 21 days. Episodes are induced by the same environmental stresses as hypokalemic periodic paralysis, although not by a high carbohydrate intake. The attacks occur, as do those of hypokalemic periodic paralysis, in the morning on awakening. A major problem during attacks is the occurrence of cardiac arrhythmias, usually multifocal ectopic beats.[4]

Drugs have unusual effects here. Digitalis preparations cause weakness, whereas quinidine reverses this effect, as does sodium loading. An increase in potassium provokes attacks. The use of 9-alpha fluorohydrocortisone and sodium loading is prophylactic against attacks.

Owing to the nature of the spontaneous paralytic episodes, it would seem wise to protect the airway with an endotracheal tube. The same problems mentioned above apply to anesthetic management, although the ECG monitor is now used not to diagnose paralysis but to watch for arrhythmias. If arrhythmias occur during anesthesia, this may be due to the anesthetic or the primary disease. Use of large doses of sodium to correct or prevent both the paralysis and cardiac arrhythmias would seem indicated, although care must be taken not to overload these patients. The effects of quinidine make one wonder whether procainamide or intravenous lidocaine would be helpful in counteracting arrhythmias.

REFERENCES

Muscular Dystrophies

1. Baldwin, B. J., Talley, R. C., Johnson, C., and Nutter, D. O.: Permanent paralysis of the atrium in a patient with facioscapulohumeral muscular dystrophy. Am. J. Cardiol. *31*:649, 1973.
2. Baraka, A., et al.: Control of succinylcholine induced myotonia by d-tubocurarine. Anesthesiology *33*:669, 1970.
3. Benaim, S., and Worster-Drought, C.: Myotonic dystrophy with myotonia of the diaphragm causing pulmonary hypoventilation with anoxaemia and secondary polycythemia. Medical Ill. *8*:221, 1954.
4. Boba, A.: Fatal postanesthetic complications in two muscular dystrophic patients. J. Pediatr. Surg. *5*:71, 1970.
5. Bourke, T. D., and Zuck, D.: Thiopentone in dystrophica myotonia. Brit. J. Anaesth. *29*:35, 1957.
6. Brown, G. L., and Harvey, A. M.: Congenital myotonia in the goat. Brain *62*:341, 1939.
7. Bush, G. H.: Pharmacogenetics and anesthesia. Proc. Roy. Soc. Med. *61*:171, 1968.
8. Cannon, P. G.: The heart and lungs in myotonic muscular dystrophy. Am. J. Med. *32*:765, 1962.
9. Carlson, C. B., and Swanson, A. G.: Genetics on neuromuscular disease. Pediat. Clin. North Amer. *14*:949, 1967.
10. Caughey, J. E., and Myrianthopoulas, N. C.: Dystrophic Myotonia and Related Disorders. Springfield, Ill., Charles C Thomas, 1963.
11. Cobham, I. G., and Davis, H. S.: Anesthesia for muscular dystrophy patients. Anesth. Analg. *43*:22, 1964.
12. Coccagna, G., Mantovani, M., Parchi, C., Mironi, F., and Lugaresi, E.: Alveolar hypoventilation and hypersomnia in myotonic dystrophy. J. Neurol. Neurosurg. Psychiat. *38*:977, 1975.
13. Cwizewicz-Adamska, J., and Wilmowska-Pietruszynska, A.: Anaesthesiological problems in myotonic syndromes (description of two cases). Anaesth. Resus. Inten. Ther. *2*:93, 1974.
14. Dalal, F. Y., et al.: Dystrophica myotonica: a

multisystem disease. Canad. Anaesth. Soc. J. 19:436, 1972.

15. de Backer, M., Bergmann, P., Perissino, A., Gottignies, P., and Kahn, R. J.: Respiratory failure and cardiac disturbances in myotonic dystrophy. Eur. J. Int. Care Med. 2:63, 1976.

16. Denny-Brown, D., and Nevein, S.: The phenomenon of myotonia. Brain 64:1, 1941.

17. Desnoyers, Y.: A propos de la dystrophie myotonique. Canad. Anaesth. Soc. J. 16:377, 1969.

18. Dundee, J. W.: Thiopentone in dystrophia myotica. Curr. Res. Anes. 31:257, 1952.

19. Engel, W. K., et al.: Clinical approach to the myopathies. Clin. Orthop. Rel. Res. 39:4, 1965.

20. Engel, W. K.: Muscle biopsy in neuromuscular diseases. Pediat. Clin. North Amer. 14:963, 1967.

21. Gardy, H. H.: Dystrophia myotonica in pregnancy. Report of a case. Obstet. Gynec. 21:441, 1963.

22. Genever, E. E.: Suxamethonium-induced cardiac arrest in unsuspected pseudohypertrophic muscular dystrophy. Case report. Br. J. Anaesth. 43:984, 1971.

23. Geschwind, N., and Simpson, J. A.: Procainamide in the treatment of myotonia. Brain 78:81, 1955.

24. Gilbertson, A., and Boulton, T. B.: Anesthesia in difficult situations. 6. Influence of disease on the preoperative preparation and choice of anesthesia. Anaesthesia 22:607, 1967.

25. Gillam, P. M. S., et al.: Respiration in dystrophia myotonica. Thorax 19:112, 1964.

26. Greene, N.: Commenting on a paper by Cobham. Anesth. Analg. 43:29, 1964.

27. Greenspan, L.: Myopathies. Mod. Treat. 5:1036, 1968.

28. Griggs, R. C., Reeves, W., and Moxley, III, R. T.: The heart in Duchenne dystrophy. In Pathogenesis of Human Muscular Dystrophies. Proceedings, Fifth International Scientific Conference of the Muscular Dystrophy Association, Colorado, 1976. Amsterdam, Excerpta Medica, 1977, p. 661.

29. Hakim, C. A., and Thomlinson, J.: Myotonia congenita in pregnancy. J. Obstet. Gynaec. Brit. Cwlth. 76:561, 1969.

30. Haley, F. C.: Anaesthesia in dystrophic myotonia. Canad. Anesth. Soc. J. 9:270, 1962.

31. Harvey, J. C., Sherbourne, D. H., and Siegel, C. I.: Smooth muscle involvement in myotonic dystrophy. Am. J. Med. 39:81, 1965.

32. Hewer, C. L.: Correspondence. Brit. J. Anaesth. 29:180, 1957.

33. Hook, R., Anderson, E. F., Noto, P.: Anesthetic management of a parturient with myotonia atrophica. Anesthesiology 43:689, 1975.

34. Huff, T. A., et al.: Abnormal insulin secretion in myotonic dystrophy. N. Engl. J. Med. 2:837, 1967.

35. Huff, T. A., and Lebovitz, H. E.: Dynamics of insulin secretion in myotonic dystrophy. J. Clin. Endocrin. Metab. 28(12):992, 1968.

36. Hunter, A. R.: Commenting on a paper by Kaufman. Proc. Roy. Soc. Med. 53:187, 1959.

37. Jacob, J. G., and Varkey, G. P.: Curare sensitivity in ocular myopathy. Canad. Anaesth. Soc. J. 13:449, 1966.

38. Kaufman, L.: Anesthesia in dystrophia myotonica: a review of the hazards of anesthesia. Proc. Roy. Soc. Med. 53:183, 1959.

39. Kepes, E. R., Martinez, L. R., Andrews, C. I., Arkins, R. E., Jadwat, C. M., Radney, P. A., and Stark, D. C. C.: Anesthetic problems in hereditary muscular abnormalities. Clinical Anesthesia Conference. N. Y. State J. Med. 72:1051, 1972.

40. Kilburn, K. H., et al.: Cardiopulmonary insufficiency in myotonic and progressive muscular dystrophy. N. Engl. J. Med. 261:1089, 1959.

41. Kilburn, K. H., et al.: Cardiopulmonary insufficiency associated with myotonic dystrophy. Am. J. Med. 26:929, 1959.

42. Lanari, A.: Mechanism of myotonic contraction. Science 104:221, 1946.

43. Landau, W.: Essential mechanism in myotonia: an electromyographic study. Neurology 2:369, 1952.

44. McClelland, R. M. A.: Myasthenic state and myotonic syndrome. Brit. J. Anaesth. 32:81, 1960.

45. MacDermot, V.: The history of the neuromuscular junction in dystrophia myotonica. Brain 84:75, 1961.

46. Merritt, H. H., and Rowland, L. P.: Muscle. In Merritt, H. H. (ed.): A Textbook of Neurology, 6th ed. Philadelphia, Lea & Febiger, 1979, pp. 576–596.

47. Meyers, M. B., and Garash, P. G.: Case history number 90: Cardiac decompensation during enflurane anesthesia. A patient with myotonia atrophica. Anesth. Analges. 55:433, 1976.

48. Miller, E. D., Jr., Sanders, D. B., Rowlingson, J. C., Berry, F. A., Sussman, M. D., and Epstein, R. M.: Anesthesia-induced rhabdomyolysis in a patient with Duchenne's muscular dystrophy. Anesthesiology 48:146, 1978.

49. Mitchell, M. M., Ali, H. H., and Savarese, J. J.: Myotonia and neuromuscular blocking agents. Anesthesiology 49:44, 1978.

50. Muller, J., and Suppan, P.: Case report: anaesthesia in myotonic dystrophy. Anaesth. Intens. Care 5:70, 1977.

51. Munsat, T. L., and Pearson, C. M.: Differential diagnosis of neuromuscular weakness in infancy and childhood. Devel. Med. Chid. Neuro. 9:222, 319, 1967.

52. Norris, F. H., Jr.: Intracellular recording from human striated muscle. In Enslein, K. (ed.): Data Acquisition and Processing in Biology and Medicine. New York, Macmillan, 1962, Vol. II, p. 59.

53. Orndahl, G.: Myotonic human musculature; stimulation with depolarizing agents. 1. Mechanical registration of the effects of acetylcholine and choline. Acta Med. Scand. 172:739, 1962. 2. Clinicopharmacologic study. Acta Med. Scand. 172:753, 1962.

54. Paterson, I.: Generalized myotonia following suxamethonium. Brit. J. Anaesth. 34:340, 1962.

55. Pruzanski, W., and Profis, A.: Pulmonary disease in myotonic dystrophy. Ann. Rev. Resp. Dis. 91:874, 1965.

56. Ravin, M., Newmark, Z., and Saviello, G.: Myotonia dystrophica — an anesthetic hazard: two case reports. Anesth. Analges. 54:216, 1975.

57. Richards, W. C.: Anaesthesia and serum creatine

phosphokinase levels in patients with Duchenne's pseudohypertrophic muscular dystrophy. Anaesth. Intens. Care 1:150, 1972.

58. Ross, R. T.: Ocular myopathy sensitive to curare. Brain 86:67, 1963.

59. Rowland, L. P., and Eskenazi, A. N.: Myasthenia gravis with features resembling muscular dystrophy. Neurology 6:667, 1956.

60. Samolia, F. J., and Gengley, J.: Biochemical abnormalities of sarcoplasmic reticulum in muscular dystrophy. N. Engl. J. Med. 280:184, 1969.

61. Seay, A. R., Ziter, F. A., and Thompson, J. A.: Cardiac arrest during induction of anesthesia in Duchenne muscular dystrophy. J. Pediatr. 93:88, 1978.

62. Suppan, P.: Althesin in dystrophia myotonica. Anaesthesia 30:95, 1975.

63. Taverner, D.: Neurologic aspects of anesthesia. Brit. J. Anaesth. 32:514, 1960.

64. Thiel, R. E.: Myotonic response to succinylcholine. Brit. J. Anaesth. 39:815, 1967.

65. Tsueda, K., Shibutani, K., and Lefkowitz, M.: Postoperative ventilatory failure in an obese myopathic woman with periodic somnolence: A case report. Anesth. Analges. 54:523, 1975.

66. Tyler, F.: Muscular dystrophies. In Stanbury, J. B., et al. (eds.): In Metabolic Basis of Inherited Disease. 2nd ed., New York, McGraw-Hill, 1966.

67. Waters, D. D., Nutter, D. O., Hopkins, L. C., and Dorney, E. R.: Cardiac features of an unusual X-linked humeroperoneal neuromuscular disease. N. Engl. J. Med. 293:1017, 1975.

68. Watson, B. M.: Pharmacogenetics. Anaesthesia 24:230, 1969.

69. Welsh, J. D., et al.: Myotonic muscular dystrophy. Arch. Intern. Med. 114:669, 1964.

70. Wheeler, A. S., and James, F. M.: Local anesthesia for laparoscopy in a case of myotonia dystrophica. Anesthesiology 50:169, 1979.

71. Wislicki, L.: Anesthesia and postoperative complication in progressive muscular dystrophy. Anaesthesia 17:482, 1962.

72. Zatuchni, J., et al.: The heart in progressive muscular dystrophy. Circulation 3:846, 1951.

73. Zundel, W. S., and Tyler, F. H.: Muscular dystrophies. N. Engl. J. Med. 273:537, 596, 1965.

Glycogen Storage Diseases

1. Casson, H.: Anaesthesia for portacaval bypass in patients with metabolic diseases. Br. J. Anaesth. 47:969, 1975.

2. Cox, J. M.: Anesthesia and glycogen storage disease. Anesthesiology 29:6, 1968.

3. DiMauro, S., et al.: Genetic heterogeneity of glycogen diseases. In Pathogenesis of Human Muscular Dystrophies. Proceedings, Fifth International Scientific Conference of the Muscular Dystrophy Association, Colorado, 1976. Amsterdam, Excerpta Medica, 1977, p. 341.

4. Edelstein, G., and Hirshman, C. A.: Hyperthermia and ketoacidosis during anesthesia in a child with glycogen-storage disease. Anesthesiology 52:90, 1980.

5. Engel, A. G.: Acid maltase deficiency in adults. Brain 93:599, 1970.

6. Engel, W. K., et al.: Clinical approach to the myopathies. Clin. Orthop. Rel. Res. 39:4, 1965.

7. Engel, W. K.: Muscle biopsy in neuromuscular diseases. Pediatr. Clin. North Amer. 14:963, 1967.

8. Fattah, S. M., et al.: McArdle's disease — review of previous 23 cases + 1 new case. Am. J. Med. 48:693, 1970.

9. Field, R. A.: Glycogen storage diseases. In Stanbury, J. B., et al. (eds.): Metabolic Basis of Inherited Disease. 2nd ed. New York, McGraw-Hill, 1966.

10. Field, R. A.: The glycogenoses: von Gierke's disease, acid maltase deficiency, and liver glycogen phosphorylase deficiency. Am. J. Clin. Pathol. 60:20, 1968.

11. Hohn, A. R., Lowe, C. U., Sokal, J. E., and Lambert, E. C.: Cardiac problems in the glycogenoses with specific reference to Pompe's disease. Pediatrics 35:313, 1965.

12. Kaplan, R.: Pompe's disease presenting for anesthesia. Anesth. Rev. 7:21, 1980.

13. Layzer, R. B.: Glycolysis and glycogen. In Pathogenesis of Human Muscular Dystrophies. Proceedings, Fifth International Scientific Conference of the Muscular Dystrophy Association, Colorado, 1976. Amsterdam, Excerpta Medica, 1977, p. 351.

14. Pearson, C. M.: Glycogen metabolism and storage disease of types III, IV and V. Am. J. Clin. Pathol. 50:29, 1968.

15. Ryan, J. F., and Papper, E. M.: Malignant fever during and following anesthesia. Anesthesiology 32:196, 1970.

16. Satoyoshi, E., and Kowa, H.: A new myopathy. Am. Neur. Assoc. Trans. 1965, p. 46.

17. Tauri, S., et al.: Phosphofructokinase deficiency in skeletal muscle. A new type of glycogenosis. Biochem. Biophys. Res. Comm. 19:517, 1965.

Lipid Storage Myopathies

1. Angelini, C.: Lipid Storage Myopathies: a review of metabolic defect and of treatment. J. Neurol. 214:1, 1976.

2. Bank, W. J., DiMauro, S., Bonilla, E., Capuzzi, D. M., and Rowland, L. P.: A disorder of muscle lipid metabolism and myoglobinuria: Absence of carnitine palmityl transferase. N. Engl. J. Med. 292:443, 1975.

3. Cornelio, F., DiDonato, S., Peluchetti, D., Bizzi, A., Bertagnolio, B., D'Angelo, A., and Wiesmann, U.: Fatal cases of lipid storage myopathy with carnitine deficiency. J. Neurol. Neurosurg. Psychiatry 40:170, 1977.

4. Engel, A. G., and Angelini, C.: Carnitine deficiency of human skeletal muscle with associated lipid storage myopathy: A new syndrome. Science 1173:899, 1973.

Myositis Ossificans

1. Merritt, H. H., and Rowland, L. P.: Muscle. In Merritt, H. H. (ed.): A Textbook of Neurology. 6th ed. Philadelphia, Lea & Febiger, 1979, pp. 576–596.

2. Russell, R. G. G., et al.: Treatment of myositis ossificans progressiva with a diphosphonate. Lancet 1:10, 1972.

Mitochondrial Myopathies

1. Affifi, A. K., Ibrahim, M. Z. M., Bergman, R. A., et al.: Nonpathologic features of hypermetabolic mitochondrial disease. J. Neurol. Sci. 15:271, 1972.
2. Coleman, R. F., et al.: New myopathy with mitochondrial enzyme hyperactivity. J.A.M.A. 199:624, 1967.
3. Engel, W. K.: A critique of congenital myopathies and other disorders. *In* Milhorat, A. T. (ed.): Exploratory Concepts in Muscular Dystrophy and Related Disorders. Baltimore, Williams & Wilkins, 1967.
4. Haydar, N. A., et al.: Severe hypermetabolism with primary abnormality of skeletal muscle mitochondria. Ann. Intern. Med. 74:548, 1971.
5. Luft, R., et al.: A case of severe hypermetabolism of n-thyroid origin with a defect in maintenance of mitochondrial respiratory control: correlated clinical, biochemical and morphological study. J. Clin. Invest. 41:16, 1962.
6. Luft, R.: Personal communication.
7. Padykala, H., and Gauthier, G.: Morphological and cytochemical characteristics of fiber type in normal mammalian skeletal muscle. *In* Milhorat, A. T. (ed.): Exploratory Concepts in Muscular Dystrophy and Related Disorders. Baltimore, Williams & Wilkins, 1967.
8. Shy, G. M, et al.: Two childhood myopathies with abnormal mitochondria. Brain 89:133, 1966.
9. van Wijngaarden, G. K., et al.: Skeletal muscle disease with abnormal mitochondria. Brain 90:577, 1967.
10. Yadell, A.: Newly defined muscular dystrophies. Arizona Med. Rev. 24:950, 1967.

Sarcoplasmic Myopathies

1. Denborough, M. A., et al.: Central core disease and malignant hyperpyrexia. Br. Med. J. 1:272, 1973.
2. Engel, W. K., et al.: Central core disease: An investigation of a rare muscle abnormality. Brain 84:167, 1961.
3. Engel, W. K.: A critique of congenital myopathies and other disorders. *In* Milhorat, A. T. (ed.): Exploratory Concepts in Muscular Dystrophy and Related Disorders. Baltimore, Williams & Wilkins, 1967.
4. Harriman, D. G. F., and Ellis, F. R.: Central core disease and malignant hyperpyrexia (correspondence). Br. Med. J. 3:545, 1973.
5. Hopkins, I. J., et al.: Nemaline myopathy: a long term clinico-pathological study of affected mother and daughter. Brain 89:299, 1966.
6. Lindsey, J. R.: Pathology of nemaline myopathy. John Hopkins Hosp. Bull. 119:378, 1966.
7. Shy, G. M.: Central core disease and nemaline myopathy. *In* Stanbury, J. B., etal. (eds.): Metabolic Basis of Inherited Disease. 2nd ed., New York, McGraw-Hill, 1966.
8. Tizard, J. P. M.: Neuromuscular disorders in infancy. *In* Walton, J. N. (ed.): Disorders of Voluntary Muscle. 3rd ed., Edinburgh, Churchill, 1974.
9. Yadell, A.: Newly defined muscular dystrophies. Arizona Med. Rev. 24:950, 1967.

Malignant Hyperthermia

1. Britt, B. A.: Recent advances in malignant hyperthermia. Anesth. Analg. (Cleve.) 54:841, 1972.
2. Fraser, J. G., Crumrine, R. S., and Izant, R. J.: A pre-planned treatment for malignant hyperthermia. Anesth. Analg. 55:713, 1976.
3. Relton, J. E. S., Britt, B. A., and Steward, D. J.: Malignant hyperthermia. Brit. J. Anaesth. 45:269, 1973.
4. Britt, B. A., and Kalow, W.: Malignant hyperthermia: a statistical review. Canad. Anaesth. Soc. J. 17:293, 1970.
5. Gatz, E. E., Kerr, D. D., and Wingard, D. W.: Earlier diagnosis of malignant hyperthermia. *In* Aldrete, J. A., and Britt, B. A. (eds.): Second International Symposium on Malignant Hyperthermia, 1977. New York, Grune & Stratton, 1978, pp. 147–157.
6. Denborough, M. A., Hudson, M. C., Forster, J. F. A., et al.: Biochemical changes in malignant hyperthermia. Lancet 2:1137, 1970.
7. Donlon, J. V., Newfield, P., Sreter, F., and Ryan, J. F.: Implication of masseter spasm after succinylcholine. Anesthesiology 49:298, 1978.
8. Isaacs, A., and Heffron, J. J. A.: Morphological and biochemical defects in muscles of human carrier of the malignant hyperthermia syndrome. Brit. J. Anaesth. 47:475, 1975.
9. Denborough, M. A., Hird, F. J. R., King, J. O., et al.: Mitochondrial and other studies in Australian Landrace pigs affected with malignant hyperthermia. *In* Gordon, R. A., et al. (eds.): International Symposium on Malignant Hyperthermia, 1971. Springfield, Ill. Charles C Thomas, 1973, pp. 229–237.
10. Hall, G. M., Lucke, J. N., and Lister, D.: Porcine malignant hyperthermia V: Fatal hyperthermia in the Pietrain pig, associated with the infusion of α-adrenergic agonisits. Brit. J. Anaesth. 49:855, 1977.
11. Anderson, I. L., and Jones, E. W.: Porcine malignant hyperthermia: Effect of dantrolene sodium on in-vitro halothane-induced contraction of susceptible muscle. Anesthesiology 44:57, 1976.
12. Gronert, G. A., Milde, J. H., and Theye, R. A.: Dantrolene in porcine malignant hyperthermia. Anesthesiology 44:488, 1976.
13. Harrison, G.: Control of the malignant hyperpyrexia syndrome in MHS swine by dantrolene sodium. Brit. Med. J. 47:62, 1975.
14. Short, C. E., and Paddleford, R. R.: Malignant hyperthermia in the dog. (Letter to the Editor.) Anesthesiology 39:462, 1973.
15. de Jong, R. H., Heavner, J. E., and Amory, D. W.: Malignant hyperpyrexia in the cat. Anesthesiology 41:608, 1974.
16. Klein, L. V.: Case report: A hot horse. Vet. Anesth. 2:41, 1975.
17. Kalow, W., Britt, B. A., Terreau, M. E., et al.: Metabolic error of muscle metabolism after recovery from malignant hyperpyrexia. Lancet 2:895, 1970.
18. Isaacs, H., Heffron, J. J. A., and Badenhorst, M.: Predictive tests for malignant hyperpyrexia. Brit. J. Anaesth. 47:1075, 1975.
19. Dykes, M. H. M.: Evaluation of a muscle relax-

ant: Dantrolene sodium (Dantrium). J.A.M.A. 231:862, 1975.

20. Morgan, K. G., Bryant, S. H.: The mechanism of action of dantrolene sodium. J. Pharmacol. Exp. Ther. 201:138, 1977.

21. Van Winkle, W. B.: Calcium release from skeletal muscle sarcoplasmic reticulum: Site of action of dantrolene sodium? Science 193:1130, 1976.

22. Lee, C.: Personal observations.

Myasthenias

1. Bell, C. M. A., and Lewis, C. B.: Effect of neostigmine on integrity of ileorectal anastomoses. Brit. Med. J. 3:587, 1968.

2. Greene, L. F., Ghosh, M. K., and Howard, F. M., Jr.: Transurethral prostatic resection in patients with myasthenia gravis. J. Urol. 112:226, 1974.

3. Dalal, F. Y., Bennett, E. J., and Gegg, W. S.: Congenital myasthenia gravis and minor surgical procedures. Anaesthesia 27:61, 1972.

4. Davies, D. W., and Steward, D. J.: Myasthenia gravis in children and anaesthetic management for thymectomy. Canad. Anaesth. Soc. J. 20:253, 1973.

5. Drachman, D. B., Kao, I., Pestronk, A., Toyka, K. V., Griffin, D. E., and Winkelstein, J. A.: Myasthenia gravis: a human disorder of acetylcholine receptors. In Pathogenesis of Human Muscular Dystrophies. Proceedings, Fifth International Scientific Conference of the Muscular Dystrophy Association, Colorado, 1976. Amsterdam, Excerpta Medica, 1977, p. 111.

6. Elmquist, D., and Lambert, E. H.: Detailed analyses of neuromuscular transmission in a patient with myasthenic syndrome sometimes associated with bronchogenic carcinoma. Mayo Clin. Proc. 43:689, 1968.

7. Engel, A. G., Tsujihata, M., Sakakibara, H., Lindstrom, J., and Lambert, E. H.: Ultrastructural evidence for acetylcholine receptor dysfunction in myasthenia gravis and in its autoimmune model. In Pathogenesis of Human Muscular Dystrophies. Proceedings, Fifth International Scientific Conference of the Muscular Dystrophy Association, Colorado, 1976. Amsterdam, Excerpta Medica, 1977, p. 132.

8. Girnar, D. S., and Weinreich, A. I.: Anesthesia for transcervical thymectomy in myasthenia gravis. Anesth. Analg. 55:13, 1976.

9. Lake, C. L.: Curare sensitivity in steroid-treated myasthenia gravis: A case report. Anesth. Analg. 57:132, 1978.

10. Lambert, E. H., and Rooke, E. D.: Myasthenic state and lung cancer. In Brain, R. L., and Norris, F. H. (eds.): Remote Effects of Cancer on the Nervous System. New York, Grune & Stratton, 1965, p. 67.

11. Leventhal, S. R., Orkin, F. K., and Hirsh, R. A.: Predicting postoperative ventilatory need in myasthenia. Anesthesiology 51:S 151, 1979.

12. Lindstrom, J.: Autoimmune response to acetylcholine receptors in myasthenia gravis and its animal model. In Pathogenesis of Human Muscular Dystrophies. Proceedings, Fifth International Scientific Conference of the Muscular Dystrophy Association, Colorado, 1976. Amsterdam, Excerpta Medica, 1977, p. 121.

13. Loach, A. B., Young, A. C., Spalding, J. M. K.,

and Smith, A. C.: Postoperative management after thymectomy. Brit. Med. J. 1:309, 1975.

14. Merritt, H. H., and Rowland, L. P.: Muscle diseases. In Merritt, H. H. (ed.): A Textbook of Neurology, 6th ed. Philadelphia, Lea & Febiger, 1979, pp. 597–605.

15. Rolbin, S. H., Levinson, G., Shnider, S. M., and Wright, R. G.: Anesthetic considerations for myasthenia gravis and pregnancy. Anesth. Analg. 57:441, 1978.

16. Samaha, F. J.: Electrodiagnostic studies in neuromuscular disease. N. Engl. J. Med. 285:1244, 1971.

17. Thoulon, J. M., Galopin, G., Seffert, P., Garin, J. P., and Dumont, M.: Myasthenie et grossesse. J. Gyn. Obst. Biol. Repr. 7:1395, 1978.

18. Wahlin, A., Havermark, K. G.: Enflurane (Ethrane) anesthesia on patients with myasthenia gravis. Acta Anaesth. Belg. 2:215, 1974.

Familial Periodic Paralysis

1. Bashford, A. C.: Case report: anaesthesia in familial hypokalaemic periodic paralysis. Anaesth. Int. Care 5:74, 1977.

2. Caughey, J. E., and Myrianthopoulas, N. C.: Dystrophic myotonia and related disorders. 1963.

3. Egan, T. J., and Klein, R.: Hyperkalemic familial periodic paralysis. Pediatrics 24:761, 1959.

4. Engel, A. G.: Treatment of metabolic and endocrine myopathies. Mod. Treat. 3:313, 1966.

5. Engel, W. K., et al.: Clinical approach to the myopathies. Clin. Orthop. Rel. Res. 39:4, 1965.

6. Gordon, A. M., and Kas, I.: Membranes, electrolytes, periodic paralysis. In Rowland, L. P. (ed.): Pathogenesis of common muscular dystrophies. Amsterdam, Excerpta Medica, p. 762, 1972.

7. Hofmann, W. W., and Smith, R. A.: Hypokalemic periodic paralysis in vitro. Brain 93:445, 1970.

8. Horton, B.: Anesthetic experiences in a family with hypokalemic familial periodic paralysis. Anesthesiology 47:308, 1977.

9. McArdle, B.: Adynamia episodica hereditaria. Brain 85:121, 1962.

10. Merritt, H. H., and Rowland, L. P.: Muscle. In Merritt, H. H. (ed.): A Textbook of Neurology. 6th Edition. Philadelphia, Lea & Febiger, 1979, pp. 606–612.

11. Norris, F. H., Jr.: Intracellular recording from human striated muscle. In Data Acquisition and Processing in Biology and Medicine. New York, Macmillan, 1962, Vol. 11, p. 59.

12. Siler, M. N., and Discavage, W. J.: Anesthetic management of hypokalemic periodic paralysis. Anesthesiology 43(No. 4):489, 1975.

13. Streeten, D. J.: Periodic paralysis. In Stanbury, J. B., et al. (eds.): 2nd ed., New York, McGraw-Hill, 1966.

14. Viskopfer, R. J., Licht, A., and Fidelchaco, J.: Acetazolamide treatment of hypokalemic periodic paralysis. A metabolic and electromyographic study. Am. J. Med. Sci. 266:119, 1973.

15. Vroom, F. Q., Jarrell, M. A., and Maren, T. H.: Acetazolamide treatment of hypokalemic periodic paralysis. Probable mechanism of action. Arch. Neurol. 32:385, 1975.

16. Wise, R. P.: Muscle disorders and the relaxants. Brit. J. Anaesth. 35:558, 1963.

17. Zundel, W. S., and Tyler, F. H.: Muscular dystrophies. N. Engl. J. Med. 273:537, 596, 1965.

15

Skin and Bone Disorders

By RICHARD E. BERRYHILL, M.D.

Epidermolysis Bullosa
Pemphigus and Pemphigoid
Erythema Multiforme
Toxic Epidermal Necrolysis
Staphylococcal Scalded Skin Syndrome
Behçet's Disease
Scleroderma
Psoriasis
Neurofibromatosis
Erythema Nodosum
Mastocytosis
Malignant Atrophic Papulosis

Hereditary Anhidrotic Ectodermal Dysplasia
Fabry's Disease
Incontinentia Pigmenti (Bloch-Sulzberger Syndrome)
Osteoporosis, Osteomalacia, and Osteopetrosis
Osteogenesis Imperfecta
Dwarfism
Craniofacial and Mandibulofacial Dysostoses
Paget's Disease (Osteitis Deformans)
Fibrous Dysplasia

INTRODUCTION

This chapter presents uncommon diseases of both skin and bone and their associated anesthesia considerations and problems. At the end of each disease presentation, management guidelines are listed which are intended to aid the reader in the safe conduct of anesthesia for his or her patients. The skin diseases are closely related to one another in that their anesthetic management considerations involve special measures to avoid skin trauma, special difficulties in maintenance of an airway, the need for perioperative corticosteroid coverage, and difficulties associated with general debilitation. The anesthetic management considerations for the bone diseases are also closely related to one another in that most of these diseases involve the need for careful movement, transfer and positioning of these fracture susceptible patients, conduction anesthesia and ventilatory difficulties associated with kyphoscoliosis, airway management difficulties, and difficulties associated with concomitant congenital anomalies.

EPIDERMOLYSIS BULLOSA

Epidermolysis bullosa is a group of rare mucocutaneous disorders whose common primary feature is the formation of blisters following even trivial trauma. A recent reclassification divides the several forms into two major groups, nonscarring and scarring.[1]

Included in the *nonscarring category* are the following: epidermolysis bullosa simplex, generalized (Koebner) or localized (Weber-Cockayne); junctional epidermolysis bullosa (letalis); and localized absence of skin with blistering and nail dystrophy (Bart's syndrome).

With *epidermolysis bullosa simplex* types, onset may occur from birth to adulthood, and is inherited as an autosomal dominant trait. Blistering may be limited to the hands and feet (Weber-Cockayne), or involve much of the skin surface (Koebner), but rarely produces oral or nailbed lesions, and heals without scarring. Incidence of the disease is increased in frequency with patient exposure to warmer ambient temperature (summer months), and results from cytolysis of basal and suprabasal layers of the epidermis.

Junctional epidermolysis bullosa, formerly described as epidermolysis bullosa letalis, is inherited as an autosomal recessive trait. It is characterized by onset at birth of severe generalized blistering involving the skin, oral cavity, and esophagus. Moderate to severe refractory anemia is common. The majority of patients die within the first two years of life. Patients who survive infancy usually develop the complications associated with the scarring recessive dystrophic type. High dose systemic corticosteroid therapy during life-threatening periods appears to be useful.

Included in the *scarring category* are the following: dystrophic epidermolysis bullosa, autosomal dominant (hyperplastic Cockayne and Torraine or albopapuloid Pasini); dystrophic epidermolysis bullosa, autosomal recessive (polydysplastic); acquired epidermolysis bullosa (acquisita).

Dominant dystrophic epidermolysis bullosa occurs in infancy. Blistering may be localized to the extremities or become generalized. Oral lesions when present are mild.

Recessive dystrophic epidermolysis bullosa has its onset at birth or early infancy. The almost ever-present oropharyngeal, esophageal, and anal mucosal lesions present nutritional problems. Ocular and genitourinary involvement may occur. Chronic anemia may be present. A recent report suggests that dystrophic recessive epidermolysis bullosa is a disease of stratified squamous epithelium and that this is therefore the reason for no reports of tracheal involvement.[2] Laryngeal involvement with scarring and airway obstruction has been recently reported (the mucosa of the true vocal cords is stratified squamous epithelium).[3]

Acquired epidermolysis bullosa occurs in adulthood without evidence of genetic disease, tends to be localized to the extremities, and has variable oropharyngeal involvement.

Treatment for all forms of epidermolysis bullosa is largely supportive and generally less than satisfactory. Local skin care, avoidance of mucosal and cutaneous trauma, control of secondary bacterial infections with appropriate antibiotics and the use of corticosteroid therapy during life-threatening periods constitute conservative conventional treatment. Surgery for most of these patients consists primarily of dental restoration or superficial reconstructive operations to alleviate severe scarring. Intra-abdominal and thoracic operations have been performed for the usual indications.

Although epidermolysis bullosa includes a broad spectrum of disease with minimal to severe systemic involvement, general guidelines for the anesthetic and perioperative management of patients with this disease are as follows:

1. The prevention of friction and trauma is essential. Avoid rubbing the skin and mucosal surfaces. Any friction can produce bullae. When possible patients should move themselves to and from the operating table, otherwise they must be transferred with great care. Tape of any type should be avoided. Blood pressure cuffs, tourniquets, precordial and esophageal stethoscopes, esophageal and rectal temperature probes, and adhesive ECG electrodes should be used only when specific instances dictate their use. When they are necessary, the skin and mucosal surfaces must be well protected by the generous use of lubricant and/or lubricant soaked gauze or cotton sponges. Monitoring in the recovery room should also be limited to the essential. Care must be exercised in establishing and securing intravenous cannulae (e.g., spray antiseptic skin preparation and gauze wrap). The eyes should be protected with an appropriate ophthalmic ointment and not taped shut.

2. Airway management may be extremely difficult. A general principle should be to avoid all airway manipulation whenever possible. Although laryngoscopy and endotracheal intubation have been performed in some patients without sequelae,[4] life-threatening oropharyngeal bullae and hemorrhage have occurred in other patients.[5] Laryngeal scarring has recently been reported.[3, 6] Tracheal involvement has not been reported. This may be due to the difference between the mucosa of the upper and lower airway.

If there is a clear airway and spontaneous ventilation and inhalation drugs are used, large fresh gas flows delivered by a mask held first above the skin surfaces of the face and nose will provide anesthesia while avoiding facial trauma. If a tight mask fit becomes necessary, the face must be protected by lubricant soaked cotton or gauze sponges. Various types of head bags and boxes and insufflation techniques have also been used.[7, 8] The use of oropharyngeal and nasopharyngeal airways and esophageal stethoscopes and temperature probes should be avoided.

If endotracheal intubation is necessary, a laryngoscope and a small endotracheal tube, both literally "dripping" with lubricant, should be used to minimize friction when instrumenting the airway. Under these controlled conditions, tracheal intubation may be a less threatening procedure than insertion of oral or nasal airways. In some patients tracheostomy may ultimately be required to secure the airway; however, tracheostomy may also produce subsequent airway management problems. A surgeon and equipment to perform a tracheostomy should be present during the induction of anesthesia as well as postoperatively. Extubation of the trachea requires the same gentleness as intubation. Postoperatively, patients must be closely observed for the development of airway obstruction.

3. Most patients will be taking or will have taken corticosteroid drugs at some time prior to surgery; therefore, appropriate perioperative therapy with corticosteroids is indicated.

4. Other associated disease states include general debilitation with malnutrition, electrolyte imbalance, and anemia. Congenital pyloric atresia, porphyria, amyloidosis, multiple myeloma, enteritis, diabetes mellitus, and hypercoagulable states are also reported.[9] Secondarily, skin wounds may be infected and sepsis may occur. These complications must be diagnosed and corrected prior to the administration of anesthesia and surgery.

5. Anesthetic drugs and techniques: The use of potent inhalation drugs is discussed above. Intravenous barbiturate induction has been used satisfactorily; however, the possibility of associated porphyria must be remembered. Ketamine, intramuscularly and intravenously, has been used as the sole anesthetic drug.[10] The induction of anesthesia must be smooth, and struggling must be avoided. Local infiltration is to be avoided because of the potential for skin sloughing. There are no reports of regional techniques having been used.

6. All members of the medical team must be alerted to the special problems of these patients. Meticulous care in the operating room is negated if the patient is mishandled in the postoperative period.

PEMPHIGUS AND PEMPHIGOID

Pemphigus comprises a group of mucocutaneous diseases that have a possible autoimmune etiology and are characterized by bullous eruptions of the skin and mucous membranes. Various forms include pemphigus vulgaris, pemphigus vegetans, pemphigus foliaceus, pemphigus erythematosus (Senear-Usher syndrome), and Brazilian pemphigus foliaceus. Pemphigoid is considered to be a separate clinical entity. Differentiation is determined by histologic and immunologic tests.[1]

Pemphigus vulgaris, the most common form of the disease, occurs predominantly in Jewish or Mediterranean peoples usually in the fourth to sixth decades of life, although occurrence from 3½ years to 70 years of age has been reported. The tender, painful bullous eruptions and erosions are located within the epidermis and heal without scarring. Nikolsky's sign, which is separation of the epidermis with lateral finger pressure, is frequently present. Mucous membranes are commonly involved, and oral lesions may precede cutaneous lesions by several months. Severe oropharyngeal lesions may interfere with adequate nutrition. Lesions of the pharynx and larynx may produce hoarseness. Nasal, vaginal, and anal mucosa may be affected. With extensive disease, electrolyte imbalance and hypoalbuminemia are common. High dose corticosteroid therapy has markedly reduced the once existent 90 per cent mortality of the untreated disease. Immunosuppressive drugs, methotrexate, cyclophosphamide, and azathioprine are used.[2] Gold therapy has also been effective. A recent report suggests plasma exchange for patients with acute exacerbation of the disease.[3]

Other organ systems do not appear to be primarily involved. However, degeneration of the adrenal glands, pulmonary edema, pneumonia, atelectasis, and focal myocardial degeneration have been found at autopsy in patients who died with fulminant pemphigus.

Pemphigus vegetans differs from pemphigus vulgaris in that with healing of the denuded skin and mucosa, hypertrophic verrucoid granulations occur, occasionally with pustular areas (intraepidermal eosinophilic abscesses) at the periphery of these lesions. Otherwise, the clinical presentation and course closely resemble that of pemphigus vulgaris.

Pemphigus foliaceus and *pemphigus erythematosus* represent the less severe forms of the disease. Pemphigus erythematosus is a localized variant of the more generalized pemphigus foliaceus in which the seborrheic-like eruptions are confined primarily to the anterior chest and the "butterfly" distribution of the face. *Brazilian pemphigus* is a variant of pemphigus foliaceus that is endemic to south central Brazil. In contrast to pemphigus vulgaris, oropharyngeal lesions are not frequently present.

Benign familial pemphigus (Hailey-Hailey disease) is a hereditary vesiculobullous eruption having recurrent lesions in intertriginous areas of the skin.[4] The disease is autosomal dominant and usually occurs in early adult life, becoming less severe with increasing age. Oropharyngeal lesions are unusual, and when present make the diagnosis questionable. Topical and systemic corticosteroids are the treatment of choice.

Pemphigoid is distinguished from pemphigus by virtue of the fact that the bullous eruptions occur subepidermally rather than intraepidermally.[5]

Bullous pemphigoid is characterized by large, tense bullae occurring primarily in intertriginous areas. It can also involve oropharyngeal, esophageal, anal, and vaginal mucosa, although to a lesser extent than pemphigus. It is a disease of the elderly, but has been documented in childhood.[6] The clinical course is one of exacerbations and remissions.

Cicatricial pemphigoid (benign mucous membrane pemphigoid) is characterized by bullous eruptions that heal with scarring and involve primarily mucous membranes of the oropharynx, nasopharynx, conjunctiva, larynx, esophagus, genitalia, and anus. Intertriginous areas of the skin may be affected. Because of scarring, stenosis of the various mucosal orifices can result in airway, genitourinary, and gastrointestinal obstruction.

Therapy of pemphigus consists of cortico-steroids, immunosuppressives (methotrexate, cyclophosphamide, azathioprine), sulfapyridine, and sulfones. However, the treatment of cicatricial pemphigoid is for unknown reasons less than satisfactory.

Benign chronic bullous dermatosis of childhood affects children of preschool age, is characterized by large, tense bullae of the skin, and clinically resembles adult bullous pemphigoid. The disease does not persist into adult life and has a clinical course of exacerbations and remissions with spontaneous remission usually occurring within two to three years of onset. Therapy may include corticosteroids, sulfapyridine, and sulfones.

Guidelines for the anesthetic management of patients with pemphigus and/or pemphigoid are as follows:

1. Airway management may be difficult because of cutaneous, oropharyngeal, and laryngeal involvement; therefore, the principles of airway management discussed under epidermolysis bullosa should be considered.

2. Other disease states associated with pemphigus and pemphigoid include myasthenia gravis, systemic lupus erythematosus, rheumatoid arthritis, pernicious anemia,[7] and primary hepatic cirrhosis,[8] suggesting an autoimmune mechanism for the disease. In addition, increased levels of autoantibodies, complement, and immune complexes are found in these patients and support the autoimmune hypothesis. Since each of these associated diseases has serious anesthetic management implications (e.g., muscle relaxants and myasthenia gravis), preanesthetic diagnosis of these conditions is extremely important.

3. The potential toxic bone marrow and hepatic effects of the drugs used for treatment dictate that preoperative laboratory evaluation of hematologic and hepatic function be performed. Dapsone (sulfone) has also been implicated in causing a peripheral neuropathy.[9]

4. Since water and salt can be lost through the mucocutaneous lesions, the degree of hydration and electrolyte balance should be assessed.

5. Many patients will be taking or will have taken corticosteroid drugs at some time prior to surgery; therefore, appropriate perioperative therapy with corticosteroids is indicated.

6. Anesthetic drugs and techniques: No particular anesthetic drug or technique is recommended. Local infiltration should be avoided because of the potential for skin sloughing. Airway management remains the primary concern. In the only reported case of anesthetic management of this disease, the authors utilized continuous thoracic epidural anesthesia supplemented with ketamine intravenously for cholecystectomy. The patient did not have any complications.

ERYTHEMA MULTIFORME

Erythema multiforme describes a spectrum of acute inflammatory diseases ranging from a mild illness referred to as erythema multiforme minor to a severe, life-threatening condition known best as Stevens-Johnson syndrome.

Many precipitating factors have been implicated in erythema multiforme, although in approximately half the cases no specific etiology is found. Drug associations have been prominent and include barbiturates, sulfonamides, penicillin, salicylates, antipyrine, phenytoin, hydralazine, digitalis, and others. Erythema multiforme may be a manifestation of dermatomyositis, lupus erythematosus, polyarteritis nodosa, rheumatoid arthritis, or Wegener's granulomatosis. Viral, bacterial, fungal, and parasitic infections and malignancy have also been implicated. *Mycoplasma pneumonia* is frequently concomitantly present.[2]

Erythema multiforme minor accounts for up to 1 per cent of dermatologic outpatient visits. The disease rarely occurs in persons over 50 years of age and is commonly seasonal (spring and fall).[1] A mild prodrome of low grade fever, malaise, arthralgia, and upper respiratory tract symptoms frequently precedes the characteristic rash. The rash is generally symmetrical, present on the extensor surfaces of extremities, and can involve palms, soles, oral mucosa, and conjunctiva. The lesions are characteristic and appear as circumscribed concentric rings of alternating pale and erythematous zones with a central dusky papule or vesicle, and are thus known as "targets" or as an "iris." The lesions appear in crops over a period of two to three days, last about one week, and then heal. Recurrences are common.[2] Erythema multiforme minor generally requires little treatment. Corticosteroid therapy may be necessary for short periods when cutaneous or mucosal involvement is extensive.

Stevens-Johnson syndrome is the most severe form of erythema multiforme, occurs infrequently, usually within the first three decades, and has a peak occurrence in v inter. The disease is an extremely serious one and has a 10 to 20 per cent mortality rate. Prodromal illness typically consists of fever, malaise, cough, sore throat, chest pain, vomiting, diarrhea, myalgia, and arthralgia. This is followed by an explosive appearance of inflammatory bullous lesions of the skin and mucous membranes. The severe cutaneous lesions result in sloughing of the epithelium, leaving large denuded areas of skin. The severe mucosal lesions cause ulceration of the nose, oropharynx, larynx, trachea, and bronchi.[2] Oral lesions may interfere with adequate nutrition. The eyes are also commonly affected with conjunctivitis, corneal ulceration, anterior uveitis, or panophthalmitis. Bullae of visceral pleura have resulted in bronchiolar-alveolar-pleural fistulas and bilateral pneumothoraces with subcutaneous emphysema.[3] Ulceration of the esophagus and colon has caused perforation and fatal gastrointestinal hemorrhage.[4] Anemia secondary to bleeding, infection, and/or poor nutrition is common. Acute atrial fibrillation has been reported,[5] and acute myocarditis has been found at autopsy. An acute inflammatory renal lesion may cause acute renal failure. Stevens-Johnson syndrome has a protracted clinical course of two to seven weeks, with recurrences in up to 20 per cent of cases. There is no specific therapy. Associated conditions such as the collagen diseases or infection should be treated. Any drugs associated with the disease should be discontinued. Corticosteroids should be administered until the lesion heals. Appropriate antibiotics are used to treat secondary bacterial infection. Careful attention to fluid and electrolyte balance is imperative. Local skin care, ocular care, and oral hygiene are important. Pulmonary complications and severe infections are the most common causes of death.

Guidelines for anesthetic management of patients with erythema multiforme are as follows:

1. The patient with erythema multiforme minor usually presents no major problems

for the anesthesiologist. The patient with Stevens-Johnson syndrome, however, presents a significant challenge. Because many of the anesthetic considerations for this disease are similar to those of epidermolysis bullosa, the reader is additionally referred to that section.

2. If significant oropharyngeal and laryngeal edema is present, a tracheostomy prior to the administration of anesthesia and surgery should be considered. Placement of endotracheal tubes, oral or nasopharyngeal airways, and esophageal stethoscopes or temperature probes may result in hemorrhagic bullae that can rupture and severely compromise the airway. If a mask is used, the face should be protected by lubricated cotton or gauze sponges.

3. The possible occurrence of visceral pleural blebs and pneumothorax suggests that positive-pressure ventilation be avoided if possible.

4. The frequent presence of *Mycoplasma pneumonia* and other pulmonary infections necessitates careful decontamination and isolation of anesthetic equipment. When possible the use of disposable equipment is recommended.

5. The skin should be protected from blood pressure cuffs and precordial stethoscopes.

6. Because of the potential for dysrhythmias and myocarditis, ECG monitoring is recommended; however, care must be used in placing and removing electrodes.

7. The use of a cooling blanket is recommended because of the frequency of febrile episodes. The axilla is a convenient and generally atraumatic site for monitoring temperature.

8. The state of hydration and electrolyte balance must be assessed and appropriately corrected.

9. Anesthetic drugs and technique: No specific drugs or techniques are recommended. Local anesthetic infiltration is appropriate when possible. Regional anesthesia may be used depending upon the condition of the skin overlying the site of entry and the presence of systemic infection. Barbiturates should be used with caution because of their association as a precipitating factor of the disease. In patients who have renal insufficiency, potentially nephrotoxic drugs (methoxyflurane, enflurane)[6] and drugs eliminated via the kidney (gallamine, metocurine, and, to a lesser extent, curare and pancuronium) should be used with caution or avoided. Ketamine intramuscularly and intravenously has been used as the sole anesthetic with success.[4]

10. Most patients with this disease will be taking or have taken corticosteroids at some time prior to surgery; therefore, appropriate perioperative therapy with corticosteroids is indicated.

TOXIC EPIDERMAL NECROLYSIS (LYELL'S DISEASE)

Toxic epidermal necrolysis is a severe mucocutaneous disorder characterized by the sudden onset of widespread erythema and detachment of epidermis.

The large majority of cases occur in adults. A prodrome of conjunctival irritation, skin tenderness, fever, malaise, and arthralgia may precede the onset of a morbilliform rash. The rash often becomes confluent and is accompanied by diffuse erythema and vesiculation that can involve the entire skin surface.[1] Nikolsky's sign, which is separation of the epidermis with lateral finger pressure, is present in the erythematous areas. Mucous membranes may be severely involved, including the oropharynx, tongue, esophagus, larynx, and tracheobronchial tree, and may result in esophageal and gastrointestinal hemorrhage and tracheitis with cicatricial healing of the mucosa. Hypovolemia, electrolyte imbalance, and albuminuria may proceed to hypoperfusion, renal failure and pulmonary edema.[2]

Most often, drugs have been implicated as etiologic factors and include barbiturates, sulfonamides, antibiotics, pentazocine, and hydantoins.[3, 4] Other diseases that have been associated with toxic epidermal necrolysis include viral, bacterial (*E. coli*), and fungal (pulmonary aspergillosis) infections. Vaccinations and neoplastic disease have also been implicated.[5] An idiopathic form of the disease has been described. Histologic examination reveals selective necrosis (necrolysis) of the basal layers of the epidermis, which distinguishes this disease from other necrotic skin (full thickness) maladies such as the staphylococcal scalded-skin syndrome.[1] Mortality has ranged from 20 to 45 per cent.

There is no specific therapy. Fluid and

electrolyte balance must be maintained. Specific antibiotic therapy for identified pathogens is indicated. Skin care, oral hygiene, and ocular care are important. Early administration of high dose corticosteroids appears to help.

Guidelines for the anesthetic management of patients with toxic epidermal necrolysis are similar to those for patients with epidermolysis bullosa and erythema multiforme, and the reader is referred to those sections. In addition, it should be noted that pentazocine has been questionably implicated as producing this disease as well as reversible renal insufficiency.[6]

STAPHYLOCOCCAL SCALDED-SKIN SYNDROME (RITTER'S DISEASE)

Staphylococcal scalded-skin syndrome is a mucocutaneous disorder ranging from localized bullous impetigo to widespread epidermolysis and superficial desquamation.[1] The etiology has been identified as group 2 *Staphylococcus aureus* and is now recognized as distinct from toxic epidermal necrolysis.

The disease occurs primarily in neonates and children and occasionally in adults. A prodrome of purulent conjunctivitis, otitis media, occult nasopharyngeal infection, and classically cutaneous tenderness precedes the onset of a scarlatiniform rash. Nikolsky's sign (separation of the epidermis with lateral finger pressure) is often present. Large flaccid bullae then appear with separation of the epidermis and superficial desquamation. Necrolysis does not occur.[2] Mucosal involvement is rare, and healing occurs usually within five to seven days.

Therapy includes penicillinase-resistant antistaphylococcal antibiotics, skin care, hydration, and maintenance of electrolyte balance. Routine corticosteroid therapy is contraindicated because of the bacterial etiology. Mortality is 2 to 3 per cent.[3]

Guidelines for the anesthetic management of patients with staphylococcal scalded-skin syndrome are as follows:

1. Mucosal involvement is rare; however, the potential for traumatic bullae formation remains; therefore, any airway manipulation must be gentle.

2. Because of the bacterial etiology of the disease, equipment must be appropriately cleansed and clothing changed to avoid pathogen transfer to other patients (e.g., epidemic impetigo).

3. Corticosteroid therapy is relatively contraindicated.

4. Anesthetic drugs and techniques: No particular anesthetic technique is recommended. The use of regional anesthesia will depend upon the absence of involvement of the site of injection.

BEHÇET'S DISEASE

Behçet's disease, once described as a symptom complex triad of recurring iritis, ulceration of the mouth and ulceration of the genitalia, is now recognized as involving additional organ systems, including the skin, central nervous system, heart, vasculature, lungs, and joints. Fibrinolysis is altered in some patients. Possible etiologies of the disease include viral, parasitic, and bacterial infections, defective fibrinolytic activity, and most recently an autoimmune mechanism. Males are affected much more often than females (5:1). The diagnostic criteria have been divided into major criteria (oral, genital, ocular, and skin lesions) and minor criteria (gastrointestinal, thrombophlebitis, cardiovascular, arthritis, central nervous system lesions, and family history). The diagnosis of Behçet's disease is based upon the presence of the three original major criteria or the combination of two major and two minor criteria.[1]

Oral, genital, or ocular lesions are the most common initial manifestations of the disease. The mucosal lesions are recurrent, painful 2 to 10 mm. in diameter ulcers, which have a yellowish necrotic base and which may be shallow or deep, and last 7 to 14 days. The oral ulcerations may involve the lips, gums, tongue, mucosa, tonsils, and larynx and can interfere with adequate nutrition. Healing with severe oropharyngeal scarring is reported.[2] Ocular manifestations include anterior chamber changes (iridocyclitis and hypopyon), optic atrophy, choroiditis, and relapsing conjunctivitis. Blindness may result. Skin lesions include papules, vesicles, pustules, pyoderma, folliculitis, acne, furuncles, abscesses, and erythema nodosum-like lesions. Characteristic is nonspecific inflammatory reactivity to any scratches or intracutaneous lesions. The central nervous system may be affected in many ways including hemiparesis, quadriparesis, dementia, ataxia, meningitis, seizures, pseudobulbar palsy, spinal cord lesions, cauda equina syndrome, hyperreflexia and coma.[4] These symptoms may resolve and then recur. Cardiovascular manifestations include pericarditis, recurrent thrombophlebitis, superior and inferior venae caval obstruction, and arterial aneurysms.[4, 5] Pulmonary vasculitis, hemoptysis, and obstructive airways disease have been reported.[6]

Arthritis is usually recurrent and limited to the large joints, and generally does not cause deformities or roentgenographic changes. Small joints such as of the finger are usually spared. The arthritis is usually accompanied by low grade fever. A relative inhibition of the fibrinolytic system can be demonstrated in patients during periods of thrombophlebitis; however, this defect returns to normal during periods of remission. The natural history of Behçet's disease is one of recurrent exacerbations and remissions with a gradual overall deterioration.

Treatment for Behçet's disease has included systemic and topical corticosteroids, immunosuppressive drugs (cyclophosphamide), and fibrinolytic drugs (streptokinase, streptodornase) but the results have been generally unsatisfactory and the treatment does not appear to alter the natural history of the disease.[3]

Guidelines for the anesthetic management of patients with Behçet's disease are as follows:

1. Scarring from recurrent ulceration of the oropharyngeal and nasopharyngeal mucosa (though not the usual circumstance) can result in complete obliteration of the nasopharynx and extreme difficulty in endotracheal intubation.[3] In such instances, the trachea should be intubated while the patient is awake with the aid of topical anesthesia, regional nerve blocks (glossopharyngeal, superior laryngeal), and/or sedation when appropriate. Use of a fiberoptic bronchoscope should be considered. Tracheostomy may be necessary.

2. Organ systems that may be involved need the appropriate preoperative evaluation.

3. Needle punctures should be kept to a minimum because of the diffuse inflammatory skin changes and pyodermas that can occur. The potential site for an injection or

intravenous catheter must be inspected closely for signs of early infection.

4. Anesthetic drugs and techniques: Other than the potential difficulties in airway management, no particular technique is recommended. The advantages of regional anesthesia must be weighed carefully against subsequent central nervous system complications that may develop during the natural course of the disease. The use of succinylcholine in patients with neurological involvement may result in sudden hyperkalemia and cardiac dysrhythmias.[8]

5. Autonomic hyperreflexia resulting in acute severe hypertension is a potential problem in patients with spinal cord involvement.[9]

SCLERODERMA

Scleroderma (progressive systemic sclerosis) is a chronic, progressive multisystem disorder characterized by varying degrees of vascular change, inflammation, and fibrosis of the skin and internal organs (lungs, kidneys, heart and gastrointestinal tract).[1] The etiology is thought to involve both immune and connective tissue system abnormalities.[2]

Three principal forms of scleroderma exist. First, acrosclerosis, involving 90 to 95 per cent of patients, has a peak onset between the third and fifth decades and is characterized by involvement of the skin (face and hands) and the presence of Raynaud's phenomenon. The CREST syndrome, consisting of calcinosis, Raynaud's phenomenon, esophageal motility disorder, sclerodactyly, and telangiectasia, is present in only about 5 per cent of patients. Visceral involvement usually does not occur in these patients, although Sjögren's syndrome or biliary cirrhosis may be present in a few. Fulminant pulmonary fibrosis and pulmonary hypertension have developed late in the disease. Second, diffuse scleroderma is a more aggressive form of the disease and has severe, fulminant visceral involvement. Raynaud's phenomenon is rare, and skin involvement is predominantly truncal. Third, localized scleroderma (morphea) is a benign variant with localized cutaneous involvement of the trunk, extremities, and scalp.

The majority of patients can expect prolonged survival; decreased survival is clearly related to pulmonary, cardiac, and renal involvement.

Cutaneous involvement is manifested by the appearance of stiff, indurated skin which progresses to atrophied, smooth, tense, "hidebound" skin. Inability to open the mouth is due to constriction of the perioral skin and soft tissues and dysfunction of the temporomandibular joint.[3]

Pulmonary involvement may include either pulmonary interstitial fibrosis or pulmonary arterial sclerosis or both.[4] Small airways disease is frequently present and is an early pulmonary function abnormality that precedes the characteristic development of restrictive lung disease and impairment of gas diffusion.[5] Pulmonary arterial disease and, to a lesser extent, pulmonary fibrosis can result in pulmonary hypertension, right ventricular hypertrophy, failure, and cardiac death.

Cardiac involvement may be primary or secondary. Angina pectoris, contraction band myocardial necrosis, dysrhythmias, and sudden death have recently been reported in these patients.[6] Since autopsy findings have revealed morphologically normal coronary arteries, the myocardial abnormalities may result from a primary Raynaud's phenomenon of the coronary arteries. Pericarditis with chronic pericardial effusion may occur.[1] Pulmonary and systemic hypertension can result in secondary right and left ventricular failure.

Renal failure is not infrequent and commonly causes systemic hypertension. However, successful renal transplantation has been performed.[7]

Telangiectasias of the oral mucous membranes may result in epistaxis.[8] Dysphagia, gastroesophageal reflux with esophagitis, esophageal stricture, and bowel perforation are not uncommon. An abnormal, involuntary vocalization called "scleroderma bark" is probably due to aerophagia in the presence of an incompetent gastrointestinal junction.[3] Bacterial overgrowth in atonic areas of the bowel leads to malabsorption, weight loss, and malnutrition. Malabsorption of vitamin K may lead to clotting abnormalities. Biliary cirrhosis (Sjögren's syndrome) may occur in a few patients.

Guidelines for the anesthetic management of patients with scleroderma are as follows:

1. Careful evaluation of the airway is important. Because of the constricted perioral soft tissues and dysfunction of the temporomandibular joint, laryngoscopy and tracheal intubation may prove difficult. Gentle "awake" oral or nasotracheal intubation may be necessary. A fiberoptic laryngoscope or optical stylet may be useful aids. Tracheostomy may occasionally be necessary. Since the airway will be manipulated, the oropharynx should always be evaluated for oral telangiectasis.

2. The operating room should not be cold because of the risk of Raynaud's phenomenon. The hands may additionally be wrapped. If possible, drawing arterial blood gas samplings from the radial or ulnar arteries should be avoided.

3. Pulmonary function testing should be performed preoperatively.

4. The cardiovascular system should be evaluated for the presence of pulmonary or systemic hypertension, right or left ventricular failure, pericarditis, pericardial and pleural effusion, and angina pectoris. Most of these abnormalities are correctible and preoperative treatment should be considered.

5. Renal, liver, and coagulation functions should be evaluated preoperatively.

6. Because of gastroesophageal junction incompetence, there is an increased risk of regurgitation and aspiration. Preoperative use of antacids and/or cimetidine is recommended. Cricoid pressure (Sellick maneuver) should be used prior to securing the airway with an endotracheal tube in patients who receive general anesthesia.

7. Perioperative corticosteroid treatment is recommended for those patients who are taking or who have recently taken corticosteroids. Phenoxybenzamine and reserpine are used to ameliorate Raynaud's phenomenon.

8. Anesthetic drugs and techniques: No particular technique is recommended. Enflurane[9] should probably be avoided because of potential nephrotoxicity. In the presence of chronic renal failure, gallamine and metocurine should be avoided. Prolonged regional analgesia following the use of lidocaine, one per cent, has been reported.[10, 11] The use of an ester-linked local anesthetic rather than an amide-linked local anesthetic for regional nerve block is recommended.[10]

PSORIASIS

Psoriasis is a chronic skin disease which is characterized by an accelerated epidermal turnover and epidermal hyperplasia. The disease appears to have both genetic and environmental etiologic components. The initial appearance of the disease is often associated with superficial cutaneous trauma (burn, cut, scratch) and exposure to low humidity, chemical injury, and drugs (corticosteroids). Sites of skin involvement are usually the sacral region, elbows, knees, and scalp. The palms, soles, oral mucosa, and entire integument are occasionally affected.[1] The cutaneous lesions of psoriasis consist of hypertrophied dermal papillae and epidermis, which form thick loosely adherent scales with increased vascularity. Arthritis and hyperuricemia are associated with psoriasis.

Psoriatic erythroderma, a more fulminant form of the disease, is characterized by involvement of the entire skin, fever, leukocytosis, and prostration. High output congestive heart failure has been reported as a result of greatly increased cutaneous blood flow.[2]

In 20 to 50 per cent of patients, the psoriatic lesions are culture positive for *Staphylococcus aureus*.[3, 4] However, most of these patients do not have a clinical pyoderma. The carriage rate for *S. aureus* on the skin of the normal population is less than 10 per cent. In one report an epidemic of staphylococcal wound infection was traced to an anesthetist with psoriasis who was a *S. aureus* carrier.[5]

Treatment includes low dose ultraviolet light, topical tars, psoralen, anthralin, methotrexate, and hydroxyurea.

Guidelines for the anesthetic management of patients with psoriasis are as follows:

1. Specific efforts should be taken to avoid any type of trauma to the skin, particularly in the areas of existing psoriatic lesions. Likewise, tape should be used on skin surfaces only when necessary.

2. Because of the increased presence of *S. aureus* in psoriatic lesions, these areas should be avoided as administration sites for regional anesthetics or intravenous cannulae.

3. Anesthetic drugs and techniques: Keeping in mind the first two recommenda-

tions, there otherwise appears to be no contraindication to any particular technique or drug.

4. In patients with psoriatic erythroderma, evaluation of the cardiovascular system for undiagnosed high output congestive heart failure is recommended.

NEUROFIBROMATOSIS

Neurofibromatosis of von Recklinghausen is an autosomal dominant disease (1 per 3000 births) in which the skin, nervous system, bones, endocrine glands, and sometimes other organs are the sites of a variety of congenital abnormalities, tumors, and hematomas.[1]

Clinical diagnosis in most patients is based upon the presence of spots of cutaneous hyperpigmentation (café au lait nevi) and cutaneous and subcutaneous tumors (neurofibromas). A presumptive diagnosis of the disease is made by the presence of five or more café au lait nevi with one dimension of the spot greater than 1.5 cm. Freckling in the axillary folds is particularly characteristic. Neurofibromas may affect all areas of the skin including genitalia, palms, and soles. The neurofibromas may be soft or hard, and may coalesce to form large plexiform neurofibromas. These tumors are thought to derive from the neurilemmal sheath (Schwann cells) or fibrocytes of peripheral nerve coverings.

Central nervous system involvement in neurofibromatosis is common, and in one series the prevalence was as high as 66 per cent. There is also an increased incidence of meningiomas and gliomas. The cranial nerves are commonly affected by the neurofibromas. Acoustic neuromas may produce deafness and other symptoms of cerebellopontine angle tumors. Involvement of the optic nerve may result in visual impairment. Cranial nerves V and X may also be affected. Fibromatous growth near the pituitary gland or hypothalamus can produce a variety of endocrine abnormalities, including stunted growth and precocious sexual development.[1] Mental retardation is not uncommon. Fibromas of the spinal cord can mimic cord transection. Intrathoracic fibromas and meningocele have been reported.[2]

Pharyngeal and laryngeal neurofibromatosis have occurred, resulting in airway obstruction, dyspnea, dysphonia, dysphagia, and the occasional need for tracheostomy.[4] Respiratory distress in a child of an affected parent should suggest this possibility.[5]

In patients with neurofibromatosis between 35 and 60 years of age, there can be as much as 20 per cent incidence of interstitial lung disease (fibrosing alveolitis). Pulmonary involvement may result in hypoxemia from ventilation-perfusion and diffusion abnormalities. Cor pulmonale, progressive respiratory failure, and death may occur.[6]

Visceral hypertrophy may result from plexiform neuromas of the autonomic nervous system. Pheochromocytoma occurs in as many as 1 per cent of patients. Involvement of the genitourinary system can result in obstruction and uremia. In obstetrical patients, obstructed labor from neurofibromas preventing vaginal delivery has been reported.[7]

In children, hypertension associated with neurofibromatosis is generally due to renal artery stenosis. In adults, hypertension associated with neurofibromatosis is generally due to pheochromocytoma.[1]

Subperiosteal fibromas can produce bone resorption and cyst formation with resultant fracture. Abnormalities of the vertebral column such as scoliosis or kyphoscoliosis are common.[3] Prolonged neuromuscular block in response to administration of succinylcholine, d-tubocurarine, and pancuronium has been reported in three patients.[8, 9]

Although the quality of life may be greatly altered, a normal life span is generally the rule unless malignancy develops, e.g., sarcomatous degeneration. Many patients with this disease require surgery for cosmetic reasons or excision of malignancy. Nerve decompression for paresthesias or pain may be required. Obstructive uropathy, renal artery stenosis, and pheochromocytoma require surgery. Reduction of pathologic fractures is sometimes necessary.

Guidelines for the anesthetic management of patients with neurofibromatosis are as follows:

1. Because of possible laryngeal involvement, meticulous evaluation of the airway is important preoperatively, including indirect laryngoscopy if necessary. Tracheostomy may be necessary.

2. Preoperative pulmonary evaluation is indicated in patients with kyphoscoliosis or chronic lung disease, and includes arterial blood gases and static and dynamic lung volumes and gas flow rates. Intraoperatively, frequent blood gas analysis may be necessary.

3. Examination of the back for deformities is essential when regional anesthesia is considered. Additionally, the anesthetist should consider the implications of the natural history of the disease, which includes the development of neurologic abnormalities. Asymptomatic intraspinal neurofibroma can make the identification and entry into the epidural or subarachnoid space difficult or impossible. Careful positioning and padding of pressure areas is important.

4. Preoperative determination of urinary catecholamine levels is recommended in all patients because of the association of pheochromocytoma. Appropriate drugs to treat a hypertensive crisis should be readily available.

5. The evaluation of pituitary function may be indicated.

6. Anesthetic drugs and techniques: No particular anesthetic drug or technique is recommended. In patients with spinal cord lesions above the mid-thoracic level, autonomic hyperreflexia is a potential complication.[10] In patients with muscle atrophy, avoidance of succinylcholine is recommended.[11] The reports of prolonged neuromuscular block following succinylcholine, d-tubocurarine, and pancuronium suggest careful evaluation of neuromuscular function postoperatively. Regional anesthesia (subarachnoid) has been used successfully.[12]

ERYTHEMA NODOSUM

The primary manifestation of erythema nodosum is the appearance of inflammatory cutaneous nodules on the extremities. The disease occurs most often between 15 and 30 years of age, affects females more than males (3:1), and is felt to be a hypersensitivity response to a variety of antigens.

There have been numerous antigens proposed for erythema nodosum, including infections such as streptococcus, tuberculosis, brucellosis,[1] leptospirosis,[2] toxoplasmosis, coccidioidomycosis, psittacosis,[3] and viruses; drugs (sulfonamides, oral contraceptives, phenytoin, and salicylates); and enteropathies. Behçet's syndrome has also been implicated.[3]

The clinical presentation includes a prodrome of fever, malaise, arthralgia, pain, and gastrointestinal disturbances. The nodules, which are multiple, bilateral, extremely tender, red, and slightly elevated, occur over the extensor surfaces of the limbs, particularly the lower extremities. Over a two to three week period the color changes from red to purple, resembling a bruise, and then to a yellow-green color. Ulceration of the nodules is rare, and healing occurs without a scar.[5] No mucosal involvement is reported.

In patients with joint involvement, effusion, swelling, and tenderness usually occur, although crippling arthritis is rare. Knees, ankles, wrists, fingers, elbows, shoulders, and hips may be involved.

Erythema nodosum is a self-limited disease resolving three to five weeks after onset. Any mortality is due to the associated underlying disease.

Treatment of erythema nodosum is directed at the cause, when known. Thus, appropriate antibiotics are indicated for bacterial, fungal, and viral infections. Known associated drugs should be discontinued. Bed rest, wet dressings to areas of nodule formation, and administration of salicylates (if not the cause) are important. Corticosteroids should be avoided if the cause is unknown. Potassium iodide has also been used.

Guidelines for the anesthetic management of patients with erythema nodosum are as follows:

1. Because of the possible infectious etiology of the disease, careful cleansing of all anesthetic equipment is mandatory. If possible, use disposable equipment.

2. Corticosteroids, unless specifically indicated, should be avoided because of the potential for an underlying infection.

3. If arthritis is present, careful evaluation of the airway is important. Care in positioning the patient is necessary.

4. Anesthetic drugs and techniques: No particular technique is recommended.

MASTOCYTOSIS

Mastocytosis is a disease in which there is an abnormal accumulation of mast cells in various organs of the body. Most commonly the mast cell proliferation occurs in the skin, appears as multiple reddish-brown or yellow macules, papules, or nodules, and is identified as *urticaria pigmentosa*.[1] Isolated dermal infiltrates (mastocytomas) can occur. Vesiculation and bulla formation in the skin are seen in lesions of children less than two years of age. Systemic mastocytosis involves multiple organs including bone, liver, spleen, lymph nodes, gastrointestinal tract, and skin. Mast cell leukemia can be a malignant form of this disease.

The pathophysiology of the disease is related to the substances that are stored in the mast cell, namely histamine and heparin. Histamine release in these patients can result in urticaria, pruritus, flushing, headache, abdominal cramps, vomiting, diarrhea, febrile episodes, or grand mal seizures. Systemic vascular dilatation can result in hypotension, tachycardia, dizziness, syncope, and cardiovascular collapse that may be profound and intractable. However, bronchospasm is unusual. Stimuli that may produce these signs and symptoms include mechanical irritation of the lesion, psychological stress, temperature change, alcohol consumption, vomiting, exercise, and histamine-releasing drugs.[1] Systemic heparin release may be responsible for the occasional hemorrhagic diathesis observed in patients with or without systemic mastocytosis.[2]

The development of mast cell leukemia results in severe anemia and thrombocytopenia, and is rapidly fatal. Hepatosplenomegaly occurs as a result of accumulation of mast cells in the liver and spleen. Hepatic involvement and gastrointestinal malabsorption results in decreased synthesis of coagulation factors. Diffuse lymphadenopathy may occur. Bone lesions can be osteoporotic or osteosclerotic, painful, commonly involve the pelvis, ribs, vertebrae, skull and long bones, and result in pathologic fractures. Lung tumors and pulmonary eosinophilic granuloma have been reported. Pulmonary function, however, is usually normal.[3]

Because there is no specific treatment for mastocytosis, therapy is directed toward relief of symptoms. Corticosteroids, ACTH, antihistamines, and antimetabolites have been used with variable results. Beta$_2$-adrenergic stimulants have proved useful in the treatment of chronic urticaria. Local irradiation for bone pain is sometimes helpful.[2]

Patients with mastocytosis may present for gastrointestinal surgery, splenectomy, thoracotomy and pulmonary resection, excision of isolated cutaneous lesions, and reduction of pathologic fractures as a result of the disease.

Guidelines for the anesthetic management of patients with mastocytosis are as follows:

1. In patients who have unexplained episodes of pruritus, urticaria, flushing, dizziness, and syncope, this disease must be suspected.

2. Preoperative laboratory data should include hemogram, platelet count, and evaluation of coagulation. Platelet transfusion, vitamin K and/or fresh frozen plasma may be necessary. Serum electrolyte values should be determined in patients with gastrointestinal disturbances.

3. Appropriate perioperative corticosteroid coverage is indicated in patients taking corticosteroids.

4. When bone involvement exists, movement and positioning of the patients must be accomplished with care because of the potential for fracture.

5. No specific anesthetic drugs or techniques are recommended owing to insufficient data in these patients. The prime concern, however, is avoidance of histamine release. Histamine release can occur spontaneously or from psychological, chemical, or physical stimuli. Therefore, adequate premedication to reduce anxiety and produce sedation is important and an antihistamine drug may be used as part of the premedication. Occasionally an antihistamine drug precipitates the release of histamine. Use of histamine-releasing drugs such as opiates, decamethonium, metocurine, curare, and dextran should be avoided. A histamine reaction has been reported with the use of a regional perfusion block of the upper extremity using lidocaine.[1] Sodium thiopental[4] and pancuronium[5] have been implicated in histamine release. Inhalational anesthetics do not appear to release histamine.

6. Rubbing of the skin should be minimized. Fluctuations in temperature should be avoided. Transfusion reactions that are minor in normal patients may be life-threatening in patients with mastocytosis.

7. Appropriate drug therapy to treat a histamine reaction, such as the catecholamines, antihistamines, bronchodilators and intravenous fluids, should be immediately available. Equipment for airway management is also necessary.

8. Although involvement of oral mucosa may occur, bulla formation has not been reported. Therefore, airway management should not be a problem.

MALIGNANT ATROPHIC PAPULOSIS (DEGO'S DISEASE)

Malignant atrophic papulosis (Dego's disease) is a rare, almost always fatal, multisystem disease characterized by multiple infarctions of the skin, gastrointestinal tract, and central nervous system. The heart, pericardium, lungs, pleura, eyes, and kidneys may also be involved. The vascular lesion is thought to be thromboangiitis obliterans, the etiology of which is unknown.[1]

The skin lesions appear as porcelain-white papules 2 to 5 mm in size, which subsequently form an atrophic scar. Gastrointestinal tract involvement usually results in perforation of the gut, peritonitis, and death. Lung and pleural involvement can result in pleuritis and pleural effusion with subsequent severe restrictive pulmonary disease. Constrictive pericarditis with calcification can occur.[2] Progressive central nervous system infarctions can result in cerebral edema, increased intracranial pressure, and uncal herniation.[3]

The patient with malignant atrophic papulosis usually presents as a surgical emergency with a perforated viscus and peritonitis. In some instances pulmonary decortication or pericardiectomy may be necessary.

Guidelines for the anesthetic management of patients with malignant atrophic papulosis are as follows:

1. Because of frequent peritonitis, large volumes of intravenous fluid may be required for adequate perioperative fluid resuscitation. Invasive cardiovascular monitoring may be necessary.

2. Because of potential pleural or pericardial involvement, these patients require special attention to the preoperative evaluation of pulmonary and cardiac function.

3. Anesthetic drugs and techniques: With extensive central nervous system involvement, cerebral edema may occur, with subsequent increased intracranial pressure. Under these circumstances anesthetic drugs and techniques that decrease intracranial

pressure should be used. Otherwise, no particular anesthetic drug or technique is recommended.

HEREDITARY ANHIDROTIC ECTODERMAL DYSPLASIA

Hereditary anhidrotic ectodermal dysplasia is a sex-linked recessive disorder characterized by ectodermal atrophy and malformations. Absent or decreased numbers of sweat glands result in hypohidrosis or anhidrosis and altered thermoregulation. Hypotrichosis (decreased amount of hair) and anodontia (absence of teeth) are characteristic. Underdeveloped maxillas and mandibles may be present. Lacrimation may be decreased or absent. An associated entodermal defect may result in absence of seromucous glands throughout the respiratory tract; this defect may result in frequent respiratory infections. Recurrent unexplained fever in infants and children may result from this disease.[2]

Guidelines for the anesthetic management of patients with hereditary anhidrotic ectodermal dysplasia are as follows:

1. The anesthesiologist should have a high index of suspicion that airway management, including an adequate mask fit and tracheal intubation, may be difficult because of the dental, maxillary, and mandibular abnormalities; appropriate alternative plans should be made in advance.

2. Hyperthermia may be a problem, owing to decreased thermoregulation. The patient's temperature should be monitored and the environment kept cool. In patients with hypohidrosis, use of anticholinergic drugs such as atropine, scopolamine, or glycopyrrolate with premedication should be avoided, and atropine or glycopyrrolate use with an anticholinesterase to reverse a nondepolarizing neuromuscular block could theoretically create additional heat loss problems.

3. The use of an ophthalmic ointment and taping the eyes closed are recommended because of decreased lacrimation.

4. The humidification of inspired gases is recommended because of associated decreased or absent respiratory tract mucous glands. Vigorous postoperative pulmonary care is necessary.

5. Anesthetic drugs and techniques: No particular anesthetic technique is recommended.

FABRY'S DISEASE: α GALACTOSIDASE A DEFICIENCY (ANGIOKERATOMA CORPORIS DIFFUSUM)

Fabry's disease is a sex-linked disease characterized by widespread deposition of glycosphingolipid in the vasculature of multiple organ systems including the skin, mucous membranes, eye, brain, heart, liver, and kidneys. Life expectancy is significantly reduced.

The cutaneous lesions, angiokeratomas, are ectasias of small vessels in the dermis and are found primarily in the scrotal, sacral, and umbilical areas, the thighs, fingers, toes, lips, and oral mucosa. Burning pain of the hands and feet is a cardinal symptom and is not usually relieved by analgesics.[1] Hypohidrosis and hypotrichosis (loss of hair) are also features of this disease. Acute febrile episodes have also occurred.

Ocular symptoms include corneal opacities, lens involvement, and tortuosity of conjunctival and retinal vessels. Central nervous system involvement causes presenile dementia, vertigo, myoclonic seizures, and pontine hemorrhages.[2] Cerebrovascular accidents occur often in early adult life. Cardiac involvement includes hypertension, angina pectoris, myocardial infarction,[3] and valvular disease (mitral insufficiency).[4] Accelerated atrioventricular conduction and paroxysmal atrial tachycardia have been reported.[5] Renal damage is frequently the most serious complication of the disease, resulting in proteinuria, edema, renal failure, uremia, and hypertension.

No specific therapy will correct the biochemical defect of the disease. Cardiac and renal failure must be treated symptomatically. Paresthesias and pain of the extremities have been controlled with oral administration of phenytoin.[1] Most males die between 40 and 50 years of age from renal failure or cerebrovascular accident. In females the course appears to be more benign.

Guidelines for the anesthetic management of patients with Fabry's disease are as follows:

1. Preoperative evaluation of cardiovascular and renal functions is necessary. Recent onset of peripheral edema or weight gain suggests either cardiac or renal failure. Angina pectoris is indicative of coronary artery involvement resulting in insufficient

myocardial oxygen supply and possible impending myocardial infarction. Cardiomegaly and ventricular hypertrophy may be demonstrated by chest roentgenogram and ECG. Laboratory tests including BUN, serum creatinine, and electrolytes, and the presence of albuminuria may indicate significant renal impairment.

2. Because of central and peripheral nervous system involvement, any preoperative neurological deficit should be well documented and considered before using regional anesthesia techniques.

3. Anesthetic drugs and techniques: No particular anesthetic technique is recommended. Lesions of the mouth are not sufficiently extensive to cause difficulty during airway instrumentation. If coronary artery disease is present, efforts to prevent large changes in blood pressure and heart rate are necessary. In patients with renal disease the avoidance of potentially nephrotoxic drugs such as methoxyflurane and enflurane[6] is recommended.

4. Stable environmental temperatures are recommended because of possible precipitation of extremity pain and acute febrile episodes in the presence of hypohidrosis. The avoidance of anticholinergic drugs is also recommended if hypohidrosis exists.

INCONTINENTIA PIGMENTI (BLOCH-SULZBERGER SYNDROME)

Incontinentia pigmenti is a hereditary disease that consists of dermatological, neurological, skeletal, ocular and dental defects. Inheritance is either by an autosomal dominant gene or by a sex-linked dominant gene, both of which are almost always lethal in males. Female patients are therefore far more common than males (37:1). The onset of the disease is from birth or within two weeks thereafter in 90 per cent of cases.[1]

Skin involvement, the most visible but least compromising organ pathology, is manifested by occurrence of trunk and extremity erythematous vesicular eruptions, followed by verrucous lesions and finally by irregular macules that have streaks and splashes of brown to slate-gray pigmentation. These skin lesions gradually resolve and are usually absent by adulthood.

Central nervous system involvement includes motor and psychomotor retardation, spastic paralysis of the diplegic, hemiplegic, and tetraplegic types, and seizures. Microcephaly, hydrocephalus, and cortical atrophy are reported.[1]

Ocular manifestations include strabismus, cataracts, retinitis proliferans, retrolental fibroplasia (without oxygen therapy as the cause), chorioretinitis, metastatic ophthalmitis, uveitis, retinal detachment, and optic nerve atrophy. Blindness is the usual result.

Skeletal abnormalities, though infrequent, include skull deformities, dwarfism, spina bifida, cleft lip and/or cleft palate, and chondrodystrophy. Growth of the mandible appears normal. Characteristic defects are partial anodontia and pegged (conical) deformity of the teeth.

Guidelines for anesthetic management of patients with incontinentia pigmenti are as follows:

1. Despite numerous physical abnormalities, technical difficulties relating to the administration of anesthesia are not reported. Because of the dental abnormalities, airway instrumentation must be performed gently. Since mandibular development is normal, laryngoscopy and tracheal intubation should not be unusually difficult.

2. Anesthetic drugs and techniques: No particular technique is recommended. With central nervous system involvement of spastic paralysis, succinylcholine should be used with caution because of the potential for serum potassium increases and dysrhythmias. Any preoperative neurological deficit should be well documented and considered before using regional anesthesia.

3. Autonomic hyperreflexia (mass reflex), which can result in acute severe hypertension, has not been previously reported in this disease. However, this complication remains a potential problem in patients with spinal cord injury.[2]

OSTEOPOROSIS, OSTEOMALACIA, AND OSTEOPETROSIS

Osteoporosis is a disorder of bone in which the overall quantity of bone substance is reduced without an alteration of the normal bone shape, composition, and morphology.[1] Other diseases with which osteoporosis is associated include hyperthyroidism, hyperparathyroidism, Cushing's syndrome, acromegaly, malabsorption, and malnutrition.[2] Long term corticosteroid therapy can also be an etiologic factor. The etiology is unknown. The defect usually requires several years to develop and occurs primarily and almost universally in the elderly and also in postmenopausal women.

The pathophysiology appears to be an imbalance between bone resorption and formation. As a result of the loss of bone substance, bone fractures occur more easily. The more common fractures include vertebral body with vertebral column compression, neck of the femur, distal radius, proximal humerus, and pelvis. Bone pain is a frequent symptom.[3] Severe kyphosis is not uncommon. Significant neurologic sequelae rarely occur.

Treatment is less than satisfactory, for long term results fail to show an increase in bone density. Drugs that have been used in therapy include estrogens, anabolic steroids, vitamin D, calcium, calcitonin, diphosphonates, and sodium fluoride. Patients may require surgical stabilization of fractures, but immobilization, other than local splinting, should be kept to a minimum, since it will worsen the condition.

Osteomalacia is a metabolic bone disorder in which normal bone is replaced by nonmineralized osteoid tissue. The soft resultant pliable bones are easily deformed or fractured. Etiologic factors include vitamin D deficiency (malabsorption, abnormal liver and/or kidney metabolism), hypocalcemia, hypophosphatemia, and hypophosphatasia. Major symptoms include bone pain, bone tenderness, and muscle weakness. Paresthesias, muscle cramps, and tetany may occur as a result of severe associated hypocalcemia. Scoliosis and kyphosis may be present. Roentgenographic signs include a nonspecific decrease in radiodensity of bone and pseudofracture (Looser's zone). Therapy includes adequate nutrition, calcium, phosphate, vitamin D, sun exposure, correction of abnormalities of the gastrointestinal and biliary tracts if present, removal of tumors if present, and renal transplantation if renal failure is present.[4] Unlike osteoporosis, the response to treatment in osteomalacia is usually good. Previously incapacitated patients may become asymptomatic in two or three months. If, however, osteoporosis is also present, skeletal recovery may not be complete and the risk of fractures remains.

The *osteopetroses* (abnormally dense bone) are now recognized as a hereditary group of disorders characterized by various combinations of bony sclerosis and modeling defects. Inheritance can be autosomal dominant or recessive. Present classification into four major categories includes: 1) osteosclerosis (hard, dense bone); 2) craniotubular dysplasia; 3) craniotubular hyperostoses and hypertrophy of bone; and 4) miscellaneous sclerosing and hyperostotic disorders.[5] Knowledge of the variable degrees of bone fragility, muscle weakness, scoliosis, and cranial, facial bone, and mandibular (micro- or macrognathia) involvement is important. In *sclerosteosis*, progressive overgrowth of the skull may cause increased intracranial pressure. Sudden death from brainstem herniation through the foramen magnum has been reported in adults.[6]

Guidelines for the anesthetic management of patients with osteoporosis, osteomalacia, or osteopetrosis are as follows:

1. Because of the increased risk of bone fracture, these patients must be moved and positioned carefully. Padding of all pressure areas is recommended.

2. The knowledge of any existing metabolic or endocrine disorders and their anesthetic implications in these patients prior to surgery is important.

3. If kyphoscoliosis is present, an evaluation of the patient's pulmonary function is recommended.

4. In patients with sclerosteosis, the potential for increased intracranial pressure must be remembered, and anesthetic techniques that will either decrease or not cause an increase in intracranial pressure should be considered.

5. Anesthetic drugs and techniques: With the exception of sclerosteosis, no particular anesthetic drugs or techniques are recommended. The presence of vertebral compression may make the use of regional techniques (e.g., subarachnoid, epidural) difficult. Any preoperative neurologic deficit should be well documented.

OSTEOGENESIS IMPERFECTA

Osteogenesis imperfecta is a rare inherited disease with many different systemic manifestations. Although the disease is a generalized connective tissue disorder with many organs affected, it is considered primarily a dwarfing syndrome. The primary bone lesion is the lack of normal ossification of the endochondral bone, resulting in very fragile bones. Classically two major clinical types are recognized: 1) osteogenesis imperfecta congenita (fetal type), in which skeletal fractures with resulting deformities occur in utero and therefore are present at birth, and 2) osteogenesis imperfecta tarda, in which skeletal fractures and deformities occur after birth. Further classification depends in part upon the presence of blue sclera and/or hearing loss.[1] Of particular interest to anesthesiologists is the fact that mandibular fractures occur more frequently in these patients than in the normal population; however, facial bone fractures do not.[2]

Other abnormalities associated with osteogenesis imperfecta include hyperthermia, hyperhidrosis, platelet cell dysfunction,[3] easy bruisability, bleeding, kyphoscoliosis, cor pulmonale, congenital heart disease, valvular heart disease,[4] joint laxity, thin skin, and dentinogenesis imperfecta.[5] Hyperthermia and hyperhidrosis appear to be secondary to either an abnormal central nervous system temperature regulating mechanism or abnormal cellular energy metabolism.[3] Platelet dysfunction is due to decreased release of platelet factor 3 and platelet adhesiveness; this may be due to immature platelets,[3] since the platelet count is normal. Kyphoscoliosis may cause significant mechanical pulmonary disease resulting in cor pulmonale.[2] Additional thoracic deformities may include pectus carinatum and pectus excavatum. Cardiac lesions include patent ductus arteriosus, atrial septal defect, ventricular septal defect, and mitral and/or aortic insufficiency.[5] Usually valvular stenosis occurs only following a bacterial endocarditis.[4]

Guidelines for the anesthetic management of patients with osteogenesis imperfecta are as follows:

1. When moving the patient to and from the operating table or turning and positioning the patient, care must be exercised to avoid fractures. Padding all pressure areas is recommended.

2. If airway management requires the use of a face mask or laryngoscopy and tracheal intubation, care must be exercised to avoid mandibular or facial bone fracture.

3. Unusual bleeding may require platelet transfusion.

4. Elective surgery should be postponed in patients with preoperative hyperthermia. One report demonstrated a rise in temperature to 102° F following induction of anesthesia without muscle rigidity which was controlled by use of a cooling blanket, cold intravenous solutions, and high fresh gas flows. Following operation, temperatures returned to preanesthetic levels.[6] Thus, even if a patient is normothermic preoperatively, he or she should be closely monitored for temperature elevation intraoperatively. A cool environment is recommended. A cooling blanket should be placed on the operating table. Cold solutions for intravenous administration should be available.

5. The presence of cardiac lesions and thoracic cage deformities requires careful cardiac and pulmonary function evaluation.

6. Anesthetic drugs and techniques. No particular anesthetic technique is recommended. Use of anticholinergic drugs should be avoided because of the possible exacerbation of hyperthermia. Ketamine has been used both intramuscularly and intravenously with success.[7]

DWARFISM

Dwarfism is a disease with a variety of presentations so that more than 55 distinct syndromes with many subtypes have been described. Many cases of dwarfism have not yet been classified. Patients with these syndromes are placed into two major categories: those with disproportionate short stature, "dwarfs," and those with proportionate short stature, "midgets." Further subdivision is made according to the abnormal development of bone and/or cartilage (osteochondrodysplasias) or malformations of individual bones (dysostoses). The distinction is made between involvement of the appendicular skeleton (short limbs) and the axial skeleton (short trunk). Classification according to the roentgenographic evidence of bone involvement (epiphyseal, metaphyseal, or diaphyseal) is used. The prefix spondylo- refers to spine involvement. Rhizomelic (proximal segment), mesomelic (middle segment), and acromelic (distal segment) shortening refers to the affected segments of long bones. A distinction is made according to mode of inheritance, e.g., X-linked versus autosomal.[1]

The etiology for most of the skeletal dysplasias is unknown. Known etiologic factors include nutritional disorders, chromosomal aberrations, primary metabolic abnormalities, and endocrine, hematologic, neurologic, renal, gastrointestinal, and cardiopulmonary disorders.[2, 3] Diagnosis is based primarily upon clinical and roentgenographic findings. Except for a few syndromes (e.g., mucopolysaccharidoses, hypophosphatasia, mucolipidoses, and hypercalciuria), biochemical procedures are of little value in the diagnosis.

Major abnormalities that may be present in patients with dwarfism and that the anesthesiologist should be aware of are as follows:

1. Atlantoaxial instability
2. Spinal stenosis
3. Airway and facial abnormalities
4. Thoracic dystrophy
5. Scoliosis, kyphosis, lordosis
6. Congenital cardiac disease
7. Hydrocephaly
8. Mental retardation
9. Seizure disorders

Dwarfed patients may require anesthesia for the surgical correction of many of these abnormalities.

1. *Atlanto-axial instability* can result from a normal, hypoplastic, aplastic, or detached odontoid process and varying degrees of ligamentous laxity. Dwarfing syndromes in which odontoid dysgenesis[2-4] has been found are as follows:

a. Spondyloepiphyseal dysplasia tarda
b. Spondyloepiphyseal dysplasia congenita
c. Achondroplasia
d. Pseudoachondroplasia
e. Pseudo-Morquio's syndrome (non-keratin secreting)
f. Multiple epiphyseal dysplasia congenita
g. Morquio's mucopolysaccharidosis
h. Metatrophic dwarfism
i. Spondylometaphyseal dysplasia (Murdock)
j. Spondylometaphyseal dysplasia (Kozlowski)
k. Metaphyseal chondrodysplasia (McKusick, cartilage-hair hypoplasia)
l. Kniest dwarfism

The classic symptoms of atlantoaxial instability are progressive weakness, hypotonia, neuromuscular disturbances (spasticity, clonus, hyperreflexia, Babinski sign), para-

plegia, quadriplegia, and on occasion sudden death. An evaluation of the atlantoaxial joint should be made in the dwarf who exhibits any of the following:[2] a) dwarfism of the osteochondrodystrophy group; b) a disproportionately short trunk; c) vertebral body involvement seen roentgenographically; d) congenital stippled epiphyses; e) decreasing physical endurance. Present recommended treatment is surgical fusion.[5, 6]

2. *Spinal stenosis* describes a syndrome that results from a narrowed spinal canal such that the contents of the canal completely fill the available space.[7, 8] As a result, symptoms and signs of spinal cord and nerve root compression occur, for example, weakness, paralysis, cauda equina syndrome. High cervical cord compression due to stenosis of the foramen magnum may occur. Treatment is decompression laminectomy and/or decompression of the foramen magnum. Spinal stenosis most often occurs in achondroplastic dwarfism but may also occur in Morquio's syndrome and diastrophic dwarfism.

3. *Airway management difficulty* may result from hypoplasia of the mandible or micrognathia, cleft palate, and cleft lip. Hypoplastic mandible is associated with the following dwarfing syndromes:[2, 3]

a. Acrocephalopolysyndactyly type II (Carpenter)
b. Idiopathic hypercalcemic syndrome
c. Mesomelia (Langer)
d. Metaphyseal chondrodysplasia (Jansen)
e. Cri du chat
f. Antimongolism
g. Oculomandibulodyscephaly (Hallermann-Streiff)
h. Ring-4 chromosome syndrome
i. Trisomy 22
j. Craniocarpotarsal dystrophy (Freeman-Sheldon, whistling face syndrome)

4. *Thoracic dystrophy* is a deformity of the trunk characterized by a small narrow contracted chest cage, marked shortening of the ribs, thoracic lordosis, and segmentation defects of the vertebrae. The dwarfing syndromes involving lethal thoracic dystrophy include thanatophoric dwarfism, achondrogenesis and short rib, thoracic dystrophy polydactyly syndrome (Majewski, Salvino-Noonan). In these syndromes death occurs in the newborn period. A second group denoted as surviving thoracic dystrophy in-

cludes asphyxiating thoracic dystrophy (Jeune), metatrophic dwarfism, chondroectodermal dysplasia (Ellis-van Creveld), and spondylothoracic dysplasia. These infants are plagued with ventilatory problems from birth, frequent pneumonias and a high mortality. However, several of the second group have survived and often present severe problems of management because of the spinal curves and decreased ventilatory capacity.[5]

5. *Scoliosis* and kyphoscoliosis occur frequently and vary from mild to severe. The short trunk causes severe crowding of the normal sized abdominal viscera and general congestion of the intrathoracic and intra-abdominal contents. Severe scoliosis compounds these problems. As a result, pulmonary and cardiovascular functions in the dwarf can be severely impaired.[5, 9] Kyphosis and lordosis may progress to produce spinal cord compression. These conditions may require surgery for correction or stabilization.

6. *Congenital cardiac disease* (patent ductus arteriosus, atrial septal defects, coarctation of the aorta) is associated with thanatophoric dwarfism and achondrogenesis. Chondroectodermal dysplasia (Ellis-van Creveld syndrome) is associated with large atrial septal defects.[3]

7,8,9. *Central nervous system* involvement can include mental retardation, hydrocephaly and seizure disorders.[1, 3]

Guidelines for the anesthetic management of patients with dwarfing syndromes are as follows:

1. Stability of the atlantoaxial joint should be evaluated by history, neurologic examination, and appropriate lateral flexion and extension roentgenographic views of the cervical spine. Tomography, cineradiography, and gas myelography may be necessary. Should atlantoaxial instability be present, procedures to insure protection of the spinal cord must be used.[10] Cervical spine extension is generally maintained in symptomatic patients. Efforts to keep this position during the induction and maintenance of anesthesia should be made. Application of cervical stabilizing devices such as a halo cast or plaster bed should be considered.[11]

2. Regional anesthesia (subarachnoid and epidural) has been used successfully in dwarfs without apparent neurologic sequelae. However, because of the potential for development of neurologic problems due to spinal stenosis and vertebral malalignment, regional anesthesia should be reserved for patients in whom there is a specific indication and in whom the immediate advantages of regional techniques outweigh other alternatives.[12] Any preoperative neurologic deficit should be well documented.

3. Careful evaluation of the patient's airway must be made to assess the ease or difficulty with which tracheal intubation could be performed if necessary. Appropriate equipment must be available (fiberoptic bronchoscope) for tracheal intubation in the patient with a "difficult airway."[13]

4. Ventilatory problems may occur in patients with thoracic dystrophy and/or vertebral malalignment. These patients may need mechanical ventilatory assistance and may be difficult to wean from it.

5. Cardiac defects, mental retardation, hydrocephaly, or seizures must be considered in the design of the anesthetic technique to be used.

6. Autonomic hyperreflexia is a potential problem in patients who have spinal cord lesions resulting from spinal stenosis or vertebral malalignment.[14] Appropriate drugs (α and β blockers, vasodilators) must be immediately available.

7. Anesthetic drugs: no particular anesthetic drug appears to be contraindicated for use in patients with dwarfing syndromes.

Comment: The major complications of dwarfism with implications for the anesthetic management of these patients have been considered. For a more detailed discussion of the individual syndromes, the reader is referred to three recent publications.[1, 2, 3]

CRANIOFACIAL AND MANDIBULOFACIAL DYSOSTOSES

Several syndromes that are characterized by abnormalities of the skull, facial bones, and mandible are frequently not associated with dwarfism. Most of these patients are from the pediatric population.

Apert's syndrome (acrocephalosyndactyly) is characterized by craniosynostosis, high forehead, flat bridge of the nose, maxillary hypoplasia, relative mandibular prognathism, synostosis of the cervical spine, visceral malformations, and congenital heart defects.[1, 2]

Crouzon's syndrome is characterized by

craniosynostosis, maxillary hypoplasia, relative mandibular prognathism, and a prominent nose, "parrot beak." Increased intracranial pressure has been found in these patients.[2]

Goldenhar's syndrome (oculoauriculovertebral dysplasia) is characterized by eye and ear abnormalities, micrognathia, maxillary hypoplasia, cleft or high arched palate, synostosis of the cervical spine, and congenital heart defects.[1, 3]

Treacher Collins syndrome (Franceschetti-Zwahlen-Klein) is characterized by antimongoloid obliquity of the palpebral fissures, coloboma, microphthalmia, choanal atresia, hypoplasia of the zygoma, maxillary, and mandibular bones, deafness, congenital heart defects, and occasionally dwarfism.[1, 4]

Pierre Robin syndrome is characterized by severe micrognathia, cleft palate, and glossoptosis (tongue forced back into the airway channel) resulting in life threatening airway obstruction. Respiratory distress and cyanosis occur most frequently when the infant is placed supine and are generally relieved when the infant is placed prone or up on its side. Nasoesophageal intubation has been effective in attenuating the respiratory distress.[5] As the child grows older, the glossoptosis decreases and the respiratory distress resolves owing to a relatively increased rate of growth of the mandible.

Meckel syndrome consists of microcephaly, cleft palate, cleft tongue and epiglottis, micrognathia, congenital heart defects, and renal abnormalities, and is usually fatal in infancy as a result of renal insufficiency.[6]

Osteodysplasty (Melnick-Needles syndrome) is characterized by exophthalmos, full cheeks, micrognathia, and malalignment of the teeth.[6]

Hanhart syndrome is characterized by micrognathia and a variety of limb abnormalities.[6]

Aglossia adactylia consists of a small or absent tongue, micrognathia, and variable limb abnormalities.[6]

Oral-facial-digital syndrome is characterized by hypoplasia of the nasal alae, micrognathia, lobate tongue, cleft lip, and a high arched cleft palate.[6]

Hemifacial microsomia is characterized by unilateral facial involvement. One side of the mandible may be hypoplastic or absent. The mouth and face show marked asymmetry. Hypoplasia or agenesis of the lung on the affected side may occur.[1]

Guidelines for the anesthetic management of patients with various craniofacial dysostoses are as follows:

1. The necessity for careful evaluation of the airway is usually very obvious by simply observing the patient. Hypoplasia of the maxillary bones (midface) may result in a difficult mask fit. Micrognathia with the receding chin can make the visualization of the larynx impossible during attempted direct laryngoscopy. Temporomandibular joint dysfunction may prevent wide opening of the jaws. Cervical vertebral synostosis may prevent flexion or extension of the neck. Choanal atresia or hypoplasia may be present, preventing the use of blind nasotracheal intubation.

Methods for tracheal intubation may include the use of the fiberoptic laryngoscope, the optical stylet, direct palpation of the epiglottis followed by "blind" oro- or nasotracheal intubation and transtracheal passage of a "guidewire" retrogradely into the oropharynx.

2. Evaluation of the patient for abnormalities of the heart, lungs, and other visceral organs must be done.

3. Patients with craniosynostoses may also have increased intracranial pressure.[2]

4. Anesthetic drugs and techniques: No particular drug is recommended. Techniques that allow spontaneous ventilation by the patient until the anesthetist is certain the airway can be managed (with a mask if necessary) are recommended. Only then, if at all, should muscle relaxants be used to facilitate tracheal intubation.[1] Awake oral or "blind" nasotracheal (when the nares are patent) intubation is a viable alternative. The surgeon and tracheostomy equipment should be present during the induction of anesthesia. Tracheostomy with local anesthesia prior to the induction of anesthesia may be necessary.

PAGET'S DISEASE (OSTEITIS DEFORMANS)

Paget's disease is a metabolic disorder of unknown etiology characterized by excessively rapid remodeling of bone.[1] Three phases are recognized in this remodeling process. First, an intense resorption of existing bone occurs by increased osteoclast activity. Second, the deposition of new bone occurs by increased osteoblast activity.

Third, as bone resorption begins to decrease, continued bone formation results in sclerotic areas of bones (the roentgenographic "cotton wool" appearance of bone) which are weak and fracture easily.

Most patients present with bone pain and fractures at the sites of involvement. Areas most frequently affected include the pelvis, femur, skull, tibia, and vertebrae. Symptoms and signs of spinal cord compression can occur from vertebral fracture, atlantoaxial instability,[2] and basilar invagination of the skull. Hydrocephalic dementia[3] and death from cerebellar tonsillar herniation[4] resulting from basilar invagination of the skull have occurred. Hearing loss is common. Severe kyphosis may be present.

Cardiac output may be greatly increased owing to the increased vascularity of the affected areas of bone, and high output congestive heart failure may result. Arteriovenous anastomotic shunting does not appear to be the cause of the increased cardiac output.[5] With treatment and resolution of Paget's disease, cardiac output may return to normal.[6]

Treatment of Paget's disease has included high dose salicylates and corticosteroids for short periods (side effects have precluded long term use of these drugs). Calcitonin, mithramycin, and diphosphonates are also used.

Guidelines for the anesthetic management of patients with Paget's disease are as follows:

1. Careful moving and positioning of the patient is required because fractures may occur with even mild trauma. Padding of all pressure areas is recommended.

2. Preoperative evaluation of atlantoaxial stability is recommended. If instability is present, extreme care must be used to maintain a neutral position of the cervical spine, particularly if laryngoscopy and tracheal intubation are performed.

3. In patients with kyphosis, pulmonary function should be evaluated. Patients with decreased pulmonary reserve may require postoperative mechanical ventilatory assistance.

4. Evaluation of the cardiovascular system for the presence of high output congestive heart failure should be performed. If heart failure is present, elective operations should be postponed until the failure can be corrected.

5. Anesthetic drugs and techniques: No particular anesthetic drug or technique is recommended. The presence of vertebral compression may make the use of regional techniques (e.g., subarachnoid, epidural) difficult.

6. Autonomic hyperreflexia is a potential complication in patients with spinal cord injury.[7]

7. Appropriate perioperative corticosteroid coverage is recommended for those patients taking corticosteroids preoperatively.

8. Platelet function should be evaluated in patients taking salicylates.

FIBROUS DYSPLASIA

Fibrous dysplasia is a disorder of unknown etiology characterized by expanding fibro-osseous lesions in bone. The three major types are: 1) monostotic, single bone involvement; 2) polyostotic, multiple bone involvement; and 3) Albright's syndrome with multiple bone involvement, cutaneous pigmentation, endocrine dysfunction, and precocious puberty in females.[1, 2] The major skeletal defect in fibrous dysplasia is a weakened structural integrity, and fractures are produced frequently by mild trauma. Clinical features include pain, fracture, deformity, or an enlarging mass. A painful lesion signals impending fracture, enlargement of the fibrino-osseous mass, or a malignant change, which is rare.

Craniofacial involvement with grotesque facial deformity is not uncommon.[3, 4] Spine involvement, although unusual, includes vertebral collapse or an expanding fibro-osseous mass.[1, 5] Weakness, spasticity, and paralysis may result. Associated endocrine dysfunction includes acromegaly, hyperparathyroidism, hyperthyroidism, and Cushing's syndrome. Treatment is symptomatic, e.g., fracture reduction and stabilization and reconstruction for deformity and treatment of endocrine dysfunction.

Guidelines for the anesthetic management of patients with fibrous dysplasia are as follows:

1. Careful movement, turning, and positioning of the patient are required because fractures occur with even mild trauma. Padding of all pressure areas is recommended. Laryngoscopy and tracheal intubation must

be performed gently to avoid mandibular fracture.

2. With extensive maxillomandibular involvement, airway management may prove to be difficult. Direct laryngoscopy may be impossible. Indirect laryngoscopy is recommended to evaluate the epiglottis and laryngeal inlet. Awake "blind" nasotracheal intubation, fiberoptic laryngoscopy, or use of an intubating bronchoscope[4] may be necessary. Tracheostomy may be required.

3. Any existing endocrine disorder must be evaluated preoperatively and the anesthetic implications considered.

4. Anesthetic drugs and techniques: No particular technique is recommended. In patients with spinal cord injury, regional anesthesia (subarachnoid, epidural, regional nerve block) should be used with extreme caution. Any preoperative neurologic deficit should be well documented.

5. Autonomic hyperreflexia is a potential complication in patients with spinal cord lesions.[6]

REFERENCES

Epidermolysis Bullosa

1. Bauer, E. A., and Briggaman, R. A.: The mechanobullous diseases (epidermolysis bullosa). *In* Fitzpatrick, T. B. (ed.): Dermatology in General Medicine. 2nd ed., New York, McGraw-Hill Book Co., 1979, p. 334.
2. Berryhill, R. E., Benumof, J. L., Saidman, L. J., et al.: Anesthetic management of emergency cesarean section in a patient with epidermolysis bullosa dystrophica polydysplastica. Anesth. Analg. 57:281, 1977.
3. Cohen, S. R., Landing, B. H., and Issacs, H.: Epidermolysis bullosa associated with laryngeal stenosis. Ann. Otol. Rhinol. Laryngol. 87:25, 1978.
4. Reddy, A. R. R., and Wong, D. H. W.: Epidermolysis bullosa, a review of anaesthetic problem and case reports. Canad Anaesth. Soc. J. 19:536, 1972.
5. Pratilar, V., and Biezumski, A.: Epidermolysis bullosa manifested and treated during anesthesia. Anesthesiology 45:581, 1975.
6. Ramadass, T., and Thangavelu, T. A.: Epidermolysis bullosa and its ENT manifestations. J. Laryng. Otol. 92:441, 1978.
7. Petty, W. C., and Gunther, R. C.: Anesthesia for nonfacial surgery in polydysplastic epidermolysis bullosa (dystrophic). Anesth. Analg. 49:246, 1970.
8. Fisk, G. C., and Kern, I. B.: Anesthesia for oesophagoscopy in a child with epidermolysis bullosa — a case report. Anaesth. Intens. Care 1:297, 1973.

9. Tio, T. H., Waardenberg, P. J., and Vermeullen, H. J.: Blood coagulation in epidermolysis bullosa hereditaria. Arch. Derm. 88:76, 1963.
10. LoVerne, S. R., and Oropollo, A. T.: Ketamine anesthesia in dermolytic bullosus disease (epidermolysis bullosa). Anesth. Analg. 56:398, 1977.

Pemphigus

1. Jordan, R. E.: Pemphigus. *In* Fitzpatrick, T. B. (ed.): Dermatology in General Medicine. 2nd ed., New York, McGraw-hill Book Co., 1979, p. 310.
2. Lever, W. F., and Schaumburg-Lever, G.: Immunosuppressants and prednisone in pemphigus vulgaris. Arch. Derm. 113:1236, 1977.
3. Cotterill, J. A., Barker, D. J., Millard, L. G., and Robinson, E. A.: Plasma exchange in the treatment of pemphigus vulgaris. Brit. J. Derm. 98:243, 1978.
4. Lever, W. F.: Familial benign pemphigus. *In* Fitzpatrick, T. B. (ed.): Dermatology in General Medicine. 2nd ed. New York, McGraw-Hill Book Co., 1979, pp. 331–334.
5. Jordan, R. E.: Bullous pemphigoid, cicatricial pemphigoid and chronic bullous dermatosis of childhood. *In* Fitzpatrick, T. B. (ed.): Dermatology in General Medicine. 2nd ed. New York, McGraw-Hill Book Co., 1979 p. 318.
6. Piamphongsant, T.: Bullous pemphigoid in childhood: Report of three cases and a review of literature. Int. J. Dermatol. 16:126, 1977.
7. Obasi, O. E., and Savin, J. A.: Pemphigoid and pernicious anaemia. Brit. Med. J. 2:1458, 1977.
8. Hamilton, D. V., and McKenzie, A. W.: Bullous pemphigoid and primary biliary cirrhosis. Brit. J. Derm. 99:447, 1978.
9. Epstein, F. W., and Bohn, M.: Dapsone-induced peripheral neuropathy. Arch. Derm. 112:1761, 1976.
10. Jeyaram, C., and Torda, T. A.: Anesthetic management of cholecystectomy in a patient with buccal pemphigus. Anesthesiology 40:600, 1975.

Erythema Multiforme

1. Elias, P. M., and Fritsch, O. P.: Erythema multiforme. *In* Fitzpatrick, T. B. (ed.): Dermatology in General Medicine. 2nd ed., New York, McGraw-Hill Book Co., 1979, pp. 295–303.
2. Chanda, J. J., and Callen, J. P.: Erythema multiforme and the Stevens-Johnson syndrome. South. Med. J. 71:566, 1978.
3. Broadbent, R. V.: Stevens-Johnson disease presenting with pneumothorax. Rocky Mountain Med. J. 64:69, 1967.
4. Cucchiara, R. F., and Dawson, B.: Anesthesia in Stevens-Johnson syndrome: Report of a case. Anesthesiology 35:537, 1971.
5. Schartum, S.: Stevens-Johnson syndrome with cardiac involvement. Acta Med. Scand. 179:729, 1966.
6. Eichhorn, J. J., Hedley-Whyte, J., Steinman, T., Kaufman, J. M., and Laasberg, L. H.: Renal failure following enflurane anesthesia. Anesthesiology 45:557, 1976.

Toxic Epidermal Necrolysis

1. Lyell, A.: Toxic epidermal necrolysis (the scalded skin syndrome): A reappraisal. Brit. J. Derm. *100*:69, 1979.
2. Krumlovsky, F. A., Del Greco, F., Herdson, P. B., and Lazar, P.: Renal disease associated with toxic epidermal necrolysis (Lyell's disease). Amer. J. Med. *57*:817, 1974.
3. Stuttgen, G.: Toxic epidermal necrolysis provoked by barbiturates. Brit. J. Derm. *88*:291, 1973.
4. Pollack, M. A., Burk, P. G., and Nathanson, G.: Mucocutaneous eruptions due to antiepileptic drug therapy in children. Ann. Neurol. *5*:262, 1979.
5. Fritsch, O. P., and Elias, P. M.: Toxic epidermal necrolysis. *In* Fitzpatrick, T. B. (ed.): Dermatology in General Medicine. 2nd ed., New York, McGraw-Hill Book Co., 1979, pp. 303–306.
6. Hunter, J. A. A., and Davison, A. M.: Toxic epidermal necrolysis associated with pentazocine therapy and severe reversible renal failure. Brit. J. Derm. *88*:287, 1973.

Staphylococcal Scalded Skin Syndrome

1. Melish, M. E., and Glasgow, L. A.: Staphylococcal scalded skin syndrome. The expanded clinical syndrome. J. Pediatr. *78*:958, 1971.
2. Lyell, A.: Toxic epidermal necrolysis (the scalded skin syndrome): A reappraisal. Brit. J. Derm. *100*:69, 1979.
3. Elias, P. M., and Fritsch, P. O.: Staphylococcal scalded-skin syndrome. *In* Fitzpatrick, T. B. (ed.): Dermatology in General Medicine. 2nd ed., New York, McGraw-Hill Book Co., 1979, pp. 306–310.

Behçet's Disease

1. Mason, R. M., and Barnes, C. G.: Behçet's syndrome with arthritis. Ann. Rheum. Dis. *28*:95, 1969.
2. Turner, M. E.: Anesthetic difficulties associated with Behçet's syndrome. Brit. J. Anaesth. *44*:100, 1972.
3. Chajeh, T., and Fainarn, M.: Behçet's disease. Report of 41 cases and a review of the literature. Medicine *54*:179, 1975.
4. Kozin, F., Haughton, V., and Bernhard, G. C.: Neuro-Behçet disease: Two cases and neuroradiologic findings. Neurology *27*:1148, 1977.
5. Roguin, N., Haim, S., Reshef, R., Peleg, E., and Riss, E.: Cardiac involvement and superior vena caval obstruction in Behçet's disease. Thorax *33*:375, 1978.
6. Cadman, E. C., Lundberg, U. B., and Mitchell, M. S.: Pulmonary manifestations in Behçet's syndrome. Arch. Int. Med. *136*:944, 1976.
7. Ahonen, A. V., Stenius-Aarniala, B. S. M., Viljanen, B. C., et al.: Obstructive lung disease in Behçet's syndrome. Scand. J. Resp. Dis. *59*:44, 1978.
8. Cooperman, L. H.: Succinylcholine-induced hyperkalemia in neuromuscular disease. J.A.M.A. *213*:1867, 1970.

9. Basta, J. W., Niedjadlik, K., and Pallares, V.: Autonomic hyperreflexia: Intraoperative control with pentolinium tartrate. Brit. J. Anesth. *49*:1087, 1977.

Scleroderma

1. Siegel, R. C.: Scleroderma. Med. Clin. North. Am. *61*:283, 1977.
2. Fleilschmajer, R.: The pathophysiology of scleroderma. Int. J. Derm. *16*:310, 1977.
3. Weisman, R. A., and Calcaterra, T. C.: Head and neck manifestations of scleroderma. Ann. Otol. *87*:332, 1978.
4. Young, R. H., and Mark, G. J.: Pulmonary vascular changes in scleroderma. Am. J. Med. *64*:998, 1978.
5. Guttadauria, M., Ellman, H., Emmanuel, G., Kaplan, D., and Diamond, H.: Pulmonary function in scleroderma. Arthritis Rheum. *20*:1071, 1977.
6. Bulkley, B. H., Klacsmann, P. G., and Hutchins G. M.: Angina pectoris, myocardial infarction and sudden cardiac death with normal coronary arteries: A clinicopathologic study of 9 patients with progressive systemic sclerosis. Am. Heart J. *95*:563, 1978.
7. LeRoy, E. C., and Fleischmann, R. M.: The management of renal scleroderma: Experience with dialysis, nephrectomy and transplantation. Am. J. Med. *64*:974, 1978.
8. Winterbauer, R. H.: Multiple telangiectasis, Raynaud's phenomenon, sclerodactyly, and subcutaneous calcinosis: A syndrome mimicking hereditary hemorrhagic telangiectasia. Johns Hopkins Hosp. Bull. *114*:361, 1964.
9. Eichhorn, J. H., Hedley-Whyte, J., Steinman, T. I., Kaufmann, J. M., and Laasberg, L. H.: Renal failure following enflurane anesthesia. Anesthesiology *45*:557, 1976.
10. Eisele, J. H., and Reitan, J. A.: Scleroderma, Raynaud's phenomenon and local anesthetics. Anesthesiology *34*:386, 1971.
11. Lewis, G. B. H.: Prolonged regional analgesia in scleroderma. Canad. Anaesth. J. *21*:495, 1974.

Psoriasis

1. Farber, E. M., and VanScott, E. J.: Psoriasis. *In* Fitzpatrick T. B. (ed.): Dermatology in General Medicine, 2nd ed., New York, McGraw-Hill Book Co., 1979, pp. 233–247.
2. Fox, R. H., Shuster, S., Williams, R., Marks, J., Goldsmith, R., and Condon, R. E.: Cardiovascular, metabolic and thermoregulatory disturbances in patients with erythrodermic skin diseases. Brit. Med. J. *1*:619, 1965.
3. Raza, A., Maiback, H. I., and Mandel, A.: Bacterial flora in psoriasis. Brit. J. Derm. *95*:603, 1976.
4. Marples, R. R., Heaton, C. L., and Kligman, A. M.: *Staphylococcus aureus* in psoriasis. Arch. Derm. *107*:568, 1973.
5. Payne, R. W.: Severe outbreak of surgical sepsis due to *Staphylococcus aureus* of unusual type and origin. Brit. Med. J. *4*:17, 1967.

Neurofibromatosis

1. Wander, J. V., and Das Gupta, T. K.: Neurofibromatosis. Curr. Prob. Surg. *14*:11, 27, 51, 70, 1977.
2. Leech, R. W.: Intrathoracic meningocele and vertebral anomalies in a case of neurofibromatosis. Surg. Neurol. *9*:55, 1978.
3. Chaglassian, J. H., Riseborogh, E. J., and Hall, J. E.: Neurofibromatous scoliosis. J. Bone Joint Surg. *58A*:695, 1976.
4. Chang-lo, M.: Laryngeal involvement in Von Recklinghausen's disease: A case report and review of the literature. Laryngoscope *87*:435, 1977.
5. Cohen, S. R., Landing, B. H., and Isaacs, H.: Neurofibroma of the larynx in a child. Ann. Otol. Rhinol. Laryngol. *87*:29, 1978.
6. Sagel, S. S., Foreest, J. V., and Askin, F. B.: Interstitial lung disease in neurofibromatosis. South. Med. J. *68*:647, 1975.
7. Griffiths, M. L., and Theron, E. J.: Obstructed labor from pelvic neurofibroma. South. Afr. Med. J. *53*:781, 1978.
8. Magbagbeola, J. A. O.: Abnormal responses to muscle relaxants in patients with von Recklinghausen's disease. Brit. J. Anaesth. *42*:710, 1970.
9. Yamashita, M.: Anaesthetic considerations in von Recklinghausen's disease (multiple neurofibromatosis). Abnormal response to muscle relaxants. Anaesthetist *26*:317, 1977.
10. Basta, J. W., Niedjadlik, K., and Pallares, V.: Autonomic hyperreflexia: Intraoperative control with pentolinium tartrate. Brit. J. Anaesth. *49*:1087, 1977.
11. Cooperman, L. H.: Succinylcholine-induced hyperkalemia in neuromuscular disease. J.A.M.A. *213*:1967, 1970.
12. Fisher, M. M.: Anesthetic difficulties in neurofibromatosis. Anaesthesia *30*:648, 1975.

Erythema Nodosum

1. Goldstein, R. S.: Erythema nodosum and brucellosis. Brit. Med. J. *1*:809, 1976.
2. Buckler, J. M. H.: Leptospirosis presenting with erythema nodosum. Arch. Dis. Child. *52*:418, 1977.
3. Longmore, H. J. A.: Toxoplasmosis and erythema nodosum. Brit. Med. J. *1*:490, 1977.
4. Reece, R. M.: Erythema nodosum. Am. Fam. Phys. *13*:99, 1976.
5. de Moragas, J. M.: Panniculitis (erythema nodosum). *In* Fitzpatrick, T. B. (ed.): Dermatology in General Medicine. 2nd ed., New York, McGraw-Hill Book Co., 1979, pp. 784–789.

Mastocytosis

1. Rosenbaum, K. J., and Strobel, G. E.: Anesthetic consideration in mastocytosis. Anesthesiology *38*:398, 1973.
2. Parker, F., and Odland, G. F.: The mastocytosis syndrome. *In* Fitzpatrick, T. B. (ed.): Dermatology in General Medicine. 2nd ed, New York, McGraw-Hill Book Co., 1979, pp. 772–783.
3. Wyre, H. W., and Henrichs, W. D.: Systemic mastocytosis and pulmonary eosinophilic granuloma. J.A.M.A. *239*:856, 1978.
4. Brown, T. P.: Thiopentone anaphylaxis — case report. Anaesth. Intens. Care *3*:257, 1975.
5. Buckland, R. W., and Avery, R. F.: Histamine release following pancuronium: A case report. Brit. J. Anaesth. *45*:518, 1973.

Malignant Atrophic Papulosis

1. Black, M.: Malignant atrophic papulosis (Dego's Disease). Int. J. Derm. *15*:405, 1976.
2. Pierce, R. N., and Smith, G. J. W.: Intrathoracic manifestations of Dego's disease (malignant atrophic papulosis). Chest *73*:79, 1978.
3. Horner, F., Myers, G., Stumpf, D., et al.: Malignant atrophic papulosis (Kohlmeier-Dego's disease) in childhood. Neurology *26*:317, 1976.

Hereditary Anhidrotic Ectodermal Defect

1. Capitanio, M. A., Chen, J. T. T., Arey, J. B., and Kirkpatrick, J. A.: Congenital anhidrotic ectodermal dysplasia. Amer. J. Roentgenol. *103*:168, 1968.
2. Ramchander, V., Jankey, N., Ramkissoon, R., and Rajn, G. C.: Anhidrotic ectodermal dysplasia in an infant presenting with pyrexia of unknown origin. Clin. Pediatr. *17*:50, 1978.

Fabry's Disease

1. Frost, A., and Spaeth, G. L.: α-Galactosidase A deficiency: Fabry's disease (angiokeratoma corporis diffusum universale). *In* Fitzpatrick, T. B. (ed.): Dermatology in General Medicine. 2nd ed., New York, McGraw-Hill Book Co., 1979, pp. 1125–1134.
2. Taaffe, A.: Angiokeratoma corporis diffusum: The evolution of a disease entity. Postgrad. Med. J. *53*:78, 1977.
3. Ferrans, V. J., Hibbs, R. G., and Burda, C. D.: The heart in Fabry's disease. Am. J. Cardiol. *24*:95, 1969.
4. Desnick, R. J., Blieden, L. C., Sharp, H. L., Hofschire, P. J., and Moller, J. H.: Cardiac valvular anomalies in Fabry disease. Circulation *54*:818, 1976.
5. Rowe, J. W., and Caralis, D. G.: Accelerated atrioventricular conduction in Fabry's disease. Angiology *29*:562, 1978.
6. Eichhorn, J. H., Hedley-Whyte, J., Steinman, T. I., Kaufman, J. M., and Laasberg, L. H.: Renal failure following enflurane anesthesia. Anesthesiology *45*:557, 1976.

Incontinentia Pigmenti

1. Carney, R. G.: Incontinentia pigmenti, a world statistical analysis. Arch. Dermatol. *112*:535, 1976.
2. Basta, J. W., Niedjadlik, K., and Pallares, V.: Autonomic hyperreflexia: Intraoperative control with pentolinium tartrate. Brit. J. Anesth. *49*:1087, 1977.

Osteoporosis, Osteomalacia, and Osteopetrosis

1. Chalmers, G. L.: Disorders of bone. Practitioner 220:711, 1978.
2. Wheeler, M.: Osteoporosis. Med. Clin. North Amer. 60:1213, 1976.
3. Khairi, M. R. A., and Johnston, C. C.: What we know and don't know about bone loss in the elderly. Geriatrics 33:67, 1978.
4. Frame, B., and Parfitt, A. M.: Osteomalacia: current concepts. Ann. Intern. Med. 89:966, 1978.
5. Beighton, P., Horan, F., and Hamersma, H.: A review of Osteopetroses. Postgrad. Med. J. 53:507, 1977.
6. Beighton, P., Durr, L., and Hamersma, H.: The clinical features of sclerosteosis. Ann. Intern. Med. 84:393, 1975.

Osteogenesis Imperfecta

1. Bailey, J. A. II: Disproportionate Short Stature: Diagnosis and Management. Philadelphia, W. B. Saunders Co., 1973, pp. 223–231.
2. Bergstrom, L.: Osteogenesis imperfecta: Otologic and maxillofacial aspects. Laryngoscope 87 (supp 6):1, 1977.
3. Solomons, C. C., and Nillar, E. A.: Osteogenesis imperfecta—new perspectives. Clin. Orthop. 96:299, 1973.
4. Stein, D., and Kloster, F. E.: Valvular heart disease in osteogenesis imperfecta. Amer. Heart. J. 94:637, 1977.
5. Shoenfeld, Y., Fried, A., and Ehrenfeld, N. E.: Osteogenesis imperfecta; review of the literature with presentation of 29 cases. Am. J. Dis. Child. 129:679, 1975.
6. Solomons, C. C., and Myers, D. N.: Hyperthermia of osteogenesis imperfecta and its relationship to malignant hyperthermia. In Gordon, R. A., Britt, B. A., and Kalow, W. (eds.): Malignant Hyperthermia. Springfield, Ill., Charles C Thomas, 1971, pp. 319–330.
7. Oliverio, R. N.: Anesthetic management of intramedullary nailing in osteogenesis imperfecta: Report of a case. Anesth. Analg. 52:232, 1973.

Dwarfism

1. Sillence, D. O., Rimonin, D. L., and Lachman, R.: Neonatal dwarfism. Ped. Clin. North Amer. 25:453, 1978.
2. Bailey, J. A., II: Disproportionate Short Stature: Diagnosis and Management. Philadelphia, W. B. Saunders Co., 1973, pp. 13–25, 36–56.
3. Rimoin, D. L.: The chondrodystrophies. Adv. Hum. Genet. 5:1, 1975.
4. Gulati, D. R., and Ront, D.: Atlantoaxial dislocation with quadriparesis in achondroplasia. J. Neurosurg. 40:394, 1974.
5. Goldberg, M. J.: Orthopedic aspects of bone dysplasias. Orthop. Clin. North Amer. 7:445, 1976.
6. Lipson, S. J.: Dysplasia of the odontoid process in Morquio's syndrome causing quadriparesis. J. Bone Joint Surg. 59A:340, 1977.
7. Kopits, S. E.: Orthopedic complications of dwarfism. Clin. Orthop. 114:153–179, 1976.
8. Lutter, L. D., Lonstein, J. E., Winter, R. B., and

9. Langer, L. O.: Anatomy of the achondroplastic lumbar canal. Clin. Orthop. 126:139, 1977.
9. Hope, E. O. S., Farebrother, M. J. B., and Bainbridge, D.: Some aspects of respiratory function in three siblings with Morquio-Brailsford disease. Thorax 28:335, 1973.
10. Jones, A. E. P., and Croley, T. F.: Morquio syndrome and anesthesia. Anesthesiology 51:261, 1979.
11. Birkinshaw, K. J.: Anesthesia in a patient with unstable neck: Morquio's syndrome. Anesthesia 30:46, 1975.
12. Waltz, L. F., Finerman, G., and Wyatt, G. M.: Anesthesia for dwarfs and other patients of pathological small stature. Canad. Anaesth. Soc. J. 22:703, 1975.
13. Ravindran, R., and Stoops, C. M.: Anaesthetic management of a patient with Hallermann-Streiff syndrome. Anesth. Analg. 58:254, 1979.
14. Basta, J. W., Niejadlik, K., and Pallares, V.: Autonomic hyperreflexia: Intraoperative control with pentolinium tartrate. Brit. J. Anaesth. 49:1087, 1977.

Craniofacial and Mandibulofacial Dysostoses

1. Gravenstein, J. S.: Congenital malformation. In Saidman, L. J., and Moya, F. (eds.): Complications of Anesthesia. Springfield, Ill., Charles C Thomas, 1970, pp. 100–109.
2. Cohen, M. M., Jr.: Craniofacial dysostoses. Birth Defects 11(2):145, 1975.
3. Feingold, M., and Baum, J.: Goldenhar's syndrome. Am. J. Dis. Child. 132:136, 1978.
4. Sklar, G. S., and King, B. D.: Endotracheal intubation and Treacher Collins syndrome. Anesthesiology 44:247, 1976.
5. Gershanik, J. J., and Nervez, C.: Nasoesophageal intubation in the Pierre Robin syndrome. Clin. Pediatr. 15:173, 1976.
6. Goldberg, M. J., and Ampola, M. G.: Birth defect syndromes in which orthopedic problems may be overlooked. Ortho. Clin. North Amer. 7:411, 1976.

Paget's Disease

1. Krane, S. M.: Paget's disease of bone. Clin. Orthop. 127:24, 1977.
2. Brown, H. P., La Rocca, H., and Wickstrom, J. K.: Paget's disease of the atlas and axis. J. Bone Joint Surg. 53A:1441, 1971.
3. Goldhammer, Y., Braham, J., and Kosary, I. Z.: Hydrocephalic dementia in Paget's disease of the skull: Treatment by ventriculoatrial shunt. Neurology 29:513, 1979.
4. Epstein, B. S., and Epstein, J. A.: The association of cerebellar tonsillar herniation with basilar impression incident to Paget's disease. Amer. J. Roentgenol. 107:535, 1969.
5. Rhodes, B. A., Greyson, N. D., Hamilton, C. R., White, R. I., Giargiana, F. A., and Wagner, H. N.: Absence of anatomic arteriovenous shunts in Paget's disease of bone. N. Engl. J. Med 287:686, 1972.
6. Woodhouse, N. J. Y., Crosbie, W. A., and Mohamedally, S. M.: Cardiac output in Paget's dis-

ease: response to long-term salmon calcitonin therapy. Brit. Med. J. 4:686, 1975.

7. Basta, J. W., Niejadlik, K., and Pallares, V.: Autonomic hyperreflexia: Intraoperative control with pentolinium tartrate. Brit. J. Anaesth. 49:1087, 1977.

Fibrous Dysplasia

1. Grabias, S. L., and Campbell, C. J.: Fibrous dysplasia. Ortho. Clin. North Amer. 8:771, 1977.
2. Albright, F., Butler, A., Hampton, A., and Smith, P.: Syndrome characterized by osteitis fibrosa disseminata, areas of pigmentation and endocrine dysfunction, with precocious puberty in females. Report of five cases. N. Engl. J. Med. 216:727, 1937.
3. Caudill, R., Saltzman, D., Guarm, S., and Granite, E.: Possible relationship of primary hyperparathyroidism and fibrous dysplasia: Report of case. J. Oral. Surg. 35:483, 1977.
4. Kunder, J. P., and Pan, A. K.: Congenital fibroosseous dysplasia of jaws ("hippopotamus face"), an anesthetic problem. Brit. J. Anaesth. 51:465, 1979.
5. Montoya, G., Evart, C. M., and Dohn, D. F.: Polyostotic fibrous dysplasia and spinal cord compressions. J. Neurosurg 29:102, 1968.
6. Basta, J. W., Niedjadlik, K., and Pallares, V.: Autonomic hyperreflexia: Intraoperative control with pentolinium tartrate. Brit. J. Anaesth. 49:1987, 1977.

16

Infectious Diseases

By THOMAS B. CALDWELL III, M.D.

The Human Metabolic Response to Infection
Effects of Anesthesia on Resistance to Infection
Interaction of Antibiotics with Drugs Employed During Anesthesia
  Antibiotics Causing Respiratory Depression
  Infrequent Adverse Effects of Antibiotic Therapy During Anesthesia
Choice of Anesthesia for Patients with Infections but not in Shock

Anesthesia and Septic Shock
  Epidemiology of Septic Shock
  Pathophysiology of Septic Shock
  Bacteremic Shock: The Syndrome in Man
  Cardiovascular Dynamics of Septic Shock
  Controversial Areas in the Pathophysiology of Septic Shock
  Therapy of Septic Shock
  Experimental Drugs and Adjuncts to Therapy in Septic Shock
  Anesthesia for Patients with Septic Shock

The anesthesiologist often encounters patients with infectious disease, ranging from mild respiratory infections to potentially lethal bacteremic shock. Despite advances in antibiotic therapy, surgery for drainage of abscesses or resection of infected tissues is still the basic treatment for many patients with infections. Infections acquired in hospitals remained a great problem in the 1970's, since it is estimated that in the United States there are approximately 71,000 iatrogenic infections annually, resulting in about 18,000 deaths each year.[1] The problem of iatrogenic infections is discussed in a recent editorial by Riley,[2] while iatrogenic infections resulting from anesthesia are covered in a review by Johanson and Sanford.[3]

The metabolic response to infection has been restudied, with the aid of radioisotope and computer techniques. There has been considerable research into the effects of general anesthetics on host mechanisms of defense against infection. Today much is known about interactions between antibiotics and the drugs employed during anesthesia, and some information on the cardiac depressant effects of certain antibiotics is available.

The syndrome of septic shock in man and the hemodynamic changes occurring in septic shock have been described extensively in the surgical and anesthetic literature. Much information concerning regional circulatory changes in the lung, kidney, and brain during bacteremic shock is now available from studies in animals, and especially in primates. Considerable progress has been made in analyzing the effects of sepsis on the blood, and on the endocrine and reticuloendothelial systems. There is even some information available concerning the effects of sepsis on metabolism at the cellular level.

It seems useful to examine the following topics: the metabolic response to systemic infection in man; the effects of anesthesia on mechanisms of defense against infection; the interaction of antibiotics with drugs employed during anesthesia, and the circulatory effects of some antibiotics; the clinical syndrome of septic shock, including its pathophysiology; the cardiovascular dynamics of septic shock, and the effects of septic shock on regional blood flow in lung, kidney, and brain; the metabolic effects of bacteremia on cellular metabolism during shock; the therapy of septic shock; experimental approaches to the treatment of bacteremic shock; and the anesthetic management of patients with septic shock.

THE HUMAN METABOLIC RESPONSE TO INFECTION

The studies of Beisel and his coworkers have accurately quantitated many of the changes that occur in man during the course of systemic infections — infections not progressing to septic shock.[4] They used healthy males voluntarily infected with one of three organisms: Pasteurella tularemia, a gram-negative rod; phlebotomus fever, a virus; and *Coxiella burnetti*, a member of the rickettsiae.

Within 24 to 48 hours after the onset of infection with all three organisms, negative nitrogen, sodium, and potassium balance developed. Beisel and his group also observed negative phosphorus, magnesium, and calcium balances, but the net change in calcium was small. The sodium deficit reached a maximum during the most severe phase of the volunteers' illnesses. As the disease process resolved, renal sodium retention occurred, partially restoring the deficit. The changes in chloride paralleled those in sodium. The negative potassium balance, which first appeared with the onset of symptoms, could be accounted for by decreased dietary intake; little potassium was excreted in the urine. A decreased intake of magnesium and nitrogen also explained the negative balances of these elements. The pattern of potassium deficit closely paralleled that of nitrogen. One might infer that tissue catabolism during infection explains the similar changes that occur in the nitrogen and potassium balances. Slight increases in serum and urine glucocorticoids were observed, but these increases were much too small to account for the potassium and nitrogen deficits on the basis of increased glucocorticoid activity.

It is generally appreciated that protein catabolism after uncomplicated major surgery is only slightly in excess of that observed in persons with a dietary intake equivalent to that received by surgical patients. The presence of significant infection in a surgical patient intensifies protein catabolism and increases deficits of potassium, sodium, chloride, and magnesium. Moreover, when infection is present, the period of inadequate dietary intake may be prolonged because of ileus or anorexia.

The use of total parenteral hyperalimentation (TPA), which has developed in the past decade, can replete the metabolic deficits seen with moderate systemic infections or in postoperative patients with prolonged ileus. The normal daily adult requirement of 30 kcal per k of body weight per day as dextrose and the basal adult requirement of 5 grams of nitrogen per day as protein hydrolysate can be given parenterally. Double and triple these amounts may be required and can be given, if the infection becomes severe. Sodium, potassium, calcium, magnesium, and phosphate may be added to replenish losses that occur during mild to moderate systemic infections.[5] The radical changes in metabolism that occur when septic shock develops will be discussed below.

EFFECTS OF ANESTHESIA ON RESISTANCE TO INFECTION

As early as 1904 Rubin had demonstrated an increased susceptibility to infection with streptococcus or pneumococcus, when rabbits were anesthetized with diethyl ether or ethyl alcohol.[6] In 1911 Graham observed a decrease in the ameboid motion of polymorphonuclear leukocytes in vivo in rabbits during diethyl ether anesthesia.[7] He looked for but did not find changes in the capability of the serum to agglutinate and lyse bacteria during anesthesia in rabbits and in man. No further work was done in this field until 1935, when Andrewes and his group reported that ether anesthesia made mice more susceptible to pneumonia upon exposure to swine influenza virus.[8] Dubin found that there was no significant difference in infection rates between mice anesthetized with ether or with pentobarbital, thus casting doubt on the earlier explanation that ether increased susceptibility by irritating the mucous membranes of the respiratory system.[9] He suggested that the anesthetics depressed the animals' cough reflexes, in effect increasing the number of viruses with which the animals were challenged.

After an interval of 20 years since the

work of Dubin, Bruce reopened the study of the role of anesthesia in resistance to infection.[10] With phase microscopy he observed decreased cytoplasmic streaming and decreased motility in leukocytes in vivo during halothane anesthesia in the bat. Using the method of Fruhman, he also showed a very large decrease in leukocyte migration into the peritoneum of rats anesthetized with 1 per cent halothane and injected intraperitoneally with 0.1 μg of pseudomonas lipopolysaccharide. Leukocyte counts in peritoneal fluid dropped from 3.5 million to about 300,000 to 400,000 per cubic millimeter, but rose to normal within four hours after anesthesia had been discontinued. Bruce demonstrated the biological significance of this effect by injecting live salmonella into mice subsequently anesthetized with halothane for six hours. None of the controls but 70 per cent of the anesthetized mice had died by the seventh hour after injection.[10] Similar results were obtained by Duncan and coworkers, who found an 81 ± 7 per cent 14 day mortality in mice given 0.6 per cent halothane for four hours before or after they were injected intraperitoneally with colonic contents.[12] The mortality in controls given only oxygen for four hours was 44 ± 16 per cent (p of difference <0.005). In a second set of experiments in which mice were given intramuscular *Candida albicans* to create an abcess in the thigh before or after exposure to 1.17 per cent halothane for four hours, Duncan's group found no difference in mortality rate or in the size of the abscesses when mice exposed to halothane were compared with similarly infected mice given oxygen for four hours. The anesthetic had no effect upon the mobilization and deposition of inflammatory cells at the abscess site. They postulate that reduced phagocytosis by the reticuloendothelial system might account for the difference in mortality during intraperitoneal infection between mice given halothane and control mice.[12] Other factors, such as reduced splanchnic blood flow during halothane anesthesia, might modify the animals' response to intraperitoneal infection.[13]

Cullen and coworkers found small reductions in phagocytosis of latex particles by polymorphonuclear leukocytes and by monocytes in blood samples from patients after induction of halothane or thiopental–Innovar-nitrous oxide anesthesia.[13] Cullen's study compared phagocytosis prior to anesthesia with phagocytosis after induction of anesthesia but prior to starting surgery, using each patient as his own control. Also, the reduction of nitroblue tetrazolium in leukocytes of patients after induction of anesthesia was inhibited. Cullen noted that the amount of the decreases in leukocyte function, although statistically significant, was rather small and should be well tolerated by most patients.[13]

Cullen and Chretien also studied the transformation of lymphocytes — the process by which contact with an antigen causes the lymphocyte to enlarge, synthesize desoxyribonucleic acid, and divide into daughter cells.[14] Phytohemagglutinin also can cause transformation of lymphocytes; this transformation can be inhibited by halothane, but not by ketamine, at 0.5 to 2.0 μg per ml concentrations — concentrations similar to those achieved clinically.[14] Wilson and coworkers demonstrated that ketamine anesthesia had no effect on ribonucleic acid synthesis rates in human lymphocytes.[15]

Stanley and his group measured neutrophil chemotaxis in blood samples from patients before anesthesia, after induction of anesthesia, and 24 hours postoperatively. They found that neutrophil chemotaxis was reduced 36 per cent by halothane and nitrous oxide, 32 per cent by enflurane and nitrous oxide, and 21 per cent by morphine and nitrous oxide. Neutrophil chemotaxis returned to normal by 24 hours postoperatively after all three anesthetic combinations tested.[16]

The effects of cyclopropane, methoxyflurane, halothane, and pentobarbital on the bactericidal activity of murine lungs was studied by Goldstein and coworkers.[17] Using aerosols of *Staphylococcus aureus* to seed the lungs of mice, using a ^{32}P label to quantitate the bacterial content of the lungs, and using quantitative cultures to measure surviving bacteria, they found that cyclopropane reduced bactericidal activity to 74 per cent (versus 91 per cent for controls), and methoxyflurane reduced bactericidal activity to 78 per cent (versus 87 per cent for controls), while halothane and pentobarbital had no effect on pulmonary bactericidal activity during four hours of anesthesia.

It is apparent that a variety of inhalational

agents — diethyl ether, enflurane, halothane, and cyclopropane — can depress specific leukocyte functions to a mild or moderate degree, and can make experimental animals more susceptible to death from infection. Halothane, for example, can depress cytoplasmic streaming, chemotaxis, phagocytosis, and transformation in leukocytes. Halothane's effect on neutrophil chemotaxis disappears within 24 hours after anesthesia,[16] and it is not unlikely that its other effects on leukocyte function are also transient. Thiopental, morphine, and Innovar as supplements to nitrous oxide also slightly depress phagocytosis.[13] Many drugs employed during anesthesia have not yet been tested for their effects on the immune system.

There still is no published data proving any effect of anesthetic drugs on the incidence of postoperative infection in man. Cruse reports that the infection rate for clean wounds increases from 1.4 per cent for operations lasting less than an hour to 4.4 per cent for operations lasting two to three hours.[18] This Canadian study confirms the earlier conclusions of the United States National Research Council study of postoperative wound infections that longer operative times in elective herniorrhaphies correlated with a higher rate of infections.[19] Regional anesthesia did not result in a lower postoperative infection rate. However, Bruce points out that the frequent use of prophylactic antibiotics might lead one to discount the negative finding of this one attempt to relate anesthetic technique to incidence of infection in man.[10, 11]

INTERACTIONS OF ANTIBIOTICS WITH DRUGS EMPLOYED DURING ANESTHESIA

Antibiotics may interact with anesthetic agents and muscle relaxants, resulting in prolonged apnea. With the increasing use of muscle relaxants and with the development of new antibiotics, the possibility of encountering such interactions is increasing. There are occasional reports of other complications of antibiotics that are of concern to anesthesiologists — anaphylaxis, potassium overdose, convulsions, methemoglobinemia, cardiac depression, and ototoxicity — but complications of this type are infrequent.

Table 16–1   Neuromuscular Blocking Actions of Antibiotics

Drug	Dose/kg.	Per Cent Blockade
d-Tubocurare	40 mcg.	23
Polymyxin B sulfate	10 mg.	50
Neomycin sulfate	25 mg.	40
Streptomycin sulfate	25 mg.	10
Dihydrostreptomycin sulfate	50 mg.	23
Kanamycin sulfate	100 mg.	23

ANTIBIOTICS CAUSING RESPIRATORY DEPRESSION

The earliest report of antibiotics causing paralysis is that of Pridgen, who in 1956 collected four cases of apnea occurring shortly after peritoneal irrigation with neomycin.[20] Two of his patients were infants, ages 14 and 17 months, who became apneic within 20 minutes after lavage with neomycin 0.5 gm. In both cases diethyl ether was the primary anesthetic agent, and both infants died in spite of artificial ventilation. His two other cases were adults in whom 3-gm doses of neomycin resulted in postoperative apnea lasting three to 30 hours.

There have been many subsequent reports of antibiotics causing neuromuscular blockade in man and in experimental animals. The reader may gain a rough idea of the degree of neuromuscular blockade of several antibiotics from the data of Timmerman and others, which are reproduced in Table 16–1.[21] Gentamicin, which is frequently used today, falls between neomycin and streptomycin in the degree of blockade it produces.[22]

Pittinger and Adamson, in a review article, state that the following antibiotics have caused neuromuscular blockade in man: colistin and colistin methanesulfonate; kanamycin, neomycin, streptomycin and dihydrostreptomycin; oxytetracycline and rolitetracycline; and polymyxin B.[23] Although human neuromuscular blockade by gentamicin — an aminoglycoside similar to kanamycin — has not yet been reported, it seems likely that cases of gentamicin paralysis in man will soon appear; gentamicin is now in widespread use, and it is reported to reduce twitch height in cats more than streptomycin does.[22]

Lincomycin has caused respiratory paralysis in a healthy patient recovering from anesthesia with nitrous oxide and curare.[24] After reversal of the curare, lincomycin, 600 mg intravenously, caused ten minutes of apnea. Samuelson and coworkers demonstrated in cats that lincomycin given during recovery from d-tubocurarine significantly increased neuromuscular blockade.[24] Any effect that lincomycin might have in myasthenics, Wullen et al. ascribed mainly to the magnesium in the solvent.[25]

Tetracycline administered intravenously is reported to have made patients with myasthenia gravis weaker;[26] and tetracycline, 50 mg per k, did cause a 45 per cent neuromuscular blockade in rabbits.[27] To date, there are no reports that tetracycline causes paralysis in man except in myasthenics. McQuillen and coworkers state that a very weak neuromuscular blockade might occur with tetracycline in man, but they doubt its clinical significance.[28]

Neuromuscular blockade probably does not occur with penicillin, chloramphenicol, or bacitracin, and there is no evidence whatever for blockade with erythromcyin, oleandomycin, vancomycin, ristocetin, and tyrothricin.[28] For a list of antibiotics causing neuromuscular blockade in laboratory preparations but not yet implicated in paralysis in man, the reader is referred to the reference by Pittinger and Adamson.[23] Included in this list are aminosidine, gentamicin, polymyxin A, rolitetracycline, viomycin, clindamycin, and others.

Enflurane, methoxyflurane, diethyl ether, curare, gallamine, pancuronium, and succinylcholine can synergize with those antibiotics described above as having a neuromuscular blocking action.[28, 29] Promethazine, procaine amide, and quinidine have been reported to enhance the effects of antibiotics with neuromuscular blocking properties.[23]

The fundamental treatment for respiratory paralysis from antibiotics is mechanical ventilation until the drug effect wears off and the patient can sustain adequate ventilatory volumes. Lee and coworkers point out that reversal of neuromuscular blockade with calcium or with anticholinesterases in cases of paralysis from neomycin or from polymyxin is often incomplete.[30, 31]

An attempt to reverse antibiotic neuromuscular blockade in order to shorten the period of mechanical ventilation is worth while in occasional cases. Pittinger states that blockade by antibiotics resembling streptomycin — aminosidine, dihydrostrep-

tomycin, gentamicin, kanamycin, neomycin, and viomycin (the aminoglycosides) — can be reversed by calcium salts.[23] McQuillen and coworkers and Pittinger both note the similarity between the block produced by magnesium and the block produced by kanamycin and neomycin.[23, 28] Brazil and coworkers proved that neomycin and gentamycin greatly decreased the prejunctional release of acetylcholine — an effect similar to that of magnesium on the nerve terminal.[32] Addition of calcium ions to the preparation restored the amount of acetylcholine liberated nearly to control values. Some post-junctional desensitization with both neomycin and gentamicin was also noted.[32] When calcium is given to reverse antibiotic blockade, it should be administered slowly so as not to precipitate cardiac arrhythmias, and its effect should be followed by monitoring both the twitch response and the cardiac rhythm. Pittinger cautions against the use of calcium in digitalized patients, and he suggests that neostigmine be tried, if reversal with calcium appears incomplete. Timmerman and coworkers suggest that neostigmine can be used to counteract the neuromuscular blockade of streptomycin sulfate and dihydrostreptomycin sulfate.[21] McQuillen noted a transient improvement with neostigmine of blockade by kanamycin in man.[28] Lee and coworkers warn that complete antagonism of neomycin blockade often does not occur with either neostigmine or pyridostigmine or calcium.[30] They also noted that when neostigmine blockade was present, tetanic contractions did not fade, even when twitch was 95 per cent depressed. They consider post-tetanic exhaustion of twitch to be the most reliable sign of neomycin blockade. Although they reported complete reversal of neomycin paralysis with germine monoacetate, 0.5 to 3 mg per kg in laboratory preparations, they recommend that mechanical ventilation and not pharmacologic reversal be the treatment of choice for neuromuscular blockade induced by neomycin.[30]

The polymyxins A through E and colistimethate sodium are polypeptide antibiotics whose neuromuscular blockade is not fully reversible with antagonists presently available for clinical use. Their exact mechanism of action on the myoneural junction is not known.[31] Competition with calcium, resulting in decreased prejunctional acetylcholine release — the mechanism of blockade by the aminoglycosides — does not appear to play a role in polymyxin paralysis.[33] Lee and coworkers note that the polymyxins are cationic detergents that can alter membrane permeability. They found that calcium and small doses of edrophonium, neostigmine, and pyridostigmine only partly antagonize polymyxin blockade, while larger doses increase the degree of blocks. Their findings confirm the earlier work of Van Nyhuis and coworkers that neostigmine enhances neuromuscular blockade induced by polymyxin.[34] Naiman and Martin also found that neither calcium nor neostigmine reverses polymyxin blockade.[35] Lee and coworkers proved that 4-aminopyridine, a drug which facilitates neuromuscular transmission but can cause convulsions, completely reverses polymyxin in cats.[36] This drug, which was first used by Foldes to antagonize nondepolarizing muscle relaxants, is not available for clinical use.

The final resolution of neuromuscular blockade induced by antibiotics depends ultimately on renal excretion of the drugs causing it; however, many of these antibiotics are excreted rather slowly in the urine. Fogdall and coworkers point out that urinary levels of polymyxin peak 24 hours after an intramuscular dose of the drug.[37] Lindesmith, McQuillen, and others emphasize the role of underlying renal disease in antibiotic-induced neuromuscular blockade.[28, 31] Renal disease predisposes to slow excretion of the antibiotics and to a low total body calcium. Many of the patients reported with paralysis from antibiotics were being treated for urinary tract infection or were anesthetized for urologic surgical procedures.

In any case of respiratory depression from antibiotics, close observation for 24 hours is mandatory, and mechanical ventilation is usually necessary.

INFREQUENT ADVERSE EFFECTS OF ANTIBIOTIC THERAPY DURING ANESTHESIA

Rather infrequent complications of antibiotic therapy during anesthesia are anaphylaxis, convulsions, potassium overdose leading to cardiac asystole, direct cardiac depression from certain antibiotics, ototoxicity, methemoglobinemia, and nephrotoxicity. The nephrotoxicity of the aminoglycosides is well known, and the reader can refer to the review article by Alford for a discussion of this problem.[38]

Anaphylactic shock can result from penicillin, ampicillin, amphotericin B, streptomycin, the sulfonamides, and vancomycin.[39] It also occurs with the cephalosporins. The anesthesia community is well aware of the anaphylactic hazard of penicillin; the possibility of adverse reaction should be kept in mind, especially during surgery on patients who are unconscious or otherwise unable to give a medical history.

Weinstein and coworkers have reported generalized convulsions associated with high serum levels of penicillin in a child and in adults. Impaired renal excretion of drug was present in these patients.[40] Seizures have also occurred when massive doses of penicillin were used during cardiopulmonary bypass.[41]

Since each million units of penicillin G contains 1.5 mEq of potassium, fast "massive" intravenous doses during anesthesia can lead to cardiac asystole.[40] There is also the possibility of precipitating tachycardia in patients with atrial flutter or fibrillation whose ventricular response has been controlled with digitalis. Patients with renal diseases are particularly sensitive to intravenous potassium.[40] The sodium salt of penicillin G may be used, but it will add to the salt load in patients with actual or incipient congestive heart failure.

At least seven antibiotics are known to cause direct dose-related myocardial depression. These include colistimethate sodium, erythromycin, lincomycin, kanamycin, streptomycin, tetracycline, and vancomycin.[42, 43] Cohen and his group described a postoperative cardiac surgical patient with persistent hypotension because of streptomycin.[42] They found that after up to 40 mg per kg of intravenous streptomycin in dogs, mean arterial blood pressure declined 44 ± 5 per cent, and left ventricular dp/dt declined 37 ± 4.9 per cent (Fig. 16–1). After intravenous tetracycline given as 100, 200, and 300 mg boluses, left ventricular dp/dt decreased by 9, 14, and 21 per cent, respectively, and mean arterial pressure decreased by up to 22 ± 6 per cent (Fig. 16–2). Left atrial pressure rose. After intravenous kanamycin, 333 mg, left ventricular dp/dt decreased by 16 ± 3 per cent, and mean arterial pressure declined 17 ± 2 per cent (Fig. 16–3). Similar reductions in left ven-

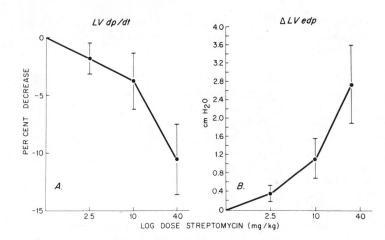

Figure 16–1. Decrease in left ventricular dp/dt (left) and increase in left ventricular end-diastolic pressure (right) in dogs after administration of streptomycin 2.5, 10, and 40 mg/kg. (From Cohen, L. S., Wechsler, A. F., Mitchell, J. E., and Glick, G.: Amer. J. Cardiol. 26:508, 1970.)

tricular dp/dt and mean arterial pressure were noted with colistimethate, erythromycin, and vancomycin. No depression of myocardial performance was noted with sodium penicillin, cephalothin, or chloramphenicol. Cohen and his group point out that the blood levels of antibiotics in their study are within the range of levels attained in patients with moderate impairment of renal function.[42]

Lincomycin given as an intravenous bolus has caused cardiac arrest during anesthesia in man.[43] An overdose — 12 gm — resulted in asystole for 45 minutes and then ventricular fibrillation for 45 minutes in a previously healthy 20 year old man.[43] Daubeck and coworkers were able to cause either ventricular fibrillation or asystole in dogs, depending on the rate of administration and the dose employed. They believe that lincomycin's principal effects are on excitability and conduction, rather than on

contractility.[43] Waisbren[44] reported four cardiac arrests following high dose lincomycin in man and noted some structural similarity between lincomycin and quinidine.

Ototoxicity, including both cochlear and vestibular damage, occurs as a direct effect of aminoglycoside antibiotics. The amount of damage depends on serum levels, duration of therapy, and prolonged presence of aminoglycoside in the endolymph.[38] Elevated trough serum levels may contribute to ototoxicity. Advanced age, renal impairment, and concurrent use of other ototoxic drugs, such as large doses of furosemide or ethacrynic acid, all predispose to aminoglycoside ototoxicity. Amikacin and kanamycin may be somewhat more ototoxic than gentamicin. Streptomycin is particularly toxic to the vestibular apparatus.[38] The administration of these drugs intramuscularly or by intravenous drip over 20 to 30 minutes can prevent high peak serum levels and may

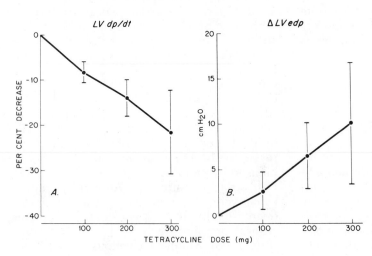

Figure 16–2. Decrease in left ventricular dp/dt (left) and increase in left ventricular end-diastolic pressure (right) in dogs, after administration of tetracycline, 100, 200, and 300 mg. (From Cohen, L.S., Wechsler, A.F., Mitchell, J.E., and Glick, G.: Amer. J. Cardiol. 26:508, 1970.)

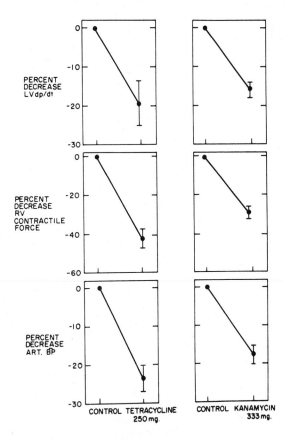

Figure 16–3. Per cent decreases in left ventricular dp/dt, in right ventricular contractile force measured by a strain gauge arch, and in mean arterial blood pressure in dogs following the administration of tetracycline, 250 mg (left), and kanamycin, 333 mg (right). (From Cohen, L.S., Wechsler, A.F., Mitchell, J.E., and Glick, G.: Amer. J. Cardiol. 26:507, 1970.)

avoid the occurrence of ototoxicity as well as other undesirable effects of bolus administration.

Clinically significant methemoglobinemia can occur with antimalarial chemoprophylaxis with chloroquine, primaquine, or diaminodiphenylsulfone (Dapsone). Cohen et al. claims that Dapsone is the worst of the three; they suggest that a heterozygous methemoglobin reductase deficiency is present in these cases.[45]

Hemolysis can occur in patients with glucose–6–phosphate dehydrogenase deficiency during treatment with certain antibiotics. In a review of this subject, Beutler lists quinine, quinacrine, pamaquine, and primaquine, and also chloramphenicol, nitrofurantoin, para-amino salicylate, and the sulfonamides as etiologic agents in this type of hemolytic anemia.[46] Methemoglobinemia or hemolysis resulting from antimicrobials is important in anesthesia because of the reduced oxygen-carrying capacity of the blood. Quinine and its derivatives can also potentiate nondepolarizing muscle relaxants.

CHOICE OF ANESTHESIA FOR PATIENTS WITH INFECTIONS BUT NOT IN SHOCK

For patients with localized infections or with mild to moderate systemic infections who are not in septic shock, the anesthesiologist has a wide range of agents and techniques from which to choose.

Either general or regional anesthesia may be used. For general anesthesia, any agent currently in clinical use seems acceptable — enflurane, halothane, nitrous oxide, and the adjunct drugs employed with nitrous oxide, i.e., ketamine, thiobarbiturates, narcotics, diazepam, and droperidol. For short cases, methoxyflurane in low concentrations still seems acceptable. The older agents ethylene, diethyl ether, and cyclopropane are acceptable in patients with infections who are not in shock, but their flammability limits the use of cautery and adds an additional risk. Although there is some evidence of mild depression of certain leukocyte functions by cyclopropane, diethyl ether, enflurane, halothane, nitrous oxide, thiopental, and Innovar, this depression of function seems to be transient; so far no anesthetic agent or adjunct drug has been proved to have a harmful effect on the course of clinical infections in man.

The choice among general anesthetic agents may be affected by the site of the infection or by the presence of coexisting disease. For example, one might avoid using halothane in patients with hepatitis, cholecystitis, or cholangitis, simply because it might confuse the differential diagnosis of jaundice postoperatively. One might avoid using methoxyflurane or enflurane in patients with renal disease, particularly during lengthy surgical procedures. In patients with pneumonia and significant right to left shunt, one might avoid using ethylene or nitrous oxide; while in patients with bronchitis or secretion problems, one might avoid diethyl ether. The reader should bear in mind that none of these examples is to be regarded as an absolute contraindication. An acceptable choice of anesthetic agent depends on many factors — disease and anatomical problems in the patient, surgical requirements, availability of safe postoperative mechanical ventilation, and the familiarity of the anesthesiologist or nurse anesthetist with the agent.

If general anesthesia is used for patients with localized infections or mild to moderate systemic infection, the anesthesiologist must watch for interactions between antibiotics that cause paralysis and drugs employed as muscle relaxants during anesthesia. The doses of muscle relaxants should be decreased, and mechanical ventilation must be available, if antibiotic-induced respiratory paralysis occurs.

In patients with localized infections of the extremities or perineum, regional anesthesia is often preferable to general anesthesia. The use of regional anesthesia for patients who have abscesses on the extremities and who have full stomachs avoids the hazards of a rapid induction; and patients having amputations of gangrenous legs often have vascular disease involving the heart, brain, and splanchnic organs which increases their risk with general anesthesia.

Sciatic-femoral block can be used for drainage of abscesses of the foot, while epidural, caudal, or spinal anesthesia can be used for surgery on the thigh or perineum.

Intravenous regional block (Bier block) may be used for drainage of localized abcesses on the fingers, hand, or forearm, while axillary or brachial block may be used for any procedure on the hand or arm. Spinal anesthesia may be used for drainage of infections in the perineum, provided the patient does not have bacteremia (a chill followed by a temperature spike) when the spinal is given,[47] and provided there is no tenderness or erythema at the site where the spinal needle is to be inserted. Similarly, axillary or femoral blocks should be avoided if there is significant adenopathy and tenderness at the site of injection. Field blocks done around abscesses are satisfactory, but local anesthetic drugs injected directly into infected tissues do not work; the low pH of necrotic tissue prevents the liberation of the free base, which is the form of the drug that actually penetrates the nerve fiber.

During anesthesia in patients with either systemic or localized infection, temperature should be monitored. Patients with high fevers (102°F and above) should be treated with alcohol sponges or a cooling mattress preoperatively and with antipyretics (aspirin suppositories). If these measures do not work, small doses of chlorpromazine (0.3 mg per kg) intramuscularly will usually reduce the fever in conjunction with external cooling. A temperature within two degrees of normal, Fahrenheit, keeps tissue oxygen demand and carbon dioxide production fairly close to normal. Reducing high fevers preoperatively contributes to the patient's safety if hypoxemia or hypercarbia occurs during anesthesia and surgery. Temperature spikes during anesthesia should be treated with external cooling. Historically, "ether convulsions" resulted from the effects of fever, dehydration, acidosis, carbon dioxide retention, and hypoxia on the central nervous system, commonly in children.[48] "Ether convulsions" were seen with other anesthetic agents besides diethyl ether, and control of fever and good hydration, preoperatively and intraoperatively, together with improvements in the management of ventilation during anesthesia, have almost eliminated this complication in patients with infectious disease.

Finally, the anesthesiologist must be alert for the infrequent side effects of antibiotics — anaphylaxis, convulsions, cardiac depression, and ototoxicity — that can appear during anesthesia for patients with localized infections or moderate systemic infections.

ANESTHESIA AND SEPTIC SHOCK

The anesthesiologist is frequently called upon to manage patients who have severe bacteremia or who are in septic shock. There is general agreement that surgical intervention for drainage of abscesses or removal of infected tissue is often decisive in the survival of the septic patient.[49, 55] At present, about one third of the cases of bacteremic shock are due to gram-positive organisms, while about two thirds are due to gram-negative bacteria.[2, 53, 55] A small percentage of cases of septic shock are of fungal etiology.[56] The incidence of staphylococcal infections in the hospital population has decreased from nearly 50 per cent in the early 1960's to less than 20 per cent at present.[2, 56] The incidence of sepsis with gram-negative organisms is increasing,[2] and rates of infection with *Klebsiella* and *Pseudomonas* in particular are increasing.[56] Matson points out that the recent increase in nosocomial infection correlates with an increase in the percentage of elderly and poor risk patients currently in hospital.[56] The average rate of hospital-acquired infection is now approximately five infections per 100 discharged patients.[2] As an example of the increased incidence of septicemia during the past quarter century, Altemeier found only eight cases of septicemia at the Cincinnati General Hospital in 1957, but in 1966 found 115 cases.[57] Alexander notes a current infection rate of 5.5 per cent in surgical patients at Cincinnati.[58] Data on foci of infection and pathogens in sepsis are listed in Table 16–2. The incidence of shock in cases of septicemia ranges from 24 per cent[59] to 40 per cent;[49, 57] Weinstein notes that while some hypotension will occur in 80 per cent of patients with gram-negative bacteremia, the complete syndrome of septic shock develops in about 20 per cent.[53]

The mortality rates in septicemia vary with age. Mortality rates in infants are about 20 per cent;[57, 60] in children and in adults below 40 years old, 26 per cent; and in adults over 40 years of age, 67 per cent.[57] When shock appears in a bacteremic

Table 16–2 Foci of Infection and Pathogens in Sepsis–Statistics from Cincinnati General Hospital*

Organisms		Portal of Entry
E. coli	34.9%	GU tract — 56.7%
Klebsiella	22.4%	Respiratory tract — 16.3%
Proteus	13.3%	GI tract — 10.9%
Pseudomonas	14.0%	Skin — 15.1%
Paracolon	6.7%	Vascular catheters — 2.4%
Bacteroides	4.5%	
Serratia	1.8%	
Others	7.5%	

*From Altemeier, W. A., Todd, J. C., and Inger, W. W., Ann. Surg., *166*:530, 1967. In occasional patients there was more than one organism or portal of entry.

patient, the mortality rate increases significantly. Death rates of from 40 to 80 per cent are reported in the larger series.[49, 55, 57, 59, 61, 62, 63, 64, 70] Many authors report death rates close to 70 per cent.[49, 57, 59, 65, 66, 67] Factors contributing to high mortality rates in many series were pre-existing heart disease,[65] advanced age,[57] severity of underlying disease,[66] and low initial cardiac index.[54] In certain studies where cases were included because of sepsis presenting as respiratory failure,[68] or because of pseudomonas bacteremia[66] or tetanus,[69] mortality rates were 68, 67, and 77 per cent, respectively. The death rate in acute leukemics who develop pseudomonas septicemia is close to 90 per cent.[70]

Septicemia in man — and particularly gram-negative septicemia — often results from surgery on the gastrointestinal or urinary tracts, or occurs during mechanical ventilation. Predisposing causes of sepsis include agammaglobulinemia, asplenism,[71] extensive burns, immunosuppression, perforated intra-abdominal viscus, infection in utero,[54] cirrhosis with ascites, leukemia or lymphoma,[54] and neoplasms,[70] as well as therapy with antimetabolites, radiation, steroids,[54] and prophylactic antibiotics.[53] Major trauma may also predispose to sepsis.[72] Procedures predisposing to sepsis include abortion,[54] gastrointestinal and biliary tract surgery[53, 54] and urinary tract surgery, especially in the presence of bacteriuria.[53]

The presence of intravascular catheters, urinary catheters, or artificial airways such as endotracheal tubes[60, 73] or tracheostomy is associated with an increased incidence of sepsis. Contaminated intravenous solutions[74] and contaminated drugs[75] used during anesthesia have also caused bacteremia.

It seems useful to examine the physiology of septic shock first in laboratory animals and then in man, emphasizing recent studies of the hemodynamics of septic shock in man. The anesthetic management of patients with bacterial shock depends on a knowledge of the effects of sepsis on many organ systems; an understanding especially of cardiopulmonary and vascular problems during septic shock is fundamental to the successful anesthetic management of these severely ill patients.

PATHOPHYSIOLOGY OF SEPTIC SHOCK

Sepsis, whether the result of gram-positive or gram-negative organisms, is characterized by fever, prostration, and ultimately circulatory collapse. What is currently known about the pathophysiology of septic shock on the cells and tissues, on the microcirculation, and on regional blood flow may be outlined as follows:

Fever. Exotoxins from gram-positive organisms may cause fever directly by acting on the thermoregulatory center in the hypothalamus, whereas in gram-negative sepsis the endotoxins released by lysed bacteria cause endogenous pyrogen to be released from the patient's leukocytes, and this endogenous pyrogen acts upon the hypothalamus to produce fever.[76] Endogenous pyrogen — a protein with a molecular weight between 10,000 and 20,000 — has been discovered in alveolar macrophages, in Kupfer cells, and in mononuclear cells in peritoneal exudates in rabbits.[77] Lymphocytes themselves do not release endogenous pyrogens but can release a substance that activates granulocytes in vitro to produce endogenous pyrogen. Endogenous pyrogen and gram-positive exotoxins act on the thermoregulatory center in the anterior hypothalamus to bring about vasoconstriction in the skin and increased heat production by somatic muscle.[77] When exotoxins or pyrogens act on the thermoregulatory center, the patient experiences a hard shaking chill.

Effects on Platelets and Leukocytes. Immediately after intravenous endotoxin, blood platelet counts and leukocyte counts decrease sharply. Myrvold, using *Pseudo-*

monas aeruginosa, which makes both exo- and endotoxins, found a 97 per cent decrease in canine platelet count and a 90 per cent decrease in canine leukocyte counts within two minutes after intravenous *Pseudomonas* injection.[78] Biopsies showed massive aggregation of platelets in pulmonary vessels, but intravascular coagulation was not involved. Rowe and coworkers, using live *E coli* intravenously in pigs, found only small amounts of platelet aggregates in pulmonary vessels, no change in platelet production, and no increased sequestration in the spleen, but did find massive injury and destruction of platelets two to five hours after bacteremia.[79] Platelets developed large cytoplasmic vacuoles, became depleted of glycogen, and disintegrated. Myrvold noted that platelet trapping in the lung was a transient phenomenon; by one to two hours after intravenous injection of pseudomonas, many platelets had gone back into circulation.[78] *Salmonella* endotoxin can release 5-hydroxytryptamine (serotonin) from platelets without lysing them.[80] Endotoxins can react with mast cells as well as with platelets, releasing both histamine and 5-hydroxytryptamine.[108] They also cause leukocytes to adhere to capillary walls — an effect that can be prevented by pretreatment with hydrocortisone or phenoxybenzamine.

While endotoxins have no known direct effect on arteriolar tone in isolated, perfused limbs which quickly become depleted of catecholamines,[49] they do cause a marked increase in the sensitivity of small blood vessels to catechols in whole animals.[83] *Pseudomonas* endotoxin can even sensitize the pulmonary artery to acetylcholine.[84] It may well be that the initial rise in pulmonary artery resistance seen immediately after intravenous injection of endotoxins or of live organisms in most species,[78] including primates,[84] is mediated mainly through vasoactive substances released from platelets, since Myrvold showed that the increase in pulmonary vascular resistance was nearly abolished by pretreatment with anti-platelet antiserum.[78]

Effects on Plasma. Human plasma apparently has a strong potentiating effect on endotoxin. Clark[85] reported a 2000-fold increase in virulence of endotoxin mixed with human plasma, using the rabbit as a test system. Here no release of intracellular vasoactive substance is involved. Nies and his coworkers studied *E. coli* and *Pseudomonas pseudomallei* endotoxin in subhuman primates. Twenty minutes after the infusion of endotoxin they noted decreases in systemic blood pressure that could be explained by decreased peripheral vascular resistance.[86] A plasma kinin level of 6 to 7 μg per ml corresponded with a 20 mm Hg decrease in blood pressure; the rise in plasma kinin level preceded the drop in peripheral vascular resistance. The concentration of kinins measured was enough to account for the cardiovascular changes observed. Animals that died had greater drops in peripheral resistance and tended to have higher circulating levels of kinins over a six hour period than did animals that lived.[86] Miller and his group state that kininogens, which are α-2-globulins found in human blood, can split off three kinins: bradykinin, a nonapeptide; kallidin, a decapeptide; and methionyl-lysl-bradykinin, a decapeptide.[87] In the primates — man and money — larger amounts of kinins are generated than in other species. Kallikreins, which are found in plasma, in granulocytes, and in pancreas, gut, and kidney, act as proteases to release kinins from kininogen. Prekallikrein can be converted to kallikrein by Hageman factor (Factor XII), and endotoxin and damaged endothelium can activate Hageman factor (Fig. 16–4). Much more kinin is generated when Hageman factor and plasmin interact. Streptokinase and staphylokinase can activate plasminogen to plasmin directly. Also, complement together with an S-19 macroglobulin antibody to endotoxin will generate kinin when incubated with endotoxin. Finally, phagocytosis of endotoxin by leukocytes can result in release of enzymes from leukocytes, which in turn generate kinins.

Although the half-life of kinins is measured in seconds because of inactivation by kininases, primates exposed to endotoxin generate sufficient kinin to be detectable in peripheral venous blood. Figure 16–4, from Miller and coworkers, summarizes the mechanisms for generating kinins and indicates several interactions between the kinins, the humoral immune system (complement), and the clotting system (Hageman factor).[87] Kinins and other vasoactive substances are present in increased amounts in human plasma during bacteremic shock. In the patients in Wilson's series, bradykinin was elevated in 60 per cent, TAME esterase in 19 per cent, and histamine in 19 per cent, while the Oxford carotid strip test was positive in 81 per cent of cases tested.[50] Although kinins may account for the reduced peripheral resistance and hypotension in septic shock, Miller and coworkers point out that they do not account for the fatal outcome of the syndrome.[87]

Effects on Serum Complement. McCabe[88] demonstrated reduced levels of serum complement (C3) in patients with bacteremic shock due to gram-negative organisms. In his series, C3 levels in patients with bacteremia who were not in shock were normal. Increased mortality correlated with lower C3 levels. Of 24 patients with C3 levels below 100 mg per 100 ml, 15 developed shock (63%), and 11 died (46%), whereas the mean C3 level in 41 patients who did not develop shock was 150 ± 50 mg per 100 ml.[89] McCabe notes that significant consumption of complement occurs in bacteremic shock, and especially in lethal bacteremic shock.[88, 89] Bjornson and coworkers demonstrated consumption of complement in infected burn patients.[90]

Figure 16–4. Possible mechanisms of kinin generation. The bold arrows represent major paths of kinin generation. The circled numbers are steps at which endotoxin might initiate the generation of kinins. (From Miller, R.L., Reichgott, M.J., and Melmon, K.L.: J. Infect. Dis. *128* [Suppl. S–144] 1973.)

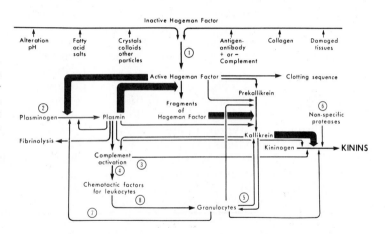

Effects on Cell Metabolism. Considerable evidence for inhibition of oxidative metabolism during severe sepsis has appeared. Although many workers in the field realized that, in the latter stages of septic shock, tissue hypoxia resulting from failing circulation produced anaerobic metabolism and increased lactate production, there is now evidence for inhibition of oxidative metabolism at an earlier stage in shock before the circulation has failed. Moss and coworkers tested the effect of *E. coli* lipopolysaccharide on the metabolism of several substrates by rat liver mitochondria and found that the oxidative metabolism of pyruvate was halved, that of citrate was reduced by a factor of eight, and that of alpha-ketoglutarate was reduced by a factor of five.[91] Mela and coworkers found that *E. coli* endotoxin, 125 μg per mg of mitochondrial protein, inhibited the reduction of cytochrome B by succinate in rat liver mitochondria in the presence of organic phosphate.[92] They also found that mitochondrial glutamate-malate oxidation and mitochondrial ATPase activity were inhibited by 119 and 45 μg per mg and per gm of mitochondrial protein respectively. They also noted mitochondrial swelling and inhibition of mitochondrial calcium uptake. Their dose of 80 to 100 μg per mg of mitochondrial protein was close to the LD_{80} of *E. coli* endotoxin for the rat, 100 μg per gm of body weight.[92] Ryan and coworkers found that pyruvate dehydragenase activity in rat diaphragm was decreased about threefold in fasting rats made septic by cecal ligation. Pyruvate dehydrogenase catalyzes the conversion of pyruvate to acetyl-CoA as pyruvate enters the citric acid cycle.[93] Seyfer and coworkers demonstrated a fall in oxygen consumption in dogs given endotoxin and kept on cardiopulmonary bypass at a constant flow. Oxygen consumption began to fall about 15 minutes after endotoxin administration and reached its lowest value after 90 minutes.[94]

As circulation fails, cells become anoxic. The changes in cell metabolism as outlined by Schumer and Sperling[95] are as follows: In the absence of oxygen, glucose is metabolized via the Embden-Meyerhof pathway as far as acetyl-CoA, which cannot be metabolized via the citric acid cycle. An excess of lactic acid is produced, and a portion of it diffuses out into the capillaries. Some glucose and amino acids are metabo-lized only to pyruvate. At a later stage, the pathway for glucose, which is a series of chemical equilibria, is partly reversed as glycogen is utilized; glucose and amino acids accumulate and diffuse out into the capillaries. Since ATP is no longer being formed, phosphates accumulate in the cell. The sodium pump fails, and sodium diffuses into the cells, while potassium diffuses out into the extracellular fluid.[95] Serum ionized calcium decreases, and serum magnesium and phosphate levels rise during septic shock in man and other primates.[96] The transmembrane potential in skeletal muscle becomes less negative.[97] Intracellular acidosis leads to disruption of lysosomes, and cellular substructures made of lipids and proteins dissolve.[95] Hydrolases, acid phosphatase, and other enzymes escape into the extracellular fluid and blood. Glenn[98] and coworkers demonstrated increases in serum levels of the lysosomal enzymes beta glucuronidase and cathespin during shock in cats — increases that could be blocked by pretreatment with methylprednisolone, 20 mg per kg. Infusions of lysosomal extracts have been shown to decrease cardiac output by 60 per cent and to increase peripheral arterial resistance, especially in the mesenteric arteries.[99] Plasma dopamine beta hydroxylase activity is also decreased in man during septic shock.[100] Inhibitors of this enzyme have been found in cultures of gram-negative organisms. The lysosomal enzymes are cleared from the plasma by reticuloendothelial cells in the liver.[99]

Effect on the Reticuloendothelial System. Overload of the reticuloendothelial system can lead to sepsis and death. Woodruff and coworkers found that 20 of 35 patients dying with liver, lung, or gastrointestinal disease had endotoxemia, demonstrated by the Limulus-lysate test.[101] Since many of these patients had no identifiable focus of infection, Woodruff and his group postulate that endotoxomia of intestinal origin appeared because of failure of the liver's reticuloendothelial system to detoxify the portal venous blood. Brief superior mesenteric artery occlusion — a lesion producing volume loss and bacteremia — will increase phagocytic index for carbon colloids in rats.[102] Alexander has demonstrated a relation between poor polymorphonuclear leukocyte function and incidence of bacteremia.[58] It is of interest that hemoglobin from damaged erythrocytes can seriously depress neutrophil function. The reticuloendothelial system removes toxins, bacteria, and lysed fragments of erythrocytes, leukocytes, and platelets from the circulation.

Effect on Erythrocytes. Johnson and his group found small decreases in erythrocyte 2,3-diphosphoglycerate during *E. coli* endotoxin shock in primates. They estimated that the small decrease in 2,3-diphosphoglycerate would result in an 11 per cent decrease in oxygen delivery — not nearly enough to account for the large amounts of lactic acid produced by these primates during septic shock.[103] Sugerman and coworkers[104] found an inverse relation between 2,3-diphosphoglycerate concentration and central venous oxygen content in man during sepsis, but other investigators[105] have not found altered affinity of hemoglobin for oxygen during septic shock. It may well be that decreased 2,3-diphosphoglycerate plays a small but definite role in decreased oxygen delivery during septic shock, but further investigation of this problem appears necessary.

Effects on the Sympathetic System. Endotoxins cause increased secretion of epinephrine and norepinephrine by sympathetic nerves and by the adrenals.[106, 107] Serum levels of angiotensin II also rise early in septic shock.[109] Clowes noted catecholamine levels as high as 75 μg per liter in sepsis when the cardiac index was below normal. Clowes also attributes the decreased insulin secretion seen in low output septic shock to high catecholamine levels; alpha stimulation reduces both insulin secretion and pancreatic blood flow.[120] Animals rendered tolerant to epinephrine have a lower mortality from intravenous endotoxin than do controls.[121]

Effects on the Microcirculations. Orkin[111] described the following sequence of events as septic shock progresses: Catechols and vasoactive amines together with increases in sympathetic tone cause an initial decrease in blood flow into capillary beds throughout the body. After about two hours the effect of local accumulation of anaerobic metabolites overrides the vasoactive factors, and the precapillary sphincters dilate. Yet the postcapillary sphincters, which are more resistant to hypoxemia, remain constricted. The rate of blood flow through the capillaries decreases, and sludging of blood and rouleaux formation

begin. Fluid is lost from the capillaries into the tissue spaces.[111]

The sequence of events described by Orkin somewhat resembles lethal shock produced in experimental animals by catechol infusions. Hermreck and Thal have shown that arterioles even in infected tissues respond normally to alpha constrictors — norepinephrine, phenylephrine, and angiotensin.[112] Weinstein indicated that acidosis affects venous smooth muscle less than it affects arterial smooth muscle.[53] Mellander and Lewis demonstrated that sympathetic stimulation for over one and two thirds hours will cause the loss of 0.035 ml of fluid per minute from the capillaries into the tissue space in cat skeletal muscles.[113] However, more recent work challenges portions of this sequence of events. Hinshaw and coworkers and Weidner and coworkers found *decreases* in the weight of innervated or denervated limbs of dogs given lethal doses of live *E. coli* or its endotoxin.[114, 115] There was no evidence for loss of fluid into skin or muscle that could account for the diminished venous return seen in endotoxin shock. In his review of the interactions between the sympathetic system and the microcirculation, Emerson[109] points out that alpha blockade with phenoxybenzamine did not prevent pooling of blood, decreases in venous return and cardiac output, and acidosis in dogs given *E. coli* endotoxin. Nor did bilateral adrenalectomy or splanchnic sympathectomy prevent these changes.[109] Although fluid loss into capillary beds in skeletal muscle may not occur through the sequence of steps involving changes in sympathetic tone in pre- and postcapillary sphincters described above by Orkin, there is a great deal of evidence that fluid loss in many organs does occur during septic shock, probably because of damage to capillary endothelium. Seyfer and coworkers, perfusing dogs at a constant flow, found that animals given endotoxin required twice as much fluid as did the control dogs in order to maintain a constant venous pressure and a constant pump flow rate.[94] Dogs given endotoxin developed ascites. Coalson and coworkers noted edema in capillary walls and in inter- and intrafiber compartments in hearts of primates six hours after *E. coli* endotoxin administration.[116] Postel and coworkers also found myocardial edema.[117] Adair and his group found fluid accumulation in the lungs of sheep that had low cardiac indices secondary to burn wound sepsis.[118] Clowes notes that interstitial edema is present early in the development of "septic lung" in man.[119] Pang found increased lung lymph flow during bradykinin infusion, and suggested that bradykinin increases pulmonary vascular permeability.[124] Pulmonary edema not due to low serum albumin levels was found in all patients who died with sepsis in the study of Vito and his group.[68]

Effects on Capillary Morphology. Anatomic changes occur in the capillary walls during sepsis. When the shock is still reversible, capillary endothelial cells show edema, some disarray in the pattern of the myofibrils, and the formation of minute vesicles that project outward from the cytoplasmic membrane. These changes can be reversed by dexamethasone.[122] Reduced electron density of capillary endothelial cell hyaloplasm has also been reported.[78] In later, irreversible stages of shock, the endothelium of capillaries and small vessels is disrupted, and fibrin deposits and microscopic hemorrhages appear.

Effects on Regional Blood Flow. Blood flow in the outer cortex of the kidney dropped to one fourth of control values within two minutes of E. coli endotoxin injection in dogs.[125] Cronenwett and coworkers[126] found a similar decrease in blood flow to the outer renal cortex, but an increased flow to the juxtamedullary cortex, using live Pseudomonas organisms in dogs. Urine output and sodium excretion doubled. The shift in intrarenal blood flow can cause an inappropriately high urine output in spite of hypovolemia and hypotension. They warn against fluid restriction in septic patients simply on the basis of normal or increased hourly urine output.[126] Hinshaw reported fibrin thrombi in renal vessels in primates given live E. coli organisms; although pretreatment with heparin prevented the thrombi, it did not prevent changes in renal function.[127]

Regional blood flow in the brain is reduced by 30 per cent or more, two to four hours after E. coli endotoxin administration in dogs. Increased cerebral vascular resistance rather than changes in arterial carbon dioxide tension or mean blood pressure appeared to cause the decrease in flow. Blood flows in the pons, medulla, hypothalamus, and thalamus were decreased, but pretreatment with methylprednisolone, 20 mg per kg, prevented the reduction in flow.[128]

Pulmonary circulation is altered during septic shock. Harrison and coworkers noted increases in pulmonary vascular resistance and decreased pulmonary venous oxygen tension in dogs following intravenous administration of live E. coli. They suggested that as pulmonary artery pressure rose, right to left shunts opened up within the lung. They also noted a 30 per cent reduction in pulmonary surfactant.[129] Vito and his group noted an association between high pulmonary vascular resistance and a fatal outcome.[68] Clowes noted right to left shunts of up to 21 per cent in 30 patients with sepsis but with normal to increased cardiac index. Right to left shunt in these patients increased to 30 per cent over several days. In his patients with sepsis and low cardiac output, pulmonary right to left shunt rose to an average of 34 per cent, and values up to 51 per cent were observed in individual patients prior to death.[119] Clowes noted that as the heart responds to therapy with inotropic drugs, pulmonary artery pressure and right to left shunt decrease. Adair and Traber found increased pulmonary artery pressures, increased pulmonary vascular permeability, and arterial desaturation in animals with hypodynamic septic shock.[118]

Effects on Veins. As early as 1966, Hinshaw and coworkers had noticed a progressive decrease in venous return following intravenous endotoxin injection.[130] This was a somewhat different response than the species-specific splanchnic pooling seen after endotoxin administration in dogs. Using cannulae in the vena cavae, Hinshaw collected, measured and reinfused the venous return in monkeys given E. coli endotoxin, 10 mg per kg. The venous return decreased progressively with time after endotoxin administration, and the systemic arterial hypotension that developed closely paralleled the reduction in venous return. The plot of venous return versus mean arterial blood pressure was virtually a straight line (Fig. 16–5). The hematocrits did not change, making the possibility of major fluid shifts from the vascular space rather unlikely. Infusion of angiotensin II after an hour of hypotension increased venous return in three animals by 10 to 20 per cent, indicating that the dilated capacitance vessels still could react.[130] Thomas and coworkers, using washed (endotoxin free)

Figure 16–5. Mean systemic arterial pressure vs. venous return in seven monkeys given endotoxin. The venous return was collected from caval cannulae, measured, and reinfused. Each numbered point represents the average value for arterial pressure and venous return for the group of seven animals. The points are five minutes apart in time, and are numbered sequentially 1 to 13. A progressive decrease in venous return resulting in hypotension was observed. (From Hinshaw, L.B., Emerson, T.E., Jr., and Raines, D.A.: Amer. J. Physiol. 210:335, 1966.)

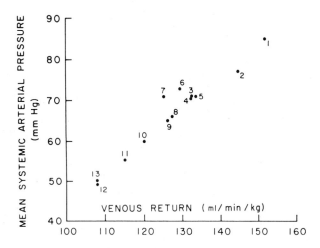

live *E. coli*, also found systemic hypotension related to decreased venous return in dogs and monkeys. Thomas noticed no change in myocardial performance and suggested that venous pooling contributes to irreversible shock in several species.[84]

Effects on the Clotting System. While disseminated intravascular coagulation may occur during sepsis, it is not necessarily a part of the clinical syndrome of septic shock. Intravascular coagulation not infrequently appears during severe sepsis with *Aerobacter aerogenes, Escherichia coli, Proteus vulgaris* and *Pseudomonas aeruginosa.*[131] It may also be seen with *Clostridia perfringens* infections (gas gangrene), and in meningococcal infections. Holcroft and his group found evidence of intravascular coagulation in primates after live *E. coli* infusion.[132] Fibrinogen concentration fell to 20 per cent of control levels, prothrombin time and partial thromboplastin times more than doubled, and the test for fibrin degradation products became positive. Holcroft stated that fibrin deposition in the lungs of septic animals was three times that found in control animals. He points out that fibrin deposition was best demonstrated by electron microscopy; much of the fibrin was too small to see by light microscopy.[132] Corrigan emphasizes that the diagnosis of intravascular coagulation in septic patients requires proof of elevation of fibrin split products or of low levels of fibrinogen or Factors V and VII.[133] A prolonged prothrombin time or partial thromboplastin time is a nonspecific finding present in roughly 25 per cent of patients with bacteremia. Low platelet counts do not imply intravascular coagulation; as mentioned above, endotoxins can

cause platelet destruction. Corrigan analyzed 222 cases of septicemia and found no improvement in survival from therapy with heparin. He points out that with successful treatment of the shock state, the intravascular coagulation will usually resolve spontaneously. If the patient is bleeding, platelets may be given for thrombocytopenia, cryoprecipitate may be given for hypofibrinogenemia, and fresh frozen plasma may be given for deficits of other coagulation factors.[133]

Whether intravascular coagulation develops or not, as septic shock progresses, circulating blood volume decreases as blood is sequestered in veins and in capillary beds. Fluids, proteins, and red cells leak through damaged capillary endothelium. Peripheral resistance increases as cardiac output declines, resulting in less perfusion to the kidneys and abdominal viscera. Heart failure develops and metabolic acidosis, present earlier in bacteremic shock, grows worse.

In the later stages of shock, vasopressors merely serve to increase venous tone.[111] Alpha adrenergic drugs are of little or no benefit, since catechol levels tend to be high as cardiac output falls in the terminal phase of septic shock.[120] Clowes advises the use of inotropic therapy instead of alpha adrenergic drugs late in septic shock.[120] Since precapillary sphincter tone is more depressed by acidosis than is the tone of postcapillary vascular smooth muscle, Orkin states that the use of alpha adrenergic drugs can increase fluid loss from the circulation by raising venous back pressure on the capillary beds. He suggested that vasodilators and volume replacement are indicated in an attempt to increase flow rate through the capillary beds in this late stage of shock.[111] Sludging of blood, rouleaux formation, and abnormalities in coagulation appear; low molecular weight dextran or other agents that alter blood viscosity may be indicated. Terminally, mucosal ulceration and hemorrhage as well as centrilobular necrosis of the liver occur.

Much of the data on the pathophysiology of septic shock has been derived from animal studies using analytic methods that cannot be employed in man. Orkin points out that such parameters as urine output and blood lactate levels are late indicators of changes that have occurred in the microcirculation. He suggests that it is even "difficult to interpret specific descriptions of successful treatment"[111] for patients in shock until better techniques are available for measuring microcirculatory changes.

Before reviewing the recent data analyzing the altered hemodynamics of patients with bacterial shock, a brief description of clinical manifestations of sepsis is necessary.

BACTEREMIC SHOCK: THE SYNDROME IN MAN

The shock states resulting from gram-negative and gram-positive organisms, and even from certain viruses, have many similarities. Differences among them appear to be more a matter of degree or of altered timing in the development of the clinical features and the hemodynamic abnormalities. Since septicemia from gram-negative organisms is encountered much more frequently in clinical medicine than is bacterial shock from gram-positive organisms or from mixed infections, gram-negative sepsis will be described first, followed by a discussion of how sepsis with gram-positive organisms and viruses differs from it.

The first sign of gram-negative sepsis may simply be mental confusion, hyperventilation, oliguria, or a chill. Sepsis may also present as respiratory failure, especially in postoperative surgical patients with occult infection below the diaphragm.[68] Fever above 101° F occurs shortly thereafter in adults, but not necessarily in infants or debilitated patients or the elderly. The skin soon becomes warm and dry, the pulse may feel full or bounding, and urine flow may appear adequate despite arterial hypoten-

sion. Weinstein has termed this early phase "warm shock."[53] When an increase in sympathetic tone occurs, the skin becomes cold and moist. Nausea and vomiting appear in about half the patients.[134, 142] In man, a leukopenia occurs after the endotoxin enters the blood, but before the onset of chills. In sepsis caused by *Pseudomonas* the leukopenia is often severe and prolonged.[135] Oliguria is often present before the arterial pressure drops to levels too low for glomerular filtrate formation.[49] There are no consistent hematocrit changes early in gram-negative shock.

In studies of the effects of endogenous pyrogen in man, Moser and his group showed that there was a 27 per cent increase in cardiac output immediately after intravenous pyrogen injection and before fever developed.[136] Mild hyperventilation occurred during the chill — probably as an effect of endotoxin on the central nervous system, because metabolic acidosis was not yet present.[50, 136] Total peripheral resistance declined during the flush that followed the chill, and pulmonary artery pressures increased slightly. The heart rate was proportional to the fever. From this study it is evident that increased cardiac output and increased cardiac work occur early in gram-negative sepsis, even before fever develops. This finding of Moser and his group may explain the occasional patient in whom gram-negative sepsis presents as dyspnea or frank pulmonary edema. In most cases skin pallor or mottled cyanosis is a late sign.

According to Dietzman et al., the increased in temperature, pulse, and respiration closely parallel the increased circulating catecholamine levels.[137] The electrolyte pattern most frequently encountered consists of hyponatremia (a mean of 10.9 mEq L below normal), hypochloremia (3.7 mEq/L below normal), an increased potassium (0.54 mEq/L above normal), and an elevated BUN (16.5 mEq/L above normal).[134] Arterial gases show an initial respiratory alkalosis, followed by the development of progressive metabolic acidosis. Terminally, there may be a marked rise in potassium. Increased levels of serum catechols seen in septic shock with low cardiac output cause decreased secretion of insulin. In the series of Clowes, blood insulin averaged 42 ± 6 μU per ml in patients whose cardiac index averaged 4.6 liters per minute, but averaged only 12 ± 3 μU per ml in patients whose cardiac index averaged 2.4 liters per minute.[120] Blood glucose is elevated early in sepsis but drops to very low values terminally as serum potassium rises. The vasoconstriction that appears is most intense in the skin, the skeletal muscle, and the extremities. Renal perfusion decreases, although to a lesser degree than the perfusion of peripheral tissues; and splanchnic blood flow decreases, but to a lesser degree than renal blood flow.[111] Oliguria and anuria develop. Lactic acidosis increases as the shock state grows worse. Lactate levels have some value as a prognostic sign. Schweizer and Howland[138] found that four of five septic patients with blood lactates over 10 mEq per liter died. Winslow and Loeb[67] found that initial arterial lactate was 31 mg per 100 ml in patients in their series who survived, while in those who died initial arterial lactate was 63 mg per 100 ml. A diabetic type of glucose tolerance curve is often observed during severe infections in man,[120] and during septic shock but prior to its terminal state, insulin levels are high enough to prevent lipolysis.[139] Hence, the patient resorts to catabolism of muscle, with gluconeogenesis of branch chain amino acids (valine, leucine, and isoleucine) by the liver as a source of energy. Freund et al. note that blood levels of aromatic amino acids (phenylalanine and tyrosine) and sulfur containing amino acids (taurine, cystine, and methionine) rise during septic shock since they do not participate significantly in gluconeogenesis. Freund associates elevation of these particular amino acids with encephalopathy and coma that occurs as septic shock progresses.[139] Several authors describe insulin resistance in skeletal muscle during septic shock,[120, 139] but Wichterman did not find this effect.[140] Further research appears to be needed into the problem of resistance to insulin during septic shock. Clowes noted twice the lactate production in muscle of hypodynamic animals than in hyperdynamic animals, even though minute oxygen uptake by the muscle did not differ between the two groups, and suggested that this increased lactate production may result from pyruvate dehydrogenase inhibition, as described above in the study of Ryan and coworkers,[93] and by Schumer.[141] Serum SGOT may rise because of damage to heart, liver, and other tissues, and serum amylase may rise because renal clearance of amylase is reduced.[142]

Cycles of hypercoagulation alternating with hypocoagulation may appear in gram-negative sepsis.[143] The prothrombin time is initially prolonged in 64 per cent of patients with septic shock,[50] and abnormalities of Factors V and VIII have been reported in about one fifth of the cases.[50] Fibrinogen levels rise abruptly and then slowly decline over two or three weeks. Platelet counts may be severely depressed,[144] as described previously.[78, 79] The changes in the clotting mechanism are more apparent in shock of greater severity or longer duration, and are often associated with a hemorrhagic diathesis. A drop in fibrinogen may occur if intravascular coagulation appears,[131, 132] or it may be associated with sludging of blood and fibrin deposition in capillary beds. In addition, in cases of septic abortion with a bleeding diathesis and shock prior to death, a pattern of fibrin deposition in the glomerular vessels resembling that of a generalized Shwartzman reaction has been discovered.[145] Fibrinolysins may cause hemorrhagic diatheses in septic shock, and can also activate bradykininogen to bradykinin.[146] In Wilson's series of 25 patients with "pure" septic shock, bradykininogen was decreased in 52 per cent, and bradykinin was elevated in 60 per cent, although in his patients the euglobulin lysis time was normal.[50]

As septic shock intensifies, severe, uncompensated metabolic acidosis develops, progressive arterial desaturation occurs, heart failure appears and cardiac output decreases; dilated pupils, Cheyne-Stokes respiration, and hypothermia may appear; and the patient dies in coma from cardiac failure.

Certain physical and laboratory findings may be seen often enough in gram-negative shock to be considered a part of the syndrome. When sepsis presents as respiratory failure, as Clowes points out, there may be an initial phase of arterial hypoxemia (right to left shunt) in the presence of a clear chest x-ray. Histologically interstitial edema, septal invasion by leukocytes, and diffuse alveolar collapse are present.[119, 120] This phase may be followed by bronchopneumonia, the typical pulmonary lesion in septic shock.[120] Vito and coworkers noted decreased compliance in patients whose sepsis presented as respiratory failure.[68] Elevated pulmonary artery pressures and a tendency toward right heart failure may be present. Sixty per cent of the patients who had sepsis presenting as respiratory distress in the series of Sibbald[147] and his group had elevated pulmonary artery pressures. The use of mechanical ventilation and positive end expiratory pressure can improve arterial desaturation and compensate for the increased work of breathing. Improvement in cardiac performance can lead to decreased pulmonary artery pressures and to a decrease in right to left shunt, as noted above.[119] Pleural effusions are frequent in sepsis resulting from intra-abdominal inflammation.[50] Any sizeable effusions should be tapped to improve ventilation. Lung compliance is reduced because of vascular congestion and interstitial edema, and higher airway pressures than normal will often be necessary during mechanical ventilation of patients with septic shock. Vito et al. found that in their series lung compliance was lower in patients who died.[68] The data of Clowes and his group showing cardi-

ac index, pulmonary artery mean and wedge pressures, per cent right to left pulmonary shunt, peak inspiratory airway pressure, and alveolar-arterial pO_2 gradient in patients with hyperdynamic septic shock and in patients after hemorrhagic shock are reproduced in Figure 16–6.[119]

Even when septic shock does not present as respiratory failure, ventilatory insufficiency frequently develops.[50, 164, 165] While the pathologic changes in the lung described above are the main causes of respiratory insufficiency in sepsis, neural or muscular defects that interfere with chest bellows action,[164] or simple physical exhaustion[165] may hinder ventilation. Nor should ventilatory insufficiency from simple upper airway obstruction in the debilitated patient be overlooked. Ledingham and McArdle consider earlier and more frequent use of mechanical ventilation one of the main reasons for the 20 per cent reduction in the mortality rate from septic shock in

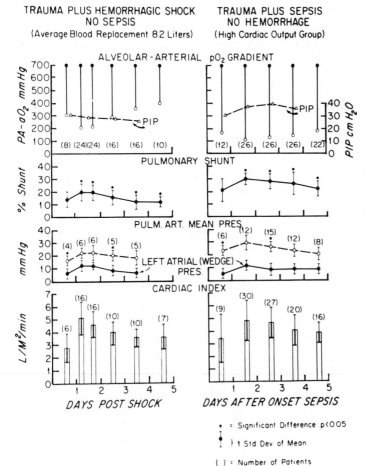

Figure 16–6. A comparison of alveolar-arterial oxygen gradient, peak inspiratory pressure, pulmonary shunt, pulmonary artery mean and wedge pressures, and cardiac output in patients after hemorrhagic shock (left) and during sepsis. Note that an elevated peak inspiratory pressure corresponds with increased pulmonary shunt and increased mean pulmonary artery pressure during sepsis. (From Clowes, G.H.A., Jr., Hirsch, E., Williams, L., Kwasnik, E., O'Donnell, T.F., Cuevas, P., Saini, V.K., Moradi, I., Saravis, C., Stone, M., and Kuffler, J.: Ann. Surg. 181:689, 1975.)

their patients.[55] Mortality rates above 65 per cent have been reported in patients with septic shock and respiratory failure.[50, 68]

Jaundice often appears late in septic shock, although it may appear earlier in patients having hemolysis or intraperitoneal leakage of bile.[106] The electrocardiogram may show either nonspecific ST changes,[49] usually on the basis of electrolyte imbalance, or ischemic changes, especially in older patients[59] and in patients with heart disease.[54] Since elderly patients may not develop fever or significant leukocytosis when septic, they may present only with signs and symptoms of congestive heart failure. A differential diagnosis between septic shock and myocardial infarction may be difficult to make. Measurement of serum creatinine phosphokinase enzyme (CPK-2), which is elevated in myocardial infarction, can aid in the diagnosis. The history may be of value in this differential, and the diagnosis will soon become apparent from the clinical course. Appropriate diagnostic studies should be obtained.

Sepsis and septic shock in infants may be difficult to diagnose, especially in the early postoperative period. In the series of Pierce and others, only 2 per cent of septic infants had rectal temperatures over 39°C (102.2°F), and only 45 per cent had leukocyte counts above 15,000 per mm³. None of the infants had jaundice or splenomegaly. Respiratory distress, oliguria, acidosis, and episodes of bradycardia were present, but these are nonspecific signs in any severely ill infant. The diagnosis of sepsis was not made until autopsy in 70 per cent of their cases.[60] A high index of suspicion and the use of frequent blood cultures are necessary to make the diagnosis of sepsis in infants. The reason for the increased susceptibility of infants less than six months of age to sepsis is not known at present.

Sepsis with gram-positive organisms follows the same basic course as gram-negative sepsis but differs from it in the timing of the physiologic changes. In gram-positive sepsis, the period of "hot shock," characterized by a high cardiac output and warm extremities, lasts much longer on the average than it does it gram-negative sepsis. Oliguria appears later, and intravascular coagulation appears less frequently. Hemodynamic measurements made when shock is first diagnosed are more likely to show a high cardiac output and a low systemic vascular resistance in gram-positive shock. The per cent of right to left pulmonary shunting is often less than it is in patients with gram-negative sepsis.

The time course of septic shock with rickettsial and viral organisms resembles that of shock with gram-positive organisms, and is characterized by the development of a great deal of peripheral edema in skin, muscle, and other tissues.[54] Edema formation and vasodilatation lead to major deficits in intravascular volume in these diseases.[54] Weinstein notes that cardiac failure secondary to myocarditis is a feature of septic shock with influenza and Coxsackie-B viruses, Rickettsiae, and diphtheria.[53]

The clinical course of patients with tetanus appears to differ from sepsis with other organisms in that their course is characterized by erratic changes in the cardiovascular system, rather than by a steady downward progression. According to Tsueda and coworkers, hypertension, tachycardia, vasomotor instability, and cardiac arrest occur in paralyzed tetanus patients during mechanical ventilation, in the absence of electrolyte imbalance, acidosis, or hypoxemia.[69] Unexplained bradycardia can also occur. Histologic evidence of myocarditis or lesions in the conduction system are seen in some of these cases. A syndrome of sympathetic nervous system hyperactivity with high but labile blood pressure, tachyarrhythmias, fever, a high metabolic rate, sweating, peripheral vascular constriction, and high urinary norepinephrine occurs in some cases of tetanus. An effect of tetanus toxin on the sympathetic nervous system has been suggested. Continuous sedation with a thiopental sodium drip has been used in tetanus patients, and propranolol and other peripheral blocking agents have been used successfully.[69]

The principal clinical findings in septic shock are listed in Table 16–3.

Hemodynamic Changes in Patients with Sepsis

Although there are wide variations in the published data of different investigators doing research into the hemodynamic effects of septicemia, a general pattern for these effects has emerged. Many of the apparent discrepancies among the findings of the various research groups can be explained in terms of patient selection by considering the type of organism involved (gram-positive or gram-negative), the volemic state of the patient, the presence of other diseases in the patient, and the progression of the disease process at the time when the patient was studied.

Blain and others studied the initial phases of bacteremic shock by measuring hemodynamics in patients having urologic surgery and correlating their measurements with blood cultures taken during and after surgery.[148] There were 10 gram-positive, eight gram-negative, and three mixed bacteremias. When bacteremia first occurred, cardiac output was elevated an average of 1.6 liters per minute in the gram-negative patient group, but showed virtually no change for the gram-positive patients when compared with measurements made the day prior to surgery. Systemic vascular resistance dropped farther in the gram-negative patients (mean decrease — 10 mm Hg/L/min) than it did in the gram-positive patients (mean decrease — 2 mm Hg/L/min). The central venous pressure tended to decrease more in the gram-negative group, but the degree of mild arterial hypotension was the same in both groups. In the two patients who developed clinical gram-negative shock, cardiac output increased 2.9 liters per minute and systemic vascular resistance dropped by 67 per cent, compared with control measurements.[148]

Early reports in the literature by Lillehei and coworkers and by Dietzman and coworkers indicated some increases in total peripheral resistance during gram-negative shock in man.[137, 149] Udhoji and Weil reported a high vascular resistance (1987 ± 1168 dyne sec cm^{-5}) and a low cardiac index (1.42 ± 0.54 L/m^2) in seven patients with gram-negative septic shock whose CVP was normal (10 ± 6.1 cm H_2O).[150] More recently, Winslow and coworkers studied 50 medical patients with positive blood cultures who developed shock, 19 with gram-positive and 31 with gram-negative infection.[67] They found that patients with gram-positive shock had more tachycardia (119 ± 4/min vs. 100/min, p<0.01) and greater cardiac indices (3.8 ± 0.3 L/min/m^2 vs. 2.9 ± 0.2 L/min/^{2}, p<0.05) than did patients with

Table 16–3 *Principal Clinical Findings in Septic Shock (in Approximate Order of Appearance)*

	Clinical	Laboratory
Early	Confusion	Respiratory alkalosis
	Tachypnea	Mild to moderate lactic acidosis
	Oliguria	Leukopenia, then leukocytosis
	Bounding pulses	Slight BUN elevation
	Hypotension	Low serum Na^+ and Cl
	Fever	Slightly increased K^+
	Tachycardia	Reduced CO_2 combining power
	Chills	Prolonged prothrombin time
	Nausea or vomiting	Elevated fibrinogen
	Diarrhea	Low peripheral resistance
	Warm, moist skin	High cardiac output, if normovolemic
Late	Lethargy or coma	Significant lactic acidosis
	Weak pulse	Leukocytosis
	Anuria	Rising BUN
	Pallid, cold limbs	Fibrinogen variable
	Shallow tachypnea	CVP variable
	Cyanosis	Higher peripheral resistance
	Metabolic acidosis	Normal or low cardiac output
Terminal	Coma	Severe lactic acidosis
	Cheyne-Stokes respiration	Combined respiratory and metabolic acidosis
	Severe cyanosis	Terminal K^+ rise
	Hyporeflexia	Desaturation — over 30% R-L shunt
	Hypothermia	Low platelet count
	Dilated, sluggish pupils	Low fibrinogen
	Jaundice	Circulating fibrinolysins
	Hemorrhagic diathesis	Elevated bradykinin (>20 μ/cc.)
		CVP low, until CHF occurs
		Low peripheral resistance
		Very low cardiac output

gram-negative shock. Moreover, 12 of 13 patients with initial cardiac indices less than 2.5 L/min had gram-negative bacteremia.[67] Kwaan and Weil had previously reported a difference in the hemodynamic patterns of patients with shock from gram-negative or gram-positive organisms.[151] Both gram-positive and gram-negative groups had equally low systemic pressures, but patients with gram-negative infections had lower cardiac indices, higher peripheral resistances, and higher lactate levels than patients with gram-positive sepsis. The gram-negative patients were more oliguric and had cooler extremities than the gram-positive patients. The arterial oxygen saturations and arterial pCO_2 values were equal in both groups, and no patients were clinically terminal when studied. The higher serum lactates in the gram-negative patients suggest either poorer tissue perfusion or, perhaps, a greater inhibition of oxidative metabolism. The data of Kwaan and Weil are reproduced in Table 16–4.[151] The findings of Gunnar and coworkers[152] were very similar to those of Kwaan and Weil.

There is some variation in published reports concerning hemodynamic differences between gram-positive and gram-negative septic shock. Wilson and others reported normal or low total peripheral resistance in 88 per cent (28 of 32) of his patients with septic shock, The incidence of gram-negative infection in his series was 65.3 per cent.[50] Cohn and his group report similar values.[153] As Blain and coworkers demonstrated in the study referred to previously, early in gram-negative septic shock, there is usually high cardiac output and low peripheral resistance.[148] Most investigators have found higher peripheral resistance and lower cardiac output in patients with gram-negative sepsis than in patients with gram-

positive infections. It appears likely that the pattern of low resistance, high cardiac output changes to a low cardiac output, high resistance pattern earlier in the course of sepsis with gram-negative organisms than it does in the gram-positive infections. Some groups (Wilson,[50] MacLean,[51] and Cohn[153]) report normal or low resistance and normal or high cardiac output in patients with gram-negative septic shock, and one wonders if their patients are being studied earlier in the disease process. It must also be remembered that there is a great deal of individual variation in patients. Siegel and coworkers point out the fallacy of trying to compare peripheral resistance data in patients with different cardiac indices, because the relationship between blood flow and mean arterial pressure is not linear.[154] They found a generally lower value for peripheral resistance in 30 patients with septic shock than in 26 patients in shock for other reasons. Their data, plotting cardiac index against total peripheral resistance, are shown in Figure 16–7. Gram-positive shock usually has a low peripheral resistance throughout most of its course, until the terminal stage is reached. Gram-negative shock has an early phase with high cardiac output and low resistance that usually soon changes to the low cardiac output, high resistance pattern typically found with gram-negative bacterial shock. However, occasional patients with gram-negative sepsis stay in a high output, low resistance state during most of their course.

The blood volume of the patient when septic shock begins frequently determines the patient's hemodynamic response. Wilson and coworkers[155] found that in eight patients with both septic shock and hypovolemia (CVP 0 to 7.5 cm H_2O, mean 3.6 cm H_2O) the total peripheral resistance (TPR)

Table 16–4 *Comparison of Gram-Negative and Gram-Positive Septic Shock**

	Gram-Positive, 6 Patients	Gram-Negative, 8 Patients	P Value of Difference
Cardiac index (L./min./m.²)	2.81 ± 0.24	1.85 ± 0.21	0.02
Systemic resistance (dyne sec. cm.⁻⁵)	1058 ± 52	1649 ± 172	0.02
pH	7.44 ±	7.32 ± 0.03	0.02
Urine (cc./hr.)	26.5 ± 1.10.6	5.7 ± 1.8	0.05
Lactate (mM./L.)	2.54 ± 1.07	10.28 ± 2.36	0.02
Bicarbonate (mEq./L.)	20.5 ± 1.5	13 ± 1.7	0.01

*No significant differences were found in systolic and diastolic blood pressure, central venous pressure, hemoglobin, hematocrit, arterial pCO_2 or hemoglobin saturation.

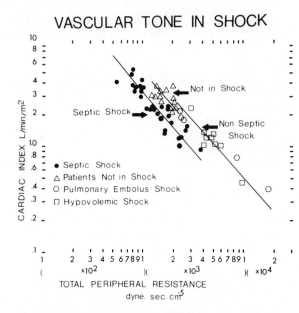

Figure 16–7. For a given cardiac index, total peripheral resistance is lower in patients with shock from sepsis than from other causes. (From Siegel, J.H., Greenspan, M., and Del Guercio, L.R.M.: Ann. Surg. *165*:504, 1967.)

tended to be higher (1156 dyne sec cm^{-5}) than in patients with "pure" septic shock unaccompanied by hypovolemia whose resistance was lower (1000 dyne sec cm^{-5} or less in 11 of 12 cases). The cardiac indices were also lower (mean 2.8 L/min/m^2).[155] MacLean's group, categorizing their cases according to the initial venous pressure, found that 39 patients with normal or high CVP had cardiac indices of 4.1 L per min per m^2, and low TPR values (640 dyne sec cm^{-5}), whereas 17 patients in septic shock with a low CVP (mean 3.5 cm H$_2$O) had low cardiac indices (mean 2.1 L/min/m^2) and a higher TPR (1243 dyne sec cm^{-5} — within the normal range.)[51] Thus hypovolemia superimposed upon gram-negative shock results in a low cardiac output with a reflex arterial vasoconstriction. A low CVP may be associated with a TPR higher than normal during sepsis.[57] Blood volumes much greater than normal are required to sustain cardiac output and return arterial pressure toward normal in bacteremic shock (Fig. 16–8).[61]

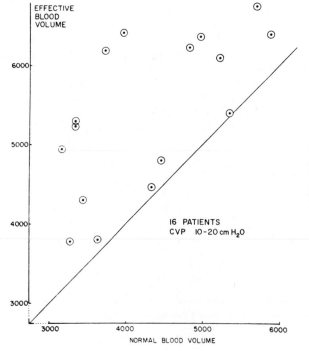

Figure 16–8. Increased "effective" blood volume required to attain a CVP of 10 to 20 cm H$_2$O and to restore arterial pressure, urine output, and tissue perfusion in patients with septic shock. (From MacLean, L.D., Duff, J., Scott, H.M., and Peretz, D.I.: Surg. Gynec. Obstet. *120*:282, 1965.)

Survival during septic shock has been associated with increased blood volumes.[54] A 20 per cent depletion of extracellular fluid as measured by radioactive sulfate has been observed in experimental endotoxin shock.

The presence of several additional diseases may alter the patient's hemodynamic response to septic shock. Udhoji and Weil have shown that in eight patients, seven of whom had cirrhosis and one of whom had multiple sclerosis, the hemodynamic response to gram-negative shock included a high cardiac output (4.09 ± 1.45 L/min/m²) and a low TPR (668 ± 200 dyne sec cm⁻⁵). The O_2 saturation was 93 ± 7.1 per cent in these patients, indicating considerable right to left shunt in the lungs in the presence of a high cardiac output state.[150] The cirrhotic with septic shock is more likely to develop high output congestive heart failure than the average patient because cirrhosis is accompanied by arteriovenous shunting.

Some arteriovenous shunting of blood through inflamed tissue apparently does occur during bacteremic shock. Wilson and his group noted an increased saturation in iliac venous blood in two patients with pelvic inflammation.[50] Albrecht and Clowes were among the first to recognize that an inflamed region might act as an A-V fistula.[157] Dietzman and others attributed low peripheral resistance seen in many patients with shock to shunting of blood through large inflamed regions, as in generalized peritonitis, and believed that such shunting could mask the presence elsewhere in the body of capillary beds that are underperfused because of vasoconstriction of their afferent arterioles.[137] Cronenwett and coworkers created localized abscesses on the legs of dogs and found that after four days, arteriovenous shunting in the infected limb was 10 per cent of limb blood flow versus 2 per cent for the uninfected control limb.[158] Archie, using a radioactive microsphere technique, studied dogs with septic shock from cecal ligation.[159] He found that A-V shunt was 36 per cent in the splanchnic bed of the animals with peritonitis versus 18 per cent in the control group. He found no evidence of increased A-V shunt in other tissues. It appears that arteriovenous shunting does occur through infected regions of the body, and this shunting may contribute somewhat to lowering resistance and increasing the central venous oxygen saturation.

Currently, there is a growing understanding of the importance of heart failure during septic shock in man, not just during the terminal phase of sepsis but also during the transition from high output low resistance shock to the phase of low output with higher resistance. MacLean et al. first called attention to the high incidence of treatable occult heart failure in patients with septic shock when they reported its presence in 10 patients of a group of 30 studied.[61] Occult heart failure may be difficult to diagnose clinically. Rales and a gallop rhythm are absent, but the patient has hypotension, tachycardia, oliguria, and a low cardiac index, together with a CVP that is either normal or elevated. The history may not suggest that the patient is likely to develop cardiac failure; he may be young and have no history of hypertension, decreased exercise tolerance, or myocardial infarction. Weisel and coworkers calculated left ventricular performance curves while the patients' blood volume was increased by 500 ml.[65] Half of the 50 patients in their series showed evidence of heart failure — developed a downslope in their performance curve (Fig. 16–9). No patient survived with an upslope of less than 2 gm·m/m². When remeasured several days later, 10 patients showed improved upslopes, demonstrating that the myocardial depression of sepsis is potentially reversible. Septic patients who developed postoperative heart disease (ischemia or infarction) had poor upslopes (2.21 gm·m/m²) and a uniformly fatal outcome (9 of 9), emphasizing the importance of myocardial performance to survival in sepsis. Weisel looked for but did not find elevated right heart pressures, and noted a very poor correlation between central venous and pulmonary artery wedge pressures.[65] In about half the septic patients in the series of Krausz and coworkers, left heart failure was evident from rises in pulmonary wedge pressure during fluid infusion.[160] In animals, Postel and coworkers demonstrated decreases in cardiac output and stroke volume and increases in pulmonary wedge pressure as early as one hour following infusion of *Pseudomonas aeruginosa* organisms.[161] These changes imply the onset of left ventricular failure. At post, the myocardial capillaries appeared congested, and the muscle showed separation of the fibers by edema, intracellular edema, and foci of inflamma-

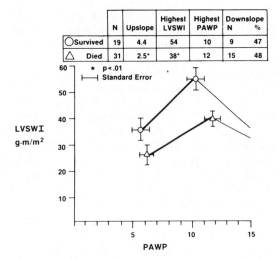

	N	Upslope	Highest LVSWI	Highest PAWP	Downslope N	%
○ Survived	19	4.4	54	10	9	47
△ Died	31	2.5*	38*	12	15	48

Figure 16-9. Left ventricular stroke work index vs. pulmonary artery wedge pressure during fluid challenge in survivors (circles) and nonsurvivors (triangles) of septic shock. Survivors showed greater increases in stroke work index and had a higher stroke work index for a given wedge pressure. Stroke work index and wedge pressure before fluid challenge were not significantly different between survivors and nonsurvivors. Note that downslopes occur at a wedge pressure of only 10 to 12 mm Hg. (From Weisel, R.D., Vito, L., Dennis, R.C., Valeri, C.R., and Hechtman, H.S.: Amer. J. Surg. 133:514, 1977.)

tion. However, Thomas et al.[84] and Buckberg et al.[162] did not find evidence of heart failure in their studies. Clowes and coworkers documented right heart failure during septic shock in patients with large right to left pulmonary shunts and high pulmonary vascular resistance.[119] Some of the patients in the study of Winslow et al. demonstrated heart failure.[67] There is general agreement that heart failure always occurs in terminal septic shock when hypotension, marked acidosis, and poor coronary perfusion have been present for a number of hours.[153]

Inotropic therapy is indicated in patients with heart failure and septic shock. Isoproterenol had been recommended,[61] but dopamine now appears to be the drug of choice.[67] Winslow and his group used three different catecholamines to titer patients in septic shock to a mean arterial pressure of 70 to 80 mm Hg when possible. Doses used averaged 25 μg per minute for norepinephrine, 750 μg per minute for dopamine, and 5.9 μg per minute for isoproterenol. They noted no significant difference in heart rate or cardiac index between isoproterenol and dopamine, but found that for the same cardiac index and pulse rate, dopamine achieved a higher arterial pressure and systemic vascular resistance than isoproterenol. They stated that isoproterenol increased blood flow to skeletal muscle but that dopamine produced a more favorable clinical response. Their data comparing hemodynamic effects of these three drugs during septic shock are shown in Figure 16-10.[67] If tachycardia or other arrhythmias occur during therapy with dopamine or isoproterenol,

digitalis is indicated. With inotropic drug therapy, the cardiac index may achieve greater than normal values. A high cardiac index is necessary for survival in septic shock.[54]

Figure 16-11 is a plot of left ventricular stroke work versus CVP in a young woman in septic shock following abortion. Stroke work was low initially. Treatment with volume replacement, antibiotics, and steroids had been unsuccessful, but she responded well to inotropic therapy with digitalis, and even became mildly hyperdynamic over the next 48 hours.

Therapy with glucose, insulin, and potassium can be of great hemodynamic benefit when cardiac failure and a low cardiac output state have developed during septic shock. This therapy appears to provide an inotropic effect of great magnitude, especially late in shock when blood insulin levels are low and catechol levels are high. It may benefit patients who have not responded to therapy with fluids, steroids, and inotropic catechols. Clowes and his group report that in 10 patients with bacteremic shock whose cardiac outputs averaged 3.0 ± 0.3 L/min., whose CVP averaged 14 cm H_2O, and whose mean arterial pressure was 59 ± 7 mm Hg on isoproterenol, the administration of a solution containing glucose, insulin, and potassium caused the cardiac output to increase to 8.6 ± 0.5 L/min., mean arterial pressure to rise to 76 ± 4 mm Hg, and CVP to fall to 9 cm H_2O. The data of Clowes and his group are shown in Table 16-5, and in Figure 16-12.[120] Archer and coworkers demonstrated failure in animal heart preparations after endotoxin

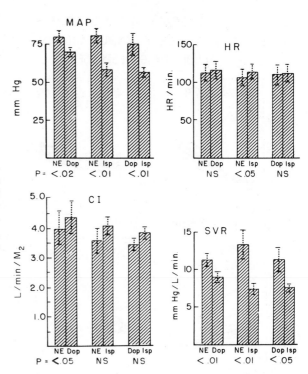

Figure 16-10. Comparisons between norepinephrine (NE) and dopamine (Dop), norepinephrine and isoproterenol (Isp), and isoproterenol and dopamine in patients during septic shock. Effects of these drugs are shown on mean arterial pressure (MAP), heart rate (HR), cardiac index (CI) and systemic vascular resistance (SVR). P values are calculated by paired T test. P greater than 0.05 was not significant (NS). (From Winslow, D.J., Loeb, H.S., Rahimtoola, S.H., Kamath, L., and Gunnar, R.M.: Amer. J. Med. *54*:429, 1973.)

administration and three hours of hypotension (mean b.p. 50 mm Hg), even though blood glucose was 111 mg per 100 ml. They then showed improved myocardial performance by administering insulin.[163]

The clinician who has no access to equipment for measuring cardiac output and therefore cannot calculate arterial resistance might wonder whether resistance can be estimated from the physical findings in patients with septic shock. MacLean et al. noted warm, pale, dry skin in 39 patients

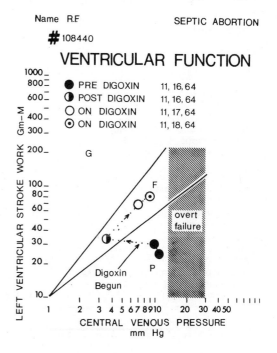

Figure 16-11. Response to inotropic therapy with digitalis in a young woman with septic shock following abortion. (From Siegel, J.H., Greenspan, M., and Del Guercio, L.R.M.: Ann. Surg. *165*:504, 1967.)

CLINICAL SEPSIS: LOW OUTPUT STATE
EFFECTS OF GLUCOSE, POTASSIUM AND INSULIN
HEMODYNAMIC RESPONSES

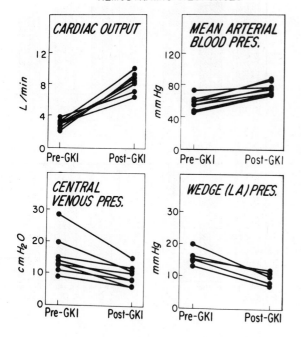

Figure 16–12.   Early hemodynamic effects of therapy with glucose, insulin, and potassium in patients with hypotension resulting from septic shock with a low cardiac output. (From Clowes, G.H.A., Jr., O'Donnell, T.F., Ryan, N.T., and Blackburn, G.L.: Ann. Surg. *179*:690, 1974.)

with a low TPR.[51] Kwaan and Weil found that the temperature gradient between thigh and toe in gram-negative septic shock patients with elevated TPR values was 4° C larger than the gradient in gram-positive patients with lower resistances.[151] However Udhoji and Weil[150] reported cyanotic ex-

tremities in 17 patients whose peripheral arterial resistance was normal or low; in four patients with cold and clammy skin, Wilson and coworkers[50] reported TPR values below 680 dyne sec cm^{-5}. The pulse pressure is more an index of peripheral resistance than of cardiac output. It seems

Table 16–5   *Clinical Response to Glucose, Potassium, and Insulin in Low Output Septic State*
Values ± SEM

	Pre GKI	Post GKI
Hemodynamic		
Cardiac Output (L/min)	3.0 ± 0.3(8)	8.6 ± 0.5(7)
Pulse (beats/min)	124 ± 4 (10)	115 ± 4 (10)
Mean Arterial Pres. (mm Hg)	59 ± 7 (10)	76 ± 4 (10)
Centr. Venous Pres. (cm H$_2$O)	14 ± 3 (8)	9 ± 2 (8)
Pulm. Wedge Pres. (mm Hg)	16 ± 3 (5)	12 ± 2 (5)
Metabolic		
Rectal Temperature (°F)	100.6 ± 0.6 (7)	101.2 ± 0.5(7)
Blood Glucose (uM/ml)	10.2 ± 2.3 (8)	16.3 ± 3.1(6)
Lactate (uM/ml)	2.6 ± 0.8 (6)	1.9 ± 1.1(6)
FFA (uM/ml)	971 ± 124(7)	432 ± 78 (6)
Blood Insulin	12 ± 3 (4)	230 ± 56 (4)
Blood Gases		
Resp. O$_2$ Gas Mixture (%)	40 ± (7)	40 ± (7)
Arterial pO$_2$ (mm Hg)	89 ± 12 (8)	109 ± (8)
Arterial pCO$_2$ (mm Hg)	35 ± 3 (7)	38 ± 4 (7)
Hydrogen Ion (pH units)	7.41 ± .03 (10)	7.44 ± .04(9)
Urine Output (ml/br)	18 ± 6 (6)	61 ± 14 (6)

Number of observations in parentheses.
(From Clowes, G. H. A. Jr., et al.: Energy metabolism in sepsis. Ann. Surg. *179*:684, 1974.)

far preferable to measure the hemodynamics (including the capillary wedge pressure) in patients with septic shock and to use hemodynamic measurements as a guide to therapy, rather than to base treatment only on the physical signs, urine output, and central venous pressure.

CONTROVERSIAL AREAS IN THE PATHOPHYSIOLOGY OF SEPTIC SHOCK

At present there are several controversies concerning the pathophysiology of septic shock. We shall discuss three controversies: first, the existence of major systemic arteriovenous shunting; second, the meaning of lactic acidosis; and third, the role of the myocardial depressant factor discovered by Glenn, Lefer, and others.

Systemic A-V Shunting

Early in bacteremic shock cardiac output increases and saturation of central venous blood rises. The arteriovenous oxygen difference narrows, and less oxygen is extracted from circulating blood; yet at the same time, tissues are apparently hypoxemic, as indicated by their production of lactic acid and by dysfunction in many organs. Three explanations are possible: blood is shunted by capillary beds, oxygen release is inhibited, or cellular oxidation is blocked. As noted above in reports by Albrecht and Clowes[157] and Dietzman[137], some shunting of blood through specific inflamed regions does occur; but the amount of regional shunting — even with peritonitis — can not account for the magnitude of the increase in central venous oxygen saturation. Some decrease in availability of oxygen due to hyperventilation and a low arterial pCO_2 resulting in a shift of the hemoglobin dissociation curve does occur. Moreover, erythrocyte 2,3-DPG is somewhat reduced during septic shock. These effects are of small magnitude and do not appear to account for the increased central venous oxygen saturation. Cohen and coworkers found an average A-V O_2 difference of 2.92 ±0.48 vol. per cent in patients with peritonitis or septicemia, while the normal A-V O_2 difference is 4.50 vol. per cent.[153] Minute oxygen consumption was also reduced in Cohen's patients (192.7 ± 29.9 ml/min vs. the predicted normal 250 ml/min). Either cellular

oxidation is blocked to a great extent or considerable arteriovenous shunting must occur. MacLean and coworkers found that A-V O_2 difference correlated directly with peripheral resistance and inversely with cardiac output, as shown in Figure 16–13. It is apparent that patients in septic shock who have the highest cardiac output also have the lowest arteriovenous oxygen differences.[166] Siegel and coworkers studied oxygen consumption in shock of different etiologies and found that in patients with hyperdynamic septic shock, cardiac output showed very little relation to oxygen consumption (Fig. 16–14). Siegel and his group point out the inefficiency of this circulatory response, which could result in death from high output cardiac failure. They also found that the amount of shunt is proportional to total aortic blood flow, suggesting paralysis of regulatory mechanisms that normally keep these shunts closed.[154] They suggested that the primary pathology in septic shock is a vascular tone defect, probably at the precapillary level. Hermreck and Thal have shown that venous blood from septic limbs of dogs contains a substance that causes arterial dilatation in animal limbs and could conceivably dilate arteriovenous connections.[167]

Wilson et al. have a different interpretation of the pattern of hyperdynamic septic shock.[155] Although they state that low peripheral resistance does not imply good tissue perfusion, they claim that it is difficult to imagine inadequate tissue perfusion in patients with septic shock but with warm, dry skin.[50] Wilson and his group wondered whether utilization of oxygen by cells is blocked in patients with bacteremic shock.[155] Wright and his group studied tissue blood flow in dogs made septic by cecal ligation. Using radioactive ^{133}xenon injected into the anterior tibial compartment, they found a good correlation between blood flow through muscle tissue and cardiac index in hyperdynamic septic animals (Fig. 16–15). Wright's animals had narrowed A-V O_2 differences and displayed the same correlations of A-V O_2 difference directly with peripheral resistance and inversely with cardiac output that MacLean had found in their hyperdynamic septic shock patients (Fig. 16–13). Wright suggests that the high cardiac output seen in septic shock may represent an attempt to compensate for a primary defect in cellular oxygen utiliza-

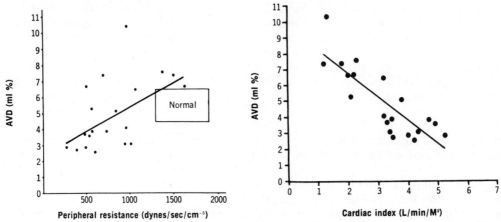

Figure 16–13. AV O₂ difference vs. peripheral resistance and cardiac index in normals and in patients with septic shock. The line drawn through the points represents the response in patients with septic shock. The line having no points along it represents the normal response. AV O₂ difference correlated directly with peripheral resistance and inversely with cardiac index during septic shock. (From MacLean, L.D., McLean, A.P.H., and Duff, J.: Postgrad. Med. *48*:114, 1970. Copyright by McGraw-Hill, Inc.)

tion.[168] Thus, it appears that generalized arteriovenous shunting does not occur in septic shock, but that a decrease in cellular utilization of oxygen causes the narrowed A-V O₂ difference and leads to a hyperdynamic circulatory state.[168]

When the hyperdynamic circulatory state fails, a low flow state with increased peripheral resistance develops, and then poor blood flow through capillary beds decreases availability of oxygen to cells whose ability to utilize oxygen is already hindered.

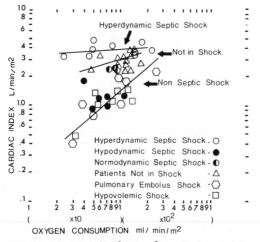

Figure 16–14. Cardiac index vs. oxygen consumption in different types of shock. Note that cardiac index bears little relation to oxygen consumption in hyperdynamic septic shock. (From Siegel, J.H., Greenspan, M., and Del Guercio, L.R.M.: Ann Surg. *165*:504, 1967.)

Lactic Acidosis and Tissue Hypoxia

A second area of controversy concerns the meaning of lactic acidosis in septic shock. An elevation of lactic acid, either in tissue or in serum, has generally been considered an indication of anaerobic metabolism, either because of anoxia or because of a block in the Krebs cycle. MacLean et al. have shown that lactate levels correlate inversely with oxygen consumption during septic shock, both in animals and in man.[166] Their data are shown in Figure 16–16. Serum lactate levels have been regarded as a prognostic indicator in both hypovolemic and septic shock in man.[51] Rosenberg and Rush have challenged the belief that lactic acid levels reflect the oxygen debt in septic shock.[171] Dogs anesthetized with thiopental, intubated, and mechanically ventilated were given intravenous *E. coli* endotoxin after a control period during which oxygen consumption was measured. Animals that became febrile were excluded from the series. Thirty minutes after the administration of endotoxin, the arterial lactate and excess lactate values rose and remained high until death. This change did not parallel the developing oxygen deficit, which was calculated as the difference in minute oxygen consumption between the control period and the period following endotoxin injection. Rosenberg and Rush postulated a cellular inhibition of oxidative metabolism and claimed that excess lactate did not correlate with oxygen

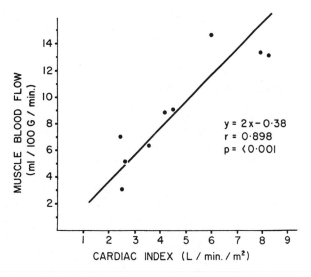

Figure 16–15. The direct correlation between capillary blood flow in skeletal muscle and cardiac index during hyperdynamic sepsis in dogs. Capillary blood flow was measured with radioactive xenon. The correlation was highly significant, r = 0.898 p<0.001. (From Wright, C.J., Duff, J.H., McLean, A.P.H., and MacLean, L.D.: Surg. Gynec. Obstet. *132*:540, 1971.)

deficit.[171] Clowes and his group found that lactic acid production in the legs of septic pigs was twice what it was prior to sepsis, but that the minute oxygen consumption by the legs was virtually the same before and after the pigs were made septic. They suggest that reduced muscle pyruvate dehydrogenase activity or the elevated fatty acid concentration they observed might have caused increased conversion of pyruvate to lactate.[120] Cain points out that tissue oxygen debt may not be a measure of tissue energy deficit.[172] More research into the effects of septicemia on cell metabolism is needed.

Myocardial Depressant Factor (MDF)

One study described in animals and in man during septic shock and other illnesses the presence of a factor in circulating blood that depresses myocardial contractility.[173] This factor is apparently a polypeptide with a molecular weight of 500 to 1000.[174] It can be made from pancreas and appears in portal venous blood. It can depress papillary muscle in vitro and apparently can be associated with poor myocardial function in man. It accumulates slowly, and its production can be blocked by the administration of

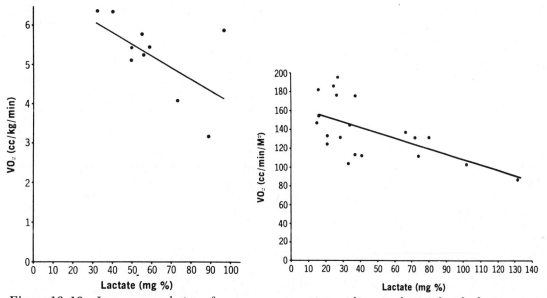

Figure 16–16. Inverse correlation of oxygen consumption with serum lactate levels during septic shock in dogs (left) and in man (right). (From MacLean, L.D., McLean, A.P.H., and Duff, J.: Postgrad. Med. *48*:114, 1970. Copyright by McGraw-Hill Inc.)

corticosteroids or by aprotinin (Trasylol). More research into myocardial depressant factor is needed.

THERAPY OF SEPTIC SHOCK

At present, there is no drug that can specifically counteract the effects of bacteria and their toxins on the circulation or that can reverse their inhibition of oxidative metabolism at the cellular level. Therapy, therefore, is directed toward controlling the infection with antibiotics and appropriate surgery, and also toward supporting the patient's circulation, respiration, and renal function until the sepsis is no longer present and these three systems are functioning normally.

The antibiotic therapy for septicemia has been described by Martin,[135] and the use of the newer aminoglycoside antibiotics for treatment of endocarditis is discussed in articles by Reyes et al.,[64, 175] Andriole,[176] and Baltch et al.[66]; the reader who is interested in this facet of the problem is referred to these articles.

A brief outline of suggested therapy for patients with septic shock is as follows. When septic shock is suspected, appropriate diagnostic studies should be obtained, repletion of fluid and blood volume deficits should begin at once, and respiratory failure should be treated with mechanical ventilation as soon as it appears. Therapy with antibiotics should be started after cultures have been obtained. When septic shock occurs, antibiotic treatment must be started without waiting for the results of cultures; the antibiotics can be changed later, if the patient survives. Pharmacologic doses of steroids should be given. If metabolic acidosis is present, initial therapy with buffers is indicated to counteract the depressing effect of acidosis on myocardial performance. If there is no response to these measures, inotropic therapy with dopamine or digitalis, or possibly with isoproterenol should be started.

If a low cardiac output should develop in spite of these measures, a trial of therapy with glucose, insulin, and potassium solution (GIK) may be indicated. Vasopressors of the alpha stimulating type are probably not indicated in septic shock. Surgery, if indicated, should be done following the initial treatment with volume replacement and, if necessary, with inotropic drugs. Vasodilators may be indicated if low cardiac output develops and the peripheral resistance rises towards or above normal.

Monitoring

When a diagnosis of septic shock is entertained, certain baseline studies should be made. The temperature and electrocardiogram should be monitored continuously. Catheters should be inserted for accurate interval measurements of CVP, venous oxygen saturation, and urine output. An arterial blood gas should be obtained to determine acid-base status and the presence or absence of respiratory failure. Cultures of urine, sputum, and blood, as well as of other sites (wounds, drainage tubes, intravenous catheters, etc.), should be obtained, and antibiotics should be started.[38, 135] Blood samples for electrolytes, BUN, creatinine, hematocrit, leukocyte count, bilirubin, and glucose should be drawn. If indicated, serum enzyme values (SGOT, SGPT, LDH, CPK-2, and amylase) or a profile of the clotting mechanism (bleeding, clotting, and clot lysis times, prothrombin and partial thromboplastin times, platelet count, and tests for levels of fibrinogen and fibrin split products) should be obtained.

A Swan-Ganz catheter should be inserted if the patient is hemodynamically unstable during initial therapy with volume and inotropic drugs, or if respiratory failure develops.[65] Other indications for inserting a Swan-Ganz catheter include the presence of heart disease in patients receiving large amounts of fluid, or oliguria with an elevated CVP, which implies cardiac dysfunction. The use of a Swan-Ganz catheter, which contains a thermistor probe, enables cardiac output* to be measured using the principle of thermal dilution. Patients sick enough to need a Swan-Ganz catheter should have a radial arterial catheter for monitoring blood pressure and for obtaining arterial blood samples. Radial artery catheters can nearly always be inserted percutaneously, but a

---

*What is actually measured is pulmonary artery blood flow. Coronary venous flow is included in this measurement, but the small fraction of aortic blood flow that enters the bronchial arteries is not included. For practical purposes, pulmonary artery blood flow approximates aortic root blood flow unless intracardiac shunts are present.

cut-down may be necessary if the patient is hypotensive or has severely constricted peripheral arteries. Dye dilution techniques may also be used to obtain cardiac output measurements. When cardiac output (CO) and mean arterial pressure ($\bar{P}$) are known, total peripheral resistance can be calculated as follows:

$$\text{Systemic resistance} = \frac{\bar{P}\text{art} - \text{CVP mm Hg}}{\text{CO ml/min}}$$
$$\times 1332 \times 60 \text{ dyne sec. cm}^{-5}$$

Note that the CVP must be expressed in millimeters of mercury (1.3 cm H_2O = 1 mm Hg). The Swan-Ganz catheter makes it possible to use what is essentially a left atrial pressure as a guide to fluid therapy and volume expansion. It also enables the anesthesiologist to follow pulmonary artery pressures which, as noted above, may be quite elevated in patients who develop large right to left shunts during sepsis. The resistance in the pulmonary circulation may also be calculated when the cardiac output, mean pulmonary arterial pressure, and left atrial pressure (pulmonary artery wedge) are known. Sibbald and coworkers point out that a large error may occur in calculating pulmonary arterial resistance, because the formula for resistance assumes fluid flow through a rigid tube; they recommend simply using the difference between pulmonary artery diastolic pressure and pulmonary artery wedge pressure as an indication of pulmonary resistance during therapy.[178] Hemodynamic measurements are useful as a guide to volume expansion and to therapy with inotropic drugs. They are probably necessary during therapy with vasodilators.

Respiratory Failure

During severe sepsis, respiratory failure often develops.[119] Mechanical ventilation should be instituted when blood gases indicate carbon dioxide retention or arterial hypoxemia. The use of positive end expiratory pressure (PEEP) can improve arterial oxygen tension when interstitial edema is present. When dyspnea and tachypnea are present, mechanical ventilation should be started immediately. Ledingham and coworkers noted that earlier institution of mechanical ventilation resulted in improved survival in their series of patients

with septic shock.[55] The work of breathing increases as "shock lung" develops during sepsis. Mechanical ventilation can decrease the demand on the myocardium by doing the work of breathing.[138] Patients comatose from septic shock may require intubation to prevent airway obstruction.[165] In addition, intubation provides a convenient way to deal with the increased secretions that accompany the pulmonary lesion during septic shock. The importance of skilled management of respiratory failure during sepsis is evident from Weil and Shubin's experience. In their series, respiratory failure was among the most frequent immediate causes of death.[164]

Volume Deficits

Replacement of the volume deficit that appears during septic shock is a fundamental step toward restoring the cardiac output. According to MacLean and coworkers, a CVP of 8 to 15 cm H_2O generally indicates a filled vascular compartment, whereas lower CVP values usually indicate a volume deficit.[61] Weisel et al. found that when the CVP was less than 5 mm Hg, the pulmonary artery wedge pressure was nearly always below 10 mm Hg; and when the CVP was above 12 mm Hg, the pulmonary artery wedge pressure was nearly always above 12 mm Hg.[65] If the CVP is above 12 mm Hg, low cardiac output or low arterial blood pressure is not caused by hypovolemia. Thus CVP values below 5 mm Hg indicated the need for volume expansion, and above 12 mm Hg indicated adequate intravascular volume in Weisel's series. CVP values 6 to 11 mm Hg were not useful as a guide to fluid therapy in Weisel's series. Wilson and coworkers found that the CVP response to volume loading was a better guide to fluid administration than were single CVP measurements. If the CVP rises more than 2 cm H_2O as 200 ml of fluid is run in over 10 minutes, fluids are discontinued.[179] Weil also recommends the use of fluid challenges.[54] The use of pulmonary artery wedge pressure as a guide to fluid administration is preferable to the use of CVP, especially when left ventricular dysfunction is present. Weisel recommends that fluids be administered to keep the left atrial (P.A. wedge) pressure at 10 to 12 mm Hg.[65] Weil suggests fluid challenges of up to 200 ml over 10 minutes; if left atrial pressure rises more than 7 mm Hg, he suggests discontinuing the infusion.[54] Krausz and coworkers found that in nearly half of their patients with septic shock, initial pulmonary wedge pressure was lower than initial CVP.[177] This group of patients was given an average of 2 liters more fluid (crystaloid and fresh frozen plasma) in the first 24 hours than patients in whom initial CVP was higher than wedge pressure. Krausz et al. emphasize that wedge pressure measurements enabled them to pick out which patients would benefit from more volume expansion when an elevated CVP or some right heart failure was present. Krausz et al. noted improvement in blood pressure and urine output in those patients given larger amounts of fluids during wedge pressure monitoring.[177] Frank noted that coexisting hypovolemia and an elevated CVP implying heart failure are more frequently encountered in elderly patients.[165] Cardiotonic drugs may be needed before more fluid can be administered.

If a fluid deficit is present and if the hematocrit is below 35, whole blood should be given; if above 35, Ringer's lactate with 5 per cent dextrose should be used.[50] However, Weisel and coworkers recommend a higher hematocrit to assure maximal oxygen transport. They suggest maintaining hemoglobin concentration between 12 and 14 grams per 100 ml of blood, using packed red cell transfusions.[65] Serum albumin or fresh frozen plasma may also be used for volume expansion. Since a low serum albumin can contribute to pulmonary interstitial edema, serum albumin should be kept within normal limits, but the use of solutions containing albumin does not prevent the development of interstitial pulmonary edema during resuscitation from septic shock. Holcraft and coworkers found no difference in extravascular lung water in primates given Ringer's lactate or Plasmanate to resuscitate them from septic shock caused by *E. coli*.[180]

If arterial hypotension or oliguria is present after blood and fluid volume deficits have been repleted, therapy with inotropic drugs may be necessary. Diuretics such as mannitol, 25 gm, or furosemide, 60 mg, may help restore urine flow. If the CVP does not rise after massive amounts of blood and fluids have been given, the prognosis is grave; either the capacitance vessels have failed or significant loss of blood and fluids into the capillary beds is occurring.[61]

Treatment of Acidosis

Among the initial steps in the therapy of septic shock is the treatment of acidosis. Acidosis should be corrected because myocardial response to endogenous catechols diminishes at or below pH 7.2. If the patient presents with acidosis and an arterial pCO_2 greater than 50 torr, part of the therapy for his acidosis is mechanical ventilation. If the patient simply has a metabolic acidosis, he should be given sodium bicarbonate according to the commonly accepted formula, mEq base needed = (0.2) (weight in kilos) (measured base deficit in mEq/L). Serial measurements of base deficit must be made because patients with septic shock often have decreased extracellular fluid and blood volumes, particularly when a third space is present, as in peritonitis. Hence, the usual assumptions concerning the size of the compartments in which base deficits are distributed do not apply in septic shock. Moreover, the patients are not stable. If hypodynamic circulatory failure occurs, lactic acid production can increase rapidly. In this low output state, when blood insulin levels are low, it appears that the administration of insulin may result in less lactic acid production, although more evidence is needed concerning this effect.[120] While buffers may be used to achieve a temporary improvement in myocardial performance, the fundamental treatment of acidosis during septic shock is the maintenance of a hyperdynamic circulation and as near normal cellular metabolism as possible.

Steroids

Most researchers in the field of septic shock advocate the use of steroids, although there are a few reports that steroids are ineffective. Weil and others reported a 79 per cent survival rate in patients with septic shock treated with over 300 mg of hydrocortisone per day versus a survival of 15 to 17 per cent in patients treated with lesser amounts of steroids.[181] Weil et al. recommended a large initial dose of dexamethasone, followed by 20 mg every four to six hours until the patient is no longer in shock. Lillehei et al. reported an excellent therapeutic effect from two grams of hydrocortisone followed two hours later by an additional two gram dose.[182] Wilson[50] advised steroids (hydrocortisone, 50 mg per kg) if a patient shows deterioration after volume replacement, cardiotonics and vasodilators have been used. He administered an additional 50 mg per kg by drip over the next 24 hours.[50] Motsay et al.[183] reported survival in 13 of 15 patients with septic shock when steroids were given within two hours of the onset of shock. They used dexamethasone, 6 mg per kg, or methylprednisolone, 30 mg per kg, or hydrocortisone, 150 mg per kg every four hours.[183] In a recent double blind study of 172 cases of bacteremic shock, Schumer[184] reports that the mortality rate of patients that received steroids was 10.4 per cent, while the mortality rate of patients receiving saline placebo was 38.4 per cent. (P of difference <0.001). They used dexamethasone, 3 mg/kg, or methylprednisolone, 30 mg/kg as an initial intravenous bolus and repeated the dose four hours later if shock was still present.[184] Cahill and others advocated the use of steroids in any patient with a fulminant septicemia, because a relative adrenal insufficiency is difficult or impossible to rule out.[188]

There are some reports that steroids are ineffective in bacteremic shock. McCabe et al.[62] and Hodgin et al.[49] found no improvement with steroid therapy. Hodgin apparently did not use massive doses, while McCabe did not publish data on dosage and methods of case selection. Nishijina and Weil and others reviewed seven studies and concluded that the use of corticosteroids was associated with increased survival if given within 24 hours of the onset of shock. In a recent article, these same authors remark that the "only securely established therapeutic maneuver" to increase survival in septic shock is augmentation of the blood volume. None the less, the current evidence favoring the use of steroids is rather impressive.

Considerable evidence has accumulated concerning mechanisms of actions of steroids during septic shock in both man and animals. Wilson and coworkers studied 23 patients in shock (22 septic) after treatment with steroids (50 mg/kg) and found an increase of approximately 20 per cent in cardiac output at 30 and 60 minutes.[187] There was an early, small decrease in peripheral resistance followed by a small increase at one and three hours. Blood pressure showed a slight initial drop, followed by a slight increase over the next five hours. The remarkable finding in this study was not the magnitude of the changes but the tendency to normalize circulatory dynamics. Patients with the lowest cardiac indices had increases in cardiac indices, whereas hyperdynamic patients showed decreases in cardiac indices.[187] Steroids have also been reported to suppress fever for up to 24 to 30 hours in patients with septic shock.[189] There are reports that steroids decrease the release of histamine and serotonin, inhibit the interaction of endotoxin and complement,[184] prevent margination and degranulation of leukocytes, inhibit pulmonary vascular endothelial damage, inhibit pulmonary edema,[190] prevent lysis of platelets,[79, 190] prevent decreases in Factors VIII and XII and in fibrinogen,[190] prevent loss of plasma volume,[192] dilate constricted venules, stabilize capillary membranes[111, 183] and lysosomes,[95, 190, 193] and increase oxygen consumption.[183] Steroids also increase mesenteric blood flow and decrease right to left pulmonary shunt in animals, and improve survival rates in animals with bacteremic shock.[194] Orkin believes that massive doses of steroids may also help in refractory shock.[111]

Inotropic Therapy

If treatment by blood volume expansion, steroids, correction of base deficits, and, if necessary, mechanical ventilation has failed to bring the patient out of septic shock, then therapy with inotropic agents to increase the cardiac output is indicated. A large increase in cardiac output during septic shock is associated with survival, according to Weil's analysis of the results of treatment of septic shock by seven groups of researchers.[186] Clowes and his group noted rapid recovery from septic shock in 12 patients whose cardiac indices rose to 3.5 liters per minute per m² — a value greater than the normal 2.8 L/min/m.²

The principal inotropic drugs currently employed are dopamine, isoproterenol, and digitalis. Dopamine now appears to be the inotropic drug of choice for patients with bacterial shock, according to most reports in the literature. Both dopamine and isoproterenol can cause large increases in cardiac output, but the distribution of blood to the kidneys and mesenteric vessels with dopamine makes it generally more useful in therapy of septic shock than isoproterenol.

Digitalis preparations are beneficial in some cases of septic shock.

Dopamine increases cardiac contractility and rate by acting directly on beta receptors and, in doses of 1 to 10 μg per kg per minute, does not cause an increase in mean arterial pressure by stimulating the alpha receptors. It also causes vasodilation in the renal and mesenteric vascular beds — a vasodilation not blocked by alpha or beta antagonists but which can be partly antagonized by haloperidol and by phenothiazides. When large doses of dopamine are administered, vasoconstriction mediated via the alpha receptors occurs in all vascular beds.[195] As early as 1966, MacCannel and Goldberg et al. reported that dopamine increased the urine output of several patients without significantly increasing their mean arterial pressure. This observation suggested to them that the vasodilating effect of dopamine they had proved to exist in animals was also present in man.[196] They used doses of 0.5 to 10.0 μg per kg per minute. Winslow and his group studied several catechols in patients with septic shock, regulating the dose to try to achieve a mean arterial pressure between 70 and 80 mm Hg.[67] Dopamine, given in whole body doses averaging 750 μg per minute, had the same effects on heart rate and cardiac index as did isoproterenol given at 5.9 μg per minute, but dopamine tended to raise mean arterial pressure and peripheral resistance more than isoproterenol (Isuprel) (see Fig. 16–10). In 12 oliguric patients in the series, dopamine caused increases in urine output greater than 1.2 ml per minute in four while isoproterenol caused such increases in only two of these same patients. Winslow used each patient as his own control and varied the sequence in which the drugs were administered. Many of these patients were quite ill, and mean arterial pressures above 70 mm Hg could not always be attained. Winslow noted that an adequate mean arterial pressure was necessary for urine formation, and attributed part of the beneficial effect of dopamine on urine output to its ability to raise blood pressure. He noted that the few patients in whom isoproterenol caused increased urine tended to have higher mean pressures before they received isoproterenol. Winslow claims that dopamine "produced a more favorable over-all response" than isoproterenol in his series of

patients.[67] Loeb and coworkers report significantly higher urine output (0.8 ml/min) in 19 patients with septic shock during therapy with dopamine infusion, 0.81 mg/min, than during isoproterenol infusion (P <0.05).[197] In this series, cardiac output was actually greater during isoproterenol infusion, but mean arterial pressure was slightly lower. With dopamine infusion, cardiac output increased an average of 37 $\pm$ 6 per cent. Dopamine and isoproterenol increased stroke work and pulse rate to the same extent at these doses. Loeb suggests that differences in regional blood flow and not simply total cardiac output be considered in choosing inotropic drugs for patients with bacteremic shock.[197] Talley and coworkers also report increases in cardiac output and peripheral resistance with dopamine in their series of 22 patients. They noted no increased urine output with isoproterenol but found that dopamine increased urine formation in some patients. In two patients, simultaneous use of dopamine and isoproterenol caused a temporary improvement not obtained by the use of each drug separately.[198] Hinshaw noted that dopamine counteracts venous pooling, and reports increased survival in endotoxic shock in animals treated with dopamine.[199, 200] Goldberg recommends administering dopamine at the lowest infusion rates that will achieve adequate patient perfusion — usually below 20 μg per kg per minute — but states that rates over 50 μg per kg per minute are occasionally necessary.[195]

Isoproterenol may be used to increase cardiac output and decrease peripheral resistance in bacteremic shock. Goldberg notes that isoproterenol may be of benefit in occasional patients with intense vasoconstriction.[195] MacLean et al. point out that isoproterenol increases cardiac output, rate, and contractility, decreases resistance in the renal and mesenteric arteries, and in the arteries supplying skeletal muscle.[61] The tachycardia and the increase in skeletal muscle blood flows are disadvantages of the drug, but the other effects are beneficial in patients with septic shock.[206] Isoproterenol also increases venous return.[181, 201] MacLean noted a marked improvement in 24 of 28 patients with hyperdynamic septic shock treated with isoproterenol to heart rates of 100 per minute. These patients had a high initial cardiac index (4.1 L/min/m²) and a low peripheral resistance, and although their CVP's were high, they remained in shock until isoproterenol was given. Cohn et al. recommend the use of inotropic agents early in septic shock.[153] Du Toit reported excellent results with isoproterenol in four young patients in septic shock after therapeutic abortion.[202] Starzecki et al. and Hershey et al. have demonstrated increased survival in septic animals treated with isoproterenol.[204, 205]

If tachycardia over 130 per minute is present, isoproterenol should not be used, since ventricular filling time will decrease and a lower cardiac output may occur. Tachycardia also increases myocardial oxygen consumption. Thal and Hermreck questioned the use of isoproterenol in shock with low resistance and high cardiac output.[207] Since dopamine is no longer experimental and since it increases arterial resistance more than isoproterenol, it could be used in hyperdynamic bacterial shock instead of isoproterenol. Digitalis might also be utilized in low resistance, high cardiac output shock.

Digitalis preparations may be used as inotropic agents in septic shock. Digitalis can be given in the presence of tachycardia and may be indicated in patients whose history suggests a diminished cardiac reserve. Even in the absence of a gallop rhythm or pulmonary edema, the presence of hypotension with elevated central venous or pulmonary artery wedge pressures is an indication for digitalis. Many authors advocate the use of digitalis in patients with shock due to bacterial sepsis.[50, 51, 153, 154, 202] Figure 16–11 shows improved cardiac function in a patient with septic shock after digitalization.[154] Studies in septic animals also show that digitalis improves cardiac function. Winslow and coworkers, however, point out that, in their experience, digitalis has not provided enough of an increase in myocardial performance, except in occasional patients.[67] There is some increased risk of digitalis toxicity when patients with septic shock are digitalized, because a diminished circulating blood volume during shock causes a higher myocardial concentration when digitalis is given on a weight basis. Digitalis is still useful as an inotropic drug during septic shock, especially when occult heart failure is present or when tachycardia limits the use of dopamine or isoproterenol.

Inotropic Therapy with GIK Solution

Clowes and his group have recently recognized that patients with septic shock whose cardiac index is lower than normal may have very low blood insulin levels that contribute significantly to myocardial dysfunction. They reported that 21 patients with a cardiac index of 4.08 ± 0.82 L/m^2/min had blood insulin levels averaging 38.4 ± 21.7 μU/ml, while 17 patients with cardiac indices averaging only 1.78 L/m^2/min had a mean insulin level as low as 9.3 ± 5.5 μU/ml.[209] Blood glucose levels did not differ significantly. Clowes and his group have had some success in improving myocardial performance with a solution containing glucose, insulin, and potassium.[120] In 1974 they reported treating eight patients with septic shock and a low cardiac output with GIK solution. The patients had an average blood insulin level of 12 ± 4 17mM/ml, a mean arterial pressure of 59 ± 7 mm Hg, and a lactate level of 2.74 ± 0.3 μMol/ml. The patients were given glucose, 1 gm/kg, and crystaline insulin, 1.5 U/kg; to that solution was added 10 mEq of potassium chloride. The mixture was given intravenously over a 10 minute period, and another set of measurements was made. The mean cardiac output increased from 3.0 ± 0.3 L/min to 8.6 ± 0.5 L/min. Blood pressure rose to a mean of 76 ± 4 mm Hg, while left atrial wedge pressure fell from 16 ± 3 to 12 ± 2 mm Hg, and CVP fell from 14 ± 3 to 9 ± 2 cm H$_2$O. The arterial pO$_2$ rose, and the hourly urine output tripled (see Table 16–5 and Fig. 16–12).[120] Clowes speculates that the low blood insulin plays some role in cardiac dysfunction in low output shock. He notes that the amount of sympathetic constriction of the peripheral vasculature appears to decrease following glucose-insulin-potassium (G.I.K.) therapy. Clowes found a similar response to G.I.K. solution in pigs with hypodynamic septic shock.[120] Manny and his group reported that G.I.K. solution significantly increased the ability of dogs to survive endotoxic shock.[211] Archer and his group, as noted previously, have reported that insulin improved myocardial function in isolated heart preparations.[163] While it is not absolutely certain that the effect of G.I.K. solution is on the heart and is not mediated through metabolic effects elsewhere in the body, the net result is an increase in cardiac function. Hence, G.I.K.

solution is listed here among the inotropic agents. While general use of G.I.K. solution should await further testing, it does appear to offer the possibility of improvement in bacterial shock with low cardiac output.

Vasopressor Drugs

In general, vasopressors are of little use in septic shock. Most of the common pressor agents decrease tissue perfusion, and large doses over a sufficient interval of time can cause shock. As part of the initial treatment for shock in patients who have been on vasopressors, Wilson et al. suggest discontinuing them.[50] If discontinuing pressors is followed by vascular collapse, Wilson suggests a dilute norepinephrine drip as a temporary measure while more effective treatment is begun. Elderly patients or patients with heart disease are more likely to require such temporary use of pressors. MacCannell et al. remark that treatment with vasoconstrictors may occasionally be needed to maintain coronary and cerebral perfusion until more definitive therapy can be effected.[196] Clowes and Orkin concur.[110, 111] A discussion of some common vasopressors and their effects in patients with bacteremic shock is in order.

Pressors with Mixed Alpha- and Beta-stimulating Actions. These include epinephrine, norepinephrine (Levophed), and metaraminol (Aramine).

Epinephrine in very low doses (10–20 μg/min) has primarily a beta effect; in higher doses it also has an alpha effect. Epinephrine increases cardiac contractility and rate, yet cardiac efficiency is decreased. Even low doses of epinephrine (3–23 μg/min) reduce renal blood flow up to 40 per cent. Because of these effects, in treating patents with septic shock, epinephrine should be used mainly during resuscitation from cardiac arrest or near arrest situations.

Norepinephrine (Levophed) is primarily alpha stimulating, although in higher doses it has a weak effect on beta receptors. It decreases renal, mesenteric, and hepatic blood flow. Weil notes that it might occasionally be used temporarily to increase coronary perfusion pressure but states that there is general agreement that norepinephrine is no longer indicated in therapy of bacteremic shock.[54]

Metaraminol (Aramine) also is mainly alpha stimulating but has a weak beta effect. It decreases renal and splanchnic flows, but it mobilizes blood pooled in the capacitance veins.[206] If metaraminol is used, Shubin and Weil advise keeping the blood pressure 20 to 30 mm Hg below the patient's normal preshock level.[59] Currently, Weil regards metaraminol as no longer indicated for routine therapy in septic shock.[54]

Pressors with alpha-stimulating action, namely angiotensin, methoxamine (Vasoxyl), and phenylephrine (Neosynephrine), have no known value in septic shock and are mentioned only so that the reader may avoid them.[59, 61]

EXPERIMENTAL DRUGS AND ADJUNCTS TO THERAPY IN SEPTIC SHOCK

Vasodilator Therapy. High levels of catecholamines and high sympathetic tone associated with low cardiac output in bacteremic shock have been recognized for many years.[121] A slow rate of blood flow through capillary beds because of sympathetic stimulation of postcapillary sphincters has also been postulated.[111] In terminal septic shock an increase in systemic arterial resistance is often present. Historically, these facts and hypotheses provided the basis for the use of vasodilating drugs in bacteremic shock. Phenoxybenzamine, the drug first used as a vasodilator in septic shock, is no longer available in the United States but may still be available abroad. Anderson et al. reported four young patients with septic shock in whom fluid and digitalis therapy were ineffective but who responded very well to phenoxybenzamine.[212] Thal and Hermreck also reported patients with elevations of TPR and CVP in spite of hypovolemia. Phenoxybenzamine was used in these patients to block alpha receptors and to enable the patients to tolerate more blood volume; then a dilute norepinephrine drip was used for its beta effect to increase cardiac output.[207] However, many authors have reported poor results with alpha blockade during septic shock. Only one of 28 patients in whom Wilson used phenoxylbenzamine survived. Eckenhoff and Cooperman reported that alpha blockade seemed to hasten death in 11 of the 25 patients in whom they used it.[50, 213] Phenoxybenzamine fell into disuse as a vasodilator for septic shock. However, interest in other drugs to reduce cardiac preload or afterload has continued.

Nitrol paste has recently been used as a vasodilator for patients with septic shock and a low cardiac output. Cerra and coworkers recently described eight patients with shock due to gram-negative infections.[214] All eight had had appropriate surgical and antibiotic therapy and initially were in shock with a high cardiac output and low total peripheral resistance. All had been treated with volume expansion and digitalis, and all were receiving isoproterenol, 0.5 to 1.0 μg/min., and dopamine, 4 to 10 μg/kg/min. Nonetheless, they developed a low cardiac output state, with cardiac index below 1.5 L/m^2/min, and peripheral arterial resistance over 3000 dyne sec cm^{-5}. Their oxygen consumption fell to less than 100 ml/m^2/min and central venous pressures rose to over 11 cm H$_2$O. They were treated with nitroglycerine paste, 12 to 18 mg (approximately 0.5 to 1.5 inches) every four hours. Three hours after therapy their cardiac index had risen to a mean of 2.5 $\pm$ 1.01 L/m^2/min, peripheral resistance had decreased to 1507 $\pm$ 322 dyne-cm^{-5}, and central venous pressure had decreased to 5.7 $\pm$ 1.7 cm H$_2$O. The changes in cardiac index and peripheral resistance were highly significant (<0.01), while the decrease in venous pressure was significantly only at the 5 per cent level. Oxygen consumption rose somewhat to 114 ml/m^2/min (<0.02). Seven of the eight patients survived the episode of shock, but one patient had an acute myocardial infarction during nitrol paste application and died. Two other patients died three or four weeks later, and the five remaining patients recovered and were discharged from the hospital. Cerra and coworkers believed that in these volume loaded patients whose cardiac contractility was being stimulated with dopamine and isoproterenol, the primary effect of the nitroglycerine was afterload reduction. Some reduction of preload also occurred, since these patients required more volume expansion during the nitroglycerine paste therapy. Cerra and coworkers recommend the use of vasodilator therapy with nitrol paste for patients with gram-negative septic shock and a low cardiac output, in the setting of an acute care unit.[214] The increases in cardiac output were not as large as those reported by Clowes using glucose, insulin, and potassium.[120] It is likely that hemodynamic improvements similar to those reported by Cerra et al. with nitrol paste could be achieved by the slow intravenous administration of nitroglycerine solution, which is now being prepared by many hospital pharmacies for use in patients with coronary heart disease. Since vasodilator therapy with nitrates in low output bacterial shock is quite new, it should only be attempted in conjunction with measurements of the cardiac output so that its effects can be closely monitored. As more groups report experience with this type of treatment, it may be accepted as a clinically useful approach to managing patients with hypodynamic septic shock.

Chlorpromazine (Thorazine). Chlorpromazine in vitro has alpha adrenergic blocking properties.[215] Pretreatment with chlorpromazine led to increased survival rates in animals in shock from superior mesenteric artery occlusion.[216] This drug has not been studied sufficiently during septic shock in man to justify its clinical use in septic shock.

Low Molecular Weight Dextran. This agent may be of some use late in shock to decrease rouleaux formation or sludging of blood.[111] Excessive amounts may result in a hemorrhagic diathesis and may make cross matching of blood difficult. Hypersensitivity reactions to macromolecular dextrans may also occur. Weil recommends that they not be used routinely in patients with septic shock.[54]

Aprotinin (Trasylol). Aprotinin, an inhibitor of proteolytic enzymes, has been suggested for use in septic shock, particularly when pancreatitis is present.[50] Massion and Blümel have shown that aprotinin, which inhibits kallikrein and trypsin, can decrease kininogen activity in treated animals during shock. Lower levels of kinins and fewer abnormalities in the clotting system were noted in pretreated animals. They suggested that aprotinin be used early in the therapy of shock.[217] Leffler et al. reported that it can prevent the formation of myocardial depressant factor (MDF).[174] Doenicke et al. report a minor inhibition of pseudocholinesterase activity by aprotinin.[218] More research appears necessary before aprotinin can be recommended for clinical use.

Anti-Inflammatory Drugs. Northover and Subramanian first studied the effects of antipyretic drugs on endotoxin shock as early as 1962.[219] Hilton et al. have improved the survival rate of animals in shock from endotoxin by treatment with indomethacin, 1 mg/kg at hourly intervals. Less loss of plasma volume was noted in the treated animals.[220] Fletcher et al. reported that pretreatment with indomethacin, 1.5 mg/kg, aspirin, 10 mg/kg, or intravenous lidocaine, 1 mg/min, prevented death in primates given an LD_{50} dose of endotoxin. The mechanism of action of these drugs in endotoxic shock is not yet understood.

Therapy to Decrease Pulmonary Fluid Filtration. Foy and coworkers measured pulmonary vascular pressures and lung lymph flow in animals given intravenous *Pseudomonas aeruginosa* organisms. Mean pulmonary artery pressure nearly doubled and lung lymph flow rose from 6.9 to 33 ml per hour. When pulmonary artery pressure was reduced nearly to control values by an intravenous drip of isoproterenol and aminophylline, the lung lymph flow returned to control value.[223] The authors point out that in Starling's law of the capillary the only quantity that can be manipulated easily is the intravascular pressure. However, they warn that aminophylline can increase right to left shunt by dilating vessels to nonventilated regions of the lung. This therapy to decrease pulmonary extravascular water has not yet been tried in man.

Therapy to Increase Reticuloendothelial Function. Opsonic α_2-surface binding globulin, which participates in phagocytosis by reticuloendothelial cells, is found with the cold insoluble globulins in human serum. Its level is reduced in sepsis and after trauma. Saba and coworkers separated the cryoprecipitate from fresh ACD plasma and gave a dose equivalent to the cryoprecipitate from 10 units of plasma to each of five patients with severe infections. They noted improved pulmonary function, decrease in fever, and stable hematological function following this therapy. All five patients survived.[224]

ANESTHESIA FOR PATIENTS WITH SEPTIC SHOCK

Anesthesia for the patient with septic shock can be difficult and challenging. The main task of the anesthesiologist is to maintain the patient's cardiovascular, respiratory, renal, and clotting systems as well as possible during the anesthetic, and, if possible, improve their function during the operative period. The administration of the anesthetic itself is only a part of the task of treating and improving a severely ill patient over an interval of time.

The anesthesiologist must ascertain whether the patient is in hyperdynamic septic shock (warm shock) or whether he has deteriorated into the hypodynamic shock with a low cardiac output and an increased peripheral resistance. He must find out whether the patient has been treated with adequate volume expansion (fluid, frozen plasma, and perhaps blood) to replete the deficit in extracellular fluid and blood volume that develops during severe sepsis. He should check the patient's filling pressures, central venous and, if possible, pulmonary wedge to be sure that filling pressure is sufficient to sustain a maximal cardiac output. He should be sure that an elevated filling pressure suggesting occult heart failure is not present. A high CVP with a low wedge pressure suggests hypovolemia in the presence of right ventricular failure or elevated pulmonary vascular resistance. The anesthesiologist should check any measurements of cardiac output and calculations of systemic and pulmonary resistance that have been made. He may need to insert a Swan-Ganz catheter in order to make such measurements. He must judge to what extent the sepsis has caused pulmonary dysfunction. Is compliance low? How much right to left shunt is there? Has positive end expiratory pressure been needed to maintain arterial oxygenation in a safe range, and will it be needed during operation? Is mechanical ventilation necessary preoperatively because of respiratory failure, or can it wait till during and after operation?

The anesthesiologist should also ascertain how badly the sepsis and shock have interfered with the patient's metabolism. How narrow is the arteriovenous oxygen difference? How high is the serum lactate? Are there elevations of bilirubin and liver enzymes? Is oliguria or anuria or azotemia present, and what diuretics have been employed? Is fever present, and if so, what measures have been taken to reduce it? Have appropriate antibiotics and large doses of steroids been given? Is the patient alert, or confused or comatose? Has he been treated with inotropic drugs such as dopamine, or digitalis, or isoproterenol? Is his blood insulin level low, and is he a candidate for therapy with GIK solution or with nitrates? Is pre-existing or acute coronary ischemia present? Are deficits in electrolytes, hemoglobin, serum albumin, platelets, or clotting factors present? What else can be done to improve the patient's condition preoperatively?

Surgery for the purpose of removing infected tissue or draining abscesses is urgent in patients with septic shock. Therapy with antibiotics often will not stop the bacteremia and toxemia that causes the downhill course. Hence, surgery should not be delayed more than a few hours.[49, 50, 51] Since it is preferable not to anesthetize and operate on patients in shock, a brief delay to treat the patient with volume expansion, steroids, and inotropic drugs is worthwhile. Fever should be reduced preoperatively, and if respiratory insufficiency is present, mechanical ventilation should be started without delay. When the patient has received maximum supportive therapy, anesthesia and operation should proceed.

Choice of Anesthetic Techniques for Patients with Septic Shock. If the site of surgery permits, local or regional anesthesia is the technique of choice. Nerve blocks — axillary, brachial, sciatic, or femoral — are very well suited for drainage of infected extremities. For cholecystostomy or other very limited work in the abdomen, multiple intercostal blocks can provide satisfactory anesthesia. In patients with septic shock, blocks should be performed with minimal doses of anesthetic agent, since cardiac depression from absorption of local anesthetic drug has been documented by intraoperative hemodynamic measurements in at least one case.[61]

SPINAL ANESTHESIA. Spinal anesthesia is relatively contraindicated in patients with bacteremia, which is likely to be present in patients actually in septic shock. Patients with infections having chills followed by fever spikes are likely to have bacteremia during the chill and as the temperature is rising. Spinal taps should be avoided at these times, since there are scattered reports in the medical literature of bacterial meningitis following spinal anesthesia in septic patients.[231] Lund and Cwik consider spinal anesthesia to be contraindicated in patients with bacteremia or with shock.[47] Although the published literature recommends against the use of spinal anes-

thesia in patients with septic shock, it may be that the use of saddle block for drainage of abscesses in the perineum or the use of a fractional spinal for debridement or amputation of an infected lower extremity is less hazardous in selected patients with bacteremic shock than general anesthesia would be. Some sympathetic blockade is unavoidable with spinal anesthesia. The anesthesiologist should limit it as much as possible in patients with bacteremic shock by using minimal doses of drug, and even by administering small doses of the local anesthetic drug at four or five minute intervals until sufficient anesthesia is achieved. Large bore intravenous catheters should be in place so that fluids can be given rapidly to offset the effect of sympathetic blockade on venous return. If arterial pressure decreases because of sympathetic blockade, it may be necessary to administer dopamine or to increase its rate of infusion. Alpha adrenergic agents may be necessary to maintain coronary artery perfusion.

EPIDURAL ANESTHESIA. Epidural anesthesia may be employed for lower extremity surgery in patients with septic shock. With the epidural technique in bacteremic patients, the risk of causing meningitis is less than with the spinal technique, unless an inadvertent dural puncture occurs. Also with the epidural technique, as compared with the spinal technique, for a given level of sensory block there is a lower level of sympathetic blockade. The minimum dose necessary to accomplish the block should be used, since myocardial depression from local anesthetic drugs in septic shock has been reported.[61] Epidural anesthesia can cause increases in splanchnic, renal, and lower extremity blood flow, but it remains to be proved whether these increased flows occur and are beneficial in patients with septic shock. The use of epidural anesthesia for laparotomy in patients during septic shock has not been reported. It is likely that the doses of local anesthetic drug needed for this technique would cause some degree of myocardial depression.

GENERAL ANESTHESIA. In patients with septic shock requiring abdominal or thoracic surgery, general endotracheal anesthesia is necessary. Intubation is often indicated as part of the management of the pulmonary effects of septic shock.

Since normal to high cardiac output appears necessary for survival of bacterial shock, and since some heart failure is often present during septic shock, moderate to deep levels of potent inhalational agents should be avoided. Operating conditions may be achieved by combining muscle relaxants with analgesic doses of potent agents, or by using nitrous oxide and adjunct drugs. Some patients will not tolerate even 0.5 per cent enflurane, 1.0 per cent diethyl ether, 5 per cent cyclopropane, or 30 per cent concentrations of nitrous oxide or ethylene. If the patient shows signs of diminished perfusion, decreased arterial pressure, or heart failure (increasing pulmonary wedge or central venous pressure), the agent should be discontinued and the patient ventilated with 100 per cent oxygen.

Amnesia may be achieved with intravenous scopolamine, 1 to 2 mg, given intravenously slowly. Unconsciousness and amnesia may also be achieved with intravenous diazepam, 10 to 20 mg, given slowly or in small increments. No cardiac depression and very little change in vascular dynamics occurs with diazepam. Ketamine, 1 to 2 mg per kg, given intravenously slowly or in increments, can provide unconsciousness and analgesia. Its disadvantages are tachycardia and transient increases in right atrial and pulmonary artery pressures. Although it should be used cautiously in patients with tachycardia or right ventricular failure, ketamine has proved to be a useful anesthetic in patients with bacterial shock. Very small doses of meperidine, morphine, or pentazocine given intravenously may help produce analgesia. With the narcotics no significant cardiac depression occurs, but slight arterial dilatation and considerable dilatation of the capacitance veins occurs. Venous return decreases transiently, but the decreased filling pressure may be compensated for by administration of fluid, plasma, or blood.

Stanley and Reddy reported good results using a fentanyl-oxygen technique in 18 patients with bacteremic shock.[225] These patients had blood pressures less than 90 mm Hg systolic, and their blood cultures had grown gram-negative organisms. The patients were given fentanyl, 100 to 300 μg per minute until they became unresponsive. They were then given 250 μg of additional fentanyl and intubated. Extra fentanyl in 150 to 250 μg increments was given for systolic blood pressure greater than 120 mm Hg, for pulse rates greater than 125 per minute, or for sweating or tearing. The in-

vestigators noticed little change in cardiovascular parameters. No cardiac depression occurred, and there were only slight increases in heart rate, stroke volume, cardiac output, arterial blood pressure, and systemic vascular resistance during the surgery. Ten patients required naloxone to reverse the narcotic and restore resiratory drive after surgery. Four of these 10 required a second dose of naloxone.[225] The fentanyl-oxygen technique appears promising for the management of patients severely ill with septic shock.

Nitrous oxide or ethylene may be used in patients with bacteremic shock, provided that the increased right to left shunt often present during septic shock does not result in arterial desaturation. The arterial pO_2 should be checked during anesthesia and the concentrations of nitrous oxide or ethylene adjusted appropriately. There is one other problem with the use of nitrous oxide in patients with septic shock. Increases in pulmonary vascular resistance have been reported during anesthesia with nitrous oxide.[226] When treating patients in whom septic shock has led to elevated pulmonary artery pressure and right ventricular failure, nitrous oxide should be avoided.

There is some evidence that diethyl ether should be avoided in patients with sepsis. Schweizer and Williams found significantly elevated lactic acid levels in septic adults having major surgery but did not find similar elevations in septic patients during anesthesia with halothane or thiopental.[227] Virtue, in animal studies, found worse survival rates with diethyl ether than with cyclopropane or thiopental.[228]

Anesthetic doses of barbiturates can cause circulatory depression and acidosis in animals during endotoxin shock. Rety and Couves reported lower blood pressures and lower arterial pH values in dogs anesthetized with pentobarbital than in awake animals.[229] However, neither their study nor the more recent work of White et al. showed that the use of barbiturate anesthesia had any effect on mortality.[230] If barbiturates are used at all in patients with septic shock, they should be given in reduced doses, because a low circulating blood volume may result in higher blood levels than when identical doses are used in normal patients.

It is obvious that no anesthesia is necessary in the patient who is comatose from severe sepsis. Except for administering muscle relaxants, the anesthesiologist may devote his attention entirely to supportive measures.

REFERENCES

1. Wolff, S. M., and Bennett, J. V.: Gram negative bacteria. N. Engl. J. Med. 291:733, 1974.
2. Riley, H. D., Jr.: Hospital-acquired infections. South. Med. J. 70:1265, 1977.
3. Johanson, W. G., Jr., and Sanford, J. P.: Problems of infection and antimicrobials relating to anesthesia and inhalation therapy. In Jenkins, M. T. (ed.): Common and Uncommon Problems in Anesthesiology. Philadelphia, F. A. Davis Company, 1968, pp. 300–320.
4. Beisel, W. R., Sawyer, W. D., Ryll, E., and Crozier, D.: Metabolic effects of intracellular infections in man. Ann. Intern. Med. 67:744, 1967.
5. Law, D. H.: Medical intelligence: Current concepts in nutrition: Total parenteral nutrition. N. Engl. J. Med. 297:1104, 1977.
6. Rubin, G.: The influence of alcohol, ether and chloroform on natural immunity in its relation to leukocytosis and phagocytosis. J. Infect. Dis. 1:425, 1904.
7. Graham, E. A.: The influence of ether and other anesthesia in bacteriolysis, agglutination, and phagocytosis. J. Infect. Dis. 8:147, 1911.
8. Andrewes, C. H., Laidlow, P. P., and Smith, W.: The susceptibility of mice to the viruses of human and swine influenza. Lancet 2:859, 1934.
9. Dubin, I. N.: The role of ether anesthesia in the production of influenza virus pneumonia in mice. J. Immunol. 51:355, 1945.
10. Bruce, D. L.: Effect of halothane anesthesia on extravascular mobilization of neutrophils. J. Cell. Physiol. 68:81, 1966.
11. Bruce, D. L.: Effect of halothane on experimental salmonella peritonitis in mice. J. Surg. Res. 7:180, 1967.
12. Duncan, P. G., Cullen, B. F., and Pearsall, N. N.: Anesthesia and the modification of response to infection in mice. Anesth. Analg. 55:776, 1976.
13. Cullen, B. F., Hume, R. B., and Chretien, P. B.: Phagocytosis during general anesthesia in man. Anesth. Analg. 54:501, 1975.
14. Cullen, B. F., and Chretien, P. B.: Ketamine and in vitro lymphocyte transformation. Anesth. Analg. 52:518, 1973.
15. Wilson, R. D., Priano, L. L., Traber, D. L., Salsai, H., Daniels, J. C., and Ritzman, S. E.: An investigation of possible immunosuppression from ketamine and one hundred per cent oxygen in normal children. Anesth. Analg. 50:461, 1971.
16. Stanley, T. H., Hill, G. E., Portas, M. R., Hogan, N. A., and Hill, H. R.: Neutrophil chemotaxis during and after general anesthesia and operation. Anesth. Analg. 55:668, 1976.
17. Goldstein, E., Munson, E. S., Eagle, C., Martucci, R. W., and Hoeprich, P. D.: The effects of anesthetic agents on murine pulmonary bactericidal activity. Anesthesiology. 34:344, 1971.
18. Cruse, P. J. E.: A five year prospective study of 23,649 surgical wounds. Arch. Surg. 107:206, 1973.
19. Follow-Up Agency, Division of Medical Sciences, National Academy of Sciences, National Research Council: Postoperative wound infections: Influence of ultraviolet irradiation of the operating room and of various other factors. Ann. Surg. 160(Suppl. 2), 1964.
20. Pridgen, J. E.: Respiratory arrest thought to be due to intraperitoneal neomycin. Surgery 40:571, 1956.
21. Timmerman, J. C., Long, J. P., and Pittenger, C. B.: Neuromuscular blocking properties of various antibiotic agents. Toxic Appl. Pharmacol. 1:299, 1959.
22. Adams, H. R., Mathew, B. P., Teske, R. H., and Mercer, H. D.: Neuromuscular blocking effects of aminoglycoside antibiotics. Anesth. Analg. 55:500, 1976.
23. Pittinger, C. B., and Adamson, R.: Antibiotic blockade of neuromuscular function. Ann. Rev. Pharmacol. 12:169, 1972.
24. Samuelson, R. J., Giesecke, A. H., Jr., Kallus, F. T., and Stanley, V. F.: Lincomycin-curare interaction. Anesth. Analg. 54:103, 1975.
25. Wullen, F., Kast, G., and Bruck, A.: Side effects of tetracycline administration in patients with myasthenia gravis. Deutsch Med. Wschr. 92:667, 1967.
26. Gibbels, E.: Deterioration of myasthenia gravis after intravenous administration of rolitetracycline. Deutsch. Med. Wschr. 92:1153, 1967.
27. Straw, R. N., Hook, J. B., Williamson, H. E., and Mitchell, C. L.: Neuromuscular blocking properties of Lincocin. J. Pharm. Sci. 54:1814, 1955.
28. McQuillen, M. P., Cantor, H. E., and O'Rourke, J. R.: Myasthenia syndrome associated with antibiotics. Arch. Neurol. 18:402, 1968.
29. Gebbie, D.: Cholistimethate and curare. Anesth. Analg. 50:109, 1971.
30. Lee, C., Chen, D., Barnes, A., and Katz, R. L.: Neuromuscular block by neomycin in the cat. Canad. Anesth. Soc. J. 23:527, 1976.
31. Lindesmith, L. A., Jr., Baines, R. D., Jr., Bigelow, D. B., and Petty, T. L.: Reversible respiratory paralysis associated with polymyxin therapy. Ann. Intern. Med. 68:318, 1968.
32. Brazil, V., and Franchesi, P.: The nature of neuromuscular block produced by neomycin and gentamicin. Arch. Int. Pharm. Ther. 179:78, 1969.
33. Lee, C., Chen, D., and Nagel, E. L.: Neuromuscular blockade by antibiotics. Anesth. Analg. 56:373, 1977.
34. Van Nyhuis, L. S., Miller, R. D., and Fogdall, R. P.: The interaction between d-tubocurarine, pancuronium, polymyxin B and neostigmine on neuromuscular function. Anesth. Analg. 55:224, 1976.
35. Naiman, J. G., and Martin, J. D.: Some aspects of neuromuscular blockade by polymyxin B. J. Surg. Res. 7:199, 1967.
36. Lee, C., di Silva, A. J. C., and Katz, R. L.: Antagonism of polymyxin B-induced neuromuscular and cardiovascular depression by 4-aminopyridine in the anesthetized cat. Anesthesiology 49:256, 1978.
37. Fogdall, R. P., and Miller, R. D.: Prolongation of pancuronium-induced neuromuscular blockade by polymyxin B. Anesthesiology 40:84, 1974.
38. Alford, R. H.: Saturday conference: A clinician looks at the aminoglycoside antibiotics. South. Med. J. 71:684, 1978.

39. Martin, M. J., and Wellman, W. E.: Clinically useful antimicrobial agents. Postgrad. Med. 33:327, 1963.

40. Weinstein, L., Lerner, P. I., and Chew, W. H.: Clinical and bacteriologic studies of the effect of "massive" doses of penicillin G on infections caused by gram-negative bacilli. N. Engl. J. Med. 271:525, 1964.

41. Seamans, K. B., Gloor, P., Dobell, A. R. C., and Wyant, J. D.: Penicillin-induced seizures during cardiopulmonary bypass. N. Engl. J. Med. 278:861, 1968.

42. Cohen, L. S., Wechsler, A. S., Mitchell, J. H., and Glick, G.: Depression of cardiac function of streptomycin and other antimicrobial agents. Am. J. Cardiol. 26:505, 1970.

43. Daubeck, J. L., Daughety, M. J., and Petty, C.: Lincomycin-induced cardiac arrest: A case report. Anesth. Analg. 53:563, 1974.

44. Waisbren, B. A.: Letter to the editor. J.A.M.A. 206:2118, 1968.

45. Cohen, R. J., Sachs, J. R., Wickler, D. J., and Conrad, M. E.: Five blue soldiers: Methemoglobinemia provoked by anti-malarial chemoprophylaxis. Clin. Res. 16:301, 1968.

46. Beutler, E.: Glucose-6-phosphate dehydrogenase deficiency. In Stanbury, J. E., Wyngaarden, J. B., and Fredrickson, D. S. (eds.): The Metabolic Basis of Inherited Disease. 2nd ed. New York, McGraw-Hill Book Co., 1966, Chap. 47.

47. Lund, P. C., and Cwik, J. C.: Modern trends in spinal anesthesia. Canad. Anaesth. Soc. J. 15:118, 1968.

48. Collins, V. J.: Principles of Anesthesiology. Philadelphia, Lea and Febiger, 1966, p. 1017.

49. Hodgin, U. G., and Sanford, J. P.: Gram negative rod bacteremia. Am. J. Med. 39:952, 1965.

50. Wilson, R. F., Chiscano, A. D., Quadros, E., and Tarver, M.: Some observations on 132 patients with septic shock. Anesth. Analg. 46:751, 1967.

51. MacLean, L. D., Mulligan, W. G., McLean, A. P. H., and Duff, J. H.: Patterns of septic shock in man — a detailed study of 56 patients. Ann. Surg. 166:542, 1967.

52. Polk, H. C., Jr., and Shields, C. L.: Remote organ failure: a valid sign of occult intra-abdominal infection. Surgery 81:310, 1977.

53. Weinstein, L., and Klainer, A. S.: Management of Emergencies IV: Septic shock — pathogenesis and treatment. N. Engl. J. Med. 274:950, 1966.

54. Weil, M.: Current understanding of mechanisms and treatment of circulatory shock caused by bacterial infections. Ann. Clin. Res. 9:181, 1977.

55. Ledingham, I. M., and McArdle, C. S.: Prospective study of the treatment of septic shock. Lancet 1(8075):1194, 1978.

56. Matsen, J. M.: The sources of hospital infection. Medicine 52:271, 1973.

57. Altemeier, W. A., Todd, J. C., and Inge, W. W.: Gram negative septicemia: A growing threat. Ann. Surg. 166:530, 1967.

58. Alexander, J. W., Stinnett, J. D., Ogle, C. K., Ogle, J. D., and Morris, M. J.: A comparison of immunologic profiles and their influence on bacteremia in surgical patients with a high risk of infection. Surgery 86:94, 1979.

59. Shubin, H., and Weil, M.: Septic shock. In Mills, L. C., and Moyer, J. H. (eds.): Shocks and Hypotension. New York, Grune and Stratton, 1965, p. 463.

60. Pierce, W. S., Peckham, G. T., and Johnson, J.: Gram negative sepsis following operation for congenital heart disease. Arch. Surg. 101:698, 1970.

61. Maclean, L. D., Duff, J., Scott, H. M., and Peretz, D. I.: Treatment of shock in man based on hemodynamic diagnosis. Surg. Gynec. Obstet. 120:282, 1965.

62. McCabe, W. R., and Jackson, G. G.: Gram negative bacteremia. Arch. Intern. Med. 110:847, 1962.

63. Rose, R., Hunting, K. S., Townsend, T. R., and Wenzel, R. P.: Morbidity/mortality and economics of hospital acquired blood stream infections. South. Med. J. 70:1267, 1977.

64. Reyes, M. P., Palutke, W. A., Wylin, R. F., and Lerner, A. M.: Pseudomonas endocarditis in the Detroit Medical Center, 1969–1972. Medicine 52:173, 1973.

65. Weisel, R. D., Vito, L., Dennis, R. C., Valeri, C. R., and Hechtman, H. B.: Myocardial depression during sepsis. Am. J. Surg. 133:512, 1977.

66. Baltch, A. L., Hammer, M., Smith, R. P., and Sutphen, N.: Pseudomonas aeruginosa bacteria. J. Lab. Clin. Med. 91:201, 1979.

67. Winslow, E. J., Loeb, H. S., Rahmintoola, S., Kamath, S., and Gunnar, R. M.: Hemodynamic studies and results of therapy in 50 patients with bacteria shock. Am. J. Med. 54:421, 1973.

68. Vito, L., Dennis, R. C., Weisel, R. D., and Hechtman, H. B.: Sepsis presenting as acute respiratory insufficiency. Surg. Gynec. Obst. 138:896, 1970.

69. Tsueda, K., Oliver, P. B., and Richter, R. W.: Cardiovascular manifestations of tetanus. Anesthesiology 40:588, 1974.

70. Spivack, M. L.: Initial antibiotic management of suspected bacteremia. Modern Medicine 47:86, 1979.

71. Gopal, V., and Bisno, A. L.: Fulminant pneumococcal infections in "normal" asplenic hosts. Arch. Intern. Med. 137:1526, 1977.

72. Fry, D. E., Pearlstein, L., Fulton, R. L., and Polk, H. C., Jr.: Multiple system organ failure: The role of uncontrolled infection. Arch. Surg. 115:136, 1980.

73. Mulder, T.: Clinical significance of bacteriologic examination of sputum in cases of acute and chronic bacterial diseases of the respiratory tract. Adv. Intern. Med. 12:233, 1964.

74. Sacks, R. A.: Epidemic of gram-negative organism septicemia subsequent to elective operation. Amer. J. Obstet. Gynec. 107:394, 1970.

75. Siboni, K., Olsen, H., Ravn, E., et al.: Pseudomonas cepacia in 16 non-fatal cases of postoperative bacteremia derived from intrinsic contamination of the anesthetic fentanyl. Scand. J. Infect. Dis. 11:39, 1979.

76. Atkins, E.: Pathogenesis of fever. Physiol. Rev. 40:580, 1960.

77. Atkins, E., and Bodel, P.: Fever. N. Engl. J. Med. 286:27, 1972.

78. Myrvold, H. E.: Experimental septic shock. Acta Chir. Scand. (Suppl.) 470:1, 1976.

79. Rowe, M. I., Marchildon, M. B., Arango, A., Malinin, T., and Gans, M. A.: The mechanisms of thrombocytopenia in experimental gram-negative sepsis. Surgery 84:87, 1978.

80. Hawiger, J., Hawiger, A., and Timmons, S.: Endotoxin-sensitive membrane components of human platelets. Nature 256:125, 1972.

81. Mee, W. M., and Walter, C. C.: Vasoactive effect

of gram-negative endotoxin on the microcirculation. Surg. Forum 18:16, 1967.

82. Hinshaw, L. B., Brala, C. M., and Emerson, T. E., Jr.: Biochemical and pathologic alterations in endotoxin shock. In Mills, L. C., and Moyer, J. H. (eds.): Shock and Hypotension. New York, Grune and Stratton, 1965, p. 431.

83. Hershey, S. G.: Current theories of shock. Anesthesiology 21:303, 1960.

84. Thomas, C. S., Jr., Melly, M. A., Koenig, M. G., and Brockman, S. K.: The hemodynamic effect of viable gram-negative organisms. Surg. Gynec. Obstet. 128:753, 1969.

85. Clark, P. T., and Cavanaugh, D.: Septic shock. Amer. J. Obstet. Gynec. 102:21, 1968.

86. Nies, A. S., Forsyth, R. D., Williams, H. E., and Melmon, K. L.: Contribution of kinins to endotoxin shock. Circ. Res. 22:155, 1968.

87. Miller, R. L., Reichgott, M. J., and Melmon, K. L.: Bacterial mechanisms of generation of bradykinin by endotoxin. J. Infect. Dis. 128(Suppl. S-144), 1973.

88. McCabe, W. R.: Serum complement levels in bacteria due to gram-negative organisms. N. Engl. J. Med. 288:21, 1973.

89. McCabe, W. R.: Discussion. J. Infect. Dis. 128(Suppl. 5–305), 1973.

90. Bjornson, A. B., Altemeier, W. A., Bjornson, S., Tang, T., amd Isekson, M. L.: Host defense against opportunistic microorganisms following trauma. Ann. Surg. 188:93, 1978.

91. Moss, G. S., Erve, P. P., and Schumer, W.: Effect of endotoxin on mitochondrial respiration. Surg. Forum 20:24, 1969.

92. Mela, L., Miller, L., Diaco, J. F., and Sugarman, H. J.: Effect of E. coli endotoxin on mitochondrial energy-linked functions. Surgery 68:541, 1970.

93. Ryan, N. T., Broge, L. E., and Clowes, G. H. A., Jr.: Enzymatic adaptations for energy production during sepsis. Physiologist 15:254, 1972.

94. Seyfer, A. E., Zajtchals, R., Hazlett, D. R., and Mologne, L. A.: Systemic vascular performance in endotoxic shock. Surg. Gynec. Obstet. 145:401, 1977.

95. Schumer, W., and Sperling, R.: Shock and its effect on the cell. J.A.M.A. 205:75, 1968.

96. Trunkey, D., and Carpenter, M. A.: Ionized calcium and magnesium. The effect of septic shock in the baboon. J. Trauma 18:166, 1978.

97. Gibbon, W. H., Cooke, J. J., Gatipon, G., and Moses, M. E.: Effects on endotoxin shock on skeletal muscle cell membrane potential. Surgery 81:571, 1977.

98. Glenn, T. M., and Lefer, A. M.: Role of lysosomes in the pathogenesis of splanchnic ischemic shock in cats. Circ. Res. 27:783, 1970.

99. Glenn, T. M., Lefer, A. M., Beardsley, et al.: Circulatory responses to splanchnic lysosomal hydrolases in the dog. Ann. Surg. 176:120, 1972.

100. Harari, A., Martin, E., Bouvier, A. M., Geteau, O., Comoy, E., and Bohuon, C.: Decreased dopamine-beta-hydroxylase activity in septic shock. Anesthesiology 51(Suppl. S155), 1979.

101. Woodruff, P. W. H., O'Carroll, D. I., Koizumi, S., and Fine, J.: Role of the intestinal flora in major trauma. J. Infect. Dis. 128(Suppl. S-290), 1973.

102. Hershey, S. G., and Altura, B. M.: Function of the reticuloendothelial system in shock and combined injury. Anesthesiology 30:138, 1969.

103. Johnson, G., McDevitt, N. B., and Proctor, H. J.: Erythrocyte 2,3-diphosphoglycerate in endotoxin shock in the subhuman primate. Ann. Surg. 180:783, 1974.

104. Sugarman, H., Miller, L. D., and Oski, F. A.: Decreased 2,3-diphosphoglycerate (DPG) and reduced oxygen (O_2) consumption in septic shock. Clin. Res. 17:418, 1970.

105. Naylor, B. A., Welch, M. H., Shafer, A. W., and Guenter, C. A.: Blood affinity for oxygen in hemorrhagic and endotoxin shock. J. Appl. Physiol. 32:829, 1972.

106. Motsay, G. J., Dietzmann, R., and Lillehei, R. C.: Treatment of endotoxin shock. Rev. Surg. 26:381, 1969.

107. Rosenberg, J. C., Lillehei, R. C., Longerbeam, J. C., and Zimmerman, B.: Studies on hemorrhagic and endotoxin shock in relation to vasomotor changes and endogenous circulating epinephrine, norepinephrine, and serotonin. Ann. Surg. 154:511, 1961.

108. Mee, W. M., and Walter, C. C.: Vasoactive effect of gram-negative endotoxin on the microcirculation. Surg. Forum 18:16, 1967.

109. Emerson, T. E.: Participation of endogenous vasoactive agents in the pathogenesis of endotoxin shock. Adv. Expl. Med. Biol. 23:25, 1972.

110. Clowes, G. H. A.: Oxygen transport and utilization in fulminating sepsis and septic shock. In Hershey, S. G., Delguercio, L. R. M., and McCann, R., (eds.): Septic Shock in Man. Boston, Little Brown. 1971.

111. Orkin, L. R.: Microcirculatory events in shock. Anesth. Analg. 46:734, 1967.

112. Hermreck, A. S., and Thal, A. P.: Effects of vasoactive drugs on blood flow and oxygen utilization in septic tissue. Surg. Forum 20:17, 1969.

113. Mellander, S., and Lewis, D. H.: Effects of hemorrhagic shock on the reactivity of resistance and capacitance vessels and on capillary filtration transfer in cat skeletal muscle. Circ. Res. 13:105, 1963.

114. Hinshaw, L. B., and Owen, S. E.: Correlation of pooling and resistance changes in the canine forelimb in septic shock. J. Appl. Physiol. 30:331, 1971.

115. Weidner, W. J., Grega, G. J., and Haddy, F. J.: Changes in forelimb weight and vascular resistance during endotoxin shock. Am. J. Physiol. 221:1229, 1971.

116. Coalson, J. J., Hinshaw, L. B., Guenter, C. A., Berrell, E. L., and Greenfield, L. J.: Pathophysiologic responses of the subhuman primate in experimental septic shock. Lab. Invest. 32:561, 1975.

117. Postel, J., and Schloerb, P. R.: Cardiac depression in bacteremia. Ann. Surg. 186:74, 1977.

118. Adair, T. H., and Traber, D. L.: Mechanism of pulmonary edema in burn wound sepsis. Anesthesiology 51(Suppl. 3, S-175), 1979.

119. Clowes, G. H. A., Jr., Hirsch, E., Williams, L., et al.: Septic lung and shock lung in man. Ann. Surg. 181:681, 1975.

120. Clowes, G. H. A., Jr., O'Donnell, T. F., Jr., Ryan, N. T., and Blackburn, G. L.: Energy metabolism in sepsis. Ann. Surg. 179:684, 1974.

121. Dietzman, R. H., Feemster, J. A., Idezuki, Y., and Lillehei, R. C.: Tolerance to lethal vasoconstriction in endotoxin shock. Surg. Forum 18:14, 1967.

122. Fine, J.: Septic shock. Pacif. Med. Surg. 75:359, 1967.

123. Berdjis, C. C., and Vick, J. A.: Endotoxin and traumatic shock. J.A.M.A. *204*:191, 1968.

124. Pang, L. M., Stalcup, S. A., O'Brodovich, H., Lipset, J. S., and Mellins, R. B.: Bradykinin and lung lymph protein and fluid flow. Anesthesiology *51*(Suppl. 3, p. S–177), 1979.

125. Passmore, J. C., Neiberger, R. E., and Eden, S. W.: Measurement of intrarenal anatomic distribution of krypton-85 in endotoxic shock in dogs. Am. J. Physiol. *232*:H–54, 1977.

126. Cronenwett, J. L., and Lindenauer, S. M.: Distribution of intrarenal blood flow during bacterial sepsis. J. Surg. Res. *24*:132, 1978.

127. Hinshaw, L. B., Benjamin, B., Holmes, D. D., Beller, B., Archer, L. T., Coalsen, J. J., and Whitsett, T.: Response of the baboon to live *Escherichia coli* organisms and endotoxin. Surg. Gynec. Obstet. *145*:1, 1977.

128. Emerson, T. E., Jr.: Total and regional cerebral hemodynamic and metabolic abnormalities during endotoxin shock: Prevention with methylprednisolone. Adv. Neurol. *20*:173, 1978.

129. Harrison, L. H., Jr., Hinshaw, L. B., Coalson, J. J., and Greenfield, L. J.: Effects of *E. coli* septic shock on pulmonary hemodynamics and capillary permeability. J. Thorac. Cardiovasc. Surg. *61*:795, 1971.

130. Hinshaw, L. B., Emerson, T. S., Jr., and Reins, D. A.: Cardiovascular responses of the primate in endotoxin shock. Am. J. Physiol. *210*:335, 1966.

131. Corrigan, J. J., Jr., Ray, W. L., and May, N.: Changes in the blood coagulation system associated with septicemia. N. Engl. J. Med. *279*:851, 1968.

132. Holcroft, J. W., Blaisdell, F. W., Trunkey, D. D., and Lim, R. C.: Intravascular coagulation and pulmonary edema in the septic baboon. J. Surg. Res. *22*:209, 1977.

133. Corrigan, J. J., Jr.: Heparin therapy in bacterial septicemia. J. Pediatr. *91*:695, 1977.

134. McCabe, W. R., and Jackson, G. G.: Gramnegative bacteremia. Arch. Intern. Med. *110*:847, 1962.

135. Martin, W. T.: Bacteremia and bacteremic shock in surgical patients. Surg. Clin. N. Amer. *49*:1053, 1969.

136. Moser, K. M., Perry, R. B., and Luchsinger, P. C.: Cardiopulmonary consequence of pyrogeninduced hyperpyrexia in man. J. Clin. Invest. *42*:626, 1963.

137. Dietzman, R. H., Manax, W. G., and Lillehei, R. C.: Shock: Mechanisms and therapy. Canad. Anes. Soc. J. *14*:276, 1967.

138. Schweizer, O., and Howland, W. S.: The prognostic significance of high lactate levels. Anesth. Analg. *47*:383, 1968.

139. Freund, H. R., Ryan, J. A., and Fisher, J. E.: Amino acid derangements in patients with sepsis. Ann. Surg. *188*:423, 1978.

140. Wichterman, K. A., Chaudry, I. H., and Baue, A. E.: Studies of peripheral glucose uptake during sepsis. Arch. Surg. *114*:740, 1979.

141. Schumer, W.: Localization of the energy pathway block in shock. Surgery *64*:55, 1968.

142. Shubin, H., Weil, H., and Carlson, R. W.: Bacterial shock. Am. Heart J. *94*:112, 1977.

143. Attar, S., Kirby, W. H., Jr., Mosaitis, C., Mansberger, A. R., Jr., and Cowley, R. A.: Coagulation changes in clinical shock. II. Effect of septic shock on clotting times and fibrinogen in humans. Ann. Surg. *164*:41, 1966.

144. Litton, A.: Haemovascular changes in septic shock. Postgrad. Med. J. *45*:551, 1969.

145. Josey, W. E., Hoch, W., Moon, E. C., and Thompson, J. D.: Analysis of twenty-one septic abortive deaths with special reference to the generalized Shwartzman phenomenon. Obstet. Gynec. *28*:335, 1966.

146. Attar, S., Tingley, H. B., McLaughlin, J. S., and Adams, C. R.: Bradykinin in human shock. Surg. Forum *18*:46, 1967.

147. Sibbald, W. J., Niegel, A. M., Paterson, M. B., Holliday, R. L., Anderson, R. A., Lobb, T. R., and Duff, J. H.: Pulmonary hypertension in sepsis. Chest *73*:583, 1978.

148. Blain, C. M., Anderson, T. O., Pietras, R. J., and Gunnar, R. M.: Immediate hemodynamic effects of gram-negative vs. gram positive bacteria in man. Adv. Intern. Med. *126*:260, 1970.

149. Lillehei, R. C., Longerbeam, J. K., Block, J. H., and Manax, W. E.: Hemodynamic changes in endotoxin shock. *In* Mills, L. J., and Mayer, J. H.: Shock and Hypotension. New York, Grune and Stratton, 1965, p. 442.

150. Udhoji, V. N., and Weil, M. H.: Hemodynamic and metabolic studies on shock associated with bacteremia. Ann. Intern. Med. *62*:966, 1965.

151. Kwaan, H. M., and Weil, M. H.: Differences in the mechanisms of shock caused by bacterial infections. Surg. Gynec. Obstet. *128*:37, 1969.

152. Gunnar, R. M., Loeb, H. S., Pietras, R. T., and Tobin, J. R.: Hemodynamic differences between gram-positive and gram-negative bacteremic shock. Circulation (Suppl. II) *35*:128, 1967.

153. Cohn, J. D., Greenspan, M., Goldstein, C. R., Gudan, A. L., Siegel, J. H., and Del Guercio, L. R. M.: Arteriovenous shunting, high cardiac output shock syndrome. Surg. Gynec. Obstet. *127*:282, 1968.

154. Siegel, J. H., Greenspan, M., and Del Guercio, L. R. M.: Abnormal vascular tone, defective oxygen transport, and myocardial failure in human shock. Ann. Surg. *165*:504, 1967.

155. Wilson, R. F., Thal, A. P., Kindling, P. H., Grifica, T., and Ackerman, E.: Hemodynamic measurements in septic shock. Arch. Surg. *91*:121, 1965.

156. Rush, B., and Sparks, R.: Extracellular fluid shifts in endotoxin shock. J. Trauma *7*:884, 1967.

157. Albrecht, M., and Clowes, G. A.: The increase in circulatory requirements in the presence of inflammation. Surgery *56*:159, 1964.

158. Cronenwett, J. L., and Lindenauer, S. M.: Arteriovenous shunting in the canine hindlimb with sepsis. Surg. Forum *27*:24, 1976.

159. Archie, J. P.: Anatomic arteriovenous shunting in endotoxic and septic shock in dogs. Ann. Surg. *186*:171, 1977.

160. Krausz, M. M., Perel, A., Eimerl, D., and Coter, S.: Cardiopulmonary effects of volume loading in patients in septic shock. Ann. Surg. *185*:429, 1977.

161. Postel, J., and Schloerb, P.: Cardiac depression in bacteremia. Ann. Surg. *186*:74, 1977.

162. Buckberg, G., Cohn, J., and Darling, C.: *E. coli* bacteremic shock in conscious baboons. Ann. Surg. *173*:122, 1971.

163. Archer, L. T., Beller, B. K., Drake, J. K., Whitsett, L. T., and Hinshaw, L. B.: Reversal of myocardial

dysfunction in endotoxin shock with insulin. Canad. J. Pharmacol. 56:132, 1978.

164. Weil, M. H., and Shubin, H.: The "VIP" approach to the bedside management of shock. J.A.M.A. 207:337, 1969.

165. Frank, E. D.: A shock team in a general hospital. Anesth. Analg. 46:744, 1967.

166. Maclean, L. D., McLean, A. P. H., and Duff, J.: Hemodynamic and metabolic abnormalities in septic shock. Postgrad. Med. 48:114, 1970.

167. Hermreck, A. S., and Thal, A. P.: Mechanisms for the high circulatory requirements in sepsis and septic shock. Ann. Surg. 170:677, 1969.

168. Wright, C. J., Duff, J. H., McLean, A. P. H., and MacLean, L. D.: Regional capillary blood flow and oxygen uptake in severe sepsis. Surg. Gynec. Obstet. 132:637, 1971.

169. Broder, G., and Weil, M. H.: Excess lactate: an index of reversibility of shock in human patients. Science 143:1457, 1964.

170. Peretz, P. I., McGregor, M., and Dossetor, J. B.: Lacticacidosis: A clinically significant aspect of shock. Canad. Med. Assoc. J. 90:673, 1964.

171. Rosenberg, J. C., and Rush, B. F.: Lethal endotoxin shock: Oxygen deficit, lactic acid levels, and other metabolic changes. J.A.M.A. 196, 767, 1966.

172. Cain, S. M.: Effect of pCO$_2$ on the relation of lactate and excess lactate to O$_2$ deficit. Amer. J. Physiol. 214:1322, 1968.

173. Lovett, W. L., Wangensteen, S. L., Glenn, T. M., and Lefer, A. M.: Presence of a myocardial depressant factor in patients in circulatory shock. Surgery 70:223, 1971.

174. Leffler, J. N., Litvin, Y., Barenholz, Y., and Lefer, A. M.: Proteolysis in formation of a myocardial depressant factor during shock. Am. J. Physiol. 224:824, 1973.

175. Reyes, M. P., El-Khatib, M. R., Brown, W. J., Smith, F., and Lerner, A. M.: Synergy between carbenicillin and an aminoglycoside (gentamicin or tobramycin) against Pseudomonas aeruginosa isolated from patients with endocarditis. J. Infect. Dis. 140:192, 1979.

176. Andriole, V. T.: Pseudomonas bacteremia: Can antibiotic therapy improve survival? J. Lab. Clin. Med. 94:196, 1979.

177. Krausz, M. M., Perel, A., Eimerl, D., and Coter, S.: Cardiopulmonary effects of volume loading in patients with septic shock. Ann. Surg. 185:429, 1977.

178. Sibbald, W. J., Niegel, A. M., Paterson, M. B., Holliday, R. L., Anderson, R. A., Lobb, T. R., and Duff, J. H.: Pulmonary hypertension in sepsis. Chest 73:583, 1978.

179. Wilson, R. F., Sarver, E., and Birks, R.: Central venous blood pressure and blood volume determinations in clinical shock. Surg. Gynec. Obstet. 132:631, 1977.

180. Holcroft, J. W., Trunkey, D. D., and Carpenter, M. A.: Sepsis in the baboon: Factors affecting resuscitation and pulmonary edema in animals resuscitated with Ringer's lactate versus plasmanate. J. Trauma. 17:600, 1977.

181. Weil, M. H., Shubin, J., Udhoji, V. N., and Rusoff, L.: Effects on vasopressor agents + corticosteroid hormones in endotoxin shock. In Mills, L. C., and Moyer, J. C. (eds.): Shock and Hypotension. New York, Grune and Stratton, 1965.

182. Lillehei, R. C., Longerbeam, J. K., Block, J. H., and Manax, W. G.: Hemodynamic changes in endotoxin shock. In Mills, L. C., and Moyer, J. C. (eds.): Shock and Hypotension. New York, Grune and Stratton, 1965, p. 62.

183. Motsay, G. J., Alho, A., Jaeger, T., Dietzman, R. H., and Lillehei, R. C.: Effects of corticosteroids on the circulation in shock: Experimental and clinical results. Fed. Proc. 29:1861, 1970.

184. Schumer, W.: Steroids in the treatment of clinical septic shock. Ann. Surg. 184:333, 1976.

185. Nishijima, H., Weil, M. H., Shubin, H., and Caranilles, J.: Hemodynamic and metabolic studies on shock associated with gram-negative bacteremia. Medicine 52:287, 1973.

186. Weil, M. H., and Nishijima, H.: Cardiac output in bacterial shock. Am. J. Med. 64:920, 1978.

187. Wilson, R. F., and Fisher, R. R.: Hemodynamic effects of massive steroids: Clinical shock. Surg. Gynec. Obstet. 127:769, 1967.

188. Cahill, G. F., Jenkins, D., and Thorn, G. W.: Diseases of the adrenal cortex. In Harrison, T. R. (ed): Principles of Internal Medicine. 4th ed., New York, McGraw-Hill Book Co., 1962, p. 616.

189. Gill, W., Wilson, S., and Long, W. B. III: Steroid hypothermia. Surg. Gynec. Obstet. 146:944, 1978.

190. Belis, J. U., Rappaport, E. S., Gerber, L., Foreed, J., Buddingh, F., and Messmore, H. L.: A primate model for prolonged endotoxin shock: Bloodvascular reactions and effects of glucocorticoid treatment. J. Lab. Invest. 38:511, 1978.

191. Rao, P. S., and Cavanaugh, D.: Endotoxin shock in the subhuman primate. Arch. Surg. 102:486, 1971.

192. Lefer, A. M., and Martin, J.: Mechanism of the protective effect of corticosteroids in hemorrhagic shock. Am. J. Physiol. 216:314, 1967.

193. Janoff, A., Weissman, G., Zweifach, B. W., and Thomas, L.: Studies on lysosomes in normal heart animals subjected to lethal trauma and endotoxemia. J. Exper. Med. 116:451, 1962.

194. Vaughn, D. L., Bersentis, T., Kirschbaum, T. M., and Assali, B. S.: Homeostatic role of the renaladrenal axis in bacteremic shock: Its therapeutic implications. Am. J. Obstet. Gynec. 99:208, 1967.

195. Goldberg, L. I.: Dopamine — clinical use of an endogenous catecholamine. N. Engl. J. Med. 291:707, 1974.

196. MacCannell, K. L., McNay, J. F., Meyer, M. B., and Goldberg, L. I.: Dopamine in the treatment of hypotensin and shock. N. Engl. J. Med. 275:1389, 1966.

197. Loeb, H. S., Winslow, E. B. J., Rahimtoola, S. H., Rosen, K. M., and Gunner, R. M.: Acute hemodynamic effects of dopamine in patients with shock. Circulation 44:163, 1971.

198. Talley, R. C., Goldberg, L. I., Johnson, C. E., and McNay, J. L.: A hemodynamic comparison of dopamine and isoproterenol in patients in shock. Circulation 39:361, 1969.

199. Lansing, E. J., and Hinshaw, L. B.: Hemodynamic effects of dopamine in endotoxic shock. Proc. Soc. Biol. Med. 130:311, 1969.

200. Shanbour, L. L., and Hinshaw, L. B.: Cardiac and peripheral effects of dopamine infusion in endotoxic shock in the dog. J. Pharmacol. Exp. Ther. 170:108, 1969.

201. Goodman, L. S., and Gilman, A.: The Pharmacological Basis of Therapeutics. 3rd ed. New York, The Macmillan Co., 1965, p. 498.

202. Du Toit, H. J.: Treatment of endotoxic shock with isoprenaline. Lancet 2:143, 1966.

203. Kardos, G.: Isoproterenol in the treatment of shock due to bacteremia with gram-negative pathogens. N. Engl. J. Med. 274:868, 1966.

204. Starzecki, B., Reddin, J. L., and Spink, W. W.: Effect of isoproterenol on survival in canine septic shock. Ann. Surg. 167:35, 1968.

205. Hershey, S. G., Burton, M., and Orkin, L. R.: Therapy of intestinal ischemic (SMA) shock with vasoactive drugs. Anesthesiology 29:466, 1969.

206. Kramer, C. F.: Puerperal shock. Int. Surg. 50:44, 1968.

207. Thal, A. P., and Hermreck, A. S.: Current Problems in Surgery. Chicago, Year Book Medical Publishers, July 1968, p. 25.

208. Archer, L. T., Black, M. R., Greenfield, L. J., and Guenter, C. A.: Prevention and reversal of myocardial failure in endotoxic shock. Physiologist 15:169, 1972.

209. Clowes, G. A., Martin, H., Walji, S., Hirsch, E., Gazitwa, and Goodfellow, R.: Blood insulin response to blood glucose levels in high output sepsis and septic shock. Am. J. Surg. 135:577, 1978.

210. Weisel, J. P., O'Donnell, T. F., Stone, M. A., and Clowes, G. H. A., Jr.: Myocardial performance in clinical septic shock: Effects of isoproterenol and glucose–potassium–insulin. J. Surg. Res. 18:375, 1975.

211. Manny, J., Rabinoviei, N., Manny, J., Schiller, M., and Hecktman, H.: Effect of glucose-insulin-potassium on survival in experimental endotoxic shock. Surg. Gynec. Obstet. 147:405, 1978.

212. Anderson, R. W., James, P. M., Bradenberg, C. E., and Hardaway, R. M.: Phenoxybenzamine in septic shock. Ann. Surg. 165:341, 1967.

213. Eckenhoff, J. E., and Cooperman, L. H.: The clinical application of phenoxybenzamine in shock and vasoconstrictor states. Surg. Gynec. Obstet. 121:483, 1965.

214. Cerra, F. B., Hassett, J., and Siegel, J. H.: Vasodilator therapy in clinical sepsis with low output syndrome. J. Surg. Res. 25:180, 1978.

215. Nickerson, M.: Drugs inhibiting adrenergic nerves and structures innervated by them. In Goodman, L. S., and Gilman, A. (eds.): The Pharmacological Basis of Therapeutics. 3rd ed., New York, The Macmillan Co., 1965, p. 546.

216. Rovenstein, E. A., Hershey, S. G., Lanza, S., Baez, A., and Baez, S.: Relationship of bowel and liver to drug protection against shock. Anesthesiology 20:290, 1959.

217. Massion, W. H., and Blümel, G.: Irreversiblity in shock: Role of vasoactive kinins. Anesth. Analg. 50:970, 1971.

218. Doenicke, A., Gesing, H., Krumey, I., and Schmidinger, S. T.: Influence of aprotinin (Trasylol) on the action of suxamethonium. Brit. J. Anesth. 42:948, 1970.

219. Northover, B. J., and Subramanian, G.: Analgesic antipyretic drugs as antagonists of endotoxin shock in dogs. J. Pathol. Bacteriol. 83:463, 1962.

220. Hilton, J. G., and Wells, C. H.: Effects of indomethacin and nicotinic acid on E. coli endotoxin shock in anesthetized dogs. J. Trauma 16:968, 1976.

221. Fletcher, J. R., Herman, C. M., and Ramwell, P.: Improved survival in endotoxemia with aspirin and indomethacin pretreatment. Surg. Forum 27:11, 1976.

222. Fletcher, J. R., and Ramwell, P. W.: Lidocaine or indomethacin improves survival in baboon endotoxin shock. J. Surg. Res. 24:154, 1978.

223. Foy, T., Marion, J., Brigham, K. L., and Harris, T. R.: Isoproterenol and aminophylline reduce lung capillary filtration during high permeability. J. Appl. Physiol. 46:146, 1979.

224. Saba, T. M., Blumenstock, F. A., Scovill, W. A., and Bernard, H.: Cryoprecipitate reversal of opsonic α-surface binding glycoprotein deficiency in septic surgical and trauma patients. Science 201:622, 1978.

225. Stanley, T. H., and Reddy, P.: Fentanyl-oxygen in septic shock. Anesthesiology 51(Suppl. S–100), 1979.

226. Lappas, D. G., Lowenstein, E., and Waller, J.: Hemodynamic effects of nitroprusside infusion during coronary artery operation in man. Circulation 54:4, 1976.

227. Schweiger, O., and Williams, H.: The prognostic significance of high lactate levels. Anesth. Analg. 47:383, 1968.

228. Virtue, R. W., Jones, B. E., and Wells, J. B.: Effects of ether, cyclopropane, and pentothal in shocked rats. Anesthesiology 17:60, 1956.

229. Rety, N. A., and Couves, C. M.: The effects of anesthesia on experimental endotoxin shock. Canad. Anesth. Soc. J. 14:112, 1967.

230. White, G. L., Archer, L. T., Beller, B. K., and Hinshaw, L. B.: Increased survival with methylprednisolone treatment in canine endotoxin shock. J. Surg. Res. 25:357, 1978.

231. Weinstein, L.: Hemophilus infection. In Harrison, T. R. (ed.): Principles of Internal Medicine. 4th ed., New York, McGraw-Hill Book Co. 1962, p. 955.

17

Uncommon Problems in Acute Trauma

By BARRY L. ZIMMERMAN, M.D.

Basic Early Care
The Exsanguinated Patient
  Fluid Volume Replacement
  Anesthetic Management
Head Trauma
  Head Trauma Accompanying Other
    Trauma
  Hypertension Following Head
    Trauma
  Basal Skull Fractures
Spinal Cord Trauma
  Low Acute Injuries
  High Acute Injuries
  Chronic Injuries

Maxillofacial Trauma
  Airway Problems
  Intraoperative Problems
  Eye Injuries
Trauma to Major Airways
Chest Trauma
  Blunt Cardiac Trauma
  Penetrating Heart Injuries
  Aortic Rupture
Trauma to the Diaphragm
Extremity Replantation
Near-Drowning
Mass Casualties

Trauma is a common facet of our lives, causing almost 10 per cent of all deaths (a much higher percentage in the age range from 10–34 years), 380,000 cases of permanent disability, and 7.5 billion dollars in incurred medical expenses in 1977.[1] All anesthetists have experience in the care of traumatized patients, and certain aspects of trauma care, such as fluid volume resuscitation, fall within the sphere of the anesthesiologist's special expertise.[2] This chapter, therefore, is not intended as a comprehensive review of the anesthetic care of the trauma patient. Rather, after a brief general introduction, emphasis will be placed on those situations that may be unusual or controversial enough to place them outside the bounds of common knowledge in the specialty. Because of their inherent nature, the problems posed for the anesthesiologist in these situations are not amenable to definitive "solutions." The clinician who is faced with one of these difficult problems may, however, gain insight, perspective, and confidence from reviewing the experiences of other clinicians who have been in similar situations.

BASIC EARLY CARE

The initial approach to a trauma victim advocated by the American College of Surgeons' Committee on Trauma is widely accepted. This approach, as illustrated in Figure 17–1, includes certain key features listed below in approximate descending order of priority.[3]

1. Make a rapid overall assessment of the patient's condition.

2. Establish a clear airway

3. Ensure adequacy of ventilation. Rapidly evaluate and treat sucking chest wounds, flail chest, obvious major external hemorrhage, hemopneumothorax, and other disorders.

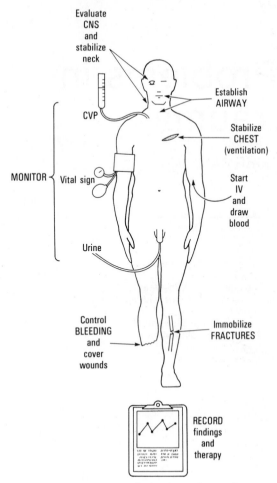

Figure 17–1. Initial steps in the evaluation and treatment of the trauma patient. Based on the guidelines of the Committee on Trauma of the American College of Surgeons.[3]

4. Establish multiple large-bore, secure intravenous lines. During insertion obtain blood for initial laboratory tests and blood cross matching. Begin infusion of balanced electrolyte solution.

5. Perform a fast but thorough examination, paying particular attention to vital signs, neurologic status, and obvious wounds. Avoid unnecessary motion of the patient.

6. Begin a medical record, and document all findings and interventions.

7. Cover open wounds, control external hemorrhage, and immobilize fractures (including the cervical spine in patients with head or neck injuries).

8. Obtain appropriate radiologic studies. Portable chest and cervical spine studies can be done in the receiving area if the patient is unstable. If the patient is transported to the radiology area, arrange to do definitive studies of all pertinent injuries at a single visit.

If the patient appears to be hypovolemic or hypotensive, the following steps are recommended in addition to the above.[4]

1. Elevate the legs to increase venous return.

2. Insert an indwelling urinary catheter and measure output every 30 minutes. Send urine for analysis.

3. If a satisfactory response is not obtained to the initial dose (1–2 liters) of balanced electrolyte solution (stable arterial pressure, falling heart rate, adequate urine output, normal blood pH) suspect continued bleeding. Insert a CVP catheter. Administer blood as needed.

In patients with severe or multiple injuries, many of these tasks may need to be done simultaneously. An anesthesiologist should become involved in the management of severely traumatized patients from the onset. Airway management and/or ventilation may be difficult and complicated, and may require application of a repertoire of techniques not possessed by the average surgeon or emergency room physician. Appropriate monitoring should take into account not only the patient's current condition but also what his condition is likely to become and the requirements of the operation likely to be performed.

Sophisticated invasive monitoring is not necessary in patients with simple injuries who respond promptly to initial therapy. Patients with massive injuries or multisystem disease or who fail to respond as anticipated to the initial volume load may require direct intravascular monitoring. The combination of central venous pressure (CVP) and intra-arterial catheters supplies the pressures on both sides of the lungs and gives the ability to obtain blood samples and to determine cardiac outputs using dye dilution techniques. If the CVP line is a short (5½ inch or 8 inch) 16 gauge catheter inserted in the external jugular, internal jugular, subclavian, or even femoral vein, it can be directly replaced at a later time by an 8-French introducer sheath using the guidewire supplied in most commercially produced introducer "kits." A pulmonary artery catheter can then be inserted with minimum time lag and without the need for another venipuncture, if it becomes necessary. Vascular access, whether for monitoring or for fluid administration, should be tailored to the individual patient depending on the location and severity of injuries. Here again, the anesthesiologist's experience and skill may be valuable in dealing with such technical problems.

THE EXSANGUINATED PATIENT

FLUID VOLUME REPLACEMENT

The physiologic sequence of events in acute, continuous hemorrhage is schematized in Figure 17–2. Upon loss of 5 per cent of the circulating blood volume, baroreceptor activity is reduced slightly, paralleling the slight decrease in stroke volume. This causes a mild increase in sympathetic tone, constriction of the venous capacitance bed, and probably secretion of renin by the kidney. This maintains stroke volume, and cardiac output is preserved with minimal or no

change in heart rate. After 10 per cent blood volume loss (BVL), stroke volume decreases further, which further decreases the output of the baroreceptors, and sympathetic tone is further augmented. Heart rate is now noticeably elevated, and cardiac output is maintained. Beyond 15 per cent BVL, cardiac output decreases, further increasing sympathetic tone and intensifying the previous changes. To maintain perfusion pressure to vital organs, precapillary sphincters constrict in skeletal muscle, skin, mesentery, and other nonvital vascular beds.[5, 6] This results in a decrease in capillary hydrostatic pressure in those structures, and interstitial fluid begins to migrate into the vascular compartment by way of the distal capillaries and venules.[7-9] This transcapillary refill slows the decrease in blood volume, but at the cost of progressive hemodilution, and hematocrit and colloid oncotic pressure decrease steadily. This phenomenon of transcapillary refill occurs almost with the onset of significant blood loss, although it may take many hours to be complete.[7, 8]

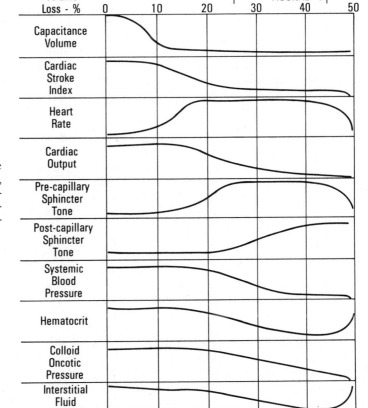

Figure 17–2. Pathophysiologic sequence of events during acute, continuous blood loss. Changes indicated are relative, and not intended to be quantitative. Sequence described in text.

Between 15 and 20 per cent BVL, all of these mechanisms are not sufficient to maintain systemic blood pressure, and hypotension occurs. This serves to intensify the increase in sympathetic tone, and extreme tachycardia and constriction of both pre- and postcapillary sphincters occurs. In acute loss of around 25 to 30 per cent of the circulating blood volume, the combination of limited cardiac output, hypotension, and vasoconstriction produces hypoperfusion of viscera, and the clinical state of "shock" occurs. Urine output ceases, mental status may deteriorate, and anaerobic metabolism results in an increasing "oxygen debt" and lactic acidosis. The failure of aerobic metabolism has further profound effects on fluid dynamics. Precapillary sphincters, being sensitive to tissue acidosis and hypoxia, dilate. However, postcapillary (venular) sphincters are less sensitive to local tissue metabolism and do not relax. This places the point of maximum resistance downstream of the capillary bed, and hydrostatic pressure in the capillary increases.[6, 9] Transcapillary filtration of fluid now reverses, and plasma volume is lost into the interstitial space. Hematocrit rises, but because of ischemic damage to the capillaries, plasma proteins leak into the interstitium, and colloid oncotic pressure does not rise. This loss of plasma volume intensifies the volume deficit, and the organism quickly decompensates and dies. In most studies death occurs after the rapid loss of 40 to 50 per cent of the total blood volume.[7]

This terminal series of events may also occur if lesser degrees of shock (e.g., 30 per cent blood volume loss) are sustained for an appropriate period of time. In these cases the progressive oxygen debt causes tissue and capillary changes that may not revert to normal upon restoration of blood volume. This results in the syndrome of so-called "irreversible shock," which means shock that leads inexorably to death despite appropriate and complete volume replacement and supportive care.[9, 10]

Before such irreversible changes take place, the sequence of events leading to death may be reversed at any point by replacement of the lost volume. In animal studies this is accomplished by reinfusing the animal's own shed blood. In clinical medicine, however, some substitute must be found. The controversy over which fluid provides the optimum combination of intra-vascular volume expansion, oxygen delivery, and restoration of normal physiology with the least risk of complications is currently one of the great debates in medicine.[11-23] Despite theoretical considerations on each side, however, clinical experience has failed to demonstrate a constant advantage for any given approach to volume replacement.

Blood Versus "Clear Fluid"

Since the basic lesion in hemorrhagic shock is the specific microcirculatory derangement caused by the combination of high resistance, low pressure, and poor flow, restoration of adequate circulation and tissue perfusion are far more important for survival than is oxygen carrying capacity.[6, 9, 10] Successful resuscitation has been reported in both animals and man with hematocrits lowered acutely by hemorrhage and hemodilution to the range of 10 to 15 per cent, without evidence of peripheral oxygen debt, as long as adequate circulation was maintained.[24-27] When available, blood is the optimum fluid for massive transfusion. However, volume restoration should not be delayed because of fears of excessive hemodilution. The "optimum hematocrit" for the patient in shock is probably lower than has been thought in the past. Nunn emphasized the importance of hemoglobin in resuscitation and considered the "optimum hematocrit" to be around 42 per cent.[28] Bland, et al, however, emphasizing circulatory dynamics, found a hemoglobin of less than 9.5 gm/100 ml to be more predictive of survival.[29]

Type of Blood. Fresh, whole, cross-matched blood would appear to be the ideal form of fluid for resuscitation, but it is in severely limited supply and is thus not available for most cases of massive transfusion. Whole banked blood is the closest approximation from the point of view of completeness (volume plus colloid plus hemoglobin) and ease of administration, and is the mainstay of current therapy. Packed (refrigerated or frozen) red cells can be used successfully,[30] but are slower to administer and require additional volume infusion. Component therapy becomes more attractive once the patient is initially resuscitated, as it allows administration of volume, hemoglobin, and coagulation factors tailored to each patient's needs. Whole blood should be cross matched if possible, but type-specific blood is almost as satisfactory.[31] The problems associated with transfusion of several units of type O-negative whole blood have been reviewed recently[32] and appear to militate strongly against this usage. If used for any reason, screening for high titers of anti-A isoagglutinin is necessary to prevent hemolysis of the recipient's native cells if he happens to be type A. This test is not done routinely in most blood banks today. Also, if more than about 4 or 5 units of O-negative blood are used, the patient should not be given his native type for about a week, to prevent an immediate hemolytic transfusion reaction.[32, 33, 34] Type O-negative packed or washed red cells avoid some of these problems,[32] but are subject to the same limitations as typed packed cells. Therefore, the use of O-negative "universal donor" blood has little justification for the individual patient. Blood is not necessary in the first minutes of resuscitation,[11, 14] and type-specific blood can be obtained in about 15 to 20 minutes. This situation is reversed, however, when dealing with more than one casualty simultaneously, as will be discussed later.

Acid-Base Status.   Stored blood is acidic, with a pH of 6.6 to 6.9 after 14 days.[35] However, the actual amount of hydrogen ions infused is small, and massive amounts of stored blood can be infused without producing significant acidosis. Whenever systemic acidemia is present with massive transfusion, it is almost always due to inadequate resuscitation, and responds to additional volume. Bicarbonate should not be given routinely during transfusion when facilities are available for blood gas and acid-base determination.[35, 36]

Citrate Intoxication.   The citrate in banked blood binds calcium, and potentially could produce significant hypocalcemic cardiac depression. This appears to be a problem only with very rapid infusion of whole blood,[35, 36] such as 150 ml per minute. Since calcium administration is not benign, it should be reserved for those situations with specific indications, such as continuous blood infusion at high rates, or evidence of direct myocardial depression. Small doses (3-4 mg/kg of the chloride) are sufficient.

Temperature.   Hypothermic cardiac arrest has been reported with infusion of large amounts of cold blood.[37] Under normal conditions, the metabolic cost to the body of warming a 500 ml unit of blood from 4° C to 37° C would amount to less than 20 kcal; or the energy provided by eating one medium carrot. However, in shock states the blood volume is restricted to the central circulation, and indeed selectively perfuses the heart before other organs. Therefore, cardiac hypothermia is a real problem in such cases. Up to about 4 to 5 units of cold blood can apparently be given quickly without great risk,[35, 37] but beyond that, warming the blood before infusion becomes increasingly important.

Filtration.   The particulate debris that accumulates in banked blood has been implicated as a causative factor in the pulmonary insufficiency that may occur after trauma and massive blood transfusion.[35, 38] Microthrombi consisting of fibrin strands and enmeshed cellular debris have been identified in sections of lungs of subjects with post-transfusion respiratory insufficiency.[38] Passing blood through a micropore (20–50 μm pore size) filter before infusion is advocated as a way of reducing pulmonary damage.[35, 36, 38] However, the evidence for the actual clinical importance of blood microfiltration is scanty. Some studies have purported to show a reduction in respiratory complications when blood was filtered, but others have not.[39] It seems to be much easier to correlate respiratory insufficiency with the severity of the initial injury or the presence of direct chest trauma, and less simple to implicate the number of unfiltered units of blood.[39] On the other hand, it is hard to see how filtering blood could be harmful. It does slow the infusion process, but probably not as much as warming does. Therefore, even though it must be admitted that some of the benefits of blood microfiltration remain speculative, it is a reasonable recommendation at this time.

Acellular Fluid Resuscitation

The largest controversy centers around whether or not "clear fluid" given as a blood substitute must contain large molecules, such as albumin, to maintain the colloid oncotic pressure in the circulation. The extent of this debate exceeds the scope of this article but certain points are reasonably clear.

"Crystalloid" Versus "Colloid."   Adequate cardiac output may be restored with

the use of either synthetic salt solutions ("crystalloid") or solutions containing natural or synthetic large molecules ("colloid"). Because a given volume of crystalloid equilibrates more readily throughout the total extravascular space, however, larger volumes must be given for the same amount of intravascular volume expansion. Studies that have suggested that resuscitation with crystalloids is inadequate have usually used a fixed ratio of crystalloid volume administered to blood shed, such as two to one or three to one.[13, 17, 23, 25] Other studies that have used normal hemodynamic indices as the endpoints for crystalloid administration demonstrated that quite adequate resuscitation was possible, even from hemorrhage of 50 to 70 per cent of the animal's blood volume.[20, 24, 27, 40] The volume used in such studies was often as high as five to 11 times the volume of shed blood. Such subjects were indeed quite "waterlogged," with large weight gains and obvious edema, but appeared to suffer no ill effects on organ function. The extra whole body fluid appeared to be readily mobilized and excreted by the kidneys within 48 to 72 hours. There is intense disagreement as to whether such edema is actually dangerous in and of itself, particularly with regard to causing pulmonary dysfunction,[14, 16, 18-21, 41] but there is no longer any doubt that crystalloid fluid given in adequate amounts is capable of restoring organ perfusion after acute hemorrhage. There is no consistent evidence that crystalloid fluids are more dangerous in patients with preexisting cardiopulmonary disease, but the best case for restricting the volume of fluid administered, particularly crystalloid, occurs in situations where the lung parenchyma has sustained a direct injury, such as fat embolization, gastric acid aspiration, or direct pulmonary contusion.[14, 41]

Saline Versus Balanced Electrolytes. Isotonic sodium chloride solutions contain an excess of the chloride ion compared with blood, and solutions such as Ringer's lactate solution (Hartman's solution) contain an excess of other anions such as lactate.[24] The other ions in such "balanced" solutions (potassium, calcium, etc.) have insignificant impact on blood chemistry. Isotonic saline tends to produce a slight hyperchloremic acidosis, while Ringer's lactate tends to produce a degree of metabolic alkalosis. The clinical significance of these changes is not clear, however, and large volumes of either solution may be used without producing serious acid-base disturbances.[24]

Human Plasma. Single-donor plasma is the cell-free supernate resulting from the concentrating process employed to produce packed red blood cells. If collected from stored, banked blood, it is called single-donor plasma (SDP); if collected from fresh blood and immediately frozen, it is called fresh frozen plasma (FFP). FFP is more "complete" than SDP in that it may be presumed to contain adequate amounts of the labile coagulation factors, but otherwise the two products are identical. Both may be used for acute volume expansion, although SDP, when available, is ready for use and does not require additional processing. Both contain the same hepatitis risk, which is almost the same as that for a unit of whole blood. Because of problems with availability, neither may be appropriate for use in acute resuscitation, but may find use later in the course of fluid management. Because of the limited supply of FFP, its use should be reserved for cases in which coagulation factors are specifically indicated.

Processed Plasma. Plasma protein fraction, 5 per cent (PPF) is human plasma that has been "pasteurized" (heat-treated) to inactivate the hepatitis virus. It is shelf-stable for up to two years and thus is ideal to store in emergency areas for rapid use. It does not contain labile coagulation factors. PPF is readily available and is usually safe. However, it suffers from several disadvantages in rapid, massive volume resuscitation. First, it is expensive.[16] The patient cost for 250 ml of PPF at our hospital is $93.50, compared to $32.50 for 250 ml of SDP. Second, systemic vasodilatation with hypotension has been reported with the rapid administration of PPF. This effect, which is proportional to the speed of administration, has been blamed on the presence of the vasoactive amines found in PPF (bradykinins, kininogens, etc.), which result from the heat processing of the globulin fraction.[42, 43] Recently, however, it has been suggested that the vasodilatation can be accounted for by the acetate content of PPF; infusion of the acetate alone in comparable concentrations causes the same amount of vasodilatation.[44] Whatever the cause, it would appear that PPF should not be infused rapidly in a patient with hemorrhagic hypotension.

Human serum albumin solutions (HSA). either 5 per cent or 25 per cent (salt-poor albumin, or SPA), have a much lower potential for causing hypotension, because they contain lower concentrations of both the vasoactive amines and acetate.[42, 44] For this reason 5 per cent HSA has become the preferred colloid solution for rapid emergency infusion in some centers.[42] The cost is approximately equal to PPF. 25 per cent HSA (SPA) has a greater oncotic effect but is slow and difficult to infuse in emergency situations.

Non-protein Colloids. Solutions containing other large non-protein molecules (dextrans, starch, etc.) have been in common use in Europe for many years, but because of adverse immunohematologic effects (e.g., coagulopathies, anaphylactoid reactions) they have never gained widespread use in the United States.[36, 45] These complications occur most often when large volumes are infused rapidly, so that their use is particularly restricted in situations of rapid, massive blood loss. At present, the most useful of these plasma substitutes would appear to be hydroxyethyl starch.[22, 46] However, it is unlikely that it will gain widespread use, especially in light of the imminent development of newer solutions that also increase oxygen carrying capacity in addition to blood volume.[23]

Ancillary Measures

Position. The Trendelenburg position is widely used to treat hypotensive patients, but the evidence for its effectiveness is scanty. It does not increase cerebral blood flow, and may enhance the formation of intracranial edema.[47] Some studies have shown an increase in afterload and a decrease in cardiac output with the assumption of the Trendelenburg position.[47] If an increase in preload and venous return is desired, it is more rational to raise the legs and leave the torso level.[4, 47]

Lower-Body Compression. "MAST" suits or "anti-gravity trousers" are logical options, especially when bleeding is in the abdomen, retroperitoneum, or pelvis. These treatments decrease blood loss and increase venous return.[48, 49] The suits may be used while diagnostic tests are underway, while transporting patients, and during resuscitation. Fluid resuscitation must be almost complete before removing the suits or severe hypotension may result.

Vasopressors/Dilators. Some of the controversy and confusion over the use of vasoactive drugs in hemorrhagic shock has undoubtedly arisen because it is difficult to determine exactly where in the natural evolution of the physiologic syndrome any given patient is at any given time.[9, 10] At various points in this evolution the patient's clinical presentation may appear to be similar yet the pathophysiology may be very different.

It seems rational to use a catecholamine, such as epinephrine, if the patient is in the "agonal" state of depressed sympathetic tone and impending cardiovascular collapse. On the other hand, it seems appropriate to use a vasodilator if the patient appears to have an adequate central blood volume as determined by a high central venous or pulmonary capillary wedge pressure, but still shows sluggish peripheral flow or low cardiac output. It would appear, then, that the routine use of a dilator or pressor could not be advocated without some determination of blood volume and/or cardiac filling pressure, cardiac output, and state of vascular tone.

Diuretics. The powerful loop diuretics such as furosemide and ethacrynic acid have the capacity to increase urine volume and salt excretion even in the face of systemic hypovolemia.[50-52] For this reason their indiscriminate use in the oliguric patient must be condemned, for they can mask the prerenal oliguria caused by inadequate volume replacement and promote a sense of false security.[50, 52] However, there is some evidence that use of furosemide may convert an oliguric acute renal failure to the nonoliguric form, which is associated with an improved prognosis.[51, 52] The drugs should not be used, however, until there is evidence of adequate volume replacement such as a high CVP, pulmonary artery wedge pressure, or a high cardiac output.

If diuretics are administered, urine for laboratory studies (creatinine clearance, free-water clearance, sodium excretion, etc.) should be obtained first, for the results of these tests will be altered by the drugs.[50, 53]

ANESTHETIC MANAGEMENT

It is extremely desirable that a bleeding patient be stabilized and resuscitated before the induction of anesthesia. However,

in some cases it is not possible to completely accomplish this goal. The anesthesiologist must than choose the agent and technique that are most appropriate to the
individual patient.

The goal in such situations is to maintain
as much tissue perfusion as possible; the
chosen anesthetic must not interfere with
cardiac output or perfusion pressure, or increase regional organ vascular resistance.
General anesthetics have profound effects
on systemic and regional hemodynamics,
but the effects are not simple to characterize.[54-58] The effects on isolated organ vascular beds may be different from effects in the
intact organism, and those effects will be
modified by pathology or pre-existing state
of sympathetic tone, volume status, and
other factors. Clearly, general anesthetics
are capable of altering or abolishing normal
compensatory responses to stress, including
blood loss.[5, 58-61] Barbiturate anesthesia can
markedly reduce renal blood flow during
hemorrhage by selectively increasing renal
vascular resistance.[5] Halothane can reduce
renal vascular resistance in isolated kidneys,[56, 57] but also blocks the compensatory
tachycardia and systemic vasoconstriction
usually seen with hemorrhage, and results
in greatly reduced cardiac outputs and systemic arterial perfusion pressures.[59] The net
effect can be a significant reduction of renal
blood flow.

Thus, it would seem desirable to use a
"vasodilating" anesthetic technique to improve organ perfusion, but only if perfusion
pressure and cardiac output can be maintained. On the other hand, while it is desirable to maintain tissue perfusion pressure,
it should not be at the expense of constricting vital nutrient circulatory beds.

The natural compensatory mechanisms
demonstrated by intact animals subjected to
hemorrhage are adaptive: they reduce perfusion of non-critical organs and maintain
perfusion of critical ones.[5, 6] Anesthesia
should interfere minimally with this natural
adaptation. In practice this is accomplished,
not by selecting a certain drug over another,
but by using all drugs cautiously and in the
smallest amount necessary to obtain a desired effect.

Many authors have stated a preference for
certain drugs in various circumstances,[62-73]
but the actual evidence for the superiority
of any given technique in hemorrhagic
shock is sparse. The choice is often perceived to be between "sympatholytic"
agents that reduce sympathetic tone and
hopefully improve organ flow by preventing
regional vasoconstriction, and "sympathomimetic" agents that support perfusion
pressure and cardiac output. Theye[71] reported improved survival in shocked dogs
anesthetized with halothane (potential vasodilator) as opposed to those given cyclopropane (vasoconstrictor). However, Longnecker[67] reported improved survival in rats
given ketamine and hemorrhaged, compared with rats given either halothane or
fluroxene. Ketamine has gained great popularity as a "sympathomimetic" agent, as
it is nonflammable, easily and rapidly administered, controllable, and provides intense analgesia and amnesia in small
doses.[62, 63, 65, 67, 73-77] However, ketamine increases blood pressure by indirect mechanisms[73] and must not be relied upon to support the circulation in seriously ill patients.
In both animals and man, ketamine may fail
to support, and may even depress, the circulatory system that is under maximal stress or
is bordering on failure.[75-77] This is probably
related either to catecholamine depletion or
to a relative insensitivity to catecholamines
in such patients.[77]

Diazepam has been advocated as a relatively safe, nondepressant drug in ill patients.[65, 66, 73] However, there is some evidence to indicate that it, too, can depress
compromised and extremely stressed circulations, and must be used with caution.[73]
Narcotics are often used to produce some
degree of vasodilatation without profound
sympathectomy or depression of the heart,
but there is little clinical evidence that they
are superior to other drugs in hemorrhagic
shock.[70] Halothane is mistrusted by many
clinicians,[64-66, 68, 69] but the evidence against
it is inconclusive, and it has been used in
many casualty situations over the years with
good success.[26, 70, 72] There is insufficient
clinical experience reported with use of
enflurane or isoflurane in shocked patients
to make meaningful comparisons with halothane possible.

In the trauma setting, sodium thiopental
has a notorious reputation. Halford's[78]
famous comment on the experience with
thiopental at Pearl Harbor (". . . an ideal
method of euthanasia") is widely quoted,
and many sources feel that the drug is
highly dangerous.[65, 66, 69] In the same issue
of Anesthesiology that contained Halford's

comments, indeed on the very next page, appeared an article by Adams and Gray,[79] who reported a favorable outcome with the use of thiopental following a severe gunshot wound with hemorrhagic shock. Details of the use of the drug in each article are revealing. Halford referred to deaths following the administration of "...doses *as low as 0.5 gm*" (italics added).[78] Adams and Gray administered the drug as a 2.5 per cent solution, giving single milliliter doses (25 mg) slowly over several minutes. The patient was intubated without relaxant after 125 mg had been given, and a total of 400 mg was used for the entire 105 minute case.[79]

An unsigned editorial that followed these articles placed the issue in perspective, and the comments are as valid now as they were in 1943. Referring to experience with Evipal, the editor noted, "...the drug was not dangerous but the method of administration was...".[80] With regard to thiopental, "(small) doses...administered slowly, with intervals between injections of sufficient length to allow the full effect to take place, is the only rational scheme of dosage."[80] In the last three decades, thiopental has been used extensively in work with military combat casualties, and has proven to be satisfactory when used in selected patients with the appropriate degree of caution and care.[26, 64, 68, 75]

Occasionally methohexital is recommended over thiopental because of early data indicating that the oxybarbiturates caused less hypotension than thiobarbiturates.[69] This has not been confirmed by subsequent work, however, and the two classes of drugs must be considered to be equally depressant.[84]

Regional anesthesia is often used in military situations. but probably has little role in the routine management of the exsanguinated, shocky patient. Regional techniques are most useful in surgery on isolated extremity injuries, and these injuries do not usually create hemorrhage that cannot be controlled and corrected before induction. Major regional blocks for body cavity surgery are less controllable than general anesthesia and may have catastrophic effects because of the abrupt sympathectomy they produce.[81-83] It is important to note that Halford's comment about thiopental was borrowed from one by Admiral Gordon-Taylor of the British Navy, whose original state-

ment was "(spinal) anesthesia is the ideal form of euthanasia in war surgery."[78]

A reasonable approach to the care of an exsanguinated patient might be constructed as follows. First, the patient who is unconscious because of shock does not need "induction" of anesthesia.[66, 69] The trachea should be intubated with or without relaxant, alveolar ventilation established, and the surgeon's approach to the bleeding site facilitated by appropriate positioning and neuromuscular blockade. Pancuronium bromide is usually preferred for this because of the hemodynamic stability associated with its use,[62] but succinylcholine may also be used, since succinylcholine-induced potassium release in the trauma patient does not occur appreciably in the first 24 hours.[85] If these manipulations cause undesired cardiovascular reflex activity or if the patient shows signs of awareness, an anesthetic drug may be slowly introduced at this point. Concerns of humanitarianism should not cause haste, but the response to graded increments of anesthesia should be carefully observed before the next increment is given. Inhalation agents have the advantages of fine control and reversibility of dosage, ability to produce unconsciousness at relatively light planes of anesthesia, ability to administer very high inhaled oxygen concentration, and independence of hepatic and renal routes of excretion to terminate their effect. Ventilation should be controlled, but with the minimum practical volumes and pressures to prevent further cardiovascular compromise.[61, 66]

If the patient's status appears to justify it, a formal induction sequence may be carried out. An intravenous technique is probably preferable for reasons of speed; even small children will probably have an intravenous line established before induction in these circumstances. Because most patients will be considered to have full stomachs, a rapid-sequence ("crash") induction is indicated. There are two forms of rapid-sequence induction. One form, as reported by Stept and Safar[86]:

1. Administer 100 per cent oxygen for at least three minutes (if practical).

2. At the same time, administer a small dose of non-depolarizing relaxant; e.g., 3 mg *d*-tubocurarine, or 0.5–1.0 mg pancuronium.

3. At the end of three minutes, administer *without pause* a dose of a chosen anes-

thetic drug and a dose of 1.5 mg/kg of succinylcholine.

4. As the patient loses consciousness, an
assistant exerts firm anteroposterior pressure on the patient's cricoid cartilage to
occlude the esophagus. The anteroposterior
pressure should not be released until after
step 5.

5. No attempt is made to ventilate the
patient by mask. As the patient relaxes, the
trachea is quickly intubated and the cuff on
the tube inflated.

6. After tracheal position of the tube is
confirmed (chest expansion, breath sounds),
the assistant releases the cricoid pressure.
The alternative form has been reported by
Brown et al.:[87]

1. Pre-oxygenate as before.

2. After three minutes administer *without
pause* 0.15 mg/kg pancuronium and the chosen dose of anesthetic.

3. Continue the sequence as before.
The latter form is particularly useful in
situations in which the muscle fasciculations caused by succinylcholine are not desired.

Which anesthetic drug to use for induction is a matter of personal clinical judgment. A more important issue is the dose
used, which may be as small as none for the
patient with impending collapse. Ketamine
probably has the advantage of producing
more profound amnesia and analgesia in
smaller doses, such as 20 to 50 mg,[73, 88, 89]
but the beneficial effects on intracranial
dynamics of thiopental or a similar drug
might be more useful in a patient with head
trauma (see section on head trauma).

HEAD TRAUMA

Cerebral trauma is not uncommon, but its
proper anesthetic management requires application of concepts and technics that may
not be common knowledge outside the rapidly emerging subspecialty of neuroanes-
thesia. The extensive literature dealing with
the interactions between intracranial fluid
dynamics, circulatory responses, and anesthetic pharmacology cannot be reviewed in
detail here.[90-99] However, selected aspects
of these interactions will be discussed that
would be of value to the anesthesiologist
called upon to anesthetize the patient with
acute intracranial trauma.

HEAD TRAUMA ACCOMPANYING OTHER TRAUMA

Head trauma frequently coexists with and
complicates trauma to other parts of the
body, particularly the chest.[100] Often the
head trauma is not serious, and attention is
focused on the other injuries. In such cases
it is important to appreciate that secondary
brain damage may occur if attention is not
paid to the changes in intracranial fluid
dynamics that occur after even minor injuries. Many authors have emphasized the
importance of giving a "neuroanesthetic" to
a patient with any degree of head injury,
even if it is not felt to be a threat to the
patient at the time.[94, 97, 101, 102] Detailed discussions of anesthesia for the patient with
head trauma or increased intracranial pressure can be found in the recent literature.[90, 92, 93, 103, 104] However, the most important anesthesia related aspects that bear
directly on the care of patients with incidental head injury who are being anesthetized for repair of other lesions will be discussed here.

Airway and Ventilation. Rapid control
of the airway and alveolar hyperventilation
are of paramount importance in dealing
with head injuries.[94, 97, 105-108] Hypocarbia
not only constricts cerebral vessels and reduces intracranial pressure (ICP) but also
restores some measure of ability to autoregulate flow to areas of the brain that had lost
this power because of injury.[92, 96-98] In normal brain, cerebral blood flow is nearly
linearly related to arterial Pa_{CO_2} in the normal clinical range.[92, 95, 96] In damaged brain,
the blood flow response to hypercapnia may
be exaggerated, and small increases in
Pa_{CO_2}, such as those associated with the
cycles of Cheyne-Strokes respirations, may
precipitate large increases in ICP.[109,110]
Therefore, it is important not to allow any
degree of airway obstruction or hypercarbia
to develop from any cause. Ventilation during general anesthesia should be controlled
even if a peripheral operation is being performed.[92]

These concepts become critical in cases
in which alternative forms of airway management are contemplated to facilitate other
surgery. For instance, operations on thoracic structures are often done more easily with
single-lung anesthesia, employing a double-lumen endotracheal tube. The delays in

ventilation that may accompany insertion and positioning of such tubes may have very adverse effects on cerebral hemodynamics.[104, 109] Therefore, the benefits to be gained from single-lung anesthesia in any particular situation must be very carefully weighed against the risks of increasing ICP. Clinicians skilled and experienced in the use of double lumen tubes may elect to use them, with careful prior hyperventilation. However, should difficulty be encountered in obtaining proper positioning, the technique should be abandoned. Whatever technique is employed, ventilation must be maintained throughout the case to provide a Pa_{CO_2} of approximately 30 torr. Thus, the need to provide a "quiet thoracic field" by reducing ventilation must be weighed against the heavy necessity of protecting the brain and the fact that associated head injury is one of the most common causes of mortality in patients with chest trauma.[111]

Positioning. Venous drainage of the head must not be impeded, or else increased cerebral blood volume, increased ICP, and cerebral edema may result.[96, 97, 105] The head injured patient should be positioned for *any* procedure with the head slightly elevated. This may call for a modification of standard practices in such operations as liver explorations or hip repairs and may prohibit entirely procedures such as percutaneous subclavian or internal jugular vein cannulation. In addition, to prevent kinking of the veins in the neck, the head should be maintained in a neutral position relative to all planes, without rotation or flexion in any direction.[105] This may require great care while turning the patient to the prone or lateral position. After the patient is positioned, the head should be inspected and any flexion or rotation corrected with appropriate support.

Changes in position may precipitate changes in cerebral dynamics, some of which may be unexpected. Magnaes[112] has demonstrated that a rapid change from supine to the sitting position is followed in subjects with intracranial pathology by two distinct events. First is a rapid fall in ICP, which is a pure hydrostatic effect. After 15 to 20 seconds, however, a reflex increase in systemic blood pressure occurs that may increase cerebral blood volume above baseline levels. This second event may result in a higher ICP than was present in the initial

supine position. The secondary reflex effect can be prevented by changing position slowly over a two to three minute period.

Choice of Anesthetic Agent and Technique. Anesthetic drugs must be selected for the head injured patient with due regard for their effects on intracranial dynamics. Ketamine increases intracranial pressure by both direct and indirect effects, and is contraindicated in patients with significant head injury.[92, 97, 102] Volatile anesthetic agents are potent cerebral vasodilators, and predictably increase ICP.[93, 97, 113] This action is moderated, but not abolished, by hyperventilation before the agent is introduced.[93, 102, 113] Most authors feel that halothane and enflurane may be hazardous to patients with disordered cerebral dynamics, and should be avoided when possible.[93, 102] If they are used at all, the patient must not be allowed to breathe spontaneously, and the Pa_{CO_2} should be reduced to 30 torr at least 10 minutes before the volatile agent is begun.[92, 113] The primary agents used for patients with elevated ICP are the intravenous narcotics and sedative-hypnotics, particularly barbiturates.[90, 92, 93, 97, 102-104] These pharmacologic requirements may raise competitive considerations for the anesthetist attempting to tailor an anesthetic to a patient with head trauma and, for instance, who also has hemorrhagic shock or severe pulmonary contusion. Often compromises must be made, but the head injury should be accorded as much consideration as possible, understanding that it is a bad bargain to save a kidney at the cost of a brain.

ICP Monitoring. Much of the previous theoretical and speculative discussion could be rendered moot if the physician simply knew what the ICP was at any given point in time. Techniques of ICP monitoring have advanced to the point where it can be considered almost routine for certain patients.[114] Certainly patients who are comatose and will require intensive therapy to control ICP need ICP monitoring. However, patients who do not appear to have very severe intracranial damage but who present with evidence of some impairment in neurologic status attributed to cerebral trauma, might also benefit from ICP monitoring if they must undergo an operation on another site. In these cases, ICP is considered to be another physiologic variable, similar to urine output or arterial pH, that can give valuable information on which to base sound clinical decision-making. It is the policy in our hospital to insert an ICP monitor (usually a fluid-filled ventricular catheter) in any patient with a preoperative neurologic deficit and evidence on computerized tomographic scanning of cerebral contusion or edema, if he is going to have an operation involving a body cavity or other procedure requiring position change or major physiologic trespass. Patients with significant neurologic deficits who require immediate operation for injuries that prohibit the completion of a neurodiagnostic evaluation will also be monitored. In these cases the ventriculostomy may be performed in the operating room while the other surgery is in progress.

HYPERTENSION FOLLOWING HEAD TRAUMA (CUSHING RESPONSE)

The classical "Cushing triad" of hypertension, bradycardia, and breathing disturbances (or apnea) rarely occurs as described.[94, 96, 115] However some degree of sympathetic activation is the rule in patients with increased intracranial pressure, although it may be inconspicuous enough to be unappreciated until surgical decompression of a "tight" head causes an abrupt decrease in arterial blood pressure.[94, 96, 116, 117] When Cushing described the "reflex," he stated that it was apparently an adaptive response which maintained cerebral perfusion pressure and prevented medullary ischemia. Hence, ". . . the rise is a conservative act and not . . . a mere reflex sensory irritation."[115] With a better appreciation of intracranial circulatory dynamics, however, has come the realization that the Cushing reflex is not necessarily adaptive and often becomes counterproductive.[130] The reflex itself is not a response to an elevated intracranial pressure (ICP), *per se*, but rather to a distortion or compression of the vasomotor centers in the medulla.[116] Hence, local trauma to the brainstem may cause hypertension while ICP is still normal; on the other hand, there may be marked swelling and local congestion in an area of the brain that does not impinge on the brainstem, and no hypertension will result. Therefore, the presence or absence of hypertension cannot be used as a guide to

the severity or extent of intracranial damage.[116]

In addition, in the presence of an elevated ICP and brain ischemia, the rise in systemic blood pressure is not usually as great as the rise in ICP, so that the cerebral perfusion pressure (CPP, defined as the mean systemic arterial pressure minus the ICP or the CVP, whichever is greater) usually falls, despite major increases in systemic arterial pressure (SAP). This has led Miller and Sullivan to refer to the Cushing reflex as a "cry of distress rather than a means of rescue. . . ."[96]

The increased SAP may also cause secondary problems in both the brain and the systemic circulation. In normal brain, increased SAP does not cause an increase in cerebral blood volume because cerebral vasoconstriction takes place to maintain flow and volume constant.[92, 95] However, in sick or damaged brain this ability to autoregulate flow is lost, and cerebral blood volume will vary passively with SAP.[99, 130] In a "tight" brain, an increase in SAP may then lead to an increase in cerebral blood volume, an increase in intracranial pressure (ICP), a decrease in CPP, and, thus, in an apparent paradox, a decrease in cerebral blood flow.[96, 99, 118, 130]

In the systemic circulation, catecholamine levels rise many-fold and sympathetic tone is greatly increased during the Cushing response.[96, 116, 117] This has been reported to lead to such consequences as subendocardial necrosis and congestive heart failure.[117, 119] Pulmonary edema following head trauma has been recognized as a clinical problem for many years, and many possible etiologies have been proposed.[117, 119, 120] The most commonly accepted theory today is that the increased sympathetic tone seen with head injury causes increased cardiac work with pulmonary vascular congestion, and, if severe enough, cardiac failure with cardiogenic pulmonary edema.[117, 119]

It becomes important, then, to control the Cushing reflex when it is encountered. Therapeutic efforts should be directed at the primary pathology, which is in the brain, rather than the systemic response. A patient who presents with hypertension and high ICP, or who develops progressive hypertension with signs of rising ICP, should have the ICP reduced as quickly as possible.[96, 107]

There are many good articles in the recent literature dealing with the acute control of ICP.[92, 94, 96, 97, 105, 107, 108] Basically, they revolve around two approaches: 1) Remove water from the brain tissue by the use of osmotic agents (mannitol, 0.5-1.0 gm/kg body weight over 15 minutes), loop diuretics (furosemide), or corticosteroids (dexamethasone 0.5-1.5 mg/kg); 2) reduce intracranial blood volume. This latter approach involves not only promoting cerebral vasoconstriction actively (hyperventilation to a Pa_{CO_2} of 25-30 torr, administration of barbiturates)[105] but also avoiding the use of drugs or techniques that may promote cerebral vasodilatation or otherwise increase intracranial blood volume, as discussed in the previous section. Increased airway pressure in a patient with head trauma can increase ICP, probably by retarding cerebral venous drainage.[124] Positive airway pressure used therapeutically must have specific, clear indications, and the patient must be monitored carefully for signs of rising ICP.[124-126]

If at any time it is felt to be imperative to control the systemic hypertension directly, and attempts to control ICP are unsuccessful, it appears that agents which act to reduce sympathetic tone would be more useful than direct-acting vasodilators. The latter, particularly sodium nitroprusside and nitroglycerine, act as cerebral vasodilators and tend to increase the ICP, especially if SAP is not promptly reduced.[121, 122] On the other hand, agents that reduce sympathetic tone (such as narcotics and sedatives), sympathetic transmission (trimethaphan), or receptor activity (phenothiazines/butyrophenones, alpha-receptor blockers) tend to cause less cerebral vasodilatation and produce a lower ICP.[92, 95, 97]

Whatever agent is chosen to control hypertension, it should be realized that the net effects on cerebral perfusion pressure and cerebral blood flow may be unpredictable, and depend on many factors including rate of administration, intracranial pathology, rate of fall of arterial pressure, whether or not the cerebral vessels retain any ability to autoregulate, among others.[123] For this reason, it is recommended that intracranial pressure be monitored directly in such situations, and SAP and ICP both be regulated to provide a CPP of about 40 to 50 torr.

BASAL SKULL FRACTURES

Fractures through the base of the skull may be identified radiographically or they may be suspected clinically in a patient who demonstrates bleeding or drainage of CSF from the nose or ears. These fractures imply specific considerations in the airway care of these patients. Passage of both nasogastric tubes and nasoendotracheal tubes into the cranial vault via basal skull fractures has been reported.[127] Also, a communication between the subarachnoid space and the nasal cavity predisposes to cerebritis and meningitis,[128] and it is possible that the presence of a nasotracheal tube, which may be associated with a predispositon toward the development of sinusitis and nasal infection,[129] might increase the possibility of infection of the CSF. For these reasons, orotracheal intubation might be given first consideration for acute airway management in patients with demonstrated or suspected basal skull fractures, and either orotracheal intubation or tracheostomy used for long-term airway protection.

SPINAL CORD TRAUMA

The incidence of significant spinal cord injury is approximately 30 per 1,000,000 population per year in the United States; about half are due to motor vehicle accidents and another 20 per cent are due to sports (including diving) accidents.[131] Victims who survive initially with significant loss of spinal cord function can be expected to spend the next five or six months in the hospital.[132]

Indications for early operation on the injury itself are still poorly defined. At the present time early decompression appears to be indicated only for incomplete lesions (some function remains below the level of injury), whereas early fusion and stabilization are gaining popularity for complete lesions, to permit earlier mobilization and rehabilitation.[133-135] Even if an operation is not performed on the injury, it is likely that spinal cord-injured patients will come to the operating room at some point in their hospital stay, either for associated injuries or for chronic complications such as pressure sores, spasticity, or urinary tract dysfunction.

The cord-injured patient actually presents a spectrum of pathologic changes, depending on the level of injury and the time since injury. For convenience, the injuries can be grouped according to low (below T6 motor level) versus high (above T5 motor level), and acute (up to several weeks) versus chronic.

LOW ACUTE INJURIES

Paradoxically, low cord injuries present more often in combination with associated injuries to the head and chest than do high (cervical) cord injuries.[131] Therefore, the patient with acute low cord injury is more likely to undergo surgery within 24 hours of injury. In general, anesthetic problems are relatively minor at this time, and are primarily related to positioning and preventing progression of the neurologic deficit. Circulatory disturbances are mild and usually respond promptly to moderate volume loading.[133, 136, 137] Volatile or intravenous anesthetic drugs may be used, and there should be no problem with ventilation, airway, or abnormal reflexes. Succinylcholine may be used within the first 24 to 48 hours after injury but probably not thereafter (see section on chronic cord injuries).[85] Prevention of secondary cord damage is important in the patient with an incomplete lesion, especially if he or she will be positioned prone on the operating table. An awake nasal or orotracheal intubation and positioning of such patients is often advantageous because it allows observation of neurologic function and avoids iatrogenic injury.

Depending on the level of injury and the planned operation, the surgeons may wish to awaken the patient after cord decompression and/or spinal fusion to test function. This possibility should be discussed beforehand and the anesthetic planned accordingly.[138]

Intraoperative problems may include accidental surgical entry into viscera or great vessels, especially when operating on the thoracic spine. Pneumothorax and accidental incision of the lungs, heart, and great vessels have been reported.[139]

HIGH ACUTE INJURIES

Lesions higher than T5 present entirely different problems to the anesthesiologist, and the higher the lesion the greater the difficulties. The anesthetic problems may be generalized into three groups: airway control, autonomic dysfunction, and motor dysfunction.

Airway Control. Endotracheal intubation is often imperative for such patients, but it must be accomplished in a way that will not increase the patient's risk of permanent neurologic sequelae. When the bony lesion has already been defined, the anesthesiologist and surgeon should discuss the plan for intubation, and should define in advance which maneuvers of the head and neck may be permitted and which are contraindicated. When the patient is in an external fixation device such as traction or a collar, the device *must not be removed or altered* without specific discussion with the surgeon. When intubation of any patient with known or potential high spinal injury must be done before the diagnosis is established, the anesthesiologist must presume the worst case exists and proceed accordingly. In general, *never flex*, either anteriorly or laterally, the neck of any neck-injured patient. Very slight extension is permitted and may be accomplished by gently placing a small roll under the back of the neck.[133] When it is necessary to lift the patient's head, the shoulders should also be lifted simultaneously in order to maintain the original degree of neck extension. The best protection for the cord is about 10 pounds of axial traction applied by means of a head harness or, preferably, tongs.[133] When the need for intubation is urgent and a traction device is not in place, an assistant may apply traction by standing at either the head or the side (depending on where the operator prefers to stand), grasping the patient's occiput and forehead, maintaining a neutral position or slight extension, and pulling gently but firmly in a straight line along the spinal axis. This assistant should have no other responsibilities, and should not release the traction until some alternative form of stabilization is provided.

Various techniques for endotracheal intubation have been described in such circumstances, the most popular being awake nasotracheal; less commonly, orotracheal intubation is used.[137, 140, 141] Techniques that can be used to expedite intubation and render it less traumatic to the awake patient include topical anesthesia of the nose and throat, blocks of the superior laryngeal and glossopharyngeal nerves, use of an exploring "guide" or retrograde catheter, and use of the fiberoptic bronchoscope or laryngoscope.[140, 142-145] Sedation and amnesia can be provided by a variety of drugs, including narcotics, diazepam, droperidol, and ketamine, singly or in combination.[143-146]

Selection of anesthetic technique should be based on an assessment of the overall condition of the patient. If the patient has a full stomach, heavy sedation or extensive local or topical anesthesia may not be advisable, as these may obtund airway reflexes and predispose to aspiration.[147] Children or combative patients may require induction of general anesthesia, but if this is necessary, it is absolutely essential to maintain axial traction, as the relaxation of the neck muscles that may accompany loss of consciousness may permit displacement of previously aligned injuries with subsequent loss of function.[133] The primary reason for advocating awake intubation in these patients is to provide maximum safety, and the technique should not be pursued to a point that this extra margin of safety is lost. In extreme emergencies such as apnea or upper airway obstruction the airway must, of course, be managed by whatever means are possible, and the risk of neurologic damage becomes a secondary consideration.

Autonomic Dysfunction. An acute high spinal cord lesion abruptly disconnects the central (medullary) autoregulatory mechanisms from the great bulk of capacitance and resistance vessels that ordinarily regulate pressure and flow in the body. In the acute stage of "spinal shock" that is present immediately after a high cord injury, meaning that the spinal cord below the lesion is quiescent and areflexic, the peripheral vascular bed is flaccid, and blood volume shifts passively in response to external forces such as gravity.[133, 137, 141, 148, 149] If the lesion is above T1 to T5, the sympathetic nervous system efferents to the heart are also lost, and bradycardia is common.[148] Under these circumstances the patient cannot respond to blood loss and may require vigorous fluid

resuscitation. If positive pressure ventilation is necessary, the venoconstriction that normally compensates for increased intrathoracic pressure will also be lost and the symptomatology of any volume deficit will be accentuated.[141]

This phase of autonomic dysfunction is brief, and recovery usually begins in the first 24 hours, although complete recovery may take several weeks.[149] The touchstone of recovery from spinal shock is the return of the bulbocavernous reflex; evidence of this reflex should be sought before the induction of anesthesia in the first few weeks following injury, as it gives valuable information about the state of neurogenic vascular control.[149]

Pulmonary edema in the first few days following high cord injury has been commonly reported.[141, 149, 150] In patients without aspiration, chest trauma, asphyxiation, or other obvious precipitating factors the occurrence of pulmonary edema may be due to persistence in vigorous fluid administration despite returning peripheral vascular tone, with resulting fluid overload.[141, 149] This can be avoided by recognizing the changes in the circulation that occur over time after cord injury and measuring cardiac filling pressures where appropriate.[150]

Because of the lack of cutaneous vasoconstriction or sweating, patients with high cord injuries become poikilothermic, and require careful attention to temperature regulation.[136, 137, 141]

Motor Dysfunction. The minute volume of ventilation is usually adequate with use of the diaphragm alone. However, loss of the intercostal muscles deprives the patient of two important protective mechanisms. First, loss of intercostal muscle activity may greatly diminish the ability to increase ventilatory effort to compensate for decreasing lung compliance or increasing airway resistance. Second, loss of intercostal muscle activity eliminates the ability to generate an effective cough, since this is dependent on the ability to contract the chest and abdominal wall muscles.[141] Therefore, these patients often get into a vicious downhill spiral of retained secretions, atelectasis, and decreasing vital capacity, terminating in frank respiratory failure despite initially adequate alveolar ventilation. Patients with high cord lesions should be placed as soon as possible on a regimen of pulmonary therapy designed to clear secretions and maintain compliance and lung volume. Special techniques such as artificial coughing and glossopharyngeal breathing, and equipment such as rotating beds, are very valuable adjuncts in this therapy, and their availability and skilled use constitute one of the prime reasons for regionalization of the care of high cord injuries.[132]

Injuries at the C4 level may produce some loss of diaphragmatic function, but ventilation will usually be adequate. Injuries above C4 usually require at least temporary institution of mechanical ventilatory support.[137, 141] Vital capacity will be further decreased with injuries at any level by virtually any other coexisting thoracic or abdominal pathology.

Anesthesia should be designed to interfere to the least possible degree with the patient's borderline respiratory reserves. Since the patient is insensitive and flaccid below the injury, minimal anesthesia and relaxation are required for operations below the highest involved dermatome.[137, 149] Operations on the thoracic spine pose the greatest problems, since these patients must be deeply anesthetized for an operation on sensitive structures, and they must be either turned prone for a posterior operation or have the chest opened for an anterior approach.[139] In such cases a marginal patient may totally decompensate unless the greatest care is taken to ensure complete termination of the effects of muscle relaxants and anesthetics, and a careful evaluation of respiratory mechanics is made prior to extubation. After extubation, the patient should be observed carefully and continuously for signs of decreasing lung volume or decreasing compliance (increasing respiratory rate, falling arterial PO_2) and respiratory support reinstituted promptly as indicated.

CHRONIC INJURIES

Since the problems related to both low and high chronic injuries are similar, they will be discussed together, with important differences pointed out where appropriate.

As discussed previously, the phase of areflexic "spinal shock" persists for a variable length of time but is usually resolved within several weeks of injury.[149] As the cord begins to function again, it regains the ability to transmit and coordinate reflex activity, but with complete lesions it is still disconnected from higher control centers. Problems that result from uninhibited reflex activity below the level of the lesion include the mass reflex and autonomic dysreflexia. The mass reflex is found in both high and low lesions (as long as the injury is a true upper motor neuron lesion involving the cord above T10) and the other, autonomic dysreflexia, is characteristic of lesions above T5.[137, 141, 149, 151, 152]

Autonomic Dysreflexia. This syndrome is sometimes discussed in conjunction with the mass reflex,[136] but they are actually quite different entities. Autonomic responsiveness is regained quickly after a complete cord lesion, usually within the first week, although the syndrome of autonomic dysreflexia may first present many months after injury.[152] Autonomic dysreflexia is usually triggered by a visceral stimulus, particularly bladder or rectal distention, and is a common problem in urinary tract manipulation or cystoscopy. Triggering by a somatic stimulus can also occur but is much less common.[152] The mechanism of the reflex appears to be stimulation of visceral autonomic fibers, which normally trigger vasoconstrictor impulses from the thoracolumbar sympathetic fibers.[152, 153] The blood pressure rise that accompanies the resulting rise in systemic resistance and venous return is sensed by the carotid and aortic arch baroreceptors, which act to inhibit the medullary cardioaccelerator center and stimulate the vagus nerve. This inhibition of sympathetic tone is passed via an intact cord down to the active segments, and the entire reflex damps itself out. With an interrupted cord the entire reflex takes place, except that the inhibitory signals are not passed below the lesion and the vasoconstrictor reflex continues unabated.[152, 153] The attack usually occurs abruptly and is characterized by severe hypertension, pounding vascular headache, flushing above the lesion and blanching below it, and sweating and piloerection in the upper body, and can lead to cerebrovascular hemorrhage and death if not controlled.[153] The effects on the heart are variable, depending on how many of the upper thoracic cardioaccelerator fibers remain under central control. With lesions in the T1-T5 area, bradycardia usually results from the increased vagal tone and depressed sympathetic tone in the upper thoracic segments.[152,153] With higher cervical lesions, however, tachycardia may occur if the upper thoracic segments become involved in the uninhibited sympathetic surge, and the resulting increase in cardiac sympathetic tone outweighs the effects of the increased vagal tone.[152]

The patient who is prone to attacks of autonomic dysreflexia is very aware of the syndrome, and this information should be elicited during the preoperative interview.[152] These patients may be receiving antihypertensive drugs or sympatholytics in an attempt to control the attacks, and this may cause drug interactions during the course of an anesthetic.[152] Patients who suffer from attacks of autonomic dysreflexia should probably receive anesthesia for operations on pelvic or abdominal viscera, although these patients may not require anesthesia for peripheral plastic or orthopedic procedures.[154] If general anesthesia is used, it must be made fairly deep, since light general anesthesia with thiopental and nitrous oxide will not reliably block the syndrome. Moderately deep halothane anesthesia will prevent or abort attacks of autonomic dysreflexia, but with a significant incidence of cardiac arrythmias.[155] As Naftchi et al. point out, autonomic dysreflexia is unique in that peripheral sympathetic and vagal tone may be simultaneously increased, and the effects on cardiac rhythm can be bizarre.[153] The rhythm disturbances with halothane anesthesia are usually easily managed (i.e., with lidocaine),[155] although enflurane and isoflurane remain as theoretically sound choices because of their lesser tendency to cause dysrhythmias.

Conduction anesthesia is probably the most reliable technique for preventing autonomic dysreflexia triggered from the pelvic viscera.[152, 156] Topical anesthesia of the bladder may be sufficient for cystoscopy, and a subarachnoid or epidural block may be done for more extensive work.[156] Such blocks can be technically difficult if the spine is deformed,[136] but they appear to be quite safe and are gaining in popularity.[155, 156] Certainly there should be no fear of "exacerbating" neurologic damage in a patient with a complete spinal cord lesion.

If an attack of autonomic dysreflexia occurs, it should be treated quickly to prevent cerebral complications. First remove any precipitating stimulus. Stop surgery and ensure that the bladder and rectum are emptied. Thus, even if the patient is not undergoing urinary tract surgery, check to be sure that the urinary catheter is patent, since a blocked or dislodged catheter may result in an attack of autonomic dysreflexia due to a distended bladder, independent of other stimuli.[152]

If general anesthesia is being used, deepen the level of anesthesia if possible. If a volatile inhalation agent is not being used, it may be helpful to introduce one. Rapidly acting intravenous drugs that act peripherally to reduce sympathetic tone are useful. Ganglion blockers, alpha-receptor blockers, and direct-acting vasodilators have all been used successfully.[152, 154, 155] The patient can lose as much as 10 to 15 per cent of his plasma volume during an attack of autonomic dysreflexia, owing to increased capillary filtration, so acute volume loading may be necessary.[153] This will, of course, lead to an increase in total extracellular fluid that may require diuresis at a later time. Because of these complex renal-cardiovascular interactions, invasive monitoring might be considered for patients with a history of autonomic dysreflexia who require general anesthesia.[150]

Mass Motor Reflexes. A phenomenon similar to autonomic dysreflexia involves spinal cord motor neurons in both low and high injuries. A minor sensory input may cause an uninhibited contraction of an entire protagonist muscle group, leading to severe muscle spasms.[149] Flexor spasms are more common and appear earlier than extensor spasms; flexor spasms often occur by the third month after injury.[149] The incidence of mass reflex phenomena rises steadily until about a year after injury, then levels off.[149] The mechanism is usually related to a somatic sensory input, particularly from a muscle stretch (spindle) receptor, which would normally cause reflex contraction of a single muscle unit. Because of the absence of central inhibitory tone, the reflex generalizes to an entire muscle group. For example, straightening a patient's knee would cause a reflex spasm of all of the flexors at the hip, thigh, calf, and foot.[149] The spasms are intensely painful and may be forceful enough to hurl the patient from the bed. While the spasms are usually triggered by somatic inputs from the skin and muscles, they may also be triggered or exacerbated by visceral stimuli, and the patient suffering from mass reflexes should be evaluated for bladder distention, urinary tract infection, or fecal impaction.[149]

The patient manifesting mass reflexes should be handled gently, with minimal manipulation of the limbs and position changes. The spasms are very difficult to control pharmacologically, and often constitute an indication for cordotomy or other neurolytic procedures. Complete general anesthesia or a good regional block will prevent the reflex, but sedation with drugs such as diazepam often will not.[137, 141, 149]

Succinylcholine and Spinal Cord Trauma. The ability of depolarizing neuromuscular blockers to release large amounts of potassium from chronically denervated muscle tissue is well known. The time limits for this effect are still poorly defined, but it has been reported as early as four days after complete spinal cord transection, and persists for many months.[85] Pretreatment with a small dose of a non-depolarizing blocker (3 mg *d*-tubocurarine or 1 mg pancuronium bromide) has been reported to reduce the incidence and severity of succinylcholine-induced muscle fasciculations, but in most studies the fasciculations were not completely abolished in all cases.[157-162] Also, it appears that potassium release can occur even without visible fasciculations.[162] Increasing the dose of non-depolarizing relaxant (e.g., 6 mg *d*-tubocurarine or 1.5 mg pancuronium) and using a small dose of succinylcholine (1 mg/kg) will further reduce the incidence of fasciculations,[161] but the neuromuscular blocking effects of the succinylcholine may then be so altered that it becomes unpredictable and often unsatisfactory.[157, 159, 162]

The safest recommendation would appear to be that succinylcholine may be used (with or without pretreatment) in the first 24 to 48 hours after injury but not thereafter, even with pretreatment. If a neuromuscular blocker must be used for endotracheal intubation, pancuronium is recommended.

Other Chronic Complications. Disuse atrophy and osteoporosis make the bones of the spinal-cord injured patient extremely fragile, and great care must be taken to avoid fracturing bones during position changes.[149, 151] Most patients are liable to pressure sores, and will have several areas of their skin in various states of necrosis, healing, or grafting. These areas should be identified preoperatively and protected from pressure during surgery. Chronic urinary tract infections are common and may lead to stone formation, chronic renal insufficiency, or even renal amyloidosis.[137, 149, 151] Thus, the adequacy of renal function should be defined preoperatively.

MAXILLOFACIAL TRAUMA

Although a large proportion of the morbidity associated with face and neck trauma is cosmetic rather than life-threatening, Hoehn has pointed out that maxillofacial trauma can occasionally be lethal or crippling if the true extent of injury is not appreciated.[163] The anesthesiologist must be alert to the potential for catastrophe, even if most cases of facial injury turn out to be routine.

AIRWAY PROBLEMS

Primary tracheostomy without prior endotracheal intubation is only very rarely necessary in the management of facial trauma and should be avoided whenever possible.[163, 164] Other than high-velocity missile wounds, few injuries cause such rapid and extensive edema or hematoma formation that peroral endoscopy and intubation are impossible.[164] Various techniques of endotracheal intubation have been used successfully with facial trauma, and each has its advantages and drawbacks.[147, 163, 164]

Blind Techniques. Blind nasotracheal intubation may seem attractive because of its speed, relative safety under most conditions, and relative patient comfort. However, blind intubation of a patient who has suffered facial trauma is often unwise, as various foreign bodies (bone, teeth) or considerable amounts of blood may be in the pharynx and may be introduced into the trachea during insertion of the tube.[163] In addition, if there is any anatomic disruption of the airway the damage may be compounded by blind intubation. Therefore direct layngoscopy and visual inspection of the airway are indicated during endotracheal intubation of the patient with maxillofacial or neck trauma.

"Asleep" Techniques. The patient who has experienced bleeding into the mouth will probably have a stomach full of swallowed blood as well as food; if bleeding has continued, blood will be in the pharynx also.[163, 164, 165] The traumatized airway might be held open only by voluntary muscle tone and may collapse on induction of general anesthesia. For these reasons an induction technique involving spontaneous inhalation of a volatile anesthetic could be hazardous. The alternative, a rapid intravenous induction with neuromuscular blockade, could be even more hazardous if the degree of airway damage has been underestimated and intubation is technically difficult.[147, 163] Nevertheless, both of these techniques have their places in special circumstances; for instance, in dealing with the child (inhalation induction), or when speed is essential because of other injuries (rapid intravenous induction). Whenever intubation under general anesthesia is contemplated, the airway should be evaluated beforehand in as much detail as is possible under the circumstances, including radiographs specifically obtained to reveal soft-tissue structures in the neck. Alternative forms of airway control must be immediately available in the induction area, including skilled surgeons with all of the equipment necessary for tracheostomy.[147]

"Awake" Techniques. Intubation of the trachea under direct visual control with the patient awake is the preferred method of airway control in the majority of patients with significant maxillofacial disruption.[147, 163] This may include nasotracheal intubation over a fiberoptic flexible bronchoscope, or orotracheal intubation with conventional direct laryngoscopy, or any other similar technique. Despite some objections to the use of topical or local anesthesia of the throat for intubation based on concern over the risk of aspiration through an incompetent larynx,[147] it seems reasonable from other points of view (cardiovascular reflexes, patient comfort, continuous awake neurologic assessment) to anesthetize the pharynx and larynx if possible. As long as the trachea is left sensitive the patient's ability to cough out a foreign body should not be greatly impaired.[142]

The choice of nasal versus oral intubation

should be made by the surgeon and anesthesiologist in consultation. When the jaw is to be wired together an oral tube may be inserted first but must be changed to either a nasal tube or tracheostomy.[163, 164] If the nasopharynx is not disrupted a nasotracheal tube will ordinarily be preferred. However, if the nose or nasopharynx is grossly disrupted, this may not be possible or desirable.[147] Also about 25 per cent of patients with maxillary fractures will demonstrate a cerebrospinal fluid leak,[164] and then the principles discussed in the previous section on basal skull fractures should be applied.

INTRAOPERATIVE PROBLEMS

The anesthesiologist must be alert for possible surgical interference with the airway, and should report any changes in apparent airway resistance or adequacy of ventilation to the surgeons.[166] The cuff on the endotracheal tube must remain inflated at all times, even if the patient is breathing spontaneously, to prevent aspiration of blood. During operations on or near the orbits, including the maxilla, reflex bradycardia resembling the oculocardiac reflex may occur.[167]

EYE INJURIES

Control of the intraocular pressure (IOP) is as crucial to the ophthalmologic surgeon as is control of intracranial pressure to the neurosurgeon. Many of the same hemodynamic and biochemical factors that influence intracranial pressure also affect IOP, but in general to a lesser degree.[168] The major avoidable source of increased IOP is external pressure applied to the surface of the globe, which may cause rapid extrusion of ocular contents if the globe is open, with subsequent loss of function. Since succinylcholine causes tetanic contraction of the extraocular muscles that cannot be reliably blocked by pretreatment with non-depolarizing muscle relaxants, its use is contraindicated in situations in which the globe is penetrated.[168-172] Almost all commonly used anesthetic drugs, with the possible exception of ketamine, lower IOP and are safe to use.[168-170]

Intraocular pressure is also increased by

arterial hypertension in a manner analogous to blood pressure effects on intracranial pressure.[168, 173] This may be particularly troublesome when the trachea is intubated under light general anesthesia or with the use of ketamine.[168, 170, 173]

Coughing also can cause undesirable increases in IOP, and great care should be taken to prevent unnecessary bucking or coughing during the course of eye surgery, especially while the globe is open.[168] The presence of an open globe injury constitutes a relative indication for a rapid intravenous induction of anesthesia prior to endotracheal intubation, using pancuronium as the muscle relaxant. Extubation and emergence is a relatively difficult period, as the requirement for awake extubation for airway protection in a patient with a full stomach may conflict with the desire to prevent coughing by using deep extubation or heavy sedation. With modern techniques of eye repair the actual danger of a cough causing disruption of the suture line is small, and therefore coughing may be permitted on emergence if it appears to be desirable for the patient's overall well-being.[168]

TRAUMA TO MAJOR AIRWAYS

Fracture of the larynx from any cause is a rare injury. In one recent review, 26 cases were accumulated over six years.[174] In another review, 49 cases were recorded in a 15 year period.[175]

The diagnosis of fracture of the larynx is often missed. Signs are nonspecific, and are often overlooked in a seriously injured patient.[174-177] This is particularly true when a patient is intubated or subjected to a tracheostomy for other indications; the anesthesiologist must share responsibility for examining the upper airway of any patient he intubates for any reason if there is a history of trauma to the neck, either at the time of intubation or later.[177] Signs and symptoms that should direct attention to the larynx include upper airway obstruction, cough, dyspnea, dysphagia, pain (often referred to the ear), a change in the quality of the voice, hemoptysis, subcutaneous emphysema, or palpable disruption of the cartilages. If the injury is not discovered early, the incidence of late scarring with loss of function is high.[174]

Disruption of a major intrathoracic airway is an uncommon feature of blunt chest trauma. A Danish study of 1178 fatal traffic accidents revealed 33 tracheobronchial ruptures. Another study reported 30 cases in a 10 year study period.[178, 179] Overall mortality approaches 30 per cent, half dying in the first hour after injury. Of those who reach the hospital alive, 10 per cent die. As many as half of the patients may have no other major injury. Only one third have fractured ribs identified. Ten per cent have no initial symptoms of airway trauma.[178-184]

The mechanism of injury to intrathoracic airways is obscure; one popular theory invokes a sudden increase in intrathoracic pressure when the patient is at high lung volume with a closed glottis, causing a "blow-out" in a vulnerable part of the airway. The precise set of conditions required to produce the lesion may account for its scarcity.[178, 179]

The great majority of lesions are within 2.5 cm of the carina and may be circumferential (complete or incomplete) or longitudinal.[178] If the latter, they are in the posterior membranous portion, and may be extensive, involving a considerable segment of the trachea and extending into either main bronchus. Bilateral or more distal lesions are extremely rare.[178, 183]

Clinical features that suggest intrathoracic airway disruption include cough, hemoptysis, dyspnea out of proportion to other clinical findings, a pneumothorax that does not promptly resolve with tube thoracostomy, and subcutaneous or mediastinal emphysema. Radiographic examinations are time-consuming and usually unrewarding.[177-179, 183]

Principles of management of laryngeal and tracheobronchial trauma are similar. Once suspicion is raised by any of the above features, the diagnosis must be made by endoscopy as soon as possible.[174-185] If the larynx is disrupted, tracheostomy may be necessary to secure the airway before examination. Although endotracheal intubation is generally desirable and will usually be possible, it should be attempted with great caution, and every preparation should be made for alternative forms of airway control. Ill-considered or hasty attempts at laryngoscopy and intubation are to be discouraged, as they may compound the problem and cause irreversible damage.[175-177]

If the lower airway is involved, bronchoscopy is both diagnostic and therapeutic.[178, 179, 183, 184] Rigid bronchoscopy is usually preferred, since if a major airway is ruptured, the bronchoscope may be advanced past the lesion to provide ventilation on the way to the operating room.[178, 183] If a mainstem bronchus is involved, the opposite lung may be cannulated.[178, 179] Fiberoptic flexible bronchoscopes may also be used for diagnosis, and have the advantage of being more easily tolerated by the awake patient. However, they cannot by themselves provide a patent airway, and care must be taken to have some means of airway support available. They are quite valuable to assist in placement of an endotracheal tube in selected patients.

Endoscopy can usually be accomplished with local or topical anesthesia in the cooperative patient. Some authors caution against using topical anesthesia if the patient has a full stomach,[147, 164] but if anesthesia is limited to the pharynx and larynx, tracheal reflexes will be preserved and the risk of uncontrolled aspiration should be minor.[142] In some situations, particularly with children, it may be necessary to induce general anesthesia before endoscopy. In this situation, the approach should be similar to that with other airway lesions such as epiglottitis or airway foreign body; anesthesia may be induced with halothane in oxygen with the patient in the position of comfort.[164, 176, 177, 185] Spontaneous ventilation should be maintained. A skilled surgical team with all the equipment necessary for rapid tracheostomy should be present. If an intrathoracic lesion is suspected, thoracic surgeons should also be available. Above all, it must be recognized that induction of general anesthesia may result in the loss of a marginal airway. Thus, an awake intubation (or tracheostomy) should always be considered if there is any doubt concerning the potential adequacy of the airway after induction of anesthesia.[177]

Once the lesion has been identified and evaluated, airway control must be individualized for each situation. In cases of laryngeal or cervical tracheal injury, tracheostomy may be indicated.[175, 177] The endoscope may be left in place while the stoma is being created. In cases of intrathoracic injury, the endoscope may suffice for maintenance of anesthesia, particularly where the lesion makes attempts at rein-tubation hazardous.[178, 179, 183] Where circumstances permit, however, the patient may be reintubated with a double-lumen endobronchial tube or a standard cuffed tube advanced past the lesion or even into the opposite lung. Each approach has its advocates, and the ultimate choice of airway should be made by consensus between the surgeon and anesthetist.[177-179, 181, 185]

When the chest is opened, it may become necessary for the surgeons to reintubate the trachea or one or both bronchi. Sterile tubes and appropriate adaptors and connectors should be provided on the field.[178]

CHEST TRAUMA

Direct trauma to the thoracic viscera or great vessels is highly lethal, but if the patient survives to reach the hospital, most such injuries are reparable.[186-190] In-hospital mortality of all patients with chest trauma is closely related to the presence of other injuries, particularly to the head or abdomen.[111, 186-188, 190] With the exception of direct cardiac wounds, shock in a patient with thoracic trauma is more commonly due to associated abdominal injuries.[111, 188, 190] The majority of thoracic injuries seen in the hospital do not require thoracotomy but can be managed with tube thoracostomy and appropriate respiratory support.[188, 190-193] However, injuries to the heart and great thoracic vessels tend to be unstable, and the momentary compensation that allows survival to the hospital may break down abruptly and lead to death unless appropriate and expeditious action is taken.

BLUNT CARDIAC TRAUMA

Contusion. The most common form of blunt heart trauma is myocardial contusion, but it is a diagnosis that is often missed.[186, 190, 195] A mild contusion may have no symptoms or signs, and the characteristic electrocardiographic findings may not appear for up to 48 hours.[195] These findings are similar to those with myocardial infarction or ischemia, with ST-segment elevation over the involved area. Contusions by themselves are rarely of concern, and resolve over a two to six week period.[186, 195] The most common clinical problem is a tendency to rhythm disturbances. Complete heart block is possibly the most common rhythm found immediately after contusion, but it is unstable and rarely lasts longer than 10 minutes.[195, 196] It then either reverts spontaneously to normal sinus rhythm or degenerates into ventricular fibrillation leading to death.[196] The injured area remains irritable, however, until healing occurs. This natural history strongly suggests that the electrocardiogram of a patient who has sustained blunt chest trauma within the previous six weeks should be examined for evidence of myocardial contusion before he is given anesthesia. A high index of suspicion is needed, as the signs may be subtle.[195] A history of rhythm disturbances while in the hospital, or evidence of evolving injury on the electrocardiogram, should suggest contusion. In these cases the anesthetic should be designed to minimize myocardial irritability, and if inhalation anesthesia is indicated enflurane might be preferred over halothane.

Extensive myocardial contusion or contusion superimposed on pre-existing disease may result in cardiac pump failure and require inotropic support, although this is almost never a cause of death.[186, 195] Significant heart failure from contusion is uncommon, however, so such a diagnosis must be supported by direct determination of myocardial function using a Swan-Ganz catheter or other sophisticated tests. Because of the myocardial irritability, an inotrope with reasonably low potential to produce dysrhythmias is indicated, and at the present dobutamine appears to be the best choice.[195, 197]

Myocardial Rupture. Blunt rupture of the heart is lethal, and rupture of a ventricle is a common postmortem finding in motor vehicle accident victims.[186, 198] Rupture of an atrium is more survivable, and can present as either exsanguination if the pericardium is also torn, or, more commonly, tamponade when the pericardium is intact.[186, 195] Exsanguination has been discussed in a previous section.

Pericardial tamponade must be suspected in any case of chest trauma in which evidence of low cardiac output persists despite high central filling pressures. The classical "Beck's triad" of low blood pressure, jugular venous distention, and muffled heart sounds may be present in less than half of such patients.[199, 200] The presence of pericardial blood may be identified by pericardiocentesis or echocardiography, but the diagnosis of tamponade is a hemodynamic one and is confirmed by a fall in right atrial pressure of at least 10 torr upon removal of pericardial fluid.[201]

Atrial rupture with tamponade is a true surgical emergency. The effects of pericardiocentesis will usually be transitory, and it should be viewed strictly as a temporizing measure while on the way to the operating room.[186, 198] Tamponade with cardiovascular collapse is an absolute indication for open-chest cardiac massage, and the chest of a person with chest trauma and absent pulses should be opened at once in the emergency room.[198, 202] Patients who are able to generate some spontaneous circulation may be transported to the operating room. The patient who is awake and breathing spontaneously in the emergency room may collapse suddenly and requires constant attendance in transit. If the patient is still awake upon arrival in the operating room, the surgeon may elect to drain the pericardium before induction of anesthesia. A subxiphoid pericardial window is more effective in this regard than needle pericardiocentesis, and should be done with only local anesthesia.[198, 200, 203] Such drainage may precipitate exsanguinating hemorrhage in the presence of myocardial rupture, however, and may be deferred in favor of a more definitive thoracotomy or sternotomy. The anesthesiologist is then faced with the responsibility of preparing the patient for thoracotomy while preventing hemodynamic decompensation. Cardiac arrest on induction of general anesthesia has been a common complication with such patients.[200, 203]

Pharmacologic considerations in pericardial tamponade have been reviewed recently by Fowler.[204, 205] Maintenance of the circulation in these patients is critically dependent upon the triad of tachycardia, high filling pressures (to allow diastolic ventricular filling against the pericardial restriction), and high ejection fraction (to allow generation of a stroke volume from a low end-diastolic volume). Interference with any one of these compensatory mechanisms will result in deterioration. The best first choice for support of the circulation is volume loading to high filling pressures, and the possibility of pulmonary edema must be accepted. This may be followed by the use of beta-agonist agents such as iso-proterenol, which will keep heart rate and contractility high. Systemic arterial dilators such as hydralazine or nitroprusside may also be used to decrease afterload and increase ejection fraction, but care must be taken to continue to support filling pressures. Vasoconstrictors such as levarterenol are not useful, because they increase afterload and have been found to reduce ejection fraction and cardiac output.[205]

The selection of anesthetic drugs should also be guided by these principles, along with the same reservation that applied to the discussion of hemorrhagic shock; namely, the choice of a specific agent is less important than the way in which it is used. As a general rule, drugs that depress myocardial contractility, such as the intravenous barbiturates or the inhalation agents as a group, should be avoided.[84, 206, 207] Vasodilators such as morphine or fentanyl could be used in very small doses if accompanied by appropriate volume loading. Ketamine has been used successfully in both experimental animal preparations and clinical work,[208] and it appears that the effects of this drug in augmenting preload and contractility outweigh any increased afterload that may result. As discussed before, some of these beneficial effects of ketamine may not be evident if the patient is under maximum catecholamine stress. However, ketamine remains the drug most likely to produce a desirable degree of analgesia and amnesia in a dose low enough to have minimum circulatory depression.[208]

When the chest is open and the bleeding site has been controlled with digital pressure or a clamp, the operation should stop temporarily.[198] Simple tears may often be repaired without cardiopulmonary bypass, but considerable blood loss should be anticipated. The overall status of the patient needs to be reassessed during this hiatus; blood volume should be completely replaced, oxygen and acid-base deficits corrected, and adequate monitoring established.

Septal Rupture. Rupture of the interatrial or interventricular septum occurs rarely, usually in association with other cardiac injuries.[186, 195, 198] It may present as an isolated lesion, however, in which case it is usually manifested as a large left-to-right shunt with congestive heart failure and pul-monary edema.[186] The diagnosis should be suspected in a patient with a systolic murmur following chest trauma, particularly with pulmonary vascular congestion. Sampling blood from the various chambers while passing a Swan-Ganz catheter may aid in the diagnosis by detecting an oxygen "step-up" in either the right atrium or ventricle,[186, 209, 210] but there are many pitfalls in this technique and the data should be interpreted with caution.[211] This is also a valuable way of differentiating a ruptured interventricular septum from acute mitral valvular insufficiency, which would also present with a systolic ejection murmur and pulmonary vascular congestion.[210] If a left-to-right shunt is present, remember that the cardiac output obtained by thermodilution techniques will be a right-heart output and will represent the sum of the left-heart output plus the shunt flow, thus overestimating the true left-heart output.[211] Determination of left-heart output with a dye dilution technique will also be difficult, and the curve obtained will be abnormal, with the characteristic low, "slurred" shape.[211] Anesthesia for the patient with an acute septal rupture should be designed to keep systemic resistance low in order to minimize left-to-right shunt flow and keep myocardial contractility high. Thus, intravenous narcotics, with or without supplemental vasodilators, are the agents of choice. Positive end-expiratory pressure may be desirable, not only to improve oxygenation but also to increase pulmonary vascular resistance and thereby further decrease the left-to-right shunt.[212] This approach should be used cautiously, however, since a right ventricle that is already stressed by a high volume load might fail if its afterload is also abruptly increased.

Valvular Disruption. Any valve may be involved by blunt heart trauma, but damage to the valves on the left side is more significant because of the higher pressures involved.[186, 195, 198] Trauma to a valve almost always results in acute insufficiency and, if severe enough, leads quickly to congestive failure and pulmonary edema.[186] Acute mitral insufficiency may be differentiated from ventricular septal defect by the results of right-heart catheterization.[210] Both aortic and mitral insufficiency respond to afterload reduction with intravenous vasodilators, although the response is highly variable.[213, 214] Aortic insufficiency is the more serious acute lesion, since it not only increases left ventricular work while reducing cardiac output but also decreases diastolic coronary flow by reducing diastolic aortic perfusion pressure and increasing left ventricular diastolic volume and pressure.[213, 215, 216] Elevations in heart rate have been found by some authors to be advantageous in acute aortic regurgitation, possibly by limiting diastolic time and thus the volume of regurgitant flow and the equalization of aortic and ventricular diastolic pressure.[215] An advantage for an increased heart rate is not universally accepted,[216] however, so it seems more reasonable to recommend preventing bradycardia rather than causing tachycardia. A heart rate of around 100 beats per minute appears to be adequate.

Principles of anesthetic management are similar to those with septal rupture. Afterload should be controlled with intravenous vasodilators; preload should be maintained with volume loading; oxygenation should be assisted with positive airway pressure; and drugs that depress the myocardium should be avoided.

Pericardial Rupture. Rupture of the pericardium with ventricular herniation is a very rare and dangerous result of blunt chest trauma that may present with hemodynamics that can be confused with pericardial tamponade.[200, 217] The diagnosis may be suspected but not confirmed by an unusual cardiac silhouette on chest x-ray or the failure to demonstrate pericardial fluid on echocardiography or pericardiocentesis. The patient may abruptly improve as he is turned to the right lateral decubitus position, as the heart falls back into the pericardium.[200] Definitive diagnosis and treatment are by thoracotomy.[217]

Pneumomediastinum. Mediastinal air is usually well tolerated, but following blunt chest trauma air may rarely be present under tension, and a picture very similar to tamponade will result.[218] A chest x-ray showing mediastinal air should suggest the diagnosis. Decompression of the mediastinum by needle aspiration or limited incision usually relieves symptoms.[218]

PENETRATING HEART INJURIES

When the heart has received a penetrating wound the significance of atrial and ventricular injury may be reversed; an atrial wound may lead quickly to exsanguination or tamponade, whereas a ventricular wound may seal spontaneously.[186, 198, 199, 219] With tamponade following limited penetrating wounds, such as knife or "icepick" injuries, pericardial drainage may be therapeutic and should be accomplished by local anesthesia. The circulation may stabilize then, allowing a controlled induction of anesthesia for exploration and repair. Otherwise, the pathophysiology is similar to that following blunt trauma, and anesthetic management is the same.

AORTIC RUPTURE

Disruption of the thoracic aorta is usually lethal, and fewer than 20 per cent of patients with transection of descending thoracic aorta at the isthmus, which is the most common site, will reach the hospital alive.[189, 190, 220, 221] This immediate survival falls to less than 5 per cent if the tear is at the aortic valve.[220] Most patients who do survive have tamponaded the bleeding within the adventitia or surrounding mediastinum to form a pseudoaneurysm. This situation is very unstable and sudden lethal exsanguination into the chest cavity may occur at any time. Rarely, if the diagnosis is missed, such an injury will stabilize and may present as a "coarctation" or aneurysm years later.

An extremely high index of suspicion is necessary, and in many cases the diagnosis is missed for hours or days.[189, 190, 220] Initial blood loss from the aorta may be small, and shock, when present, is very often due to associated abdominal injuries.[190] The classical "pseudocoarctation" syndrome of upper extremity hypertension, lower extremity hypotension, and a systolic murmur over the precordium or left scapula is highly suggestive of aortic rupture,[190, 220] but is often not present.[189] Frequently there will not even be signs of chest trauma such as fractured ribs or pulmonary contusion.[220] The most consistent early sign of aortic trauma is a widened upper mediastinum on chest x-ray, and this finding must always raise the suspicion of a torn aorta after blunt trauma.[189, 220] Other suggestive findings include loss of the aortic shadow, deviation of the trachea to the right, or depression of the left main bronchus on chest x-ray.[189] Definitive diagnosis is by aortography, which should be done as soon as it is possible to move the patient to radiology.

Assigning priorities in the care of the patient with a suspected or proven aortic tear is often difficult, and requires close communication among the involved services. Certainly, a very high absolute priority must be assigned to the need for thoracotomy in such patients, but in some situations other injuries may pose more of an immediate threat to life, such as intra-abdominal bleeding or an expanding intracranial hematoma. In these situations repair of a stable aortic injury may be deferred temporarily.[221] In the past there has been some reluctance to repair the aorta before exploring other injuries because of the fear that the heparinization required for the placement of a shunt or establishment of partial cardiopulmonary bypass employed to prevent ischemic injury below the level of the cross-clamp might aggravate bleeding in the abdomen or head. However, the use of the heparin-bonded shunt has allowed maintenance of adequate distal flow without systemic heparinization, and some authors now urge thoracotomy before repair of other injuries whenever possible.[220]

The anesthesiologist must share a considerable portion of the responsibility for successful outcome in patients with torn aortas. Speed and completeness of preoperative preparation are equally essential. Sufficient diagnostic workup must be done to ensure that severe associated injuries are not missed, and aortography is usually essential to define the lesion before surgery. The anesthesiologist may spend the time allotted to diagnosis in inserting intravenous and monitoring lines and correcting volume and acid-base deficits. If the patient requires neurodiagnostic studies such as computerized tomography, and is uncooperative, the anesthetic (induction, intubation, maintenance) may even be begun in the radiology suite. In general, the anesthesiologist should seek out ways by which the transition from diagnosis to surgery can be made more expeditiously, without waiting until the patient is delivered to the operating room to begin the search for veins. It is far easier to begin the anesthetic course under such relatively controlled conditions, rather than in the all-too-common manner in which the anesthesiologist finds himself at the receiving end of a frantic dash to bear a pulseless, gasping patient from the x-ray suite.

During the period of time before the surgeon achieves proximal control of the aorta, the patient's hemodynamic status requires careful monitoring and tight control. The preoperative approach is modeled after the regimen popularized by Wheat for aortic dissections.[222] The stress on the wall of the aorta (a combined effect of heart rate, systemic arterial pressure, and rate-of-rise of the pulse, dp/dt) should be controlled to prevent further disruption.[222, 223] Since these patients are often fully resuscitated before surgery, the primary problem is prevention or control of hypertension.[221] Various drugs have been used in the past to depress the circulation, usually a sympatholytic such as reserpine, trimethaphan, guanethidine or methyldopa.[222] For acute control, current practice usually relies on an intravenous vasodilator such as nitroprusside, phenothiazines, or hydralazine, with or without propranolol to prevent reflex increases in heart rate and contractility.[223]

The management of general anesthesia for the stable patient with a thoracic aortic tear follows similar principles. The volatile agents (halothane, enflurane) are excellent choices to achieve most of the effects discussed. They tend to reduce sympathetic tone, blood pressure, and myocardial contracility.[206, 207] Depending on the status of the individual patient, these agents may be used alone (particularly valuable when high FI_{O_2}'s are necessary) or as supplements to a basic intravenous narcotic technique, and with or without additional intravenous vasodilators. Invasive monitoring is particularly useful when deciding which drugs to use at various points in time. Optimally, such monitoring should be established before induction of anesthesia. While it is possible that the pain and the anxiety produced by inserting lines might precipitate dangerous increases in sympathetic tone,[224] this has not been our experience and we prefer to establish monitoring with the patient awake but comfortably sedated whenever possible. A double-lumen endobronchial tube is used for ventilation, as single-lung anesthesia facilitates exposure of the aorta.[220, 223] It is not absolutely essential, however, and in cases where speed is necessary, or where further manipulation of the airway might be hazardous (such as with head trauma), a single-lumen tube may be used.

The presence of any degree of head trauma must cause careful thought before beginning the anesthetic. Intracranial pressure monitoring is very useful in such situations, and should be considered. Use of volatile anesthetic agents and intravenous vasodilators is discouraged in head trauma, and alternative forms of blood pressure control should be used. A technique that I have found useful consists of large doses of thiopental sodium (1.5-2.0 gm) combined with narcotics in situations of combined head and aortic trauma. This anesthetic provides cerebral cellular protection against hypoxia, reduces intracranial pressure, and controls systemic blood pressure.[93, 97] Combinations of phenothiazines or butyrophenones with narcotics may also control systemic hypertension and ICP,[93, 97] but a barbiturate has the advantage of also reducing myocardial contractility and aortic dp/dt.[84] When necessary, trimethaphan may be used to acutely lower blood pressure, in preference to nitroprusside (see section on head trauma). If nitrous oxide cannot be used because of problems with oxygenation, an intravenous amnesic drug such as diazepam or scopolamine may be added.

Application of the aortic cross-clamp may increase left-ventricular afterload, and it may be necessary to give a vasodilator acutely, especially if the ventricle shows any signs of failing.[194, 221, 223] Most of the hemodynamic effects of the cross-clamp are relieved with the use of a shunt or partial bypass.[194]

TRAUMA TO THE DIAPHRAGM

Penetrating injuries to the diaphragm are probably more common than are blunt ruptures, but are usually smaller and, taken by themselves, are of less clinical significance.[225] Immediate significant herniation of abdominal contents into the chest is rare following penetrating injury but is the rule after blunt rupture.[225] Rupture of the left hemidiaphragm predominates (over 90 per cent of cases reported) and may be associated with no symptoms and minimal disability, or with massive herniation of stomach, small and large bowel, spleen, and associated omentum into the chest with respiratory and cardiovascular collapse.[225-227] Both blunt and penetrating injuries are associated with late herniation of abdominal contents, and a case that is not diagnosed at the time of injury may present years later as an incarcerated or strangulated hernia with signs and symptoms of bowel obstruction. Rupture of the right hemidiaphragm occurs in less than 10 per cent of cases and is usually associated with herniation of the liver alone.[226, 227] Rupture into the pericardium is reported but is rare.[226] Fistulous connections between herniated abdominal viscera and the tracheobronchial tree have been reported.[228]

The pathogenesis of blunt diaphragmatic rupture is unclear. Orringer and Kirsh suggest that if the glottis is open at the time of impact, the lungs will remain at atmospheric pressure and will collapse as the chest and abdomen are compressed.[227] This will allow the development of very high transdiaphragmatic pressure gradients.

The most common symptoms and signs of diaphragmatic hernia are nonspecific and consist of chest and abdominal pain, dyspnea, and loss of breath sounds at the lung base. Bowel sounds may be heard in the chest in some cases, but this is unusual and should not be relied upon. The diagnosis must be suspected in any patient who has an obscured lung base on chest x-ray following blunt thoracoabdominal trauma.[225-227] The diagnosis is made by identifying abdominal structures in the chest, such as loops of bowel, or a nasogastric tube in the stomach. Contrast studies may aid in diagnosis but are often negative. In less obvious cases, diagnostic pneumoperitoneum or lavage may demonstrate communication between the abdominal and chest cavities.

Indications for urgent reduction of the hernia include continued bleeding or respiratory or cardiovascular embarrassment. In other cases the reduction may be deferred until other injuries are attended to and the patient's condition stabilizes.[225]

The anesthetic management of patients with traumatic diaphragmatic hernia is based on the work of Loehning et al., who demonstrated hemodynamic compromise after induction of anesthesia and institution of controlled ventilation in such patients.[229] The physiologic situation is different from that seen with neonatal congenital diaphragmatic hernia, in that with traumatic hernia the underlying lung is presumably normal, and not hypoplastic and prone to rupture. However, the effect of positive pressure breathing added to the distortion and compression of mediastinal structures by the presence of abdominal viscera may have similar catastrophic effects.[227, 229, 230] Gentle airway control with awake intubation and spontaneous ventilation as long as is practical is recommended.[227, 230] If the condition of the patients demands, controlled ventilation may be instituted early, but with small tidal volumes and the lowest possible pressures. Otherwise, inhalation anesthesia is induced following intubation, and the patient breathes spontaneously until the surgeon is actually entering the abdomen, at which time the patient can be paralyzed and ventilation controlled.[227, 230] If cardiovascular problems develop, the surgeon is then in a position to rapidly reduce the hernia. At this point the patient should do well, since the lung and abdominal wall are normal, in contradistinction to congenital hernia.

EXTREMITY REPLANTATION

Replantation of severed extremities and digits has progressed over the last decade, from being a medical curiosity to the point where a cleanly amputated digit may be replanted with over an 80 per cent expectation of survival.[231, 232] Meticulous pre-, intra-, and postoperative care is necessary for that expectation to be achieved, however.[233] The most important factor influencing survival is the skill and patience of the surgeon in creating patent vascular channels. However, several secondary factors, including anesthesia, may have a strong influence on outcome. Regional anesthesia is almost universally recommended today for replantation surgery.[231-234] One source recommends regional block "... as it allows safe prolonged anesthesia, reduces bleeding, permits ... tourniquet control, provides postoperative analgesia and sympathetic block ... minimizes chest and thrombotic complications and is independent of the patient's gastric status."[231] While some of these claimed advantages are debatable at best,[235] the value of complete sympathetic

blockade to the extremity appears to be well documented.

In contrast to the situation in most organ beds, blood flow to the skin and distal extremities is regulated primarily by sympathetic vasomotor tone instead of local metabolic autoregulation.[232, 236] This is because surface blood flow serves to regulate body heat loss, and is thus under direct, continuous control of the central nervous system.[232] Sympathetic blockade can increase digital blood flow by a factor of six- to tenfold.[232] Conversely, increased sympathetic tone due to exercise, cold, fear, pain, or other stimuli might markedly reduce digital blood flow even in the presence of tissue hypoxia.

Sympathetic nervous activity in the hand may be interrupted at any point along its course from the upper thoracic spinal segments (high subarachnoid or epidural blocks), through the hypothalmus and vasomotor center (general anesthesia), via the sympathetic ganglia (stellate ganglion block), and along the course of the median and ulnar nerves (regional nerve blocks). Since halothane, for example, is known to depress hypothalamic thermoregulatory centers and cause marked cutaneous vasodilatation,[237] it might be thought to be a good choice for peripheral extremity replantation. However, halothane and other inhalation agents suffer from two major drawbacks in the eyes of the replantation surgeon. First, the abrupt restoration of thermoregulation at the end of anesthesia,[238, 239] combined with the hypothermia that usually accompanies prolonged general anesthesia,[237-239] may provoke intense peripheral vasospasm that compromises graft perfusion. Second, abrupt emergence from inhalation anesthesia, especially with shivering, may be associated with movement of the injured extremity that might disrupt anastomoses or otherwise jeopardize the repair.[234]

Scrupulous care must be taken to avoid these problems if general inhalation anesthesia is employed for replantations. Body temperature must be maintained by whatever means are available, including maintaining the operating room at a comfortably warm temperature, warming inspired gases, and using adjuncts such as warming blankets and lamps.[237-239] In addition, emergence must be smooth and controlled. This might be accomplished by the judicious administration of intravenous narcotic analgesics in the immediate pre-emergence period.

The same considerations apply if an intravenous balanced anesthetic technique is chosen, and under such circumstances the use of naloxone postoperatively to speed emergence might be relatively contraindicated.

The regional technique most often recommended for hand surgery is the axillary approach to the brachial plexus.[231-234] Some authors have expressed concern that such a proximal block might cause vasodilatation in the entire extremity and lead to a "steal" from the anastomotic sites to more proximal, normal vessels.[232] This theoretical consideration has not been tested, but it would appear to be reasonable to perform the block at a site as distal as is compatible with anesthetizing the surgical site.

If continued blockade in the postoperative period is desired, placing a catheter in the perineural tissues at the time of surgery could be considered, as almost all of these patients will be anticoagulated postoperatively, and this might increase the risk of repeating blocks.[232]

NEAR-DROWNING

Near-drowning is defined as short-term (24 hour) survival after asphyxiation or aspiration during submersion in liquid.[240-243] Many near-drowning victims succumb to late sequelae or complications, and must therefore be considered to be physiologically unstable. Even though drowning is a common cause of death, it is unusual for a near-drowning victim to be brought to surgery in the acute stages of the syndrome unless there are associated injuries.

The two basic pathologic mechanisms in near-drowning are asphyxiation and aspiration, and the two main target organs are the brain and lung. Either mechanism may be present alone, or in combinations of varying significance. About 10 per cent of near-drowning victims will have no fluid aspiration and will present as pure asphyxial insults.[242] The mechanism of this is probably related to laryngospasm or breath-holding due to the initial contact of the liquid with the upper airway.

The lung has been the traditional target organ in near-drowning studies. Most patients who die following near-drowning have serious pulmonary dysfunction, whereas patients who present with a normal chest x-ray or who do not require immediate mechanical ventilatory assistance have a low mortality.[241, 243] About half of near-drowning victims will be tachypneic and have radiographic signs of pulmonary edema on initial presentation.[241]

The issue of which type of water produces the most severe pulmonary aspiration syndrome is still subject to debate. Fresh water may produce more "wash-out" of surfactant with subsequent low compliance and lung volume loss,[241] while salt water may cause more alveolar flooding and direct damage to the alveolar-capillary membrane.[242, 243] However, other factors such as volume aspirated, time of exposure, gross bacterial (or other microorganism) contamination, or content of chemicals or physical debris probably have more impact on outcome. Since massive amounts of water may be swallowed, gastric distention, vomiting, and aspiration of gastric contents may also occur. Both types of aspiration will present similar pictures of low compliance, low functional residual capacity (FRC), high shunt fraction, and possibly altered alveolar capillary integrity. Treatment is supportive, with supplemental oxygen, endotracheal intubation, positive airway pressure, and ventilatory assistance employed as in other cases of acute respiratory insufficiency. Adrenal corticosteroids have not been shown to be useful in the treatment of the aspiration syndrome of near-drowning.[243-244]

Secondary pulmonary damage may occur as a result of the asphyxiation, owing to hypoxia, myocardial failure, or cardiac arrest with cardiopulmonary resuscitation. Pulmonary barotrauma is also quite common, possibly due to vigorous resuscitation efforts in the presence of low lung compliance.[241, 242]

Attention has been directed recently to the brain as a target organ in near-drowning.[240-242] The reported incidence of permanent, significant neurologic sequelae from near-drowning is 10 to 30 per cent.[240, 242] Neurologic outcome is strongly correlated with initial presentation; patients who are comatose on admission almost never recover fully, and patients who are initially alert rarely die.[241, 243] There is evidence that outcome can be influenced by early, aggressive treatment of potential brain swelling based on the more extensive work available on therapy of head trauma.[240] Such therapy is based on control of the monitored ICP by mechanical ventilation, hypocarbia and hyperoxia, administration of osmotic agents and diuretics, and care to prevent straining, coughing, bucking, increased CVP, or unnecessarily increased airway pressure.[92, 240, 241] As with head trauma, a patient being anesthetized immediately after near-drowning should be accorded a full-fledged "neuroanesthetic" even though his neurologic status may be satisfactory preoperatively (see section on head trauma). This would include avoiding volatile agents, ketamine, and spontaneous ventilation, and the liberal use of thiobarbiturates, narcotics, and relaxants. Adrenal corticosteroids would appear to have a more valid role in the treatment of the neurologic sequelae of near-drowning than they have in the treatment of the pulmonary injury.[240]

MISCELLANEOUS CONSIDERATIONS

Hypothermia. Near-drowning victims, especially children, may be severely hypothermic from immersion. The reduction of cellular oxygen consumption that accompanies hypothermia is felt to be protective to a degree, and permits restoration of nearly normal brain function after up to 30 minutes of submersion, and of cardiac function after even longer periods.[240] Because of the danger of cerebral edema in near-drowning it is recommended that body temperature be restored acutely only to a level compatible with cardiovascular stability (30–32° C), and that vigorous attempts to restore normal temperature may be inadvisable. However, the value of prolonged, deliberate hypothermia in the treatment of cerebral edema is questionable,[108] and treatment after initial stabilization should more properly be directed toward preventing hyperpyrexia rather than maintaining hypothermia.[240]

Associated Conditions. Near-drowning may often be precipitated by or associated with other injuries or conditions, and all near-drowning victims require a full diagnostic workup prior to anesthesia. Near-drowning associated with jumping or diving into the water may coexist with cervical spine injury or direct cerebral trauma, and appropriate neurodiagnostic studies are essential. Near-drowning in adults may be due to alcohol or drug use, which may affect anesthetic requirements.

Biochemical Disturbances. Despite theoretical considerations of differing osmolarity and electrolyte compositions, most studies of human victims have failed to identify any significant differences in clinical presentation between fresh and salt water near-drowning.[241-243] Serious electrolyte disturbances following near-drowning in either salt or fresh water are very rare and follow no particular pattern.[241, 243] Each patient must be evaluated individually. Arterial blood gas analysis usually reveals a variable degree of hypoxemia. If asphyxiation has been severe, a mixed metabolic and respiratory acidosis may be present but usually responds promptly to restoration of adequate ventilation and circulation.

Hemolysis may occur, especially with fresh water aspiration, but is rarely extensive enough to affect the hematocrit. Free hemoglobin may be detected in the urine, but the contribution of hemolysis to any renal dysfunction after near-drowning is hard to evaluate, since usually hypoxia and sometimes cardiac arrest have also occurred. Coagulation disorders resembling DIC may occur but their etiology is also unclear.[242]

MASS CASUALTIES

When more than one trauma victim presents at a time, the approaches discussed in the previous sections must undergo certain modifications.

Triage

The decision as to which patient is to receive what treatment at a given time can be the most important decision made in the overall care of all the patients. When there is a relative shortage of facilities or personnel, so that not all the patients can receive all of the necessary treatment at once, decisions as to priority must be made by a single person. Because of the difficulty and importance of this decision, the "triage officer" should ideally be the most experienced surgeon available.[3]

Fluid Resuscitation

The main difference in principles of fluid management from those outlined in the previous discussion of hemorrhage pertains to the use of "universal donor" (O-negative) blood. Experience in the military has demonstrated that most serious hemolytic transfusion reactions are due to clerical errors in identification rather than to laboratory errors.[32] Therefore, when blood is needed for more than one patient simultaneously, use of O-negative blood with low titers of anti-A isoagglutinin is recommended.[32-34] Since most O-negative blood stored in blood banks today is not routinely screened for titers of anti-A, it might be considered a desirable part of a hospital disaster plan to require the blood bank to identify and isolate low-titer units of O-negative blood immediately upon receiving notification of a multiple casualty situation. In the absence of such screening, it is safest to use O-negative packed cells with appropriate volume expanders.

Anesthetic Technique

When there are sufficient skilled personnel and equipment, multiple casualties will be handled in the operating room in the same manner as single casualties. Shortages may occur in three areas.

Drugs. Depending on local patterns of use, some drugs may be stocked in small quantities, and may be unavailable when needed. This particularly applies to special-purpose drugs such as ketamine. Part of the disaster plan of an anesthesia service should be directed toward inventory control and rationing of such items. To use the example of ketamine, requests for the drug could be cleared through the senior anesthesiologist in charge, and indiscriminate use of the drug for inductions just on general principles would be discouraged.

Equipment and Supplies. Techniques of administering anesthesia without machines, compressed gases, and other routine items of equipment have been described in detail elsewhere (most commonly derived from military experience).[245-249] Ventilation may be achieved by use of manual self-inflating bags, with or without oxygen. Volatile agents may be administered through such bags,[246, 247] or a pure intravenous technique may be used.[245, 249] Compressed oxygen is usually available in adequate supply in modern hospitals, but in its absence inhalation agents may be vaporized in "draw-over" vaporizers such as the EMO;[246-248] the Fluotec Mark II (but not newer vaporizers) may be used without compressed gas.[246, 247] Techniques of anesthesia administration using restricted resources should be taught routinely to anesthesia trainees.

Personnel. In situations involving overwhelming numbers of casualities, it may be necessary to allow patients to be attended by non-anesthesia personnel during surgery. Depending on the skill level of these people, techniques that would not be employed in more controlled situations may become attractive. Regional anesthesia might receive first consideration, as once established and stabilized it requires less supervision than general anesthesia. Where the demands on the time of the skilled personnel make it impossible to perform an effective regional block with safety, a standardized general anesthesia technique may be necessary. This usually means endotracheal intubation and controlled ventilation, since unskilled personnel should not be expected to recognize an obstructed airway or inadequate ventilation. Under these circumstances most experienced nurses and respiratory therapists are capable of ventilating a paralyzed patient with a manual, self-inflating bag.

REFERENCES

1. The World Almanac and Book of Facts. New York, Newspaper Enterprise Assoc., Inc., 1979, pp. 954-955.
2. Guidelines for Patient Care in Anesthesiology of the American Society of Anesthesiologists. *In* 1980 Directory of Members, 45th ed., p. 410.
3. Primary assessment and management of the injured. *In* Committee on Trauma, American College of Surgeons: Early Care of the Injured Patient. 2nd ed., Philadelphia, W. B. Saunders Co., 1976, pp. 1-12.
4. Shock and fluid replacement. ibid., pp. 30-43.
5. Vatner, S. F.: Effects of hemorrhage on regional blood flow distribution in dogs and primates. J. Clin. Invest. 54:225, 1974.
6. Zweifach, B. W., and Fronek, A.,: The interplay of central and peripheral factors in irreversible hemorrhagic shock. Prog. Cardiovasc. Dis. 18:147, 1975.

7. Kirimli, B., Kampschulte, S., and Safar, P.: Pattern of dying from exsanguinating hemorrhage in dogs. J. Trauma 10:393, 1970.

8. Skillman, J. J., Awwad, H. K., and Moore, F. D.: Plasma protein kinetics of the early transcapillary refill after hemorrhage in man. Surg. Gynec. Obstet. 125:983, 1967.

9. Zweifach, B. W.: Mechanisms of blood flow and fluid exchange in microvessels: Hemorrhagic hypotension model. Anesthesiology 41:157, 1974.

10. Massion, W. H.: Refractory hypotension: Mechanism and prevention. Int. Anesthesiol. Clin. 12(1):223, 1974.

11. Carrico, C. J., Canizaro, P. C., and Shires, G. T.: Fluid resuscitation following injury: Rationale for the use of balanced salt solutions. Crit. Care Med. 4:46, 1976.

12. Civetta, J. M.: A new look at the Starling equation. Crit. Care Med. 7:84, 1979.

13. Dawidson, I., Gelin, L.-E., and Haglind, E.: Plasma volume, intravascular protein content, hemodynamic and oxygen transport changes during intestinal shock in dogs: Comparison of relative effectiveness of various plasma expanders. Crit. Care Med. 8:73, 1980.

14. Giesecke, A. H. Jr.. and Jenkins, M. T.: Fluid therapy. In Giesecke, A. H. (ed.): Anesthesia for the Surgery of Trauma. Philadelphia, F. A. Davis, 1976, pp. 57-69.

15. Jelenko, C., III, Williams, J. B., Wheeler, M. L., et al.: Studies in shock and resuscitation, I: Use of hypertonic, albumin-containing, fluid demand regimen (HALFD) in resuscitation. Crit. Care Med. 7:157, 1979.

16. Lowe, R. J., Moss, G. S., Jilek, J., and Levine, H. D.: Crystalloid versus colloid in the etiology of pulmonary failure after trauma — a randomized trial in man. Crit. Care Med. 7:107, 1979.

17. Shoemaker, W. C.: Comparison of the relative effectiveness of whole blood transfusions and various types of fluid therapy in resuscitation. Crit. Care Med. 4:71, 1976.

18. Shoemaker, W. C., and Hauser, C. J.: Critique of crystalloid versus colloid therapy in shock and shock lung. Crit. Care Med. 7:117, 1979.

19. Stein, L., Beraud, J. J., Morissette, M., et al.: Pulmonary edema during volume infusion. Circulation 52:483, 1975.

20. Virgilio, R. W., Smith, D. E., and Zarins, C.K.: Balanced electrolyte solutions: Experimental and clinical studies. Crit. Care Med. 7:98, 1979.

21. Weil, M. H., Henning, R. J., and Puri, V. K.: Colloid oncotic pressure: Clinical significance. Crit. Care Med. 7:113, 1979.

22. Lazrove, S., Waxman, K., Shippy, C., et al.: Hemodynamic, blood volume, and oxygen transport responses to albumin and hydroxyethyl starch infusions in critically ill postoperative patients. Crit. Care Med. 8:302, 1980.

23. Nees, J. E., Hauser, C. J., Shippy, C., et al.: Comparison of cardiorespiratory effects of crystalline hemoglobin, whole blood, albumin, and Ringer's lactate in the resuscitation of hemorrhagic shock in dogs. Surgery 83:639, 1978.

24. Cervera, A. L., and Moss, G.: Dilutional reexpansion with crystalloid after massive hemorrhage: saline versus balanced electrolyte solution for maintenance of normal blood volume and arterial pH. J. Trauma 15:498, 1975.

25. Kirimli, B., Kampschulte, S., and Safar, P.: Resuscitation from cardiac arrest due to exsanguination. Surg. Gynecol. Obstet. 129:89, 1969.

26. Knight, R. J.: Resuscitation of battle casualties in South Viet Nam: experiences of the First Australian Field Hospital. Resuscitation 2:17, 1973.

27. Sharwood-Smith, G.: Anaesthetist in Salalah: Experience in a field surgical team. Anaesthesia 31:1049, 1976.

28. Nunn, J. F., and Freeman, J.: Problems of oxygenation and oxygen transport during hemorrhage. Anaesthesia 19:206, 1964.

29. Bland, R., Shoemaker, W. C., and Shabot, M. M.: Physiologic monitoring goals for the critically ill patient. Surg. Gynec. Obstet. 147:833, 1978.

30. Valeri, C. R.: Blood components in the treatment of acute blood loss: Use of freeze-preserved red cells, platelets, and plasma proteins. Anesth. Analg. (Cleve.) 54:1, 1975.

31. Blumberg, N., and Bove, J. R.: Un-cross-matched blood for emergency transfusion: One year's experience in a civilian setting. J.A.M.A. 240:2057, 1978.

32. Barnes, A., Jr.: Status of the use of universal donor blood transfusion. CRC Crit. Rev. Clin. Lab. Sci. 4:147, 1973.

33. Crosby, W. H., and Akeroyd, J. H.: Some immunohematologic results of large transfusions of group O blood in recipients of other blood groups: a study of battle casualties in Korea. Blood 9:103, 1954.

34. Barnes, A., Jr., and Allen, T. E.: Transfusions subsequent to administration of universal donor blood in Viet Nam. J.A.M.A. 204:695, 1968.

35. Miller, R. D.: Complications of massive blood transfusions. Anesthesiology 39:82, 1973.

36. Doenicke, A., Grote, B., and Lorenz, W.: Blood and blood substitutes. Br. J. Anaesth. 49:681, 1977.

37. Boyan, C. P., and Howland, W. S.: Blood temperature: A critical factor in massive transfusion. Anesthesiology 22:559, 1961.

38. Durtschi, M. G., Haisch, C. E., Reynolds, L., et al.: Effect of micropore filtration on pulmonary function after massive transfusion. Am. J. Surg. 138:8, 1979.

39. Collins, J. A., James, P. M., Bredenberg, C. E., et al.: The relationship between transfusion and hypoxia in combat casualties. Ann. Surg. 188:513, 1978.

40. Cervera, A. L., and Moss, G.: Crystalloid requirements and distribution when resuscitating with RBC's and noncolloid solutions during hemorrhage. Circ. Shock 5:357, 1978.

41. Peters, R. M., and Hogan, J. S.: Fluid overload and post-traumatic respiratory distress syndrome. J. Trauma 18:83, 1975.

42. Alving, B. M., Hojima, Y., Pisano, J. J., et al.: Hypotension associated with prekallikrein activator (Hageman-factor fragments) in plasma protein fraction. N. Engl. J. Med. 299:60, 1978.

43. Ellison, N., Behar, M., MacVaugh, H., III, and

Marshall, B. E.: Bradykinin, plasma protein fraction, and hypotension. Ann. Thor. Surg. 29:15, 1980.

44. Olinger, G. N., Werner, P. H., Bonchek, L. I., et al.: Vasodilator effects of the sodium acetate in pooled protein fraction Ann. Surg. 190:305, 1979.

45. Alexander, B.: Effects of plasma expanders on coagulation and hemostasis: Dextran, hydroxyethyl starch, and other macromolecules revisited. In Jamieson, G. A., and Greenwalt, T. J. (eds.): Blood Substitutes and Plasma Expanders. New York, Alan R. Liss, Inc., 1978, pp. 293-326.

46. Thompson, W. L. Jr.: Hydroxyethyl starch. In Jamieson, G. A., and Greenwalt, T. J. (eds.): Blood Substitutes and Plasma Expanders. New York, Alan R. Liss, Inc., 1978, pp. 283-292.

47. Sibbald, W. J., Paterson, N. A. M., Holliday, R. L., et al.: The Trendelenburg position: Hemodynamic effects in hypotensive and normotensive patients. Crit. Care Med. 7:218, 1979.

48. Brooks, D. H., and Grenvik, A.: G-suit control of massive retroperitoneal hemorrhage due to pelvic fracture. Crit. Care Med. 1:257, 1973.

49. Pelligra, R., and Sandberg, E. C.: Control of intractable abdominal bleeding by external counter pressure. J.A.M.A. 241:708, 1979.

50. Baxter, C. R.: Acute renal insufficiency complicating traumatic surgery. In Shires, G. T. (ed.): Care of the Trauma Patient. 2nd ed., New York, McGraw-Hill, 1979, pp. 505-517.

51. Brown, R. S.: Renal dysfunction in the surgical patient: Maintenance of the high output state with furosemide. Crit. Care Med. 7:63, 1979.

52. Shin, B., Mackenzie, C. F., McAslan, T. C., et al.: Postoperative renal failure in trauma patients. Anesthesiology 51:218, 1979.

53. Shin, B., Isenhower, N. N., McAslan, T. C., et al.: Early recognition of renal insufficiency in postanesthetic trauma victims. Anesthesiology 50:262, 1979.

54. Amory, D. W., Steffenson, J. L., and Forsyth, R. P.: Systemic and regional blood flow changes during halothane anesthesia in the Rhesus monkey. Anesthesiology 35:81, 1971.

55. Benumof, J. L., Bookstein J. J., Saidman, L. J., et al.: Diminished hepatic arterial flow during halothane administration. Anesthesiology 45:545, 1976.

56. Larson, C. P., Jr., Mazze, R. I., Cooperman, L. H., et al.: Effects of anesthetics on cerebral, renal, and splanchnic circulations: Recent developments. Anesthesiology 41:169, 1974.

57. Ngai, S. H.: Current concepts in anesthesiology: Effects of anesthetics on various organs. N. Engl. J. Med. 302:564, 1980.

58. Vatner, S. F., and Braunwald, E.: Cardiovascular control mechanisms in the conscious state. N. Engl. J. Med. 293:970, 1974.

59. Diamant, M., Benumof, J. L., and Saidman, L. J.: Hemodynamics of increased intra-abdominal pressure: Interaction with hypovolemia and halothane anesthesia. Anesthesiology 48:23, 1978.

60. Deutsch, S.: Kidney function during anesthesia and hemorrhage. Int. Anesthesiol. Clin. 12:109, 1974.

61. Massion, W. H.: Effects of anesthesia and hemorrhage on lung function. Int. Anesthesiol. Clin. 12:83, 1974.

62. Chasapakis, G., Kekis, N., Sakkalis, C., et al.: Use of ketamine and pancuronium for anesthesia for patients in hemorrhagic shock. Anesth. Analg. (Cleve.) 52:282, 1973.

63. Corssen, G., Reves, J. G., and Carter, J. R.: Neuroleptanesthesia, dissociative anesthesia, and hemorrhage. Int. Anesthesiol. Clin. 12:145, 1974.

64. Davidson, J. T., and Cotev, S.: Anesthesia in the Yom Kippur war. Ann. R. Coll. Surg. 56:304, 1975.

65. Dillon, J. B.: The use of anesthetic agents in trauma patients. Surg. Clin. North Am. 52:567, 1972.

66. Graves, C. L.: Management of general anesthesia during hemorrhage. Int. Anesthesiol. Clin. 12:1, 1974.

67. Longnecker, D. E., and Sturgill, B. C.: Influence of anesthetic agent on survival following hemorrhage. Anesthesiology 45:516, 1976.

68. Noble, M. J., Bryant, T., and Ing. F. Y. W.: Casualty anesthesia experiences in Viet Nam. Anesth. Analg. 47:5, 1968.

69. Raj, P. P., Montgomery, S. J., and Bradley, V. H.: Agents and techniques. In Giesecke, A. H. (ed.): Anesthesia for the Surgery of Trauma. Philadelphia, F. A. Davis Co., 1976, pp. 41-56.

70. Shin, B., Mackenzie, C. F., and Helrich, M.: Comparison of halothane vs. droperidol-fentanyl in traumatic shock. Anesthesiology 51(suppl.): S101 (abst), 1979.

71. Theye, R. A., Perry, L. B., and Brzica, S. M.: Influence of anesthetic agent on response to hemorrhagic hypotension. Anesthesiology 40:32, 1974.

72. Torpey, D. J.: Resuscitation and anesthetic management of casualties. J.A.M.A. 202:955, 1967.

73. Zsigmond, E. K., and Domino, E. F.: Ketamine: clinical pharmacology, pharmacokinetics and current clinical uses. Anesthesiol. Rev. 7:13, 1980.

74. Baraka, A.: Anaesthetic problems during the tragic civil war in Lebanon. M. E. J. Anaesth. 5:7, 1978.

75. Cromartie, R. S., III: Rapid anesthesia induction in combat casualties with full stomachs. Anesth. Analg. (Cleve.) 55:74, 1976.

76. Virtue, R. W., Alanis, J. M., Mori, M., et al.: An anesthetic agent: 2-orthochlorophenyl, 2-methylamino cyclohexanone HCl (CI-581). Anesthesiology 28:823, 1967.

77. Waxman, K., Shoemaker, W. C., and Lippman, M.: Cardiovascular effects of anesthetic induction with ketamine. Anesth. Analg. (Cleve.) 59: 355, 1980.

78. Halford, F. J.: A critique of intravenous anesthesia in war surgery. Anesthesiology 4:67, 1943.

79. Adams, R. C., and Gray, H. K.: Intravenous anesthesia with pentothal sodium in the case of gunshot wound associated with accompanying severe traumatic shock and loss of blood: Report of a case. Anesthesiology 4:70, 1943.

80. Editorial: The question of intravenous anesthesia in war surgery. Anesthesiology 4:74, 1943.

81. Bonica, J. J., Kennedy, W. F., Jr., Akamatsu, T. J.,

et al.: Circulatory effects of peridural block: III, Effects of acute blood loss. Anesthesiology 36:219, 1972.

82. Greene, N. M.: Present concepts of spinal anesthesia. *In* Hershey, S. G. (ed.): ASA Refresher Courses in Anesthesiology. Philadelphia, J. B. Lippincott Co., 1979, pp. 131-142.

83. Stanton-Hicks, M. d' A.: Cardiovascular effects of extradural anaesthesia. Br. J. Anaesth. 47:253, 1975.

84. Dundee, J. W., and Wyant, G. M.: Barbiturates: Effects on the body. *In* Intravenous Anaesthesia. Edinburgh, Churchill Livingstone, 1974, pp. 64-127.

85. Gronert, G. A., and Theye, R. A.: Pathophysiology of hyperkalemia induced by succinylcholine. Anesthesiology 43:89, 1975.

86. Stept, W. J., and Safar, P.: Rapid induction/intubation for prevention of gastric-content aspiration. Anesth. Analg. (Cleve.) 49:633, 1970.

87. Brown, E. M., Krishnaprasad, D., and Smiler, B. G.: Pancuronium for rapid induction technique for tracheal intubation. Canad. Anaesth. Soc. J. 26:489, 1979.

88. Akamatsu, T. J., Bonica, J. J., Rehmet, R., et al.: Experiences with the use of ketamine for parturition: I. Primary anesthetic for vaginal delivery. Anesth. Analg. (Cleve.) 53:284, 1974.

89. Slogoff, S., Allen, G. W., Wessels, J. V., and Cheney, D. H.: Clinical experience with subanesthetic ketamine. Anesth. Analg. (Cleve.) 53:354, 1974.

90. Albin, M. S.: Anesthetic management of the patient with head injury. Int. Anesthesiol. Clin. 15:297, 1977.

91. Fishman, R. A.: Brain edema. N. Engl. J. Med. 293:706, 1975.

92. Geevarghese, K. P.: Basic considerations. Int. Anesthesiol. Clin. 15:1, 1977.

93. Gordon, E.: Anesthesia for neurosurgery. *In*: A Basis and Practice of Neuroanaesthesia. Amsterdam, Excerpta Medica, 1975, pp. 173-198.

94. Gordon, E.: Management of acute head injuries. *In*: A Basis and Practice of Neuroanaesthesia, Amsterdam, Excerpta Medica, 1975, pp. 249-265.

95. Lassen, N. A.: Cerebral and spinal cord blood flow. *In* Cottrell, J. E., and Turndorf, H. (eds.): Anesthesia and Neurosurgery. St. Louis, C. V. Mosby, 1980, pp. 1-24.

96. Miller, J. D., and Sullivan, H. G.: Severe intracranial hypertension. Int. Anesthesiol. Clin. 17:19, 1979.

97. Shapiro, H. M.: Intracranial hypertension: Therapeutic and anesthetic considerations. Anesthesiology 43:445, 1975.

98. Trubuhovich, R. V.: Acute brain swelling. Int. Anesthesiol. Clin. 17:77, 1979.

99. Shalit, M. N., and Cotev, S.: Interrelationship between blood pressure and regional cerebral blood flow in experimental intracranial hypertension. J. Neurosurg. 40:594, 1974.

100. Trowbridge, A., and Giesecke, A. H., Jr.: Multiple injuries. *In* Giesecke, A. H., Jr. (ed.): Anesthesia for the Surgery of Trauma. Philadelphia, F. A. Davis Co., 1976, pp. 79-84.

101. Beck, G. P., and Neill, L. W.: Anesthesia for associated trauma in patients with head injuries. Anesth. Analg. 42:687, 1963.

102. Lassen, N. A., and Tweed, W. A.: Anesthesia and cerebral blood flow. *In* Gordon, E. (ed.): A Basis and Practice of Neuroanaesthesia. Amsterdam, Excerpta Medica, 1975, pp. 113-133.

103. Horton, J. M.: The anaesthetist's contribution to the care of head injuries. Br. J. Anaesth. 48:767, 1976.

104. McLesky, C. H., Cullen, B. F., Kennedy, R. D., et al.: Control of cerebral perfusion pressure during induction of anesthesia in high-risk neurosurgical patients. Anesth. Analg. 53:985, 1974.

105. Bruce, D. A.: Management of severe head injury. *In* Cottrell, J. E., and Turndorf, H. (eds.): Anesthesia and Neurosurgery. St. Louis, C. V. Mosby, 1980, pp. 183-210.

106. Rose, J., Valtonen, S., and Jennett, B.: Avoidable factors contributing to death after head injury. Br. Med. J. 2:615, 1977.

107. Rottenberg, D. A. and Posner, J. B.: Intracranial pressure control. *In* Cottrell, J. E., and Turndorf, H. (eds.): Anesthesia and Neurosurgery. St. Louis, C. V. Mosby, 1980, pp. 89-118.

108. Tarlof, E.: Optimal management of head injuries. Int. Anesthesiol. Clin. 14:69, 1976.

109. Marsh, M. L., Aidinis, S. J., and Shapiro, H. M.: Fluctuating intracranial hypertension due to Cheyne-Stokes respiration. Anesth. Analg. (Cleve.) 56:216, 1977.

110. Risberg, J., Lundberg, N., and Ingvar, D. H.: Regional cerebral blood volume during acute transient rises of the intracranial pressure (plateau waves). J. Neurosurg. 31:303, 1969.

111. Wilson, R. F., Gibson, D. R., and Antonenko, D.: Shock and acute respiratory failure after chest trauma. J. Trauma 17:697, 1977.

112. Magnaes, B.: Body position and cerebrospinal fluid pressure. Part 1: Clinical studies on the effects of rapid postural change. J. Neurosurg. 44:687, 1976.

113. Adams, R. W., Gronert, G. A., Sundt, T. M., et al.: Halothane, hypocapnia and cerebrospinal fluid pressure in neurosurgery. Anesthesiology 37:510, 1972.

114. Miller, J. D., Becker, D. P., Ward, J. D., et al.: Significance of intracranial hypertension in severe head injury. J. Neurosurg. 47:503, 1977.

115. Cushing, H.: Concerning a definite regulatory mechanism of the vaso-motor center which controls blood pressure during cerebral compression. Johns Hopkins Hosp. Bull. 12:290, 1901.

116. Graf, C. J., and Rossi, N. P.: Catecholamine response to intracranial hypertension. J. Neurosurg. 49:862, 1978.

117. Rossi, N. P., and Graf, C. J.: Physiological and pathological effects of neurologic disturbances and increased intracranial pressure on the lung: A review. Surg. Neurol. 5:366, 1976.

118. Marshall, L. F., Smith, R. W., and Shapiro, H. M.: The influence of diurnal rhythms in patients with intracranial hypertension: Implications for management. Neurosurgery 2:100, 1978.

119. Cohen, H. B., Gambill, A. F., and Eggers, G. W. N., Jr.: Acute pulmonary edema following head injury: Two case reports. Anesth. Analg. (Cleve.) 56:136, 1977.

120. Simmons, R. L., Martin, A. M., Jr., Heisterkamp, C. A., III, et al.: Respiratory insufficiency in combat casualties: II. Pulmonary edema following head injury. Ann. Surg. 170:39, 1969.

121. Gagnon, R. L., Marsh, M. C., Smith, R. S., et al.: Intracranial hypertension caused by nitroglycerin. Anesthesiology 51:86, 1979.

122. Marsh, M. L., Shapiro, H. M., Smith, R. W., et al.: Changes in neurologic status and intracranial pressure associated with sodium nitroprusside administration. Anesthesiology 51:336, 1979.

123. Marsh, M. L., Aidinis, S. J., Naughton, K. V. A., et al.: The technique of nitroprusside administration modifies the intracranial pressure response. Anesthesiology 51:538, 1979.

124. Aidinis, S. J., Lafferty, J., and Shapiro, H. M.: Intracranial responses to PEEP. Anesthesiology 45:275, 1976.

125. Frost, E. A. M.: Effects of positive end-expiratory pressure on intracranial pressure and compliance in brain-injured patients. J. Neurosurg. 47:195, 1977.

126. Kim, Y. D., Devereux, D. F., and MacNamara, T. E.: An unusual cardiovascular response to PEEP. Anesthesiology 48:365, 1978.

127. Horellou, M. F., Mathe, D., and Feiss, P.: A hazard of naso-tracheal intubation. (Letter) Anaesthesia 33:73, 1978.

128. Merritt, H. H.: Trauma. In: A Textbook of Neurology, 5th ed. Philadelphia, Lea & Febiger, 1973, pp. 314-400.

129. Arens, J. F., LeJeune, F. E., Jr., and Webre, D. R.: Maxillary sinusitis, a complication of nasotracheal intubation. Anesthesiology 40:415, 1974.

130. Langfitt, T. W., Weinstein, J. D., and Kassell, N. F.: Cerebral vasomotor paralysis produced by intracranial hypertension. Neurology 15:622, 1965.

131. Young, J. S.: Spinal cord injury: Associated and general trauma and medical complications. In Thompson, R. A., and Green, J. R. (eds.): Advances in Neurology. New York, Raven Press, 1979, vol 22, pp. 255-260.

132. Young, J. S.: Initial hospitalization and rehabilitation costs of spinal cord injury. Ortho. Clin. North Am. 9(2):263, 1978.

133. Pierce, D. S.: Acute treatment of spinal cord injuries. In Pierce, D. S., and Nickel, V. H. (eds.): The Total Care of Spinal Cord Injuries. Boston, Little, Brown and Co., 1977. pp. 1-51.

134. Stauffer, E. S., Wood, R. W., and Kelly, E. G.: Gunshot wounds of the spine: The effects of laminectomy. J. Bone Joint Surg. 61:389, 1979.

135. Wharton, G. W.: Stabilization of spinal injuries for early mobilization. Ortho. Clin. North Am. 9(2):271, 1978.

136. Desmond, J.: Paraplegia: Problems confronting the anaesthesiologist. Canad. Anaesth. Soc. J. 17:435, 1970.

137. Vandam, L. D., and Rossier, A. B.: Circulatory, respiratory, and ancillary problems in acute and chronic spinal cord injury. In Hershey, S. G. (ed.): Refresher Courses in Anesthesiology. Philadelphia, J. B. Lippincott Co., 1975, vol. 3, pp. 171-182.

138. Sudhir, K. G., Smith, R. M., Hall, J. E., et al.: Intraoperative awakening for early recognition of possible neurologic sequelae during Harrington-rod spinal fusion. Anesth. Analg. (Cleve.) 55:526, 1976.

139. Perry, J.: Surgical approaches to the spine. In Pierce, D. S., and Nickel, V. S. (eds.): The Total Care of Spinal Cord Injuries. Boston, Little, Brown and Co., 1977, pp. 53-79.

140. Kapp, J. P.: Endotracheal intubation in patients with fractures of the cervical spine: Technical note. J. Neurosurg. 42:731, 1975.

141. Quimby, C. W., Jr., Williams, R. N., and Greifenstein, F. E.: Anesthetic problems of the acute quadriplegic patient. Anesth. Analg. (Cleve.) 52:333, 1973.

142. Cooper, M., and Watson, R. L.: An improved regional anesthetic technique for peroral endoscopy. Anesthesiology 43:372, 1975.

143. Kopman, A. F., Wollman, S. B., Ross, K., et al.: Awake endotracheal intubation: A review of 267 cases. Anesth. Analg. 54:323, 1975.

144. Tahir, A. H.: The bronchofiberoscope as an aid to endotracheal intubation. Br. J. Anaesth. 44:1118, 1972.

145. Tahir, A. H., and Renegar, O. J.: A stylet for difficult orotracheal intubation. Anesthesiology 39:337, 1973.

146. De Falque, R. J.: Ketamine for blind nasal intubation. Anesth. Analg. (Cleve.) 50:984, 1971.

147. Sims, J., and Giesecke, A. H., Jr.: Airway management. In Giesecke, A. H., Jr. (ed.): Anesthesia for the Surgery of Trauma. Philadelphia, F. A. Davis Co., 1976, pp. 71-77.

148. Tibbs, P. A., Young, B., McAllister, R. G., et al.: Studies of experimental cervical spinal cord transection. Part I. Hemodynamic changes after acute cervical spinal cord transection. J. Neurosurg. 48:558, 1978.

149. Stauffer, E. S.: Long-term management of traumatic quadriplegia. In Pierce, D. S., and Nickel, V. H. (eds.): The Total Care of Spinal Cord Injuries. Boston, Little, Brown and Co., 1977, pp. 81–102.

150. Troll, G. F., and Dohrmann, G. J.: Anaesthesia of the spinal cord injured patient: Cardiovascular problems and their management. Paraplegia 13:162, 1975.

151. Freehafer, A. A.: Long-term management of lumbar paraplegia. In Pierce, D. S., and Nickel V. H. (eds.): The Total Care of Spinal Cord Injuries. Boston, Little Brown and Co., 1977, pp. 135-163.

152. Comarr, A. E.: Autonomic dysreflexia. In Pierce, D. S., and Nickel V. H. (eds.): The Total Care of Spinal Cord Injuries. Boston, Little, Brown and Company, 1977, pp. 181-185.

153. Naftchi, N. E., Demeny, M., Lowman, E. W., et al.: Hypertensive crises in quadriplegic patients: Changes in cardiac output, blood volume, serum dopamine-B-hydroxylase activity, and arterial prostaglandin PGE2. Circulation 57:336, 1978.

154. Ciliberti, B. J., Goldfein, J., and Rovenstine, E. A.: Hypertension during anesthesia in patients with spinal cord injuries. Anesthesiology 15:273, 1954.

155. Alderson, J. D., and Thomas, D. G.: The use of halothane anaesthesia to control autonomic hyperreflexia during transurethral surgery in spinal cord injury patients. Paraplegia 13:183, 1975.

156. Broecker, B. H., Hranowsky, N., and Hackler, R. H.: Low spinal anesthesia for the prevention of autonomic dysreflexia in the spinal cord injury patient. J. Urol. 122:366, 1979.

157. Bennett, E. J., Montgomery, S. J., Dalal, F. Y., et al.: Pancuronium and the fasciculations of succinylcholine. Anesth. Analg. (Cleve.) 52:892, 1973.

158. Brodsky, J. B., Brock-Utne, J. G., and Samuels, S. I.: Pancuronium pretreatment of post-succinylcholine myalgias. Anesthesiology 51:259, 1979.

159. Cullen, D. J.: The effect of pretreatment with nondepolarizing muscle relaxants on the neuromuscular blocking actions of succinylcholine. Anesthesiology 35:572, 1971.

160. Jansen, E. C., and Hansen, P. H.: Objective measurement of succinylcholine induced fasciculations and the effect of pretreatment with pancuronium or gallamine. Anesthesiology 51:159, 1979.

161. Konchigeri, H. N., and Tay, C.-H.: Influence of pancuronium on potassium efflux produced by succinylchline. Anesth. Analg. (Cleve.) 55:474, 1976.

162. Stoelting, R. K., and Peterson, C.: Adverse effects of increased succinylcholine dose following d-tubocurarine pretreatment. Anesth. Analg. (Cleve.) 54:282, 1975.

163. Hoehn, R. J.: Facial injury. Surg. Clin. North Am. 53:1479, 1973.

164. Clarke, R. S. J.: Trauma to face and neck. In Morrow, W. F. K., and Morrison, J. D. (eds.): Anaesthesia for Eye, Ear, Nose and Throat Surgery. New York, Churchill Livingstone, 1975, pp. 78-93.

165. Saletta, J. D., Folk, F. A., and Freeark, R. J.: Trauma to the neck region. Surg. Clin. North Am. 53:73, 1973.

166. Bowden, M.: Hazards of blind wiring of facial fracture. (Letter) Anesthesiology 48:79, 1978.

167. Robideaux, V.: Oculocardiac reflex caused by midface disimpaction. Anesthesiology 49:433, 1978.

168. Adams, A. P., and Fordham, R. M. M.: General anesthesia in adults. Int. Ophthalmol. Clin. 13:83, 1973.

169. Duncalf, D., and Foldes, F. F.: Effects of anesthetic drugs and muscle relaxants on intraocular pressure. Int. Ophthalmol. Clin. 13:21, 1973.

170. Elliott, J., and Morrison, J. D.: Anaesthesia for ophthalmic surgery. In Morrow, W. F. K., and Morrison, J. D. (eds.): Anaesthesia for Eye, Ear, Nose and Throat Surgery. New York, Churchill Livingstone, 1975, pp. 112-127.

171. Konchigeri, H. N., Lee, Y. E., and Venugopal, K.: Effect of pancuronium on intraocular pressure changes induced by succinylcholine. Canad. Anaesth. Soc. J. 26:479, 1979.

172. Meyers, E. F., Krupin, T., Johnson, M., et al.: Failure of non-depolarizing neuromuscular blockers to inhibit succinylcholine-induced increased intraocular pressure, a controlled study. Anesthesiology 48:149, 1978.

173. Joshi, C., and Bruce, D. L.: Thiopental and succinylcholine: Action on intraocular pressure. Anesth. Analg. (Cleve.) 54:471, 1975.

174. Whited, R. E.: Laryngeal fracture in the multiple trauma patient. Am. J. Surg. 136:354, 1978.

175. Harris, H. H., and Torbin, H. A.: Acute injuries of the larynx and trachea in 49 patients (observations over a 15 year period). Laryngoscope 80:1376, 1970.

176. Dalal, F. Y., Schmidt, G. B., Bennett, E. J., et al.: Fractures of the larynx in children. Canad. Anaesth. Soc. J. 21:376, 1974.

177. Seed, R. F.: Traumatic injury to the larynx and trachea. Anaesthesia 26:55, 1971.

178. Kirsh, M. M., Orringer, M. B., Behrendt, D. M., et al.: Management of tracheobronchial disruption secondary to nonpenetrating trauma. Ann. Thorac. Surg. 22:93, 1976.

179. Guest, J. L., and Anderson, J. N.: Major airway injury in closed chest trauma. Chest 72:63, 1977.

180. Chesterman, J. T., and Satsangi, P. W.: Rupture of the trachea and bronchi by closed injury. Thorax 21:21, 1966.

181. Collins, J. P., Ketharantham, V., and McConchie, I.: Rupture of major bronchi resulting from closed chest injuries. Thorax 28:371, 1973.

182. Kirsh, M. M., and Sloan, H.: Tracheobronchial disruption and injuries of the esophagus. In Kirsh, M. M. (ed.): Blunt Chest Trauma: Principles of Management. Boston, Little, Brown and Co., 1977, pp. 107-127.

183. McCleave, D. J., Fenwick, D. G., and MacDonald, R. R.: Management of tracheal rupture involving both bronchi. Anaesth. Intens. Care 1:53, 1975.

184. Olson, R. O., and Johnston, J. T.: Diagnosis and management of intrathoracic tracheal rupture. J. Trauma 11:789, 1971.

185. Donchin, Y., and Vered, I. Y.: Blunt trauma to the trachea. Br. J. Anaesth. 48:1113, 1976.

186. Gay, W. A., Jr., and McCabe, J. C.: Trauma to the chest. In Shires, G. T. (ed.): Care of the Trauma Patient. 2nd ed., New York, McGraw-Hill, 1979, pp. 259-289.

187. Gibbons, J., James, O., and Quail, A.: Management of 130 cases of chest injury with respiratory failure. Br. J. Anaesth. 45:1130, 1973.

188. Griffith, G. L., Todd, E. P., McMillin, R. D., et al.: Acute traumatic hemothorax. Ann. Thorac. Surg. 26:204, 1978.

189. Primm, R. K., Karp, R. B., and Schrank, J. P.: Multiple cardiovascular injuries and motor vehicle accidents. J.A.M.A. 241:2540, 1979.

190. Wilson, R. F., Murray, C., and Antonenko, D. R.: Nonpenetrating thoracic injuries. Surg. Clin. North Am. 57:17, 1977.

191. Cullen, P., Modell, J. H., Kriby, R. R., et al.: Treatment of flail chest. Use of intermittent mandatory ventilation and positive end-expiratory pressure. Arch. Surg. 110:1099, 1975.

192. Jette, N. T., and Barash, P. G.: Treatment of flail injury of the chest. Anaesthesia 33:475, 1978.

193. Trinkle, J. K., Richardson, J. D., Franz, J. L., et al.: Management of flail chest without mechanical ventilation. Ann. Thorac. Surg. 19:355, 1975.

194. Kouchoukos, N. T., Lell, W. A., Karp, R. B., et al: Hemodynamic effects of aortic clamping and decompression with a temporary shunt for resection of the descending thoracic aorta. Surgery 85:25, 1979.

195. Kirsh, M. M., and Sloan, H.: Closed injuries of the heart and pericardium. In: Blunt Chest Trauma: General Principles of Management. Boston, Little, Brown and Co., 1977, pp. 143-178.

196. Brennan, J. A., Field, J. M., and Liedtke, A. J.: Reversible heart block following non-penetrating chest trauma. J. Trauma *19*:784, 1979.

197. Leier, C. V., Heban, P. T., Huss, P., et al.: Comparative systemic and regional hemodynamic effects of dopamine and dobutamine in patients with cardiomyopathic heart failure. Circulation *58*:466, 1978.

198. Levitsky, S.: New insights in cardiac trauma. Surg. Clin. North Am. *55*(1):43, 1975.

199. Trinkle, J. K., Marcos, J., Grover, F. L., et al.: Management of the wounded heart. Ann. Thorac. Surg. *17*:230, 1974.

200. Moore, R. A., Jr., Herrin, T. J., and Wilson, R. D.: The anesthetic management of thoracic trauma. Anesthesiol. Rev. *6*:10, 1979.

201. Reddy, P. S., Curtiss, E. I., O'Toole, J. D., et al.: Cardiac tamponade: Hemodynamic observations in man. Circulation *58*:265, 1978.

202. Stephenson, H. E., Jr.: Present place of open-chest cardiac resuscitation. *In* Safar, P., and Elam, J. (eds.): Advances in Cardiopulmonary Resuscitation. New York, Springer-Verlag, 1977, pp. 102-106.

203. Stanley, T. H., and Weidauer, H. E.: Anesthesia for the patient with cardiac tamponade. Anesth. Analg. (Cleve.) *52*:110, 1973.

204. Fowler, N. O.: Physiology of cardiac tamponade and pulsus paradoxus. I: Mechanisms of pulsus paradoxus in cardiac tamponade. Mod. Conc. Cardiovasc. Dis. *47*:109, 1978.

205. Fowler, N. O.: Physiology of cardiac tamponade and pulsus paradoxus. II: Physiological, circulatory and pharmacological responses in cardiac tamponade. Mod. Conc. Cardiovasc. Dis. *47*:115, 1978.

206. Eger, E. I., II, Smith, N. T., Stoelting, R. K., et al.: Cardiovascular effects of halothane in man. Anesthesiology *32*:396, 1970.

207. Calverly, R. K., Smith, N. T., Prys-Roberts, C., et al.: Cardiovascular effects of enflurane anesthesia during controlled ventilation in man. Anesth. Analg. (Cleve.) *57*:619, 1978.

208. Kaplan, J. A.: Pericardial diseases. *In*: Cardiac Anesthesia. New York, Grune & Stratton, 1979, pp. 491-499.

209. Kaplan, M. A., Harris, C. N., Kay, J. H., et al.: Postinfarctional ventricular septal rupture: Clinical approach and surgical results. Chest *69*:734, 1976.

210. Meister, S. G., Helfant, R. H.: Rapid bedside differentiation of ruptured interventricular septum from acute mitral insufficiency. N. Engl. J. Med. *287*:1024, 1972.

211. Franch, R. H.: Cardiac catheterization. *In* Hurst, J. W., Logue, R. B., Schlant, R. C., Wenger, N. K. (eds.): The Heart. 4th ed., New York, McGraw-Hill, 1978, pp. 479-501.

212. Katz, A. M.: Application of the Starling resistor concept to the lungs during CPPV. Crit. Care Med. *5*:67, 1977.

213. Simpson, P. C., Jr., and Bristow, J. D.: Recognition and management of emergencies in valvular heart disease. Med. Clin. North Am. *63*:155, 1979.

214. Stone, J. G., Hoar, P. F., Faltas, A. N., et al.: Comparison of intraoperative nitroprusside unloading in mitral and aortic regurgitation. J. Thorac. Cardiovasc. Surg. *78*:103, 1979.

215. Chambers, D. A.: Acquired valvular heart disease. *In* Kaplan, J. A. (ed.): Cardiac Anesthesia. New York, Grune & Stratton, 1979, pp. 197-240.

216. Oliveros, R. A., Boucher, C. A., Groves, B. M., et al.: Myocardial supply-demand ratio in aortic regurgitation. Chest *76*:50, 1979.

217. Munchow, O. B. G., Carter, R., Vannix, R. S., et al.: Cardiac arrest due to ventricular herniation: Report of a case of two successful cardiac resuscitations. J.A.M.A. *173*:1350, 1960.

218. Van Stiegmann, G., Brantigan, C. O., and Hopeman, A. R.: Tension pneumomediastinum. Arch. Surg. *112*:1212, 1977.

219. Asfaw, I., and Arbulu, A.: Penetrating wounds of the pericardium and heart. Surg. Clin. North Am. *57*:37, 1977.

220. Kirsh, M. M., and Sloan, H.: Traumatic rupture of the aorta. *In*: Blunt Chest Trauma: General Principles of Management. Boston, Little, Brown and Co., 1977, pp. 179-211.

221. Turney, S. Z., Attar, S., Ayella, R., et al.: Traumatic rupture of the aorta: A five year experience. J. Thorac. Cardiovasc. Surg. *72*:727, 1975.

222. Wheat, M. W., Jr.: Treatment of dissecting aneurysms of the aorta: Current status. Prog. Cardiovasc. Dis. *16*:87, 1973.

223. Dunbar, R. W.: Thoracic aneurysms. *In* Kaplan, J. A. (ed.): Cardiac Anesthesia. New York, Grune & Stratton, 1979, pp. 369-376.

224. Lunn, J. K., Stanley, T. H., Webster, L. R., et al.: Arterial blood-pressure and pulse rate responses to pulmonary and radial arterial catheterization prior to cardiac and major vascular operations. Anesthesiology *51*:265, 1979.

225. Estrera, A. S., Platt, M. R., and Mills, L. J.: Traumatic injuries of the diaphragm. Chest *75*:306, 1979.

226. Brooks, J. W.: Blunt traumatic rupture of the diaphragm. Ann. Thorac. Surg. *26*:199, 1978.

227. Orringer, M. B., and Kirsh, M. M.: Traumatic rupture of the diaphragm. *In*: Kirsh, M. M. (ed.): Blunt Chest Trauma: General Principles of Management. Boston, Little, Brown and Co., 1977, pp. 129-141.

228. Quasha, A. L., and Pairolero, P. C.: Intraoperative diagnosis of a gastrobronchial fistula. Anesthesiology *52*:175, 1980.

229. Loehning, R. W., Takaori, M., and Safar, P.: Circulatory collapse from anaesthesia for diaphragmatic hernia. Arch. Surg. *90*:109, 1965.

230. Lobb, T. R., and Butlin, G. R.: Anaesthesia and traumatic diaphragmatic hernia. Canad. Anaesth. Soc. J. *21*:173, 1974.

231. Morrison, W. A., O'Brien, B. M., and MacLeod, A. M.: Evaluation of digital replantation — a review of 100 cases. Ortho. Clin. North Am. *8*:295, 1977.

232. Phelps, D. B., Rutherford, R. B., and Boswick, J. A., Jr.: Control of vasospasm following trauma and microvascular surgery. J. Hand Surg. *4*: 109, 1979.

233. Phelps, D. B., Lilla, J. A., and Boswick, J. A., Jr.: Common problems in clinical replantation and revascularization in the upper extremity. Clin. Orthop. Rel. Res. *133*:11, 1978.

234. O'Brien, B. M.: Replantation surgery. Clin. Plast. Surg. *1*:405, 1974.
235. Stark, D. C. C.: Aspiration in the surgical patient. Int. Anesthesiol. Clin. *15*:13, 1977.
236. Guyton, A. C.: An overall analysis of cardiovascular regulation. Anesth. Analg. (Cleve.) *56*:761, 1977.
237. Hall, G. M.: Body temperature and anaesthesia. Br. J. Anaesth. *50*:39, 1978.
238. Pflug, A. E., Aasheim, G. M., Foster, C., et al.: Prevention of post-anaesthesia shivering. Canad. Anaesth. Soc. J. *25*:43, 1978.
239. Benazon, D.: Hypothermia. *In* Scurr, C., and Feldman, S. (eds.): Scientific Foundations of Anaesthesia. Chicago, Year Book, 1974, pp. 344-357.
240. Conn, A. W., Edmonds, J. F., and Barker, G. A.: Near-drowning in cold fresh water: Current treatment regimen. Canad. Anaesth. Soc. J. *25*:259, 1978.
241. Fandel, I., and Bancalari, E.: Near drowning in children: Clinical aspects. Pediatrics *58*:573, 1976.
242. Hoff, B. H.: Multisystem failure: A review with special reference to drowning. Crit. Care Med. *7*:310, 1979.
243. Modell, J. H., Graves, S. A., and Ketover, A.: Clinical course of 91 consecutive near drowning victims. Chest *70*:231, 1976.
244. Calderwood, H. W., Modell, J. H., and Ruiz, B. C.: The ineffectiveness of steroid therapy for treatment of fresh water near-drowning. Anesthesiology *43*:642, 1975.
245. Boulton, T. B.: Anaesthesia in difficult situations: General anaesthesia-technique. Anaesthesia *21*:513, 1966.
246. Counts, H. K., Jr., Carden, W. D., and Petty, W. C.: Use of the Fluotec (R) Mark II for halothane-air anesthesia. Anesth. Analg. *52*:181, 1973.
247. Macartney, H. H.: Halothane-air anaesthesia using the "Pulmotec" apparatus: Preliminary report. Canad. Anaesth. Soc. J. *8*:281, 1961.
248. Pearson, J. W., and Safar, P.: General anesthesia with minimal equipment. Anesth. Analg. *40*:664, 1961.
249. Rybicki, Z.: Intravenous general anesthetic in abnormal conditions with controlled respiration using only air. Anaesth. Res. Int. Ther. *2*:13, 1974.

18

Anesthesia for Patients with Behavioral and Environmental Disorders

By THOMAS CALDWELL III, M.D.

Anesthetic Management of Narcotics Addicts
Medical Profile of the Narcotic Addict
Theories of Tolerance and Addiction to Narcotics
Anesthetic Management of the Narcotic Addict During Surgery
Management of the Postoperative Addict, Including Problems of Narcotic Withdrawal
Narcotic Addiction and Pregnancy
Therapy of Acute Narcotism
Anesthesia for Other Drug Abusers
Anesthesia for Patients Using CNS Depressants: Alcohol, the Barbiturates, and Other Sedatives
Medical Profile of the Alcoholic
Induction and Maintenance of Anesthesia for Patients with Acute and Chronic Alcoholism
Anesthesia for Patients Addicted to Barbiturates
Anesthesia for Patients Addicted to Miscellaneous Depressants
Anesthesia for Patients Addicted to Alcohol Derivatives, Paraldehyde, and Toxic Alcohols
Anesthetic Considerations in Patients Inhaling Poisonous Compounds: Glue (Acetone), Cleaning Fluids (Carbona), and Other Solvents
Anesthesia for Patients Using Psychedelic Drugs: Hallucinogens, Stimulants, Deliriants, Euphoriants, and Drugs Causing Psychoses
Hallucinogens
The Major Hallucinogens — LSD, Psilocybin, and Other Indoles (DMT and DET)
Anesthesia for Patients Taking Hallucinogens

The Sympathetic Hallucinogens, Nutmeg, and Mescaline
Anesthesia for Patients Taking Mescaline and TMA
Anesthetic Considerations In Patients Using Sympathomimetic Amines
Amphetamines and MAC of General Inhalational Anesthetics
Anesthetic Considerations in Patients Using Belladonna Alkaloids, Other Anticholinergics, and Cocaine
Anesthesia for Patients Intoxicated with Belladonna or with Other Anticholinergic Deliriants
Cocaine
Anesthetic Considerations in Patients Taking Cannabis (Marijuana)
The Cyclohexylamines: Methylphenidate, Phenmetrazine, and Phencyclidine (PCP)
Anesthesia for the Irradiated Patient
Effects of Whole Body Irradiation on the Patient
Effects of Irradiation on Specific Organs of Importance in Anesthesia
Effect of Irradiation on Anesthetic Mortality in Experimental Animals
Interactions of Irradiation and Drugs Used as Adjuncts During Anesthesia
Radioprotection of Normal and Neoplastic Tissue by Drugs, Anesthetics, and Physical Means
Anesthetic Management of Patients Having Therapeutic or Diagnostic Radiological Procedures
Management of Combined Trauma and Irradiation Injury
Some Conclusions

ANESTHETIC MANAGEMENT OF NARCOTICS ADDICTS

The use of drugs that alter mood or perception has become part of the lifestyle of several million Americans by the nineteen eighties. Estimates of the number of narcotics addicts range from 80,000 to 380,000.[1-5] Narcotics addicts have a high death rate — approximately one death per thousand addicts per year. Although most narcotics addicts are below age 40, this death rate approximates that of the American population in the fourth and fifth decades of life. Overdose, acute pulmonary edema, or anaphylactic reactions account for half to three quarters of the deaths from narcotics.[2, 5, 6] Narcotics addicts also have a higher incidence of trauma, sepsis, pulmonary disease, phlebitis, bacterial endocarditis, liver disease, tetanus, and obstetrical problems, although reliable data concerning the incidence of these complications still are not available.

The anesthesiologist often encounters the narcotics addict for one of the following problems: 1) anesthesia for elective or emergency surgery; 2) postoperative management of pain or of the narcotic abstinence syndrome; 3) obstetric anesthesia, including neonatal narcotic depression or abstinence syndrome; 4) resuscitation of addicts with acute respiratory failure.

Before discussing these four clinical problems, a consideration of the effects of narcotics on the major organ systems of the addicted patient and a brief review of the current theories of addiction will be presented.

MEDICAL PROFILE OF THE NARCOTIC ADDICT

Physicians treating narcotics addicts in the United States today should be aware that these patients may have diseases involving many organ systems. Addicts may have cellulitis, multiple abscesses, thrombophlebitis, bacterial endocarditis, multiple pulmonary emboli, atelectasis, pneumonia, mild anemia, adrenal suppression, chronic inflammatory changes in the liver, oligomenorrhea, amenorrhea, obstetrical complications, and tetanus. On rare occasions, they may have severe pulmonary hypertension or an acute transverse myelitis. They frequently have false positive VDRL's and an elevated fasting blood sugar, but the significance of these two abnormal laboratory findings is not clear.

Superficial Bacterial Infections. Cellulitis, superficial abscesses, and septic phlebitis are common in narcotics addicts in the United States at present. Louria reported that of 120 addicts admitted for treatment of medical complications, 21 had abscesses. Staphylococcus was the most common organism in the series.[7] Baker and coworkers recently reviewed septic phlebitis and found that 46 per cent of their cases resulted from intravenous drug abuse: heroin was the principal drug involved, although methylphenidate (Ritalin), amphetamines, and barbiturates also caused cases of phlebitis.[8] *Staphylococcus aureus* was still the most common organism, accounting for 41 per cent of the cases, while streptococcus accounted for 33 per cent, gram negative organisms (Klebsiella, Enterobacter, and Serratia) accounted for 17 per cent, and various organisms—Diphtheroids, Clostridia, Bacteroides, etc. — composed the remainder. Most of the cases of septic phlebitis in leg veins in this series resulted from drug abuse, but there were only three septic emboli in 46 cases of phlebitis due to drug abuse.[8]

Tetanus. This disease is seen mainly in black female addicts. As Cherubin pointed out, tetanus is seen mainly in "skin poppers" because the quinine used to adulterate heroin lowers the redox potential of tissues at the injection site, favoring the growth of anaerobes.[2] Louria found that of 120 addicts admitted to Bellevue Hospital for medical complications, 17 were admitted for tetanus, and nine of the 17 died.[7] Analyzing 762 narcotic addict deaths, Helpern reported that 8.3 per cent were from tetanus.[6] The mortality rate of about 75 per cent in cases of tetanus severe enough to require mechanical ventilation has been attributed mainly to the syndrome of sympathetic hyperactivity, although toxic myocarditis and intercurrent pneumonia account for some of this mortality.[9] (For the pathophysiology and therapy of tetanus, see Chapter 16).

Bacterial Endocarditis. Although localized abscesses and tetanus are more common in "skin poppers," bacterial endocarditis is common in "mainliners." As early as 1945, Hussey and Katz reported bacterial endocarditis with *Staphylococcus aureus* involving the tricuspid valve and presenting with multiple pulmonary infarcts in heroin addicts.[10] They stated that the triad of heroin addiction, positive blood cultures, and x-ray evidence of pulmonary infarction in the absence of peripheral venous disease was diagnostic of bacterial endocarditis of the tricuspid valve. Many of these patients had no tricuspid murmurs.[11] Endocarditis involving the left side of the heart was recognized by Luttgens, who discovered nine cases of aortic or mitral infections — principally with streptococcus — in "mainline" opium addicts.[12] Olsson and Romansky found evidence of systemic arterial emboli in addicts with staphylococcal tricuspid endocarditis; they postulated that the systemic emboli originated in areas of septic infarction in the pulmonary veins.[13] Oerther and coworkers reported four paregoric addicts with staphylococcal endocarditis of the mitral or aortic valves but with no tricuspid involvement.[14] Cherubin and Brown also noted mitral or aortic staphylococcal endocarditis in addicts with no apparent disease in the right side of the heart.[15]

Although *Staphylococcus aureus* is still the most frequent cause of endocarditis in heroin addicts, the incidence of endocarditis with pseudomonas has increased recently. Reyes and coworkers reported that 21 of 23 cases of pseudomonas endocarditis at the Detroit Medical Center were in heroin addicts — mostly black males.[16] Sixteen of these patients had tricuspid lesions and 15 showed septic pulmonary emboli, most of which cavitated. There were six aortic and four mitral lesions in the series, and the left atrial wall was heavily involved with vegetations in two cases. In these patients emboli to large arteries occurred; large emboli to major arteries are more frequently seen with fungal endocarditis than during bacterial endocarditis. Pseudomonas has occasionally been cultured from samples of heroin seized by the police, Reyes and coworkers noted.[16] Reyes recently reported a cure rate of over 50 per cent with antibiotic therapy.[17] Thirteen of the patients required surgery, and six of those operated on survived. Seven patients had excision of the tricuspid valve, one had excision of both

tricuspid and pulmonic valves, and four other patients had insertion of tricuspid or aortic prostheses after valvectomy. All six of the patients "cured" by tricuspid or tricuspid and pulmonic valvectomy have gone back to using heroin, and so are not candidates for prosthetic valves. They have mild limitation of activity and more right heart failure than they had preoperatively. In Reyes' series, mortality in lesions involving the left side of the heart was 89 per cent, but in lesions of the right side of the heart it was only 29 per cent.[16]

The anesthesiologist may become involved in respiratory support of addicts with multiple septic pulmonary infarction, in operations for excision of infected tricuspid valves, or in valve replacements in addicts with mitral or aortic endocarditis. The prognosis in these cases is still rather poor; survival rates of about 50 per cent can be expected.[8, 16] Because of the likelihood of reinfection from continued narcotic addiction, Carey and Hughes suggested that valve replacement be done in narcotic addicts only if death from congestive heart failure is imminent.[18]

Pulmonary Disease. Narcotic addicts are subject to several types of pulmonary diseases besides septic pulmonary infarctions. The syndrome of acute pulmonary edema and tachypnea immediately after an intravenous injection will be discussed in the section on treatment of narcotic overdose. Narcotic addicts are prone to develop bacterial pneumonia, atelectasis, and occasionally foreign body emboli or severe pulmonary hypertension. In Louria's series, 14 of 100 addicts with medical complications had bacterial pneumonia.[7] The organisms were mainly pneumococci, but five cases were caused by gram positive cocci, and one each by *Hemophilus influenzae* and by *Klebsiella aerobacter*. Since none of these cases followed an acute narcotic overdose or a known episode of aspiration, Louria suspected an association between chronic addiction and pneumonia.[7] Cherubin and Brown reported 13 bronchial pneumonias involving the lower lobe and suggested that these pneumonias occur in regions of the lungs affected by pulmonary edema in addicts.[15]

Asymptomatic atelectasis has been reported in 14 "mainline" addicts by Gelfand and coworkers.[19] On physical examination these addicts were apathetic and mentally "foggy." Chest x-rays showed platelike atelectasis one to three cm above the diaphragm, unilaterally or bilaterally. Although these authors could not rule out asymptomatic pulmonary infarction with scarring, they thought such an explanation unlikely and noted that Egbert and Bendixen had demonstrated a high incidence of atelectasis resulting from morphine in postoperative patients.[9, 20] Perhaps pneumonia in narcotic addicts begins in atelectatic regions of the lung.

Wendt and coworkers reported severe pulmonary hypertension with "blue velvet" addiction in Detroit. "Blue velvet" is a mixture of paregoric and tripelennamine (Pyribenzamine), an antihistamine which may contain citrate salts, wax, or talc.[21, 22] Embolization and thrombosis of the pulmonary vasculature is thought to result in pulmonary hypertension.[21] Spain reported occasional cotton fiber granulomas in the lungs of heroin addicts.[23] The "opium lung," which has a ground glass appearance in the lower lobes and results from heavy smoking of opium, thus far has been reported only in Asia.[24]

Sapira and coworkers studied respiratory function during a 34 week period of experimental addiction to morphine, 240 mg per day.[25] Pulmonary functions were done after the first month of addiction (the early stabilization period) and after the fifth month (late stabilization). They found that minute alveolar ventilation was significantly decreased early in the course of addiction ($p<0.01$), and arterial P_{CO_2} tended to be higher than during the control period. Carbon dioxide production was decreased early in addiction. The arterial oxygen saturation was significantly decreased during the entire period of addiction. After five months of addiction the arterial P_{CO_2} significantly increased ($p<0.02$), since carbon dioxide production increased. These changes are shown in Figure 18–1.[25] Martin and coworkers also studied the carbon dioxide

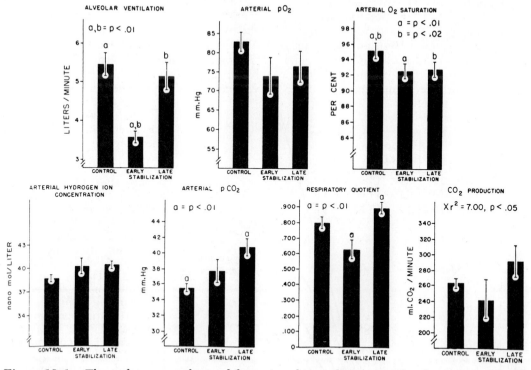

Figure 18–1. These data were obtained from six subjects during a cycle of experimental addiction to 240 mg. per day of morphine. The control values are the means of two preaddiction samples. The early stabilization values were from the first month, and the late stabilization values from the fifth month. Although the respiratory rate was depressed throughout the stabilization period, note the many parameters which changed between early and late stabilization, including alveolar ventilation. (From Sapira, J. D.: Amer. J. Med. 45:565, 1968.)

response curves in the same experimental subjects.[26] Addiction to morphine shifted the carbon dioxide response curve to the right and slightly flattened its slopes. This decrease in sensitivity to carbon dioxide persisted from the first through the eighth month of addiction. Sixteen to 20 hours following the abrupt withdrawal of morphine, there was a sudden increase in sensitivity of the respiratory center to carbon dioxide (Fig. 18–2). This hypersensitivity of the respiratory center to carbon dioxide disappeared by seven weeks following the withdrawal of narcotics. Martin and coworkers noted that respiratory rate did stay depressed all during the 34 weeks of addiction to morphine. They also noted considerable variation among individual subjects.[26]

Liver Disease. Hepatitis is the most common medical complication in narcotics addicts that necessitates hospitalization, according to Cherubin.[2] In Louria's series, hepatitis was the admitting diagnosis in 42 per cent of the patients.[7] In the series, 15 of 42 patients had SGOT's over 1000 and 17 had bilirubins over 10 mg per 100 ml. Sapira noted that 30 per cent of narcotics addicts admitted at Lexington have enlarged, firm, nontender livers.[25] Marks and Chapple, surveying 89 heroin addicts, found that 80 per cent had one or more abnormal liver func-

tion tests, 7 per cent were jaundiced, 69 per cent had SGPT elevations, 61 per cent had SGOT elevations, and 28 per cent had abnormal alkaline phosphatase values.[27] Norris and Potter found histologic abnormalities in 27 of 36 narcotics addicts they biopsied. The changes ranged from mild lymphocytic or monocytic infiltration of the portal triads to severe fibrous tissue "bridging" between the triads. Fatty changes in hepatocytes, active bile duct proliferation, and bile casts in small ducts were present in severe cases. Norris and Potter favored viral hepatitis as an explanation for these changes.[2] However, Kaplan noted that only one third of the addicts in most series in the literature had a history of hepatitis. He pointed out that the incidence of subacute hepatic necrosis in narcotics addicts was too small to explain the frequency of liver abnormalities and suggested that poor diet might explain some of these abnormalities.[29] Norkrans and coworkers reported a 10 per cent incidence of hepatitis in drug addicts during a four year period. Hepatitis A caused 32 per cent of the episodes, and Hepatitis B caused 42 per cent of the episodes, while 25 per cent were not caused by either Hepatitis A or B viruses. Cytomegalovirus and Epstein-Barr virus were excluded by serologic tests. A third type of hepatitis virus appears to be involved, and Norkrans

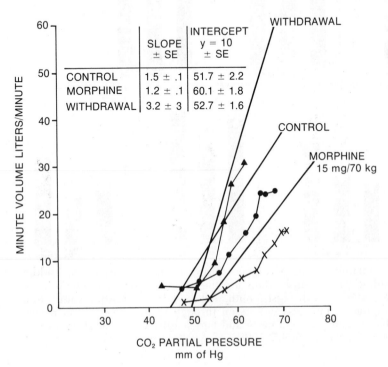

Figure 18–2. Mean calculated regression lines for $paCO_2$-VA response curves obtained during the control period, after 15 mg/70 kg of morphine, and during early withdrawal in subjects dependent on 240 mg/day of morphine. The means for each parameter were determined from values obtained in seven subjects. There was great variability in the first and last points of the response curves. The top of the regression lines represents the maximum VA obtained. A control (●), a 15 mg/70 kg dose of morphine (×), and a withdrawal (▲) $paCO_2$-VA response of one subject are presented to further illustrate these changes. (From Martin, W. R., et al.: J. Pharmacol. Expl. Ther.: 62:182, 1968.)

Figure content:

	SLOPE ± SE	INTERCEPT y = 10 ± SE
CONTROL	1.5 ± .1	51.7 ± 2.2
MORPHINE	1.2 ± .1	60.1 ± 1.8
WITHDRAWAL	3.2 ± 3	52.7 ± 1.6

MINUTE VOLUME LITERS/MINUTE

CO₂ PARTIAL PRESSURE
mm of Hg

WITHDRAWAL
CONTROL
MORPHINE 15 mg/70 kg

and coworkers doubt a toxic or nonviral etiology for the non-A and non-B cases.[30] Whatever the cause of liver disease in narcotic addicts, the anesthesiologist must be aware that hepatic problems are frequently present in these patients and must chose his anesthetic agent appropriately.

Adrenal. Narcotic addiction appears to suppress adrenal cortical function by decreasing pituitary secretion of ACTH. Eisenman and coworkers found that during experimental addiction to morphine, plasma and urine 17-hydoxycorticosteroids fell to about half normal values. During addiction, plasma 17-hydroxycorticosteroids fell from 16 to 8 gamma per cent, and urine corticosteroids fell from 7.40 to 3.49 mg per 24 hours (p<0.01). The rate of disappearance of radioactive cortisone from plasma was not changed by morphine addiction, and exogenous ACTH was able to increase plasma and urine 17-hydroxycorticosteroid values in addicts. During withdrawal from narcotics, urine and plasma hydroxycorticosteroids are greatly elevated.[31]

Central Nervous System. Except for arterial embolism to the brain in narcotic addicts with endocarditis, the most serious neurological complication is a rare transverse myelitis. Richter and Rosenberg reported myelitis in four patients with more than a 10 year history of narcotic addiction. All four had resumed the use of narcotics just prior to the onset of myelitis. Paraplegia with loss of pain, temperature, vibration, and position sense occurred. Cerebrospinal fluid and serology were normal. One of two patients who died, when autopsied, showed necrosis of both gray and white matter of the spinal cord, but the anterior spinal artery was patent and there was no evidence of arteritis. Richter and Rosenberg favored an allergic cause but could not rule out hypotension from narcotic overdose.[32]

Meperidine in large doses and in persons who have taken monoamine oxidase inhibitors within two weeks can cause convulsions and coma. Meperidine addicts can have grand mal convulsions during withdrawal; but seizures are more likely due to a mixed addiction, resulting from withdrawal of a barbiturate or other CNS depressant drug.[25] Stupor, dysarthria, and ataxia in narcotic addicts also favor a diagnosis of barbiturate intoxication. Depression of flexor and crossed extensor reflexes can occur with large doses of narcotics; these same reflexes become hyperactive during withdrawal. Hence the phrase "kicking the habit." Heroin, morphine, and codeine cause miosis, whereas meperidine may have little effect on the pupils or may cause mydriasis. It is worth emphasizing that except for the depression of the flexor and crossed extensor reflexes, addicts on maintenance doses of narcotics have no significant neurological signs or symptoms.

False Positive Serologies. Although venereal disease is common among narcotic addicts, the incidence of false positive serologies is also very high. Between a quarter and a third of addicts admitted to Lexington have positive VDRL's, but only 26.6 per cent of these are true positives.[25] Boak and coworkers reported that 94.8 per cent of 172 VDRL-positive addicts were negative when tested with *Treponema pallidum* immobilization serum.[33] Harris and Andrei, in 150 female addicts with positive serologies, found that 42 per cent were true positives.[34] The false positives did not correlate with high transaminase levels or with abnormal serum electrophoresis. In choosing an anesthetic technique, the physician should be aware that many narcotics addicts have positive serologies, but that the majority of these do not imply the presence of syphilis.

Miscellaneous Abnormalities. During experimental addiction to 500 mg of morphine per day in six adult males, Isbell found slight decreases in hemoglobin of 0.5 to 1.9 grams per 100 ml and hematocrit decreases of 3.0 to 8.5 per cent. These changes indicated a mild anemia.[35] Cherubin and Sapira found elevated glucose tolerance tests among narcotics addicts.[2, 25] Hyperglycemia due to morphine is inconstant in man; in animals it appears to be mediated by receptors near the foramen of Monro that trigger the secretion of epinephrine from the adrenal medulla, resulting in elevation of blood sugar.[36] An elevated blood glucose or a positive glucose tolerance test in a narcotic addict does not necessarily indicate diabetes mellitus.

THEORIES OF TOLERANCE AND ADDICTION TO NARCOTICS

A very brief summary of the theories of tolerance and addiction might be useful to the anesthesiologist who has to treat narcotics addicts. Some knowledge of the distribution of narcotics within the body must precede any discussion of these theories.

Heroin (diacetylmorphine) is rapidly metabolized to 6-monoacetyl morphine and then to morphine, which is an organic base. The 6-monoacetyl morphine and morphine itself are less polar compounds than heroin and can pass into the brain tissue more readily than the diacetyl form.[37] At pH 7.4, between 2 and 14 per cent of morphine is in the undissociated form. Only a minute fraction of the morphine administered enters the brain. Mice given 2 mg per kg of morphine have brain levels of only 0.04 to 0.09 μg per kg of brain tissue an hour after administration, whereas concentrations in blood, liver, and kidney are six to 80 times this amount.[38]

Way and Adler, in 1960, reviewed the evidence for increased detoxication of morphine during addiction and concluded that the observed increases are inadequate to account for tolerance to morphine.[38] Since this review, research into mechanisms of addiction and tolerance has focused on changes in the central nervous system. Important advances toward understanding the actions of narcotics within the central nervous system have occurred through tracer studies localizing sites of action of narcotics in brain, through micropipet techniques enabling the placement of small amounts of drugs at various sites in the brain, and through microelectrode techniques, by which the activity of single neurons can be measured. Studies with naloxone, a narcotic antagonist that blocks some opiate receptors, and with optical isomers of morphine have led to the realization that several different types of opiate receptors mediating different actions of morphine are present in brain. At least one opiate receptor has been identified, although its chemical composition and configuration are still not known. Finally, the discovery of the endorphins and enkephalins — opiatelike substances found in the pituitary, brain, and gastrointestinal tract in man and animals — has contributed greatly to an understanding of the effects of narcotics on the central nervous system. The following topics are of importance: 1) the effects of narcotics on the activity of single neurons; 2) evidence for opiate receptors in the brain; 3) narcotic analgesia, sedation, and tolerance within the central nervous system; 4) localization of and mechanisms for the narcotic abstinence syndrome; and 5) the effects of narcotics on acetylcholine and catecholamines in the brain.

1. Narcotic effects on single neurons. Satoh and coworkers recorded spontaneous firing rates in the sensory and motor cortex of rats.[39] In rats not dependant on narcotics, low doses of morphine applied microelectrophoretically to the neurons cause depression of spontaneous discharge activity. This depression could be antagonized by naloxone, which itself has no effect on spontaneous neuronal discharge rates in naive animals. With higher doses of morphine or with repeated doses, morphine increased rates of spontaneous firing of neurons. In chronically morphinized rats, morphine caused little or no depressant effect but instead caused an excitation or increase in spontaneous discharge rate. This excitation could not be antagonized by naloxone.[39] Thus, morphine appears to have both depressing and stimulating effects on neurons, depending on the dose and the time course of administration; and naloxone appears to block the depressing effects of morphine but not the stimulating effects.

2. Evidence for opiate receptors. Pert and Snyder first demonstrated binding of tritiated naloxone to receptors in neural tissue in 1973. They showed that the greatest amount of naloxone was bound in the microsomal fraction of brain homogenates, that the corpus striatum had four times more opiate receptors than the cortex, and that the cerebellum had no opiate receptors.[40] Lowney and coworkers, using ^{14}C levorphanol or ^{14}C dextrophan, found that these narcotics were stereospecifically bound in the rhombencephalon near the fourth ventricle in mice. The crude mitrochondrial and crude microsomal fractions of neural tissue contained most of the labeled narcotics. From these they isolated a lipoprotein-narcotic complex with a maximum molecular weight of 60,000 daltons.[41] Jacquet and coworkers made a stereoisomer of morphine that was identical to morphine chromatographically and spectroscopically but was opposite to it in optical rotation. The dextro (+) morphine they made had only 1/10,000 the ability of levo (−) morphine to displace ^3H dihydromorphine from binding sites in rat brain homogenates, and was a hundred times weaker than levomorphine in inhibiting contractions in guinea pig ileum. They found that injection of 10 μg of (−) morphine or of small doses of endorphin into the periaqueductal gray in mice causes pronounced analgesia, but that injection of 10 μg (+) morphine into the same region causes explosive motor behavior. Naloxone did not block the hyperactivity caused by optically (+) morphine. Nor did naloxone, 10 mg per kg, intraperitoneally prevent death from respiratory failure in mice given (+) morphine. Jacquet and coworkers postulated two classes of opiate receptors: first, receptors that are stereospecific, that mediate morphine analgesia, and that are blocked by naloxone; and second, a class of receptors that are *not* stereospecific, that mediate hyperexcitability of morphine at several sites in the central nervous system, and that are not blocked by naloxone.[42] In subhuman primates, Kuhar and coworkers found the greatest concentration of opiate receptors in the amygdala, and the next highest concentration in the periaqueductal gray, followed by the hypothalamus, the medial thalamus, and the head of the caudate nucleus. The frontal cortex had more opiate receptors than the pre- and post-central gyri. They also noted that in two human brains tested, the pattern of distribution of opiate receptors resembled that of subhuman primates.[43] Thus, the opiate receptors are not distributed evenly in brain tissue but are found in specific regions of the central nervous system in both animal and man.

3. *Analgesia, sedation, and tolerance within the CNS.* Kuhar and coworkers injected morphine stereotaxically into living primates and found that the analgesic response to morphine was limited to areas near the third and fourth ventricles, namely the mesencephalic and ventral diencephalic areas.[43] Jacquet and coworkers also found that marked analgesia resulted from injection of morphine into the mesencephalic periaqueductal gray areas.[42] Peters and Klemm measured multiple unit activity in rabbit brains following morphine 10, 20, and 30 mg per kg intramuscularly twice daily for three days.[44] They found the greatest depression of activity in the caudate nucleus and in the dorsal hippocampus. They suggested that these regions may play a role in the sedative or euphoric action of morphine.[44] Jacquet and Lajtha noted the rapid development of tolerance to the lethal effect of morphine in the periaqueductal gray matter. An initial dose of 40 μg of morphine injected there was fatal to half the rats given that dose; but if this dose were preceded by a dose of 20 μg injected into the periaqueductal gray matter, no rats died from the 40 μg dose. They emphasize that peripheral metabolism of opiates and changes in the blood brain barrier are not involved in tolerance to narcotics.[45] The medial thalamus also plays a part in tolerance to narcotics. Following creation of lesions in the medial thalamus of rats addicted to morphine, the rats became sleepy and lost their righting reflexes when subsequent doses of morphine were given. The medial thalamic lesions caused a dramatic reduction in the tolerance to morphine.

Teitelbaum and coworkers doubt that tolerance to narcotics is a generalized phenomenon in the central nervous system.[46] Isbell notes that inhibitors of protein synthesis such as actinomycin D or cycloheximide apparently can block the development of tissue tolerance to morphine.[3] Some years ago, Seevers and Woods proposed a "receptor occupation" theory to explain tolerance, stating that a given number of receptors for narcotics are available in the central nervous system. A narcotic exerts its effect as it occupies these receptors, and further increases in dose have little or no effect after most receptors are occupied. Supporting this thesis are the logarithmic types of dose response curves observed for analgesia and the fact that acute tolerance caused by massive intravenous doses of morphine could be explained by maximal occupation of the receptors.[47] It may well be that more opiate receptors are formed as tolerance develops, since inhibitors of protein synthesis apparently can block the development of tolerance.[3] Collier proposed the induction of "silent receptors" — receptors whose occupation by a narcotic molecule exerts no physiologic effect — as an explanation for tolerance to narcotics.[48] Although considerable information about tolerance to narcotics is available at present, still more research is needed to explain the phenomenon of tolerance.

4. *The narcotic abstinence syndrome.* Wei and coworkers studied naloxone precipitated abstinence in rats addicted to mor-

phine.[49] They applied 0.04 to 0.2 mg doses of naloxone to various regions of the brain via small implanted cannulae and looked for such signs of narcotic abstinence as wet shakes and escape behavior. They found that sites for abstinence were mainly in the medial thalamus and in medial areas of the diencephalic-mesencephalic junction. The neocortex, hippocampus, corpus striatum, and tectum were not as sensitive to naloxone abstinence.[49] Kuhar and coworkers confirmed these observations.[43]

Peters and Klemm suggested that the increase in multiple unit activity in the medial thalamus during addiction to morphine might indicate that this region participates in the narcotic abstinence syndrome.[44] Jacquet and Lajtha found that injection of morphine, 10 μg, bilaterally into the periaqueductal gray caused hyperactivity in naive rats.[45] Cheney and Goldstein found that the smaller the degree of dependence upon narcotics, the more naloxone needed to precipitate abstinence, and also showed that dependence with levorphanol does not develop if the drug is given only every 12 hours (Fig. 18–3).[50] Teitelbaum and coworkers found that the narcotic abstinence syndrome did not last as long in rats with ablative lesions in the medial thalamus as it did in animals without those lesions.[46] Jacquet and coworkers suggested that blockade of the stereospecific opiate receptors (receptors accommodating naloxone), while the nonspecific receptors remained unblocked, might cause the precipitated abstinence syndrome.[42] Jacquet et al. and Stevens and Klemm point out the resemblance between the abstinence syndrome precipitated by naloxone and the abstinence syndrome produced by deprivation of narcotics in addicted animals.[42, 51]

Stevens and Klemm hypothesize that in abstinence precipitated by naloxone the effects result from agonistic action of the narcotic on nonspecific opiate receptors, while during withdrawal of addicted animals from narcotics the effects are indirect. In naive mice given large doses of naloxone (175 mg/kg), abstinence behavior appeared after morphine, 50 mg per kg, was administered.[51] The work of Jacquet and his coworkers appears to explain the abstinence syndrome produced by the stereospecific narcotic antagonist naloxone. Whether Stevens and Klemm's hypothesis will explain the withdrawal syndrome that occurs when animals are deprived of narcotics remains to be seen.

5. *Effects of narcotics on acetylcholine and catechols in the brain.* As early as 1936 Bernheim and Bernheim discovered that morphine in concentrations of 1:30,000 inhibited by 50 per cent the action of acetylcholinesterase.[52] Wikler suggested that the morphine abstinence syndrome resulted from a surplus of acetylcholine in the central nervous system.[53] However, Young et al. and Foldes et al., using many narcotic and narcotic antagonists, were unable to show any correlation of anticholinesterase activity and analgesia.[54, 55] Domino et al. point out that although morphine does inhibit CNS acetylcholinesterase and acetylcholine transferase activity, its principal action is to reduce acetylcholine release from the cortex. The early reduction of acetylcholine release corresponds temporally with the sedative or depressant action of morphine, and can be blocked by naloxone, whereas the later stimulant action of morphine corresponds with increased utilization of acetylcholine in the cortex.[56] More research is needed to discover how the

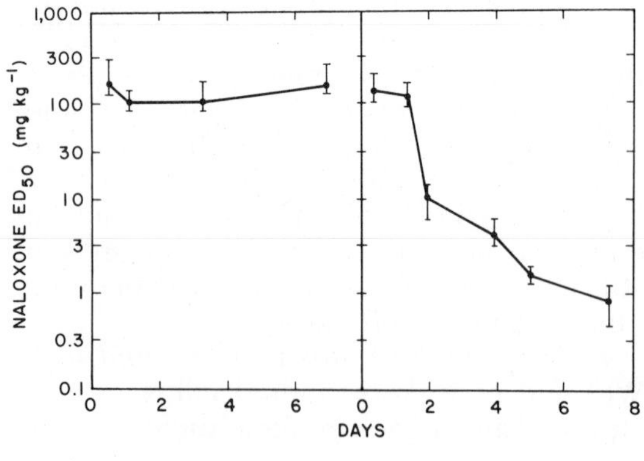

Figure 18–3. Development of physical dependence on 12 hour (left) and four hour (right) schedules of levorphanol injections (20 mg/kg^{-1}). Groups were tested with several concentrations of naloxone 12 hours or four hours, respectively, after the previous injection of levorphanol to determine the ED$_{50}$ values for naloxone-induced jumping. (From Cheney, D. L., and Goldstein, A.: Nature 232:477, 1971.)

effects of narcotics on brain acetylcholine fit into the theories of tolerance and addiction to narcotics currently being developed.

Narcotics also affect brain catechol metabolism. Maynert and Klingman suggest that tolerance to morphine may be related to an increased synthesis of catecholamines in brain, and that the severity of the narcotic abstinence syndrome is directly proportional to the rate of release of catechols.[57] A rapid drop in brain norepinephrine in cats during withdrawal or after treatment with nalorphine was discovered by Quinn and Brodie.[58] Verri and coworkers found that reserpine pretreatment abolished the analgesic effect of morphine in rats.[59] Iwamoto and coworkers found an increase in dopamine levels in the corpus striatum during naloxone precipitated withdrawal in mice addicted to morphine.[60] Physostigmine blocked the increase in dopamine levels and prevented the withdrawal jumping response. Reserpine pretreatment lowered brain dopamine levels but did not prevent either the rise in dopamine levels or the jumping response following naloxone administration. Brain noradrenaline and serotonin levels showed no changes in these experiments.[60] Smith and coworkers also found that morphine decreases the catecholamine content of brain tissue in mice, but that with repeated doses of morphine, a tolerance to this catecholamine depleting effect develops and can be blocked by naloxone.[61] Smith and his group also found that morphine increased the incorporation of ^{14}C tyrosine into norepinephrine by 106 per cent and into dopamine by 117 per cent. Yet, while morphine increased the uptake of labeled tyrosine, it also decreased the tissue content of dopamine and norepinephrine. Hence, it must increase catechol turnover. They noted the largest increases in the uptake of tyrosine in the corpus striatum and the cerebral cortex. There was considerable uptake in the diencephalon but very little in the cerebellum. Naloxone prevented the increases in uptake of labeled tyrosine. Morphine did not cause increases in tyrosine uptake by heart muscle or spleen.[61]

That brain catechols play a very important part in the narcotic abstinence syndrome is evident from the recent work of Gold and coworkers. They reported that the use of clonidine hydrochloride, an alpha-2 adren-ergic agonist, markedly reduced symptoms of withdrawal from maintenance methadone in 10 patients. They gave clonidine, 17 μg per kg per day in divided doses for a two week period, after abrupt discontinuation of methadone. The clonidine significantly ameliorated the withdrawal symptoms. Gold and his group hypothesize that clonidine replaces the narcotic mediated inhibition with an alpha-2 adrenergic inhibition of the same cells in the central nervous system whose hyperactivity causes the abstinence syndrome.[62] Gold, Redmond, and coworkers have found evidence during studies in subhuman primates that both morphine and clonidine inhibit electrical and pharmacological activation of the locus coeruleus.[63, 64] Aghajanian has also observed the depressant effect of morphine and clonidine on the neurons of the locus coeruleus.[65] Gold and coworkers have suggested that narcotic withdrawal may be due in part to increased noradrenergic activity in regions of the brain whose activity is inhibited either by narcotics via opiate receptors or by clondine through alpha-2 adrenergic receptors.[62]

ANESTHETIC MANAGEMENT OF THE NARCOTIC ADDICT DURING SURGERY

There is still fairly general agreement that the operative and postoperative period is not the proper time to withdraw an addict from narcotics. Adriani and Morton advocated giving the patient his usual maintenance dose of narcotic before surgery, and pointed out that this dose may be considerably more than the 8 to 10 mg of morphine given unaddicted patients as premedication.[66] Giuffrida and coworkers recommended either completing withdrawal prior to surgery or waiting until afterward to do so.[67] At Lexington, for addicts recently withdrawn, promazine, 25 mg, meperidine, 50 mg, and scopolamine, 0.4 mg, have been used as premedication.[68] In addicts who have had heroin less than three hours prior to operation and in addicts showing signs of respiratory depression, Giuffrida and his group recommend using only atropine as a premedication.[67] For addicts who are not fully withdrawn and who have not had heroin shortly before surgery, the narcotic dose should be greatly increased. Demerol, even in large doses, may not completely contract the abstinence syndrome in preoperative heroin or morphine addicts. Methadone will completely suppress the abstinence syndrome and is a good premedication for addicts, especially for long surgical procedures, because it is excreted slowly. For an addict showing signs of withdrawal, such as diaphoresis, lacrimation, mydriasis, piloerection, or tremors, 10 mg of intramuscular methadone is a reasonable premedication. If this dose is insufficient, another 5 to 10 mg may be given safely after one hour. With methadone, peak brain levels occur one to two hours after parenteral administration. One rarely needs to exceed 20 mg of methadone every 12 hours to suppress the abstinence syndrome, even in addicts with very large habits.[69] A few authors recommend higher doses; Giuffrida and his group often start with 20 to 40 mg of methadone, but rarely if ever exceed 80 mg per day, since much of the presently available heroin is quite adulterated.[67]

Should the anesthesiologist desire to switch the addict to methadone, he or she may find Table 18-1 useful. If the addict's preoperative dose and time schedule for maintenance on narcotics is known, the anesthesiologist can simply continue it during the surgical and recovery periods. Pentazocine should be avoided, since it is a mild narcotic antagonist and may cause the abstinence syndrome.[3, 67] An addict who has already been withdrawn from narcotics should not be premedicated with a narcotic

Table 18-1*

1 mg methadone equals:

    1 mg heroin†
    3 mg morphine†
    4 mg opium alkaloids (Pantopon)
    1 mg racemorphine (Dromoran)
    0.5 mg dihydromorphinone (Dilaudid)
    0.5 mg levorphanol (Levo-Dromoran)
    20 mg meperidine (Demerol)
    30 mg codeine
    0.3 cc laudanum (1% morphine)
    7–8 cc paregoric (0.4 mg morphine/cc)

*From Blachly, P. H.: Amer. J. Psychiat. 122:742, 1966. Copyright 1966, the American Psychiatric Association.

†Jaffe (in Goodman, L. S., and Gilman, A.: The Pharmacological Basis of Therapeutics, 3rd ed., 1965, p. 303) lists 1 mg methadone equivalent to 2 mg heroin or 4 mg morphine.

unless considerable postoperative pain is anticipated after a brief surgical procedure.

The addict who is correctly premedicated should present few problems related to narcotic abuse before or during operation. In the series of Giuffrida and coworkers, only 12 of 106 heroin addicts were agitated preoperatively, only 18 of 106 had any symptoms of withdrawal preoperatively or postoperatively, and during operation itself there were no complications related to drug abuse. Their series consisted of 54 superficial, 44 abdominal, 30 orthopedic, and 11 other cases mainly in narcotics addicts. Of their cases, 14 were for blunt trauma, 15 for gunshot wounds, and 10 for stabbings.[67]

Narcotic addicts may have some tendency toward preoperative hypotension. Although hypotension is not mentioned as a problem in most series, Eiseman et al. reported that healthy young addicts may have preoperative blood pressures as low as 50/20 mg Hg.[68] In 280 addicts who were normotensive on the ward, the mean preoperative systolic pressure was 56 mm Hg. Omission of promazine from the premedication and use of atropine instead of scopolamine made no difference in the preinduction blood pressure. Eiseman et al. had no satisfactory explanation for the hypotension they observed. Although the author has often seen young addicts with preinduction systolic pressures of 75 to 90 mm Hg, Eiseman's observation seems remarkable.

Choice of Anesthesia. General, regional, or local anesthesia may be used in narcotic addicts. The series of Giuffrida and coworkers described 145 general, 27 regional, and 9 local anesthetics in 139 patients — mainly heroin addicts, but including some patients taking other narcotics as well as ethyl alcohol, tranquilizers, and amphetamines.

Regional anesthesia — spinal, epidural, or caudal — may be used in narcotic addicts for surgery on the legs, perineum, or lower abdomen, provided that the patient has an adequate blood volume and blood pressure, and provided that he has a negative VDRL (or a positive VDRL with a negative TPI test). Transverse myelitis with paraparesis, paraplegia, and sensory changes has been reported in patients with long histories of heroin addiction who have recently resumed the habit.[31] Spinal anesthesia would appear to be contraindicated in patients with such a history who show evidence of weakness or sensory loss in the lower extremities. Spinal anesthesia is relatively contraindicated in addicts with serologic evidence of syphilis, and is definitely contraindicated if unexplained paresthesias or sensory deficits are present in the lower extremities. If a peripheral neuritis or phlebitis from injection of irritating or contaminated narcotic mixtures is present in an arm or leg, axillary or sciatic block would be ill advised.

Narcotics addicts tolerate general anesthesia very well. Years ago, the group at Lexington used mainly cyclopropane and occasionally diethyl ether because of low preinduction blood pressures in their patients.[68] Giuffrida and coworkers employed mainly cyclopropane and halothane for general anesthesia in their series, although they managed a few patients with methoxyflurane, diethyl ether, or nitrous oxide with supplements. Although 68 of their 145 general anesthetics were done with halothane, Giuffrida and his group recommended avoiding halothane in narcotic addicts because of the frequency of liver disease in these people.[63] In addicts with deranged preoperative liver functions, the anesthesiologist should avoid using halothane. One must be aware that addicts whose preoperative liver functions are normal may have recently acquired serum hepatitis. Halothane may be employed in narcotics addicts in cases where its advantages outweigh the problems that can occur if liver disease develops postoperatively. In thoracic or neurological procedures or in surgery involving the neck or the airway, the advantage of halothane may justify its use. Enflurane appears preferable to halothane as a general anesthetic agent in narcotics addicts. The author has utilized it in these patients over the past seven years and has encountered no hepatic problems with this agent. Trichlorethylene should not be used in addicts because of its hepatic toxicity. Fluoroxene is probably acceptable for use in addicts, although there is some evidence of liver damage resulting from repeated use of this agent in certain species of animals. For a few addicts receiving valve surgery because of bacterial endocarditis, the author has used large doses of intravenous morphine — up to 3 mg per kg — supplement-

ed with barbiturates and no more than 50 per cent nitrous oxide. No signs of withdrawal appeared during operation. The addicts were maintained on methadone postoperatively and were withdrawn from it after recovering from surgery.

Eiseman and coworkers had the impression that narcotic addicts needed higher doses of anesthetic agents than unaddicted persons of the same age and size. They noted that a 20 minute dilatation and curettage might require 1000 to 1500 mg of thiopental.[68] However, Giuffrida reported that only 100 to 400 mg of thiopental were necessary for induction of 123 of the 145 patients receiving general anesthesia in his series. Eleven patients needed as much as 450 to 600 mg of thiopental for induction.[67] Adriani and Morton note that inductions in narcotic addicts, unlike those in alcoholics, do not have a prolonged excitement period.[66] The use of barbiturates or tranquilizers by narcotics addicts can increase the dose of thiopental needed for induction. For one patient in Giuffrida's series, general anesthesia was chosen instead of regional because the patient was showing signs of severe narcotic abstinence preoperatively.

Maintenance of Anesthesia. Hypotension can develop during maintenance of general anesthesia in addicts because of inadequate levels of narcotic in the nervous system or because of adrenal insufficiency. More common causes of hypotension — hypovolemia and anesthetic overdose — should be ruled out before attributing hypotension to a narcotic withdrawal syndrome or to a lack of steroids.

Mark reported two cases of intraoperative hypotension in narcotic addicts.[70] In one case, a pneumonectomy under halothane–nitrous oxide–oxygen anesthesia, blood pressure dropped to 40/0 mm Hg and did not respond to intravenous epinephrine or methoxamine. Immediately after morphine sulfate, 10 mg intravenously, pressure rose to 106/50 mm Hg. This sequence occurred twice during the case. In the second case, an appendectomy under cyclopropane anesthesia in a patient on maintenance levorphanol tartrate, a blood pressure drop from 130/80 to 100/60 mm Hg was accompanied by diaphoresis and jerking motions of the legs. Levorphanol tartrate, 1 or 2 mg intravenously, restored the pressure and eliminated the signs of narcotic withdrawal. In both cases the patient's maintenance narcotic dose was known.[70] The preoperative use of an adequate dose of methadone — which has a therapeutic action lasting up to 12 hours — should nearly eliminate hypotension due to withdrawal syndrome during general anesthesia in narcotics addicts. Giuffrida and coworkers point out that in their series there were no complications related to narcotic addiction during surgery in 145 cases done with general anesthesia.[67]

Steroids may be useful in the hypotensive addict who fails to respond to volume replacement, narcotics, and vasopressors. Tinckler and Bartham believe there is probably an association between chronic opium addiction and subnormal function of the adrenal cortex.[24] As noted earlier in this section, Eisenman et al. found that 17-hydroxycorticosteroid values in plasma and urine dropped to about half of previous control values during a cycle of chronic addiction to morphine in man.[31] Prophylactic use of steroids in narcotic addicts is probably unnecessary. If hypotension from adrenal insufficiency does develop during anesthesia, it should respond within 15 minutes to hydrocortisone, 100 mg, given intravenously. In older addicts Eiseman used intravenous methoxamine 10 mg prophylactically, although he claims that addicts tolerate hypotension well.[68] The few addicts with systolic pressure below 90 mm Hg to whom the author has given enflurane, halothane, or methoxyflurane have shown little change in blood pressure during and after induction of anesthesia and have tolerated these potent agents well.

The use of curare, pancuronium, and succinylcholine presents no particular problems in narcotic addicts. Renal and hepatic function are nearly always adequate for the excretion of curare and pancuronium and for the production of pseudocholinesterase.

The anesthesiologist should be aware that addicts may have a decreased red cell mass. Isbell found reductions of 0.5 to 1.9 gm per 100 ml in hemoglobin values during experimental morphine addiction in man.[34]

Obtaining an adequate intravenous line is often difficult in narcotic addicts. While gas inductions may be done if the patient has an empty stomach, and the intravenous catheter inserted after induction, Giuffrida and coworkers recommend that an intravenous route be secured prior to induction of anesthesia, by cutdown if necessary.[67] A catheter can usually be inserted in the subclavian or internal jugular vein under local anesthesia with minimal discomfort to the patient.

MANAGEMENT OF THE POSTOPERATIVE ADDICT, INCLUDING PROBLEMS OF NARCOTIC WITHDRAWAL

No attempt at withdrawal from narcotics should be made until the patient has recovered from his surgical illness. Tinckler and Bartham emphasize that attempts to withdraw narcotics immediately after surgery only confuse the clinical picture.[24] Eiseman et al. and Giuffrida et al. recommend the use of morphine or methadone for pain and the use of methadone for gradual withdrawal of the addict from narcotics.[67, 68] Eiseman suggests that the morphine or methadone be tapered and discontinued as soon as the patient's surgical condition permits.[68]

The narcotic addict can be a difficult, hostile patient; but if the physician is firm and consistent in handling him and medicates him sufficiently to avoid most withdrawal symptoms, he will usually cooperate during the postoperative period. Addicts often exaggerate postoperative pain in order to obtain narcotics.[68]

Postoperative addicts on maintenance narcotics should be observed for evidence of atelectasis. Addicts are prone to atelectasis, as are patients maintained on narcotics postoperatively.[19, 20]

The withdrawal of narcotics when the surgical illness has resolved inevitably causes some discomfort to addicted patients. If narcotics are stopped abruptly, withdrawal symptoms occur for four to five days in meperidine addicts, seven to 10 days in morphine or heroin addicts, and 10 to 14 days in methadone addicts.[71] Good descriptions of objective signs during withdrawal are contained in papers by Blachly[69] and by Giuffrida and coworkers,[67] and in a review by Isbell.[3] (For a summary of the description by Blachly, see Table 18–2.)

Anxiety and irritability are among the first symptoms of the narcotic abstinence syndrome, and are followed by yawning, sweating, lacrimation, and rhinorrhea. A period of restless sleep ("yen") may occur followed

Table 18–2 *Abstinence Signs in Sequential Appearance After the Last Dose of Narcotic in Addicts with Well-Established Parenteral Habits**

Grade of Abstinence	Signs	Hours After Last Dose of Narcotic					
		Morphine	Heroin	Demerol	Dihydro-morphine	Codeine	Metha-done
0	Craving drug, anxiety	6	4	2–3	2–3	8	12
Grade 1	Yawning, diaphoresis, lacrimation, rhinorrhea, "yen" sleep	14	8	4–6	4–5	24	34–48
Grade 2	Increase in the above, plus mydriasis, gooseflesh, tremors, hot and cold flashes, muscle and bone aches, anorexia	16	12	8–12	7	48	48–72
Grade 3	Increase in the above, plus insomnia, elevation in blood pressure, temperature (1–2°), respiratory rate, and pulse; also restlessness and nausea	24–36	18–24	16	12	–†	–†
Grade 4	Increase in the above, plus febrile facies, curled-up position, vomiting, diarrhea, weight loss, spontaneous ejaculation or orgasm, increases in WBC and fasting blood sugar, absence of eosinophils and hemoconcentration	36–48	24–36	–†	16	–†	–†

*From Blachly, P. H.: Amer. J. Psychiat. *122*:742, 1966. Copyright 1966, the American Psychiatric Association.
†No data available.

by signs such as mydriasis, tremors, and piloerection or gooseflesh. This latter sign gave rise to the phrase "cold turkey," meaning abrupt withdrawal from narcotics. Hot and cold flashes, anorexia, and elevation of temperature, blood pressure, and respiratory rate develop; and the addict is unable to sleep. Nausea and vomiting, abdominal cramps, and diarrhea occur as well as pain in the muscles and bones of the back and extremities. Muscle spasms and jerking motions appear in the legs, giving rise to the expression "kicking the habit." Orgasm in women and ejaculation in men may occur. Leukocytosis, elevated serum and urine corticosteroid levels, dehydration, and ketosis appear; and in rare instances circulatory collapse and death may occur.[3, 67, 69, 71, 72]

The least unpleasant and most convenient way to effect withdrawal in a narcotic addict is with the use of methadone. The initial dose is 10 mg intramuscularly. If an addict still shows signs of withdrawal one to two hours after the injection, another 5 to 10 mg may be given. The maintenance dose is repeated every 12 hours. Once the maintenance dose of methadone has been ascertained, the dose should be tapered and then stopped entirely over a five day period in healthy addicts, or over a 10 day period in debilitated addicts or in addicts recuperating from major surgery.[71] Giuffrida et al.

recommend oral methadone for management of opiate withdrawal. They suggest giving enough methadone to prevent symptoms — often starting with 20 to 40 mg twice daily, and never exceeding 80 mg twice a day. The dose is then reduced 5 mg a day, unless sweating or nausea occurs. With this schedule the average time for withdrawal is seven to 10 days.[67]

Blachly points out that severe insomnia and restlessness may indicate concomitant barbiturate withdrawal. He also notes that pentobarbital, 100 to 200 mg at bedtime, is useful during withdrawal from narcotics.[69] In differentiating between dependence on narcotics or barbiturates, Giuffrida and coworkers recommend using pentobarbital, 200 mg orally, as a test dose. If the patient shows no effect in an hour, he is greatly dependent on sedatives of the alcohol or barbiturate type. If he is sleepy or has slurred speech, he is moderately dependent; and if he is asleep in an hour, he is not dependent on sedatives. Giuffrida and coworkers treat the insomnia of the opiate abstinence syndrome with chloral hydrate, since therapy with barbiturates or glutethimide, in their experience, has often led to dependence on those drugs.[67] Gay et al. recommended up to 2.5 grams of chloral hydrate or up to 60 to 90 mg of flurazepam to treat insomnia during withdrawal. They also use prochlorperazine, 10 mg. orally or by rectal suppository, for severe gastrointestinal distress, or dicyclomine (Bentyl) for mild gastrointestinal symptoms. For muscle aches and bone pain they employ propoxyphene; for nervousness they suggest phenobarbital 30 to 60 mg orally q8h, or diazepam, 5 to 10 mg q8h orally.[73]

In withdrawal from heroin or morphine, symptoms are maximal at 36 to 72 hours and abate after seven to 10 days. In withdrawal from meperidine, symptoms are maximal at about 16 hours after the last dose of the narcotic and abate after four or five days. Withdrawal from meperidine produces more muscle tremor and restlessness than withdrawal from heroin or morphine. There is little nausea, vomiting, or diarrhea in withdrawal from meperidine, and mydriasis may be absent. Withdrawal from methadone is fairly mild, reaches a peak intensity in six days, and subsides after 14 days. There is usually no vomiting or diarrhea, and the cramps and muscle aches are mild.[71] Properly managed, withdrawal from methadone resembles mild influenza.

The use of clonidine hydrochloride (Catapres) to alleviate the signs and symptoms of abrupt opiate withdrawal has recently been described by Gold and coworkers, as mentioned above. This group gave clonidine hydrochloride, 17 μg per kg per day to 10 addicts for nine days after their last dose of maintenance methadone. The doses were 7 μg per kg at 8AM, 3 μg per kg at 4PM, and 7 μg per kg at 11 PM. In some cases a dose was held if the patient's diastolic blood pressure was below 60 mm Hg. By two hours after the first dose of clonidine, none of the addicts felt the need for methadone, and none chose to return to methadone during the study. Six of the 10 patients complained of difficulty in sleeping, and there were a few complaints of bone pain, sluggishness, or a dry mouth. On the eleventh, twelfth, and thirteenth days of the study the clonidine dose was reduced by 50 per cent, and the drug was stopped on the fourteenth day. No withdrawal symptoms either of narcotic drugs or of clonidine appeared; and when tested with naloxone hydrochloride, 1.2 mg intravenously, on the fourteenth day, no signs or symptoms of narcotic abstinence appeared. Gold and coworkers suggest that clonidine might be helpful in addicts who have been unable to tolerate the symptoms

of slow withdrawal of methadone during previous attempts to detoxify. Gold et al. also mentioned that clonidine is available on the black market, and that some addicts have used it to withdraw themselves from narcotics, at the risk of serious cardiovascular side effects — dizziness, hypotension, and marked sedation.[62] Other side effects of clonidine include rare instances of congestive heart failure, ventricular trigeminy, and loss of coordination. The abrupt discontinuation of clonidine can cause an episode of severe hypertension. Obviously, therapy of narcotic abstinence syndrome with clonidine would be limited to hospitalized patients. Widespread application of clonidine should await further studies. The work of Gold and his group appears to be an important advance in managing narcotic abstinence syndrome with a single non-narcotic drug.

For addicts who have been withdrawn from narcotics prior to surgery, synthetic analgesics such as propoxyphene, ethoheptazine, or pentazocine are useful in the management of postoperative pain.[67, 73] These drugs are also useful for pain in patients in whom a clear history of narcotic addiction cannot be obtained — that is, when the physician wishes to avoid giving narcotics to a possible addict. Pentazocine is actually a weak narcotic antagonist, having 1/50 the potency of N-allylnormorphone. In large doses (240–360 mg/day), it causes unpleasant side effects when given to addicts during withdrawal from morphine.[75] In useful therapeutic doses, pentazocine (Talwin) has little tendency to precipitate morphine abstinence symptoms.[76] Cyclazocine, a cogener of pentazocine in the benzomorphan series, is a potent narcotic antagonist and should not be used for analgesia in patients with definite or possible narcotic addiction.[77] Pentazocine itself has a slight potential for addiction.[75, 76, 78]

NARCOTIC ADDICTION AND PREGNANCY

The pregnant addict presents the anesthesiologist with a high incidence of maternal obstetrical complications and the problem of neonatal narcotic addiction. Stern reported a 40.9 per cent incidence of obstetrical complications in 66 pregnant heroin

Table 18–3 *Obstetrical Conditions Encountered in Pregnant Narcotic Addicts**

Toxemia	11–15%
Premature rupture of membranes	11%
Premature labor	18.5%
Breech delivery	9–12%
Abruptio placentae	2.9%
Postpartum hemorrhage	2–9%
Stillbirths	7.1%
Neonatal mortality	3.6%

*From Perlmutter, J. F.: Obstet. Gynecol. Surv. *29*:439, 1974.

addicts, including nine cases of abruptio placentae, nine postpartum hemorrhages, and 10 cases of toxemia. There were five stillbirths and 13 premature deliveries in the series.[79] Perlmutter reported a 56 per cent incidence of prematurity in 22 heroin addicts.[80] The incidence of obstetrical complications encountered in narcotics addicts is shown in Table 18–3, taken from the review article by Perlmutter.[81] She points out that the increased incidence of breech deliveries (9–12%) is related to the high incidence of premature labor (18.5%) in addicts. The perinatal mortality — stillbirths plus neonatal mortality — is nearly 11 per cent in the offspring of mothers addicted to narcotics. Besides the medical complications of narcotic addiction described earlier in this chapter, pregnant addicts are often anemic and have an increased incidence of venereal disease, since they often support their habit by prostitution.[81]

An addict who has recently had heroin may require less analgesia for labor than the average patient.[82] Because of the high incidence of prematurity, and because of the possibility of neonatal respiratory depression from narcotics, regional anesthesia — pudendal block, spinal, epidural, or caudal anesthesia — is the technique of choice in addicts, unless abruptio placentae necessitates a rapid cesarean section. Addicts may be given just enough narcotic during labor to suppress withdrawal symptoms. For heroin addicts, small intravenous doses of morphine would seem appropriate.

The infants of heroin addicts rarely exhibit respiratory depression, implying that intrauterine tolerance to narcotics often develops.[81] Addicts note that after a dose of narcotic their fetuses often become less active for a while. Between 75 and 85 per cent

of neonates of addicted mothers will show signs of narcotic abstinence during the first six days after delivery; and approximately 90 per cent of these neonates will convulse, if not treated.[81] Even with treatment up to 3.6 per cent of these neonates may die.[83]

The narcotic withdrawal syndrome, which occurred in 83 per cent of the surviving neonates in Perlmutter's series, consists of hyperirritability, tremors, a shrill or constant cry, production of excess mucus, poor feeding, dehydration, convulsions, and even circulatory collapse (Table 18–4).[80] The syndrome usually appears within 24 hours after delivery and lasts an average of 30 days. Therapy with paregoric, phenobarbital, or chlorpromazine usually produces good results. Initial doses are elixir of paregoric, 4–6 gtt every four hours or with each feeding; phenobarbital, 5–15 mg every six hours; or chlorpromazine, 0.7–1.1 mg/kg every four to six hours. The doses are titered to alleviate signs and symptoms of abstinence and then are very slowly reduced over about 30 days. Overdose with these drugs causes shallow respirations; paregoric can decrease both rate and depth of respiration.[81] Diazepam, 1–2 mg every eight hours, can also be used for neonatal addiction. Nathenson and coworkers report that with-

Table 18–4 *Signs of Neonatal Withdrawal**

Irritability
  Hyperactivity
  Hypertonus
  Scratching face
  Trembling
  Twitching
  Convulsions
Regurgitation
Diarrhea
High-pitched cry
Sucking of fingers
Anorexia
Sneezing
Yawning
Nasal congestion
Respiratory distress
  Tachypnea
  Grunting
  Rib retraction
  Intermittent cyanosis
  Periods of apnea
Hyperpyrexia
Diaphoresis
Excessive weight loss
Incomplete Moro reflex

*From Perlmutter, J. F.: Obstet. Gynecol. Surv. *29*:439, 1974.

drawal of neonates from drugs can be accomplished safely in six days, if diazepam is used to control abstinence.[84] Therapy with morphine for neonatal addiction is rarely necessary.[85] In the offspring of addicts maintained on methadone, narcotic abstinence syndrome is usually mild, and therapy may be unnecessary. Respiratory depression in these neonates is minimal.[86]

If a neonate whose mother is a narcotic addict is apneic at birth, his respiration should be supported initially with a breathing bag and mask, and then he should be intubated and maintained with mechanical ventilation. For purposes of diagnosis and treatment, narcotic antagonists can be used, but their use will likely precipitate narcotic abstinence syndrome. Mechanical ventilation in a good neonatal intensive care unit and watchful waiting until the effect of the narcotic wears off is probably the safer course. Small doses of narcotic antagonists may be employed. Foldes recommended nalorphine, 0.2 to 0.5 mg, or levallorphan, 0.05 to 0.1 mg, given into the umbilical vein. If some response occurs but respiration still appears inadequate, one half of these doses may be repeated in five or 10 minutes. If the umbilical vein cannot be injected he recommends nalorphine, 0.5 mg, or levallorphan, 0.1 mg, intramuscularly. The maximal effect should be present in five to 15 minutes.[87] Fraser recommended an initial nalorphine dose of only 0.1 mg intravenously.[88] Both of these have largely been superseded by naloxone for the diagnosis and treatment of narcotic overdose. Naloxone, 0.01 mg per kg, may be given intravenously or intramuscularly in apneic neonates. The dose may be repeated if the response is inadequate. Close observation of these neonates is mandatory because of the likelihood of narcotic abstinence syndrome and because the effects of naloxone may wear off before the effect of the narcotic dissipates. Recurrence of respiratory depression can appear in neonates whose mothers are addicted to heroin or morphine but is more likely to occur with maternal addiction to methadone.

THERAPY OF ACUTE NARCOTISM

Much of the mortality among narcotic addicts is due to acute respiratory insuffi-ciency from overdose or from anaphylaxis with severe pulmonary edema. The anesthesiologist called on to resuscitate a narcotic addict should not assume that he is treating only the effects of hypoxia from narcotic overdose, since heart failure or arrhythmia from quinine used to adulterate the heroin may be present, and aspiration of gastric contents can still further complicate the clinical picture.

Helpern listed "overdose" as the cause of 48 per cent of the mortality among narcotic addicts in New York City from 1950 to 1961.[6] In 1966, according to Louria, narcotic overdose was the cause of 655 deaths in New York City alone.[5] At present about 35 heroin related deaths per month are reported to the Drug Abuse Warning Network of the U.S. Department of Justice, a considerable reduction from the average of 150 per month reported in 1976. In West Germany, the incidence of death from heroin overdose is nearly twice that in the United States.[89]

In Cherubin's analysis of 120 addict deaths at the Harlem Hospital, 100 of these patients presented with respiratory depression or with acute pulmonary edema on admission. The addict with a simple overdose of narcotics will have either slow respiration or apnea. Neurologic examination shows stupor or coma, miosis (but no nystagmus), flaccidity of skeletal muscles, and depression of flexor and extensor reflexes. Severe respiratory depression, cyanosis, and mydriasis may be present. There may be some rales in the lungs.

Treatment of overdose unaccompanied by hypotension consists of securing a clear airway, ventilating the patient, and using narcotic antagonists to restore spontaneous breathing. If depression is severe, controlled ventilation with tracheal intubation and 100 per cent oxygen is necessary. Gay suggests naloxone, 0.8 mg. intravenously, as an initial dose.[73] If veins are difficult to find, the antagonist may be given intramuscularly. The dose may be repeated after 10 minutes if the response to the initial dose was inadequate. Naloxone, a specific antagonist to narcotics, has virtually superseded nalorphine and levallorphan for treatment of narcotic overdose, since naloxone has no depressing effects on respiration. Louria had suggested nalorphine, 3 to 5 mg as an initial antagonist and recommended repetition of this dose at 15 minute intervals until respiration is adequate.[7] Foldes recommended somewhat higher initial doses of antagonists: naloxone 0.3 to 0.8 mg, nalorphine 5 to 12 mg, or levallorphan 1 to 3 mg. He suggested one to three subsequent doses of one third to one half the initial dose at *five or 10* minute intervals, as long as improvement in respiration continues.[87] Fraser emphasizes that the end point in antagonist therapy of narcotic overdose is adequate respiration, not the reversal of drowsiness.[88] Overdose of antagonist (e.g., 15 to 20 mg of nalorphine) as a single initial dose can precipitate the narcotic abstinence syndrome.[7] After reversal, the patient's respiration should be observed for several hours, particularly if the overdose was with methadone, since renarcotization may occur. The naloxone, which has a relatively brief duration of action, may need to be repeated several times. Therapy of narcotic overdose is quite successful. Gay notes that he has yet to lose a case of overdose if the addict arrives at his clinic with a beating heart.[73]

The narcotic addict may present with respiratory failure characterized by tachypnea and overt pulmonary edema.[5] Respiratory distress may occur during or immediately after intravenous injection of adulterated heroin. The rapid onset of symptoms makes it unlikely that narcotic depression of respiration causes this syndrome.[81] Addicts have been found dead with the needle still in a vein and with evidence of pulmonary edema. The pathophysiology of this type of respiratory failure after intravenous injection of impure narcotics may be either an acute anaphylactic reaction or possibly myocardial failure from an overdose of quinine used as an adulterant in illegal heroin preparations. A massive overdose of quinine can, on rare occasions, cause ventricular tachycardia. An allergic pulmonary edema appears to play a role in this syndrome. There is some evidence that increased pulmonary artery resistance leading to right heart failure is present in addicts with respiratory failure and pulmonary edema. Helpern was unable to find evidence of heroin in the blood of many addicts who died with fulminant pulmonary edema.[6] At autopsy the lungs are congested and hemorrhagic, and right ventricular dilatation is present.[6] Diffuse infiltrates appear on the chest x-rays, right axis deviation may be present on the electrocardiogram, and arterial gas measurements show hypoxemia, hypocarbia, and acidosis.[2]

Treatment is supportive, with tracheal intubation, mechanical ventilation with positive end expiratory pressure, and 100 per cent oxygen. Intravenous diuretics such as furosemide and nebulized ethyl alchol may help control the pulmonary edema. Hydrocortisone, 100 to 200 mg intravenously, may be given. If hypotension is present, the circulation should be supported with intravenous epinephrine.

PROPOXYPHENE (DARVON) ADDICTION

While this volume was in press, it became apparent that propoxyphene (Darvon), a drug widely employed as an analgesic, is also addicting. Structurally, propoxyphene is rather similar to methadone. Maruta and coworkers, in a study of 144 patients at the Mayo Clinic who were taking analgesics because of chronic pain, reported six patients dependent on propoxyphene. One patient who was taking 24 tablets of propoxyphene, 65 mg, daily had withdrawal symptoms as his consumption of the drug was reduced. Symptoms included agitation and abdominal cramps.[*] Salem and coworkers report the use of thioridazine, 25 mg q.i.d., to control agitation while the propoxyphene dose is decreased over a two week period.[**] Doses of propoxyphene in the range of 500 to 800 mg daily may cause physical dependence.[†]

Overdoses of propoxyphene can result in death from respiratory depression. Propoxyphene has often been combined with alcohol, sedatives, or tranquilizers to produce a "high," and such combinations have resulted in many fatalities.[†]

ANESTHESIA FOR OTHER DRUG ABUSERS

The increasing use of non-narcotic drugs that alter mood or perception is a major problem in the United States today. These drugs with psychic effects include 1) central nervous system depressants such as ethyl

---

[*]Maruta, T., Swanson, D. W. and Finlayson, R. E.: Drug abuse and dependency in patients with chronic pain. Mayo Clinic. Proc. 54:241, 1979.

[**]Salem, R. S., and Muniz, C.: Treatment of propoxyphene dependence with thioridazine. J. Clin. Psychiat. 41:179, 1980.

[†]F.D.A. Drug Bulletin 9:1, Feb. 1979, p. 2.

alcohol and the barbiturates; 2) the hallucinogens such as lysergic acid diethylamide, mescaline, and psilocybin; and 3) stimulants such as the amphetamines. Drugs within each of these three groups have similar psychological and physiological effects and display a certain degree of cross tolerance. The term "cross tolerance" for the group of CNS depressants indicates the ability of one drug to suppress the abstinence syndrome resulting from the abrupt withdrawal of another drug. For example, within the group of CNS depressant drugs, barbiturates can prevent the abstinence syndrome resulting from the abrupt withdrawal of alcohol. The term "cross tolerance" when applied to the hallucinogens

means that a user of one hallucinogenic drug who switches to another of these drugs will require higher doses to achieve the desired psychic effect than will the nonuser.

Isbell has categorized nearly all the drugs used nonmedically according to the type of dependence produced by habitual use of these drugs — strong physical dependence (Type I), mild physical dependence (Type II), or psychic dependence only (Type III) (Table 18–5). Drugs causing strong physical dependence are subdivided according to the nature of the syndrome resulting from withdrawal of the drug; drugs associated with strong physical dependence cause withdrawal syndromes that resemble either

Table 18–5 *Classification of Important Drugs Used Nonmedically**

I. Drugs causing psychic and severe physical dependence
  A. *Opiate or morphine type.* Physical dependence manifest by autonomic storm and central nervous system irritability on withdrawal. Very strong psychic dependence.
    1. Morphine and its congeners: codeine, dihydromorphinone (Dilaudid), diacetylmorphine (heroin), dihydrohydroxymorphinone (Numorphan), dihydrohydroxycodeinone (Percodan), etc.
    2. Morphinans (Levodromoran).
    3. The benzazocines: phenazocine (Prinadol).
    4. The meperidines: meperidine (Demerol), alphaprodine (Nisentil), anileridine (Leritine), pimonidine, diphenoxylate (Lomotil).
    5. Methadone and congeners: dl-methadone, l-methadone, dextropropoxyphene (Darvon).
  B. *Alcohol-barbiturate type.* Physical dependence manifest by anxiety, tremors, insomnia, convulsions, and delirium. Very strong psychic dependence.
    1. Ethyl alcohol
    2. Barbiturates
    3. Paraldehyde
    4. Chloral hydrate
    5. Meprobamate (Equanil, Miltown)
    6. Piperidinediones: gluthethimide (Doriden), methylprylon (Noludar)
    7. Benzodiazepines: chlordiazepoxide (Librium), diazepam (Valium)
    8. Ethinamate (Valmid)
    9. Ethchlorvynol (Placidyl)
II. Drugs causing mild or questionable physical dependence
  A. *Opiate agonist-antagonist type.* Mild physical dependence, resembling physical dependence on opiates, mild to moderate psychic dependence.
    1. Morphine antagonists: nalorphine (Nalline)
    2. Morphinan antagonists: levallorphan (Lorfan)
    3. Benzazocine antagonists: cyclazocine, pentazocine (Talwin)
  B. *Amphetamine type.* Physical dependence debatable but abstinence syndrome includes long sleep, hunger, apathy, and depression (may be related to cocaine).
    1. Amphetamines: dl-amphetamine (Benzedrine), d-amphetamine (Dexedrine), methamphetamine (Methedrine, Desoxyn), phenmetrazine (Preludin), diethylpropion (Tenuate), etc.
    2. Piperidines: methylphenidate (Ritalin), pipradrol (Meratran)
III. Drugs causing psychic dependence only
  A. Cocaine (may be related to amphetamines)
  B. Hallucinogens of LSD type: lysergic acid diethylamide (LSD-25) and congeners, psilocybin, mescaline, dimethyltryptamine, diethyltryptamine, hallucinogenic amphetamines (STP or DOM, TMA, etc.)
  C. Volatile solvents: "glue"
  D. Cannabis sativa: marijuana, hashish, 1-$\triangle^8$-and $\triangle^9$-*trans*-tetrahydrocannabinols
  E. Nicotine: tobacco
  F. Caffeine: coffee, tea

*Trade or popular names in parentheses following generic names.
From Isbell, H.: Anesth. Analg. *50*:886, 1971.

the pattern of opiate abstinence (Type IA) or the pattern of withdrawal from ethyl alcohol or the barbiturates (Type IB). Therapy that suppresses the abstinence syndrome from one drug in each of these two major categories (IA or IB) will generally be effective against the abstinence syndrome resulting from other drugs in the same category. Hence Isbell's classification is useful in understanding which drugs are associated with abstinence syndromes, what kind of abstinence symptoms may appear, and what therapeutic agents may be used to withdraw patients from their dependence.[1] As is apparent from the table, most sedatives and minor tranquilizers produce dependence resembling that of ethyl alcohol or the barbiturates. Isbell pointed out that pentazocine may need to be reclassified, since its withdrawal syndrome may be a variant of the opiate abstinence syndrome.[1] Nalorphine, levallorphan, and cyclazocine can cause mild physical dependence; but naloxone thus far has not been reported to cause dependence. The amphetamines and cocaine cause little, if any, physical dependence but do cause psychic dependence, as do the lysergic acid derivatives and the hallucinogens of the amphetamine type. The belladonna alkaloids (scopolamine, etc.), which were omitted from Isbell's classification, also do not cause physical dependence. Marihuana and other cannabinols, nicotine, and caffeine do not cause physical dependence but may cause a strong psychic dependence.

The anesthesiologist should be aware of the alterations in physiology resulting from the use of depressants, hallucinogens, and stimulants. He should also be aware that the use of mixtures of drugs has become popular. Combinations of LSD followed by heroin, LSD followed by barbiturates, amphetamines followed by narcotics, or alcohol followed by barbiturates are frequently encountered at present. Heroin is often used along with barbiturates or tranquilizers, particularly since the quality of heroin in the U.S. has declined during the past five years. Hallucinogenic amphetamines such as STP have been combined with chlorpromazine or other depressants, occasionally with fatal results.[2] The combination of mescaline, cocaine, and LSD in one capsule is known as the "peace pill."[2] The combination of cocaine and heroin is referred to as a "speedball."[1] These combinations of psychic drugs may present the anesthesiologist with difficult problems in diagnosis and management. Before treating patients taking combinations of drugs, the anesthesiologist must be aware of the clinical syndromes associated with each of the major groups of non-narcotic drugs that alter mood or perception: the depressants, the hallucinogens, and the stimulants.

ANESTHESIA FOR PATIENTS USING CNS DEPRESSANTS: ALCOHOL, THE BARBITURATES, AND OTHER SEDATIVES

Ethyl alcohol, the barbiturates, and sedatives such as ethinamate, flurazepam, glutethimide, meprobamate, methaqualone, methyprylon, and the benzodiazepines are all central nervous system depressants. The abrupt withdrawal of any of these compounds from an addicted patient may cause increased CNS irritability, including convulsions. Any one of these drugs is able to suppress partially or completely the abstinence syndrome resulting from the withdrawal of another of this group. During anesthesia and surgery, patients who have taken these drugs react in a similar manner, depending on the amount of drug taken, the duration of habitual use of the drug, and the interval between the last dose and the surgical procedure.

Much of the variation in descriptions of general anesthesia in alcoholics and much of the variation in reports of anesthesia in animals pretreated with alcohol or barbiturates can be explained with the aid of Figure 18-4.[3]

In a patient not habituated to a depressant drug, a single effective dose of alcohol, barbiturate, or other sedative drug will usually cause drowsiness and act additively with anesthetic agents. Some depressants, depending on the dose and the total length of time of administration, can cause an increased state of latent hyperexcitability in the central nervous system. Isbell has termed this state a "compensatory stimulating reaction to chronic depression."* This state can be unmasked during the induction

---

*Phrase coined by Harris Isbell, according to Kenneth Lampe, Ph.D., personal communication, 1971.

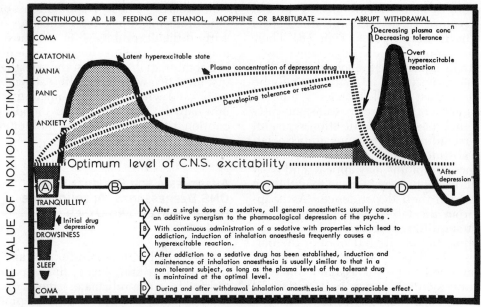

Figure 18–4. Responses during progressive development of tolerance to depressant drugs and to withdrawal. (Modified from Seevers, M. H.: Fed Proc. *13*:672, 1954.)

of general anesthesia, resulting in a prolonged excitement. With continued administration of the drug, the latent hyperexcitability declines as tolerance develops to the depressing effects of the drug. In order for tolerance to develop, maintenance of adequate plasma levels is necessary. Therefore, clinically significant tolerance does not develop with up to 200 mg of a medium-acting barbiturate (e.g., secobarbital) or with one or two alcoholic drinks per day. When tolerance to a depressant drug has developed, there is still some slight increase in the latent hyperexcitability of the CNS above preaddiction levels; but induction of general anesthesia is often uneventful, provided that blood levels of the depressant are adequate. By the peak of the abstinence syndrome, tolerance has virtually disappeared,[4] and induction times for inhalational agents and induction doses for intravenous agents become normal. Recently a question has been raised concerning the time interval needed for anesthetic dose requirements to return to normal after the chronic ingestion of alcohol is discontinued. Johnstone and coworkers found that the ED_{50} for isoflurane in mice chronically maintained on 10 per cent ethanol did not

decrease to control levels observed prior to alcohol ingestion until 55 days after the ethanol was stopped.[5] The increased tolerance for this anesthetic in this species lasted longer than the ethanol abstinence syndrome does. More research into the time course of the loss of cross tolerance to anesthetics during and after the withdrawal of ethanol in both animals and man appears necessary to clarify this question. It is of some interest that the group including Smith, Winter, and Eger has recently demonstrated auto- and cross-tolerance between nitrous oxide and several other general anesthetic agents. Chronic inhalation of 50 per cent nitrous oxide for 14 to 21 days can produce an auto-tolerance to nitrous oxide or a cross-tolerance to cyclopropane and to isoflurane in mice. This tolerance appears to resemble that seen with sedative and hypnotic drugs.[6]

We shall review the anesthetic management of patients taking ethanol, barbiturates, and other depressant drugs. Since patients indulging in alcohol may have severe pathologic changes in many organs, we shall consider anesthesia for alcoholic patients separately, and then discuss anesthesia for patients on other depressant drugs.

MEDICAL PROFILE OF THE ALCOHOLIC

Pathophysiology of the Alcoholic. Alcoholism is associated with pathological changes in many organ systems. The liver, heart, lungs, and sympathetic nerves can be affected, even in alcoholic patients who appear healthy. The diagnosis of alcoholism can be made if a blood ethanol level over 300 mg per 100 ml is present at any time, or if a blood ethanol level of 150 mg per 100 ml is present without signs of inebriation. The diagnosis may be entertained if an ethanol level of 100 mg per 100 ml is discovered during routine screening.[7]

Liver Disease. In asymptomatic chronic alcoholics liver functions may be deranged. Knott and Beard tested 30 well nourished asymptomatic alcoholics and found the incidence of abnormal liver function tests shown in Table 18–6. Serum bilirubin, total proteins, and A/G ratios were normal in all cases.[8] In a recent study of 62 middle class alcoholics, Morse and Hurt found that 39 of these patients (63 per cent) had an elevated serum gamma-glutamyl transpeptidase value, and the mean level of this enzyme in their patients was nearly four times the normal value. They point out that most alcoholics with an abnormal GGT value show hepatocellular necrosis on liver biopsy.[9] Macrocytosis without anemia appears to accompany prolonged, heavy drinking. Twenty-two per cent of their patients also had elevated serum triglycerides, and 16 per cent had elevated alkaline phosphatase values.[9] The presence of abnormal liver functions on routine screening tests may be the only indication of alcoholism in preoperative patients.

Alcoholics with fatty livers may die suddenly from massive pulmonary fat embolism, even in the absence of trauma. The annual death rate in alcoholics with fatty liver is between 1.5 and 22 per 100,000 population; the mechanism of death is unclear, although hypoglycemia, hypomagnesemia, and pulmonary fat embolization have been suggested.[10] Severe liver disease can cause a prolonged sleep when thiobarbiturates are used for anesthesia, although liver disease of such severity is seldom encountered in alcoholics who come to surgery.[11, 12]

Alcoholics with liver disease frequently require increased amounts of *d*-tubocurarine. Years ago, Dundee and Gray described seven patients with liver disease in whom approximately 1.0 mg per kg of *d*-tubocurarine was needed for adequate abdominal muscle relaxation during the first hour of surgery, whereas the 200 normal controls required only 0.5 mg per kg of curare for muscle relaxation. Baraka and Gabaldi attributed the increased requirement for curare in patients with liver disease to increased binding of the drug by gamma globulins.[14] Serum gamma globulin, produced by reticuloendothelial cells, is often increased in Laennec's cirrhosis and other liver diseases. Baraka and Gabaldi found an excellent correlation ($r = +0.604$, $p < 0.001$) between the requirement for curare and the level of serum gamma globulin. However, Ghoneim and coworkers studied the binding of tritium labeled *d*-tubocurarine in a small number of patients with hepatic disease and in normal controls and found no significant differences in the per cent of drug bound by the plasma.[15] Both equilibrium dialysis and gel filtration methods were used to determine the amount of binding. The only statistically significant difference between their groups was an increased gamma globulin in their patients with hepatic disease.[15] Thus, increased binding of curare does not explain

Table 18-6 *Percentage and Frequency of Abnormal Liver Function Tests in 30 Chronic Alcoholics**

Measurement	% Abnormal	No. Abnormal/Total	Normal Range of Test
BSP	87	26/30	0–5% retention in 45 minutes
SGOT	80	24/30	0–40 units/ml
Isocitric dehydrogenase	67	20/30	30–160 units/ml
SGPT	57	17/30	0–35 units/ml
Total bilirubin	23	07/30	0.1–1.0 mg/100 ml

*From Knott, D. H., and Beard, J. D.: Amer. J. Med. Sci. 252:261, 1966.

the increased requirement for curare in patients with cirrhosis due to alcoholism. Recent work by Duvaldestin and coworkers offers a possible explanation.[16] Duvaldestin investigated the distribution of another nondepolarizing muscle relaxant, pancuronium, in 14 patients with liver disease, 12 of whom had alcoholic cirrhosis, and in 12 normal controls. Four of the patients had up to a liter of ascites, but renal function was normal in both the patients and the controls. Most of the patients with liver disease were having portacaval shunt procedures during the study. Concentrations of bis-quaternary compounds (pancuronium and its metabolites) were measured fluorimetrically at intervals in samples of venous blood and urine, and analyzed according to the two compartment, open mathematical model described for pancuronium by McLeod et al. and by Somogyi et al.[17, 18, 19] Following a single large dose of pancuronium, 100 to 250 μg per kg, given at the beginning of the case, the volumes of the central and peripheral compartments into which the drug was distributed were calculated, the serum half-lives for the distribution and elimination phases were estimated, and the total volume of distribution of the drug was determined by the area method of Greenblatt and Koch-Weser.[20] In the patients with cirrhosis the volume of the central compartment into which the pancuronium was distributed was significantly increased (0.173 $\pm$ 0.017 L/kg, vs. 0.122 $\pm$ 0.007 L/kg, p < 0.01). The total volume of distribution of the drug was also increased in the cirrhotic patients (416 $\pm$ 58 ml/kg vs. 279 $\pm$ 15 ml/kg, p < 0.05). The serum half-lives for the distribution and elimination phases were approximately twice normal in the patients with liver disease; and the prolonged elimination phase for pancuronium in cirrhotics was consistent with an increased distribution volume of the drug. Duvaldestin and coworkers suggested that the great increase in distribution volume for pancuronium in cirrhotics might also explain the increased requirement for d-tubocurarine first noted by Dundee and Gray.[16] The possibility awaits further study.

Plasma cholinesterase decreases early in liver disease, but true cholinesterase remains normal, even in terminal cirrhosis.[14, 21] Some reduction in total dose of succinylcholine used in alcoholics with liver disease may be advisable.

Hemorrhagic problems are encountered in alcoholics most commonly because of acute gastritis, esophagitis, duodenal ulcer, or esophageal varices. Alcohol has a direct depressing effect on erythrocyte and leukocyte precursors in bone marrow, and may cause a transient thrombocytopenia.[22, 23, 24] Megaloblastic anemia caused by folic acid deficiency occurs in around 10 per cent of alcoholics, and hemolytic anemia with or without hypersplenism frequently appears.[25, 26] A mildly depressed platelet count is not likely to result in bleeding. When a hemorrhagic diathesis occurs in an alcoholic with liver disease, multiple deficiencies may be present, such as inadequate amounts of factors VII, IX, X, prothrombin, fibrinogen, and platelets.[27] Therapy with vitamin K may increase synthesis of prothrombin or factors VII, IX, or X; in the face of active bleeding, fresh frozen plasma can be used to restore these factors. Severe hypofibrinogenemia rarely is a cause of bleeding in alcoholics.[27] During hemorrhage and transfusion, the platelet count may become severely depressed, resulting in further bleeding. The administration of platelets or of fresh, whole blood, if available, is the appropriate treatment for this problem.

Heart Disease. Two forms of heart disease are associated with alcoholism — beriberi and alcoholic myocardiopathy. Beriberi, caused by thiamine deficiency, presents as congestive heart failure, and is often accompanied by paresthesias in the extremities. The pulse is usually regular, but the EKG may show T-wave inversions in the precordial leads.

Alcoholic myocardiopathy has become a well known entity. It is generally seen in well-nourished middle-aged patients, often presents as an arrhythmia — usually atrial tachycardia or atrial fibrillation — but occasionally presents as congestive heart failure. The amplitude of the T-wave may be reduced, and a "cleft" may be present at the top of the precordial T-waves.[28] Bashour et al. found a 33 per cent incidence of cardiac hypertrophy in 100 cirrhotics.[29] In 19 of these 33 cases no valvular or other lesions that might account for the hypertrophy were present. Thirteen of these cases had evidence of myocardial fibrosis, while the remaining six showed only interstitial edema of the left ventricle. In only four of these 100 patients was congestive heart failure diagnosed prior to death.[29] Alexander biopsied the myocardium of 60 alcoholics with atypical heart disease and found swollen mitochondria with degenerating cristae. He also found edema involving the myofibrils.[30] Regan and others found evidence that ingestion of moderate amounts of alcohol reduces left ventricular work index in alcoholics who have no clinical evidence of heart disease.

Klatsky noted an association between moderate to heavy ethanol intake and hypertension. Data from the Framingham Study indicate that males ingesting 60 or more ounces of alcohol per month had twice the incidence of hypertension, defined as a resting blood pressure over 165/95 mm Hg, than that found in similar males who consumed less than 30 ounces of alcohol per month.[32] Sixty ounces of ethanol per month is roughly equivalent to five ounces of 80 proof spirits, 16 ounces of wine, or five 12-ounce beers per day. Hence alcoholism apparently can contribute to hypertensive cardiovascular disease.

Lung Disease. In Laennec's cirrhosis there are no consistent changes in lung volumes or compliance, unless ascites is present.[29] When pulmonary congestion is present in severe liver disease, all ventilatory capacities are reduced. Alcoholics with cirrhosis tend to hyperventilate and often have arterial desaturation (Table 18–7). The degree of hyperventilation correlates roughly with the severity of the liver disease but not with the amount of arterial desaturation or arteriovenous admixture. The alveolar ventilation is normally around 70 per cent of the minute ventilation, but in the patients with Laennec's cirrhosis studied by Bashour and coworkers, the alveolar ventilation averaged only 58 per cent of the minute ventilation, implying an increased physiologic dead space. The cause of the hyperventilation in cirrhotics is still unknown.[29]

There is a small shift to the right in the oxyhemoglobin dissociation curve of patients with Laennec's cirrhosis, but this shift is insufficient to explain the desaturation observed in these patients.[33, 34] During breathing of 100 per cent oxygen, large alveolar-arterial oxygen gradients appear.[35] The amount of admixture is greater than can be explained by blood shunted from the portal vein to the pulmonary veins via mediastinal and periesophageal veins, so intrapulmonary right-to-left shunts must exist.[29] Berthelot et al. searched for these shunts, but found only dilatations of the smaller pulmonary artery branches in the alveolar walls and pleura.[36]

Circulation, Blood Volume, and Hydration. Cardiac output may be increased in cirrhotics or in patients with fatty infiltration of the liver who have no spider nevi.[29, 37, 38] Such patients may require more thiopental because of accelerated redistribution, as is the case in patients with thyrotoxicosis. As noted above, an increased central compartment into which pancuronium is distributed also explains the increased initial requirement for pancuronium in these patients. Cirrhotics with varices have an increased plasma volume, and with cyanosis have an increased red cell mass; but in the absence of either of these conditions, plasma volume and red cell mass are normal.[39]

While blood alcohol levels are rising, alcohol acts as a diuretic by inhibiting antidiuretic hormone. In chronic alcoholism there is an increase in total body water. Beard and Knott found that total body water in 30 alcoholics averaged 565 ml per kg on admission, but dropped to 516 ml per kg four days later.[40] The increase in total body water was both intra- and extracellular. These authors found normal serum electrolytes and normal serum magnesium and calcium values on admission but pointed

Table 18–7   *Abnormal Respiratory Parameters in 24 Alcoholic Patients with Laennec's Cirrhosis**

Parameter	24 Cirrhotics	Normal Range
Minute ventilation (L/min)	9.66 ± 2.3	6.32 ± 1.5
Arterial saturation (%)	91.6 ± 4.1	>95
Alveolar ventilation (L/min)	5.56 ± 1.5	4.44 ± 1.08
Pa_{CO_2} (mm Hg)	32.2 ± 5.2	$37 - 44$
A-a DO_2 (mm Hg)	43 ± 12	13 ± 6
pH	7.44 ± 0.4	$7.37 - 7.43$
Base excess (meq/L)	-2.4	-2 to -4

*From Bashour, F. A., et al.: Amer. Heart J. *74*:569, 1967.

out that serum values may not reflect large intracellular deficits.[40] Wadstein and Skude have recently published indirect evidence for an intracellular potassium deficit in alcoholics; they found decreases in serum potassium following the abrupt cessation of alcohol in a group of alcoholic patients prior to the onset of delirium tremens; and therapy with 160 to 240 milliequivalents of potassium per day in a few of these patients did not prevent the drop in serum potassium.[41] Lee, Giesecke, and Jenkins note that in acute intoxication in man there is an increased loss of calcium and magnesium and a decreased excretion of sodium, potassium, and chloride.[42] Of course, if vomiting appears, chloride and hydrogen ion will be lost; and if diarrhea occurs, sodium may also be lost. If hepatic function is poor, sodium retention will occur because of elevated blood aldosterone levels. Spironolactone together with thiazide diuretics is a useful combination for the management of sodium and water retention in alcoholics with cirrhosis. In chronic alcoholics the anesthesiologist should avoid overhydration and should assess and replace deficits of potassium, magnesium, and calcium.

Neurological Disease. Although Wernicke's encephalopathy or Korsakoff's psychosis occurs as a result of thiamine deficiency, of more concern to anesthesiologists is the peripheral neuropathy that leads to absence of circulatory reflexes. Barraclough and Sharpey-Schafer collected seven patients with alcoholic polyneuritis in whom sympathetic venous tone was diminished, leading to hypotension or syncope.[43] One patient with alcoholic polyneuritis became hypotensive and died under anesthesia during a breast biopsy. Hypotension in these patients is not accompanied by tachycardia, cold, clammy skin, or venous distention. The diagnosis is often mistaken for pulmonary embolus, myocardial infarction, or adrenal insufficiency. The hypotension is precipitated by ordinary doses of sedatives and narcotics, by intermittent positive pressure respiration, or by small blood losses. Plasma expander, 500 to 1000 ml, is recommended as the treatment of choice. Therapy with norepinephrine for hypotension due to peripheral dilatation may be indicated, and treatment with adrenalin may be necessary if marked bradycardia occurs or if asystole develops.

Alcoholic polyneuritis is commonly characterized by numbness, tingling, and burning pain in the extremities, as well as motor weakness, particularly in the lower extremities. Loss of sensation below the knees and loss of deep tendon reflexes may occur. Muscles may be tender to deep pressure, foot drop not infrequently occurs, and cutaneous edema and sweating may appear. Neuritis of cranial nerves may occur but follows no set pattern; neuritis of the vagal nerve can cause tachycardia.

Hypoglycemia. Significant hypoglycemia may be present during the hangover phase of acute ethanol intoxication. Vartia et al. in over 50 patients who were mainly binge drinkers found a mean blood sugar of 53 mg per 100 ml (vs. 97 mg per 100 ml in controls); in four subjects the blood glucose was below 40 mg per 100 ml.[44] Freinkel et al. reported the occurrence of hypoglycemic coma after ethanol intoxication in eight patients. This rather uncommon syndrome was not due to depleted liver glycogen. In four of the eight patients there was an abnormal glucose tolerance test, but the patients did not appear to have classic diabetes mellitus. On ethanol challenge, two patients developed blood sugars below 35 mg per 100 ml.[45] During the acute phase of ethanol intoxication, the blood sugar is above normal.[45, 46]

Paralytic Ileus and Increased Gastric Acidity. The presence of ethanol in the stomach results in gastric secretion with a high acid content, and intoxicating levels of ethanol in blood (200 to 300 mg per 100 ml) are associated with pylorospasm and with paralytic ileus.[47] Hence, the patient intoxicated with ethanol has an increased risk of aspiration.

INDUCTION AND MAINTENANCE OF ANESTHESIA FOR PATIENTS WITH ACUTE AND CHRONIC ALCOHOLISM

It is common knowledge that alcoholic patients require more anesthesia when sober but that acutely inebriated patients require less than usual anesthetic doses.[48] The effects of acute and chronic alcohol abuse on anesthetic requirement have been studied extensively, and ethanol itself has been re-evaluated for use as an intravenous anesthetic.[49] Considerable information is available concerning the effect of alcoholism on the induction of anesthesia, on minimal alveolar concentration (MAC) for maintenance of anesthesia, and on interactions of ethanol and drugs used as anesthetic adjuncts. Some information concerning the mechanism of these effects is available, along with data concerning the duration of the effect of ethanol on anesthetic requirement after cessation of alcohol intake.

Statements supporting the claim that chronic alcoholics have prolonged induction excitement or require large doses of anesthetic agents appear in many papers in the anesthesia literature.[4, 48, 50, 56] From anesthetizing patients with a history of alcoholism, this author has also received the impression that alcoholics do require larger doses of thiobarbiturates and do have longer gas induction times than nonalcoholics of the same size and age. Han has reported higher than average MAC values for halothane in chronic alcoholics.[56] Johnstone and coworkers reported that in mice chronically drinking 10 per cent ethanol in water, the ED_{50} for isoflurane rises from 1.33 per cent to 1.54 per cent after 10 days and to 1.69 per cent with more prolonged exposure to ethanol.[48] The response to application of a clamp to the tail was used to determine ED_{50}. Morton and Adriani claim that there is some degree of cross tolerance between ethyl alcohol and the following agents: chloroform, cyclopropane, diethyl ether, ethylene, halothane, methoxyflurane, nitrous oxide, and vinyl ether.[51] Thus it appears that maintenance of anesthesia in chronic alcoholics who are sober at the time of surgery requires greater concentrations of inhalation agents than are needed in nonalcoholic subjects of equivalent age and size.*

Gas inductions are prolonged in sober alcoholics. Morton and Adriani also state that chronic alcoholics who have recently imbibed show a prolonged second stage of anesthesia.[51] Abreu and Emerson, using mice pretreated with ethanol, described induction times with diethyl ether 67 per cent longer than those of the control mice.[53] Their experimental design employed weekly increases in alcohol dose up to an equivalent of 1.5 quarts daily in a 70 kilogram man. In the first several weeks of their experiment, inductions were stormy as well as prolonged; however, by the sixth week induction times became shorter. Lee et al. confirmed the findings of Abreu and Emerson and also found that rats treated with ethanol showed increased excitement when induced with 1.5 per cent methoxyflurane. There was also a trend to longer induction times when intraperitoneal methohexital, 30 mg per kg, was used as the test anesthetic. The disappearance of the prolonged, stormy inductions after several weeks of addiction to ethanol is consistent with the reduction in latent hyperexcitability that occurs when full tolerance to any of the CNS depressant drugs is achieved. Thus Figure 18–4 aids in explaining the reactions of the animals to general anesthetics in the experiments of Abreu and Emerson and of Lee and coworkers. One suspects that many of the alcoholics encountered in clinical practice do not maintain the state of complete tolerance with decreased latent hyperexcitability achieved in animal experiments. Hence stormy, prolonged inhalation inductions are often encountered in chronic alcoholics. It seems reasonable to avoid gas inductions with diethyl ether and with methoxyflurane. One should also be prepared to employ larger than average incremental doses of thiobarbiturates in alcoholics, provided that the patients' circulation tolerates such doses.

It is also worth noting that in nonalcoholics who are acutely intoxicated and in chronic alcoholics who are heavily intoxicated before induction, the alcohol and the general anesthetic agents act additively.[4, 57, 58] Keilty points out that less anesthetic is needed during emergency surgery in intoxicated patients.[50] Morton and Adriani warn that there is a real possibility of overdosing the acutely intoxicated patient with anesthetic agents, since the ethanol acts as a basal anesthetic.[52] Ramsey and Haag found a 40 per cent decrease in the lethal dose of thiopental in dogs given ethanol, 3 grams per kilogram, prior to anesthesia.[59] Johnstone and coworkers found that pretreatment with ethanol reduced the ED_{50} of

---

*It is of interest that Smith and coworkers recently demonstrated that the chronic inhalation of 50 per cent nitrous oxide can produce in mice a small but statistically significant degree of auto-tolerance.[6] They noted the similarity to the tolerance seen among the sedative and hypnotic drugs. However, they were unable to demonstrate that isoflurane produced auto-tolerance or cross-tolerance to other agents.

isoflurane in mice, but found that the combination of ethanol and isoflurane produced somewhat less the effects of the two drugs.[48] Dundee studied intravenous ethanol as an anesthetic, and demonstrated that with rapid infusion a blood level of approximately 200 mg per 100 ml sufficed to induce sleep in most patients.[60] This blood level was somewhat less than the 300 to 400 mg per 100 ml commonly accepted as necessary for light anesthesia with ethanol in nonhabituated patients.

Ethyl alcohol interacts with many drugs employed as adjuncts in anesthesia. In a review of this subject Forney and Harger categorized the interaction of ethanol and many drugs as either additive or potentiating — that is, hyperadditive.[46] Their data are reproduced in Table 18–8, which represents the conclusion of the majority of the studies of the interactions between ethanol and the drugs listed in both human and animal studies. Considerable variation was present among these studies because of differences in experimental design. There was nearly uniform agreement that ethanol prolongs the hypnotic effect of medium- and long-acting barbiturates in an additive manner. For the combination of thiopental and alcohol, three separate groups reported potentiation.[58, 59, 61] A subanesthetic dose of ethanol increased the thiopental sleeping time by a factor of 10 in dogs, and by a factor of five in rabbits, indicating a potentiation.[58, 59] Moreover, the minimal anesthetic dose of thiopental was reduced by 36 per cent (from 10.9 to 6.9 mg per kg) after ethanol, 1.5 ml per kg, and the lethal dose of thiopental was reduced by 40 per cent after

Table 18–8 *Interaction of Ethanol with Sedatives, Tranquilizers, and Morphine**

Additive	Potentiating
Amobarbital	Chlorpromazine
Barbital	Meprobamate
Diazepam	Morphine
Hexobarbital	Promethazine
Pentobarbital	Reserpine
Phenobarbital	Thiopental
Secobarbital	
Chloral hydrate	
Glutethimide	
Paraldehyde	

*Modified from Forney, R. B., and Harger, R.: Ann. Rev. Pharmacol. *9*:379, 1969.

ethanol, 3.0 ml per kg, in dogs.[59] In one of their own studies, Forney and his group found that the sedative effects of reserpine, meprobamate, chlorpromazine, and morphine were potentiated by alcohol. The degree of potentiation by ethanol in Forney's study was reserpine > chlorpromazine > morphine > meprobamate.[62] Dundee in his study of intravenous alcohol anesthesia with various premedications found some reductions in the sleep dose of ethanol with promethazine, opiates, diazepam, and barbiturates.[49] His study was not designed specifically to measure potentiation. Dundee warns that the combination of ethanol and narcotics can cause severe respiratory depression.[49] Two adjunct drugs appear to antagonize the anesthetic effects of alcohol — hydroxyzine and chlordiazepoxide. Forney demonstrated that hydroxyzine opposed the anesthetic effect of alcohol.[62] Dundee showed that after chlordiazepoxide premedication, the per cent of patients that could be induced only with intravenous ethanol and nitrous oxide did not differ from the control group. Also more of the patients premedicated with chlordiazepoxide required supplementary methohexitone to complete their surgery than did the patients of the control group.[49]

An increased resistance of the central nervous system to general depressants has been regarded as the explanation for the greater concentrations of inhalation agents required for maintenance of anesthesia in alcoholics, and for the larger doses of barbiturates required for induction in sober chronic alcoholics.[4, 63] Johnstone and co-workers found that the cross tolerance to isoflurane induced in mice by chronic ingestion of 10 per cent ethanol persisted for 55 days following the discontinuation of ethanol.[48] Amirdvani and coworkers reported that after mice were withdrawn from 15 per cent ethanol in water for 60 days, the animals' MAC for halothane rose, reaching 1.6 per cent on the eighteenth day after withdrawal.[64] It would appear from these animal studies that the effect of chronic ethanol ingestion on anesthetic requirement persists and may increase after ethanol is discontinued. No studies concerning this problem in man have appeared in the literature.

Some evidence has accumulated that increased metabolism of medium acting barbiturates may account for part of the "resistance" of chronic alcoholics to barbiturate anesthesia. Rubin and others have shown that hepatic pentobarbital hydrolase activity in human volunteers more than doubled after 12 days of ethanol ingestion. Similar changes were also found in animals.[65] Moreover, in nonalcoholic man and animals, a single dose of ethanol was associated with a twofold increase in the plasma half-life of pentobarbital and a two- to fivefold increase in the half-life of meprobamate.[66] Further work is still needed to determine whether these effects of ethanol occur for thiopental, for other barbiturates, and for nonbarbiturate sedatives.

Both Keilty, and Morton and Adriani advise using regional anesthesia in alcoholics whenever possible.[50, 52] The use of regional anesthesia may help avoid the risks of anesthetic overdose and of aspiration in alcoholic patients. Regional anesthesia might be considered relatively contraindicated in patients with signs and symptoms of alcoholic polyneuritis. However, general anesthesia in these patients has occasionally led to a fatality,[43] and the presence of significant hepatic or cardiovascular disease may justify the use of regional anesthesia — including spinal anesthesia — in this group of patients. The use of physostigmine, 2 mg intravenously, may make the acutely intoxicated alcoholic oriented and cooperative during regional anesthesia.

General anesthesia may be employed in alcoholic patients. Enflurane and nitrous oxide appear to be satisfactory for use in alcoholics. For short cases methoxyflurane may be acceptable, but gas inductions in alcoholics with either methoxyflurane or diethyl ether should be avoided. Isoflurane may prove to be a satisfactory agent for use in alcoholics. Although cyclopropane is an excellent induction agent in alcoholics, Keilty advises against its use for maintenance, because cyclopropane significantly reduces hepatic blood flow.[50, 67] Ethylene may be used but, like cyclopropane, has the disadvantage of being flammable. Trichloroethylene should not be used in alcoholics because of its hepatotoxicity. Fluoroxene can be used, although repeated use of this agent in some animal species has led to hepatic necrosis. Halothane use in alcoholics, particularly with laboratory evidence of liver dysfunction, is inadvisable. However,

in thoracic or neurosurgical procedures, or in surgery on the airway, its advantages may well justify its use. Ketamine and the barbiturates may be employed in alcoholics; in acutely intoxicated patients, the doses of barbiturates should be reduced. Narcotics such as fentanyl, meperidine, and morphine are often employed as adjunct drugs during balanced anesthesia in intoxicated patients; respiratory depression resulting from the potentiation of the narcotics by ethanol may be avoided by reducing the doses of narcotics. On occasion, mechanical ventilation or reversal with naloxone followed by close observation for several hours is necessary.

In spite of the potential dangers involved in anesthetizing alcoholics, Lee et al. reported no increased incidence of anesthetic mortality in 169 intoxicated trauma patients at the Parkland Hospital.[42] Nor was there a significant increase in anesthetic morbidity or in intraoperative hypotension. There was a nonsignificant trend toward increased mortality in patients with blood alcohol levels above 250 mg per 100 ml.

Alcohol Abstinence Syndrome

The syndrome resulting from the abrupt withdrawal of ethyl alcohol may be mild ("the shakes") or severe, with convulsions, delirium, and death. The intensity of the abstinence syndrome varies with the amount of alcohol ingested. Mild symptoms may occur if 20 ounces per day of 100 proof alcohol are consumed over seven to 16 days; severe symptoms occur if 25 to 30 ounces of 100 proof alcohol are consumed daily for one to three months.[52] Isbell considers that severe physical dependence on ethanol results from drinking a quart of whiskey a day for 30 days, or roughly 32 ounces of 100 proof alcohol daily. Withdrawal symptoms can appear with blood alcohol levels as high as 50 mg per 100 ml. Daily use of alcohol is important in creating physical dependence on it; weekend or binge drinking will not result in withdrawal symptoms.

If delirium occurs, it usually appears two to four days after the last ingestion of alcohol, although the majority of patients in Wadstein's series developed delirium one to two days after cessation of alcohol intake.[41, 68] Isbell and coworkers showed that delirium tremens can be produced only by rapidly declining blood alcohol levels.[68]

The symptoms of alcohol abstinence syndrome include tremor, diaphoresis, nausea, abdominal cramps, tachycardia, fever, and hyperreflexia. In severe cases, convulsions may occur, followed by delirium, high fever, coma, and death. When delirium and convulsions are present, the mortality rate is at least 8 per cent.[68] Mortality rates for delirium tremens as high as 15 per cent for all patients and as high as 25 per cent for patients with other major illnesses have been quoted in the literature.[69] In postoperative patients, the mortality rate is over eight per cent; wound disruption and evisceration can also occur. After several days, untreated delirium tremens usually terminates in sleep, from which the patient awakens tired but lucid.

Hypokalemia may play a role in the pathophysiology of delirium tremens. Wadstein and Skude found that serum potassium decreased from normal values on admission to a mean of 2.9 mEq. per liter in 26 patients who developed delirium. Eleven other alcoholic patients who did not develop delirium tremens showed no change in serum potassium values. As the delirium ended, serum potassium values rapidly returned to normal. The infusion of 160 to 240 mEq. of potassium per day in two patients in the group that developed delirium did not prevent the decrease in serum potassium. None of the patients developed vomiting or diarrhea prior to the onset of delirium; nor did poor nutrition appear to contribute to the potassium flux. Serum sodium, magnesium, and bicarbonate values were normal in all patients.[41] Nor could the decrease in serum potassium be attributed to alkalosis. Thompson and coworkers also noticed low serum potassium values in their 34 patients, 17 of whom developed delirium tremens.[69] Wadstein suggests that a rapid uptake of potassium by cells occurred, and speculates that a high intracellular potassium concentration might cause the hyperexcitability seen during delirium tremens.[41] More research into potassium flux during delirium tremens is obviously needed.

The management of alcohol abstinence syndrome must include adequate sedation. For mild tremulousness and agitation, chloral hydrate, 1 or 2 gm, diazepam, 10 to 20 mg, or chlordiazepoxide, 100 to 200 mg, is useful. For delirium or seizures, larger doses of diazepam or chlordiazepoxide are necessary. Intravenous administration of these drugs is convenient, because it allows the physician to titrate the agitated patient or the patient with seizures until a light sleep is achieved. The sedation is tapered over a seven to 10 day period and is then stopped.

For the treatment of delirium tremens diazepam, paraldehyde, or chlordiazepoxide may be used. Currently diazepam appears to be the drug of choice, although good results have been obtained with paraldehyde, and fair results with chlordiazepoxide. It appears that the experience of the physicians employing these different drugs has some influence on the results obtained. Thompson and coworkers recently compared the use of diazepam, 5 to 10 mg every one to four hours intramuscularly, with the use of paraldehyde, 5 to 10 ml every two to four hours rectally.[69] Doses were titered to induce and maintain a calm state. A total of 34 patients were chosen randomly for therapy with paraldehyde or with diazepam. All patients had agitation, tremulousness, disorientation, hallucinations, and urinary incontinence, and were unable to take fluids orally. A calm state was achieved in an average of one and a half hours with diazepam, and in an average of four hours with paraldehyde (p<0.01). Of the patients treated only with paraldehyde, two died, and two others had respiratory arrest that necessitated resuscitation. No untoward reactions occurred in the group treated with diazepam (p of difference <0.0005). The authors noted considerable variation in the dose required to calm these patients.[69] Golbert and coworkers employed paraldehyde, 10 ml orally or intramuscularly, every two to four hours and chloral hydrate, 0.5 to 1.0 gm. orally or intramuscularly, for the prevention of delirium tremens in alcoholics who were in a tremulous state, with agitation, confusion, and disorientation but who had not yet developed hallucinations or cloudy sensorium. Of 12 patients so treated, only one developed delirium tremens.[70] Muller also utilized paraldehyde and chloral hydrate in patients with tremor resulting from alcohol withdrawal, and none of the patients treated with these two drugs developed delirium tremens.[71] Chlordiazepoxide can be used to sedate tremulous patients and to prevent convulsions, but it does not appear to be as effective in the prevention of delirium as diazepam or paraldehyde with chloral hydrate, as described in the regimens outlined above. In the series of Golbert et al., half the patients treated with chlordiazepoxide developed delirium, while in the series of Muller, nearly half the patients treated with it had prolonged confusion and a third developed fever.[70, 71] However, chlordiazepoxide did prevent convulsions in both these series of patients and in the series of patients studied by Rothfeld.[70-72] While chlordiazepoxide can be used in patients with tremulous states, the combination of paraldehyde and chloral hydrate appears superior in preventing the development of frank delirium tremens. Paraldehyde can be used orally in mild cases and intramuscularly in more severe withdrawal. However, intravenous paraldehyde may be dangerous; the author has heard of several cases of cardiac asystole following its use to control convulsions. At present, for impending or frank delirium tremens, diazepam appears to be the drug of choice, with combination use of paraldehyde and chloral hydrate a fairly close second choice.

Several drugs have been tested for therapy of tremulous states or of delirium tremens and should be avoided. The phenothiazides, promazine and chlorpromazine, are ineffective in the therapy of tremulous states.[70, 72] These drugs do not prevent seizures or the development of delirium, and can cause side effects such as oculogyric crisis and hypotension.[70, 72] Two of the 13 patients treated with promazine in the series of Golbert et al. died — one from hypotension and one from delirium tremens.[70] Thompson and coworkers, and Isbell emphasize the point that major tranquilizers such as the phenothiazines will not suppress abstinence of the alcohol-barbiturate type and will not reliably prevent seizures or delirium tremens.[1, 69] Barbiturates have been used in delirium, but are probably a poor choice, because dangerously large doses may be necessary to control symptoms.[73] Intravenous ethanol is probably not indicated for the treatment of delirium tremens; the margin between therapeutic and lethal doses is too narrow, and the relatively rapid metabolism of alcohol makes it difficult to achieve a gradually decreasing blood alcohol level.[74] Nearly half of the tremulous patients that were treated with intravenous or oral alcohol by Golbert and coworkers developed frank delirium tremens.[70] In Golbert's hands, therapy with paraldehyde and chloral hydrate was superior to therapy with phenothiazides, ethanol, or chlordiazepoxide. Only one of 12 patients treated with paraldehyde and chloral hydrate developed delirium, as opposed to 18 of 37 patients treated with promazine, or ethanol, or chlordiazepoxide.

The reasons for death during delirium tremens are not fully known. Cerebral edema is not a satisfactory explanation. Tavel noted that there is a group of patients who become hyperthermic (104°F), convulse, and die a hypotensive death during coma. Although fluid replacement in these patients was over 6 liters per day, Tavel still believed that dehydration might have contributed to the demise of some.[74] Depletion of the adrenal cortex and of liver glycogen may also have played a role. Tavel suggests the use of steroids and external cooling in patients with delirium tremens who have temperatures over 104°F. Intravenous dextrose should also be administered.[74] The use of a Swan-Ganz catheter for measurements of pulmonary artery wedge pressures and of cardiac output should also be considered in these severely ill patients. Measurements of serum osmolarity may help in determining adequacy of hydration. If fever or convulsions are difficult to control, consideration should be given to therapy with non-depolarizing muscle relaxants and mechanical ventilation. If high output cardiac failure develops, therapy with digitalis or catecholamines may be necessary.

ANESTHESIA FOR PATIENTS ADDICTED TO BARBITURATES

Chronic Barbiturate Addiction. Patients addicted to the barbiturates generally do not present the anesthesiologist with problems as difficult as those he may encounter in narcotic addicts and in alcoholics. The chronic use of barbiturates does not cause major pathological or physiological changes in organ systems of importance to anesthesia. An acute, massive barbiturate overdose, if untreated, can result in respiratory depression, hypoxic cerebral damage, circulatory depression, and death. These complications are mainly indirect effects of the barbiturate because permanent disability and death can usually be prevented by the prompt application of measures to support respiration and circulation. The anesthesiologist also may encounter problems resulting from barbiturate abstinence, particularly anxiety, tremors, postural hypotension, convulsions, and delirium in barbiturate addicts denied access to drugs upon admission to the hospital. Barbiturate addiction causes a strong psychic and physical dependence, and abrupt withdrawal from barbiturates can lead to convulsions, delirium, and fever, which occasionally may be fatal (see Table 18–5). The anesthesiologist may also encounter problems resulting from the induction of hepatic microsomal enzymes in patients addicted to barbiturates; increased metabolism of certain volatile anesthetics and of many other drugs can be expected in these patients.

Chronic barbiturate addiction is a definite clinical entity. The existence of this entity was proved by the group at Lexington who studied experimental barbiturate addiction in man.[76-79] They found that the signs and symptoms in patients given secobarbital, 0.9 to 3.8 gm daily, resembled those of alcohol intoxication. These were confusion, emotional lability, increased irritability, paranoia, regressive behavior, and dysarthria. Nystagmus, diplopia, strabismus, ataxia, past-pointing, and decreased cutaneous reflexes were also present, but deep tendon reflexes were usually unaffected. No sensory deficits were noted. Mild hypotension was observed.[79] The patients averaged only 7½ hours of sleep each night even with massive doses. No degree of addiction sufficient to cause clinical signs of abstinence developed in patients given only 0.2 gm of secobarbital as a single daily dose. No convulsions were seen in 18 patients withdrawn from 0.4 gm of secobarbital per day, but after 0.6 gm of secobarbital per day for one to two months, a barbiturate abstinence syndrome did develop. Convulsions appeared in two of 18 patients given 0.6 gm of secobarbital daily.[79] Fraser et al. point out that in patients who appear intoxicated but lack the odor of alcohol on the breath, the physician should suspect barbiturate intoxication.[77] Tolerance to the sedative effects of barbiturates is apparent after only seven days of barbiturate intake.[78] Some tolerance to the lethal depression of barbiturates does occur, but this increased tolerance is very small indeed.[78, 80, 81] The small increase in tolerance with barbiturates makes titration of the barbiturate addict prior to withdrawal a matter of critical importance. For example, an addict may be stable on 1 gm of secobarbital per day but may be intoxicated on 1.1 gm.[82]

No histologic damage to major organs accompanies chronic barbiturate intoxication.[79] However, the intra-arterial injection of secobarbital sodium can result in ischemic necrosis or atrophy of the muscles of the forearm and hand.[86] The author has also seen a case in which this type of injury led to amputation of a hand. Chemical phlebitis and sclerosis of superficial veins because of the high pH of the barbiturates is common in barbiturate addicts who take the drug intravenously.[86]

The Barbiturate Abstinence Syndrome. The barbiturate withdrawal syndrome is well described by Fraser and his co-workers and by Wikler.[77, 83] Its intensity depends on the rate of elimination of the drug; blood clearance rates of less than 20 per cent of the drug per day were not associated with symptoms of abstinence or with EEG changes.[84] With secobarbital, an intermediate-acting barbiturate, the abstinence syndrome is as follows:[77] For the first eight to 10 hours after discontinuing the drug, patients seemed to recover from the effects of chronic barbiturate intoxication. Over the next 24 hours minor symptoms and signs such as anxiety, headache, involuntary muscle twitching, intention tremor of the hands, weakness, dizziness, and visual distortions appeared.[77] Hyperreflexia was present; insomnia, abdominal cramps, nausea, vomiting, weight loss, tachycardia, and significant postural hypotension also occurred. During the next 24 to 72 hours, one to four grand mal convulsions occurred in 79 per cent of the patients, followed in most by a psychosis resembling delirium tremens with predominant visual hallucinations. The EEG displayed high voltage spikes or spike and dome configurations. The delirium lasted from one to seven days. A rising core temperature is an ominous sign; and if hyperpyrexia appears, it must be treated vigorously.[83] A summary of the syndrome is given in Table 18–9.

Treatment of barbiturate abstinence syndrome consists of titrating the patient with a medium-acting barbiturate (e.g., pentobar-

Table 18–9 *Barbiturate Withdrawal Syndrome for Barbiturates with an Intermediate Duration of Action, e.g., Secobarbital*

Hours After Last Dose	Symptoms
12 to 36	Anxiety
	Muscle twitching
	Intention tremor of hands
	Weakness
	Dizziness
	Visual distortion (similar to DT's)
	Hyperreflexia
	Insomnia
	Nausea and vomiting
	Weight loss (up to 5 kg)
	Postural hypotension
36 to 92	One to four grand mal convulsions (in 80% of patients)
	Delirium and visual hallucinations for one to seven days
	Hyperpyrexia (occasionally)

bital) until sedation or aphasia and nystagmus appear. A reasonable initial dose is 0.2 to 0.4 gm. The patient should be examined one hour prior to each dose for signs of barbiturate abstinence and one hour after each dose for signs of barbiturate intoxication.[83] If the patient has already had a convulsion when treatment begins, the higher initial dose (0.4 gm) should be used. The initial dose may be repeated four times a day and adjusted until the patient is free of withdrawal symptoms. Titration is important, because tolerance is lost rapidly during withdrawal; use of the full barbiturate dose to which the patient has been accustomed may result in a fatality.[78] The total daily dose should then be reduced by no more than 0.1 gm per day as the patient is withdrawn, so the period of gradual withdrawal may require up to three weeks. Giuffrida and coworkers recommend reducing the dose of pentobarbital by no more than 10 per cent per day.[88] Dilantin and chlorpromazine are not effective against convulsions resulting from barbiturate withdrawal in man.[1, 83, 85] If delirium is present, the patient must receive sufficient barbiturate to suppress insomnia and hyerpyrexia.[83] Diazepam or chlordiazepoxide instead of pentobarbital may also be used to suppress the abstinence syndrome resulting from the withdrawal of barbiturates.[1]

Anesthetic Management of the Barbiturate Addict. Preoperatively the barbiturate addict will need a larger dose of barbiturate premedication than is necessary in nonaddicted patients.[52] The prolonged stormy inductions often seen in alcoholics are rare in barbiturate addicts.[52] For induction the barbiturate addict often requires elevated doses of thiopental, which can be explained by increased tolerance of the central nervous system to barbiturates.[52, 87] Support for this concept is found in the experiments of Hubbard and Goldbaum, who observed that mice tolerant to thiopental awakened at higher tissue levels of barbiturate than did the controls.[63] Many investigators have shown that pretreatment with barbiturates can lead to resistance to barbiturate anesthesia.[4, 87] However, Giuffrida and coworkers reported that unusual doses of thiobarbiturates were not required for induction in their patients. The majority of their patients were narcotic addicts or addicts taking multiple drugs, including barbiturates and ethanol. Eleven of the 145 patients did require 450 to 600 mg doses of thiopental for induction.[88] The weight of the evidence still indicates that patients addicted to barbiturates require somewhat higher doses of thiopental for the induction and maintenance of anesthesia.

To account for the shorter duration of action of sleep doses of certain short-acting barbiturates in barbiturate addicts, explanations other than the postulated increase in CNS tolerance may be necessary. Burns points out that the anesthetic action of hexobarbital and methohexital (Brevital) is terminated in part by rapid metabolism.[89] He cites data that indicate a sevenfold increase in the rate of metabolism of hexobarbital in liver microsomes of rats pretreated with phenobarbital. The increased rate of metabolism was associated with a dramatic decrease in the sleeping time of the pretreated animals (pretreated 11 minutes, vs. 216 minutes for the controls). However, it is unlikely that increases in the rate of metabolism of thiopental in barbiturate addicts would be important clinically, because redistribution rather than biotransformation terminates the anesthetic action of single induction doses of thiopental.

Rubin and others suggest that increased induction of hepatic enzymes may play a role in the development of early tolerance to barbiturates.[66] Induction of hepatic microsomal enzymes occurs both in man and in laboratory animals during chronic barbiturate use. Phenobarbital induces mixed function oxidase enzymes which metabolize numerous drugs, including some volatile anesthetics. In animals Hitt and Mazze have shown that pretreatment for four days with phenobarbital resulted in serum and urinary levels of free fluoride ion nearly double those of control animals following a two hour anesthetic with 0.25 per cent methoxyflurane (p<0.01).[90] Rice and Mazze showed in vitro that microsomal enzyme preparations from the livers of rats pretreated with phenobarbital for at least five days could remove fluoride from both isoflurane and methoxyflurane more rapidly than enzyme preparations from control animals (p of difference <0.05 for isoflurane and <0.01 for methoxyflurane).[91] Hitt and coworkers point out that patients on drugs that induce certain hepatic microsomal oxidases have a greater risk of developing nephrotoxicity after anesthesia with methoxyflurane.[90] Barbiturates did not appear to increase the rate of metabolism of enflurane in these studies.

Habitual use of phenobarbital increases the hydroxylation of cortisol to 6-β-hydroxycortisol in man,[92] and pentobarbital has been shown to inhibit reversibly the deamination of adenosine 5' monophosphate in the brains of rodents.[93]

Addiction to barbiturates does not appear to prolong induction times with inhalation anesthetics. A review of the recent anesthetic literature discloses no articles indicating that prolonged, stormy inductions occur in barbiturate addicts. Nor are there reports that barbiturate addicts require higher maintenance concentrations. In animals, Lee et al. did not find a trend toward longer induction times in rats addicted to methohexital and then anesthetized with 20 per cent diethyl ether or 1.5 per cent methoxyflurane.[4]

The anesthesiologist should have little difficulty managing barbiturate addicts, provided that he employs sufficient preoperative sedation to prevent the barbiturate abstinence syndrome, and provided that he can recognize and treat the syndrome when it appears. It may be wise to avoid using methoxyflurane because of the problem of enzyme induction in patients addicted to barbiturates.

In patients comatose from an overdose of barbiturates who also require surgery, the anesthesiologist should look for evidence of dehydration or hypovolemia. In one series of patients hospitalized for barbiturate overdose, nearly a quarter had an elevated hematocrit.[94] Hypotension was seen with all degrees of coma, and usually responded to the infusion of several liters of saline. An increased venous capacitance has been reported in patients with barbiturate overdose.[95] In cases of hypotension refractory to volume expansion with crystalloid or colloid solutions, a vasopressor drip of metaraminol, levarterenol, isoproterenol, or dopamine may be used to restore urinary output or to achieve a systolic blood pressure above 80 mm Hg.[94, 96] Barbiturate addicts who are not suffering from overdose or withdrawal may be expected to have a normal state of hydration and a normal blood volume. Their nutritional status is usually normal.[97] Small doses of secobarbital in normal, hydrated subjects result in decreases in urine flow, creatinine clearance, and solute excretion without significant changes in arterial pressure. Their inability to produce a concentrated urine suggests that altered renal perfusion rather than the action of antidiuretic hormone accounts for the water retention observed.[98]

ANESTHESIA FOR PATIENTS ADDICTED TO MISCELLANEOUS DEPRESSANTS

Many depressants other than alcohol and the barbiturates can cause addiction. Included in this group are glutethimide (Doriden) and methyprylon (Nodular), which are structurally similar to the barbiturates. Also included in this group are meprobamate (Equanil, Miltown), a carbamic ester of 2-methyl-2-n-propyl-1,3-propanediol, and methaqualone (Qualude, Sopor), a 2,3 disubstituted quinazolone. Withdrawal syndromes similar to the barbiturate abstinence syndrome have been reported in patients addicted to these drugs. Addicted patients should be kept on maintenance doses of these drugs before and after surgery, because convulsions have occurred after their abrupt discontinuation.[99, 100] Similar considerations apply to the benzodiazepine compounds chlordiazepoxide (Librium), clorazepate (Tranxene), flurazepam (Dalmane), lorazepam (Ativam), oxazepam (Serax), and diazepam (Valium). If it is desired to withdraw the patient prior to elective surgery, the amount of drug administered may be

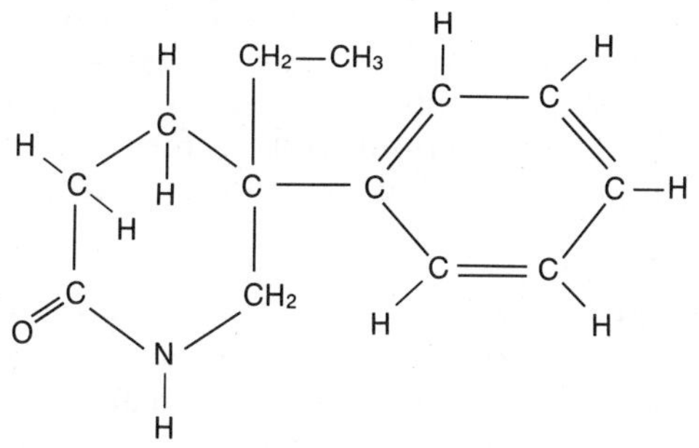

Glutethimide (Doriden)

Figure 18–5.

reduced at the rate of one therapeutic dose per day. If tremor or agitation appears, the dose must not be reduced for one to two days.[100] If the patient's type of drug or maintenance dose is not known, a barbiturate may be substituted and then slowly withdrawn. Pentobarbital, 0.2 gm every two hours, may be given until mild intoxication (nystagmus) is achieved and may then slowly be withdrawn.[100] Phenothiazines or rauwolfia alkaloids should be avoided, lest hypotension appear. Hypotension has been reported during treatment of the abstinence syndrome of ethinamate (Valmid).[100] These depressant drugs are listed in Table 18–5.

For acute overdoses of any of the depressant drugs discussed in this section, the anesthesiologist may need to apply general supportive measures such as intubation and mechanical respiration, and circulatory support with intravenous fluids and occasionally with vasopressors.

Glutethimide (Doriden) (Fig. 18–5). This sedative resembles phenobarbital structurally, but in onset and duration of action is similar to secobarbital. It has anticholinergic properties, and mydriasis is a constant feature of elevated dosage. Tolerance to its sedative effect and physical dependence have been described for doses over 1.5 gm per day,[101] although Essig suggests that a slightly higher dose (2.5 gm) is necessary.[100] Overdoses are characterized by respiratory depression, lethargy, or coma, a flushed face, mydriasis, areflexia, flaccid paralysis, and respiratory and circulatory failure. The level of consciousness may fluctuate as a result of irregular glutethimide absorption from the gastrointestinal tract. Tachypnea,

up to 50 breaths per minute, and copious tenacious bronchial secretions as well as pulmonary congestion are prominent features of glutethimide intoxication.[102] Hypotension may be severe,[103] and frequent monitoring of blood pressure is imperative. Tolerance to the sedative effects of up to 8 gm per day has been reported in addicts.[100]

The abstinence syndrome for glutethimide includes tremors, headache, nausea, vomiting, anxiety, and tachycardia. Painful muscle spasms of the back with extension of the legs and flexion of the arms have also been reported,[101] and abdominal cramps are a characteristic of glutethimide withdrawal. Convulsions may occur 15 hours to six days after discontinuation of the drug.[85] Treatment with barbiturates, as described by Essig, or by slow withdrawal of glutethimide seems acceptable.[100] If barbiturate substitution therapy is used, Wikler advises maintenance of the stabilizing barbiturate dose for several days before starting withdrawal, in order to avoid convulsions.[83]

It would appear that persons on maintenance doses of glutethimide can have a reaction resembling the abstinence syndrome. Zivin and Shalowitz describe three cases in patients taking 0.5 to 3 gm per day. The reaction consisted of mood swings, delirium, fever to 102° F, nystagmus, poor coordination, tetanic muscle spasms, and convulsions. In one patient the convulsions were controlled with Dilantin.[105] The reason for the appearance of this type of reaction in patients on maintenance doses of the drug is unknown at present.

Methyprylon (Nodular) (Fig. 18–6). Methyprylon is structurally similar to the barbiturates. The lethal dose in man is not well established, but death has been re-

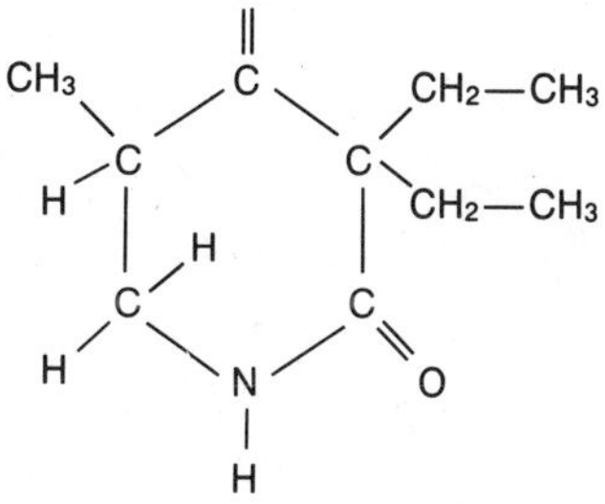

Methyprylon (Nodular)

Figure 18–6.

ported with as little as 6 gm.[100, 106] Physical dependence resulting in withdrawal symptoms has been reported with 2.4 gm per day. Withdrawal following larger doses has caused convulsions.[100] The withdrawal syndrome resembles that of barbiturates but appears two to three days after the drug has been discontinued. Polyuria and auditory and visual hallucinations are prominent features. Slow withdrawal of methyprylon or substitution of a barbiturate and its withdrawal may be used to treat this syndrome.

Convulsions after acute overdoses have occasionally been reported. Small doses of short-acting barbiturates may be used to treat this rare problem. Physostigmine may be useful in methyprylon coma. Nattel and coworkers reported some success in treating a small series of patients in coma from mixtures of depressant drugs with physostigmine; methyprylon was an agent in many of their cases, and physostigmine improved the level of consciousness in one third of their patients.[107]

Meprobamate (Miltown, Equanil) (Fig. 18–7). Meprobamate has been a very popular drug for the treatment of anxiety, and its nonprescription use by the lay public has been widespread. Therapeutic doses are 200 to 400 mg three to four times a day. The dose above which physical dependence occurs is between 1600 and 2400 mg daily.[100] Therapeutic doses of meprobamate given to normal, healthy subjects decrease postural reflexes that maintain blood pressure during continuous positive pressure breathing, as demonstrated by McGuird and Leary.[108] Systolic blood pressure fell below 100 mm Hg in four of seven subjects pretreated with meprobamate and subjected to a 65 degree tilt; in five of six subjects CPPB at 30 cm water pressure caused a 10 mm Hg decrease in arterial pressure. Patients on meprobamate should be protected against postural hypotension during anesthesia and surgery.

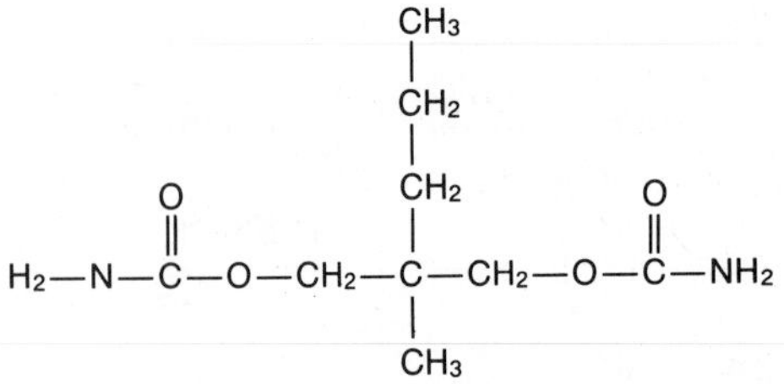

Chronic intoxication with meprobamate is characterized by drowsiness and poor coordination. Hypotension has been reported as a side effect of meprobamate addiction.[109] Tolerance to the sedative effects develops as a result of both CNS adaptation and increased metabolism (i.e., drug disposition tolerance). Philips and others using ^{14}C-labeled meprobamate found that the half-life of this drug in the brain and blood of control animals was twice that in tolerant animals (brain 3.69 vs. 1.79 hours; blood 4.34 vs. 2.18 hours).[110] About 90 per cent of ingested meprobamate is excreted as hydroxymeprobamate or as a glucuronide derivative.[111] In man, 50 per cent of the drug is excreted in 24 hours and 92 per cent is excreted in 96 hours.[112] Potentiation between meprobamate and ethanol has been documented (see above). There is little information concerning the interactions between meprobamate and general anesthetic agents, although one might anticipate both hypotensive problems and resistance to barbiturate anesthetics in chronic meprobamate users. In the nonuser who is intoxicated with meprobamate, reduced doses of thiopental should be employed.

The meprobamate abstinence syndrome has been well studied and resembles that of the barbiturates.[109, 112, 113] Insomnia, anxiety, tremors, nausea, vomiting, weakness, headache, postural hypotension, hallucinations, and convulsions appear. Symptoms are prominent from one to three days after withdrawal and subside in a week to 10 days. Convulsions appearing 36 to 72 hours after withdrawal of the drug have been reported for some patients (one of 21) taking over 3.2 gm per day.[112] Therapy with barbiturates is acceptable and would seem preferable to therapy with phenytoin, although some patients with convulsions during meprobamate abstinence apparently have responded to phenytoin.[109] Death has been reported during withdrawal in a patient addicted to 10 gm per day; hyperpyrexia (107.8° F) was a prominent feature.[114]

Methaqualone (Qualude, Sopor) (Fig. 18–8). Methaqualone is 2-methyl-3-*o*-tolyl-

Meprobamate (Miltown, Equanil)

Figure 18–7.

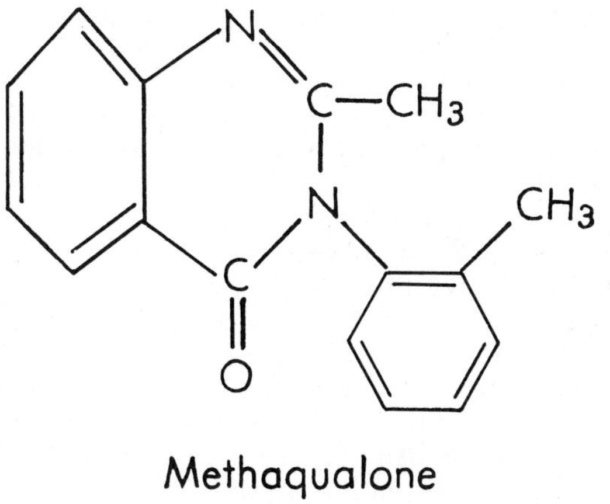

Methaqualone

Figure 18–8. Methaqualone (Qualude, Sopor).

4(3H)-quinazolinone, a 2,3 disubstituted quinazolone which has hypnotic activity in both animals and man. Its abuse has been widespread because of the mistaken ideas that it does not cause dependence and that it is effective as an aphrodisiac.[115] Methaqualone overdose results in coma accompanied by increased muscle tone, myoclonus, and flailing motions of the extremities. Twitching and shivering appear, and the deep tendon reflexes are hyperactive. The increased muscle tone and flailing motions serve as a clue to the diagnosis of poisoning with methaqualone. Increased salivation may be present. In contrast to overdoses with other depressants, respiratory depression is not characteristic of methaqualone poisoning.[116] Coma in adults occurs with oral doses of about 2400 mg of methaqualone. In severe overdoses — for example, with blood levels of methaqualone over 20 mg per 100 ml — hypotension may appear. In fatal cases of methaqualone overdose, death occurs after a prolonged series of convulsions. Treatment with non-depolarizing muscle relaxants and mechanical ventilation may be necessary to prevent exhaustion or to prevent trauma from flailing motion, as described by Abboud and coworkers.[116] Methaqualone is almost completely metabolized by hydroxylation in the liver and is eliminated quite rapidly; 80 per cent of a single dose is eliminated within 24 hours, two thirds in the urine and one third in the bile.[118] Therefore, conservative management of methaqualone overdoses has been quite successful. Matthew and coworkers reported no fatalities in 116 cases

managed without the use of dialysis.[119] Supportive therapy with intravenous fluids, tracheal intubation to secure the airway, and occasionally paralysis with muscle relaxants and mechanical ventilation to control muscular hyperactivity are necessary. Dialysis should be considered only in very severe overdoses with blood levels of methaqualone above 20 mg per 100 ml.

The abstinence syndrome with methaqualone resembles that of the barbiturates, with anxiety, insomnia, tremors, headache, delirium, fever, and convulsions. Severe symptoms can be avoided by reducing the patient's dose of methaqualone no more than 10 per cent per day during withdrawal. Therapy by substituting a barbiturate and then slowing withdrawing it also seems acceptable.

Little or no specific information regarding interactions between methaqualone and anesthetics has appeared in the literature.

Interactions of Depressants and Warfarin Anticoagulants. Three of the depressants discussed above induce hepatic microsomal enzymes that metabolize sodium warfarin (Coumadin, Dicumarol). Patients on therapeutic doses of the sedatives therefore require more sodium warfarin to maintain their Quick prothrombin times in the therapeutic range. Sudden discontinuation of the depressant drug and maintenance of the same dose of warfarin can cause the prothrombin time to become greatly prolonged, resulting in hemorrhagic problems. Udall studied this interaction between sedatives and warfarin and found that daily use of phenobarbital, 100 mg, secobarbital, 100 mg, and glutethimide, 0.5 gm, leads to a significant increase in the dose of warfarin needed to maintain anticoagulation. There was also a trend toward an altered prothrombin time with methaqualone. Chloral hydrate did not affect prothrombin times or warfarin doses. Meprobamate has a slight effect of warfarin requirement, but not enough to be significant clinically.[120] In patients using large doses of depressants, somewhat more enzyme induction can be expected. The anesthesiologist should be aware that as patients addicted to barbiturates or glutethimide and also on warfarin are withdrawn from the depressant drug, their prothrombin times may become dangerously prolonged. The warfarin dose must be reduced as the doses of depressant drug

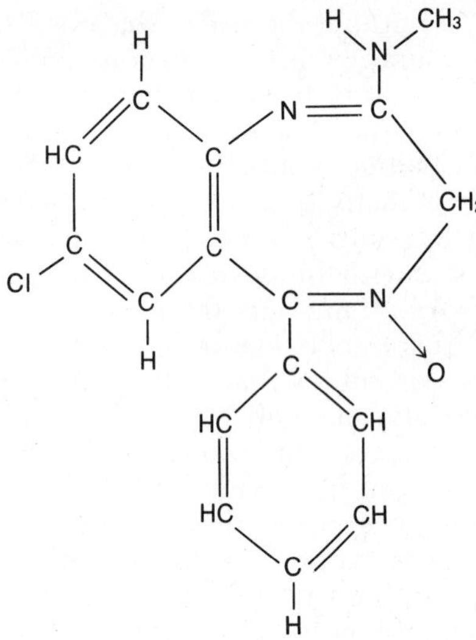

Chlordiazepoxide (Librium)

Figure 18–9.

are decreased. Frequent measurements of the prothrombin time are helpful during detoxication of patients on both warfarin and certain depressant drugs.

Benzodiazepine Compounds: Chlordiazepoxide (Librium), Chlorazepate (Tranxene), Flurazepam (Dalmane), Lorazepam (Ativam), Oxazepam (Serax), and Diazepam (Valium) (Figs. 18–9 and 18–10). When benzodiazepine derivatives are taken to obtain a "high," they are usually used in combination with another drug such as marijuana or alcohol.[121] Chronic intoxication with benzodiazepines resulting in physical dependence has been reported in man.[122] Chronic intoxication with chlordiazepoxide causes drowsiness, weakness, and vertigo; at high doses agitation may be seen.[122] Coma has been reported after as little as 300 mg but the lethal dose in man has not yet been defined.[100] The half-life of chlordiazepoxide in man is approximately two days. Abstinence reactions have been reported in patients who had been taking 300 to 600 mg daily prior to withdrawal.[122] The abstinence syndrome resulting from withdrawal from the benzodiazepines resembles that of barbiturate abstinence; anxiety, insomnia, tremors, muscle cramps, diaphoresis, abdominal cramps, and vomiting occur. Symptoms may not appear until a week after the drug is

discontinued, because the benzodiazepines and their metabolites are excreted slowly. Convulsions can occur during withdrawal in addicts using large amounts of any of the benzodiazepines. Convulsions appear late in the syndrome (seventh to twelfth day) when the benzodiazepine has nearly disappeared from the plasma.[122]

For the treatment of disorientation or hallucinations from therapeutic doses of benzodiazepines, physostigmine has been recommended. Several cases of disorientation resulting from lorazepam which responded well to physostigmine have been described in the anesthesia literature.[123] For the treatment of mild to moderate overdoses of benzodiazepines, physostigmine has also been useful. Liberti and coworkers described a 23 month old girl who ingested at least 80 mg of diazepam and became comatose. After physostigmine, 0.4 mg intramuscularly, she was awake within 20 minutes.[124] In adults with benzodiazepine intoxication, physostigmine 1 to 2 mg intravenously may be given. If the response to a second dose is still inadequate, supportive therapy is indicated. Intubation and mechanical ventilation may be necessary.

For addicts taking large amounts of benzodiazepine compounds, increased doses of barbiturates or of diazepam may be necessary for the induction of anesthesia. One benzodiazepine derivative, diazepam, is often

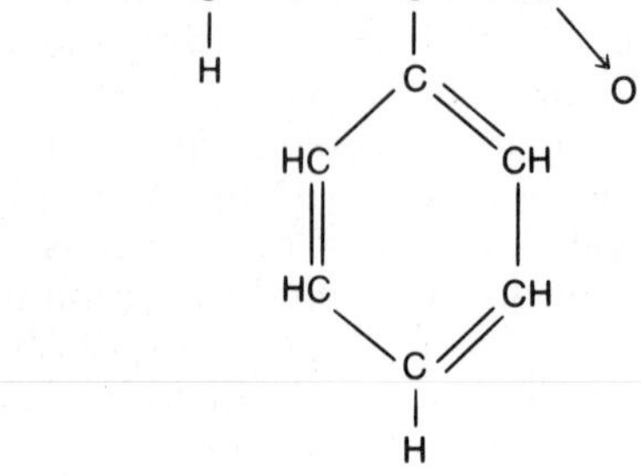

Diazepam (Valium)

Figure 18–10.

employed for sedation during regional anesthesia and as an induction agent for general anesthesia. Transient apnea but rather stable hemodynamics occur with the use of diazepam. Benzodiazepines potentiate narcotics and may act additively with general anesthetic agents. Thus far, no specific studies of minimal alveolar concentration (MAC) for general anesthetic agents in heavy users of benzodiazepine compounds have appeared.

ANESTHESIA FOR PATIENTS ADDICTED TO ALCOHOL DERIVATIVES, PARALDEHYDE, AND TOXIC ALCOHOLS

Several derivatives of tertiary alcohols or carbamic acid esters of alcohols have been used as sedatives and are addicting. Ethchlorvynol, a tertiary alcohol, and ethinamate, a carbamic acid ester of cyclohexanol, are examples of such compounds. Paraldehyde, a polymer of acetaldehyde, is also addicting. Patients taking these compounds may also present problems during anesthesia and in the postoperative period.

Ethchlorvynol (Placidyl) (Fig. 18–11). Ethchlorvynol ingestion at doses above 1500 mg per day can lead to addiction, as reported by Cahn.[125] The abstinence syndrome resembles that for barbiturates. Convulsions are seen about the fifth day. An interaction with ethyl alcohol suggesting a strong potentiation of the hypnotic effect of these drugs has been reported in two patients, but the cardiovascular effects of the combination were not described.[126]

Ethinamate (Valmid) (Fig. 18–12). Ethinamate addiction has been reported with doses of from 4 to 15 gm per day.[100, 127] The abstinence syndrome resembles that of the general depressants, but severe hypertension, arrhythmias, and syncopal episodes may occur as part of the syndrome. Hypotension from promazine therapy for

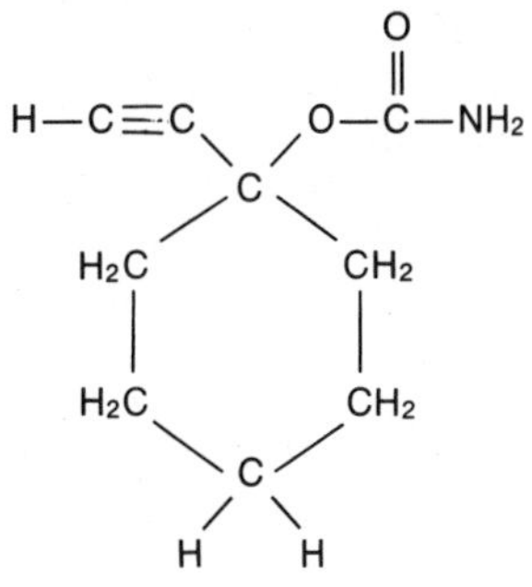

Ethinamate (Valmid)

Figure 18–12.

eth'inamate abstinence syndrome has been reported, and seizures occur fairly early during withdrawal.

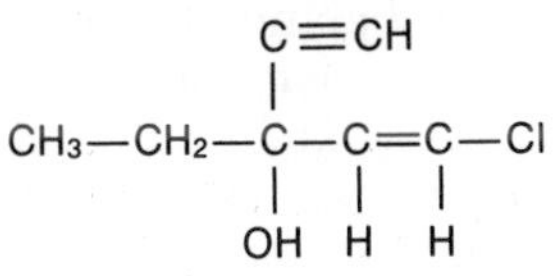

Paraldehyde (Fig. 18–13). The use of paraldehyde as an intoxicant in preference to ethyl alcohol is rather uncommon. Mendelson and others described a small group of patients who preferred paraldehyde to whiskey and who drank it regularly.[128] In patients intoxicated with paraldehyde, severe metabolic acidosis with an arterial pH 7.01 to 7.12 and a low serum bicarbonate (0.9 to 5 mEq/L) have been reported by Mendelson and his group and by Beier et al.[129] The mechanism of this acidosis remains speculative; Beier did not believe it to be acetate from decomposition of the paraldehyde or lactate from interference with oxidative metabolism. Any patient addicted to paraldehyde should be evaluated for acidosis by an arterial gas determination prior to anesthesia and surgery.

Methyl and Isopropyl Alcohols. Mendelson and others describe nine men who drank toxic alcohols regularly for periods of

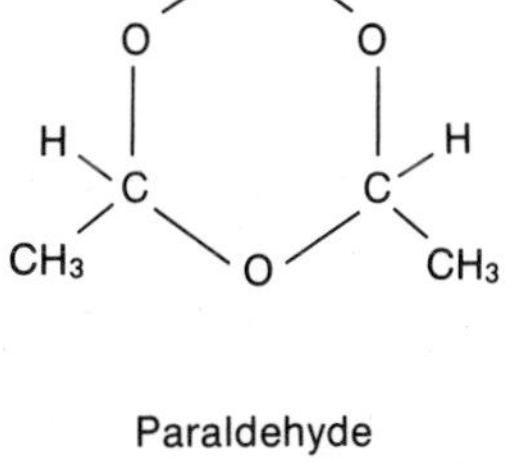

Ethchlorvynol (Placidyl)

Figure 18–11.

Paraldehyde

Figure 18–13.

from ten to 40 years. They were in surprisingly good physical condition, but hepatomegaly was present in most of them. One patient who preferred Sterno was admitted with a syndrome resembling alcoholic hallucinosis, and had a metabolic acidosis. Anesthetic management for patients with addiction to toxic alcohols should include correction of acidosis and should take into consideration the possibility that parenchymal liver and kidney damage may be present.

ANESTHETIC CONSIDERATIONS IN PATIENTS INHALING POISONOUS COMPOUNDS: GLUE (ACETONE), CLEANING FLUIDS (CARBONA), AND OTHER SOLVENTS

Patients who inhale glue or cleaning fluids are frequently in the adolescent age range and may have severe hepatic and renal damage. The fumes from many solvents may cause excitation, euphoria, vertigo, visual and sometimes auditory hallucinations, and destructive behavior. Children denied easy access to other pleasure-giving drugs may resort to "glue sniffing" or solvent abuse to gain a thrill or to escape reality. Chemicals so obtained include acetone, aliphatic acetates, alcohols, benzene, carbon tetrachloride, ethyl and vinyl ethers, naphtha, trichlorethane, trichlorethylene, toluene, and xyline.[1, 2] (See Table 18–10.) With inhalation of many of these solvents

Table 18–10 Products and Solvents Commonly Inhaled*

Products	Solvent Inhaled
Glues	Acetone, toluene
Nail polish Remover	Acetone, alcohols, aliphatic acetates
Lighter fluid	Benzene
Cleaning fluid	Naphtha, carbon tetrachloride
Lacquer thinner	Aliphatic acetates, toluene
Ethers	Ethyl and vinyl ethers
Fuels	Gasoline, kerosene
Correction fluid	Trichloroethane, xylene
Propellant	Freon-12

*Modified from Unwin, J. R.: Canad. Med. Assoc. J. 98:402, 1968.

stupor, coma, or convulsions can occur. Anorexia may result from frequent use. Renal and hepatic dysfunction frequently occurs, and hematopoietic abnormalities appear on occasion. In a survey of 8689 children, ages 11 to 19, seen in public clinics in New York City, 44 had a history of sniffing glue and 11 had inhaled cleaning fluid (Carbona). Twelve of the 44 children who had sniffed glue had abnormal liver function tests, one had postnecrotic cirrhosis proved by biopsy, and two died from hepatic necrosis. Of 11 children who had inhaled cleaning fluid, five had abnormal liver function tests and two had renal failure.[130] Anemia and depression of platelet and white blood cell counts were not seen in this series but have occasionally been reported.[2] Many of the deaths from solvent inhalation actually result from suffocating in the plastic bag used to concentrate the fumes.[2] However, deaths from pulmonary edema or from apparent cardiac arrhythmia have occurred.[2, 131] Rare fatalities have been reported from the inhalation of Freon-12 ("frost freaking"). Pulmonary edema or acute laryngeal dysfunction appears to have been involved.[2] Apparently some degree of tolerance is present in the inhalation of solvents (acetone and toluene) found in glue: many users report an increase in the number of tubes of glue necessary to obtain a "high" after several months of use. Tolerance does therefore occur in the abuse of certain solvents. As yet, no evidence for physical dependence on these substances has appeared.

The anesthesiologist may participate in resuscitating victims of solvent inhalation. The odor of a solvent on the breath of an intoxicated or comatose patient may provide a clue to the diagnosis. Anesthesia for patients with recent solvent intoxication or with a history of chronic solvent abuse should be chosen to avoid causing renal or hepatic damage. If the site of surgery permits, regional anesthesia is indicated in cooperative patients. If general anesthesia is necessary, a balanced anesthetic technique with nitrous oxide and reduced doses of barbiturates, narcotics, and relaxants would be preferable. Diethyl ether should be acceptable. Methoxyflurane, fluothane, enflurane, fluoroxene, cyclopropane, and chloroform are best avoided.

ANESTHESIA FOR PATIENTS USING PSYCHEDELIC DRUGS: HALLUCINOGENS, STIMULANTS, DELIRIANTS, EUPHORIANTS, AND DRUGS CAUSING PSYCHOSES

Numerous drugs cause alterations of mood, perception, cognitive ability, or body image. Compounds causing such alterations are referred to as psychedelic drugs. Table 18–11 lists the principal psychedelic drugs currently in use in North America, classified according to their chemical structure. The major hallucinogens — lysergic acid, psilocybin, and diethyl- and dimethyltryptamine — are derivatives of the indole nu-

Table 18–11 *Classification of Psychedelic Drugs by Chemical Structure*

	Potency (Mescaline units)‡
A. Hallucinogens	
Indoles	
Lysergic acid diethylamide (LSD)	3700
Psilocybin	31
Dimethyltryptamine (DMT)	4
Diethyltryptamine (DET)	4
B. Sympathetic Hallucinogens	
Phenylethylamines (substituted amphetamines)	
Dimethoxymethylamphetamine (DOM = STP)	80
Dimethoxyethylamphetamine (DOET)	80
Methylenedioxyphenylethylamine (MDA)	3
Methoxymethylenedioxyamphetamine (MMDA)	10
Bromodimethoxyamphetamine (DOB)	—
Trimethoxyamphetamine (TMA)	2
Trimethoxyphenylethylamine (mescaline)*	1
Nutmeg	
C. Stimulants	
Amphetamines	
Amphetamine	
Dextroamphetamine	
Methamphetamine	
D. Deliriants	
Tropanes and anticholinergics of other structure	
Atropine	
Scopolamine	
Piperidyl isomer (Ditran, Ditropan)	
Other anticholinergics (see Table 15–17)	
Cocaine†	
E. Euphoriants	
Cannabinols	
^{9}Tetrahydrocannabinol (THC) (hashish, marijuana)	
DMHP and numerous other active cannabinols	
F. Drugs Causing Psychosis	
Phenylcyclohexylamines	
Methylphenidate (Ritalin)	
Phenmetrazine (Preludin)	
Phencyclidine (PCP)	
Ethylphenylcyclohexylamine (PCE)	
Phenylcyclohexylpyrrolidine (PHP)	
Thienylcyclohexylpiperidine (TCP, TPCP)	

*Mescaline is often classified with the major hallucinogens.

†Cocaine is often classified with the sympathetic hallucinogens or with the amphetamines, which it resembles in pharmacological effects but not in chemical structure.

‡Data from Brawley, P., and Duffield, J. C.: Pharmacol Rev. *24*:31, 1972—Mescaline unit = $\dfrac{ED\ (x)}{ED\ (mescaline\ in\ mg.\ of\ the\ free\ base)}$

cleus. However, many other drugs widely used for their hallucinogenic properties are phenylethylamines — compounds derived from the amphetamine nucleus; they have certain characteristics in common with the amphetamines, but they are taken for their hallucinogenic rather than their stimulatory effects. Included in this group is mescaline, one of the oldest known hallucinogens. Members of this group (Table 18–11, B) are referred to as sympathetic hallucinogens. The amphetamines (Table 18–11, C) are taken mainly for their alerting effect on the central nervous system, and any hallucinations resulting from their use are regarded as side effects. The group of deliriants includes piperidyl isomer and the belladonna alkaloids atropine and scopolamine (Table 18–11, D). Cocaine is classified with these drugs, since it contains the tropine nucleus structurally; however, in its pharmacological effects, it more closely resembles the amphetamines or the sympathetic hallucinogens. The effects of the deliriants in man are marked amnesia and confusion. The cannabinols, which are found in marijuana, are among the most widely abused drugs in America today (Table 18–11, E). Their effects include marked euphoria, their use is not always accompanied by hallucinations, and they show no cross tolerance with the major hallucinogens. Chemically their structure differs from the indole structures of the major hallucinogens and from the phenylethylamine structure of the sympathetic hallucinogens. Hence the cannabinols are listed separately, as euphoriants. The cyclohexylamines, which include phencyclidine and its cogeners, also differ structurally from all other psychedelics and do not show cross tolerance with any of them; their abuse often results in marked feelings of depersonalization, distortion of body image, hostility, catalepsy, and a dissociated state — in sum, a psychosis (Table 18–11, F). Phencyclidine and its congeners are therefore considered separately from the other psychedelic drugs. Phenmetrazine (Preludin) and methylphenidate (Ritalin) resemble the cyclohexylamines such as phencyclidine rather closely in chemical structure, but their psychotic effects are much less prominent and they have considerable sympathetic stimulating effects; however it seems best to classify them with the cyclohexylamine compounds. The reader must bear in mind

that any classification of the psychedelic drugs, or drugs which alter mood or perception, is still empirical and somewhat arbitrary. As Brawley and Duffield point out in their review of the subject, the CNS receptor on which psychedelic drugs act has not yet been isolated and its steric configuration has not yet been described.[132] There is no reason to assume that psychedelic drugs act on only one type of receptor in the central nervous system. Furthermore, at present there is still insufficient information about possible effects that the cells of the raphe nuclei, where many hallucinogens have an inhibitory action, might have on the higher centers that mediate behavior and perception.[132] Hence, it appears that a general theory to explain the actions of the psychedelics or even of the hallucinogens must await further research into the chemistry of neurotransmission and the physiology of behavior and perception in the normal brain.

Before considering the psychedelic drugs and their effects on anesthesia individually, it might be useful to review briefly what is known concerning their mechanisms of action. There is cross tolerance among lysergic acid diethylamine (LSD), the indoles (psilocybin), and the phenylethylamines (the sympathetic hallucinogens), including mescaline.[133] This cross tolerance may suggest a common mechanism of action for these groups of drugs. There is no cross tolerance in psychic or behavioral effects between these groups of drugs and either the amphetamines or the deliriants.[1, 133] Nor is there cross tolerance between the amphetamines and the deliriants.[133] No cross tolerance has been demonstrated between phencyclidine or its cogeners and any other psychedelic drug.[134] According to Isbell, there is no cross tolerance between the cannabinols (marijuana) and LSD or the indole hallucinogens.[1] As suggested by the absence of cross tolerance to the psychic effects, several different mechanisms of action may have to be postulated to account for the psychic effects of the different groups of psychedelic drugs listed in Table 18–11.[132, 133]

LSD and the hallucinogenic indoles DET, DMT, and psilocybin have been shown to reduce the turnover of serotonin (5-HT) in the mammalian brain.[132, 135, 136] The sympathetic hallucinogen DOM also appears to retard the turnover of serotonin. Snyder and coworkers have suggested that a large receptor area is necessary for interactions with molecules, such as LSD, which have multiple ring structures.[137] Only *d*-LSD has potency as a hallucinogen; the l isomer is inert. Snyder has suggested that among the hallucinogenic indoles, the more closely the structure of a compound resembles the ring structure of LSD (Figure 18–14), the more hallucinogenic potency it will display. Snyder also suggested that in some of the substituted amphetamines and in mescaline, hydrogen bonding between the side chains could result in the formation of a functional second ring structure, making these sympathetic hallucinogens resemble *d*-LSD a bit more closely. Snyder and Richelson's calculations indicate that such hydrogen bonding within the molecule is physically possible.[137] However, even after allowing for the formation of additional rings by hydrogen bonding between the side chains, analysis of the ring structure alone cannot account for differences in hallucinogenic potency among the different indole and sympathetic hallucinogens. Snyder and Merrill also calculated the energies of the highest occupied molecular orbital for the hallucinogenic indoles and found that potency corresponded with the ability to donate electrons.[138] Kang and Greene calculated similar data for the sympathetic hallucinogens, and Brawley and Duffield recognized that for a given ring

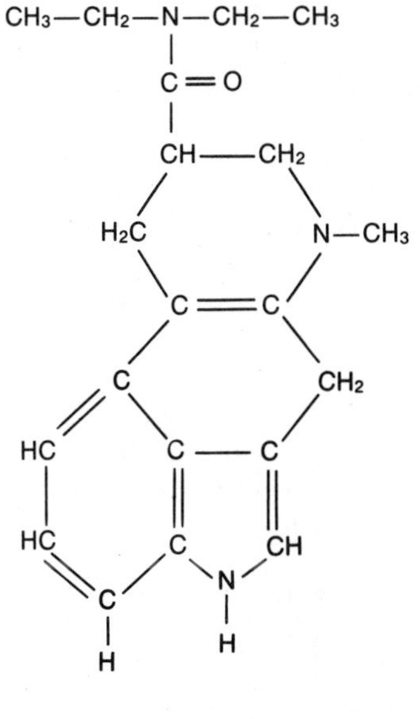

Lysergic Acid Diethylamide

Figure 18–14.

structure, hallucinogenic potency varies with the capacity to donate electrons.[132, 139] Hence, hallucinogenic potential appears to depend both on the presence of a ring structure similar to that of LSD and on the ease with which a compound can donate an electron. It would appear that the interaction between a hallucinogenic drug or between a sympathetic hallucinogen and its receptor may involve the transfer of an electron to the receptor.

The amphetamines appear to stimulate cerebral cortical activity and may also increase the activity of the reticular activating system.[132] Perception is not greatly altered, but mood is greatly affected; and after large doses confusion, delirium, and occasionally a toxic paranoid psychosis may appear. The exact mechanism of action of amphetamines in the central nervous system has not yet been elucidated, but stimulation of endogenous catechol receptors appears likely.

The deliriants atropine, scopolamine, and piperidyl isomer (Ditran) produce amnesia, auditory hallucinations, marked confusion, and delirium. These agents appear to depress cholinergic neurons in the brainstem which produce slow waves on the EEG.[133] They appear to compete with acetylcholine for receptors in the central nervous system, and can be counteracted by physostigmine or tetrahydroaminoacridine — cholinesterase inhibitors that can penetrate the blood brain barrier. For the piperidyl glycolates, Abood found that hallucinogenic potency correlated with anticholinergic activity.[140] Brawley and Duffield note that more work should be done with these compounds before a simple anticholinergic mechanism of action can be accepted.[132] Cocaine, although a tropane by chemical structure, appears to produce its effects on the central nervous system mainly by blocking the re-uptake of catechols. A syndrome not unlike amphetamine intoxication results from cocaine abuse.

Cannabinols, which are found in marijuana, depress polysynaptic cord reflexes and also depress the reticular activating system. In large doses they increase serotonin (5-HT) concentration in the brain.[133] They may reduce brain 5-HT turnover, as do the hallucinogenic indoles, including LSD. Yet the exact mechanism of action of the cannabinols is still unknown. The mechanism of action of phencyclidine and the other cyclohexylamines also is not known at present.

HALLUCINOGENS

Hallucinogens are drugs that cause central nervous system excitation, sensory distortions, delusions, alterations in mood, and depersonalization. The major hallucinogens are lysergic acid diethylamide, the infrequently used compounds psilocybin and mescaline, and the synthetic drugs dimethyltryptamine and diethyltryptamines. There are many reports of trauma associated with the use of these agents.[141, 142] Therefore, it is likely that patients will undergo anesthesia and surgery while still intoxicated by hallucinogenic drugs. Because of the absence of case reports describing how patients intoxicated by hallucinogens tolerate anesthesia and surgery, the anesthesiologist must rely on his knowledge of the pharmacology of these compounds when called upon to manage these patients.

The Major Hallucinogens — LSD, Psilocybin, and Other Indoles (DMT and DET)

Physiologic and Anesthetic Considerations. LSD is structurally similar to ergonovine, an indole amide. Psilocybin is 4-phosphoryloxy-N,N-dimethyltryptamine, an N,N-dimethyl derivative of 4-hydroxytryptamine. LSD is derived from either the ergot fungus that grows on rye or from the seeds of the morning-glory plant *Rivea corymbosa*. Much of the LSD illicitly sold is made synthetically by reacting lysergic acid with diethylamine. Psilocybin is found in *Psilocybe* mushrooms, which have been used during religious ceremonies by Indians in North and Central America. The effective dose of these agents in man is very low. For example, only 0.5 to 1 gamma per kilogram of the dextrorotatory isomer of LSD will cause psychic effects in man. Isbell notes that LSD in a dose of 0.5 μg per kg causes euphoria and mild sensory distortion, while doses of 1 μg per kg cause marked sensory distortion as well as euphoria. Doses of 2 μg per kg usually cause frightening hallucinations and illusions of a change in body image; with increased doses of LSD, "bad trips" consisting of frightening hallucinations always occur.[1] To the present day, no definite human fatality from LSD overdose has been reported; there is only one case in the literature of a suspected overdose of LSD resulting in death from respiratory arrest. The patient was thought to have taken at least 320 mg of LSD, while the lethal dose in man is estimated at 0.2 mg per kg.[143] In a few cases of massive LSD overdose, respiratory depression requiring mechanical ventilation has been reported.[143]

All of the hallucinogenic indoles have autonomic effects, mediated via the hypothalamus; whereas with cocaine and the amphetamines, stimulation of peripheral adrenergic receptors occurs. The hallucinogenic indoles cause centrally mediated sympathetic and parasympathetic effects, but the sympathetic effects are predominant. Mild tachycardia and elevations of blood pressure appear. Mydriasis, piloerection, and mild fever also occur after the use of LSD. Domino recommends that temperature be monitored in patients who have recently taken LSD.[133] Increased levels of glucose and free fatty acids in the blood resulting from adrenergic stimulation are seen after ingestion of indole hallucinogens.[1, 151] Dolphin and coworkers showed that LSD can interact with beta receptors in the central nervous system and has about as strong an affinity for these receptors as does isoproterenol.[144] Persson points out that *d*-LSD increases the in vivo hydroxylation of tyrosine to dihydroxyphenylalanine (DOPA). He also showed that psilocybin and N-N-dimethyltryptamine (DMT) caused increased DOPA levels in rat brain and believed that increased synthesis of DOPA accounted for the increased levels.[145] Thus some progress has been made toward a pharmacological explanation for the sympathetic side effects of LSD and the other hallucinogenic indoles. Parasympathetic effects of the hallucinogenic indoles include salivation, lacrimation, nausea, and vomiting, more so with psilocybin than with the other drugs in this group.[1, 151] The unpleasant autonomic effects of mescaline, a sympathetic hallucinogen sometimes considered with the indoles, are so pronounced that mescaline has become much less popular than it had been.[1]

Tolerance to the psychic and sympathetic effects develops rapidly during the use of LSD; marked tolerance occurs within three days of continuous use. Trulson and Jacobs, using tritiated 5-hydroxytryptamine (5-HT) and LSD, showed that repeated administration of LSD decreases the maximum receptor binding of 5-HT by 20 to 30 per cent in the forebrain, brainstem, and spinal cord of rats. They suggest that changes in binding may account for the profound tolerance to LSD that develops.[146] In man, ingestion of 100 gamma of LSD for three consecutive days nearly abolishes the psychic effects of the drug; and four or five drug-free days are necessary to re-establish susceptibility to these effects.[146, 152] Tolerance develops to the psychic and autonomic effects of LSD, but in animals no tolerance develops to the LD_{100}.[151] Cross tolerance is present among the major hallucinogens, LSD, psilocybin, diethyltryptamine, and mescaline. However, cross tolerance between d-LSD and either psilocybin or dimethyltryptamine is less complete than that between d-LSD and mescaline,[133, 147] and cross tolerance between the amphetamines and the hallucinogens does not occur.[1, 133]

The biological half-life of LSD in man is about 175 minutes. The onset of psychic effects occurs 40 minutes after oral ingestion, and the period of vivid hallucinations lasts another two hours, roughly corresponding to one biological half-life. Some psychic effects persist for six to eight more hours, and during this time trace amounts of the drug are still present.[149] Domino suggests that some type of protein binding between LSD and neural tissue might explain the persistence of the psychic effects of LSD for up to 12 hours after ingestion.[133] Even after the drug is no longer detectable in the patient, "flashbacks" or sudden recurrences of hallucinations can occur. It is now estimated that under stressful conditions less than 1 per cent of LSD users have "flashbacks";[148] this estimate is much less than the 5 per cent incidence reported earlier.[150] "Flashbacks" are apparently psychological in origin, since no evidence has appeared indicating that LSD can persist in the CNS for months or years.[1] Although tolerance to the hallucinogens develops quickly, there is no evidence of physical dependence; no abstinence syndrome appears with discontinuation of these drugs.[78]

The minimal effective dose that produces mild psychic effects is 25 gamma in normal volunteers; and 100 gamma (0.1 mg) will uniformly result in a psychedelic experience in all normal persons who have not developed tolerance to hallucinogens.[152] Alcoholics apparently require two to six times this dose for an experience of equal intensity.[152] At a dose of 100 gamma, a slight tachycardia, but no significant change in blood pressure, appears.[153] Increasing the dose to over 1 mg does not prolong the psychedelic experience but does intensify the physiologic changes. Hypertension has been reported with doses above 1 mg.[152] Mydriasis appears after ingestion of d-LSD, and the degree of mydriasis apparently corresponds to the intensity of the psychic experience. Increases in pupil size from 3 to 5.25 mm have been reported.[154] High doses of LSD can also cause bronchial constriction.[151] Muscle cramps may appear after ingestion, but usually resolve before the psychic effects begin. Nausea and vomiting may follow LSD ingestion, but these effects can be minimized if the drug is taken shortly after eating a full meal. Lacrimation and salivation may occur after ingestion. Prolonged psychotic reactions are rare with d-LSD, appearing in about 0.1 per cent of users; schizophrenics seem prone to such adverse reactions.[155] Muscle tremors not infrequently occur in persons who have ingested LSD, deep tendon reflexes are increased, and occasional grand mal seizures can occur after large doses.[133, 151]

A brief description of the nature and incidence of the psychic changes in 18 normal subjects given 100 to 200 gamma of d-LSD by Stefaniak and Osmond is as follows: Seven patients noted blurred vision; 11 saw images filling their entire visual field or distortions of space. Ten saw faces that appeared like caricatures or even like animals. Six noted changes in their own body image, especially alterations in the size of their hands or feet. Twelve of the 18 saw changes in colors, and many of the subjects had hallucinations of animals, people, dancing girls, castles, or infinity. The afterimages of objects moving across their visual field persisted in many of the test subjects. Six of 18 subjects had increases in visual acuity, but auditory hallucinations were rare. Eight noted anesthesia in one or more limbs, and an increase in tactile acuity was frequent. In some subjects this increased tactile acuity was painful. Most subjects lost their sense of the passage of time, and those that had taken 200 gamma showed marked impairment of association as well as some impairment of memory and of the ability to subtract serial sevens. About half of the 18 subjects became euphoric and some apparently had what was referred to by William James as a "transcendental experience."[155]

At present, the most likely explanation for the psychic effects of the hallucinogens appears to be that these compounds antagonize 5-hydroxytryptamine (5-HT) within the central nervous system. While not all 5-HT antagonists are hallucinogens, it appears that no hallucinogenic compound lacks the ability to antagonize 5-HT.[151] Boakes and coworkers, applying drugs iontophoretically to cells in the brainstems of cats, found a good correlation between antagonism to 5-HT excitation and hallucinogenic potency for LSD, for methylsergide, and for 2-bromo LSD.[156] Trulson and Jacobs indicate that other hallucinogenic indoles such as psilocybin and dimethyltryptamine, given systemically, decrease the firing rate of serotonergic neurons in the brain. They also note the similarity between the distribution of radioactively labeled LSD and 5-HT in the central nervous system, and they found that 5-HT was the most effective compound for displacing LSD from binding sites in brain tissue.[146] Giarman and Freedman as early as 1965 had suggested that the psychic effects of LSD resulted from inhibition of receptors for 5-HT in the central nervous system.[157] Berridge and Prince found that LSD can bind more tightly than 5-HT to one type of receptor normally activated by 5-HT, and suggested that the slow recovery of the receptor when occupied by LSD may play a role in its psychic effect.[158] The discovery by Aghajanian and coworkers that small systemic doses of LSD greatly depress the firing rate of serotonergic neurons in the raphe nuclei of the midbrain suggests that these neurons are a principal site of action of the hallucinogenic indoles in the CNS.[151, 160, 164] Couch has confirmed these findings using iontophoretically applied LSD.[161] Thus it appears that LSD depresses the raphe nuclei which seem to be part of an inhibitory system in the midbrain.[132] The hallucinogens also may increase sensory input into the reticular formation.[133, 162] More research into the normal function of raphe nuclei is necessary before the significance of these discoveries can be appreciated. Wong and coworkers looked for but did not find a relationship between cataleptic behavior in cats and an increased activity of choline acetyl transferase in the corpus striatum.[163] Thus far psychic effects of LSD have not been related to any interactions with cholinergic receptors. Moreover, anticholinesterases such as physostigmine and diisopropyl fluorophosphate do not antagonize LSD or the other indole hallucinogens.[132]

Considerable research has been done on the electrophysiological effects of LSD in various regions of the brain. In a quiet environment, LSD tends to cause high voltage slow waves in the cerebral cortex, and thus cataleptic or immobile behavior, while in a stimulating environment it causes fast, low voltage electrical waves in the cortex, and thus excited behavior. LSD given to animals whose brainstems are transected at the colliculi will not produce an activating effect on the cerebral cortex. Psilocybin and dimethyltryptamine do not cause cortical activation in animals sectioned just above the medulla.[132] Hence, the cortical activating effects of the hallucinogens — unlike those of the amphetamines — appear to depend on the integrity of connections to the midbrain or the medulla. Koella and Wells found that small doses of LSD increased the evoked responses in the auditory and visual areas of rabbits.[165] Schwarz and coworkers noted that LSD caused 2 to 7 Hz EEG waves in the temporal areas in man.[166] Passouant and coworkers found in cats that LSD, 50 to 200 μg/kg, caused 4 Hz waves in the septal area and neocortex.[167] Adey and coworkers found that LSD, 25 μg/kg, caused 5 Hz waves in the rostral midbrain, in the anterior ventral nucleus of the thalamus, and in the neocortex.[168] Fox and Dray recently showed that LSD, delivered iontophoretically to single neurons in the visual cortex of the cat, increased the activity of these cells.[169] Hence, it appears that the hallucinogens affect not only the dorsal raphe of the midbrain and the reticular formation but also afferent sensory tracts, the limbic system, and several cortical areas.

LSD is metabolized in rat liver mainly to 14-hydroxy-LSD-glucuronide, but some appears as 13-hydroxy-LSD-glucuronide or as 2-oxo-LSD. Less than 1 per cent is excreted unchanged.[170] It appears likely that the metabolism of LSD in man and its excretion in the bile resembles that in experimental animals. Because of problems with toxicity from the relatively large amounts of LSD needed for studies of drug metabolism, these experiments have not been done in human beings. Enzyme induction by LSD has not been demonstrated, to the present day, and appears to play no role in tolerance to LSD.[174]

The analgesic properties of LSD have been investigated by Kast and Collins.[171] Two hours after administration they found no difference in the degree of analgesia produced by meperidine, 100 mg, or by LSD, 100 gamma. The analgesia produced by LSD outlasted analgesia from dihydromorphine and from meperidine, but the psychic side effects made it unacceptable as a clinically useful analgesic.[172]

Zsigmond et al., in 1961, discovered that LSD had an in vitro anticholinesterase activity approximately one tenth that of hexafluorenium, which is used clinically to prolong the action of succinylcholine.[172, 173] Zsigmond advises that succinylcholine should be used cautiously in patients who chronically use LSD. He also suggests that the use of local anesthetics that are detoxified by plasma cholinesterase may be associated with increased toxicity in patients who have taken LSD.[172] Morton and Adriani voice similar warnings.[51, 52] LSD also has some inhibiting effect on acetylcholinesterase and on monoamine oxidase in brain.[133] It is not yet clear whether the inhibition of these two enzymes is of sufficient magnitude to contribute to the cholinergic or adrenergic side effects of LSD.

The current drug of choice for treating anxiety or panic from an LSD "trip" is diazepam.[133] Psychological support in a quiet environment is also important; patients can be "talked down" to some extent. Barbiturates, nonbarbiturate sedatives, and other tranquilizers may also be employed.[175]

Chlorpromazine is quite effective in treating patients on LSD "trips"; it causes resolution of the psychedelic and behavioral effects and also counteracts the mydriasis.[1, 176] However, there are several case reports that chlorpromazine has caused exacerbations of the motor restlessness and psychic effects of LSD.[177, 178] Although chlorpromazine has often been used for calming patients on LSD "trips," barbiturates, diazepam, or chlordiazepoxide may be preferable to chlorpromazine, particular-

ly if a mixed drug intoxication including belladonna alkaloids or the sympathetic hallucinogen dimethoxymethylamphetamine (DOM, STP) should be present. Reserpine should be avoided in the treatment of patients recovering from LSD "trips" because a marked increase in the psychic effects of LSD has been reported after reserpine therapy in both animals and man.[132, 179, 180] Depletion of brain 5-hydroxytryptamine from storage sites in nerve endings may be implicated. Amphetamines intensify and prolong the effects of d-LSD, and are often used in combination with LSD.[2] Atropine, scopolamine, and steroids have no significant effect on the LSD experience.[181] In the occasional case where LSD or another hallucinogenic indole unmasks a psychosis and the patient's "trip" fails to subside after several days, therapy with a butyrophenone tranquilizer such as haloperidol may be necessary. Such therapy is best carried out in consultation with a psychiatrist who can provide long term supervision for the patient.

The stress of surgery or the use of general anesthesia apparently can initiate "flashbacks." The author knows of one young woman in whom hallucinations recurred following a delivery. She had had a "bad trip" after LSD six months prior to delivery. After premedication with diazepam, 10 mg, and meperidine, 50 mg, she was given 30 to 40 per cent nitrous oxide for analgesia. She also received 70 per cent nitrous oxide for about one minute. After the delivery she hallucinated for 30 minutes and required sedation. On awakening, she stated that nitrous oxide seemed like marijuana.

Table 18–12 *Comparative Strength of LSD and Other Hallucinogens (Approximate)**

Marijuana (leaves and tops of *Cannabis sativa*, swallowed)		30 gm
Peyote buttons	*(Lophophora williamsii)*	30 gm
Nutmeg	*(Myristica fragrans)*	20 gm
Hashish	(resin of *Cannabis sativa*)	40 mg
Mescaline	(3,4,5-trimethoxy-phenylethylamine)	40 mg
Psilocybin	(4-phosphoryltryptamine)	12 mg
STP	(2,5-dimethoxy-4-methylamphetamine)	5 mg
LSD	(d-lysergic acid diethylamide tartrate)	0.1 mg

*From Cohen, S.: Med. Sci. *19*:30, 1968.

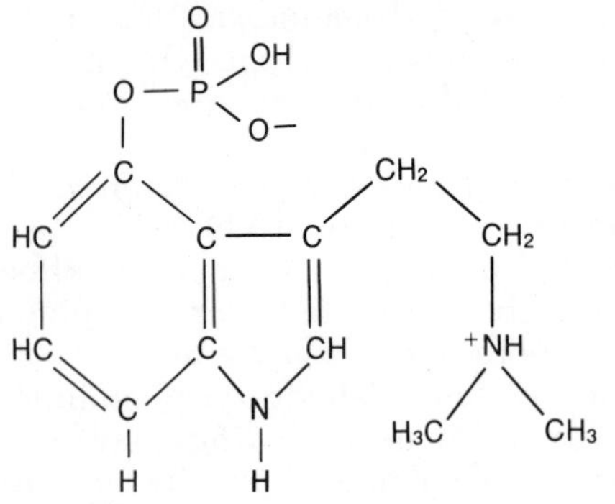

Psilocybin (4-phosphoryloxy-N,N-dimethyltryptamine)

Figure 18–15.

Psilocybin. The effects of psilocybin generally resemble those of LSD, but the drug is considerably milder than LSD (Table 18–12).[1] Its unpleasant autonomic effects may explain why it has never been widely used, and much of what is marketed as psilocybin is adulterated with belladonna alkaloids or other compounds.[182] Chemically psilocybin is 4-phosphoryloxy-N,N-dimethyltryptamine, a compound contained in the *Psilocybe* species of mushroom, which grow in Mexico. In man, 4 mg of psilocybin causes euphoria, whereas 6 to 12 mg causes an altered perception of time and space, and delusions or hallucinations similar to those experienced after the ingestion of LSD. Psilocybin causes increased activity of deep tendon reflexes, muscle twitches, nausea, mydriasis, slight increases in blood pressure and pulse rate, and some increase in body temperature. Psychedelic effects begin a half hour after oral ingestion and last for one to two hours. There may be some hangover, consisting of headache and fatigue.[183] Psilocybin is well absorbed from the gastrointestinal tract, as is LSD.[133] The LD_{50} is not known with certainty in man, but psilocybin poisoning with hyperpyrexia (102-106°F) and convulsions has resulted in the death of at least one child.[184]

The effects of psilocybin in the central nervous system generally resemble those of LSD. Psilocybin, like LSD, reduces rates of turnover of 5-hydroxytryptamine.[185] It also decreases the firing rates of serotonergic neurons in the brain — an effect similar to that of LSD.[146] The cortical alerting effect of psilocybin, like that of LSD, is also depend-ent on intact connections between the medulla and the cortex, as discussed above.[132]

Ninety-four per cent of psilocybin is excreted in the urine within 24 hours.[183] Zsigmond and others showed psilocybin to be a stronger inhibitor of plasma cholinesterase than is serotonin,[186] but to date no cases of apnea resulting from psilocybin have been reported.

The therapy for patients intoxicated with psilocybin is similar to that described above for patients who have taken LSD. Diazepam appears to be the drug of choice.[187] Chlorpromazine has also been recommended.[188] However, because of the possibility that the patient may also have taken some belladonna alkaloids or that the psilocybin had been adulterated with belladonna compounds, the physician should be very careful when using chlorpromazine in cases of alleged psilocybin intoxication. Chlorpromazine causes some CNS effects resembling those of atropine, and can exacerbate the psychic symptoms in patients intoxicated with mixtures of psilocybin and belladonna alkaloids.

Dimethyltryptamine (DMT) and Diethyltryptamine (DET). N,N-Dimethyltryptamine (DMT) and N,N-diethyltryptamine (DET) are also in the class of hallucinogenic indoles. N,N-Dimethyltryptamine is found in the Australian plant *Phalaris rundinacea* and causes the staggers in sheep. This condition presents with excitability, mydriasis, incoordination, and tetany. In severe cases death occurs from tachycardia and congestive heart failure.[189]

In man dimethyltryptamine, 75 mg, has marked sympathetic and hallucinogenic effects that appear simultaneously after parenteral administration. The hallucinogenic effects of DMT are somewhat milder

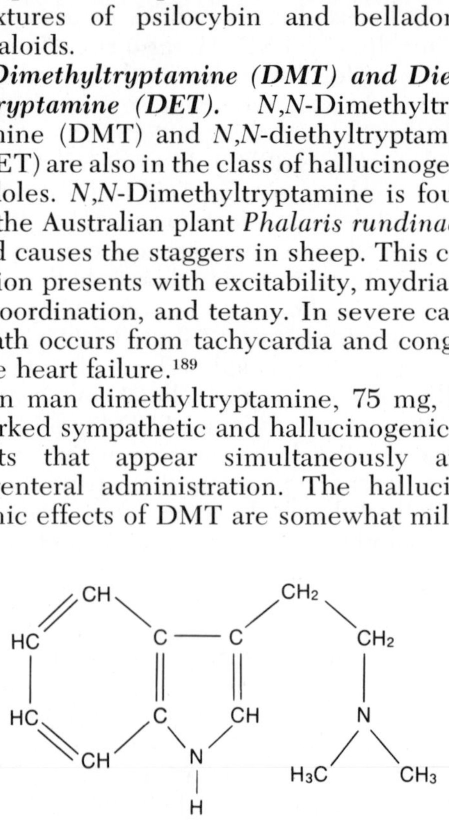

N,N-Dimethyltryptamine

Figure 18–16.

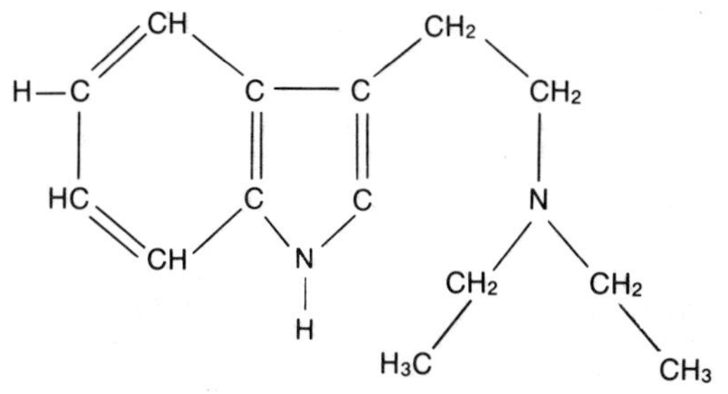

N,N-Diethyltryptamine

(DET)

Figure 18–17.

than those of LSD but a rapid onset of the drug may lead to panic.[2] The autonomic effects, however, are more pronounced than those of LSD. Mydriasis, nausea, hypertension, and tachycardia appear along with euphoria, visual distortions, and hallucinations. Szara noted these effects after taking the drug himself.[190] DMT is usually given parenterally or is inhaled; parsley, tobacco, or marijuana can be dipped into a solution of DMT and then smoked.[2, 133] With dimethyltryptamine, the effects are of brief duration, lasting only thirty minutes to an hour, whereas with diethyltryptamine, 60 mg, the effects are slower in onset but last about three hours.[2, 190]

The neuropharmacology of dimethyltryptamine and diethyltryptamine appears to resemble that of LSD. Diethyltryptamine had been shown to decrease the turnover rate of serotonin (5-HT) in brain tissue.[185] Dimethyltryptamine decreases the firing rate of serotonergic neurons in the median raphe nuclei of the midbrain.[191] Furthermore, cortical alerting by DMT depends on the integrity of connections from the medulla to the cortex.[132]

Dimethyltryptamine shows some cross tolerance with other major hallucinogens — those with an indole-amine structure (*d*-LSD, and psilocybin) and those with a phenylethylamine structure (2,5-dimethoxy-4-methylamphetamine [STP] and mescaline).[133, 192, 193, 194] There is no cross tolerance between DMT and *d*-amphetamine or scopolamine.[194]

Treatment of patients intoxicated with dimethyltryptamine or diethyltryptamine is similar to that outlined above for patients on

LSD "trips." Sedation with diazepam appears tō be the current therapy of choice.[133] However, barbiturates may also be utilized; and if one can be reasonably sure that one is not dealing with a mixture including belladonna drugs or dimethoxymethylamphetamine (DOM, STP), one may employ chlorpromazine. Furthermore, chlorpromazine should be quite effective in treating the sympathetic side effects of DMT and DET.

Mescaline. A less potent hallucinogen than LSD or psilocybin, mescaline is not an indole but resembles the vasoactive amines in chemical structure and is grouped with the sympathetic hallucinogens.

ANESTHESIA FOR PATIENTS TAKING HALLUCINOGENS

Patients who have taken hallucinogens are rather likely to become injured, and the anesthesiologist will become involved in managing these patients during surgery and in the immediate postoperative period. As premedication, sufficient diazepam should be given to control the patient's panic or anxiety. There may be little need for narcotics to control pain preoperatively, since LSD has an analgesic effect; other hallucinogenic indoles may well have analgesic effects, although their analgesic properties have not yet been studied. If patients under the influence of hallucinogens appear to be in pain, they may be treated with narcotics. If secretions are not a problem, atropine and other anticholinergics should be avoided preoperatively; hallucinogens produce a tachycardia. Although atropine and scopolamine do not affect the intensity or duration of the LSD experience, these belladonna alkaloids themselves can cause hallucinations and it seems best to avoid them in patients who have taken hallucinogenic indoles. Belladonna drugs should be employed only if the salivation caused by LSD or psilocybin becomes a problem. The psychic effects of the belladonna drugs may be reversed postoperatively by physostigmine.

Blood pressure, temperature, and the electrocardiogram should be monitored in patients intoxicated with hallucinogenic indoles, since hypertension, tachycardia, and fever are usually present. Temperature

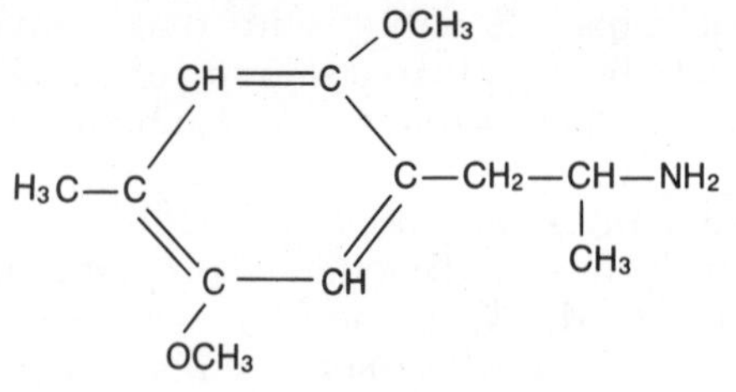

2,5-Dimethoxy-4-methylamphetamine

(DOM or STP)

Figure 18–18.

monitoring particularly should not be over-looked.[133] Hypertension and fever in these patients may respond to chlorpromazine, a drug whose sedative effects are excellent in cases of intoxication with the hallucinogen-ic indoles. However, chlorpromazine should not be administered to patients who may also have taken belladonna compounds or dimethoxymethylamphetamine (DOM-STP). If the induction of general anesthesia does not control the tachycardia and hyper-tension, peripheral alpha and beta blockers may be utilized. Intravenous propranolol, 0.5 mg, repeated at 10 minute intervals, should control the tachycardia. Intravenous phentolamine in 1.0 to 2.0 mg increments may be used to control severe hypertension. Trimethaphan camsylate (Arfonad) may be used as a slow intravenous drip to control hypertension. In patients intoxicated by hallucinogenic indoles, it should be used cautiously and in low doses, since both LSD and psilocybin inhibit to some degree the action of pseudocholinesterase, the enzyme that hydrolyzes trimethaphan.[133, 172, 173] So-dium nitroprusside may also be employed as an intravenous drip. The use of alpha-methyldopa has not been described in these patients, but no reports that it might be contraindicated have appeared.

General anesthetics may be employed in patients intoxicated by hallucinogens. In-travenous diazepam appears to be the agent of choice for induction, but barbiturates are also satisfactory. Succinylcholine may be employed for intubation; reduced doses may be advisable because of the inhibition of pseudocholinesterase by LSD and psilo-cybin, and possibly by other indole hallu-cinogens.[133, 172, 173] Prolonged apnea in man thus far has not been reported from the combination of succinylcholine and hallu-cinogenic indoles. However, if succinylcho-line is to be employed for maintenance of relaxation, monitoring of the twitch re-sponse is indicated. Nondepolarizing neu-romuscular blocking agents may be used; if tachycardia or hypertension is present, gal-lamine or pancuronium should be either avoided or used in small incremental doses. Nitrous oxide, halothane, or enflurane may be employed; and methoxyflurane may be used in low concentrations for short periods. Cyclopropane should probably be avoided if hypertension is present. Diethyl ether may be employed but is probably better avoided because of the postoperative nausea it may cause; patients who have ingested indole hallucinogens may have problems with nausea as a side effect of the hallucinogen itself.

Regional anesthesia may be possible in an occasional patient affected by hallucin-ogenic indoles. However, good control of the anxiety by diazepam or even by chlor-promazine is necessary, and the anesthesi-ologist must provide excellent psychologi-cal support or heavy sedation for the patient during surgery. General anesthesia seems preferable for most of these patients. If regional anesthesia is utilized, large doses of the ester compounds (chloroprocaine, procaine, tetracaine) should probably be avoided; inhibition of pseudocholinesterase by certain hallucinogenic indoles could theoretically lead to toxic blood levels of local anesthetics containing the ester link-age.[133, 172, 173]

THE SYMPATHETIC HALLUCINOGENS, NUTMEG, AND MESCALINE

The sympathetic hallucinogens are phen-ylethylamine compounds, and therefore have some structural resemblance to epi-nephrine and other sympathetic humors. Although they do produce euphoria and have an alerting effect on the CNS, they are taken primarily for their hallucinogenic properties. Phenylethylamine compounds produce brightly colored visual hallucina-tions with a variety of geometrical patterns. Hence they should be distinguished from the amphetamines, which are taken to achieve a feeling of increased mental prowess and euphoria. (With the amphet-amines, hallucinations may be regarded as

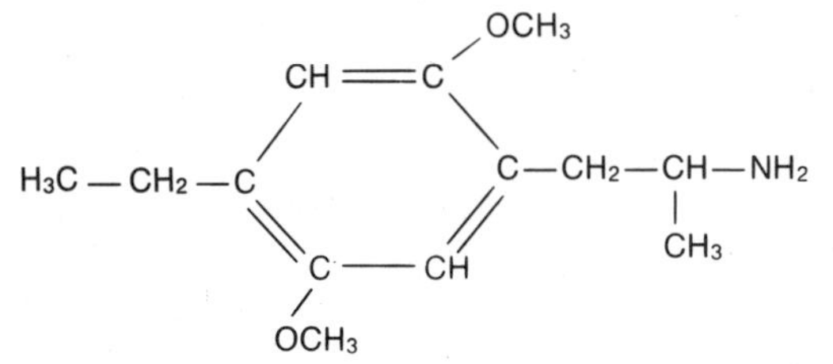

2,5-Dimethoxy-4-ethylamphetamine

(DOET)

Figure 18–19.

a side effect, a toxic psychosis.) The principal sympathetic hallucinogens are 2,5-dimethoxy-4-methylamphetamine (STP or DOM); 2,5-dimethoxy-4-ethylamphetamine (DOET); 3-methoxy-4,5-methylene dioxyamphetamine (MMDA); 3,4-methylenedioxyphenylethylamine (MDA); 4-bromo-2,5-dimethoxyamphetamine (DOB); and 3,4,5-trimethoxyphenylethylamine (mescaline) and its analogue 3,4,5-trimethoxyamphetamine (TMA). Nutmeg also contains hallucinogenic compounds whose structures resemble those of mescaline or ephedrine.[2] For a comparison of the relative potencies of these sympathetic hallucinogens in mescaline units, the reader may refer to Table 18–11.

STP or DOM. DOM, which is 2,5-dimethoxy-4-methylamphetamine, is a very potent phenylethylamine hallucinogen. Among the widely used hallucinogens it is next to LSD in potency and it is known as STP (serenity, tranquility, and peace) in the drug culture. Unwin claims that a dose of 700 μg will cause some psychic effects.[2] Doses of DOM below 3.0 mg or doses of its ethyl analogue 2,5-dimethoxy-4-ethylamphetamine (DOET) below 1.5 mg cause euphoria, increased alertness, and increased self-awareness with no hallucinations but with some closed eye imagery.[195] DOM is uniformly hallucinogenic at doses of 5 mg per 70 kg.[195] Larger doses cause convulsions. Domino notes that the subjective effects of small doses of DOM resemble those of amphetamine, while in moderate doses DOM becomes a hallucinogen, and in large doses it becomes a convulsant.[133] At low doses no significant changes in vital signs appear, and mydriasis in a few of the subjects may be the only detectable physical sign. The subjective effects of DOM begin

one to two hours after oral administration, peak at three to five hours, and are over by seven to eight hours.[196] Isbell indicates that the psychedelic experience after a moderate dose of DOM may last 12 to 16 hours, and Unwin points out that a period of insomnia lasting nearly a day and followed by a few hours of sleep usually follows the hallucinogenic experience.[1, 2] By two to three days after a single dose of DOM the user is left exhausted. DOM is slowly demethylated and then is metabolized to some extent by monoamine oxidase.[133] Its slow metabolism may explain its prolonged effects. With moderate doses of DOM, other signs and symptoms besides mydriasis appear. The mouth becomes dry, the skin becomes flushed, and tachycardia, hypertension, and delirium appear. Dysphagia, abdominal discomfort, and blurred vision occur.[2]

The intensity of the psychedelic effect is dose related, and it is estimated that black market preparations of STP contain about 10 mg per tablet. In the Palo Alto study, in which most of the subjects received doses of from 5 to 14 mg, blurred vision, optical hallucinations, slowed passage of time, euphoria, and a flooding of consciousness with thoughts occurred. The subjects were easily distracted, but their recollection of the experience was good. At these dose levels, nausea, diaphoresis, tremors, paresthesias, low grade fever, and mydriasis occurred. Pulse rate increased 25 beats per minute and systolic blood pressure rose 25 mm Hg, although diastolic values were not affected. Blood sugar did not change, but plasma free fatty acids were elevated. The sympathetic side effects peaked at four hours.[196]

Three subjects simultaneously given chlorpromazine, 200 mg, and DOM orally did develop hallucinations, but these effects seemed less intense than those of subjects given the same doses of DOM without chlorpromazine. The subjects given chlorpromazine also appeared quite drowsy.[196] The use of chlorpromazine to control the anxiety resulting from DOM is now generally considered to be contraindicated, according to Domino.[133] Unwin points out that the combination of chlorpromazine and DOM has occasionally been fatal, and even in the "drug culture" this combination is avoided.[2] The use of "downers" or sedatives and tranquilizers, which are often taken after LSD, has never become popular with persons taking DOM.[2]

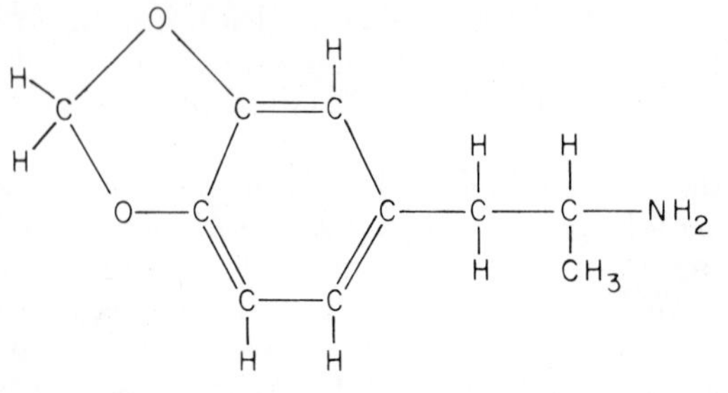

3,4 – METHYLENEDIOXYAMPHETAMINE

Figure 18–20.

Diazepam currently is the drug of choice for controlling the panic, restlessness, and tremors that may result from ingesting DOM.[133] DOM shows cross tolerance with other hallucinogens — LSD, psilocybin, DMT, and mescaline.[167]

MDA and MMDA. MDA and MMDA are 3,4-methylenedioxyphenylethyl amine and 3-methoxy-4,5-methylene-dioxyamphetamine, respectively. MDA and MMDA are three and ten times more potent than mescaline, respectively, when compared according to the weight of their free bases (see Table 18–11).[132, 198]

Shulgin reports that MMDA, 2 mg per kg, in man resembles mescaline.[199] Alles also has studied the methylenedioxyamphetamines and found euphoria, a feeling of depersonalization, changes in the intensity of sounds, and some visual hallucinations. Physiological changes included mydriasis and difficulty with accommodation. Alles notes that the methylenedioxyamphetamines differ somewhat from the amphetamines.[200]

Therapy for patients intoxicated with these phenylethylamines consists of sedation with diazepam or barbiturates. Chlorpromazine should probably be avoided in these cases, since it may be impossible to rule out intoxication with dimethoxymethylamphetamine (STP or DOM) until the results of urine chromatography are available.

Nutmeg. Nutmeg contains hallucinogenic compounds structurally similar to ephedrine and mescaline.[2] According to Unwin the dose ingested varies from a teaspoon to a whole can. The onset of psychic effects is quite slow. Two to five hours after swallowing nutmeg, hallucinations begin. Feelings of floating and depersonalization also occur.[2] Side effects characteristic of sympathetic hallucinogens occur — a dry mouth, abdominal discomfort, malaise, headache, and dizziness.[2] Therapy with diazepam or barbiturates seems appropriate.

From what is known about their chemistry and neurophysiology, the sympathetic hallucinogens resemble the hallucinogenic indoles, including LSD, in many respects. The sympathetic hallucinogens, which are phenylethyl amines, can form an additional ring through hydrogen bonding so that their structure can become a little more like the ring structure of LSD.[132, 137] Brawley and Duffield have described ring formation by hydrogen bonding among the substituents of the phenylethylamine compounds. They have shown that both ring formation and the ability to donate electrons affect hallucinogenic potency, as is the case with the hallucinogenic indoles.[132] DOM, like LSD, reduces the rate of serotonin (5-HT) turnover in the brain.[185] Aghajanian has showed that DOM, DMT, and also mescaline can inhibit serotonergic neurons in the nuclei of the dorsal raphe.[191] DOM and TMA activate the cortex only if connections between the medulla and cortex are intact.[132] Fairchild and coworkers found that DMA, MDA, MMDA, and TMA produce 3–10 Hz rhythms in the amygdala, caudate nucleus, hippocampus, supraoptic nucleus of the hypothalamus, dorsomedial nucleus of the thalamus, and the midbrain reticular formation.[201] Thus the sympathetic hallucinogens (the phenylethylamines) appear to resemble the hallucinogenic indoles, which include LSD, in many ways.

The anesthetic management of patients intoxicated by sympathetic hallucinogens (the phenylethylamines) is basically similar to that described above for patients who have taken LSD or any of the other hallucinogenic indoles. Diazepam or the barbiturates may be used for premedication or for induction. Atropine can probably be omitted from the premedication, since sympathetic hallucinogens usually decrease salivation, and cause tachycardia. Narcotics may be necessary if the patient appears to be in pain; there is little or no information available concerning any analgesic properties of the phenylethylamines. Chlorpromazine should be avoided preoperatively and intraoperatively in patients who have taken DOM. Blood pressure, temperature, and the electrocardiogram should be monitored. Hypertension and tachycardia may be treated as described above for anesthesia in patients intoxicated by LSD or other hallucinogenic indoles. Succinylcholine may be used in these patients; there is as yet no evidence that phenylethylamines inhibit pseudocholinesterase. The choice of general anesthetic agents and nondepolarizing muscle relaxants is similar to that described above for patients taking hallucinogens. General anesthesia appears preferable to regional block for most of these patients.

The sympathetic hallucinogens may alter the minimal alveolar concentration (MAC) necessary for anesthesia, an effect similar to that of the amphetamines. With the amphetamines, acute intoxication increases MAC for many inhalational agents, while chronic heavy usage of amphetamines lowers MAC. The alteration of anesthetic requirements by amphetamines is described in the following section. The effects of sympathetic hallucinogens on MAC have not yet been studied, but the practicing anesthesiologist should be aware that such effects may occur.

Anesthesia for Patients Taking Mescaline and TMA

Mescaline, an alkaloid present in the peyote cactus *Lophophora williamsii,* is another hallucinogen with stimulating effects on the sympathetic system. Mescaline, or 3,4,5-trimethoxyphenylethylamine, has the same phenylethylamine nucleus found in tyramine and the catecholamines.[170] N-methylmescaline and alpha-methylmescaline found in the peyote cactus also have psychic effects.[132, 133] The Indians in Mexico and members of the Native American Church employ peyote in religious ceremonies.

The chemistry and pharmacology of mes-

3,4,5-Trimethoxyphenylethylamine

(Mescaline)

Figure 18–21.

caline and many other alkaloids derived from the peyote cactus are described in a review article by Kapadia and Fayez.[202]

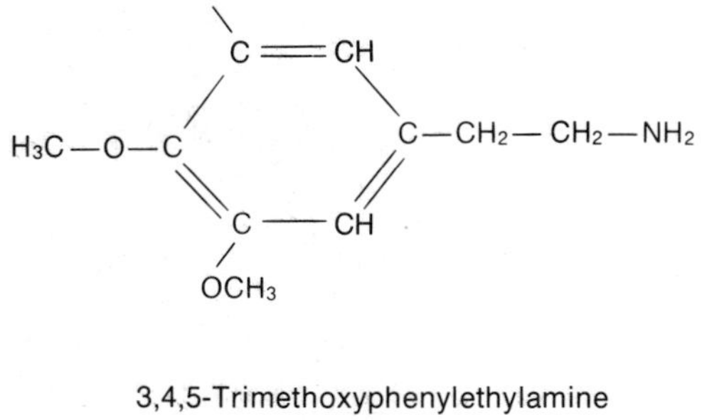

The ingestion of mescaline leads to visual hallucinations, but orientation is usually unimpaired. Auditory hallucinations are rare, but paresthesias and alteration of body image and of temperature sensation may occur. Time seems to pass more slowly.[202] Some anxiety often appears, and hyperactive reflexes and tremors may be present.[203] Initial euphoria is often followed by hostility, and the patient may appear catatonic. The hallucinations may last for 10 to 12 hours. Mescaline may be taken along with cocaine and LSD, a combination known as the "peace pill." To date, no addiction to mescaline resulting in withdrawal symptoms has been reported, and none would be expected.

After mescaline sulfate, 0.5 gm intravenously, nausea, vomiting, diaphoresis, a rise in systolic blood pressure, headache, tachycardia, and palpitations may occur. Mydriasis and some rise in temperature occur. The tachycardia may not appear if there is sufficient blood pressure rise to cause a reflex bradycardia.[202]

Many of the known pharmacological and neurophysiologic effects of mescaline resemble those of the hallucinogenic indoles and phenylethylamines. Mescaline inhibits the serotonergic neurons of the median raphe, and decreases the turnover of 5–HT.[185, 191] Mescaline also causes 3 to 10 Hz rhythms in the amygdala, caudate nucleus, hypothalamus, and midbrain reticular formation.[201] Mescaline increases primary evoked potentials, and causes a 2 to 7 Hz rhythm in the temporal lobe.[166, 204] Mescaline is oxidized by monoamine oxidase.[133]

Tolerance develops to the psychic effects of mescaline, and cross tolerance to LSD, psilocybin, STP, and other hallucinogens also develops. This tolerance disappears by four days after withdrawal of mescaline. Some tolerance to the physiological side effects may occur. The effects of mescaline are potentiated by amphetamine.[205] Prolonged psychosis can develop after the use of mescaline.[206]

For sedation in patients taking mescaline alone or in combinations, diazepam[187] or chlorpromazine has been recommended. Barbiturates have also been used with success.

The anesthesia literature contains no re-

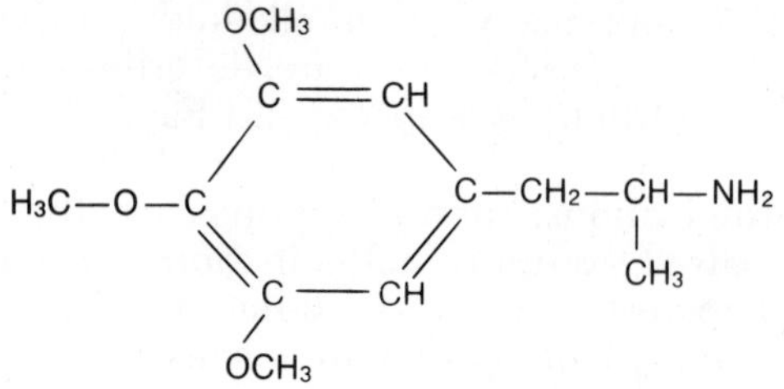

3,4,5-Trimethoxyamphetamine

(TMA)

Figure 18–22.

ports of abnormal reactions in mescaline users subjected to anesthesia and surgery. Since mescaline is not used continuously, it would seem unlikely that significant amounts of mescaline should be present in the patient's sympathetic granules. Hence, the reduction in MAC and the poor response to indirect acting vasopressors seen in chronic heavy users of amphetamines would not be expected in patients taking mescaline. The possibility that mescaline intoxication might increase MAC has not yet been investigated. The curare-like neuromuscular blockade reported for mescaline, 4 to 5 mg per kg, in dogs is transient (10–30 seconds). With larger doses it may have a somewhat longer duration,[207] but to date no significant problems with neuromuscular blockade caused by mescaline have been reported in man.

TMA, or 3,4,5-trimethoxyamphetamine, has about twice the hallucinogenic potency of mescaline (Table 18–11) and closely resembles it in structure. Doses of 50 to 100 mg orally produce hyperactivity and euphoria but no hallucinations. Doses of 200 mg orally produce tremor, vertigo, nausea, and diaphoresis followed by visual hallucinations and strong feelings of hostility.[208] Treatment is as described for mescaline.

The anesthetic management of patients who have taken mescaline or TMA is similar to that described above for patients intoxicated by sympathetic hallucinogens. Either diazepam or chlorpromazine may be used to control anxiety. General anesthesia appears preferable to regional techniques in these patients. The choice of agents has been discussed earlier, in the section Anesthesia for Patients Taking Hallucinogens.

ANESTHETIC CONSIDERATIONS IN PATIENTS USING SYMPATHOMIMETIC AMINES

The amphetamines have an alerting effect on the central nervous system and may produce a feeling of increased ability and well-being. With the amphetamines, this feeling of euphoria and power is the desired effect, and the hallucinations are merely a side effect — a part of the toxic psychosis that may develop after several days of amphetamine use. Patients on these *runs* fear the "crash" at the end and frequently try to minimize it with narcotics. The "rush" that follows an intravenous dose of amphetamine has been compared to a "total body orgasm."[209] The "rush" runs down after two or three hours, and must be renewed by another dose larger than the previous one, since tolerance develops rapidly.[1] Amphetamines are mood elevators, may increase interest in sex, and may enhance performance in athletics, unless an excessive dose causes loss of coordination.[151] With chronic abuse the euphoric effect diminishes. Currently many amphetamine abusers employ the drug only for brief weekend binges. Most amphetamine users employ the drug for three to six days or occasionally for 10 days (sprees); but chronic users may take hundreds of milligrams daily for extended periods and apparently develop some tolerance to the sympathetic effects of these drugs.[209, 210] Daily intake of 15 gm has been reported.[209] Patients intoxicated with amphetamines are hyperactive and may be confused and assaultive.[151, 211] "Speed kills." With high doses, increased reflexes and convulsions occur.[151, 212]

Sympathetic effects after moderate doses are tachycardia, hypertension, diaphoresis, flushing, palpitations, and headache; nau-

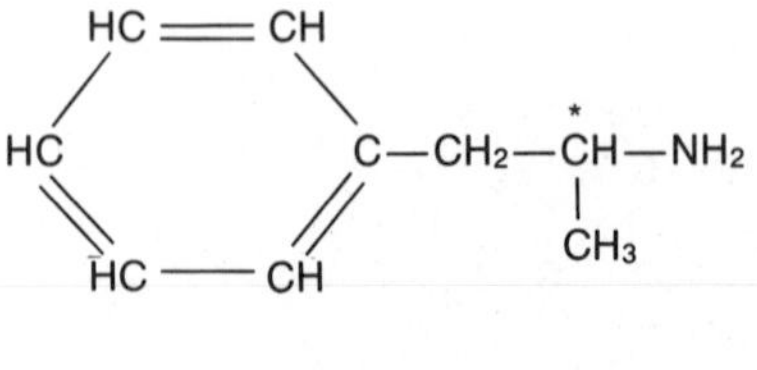

Amphetamine (Benzedrine) or Dextroamphetamine

(d-isomer)

Figure 18–23.

sea, vomiting, and fever also appear. Weight loss of 20 pounds or more caused by dehydration may occur during "runs." Ketosis appears, plasma free fatty acid rises, and the appetite is suppressed. With high doses, extreme hypertension, chest pain, cardiac arrhythmias, circulatory collapse, and coma may be seen, and cerebral hemorrhage may occur.[151, 209, 212] A toxic delirium with paranoid ideation, hallucinations (particularly auditory hallucinations), and homicidal or suicidal tendencies may appear; in the chronic amphetamine user who may have little hypertension or tachycardia, this delirium may be misdiagnosed as a paranoid schizophrenic reaction. In the patients described by Geerlings, chronic amphetamine abuse caused severe mental changes in a majority of the cases, and one third of the cases could be diagnosed as psychotic, exhibiting paranoid delusions, auditory and visual hallucinations, and occasionally aggressive behavior.[213] After amphetamines are discontinued, the toxic delirium or psychosis usually clears within a week.[214] Paranoia is more likely to occur with abuse of high doses of amphetamines; with the possible exception of angiitis, no apparent harm results from the use of up to 40 mg of Dexedrine daily.[1, 2] A summary of the signs and symptoms seen in amphetamine intoxication, as described by Ong, is shown in Table 18–13.[215]

Considerable information is now available concerning the pharmacology and

Table 18–13   Signs and Symptoms of Acute Amphetamine Intoxication*

Severity	Signs and Symptoms
1+	Restlessness, irritability, insomnia Tremor, hyperreflexia Sweating, mydriasis, flushing
2+	Hyperactivity, confusion Hypertension, tachypnea, tachycardia, extrasystoles Fever (mild) Diaphoresis
3+	Delirium, mania, self-injury Marked hypertension, arrhythmias Hyperpyrexia
4+	Convulsions and coma Circulatory collapse and death

*From Ong, B. H.: N. Engl. J. Med. 266:134, 1962.

mechanisms of action of the amphetamines. Peripherally, the amphetamines can act at sympathetic nerve endings. Hypertension with an initial reflex bradycardia may be seen after small doses.[151] With higher doses tachycardia and arrhythmias, including atrial, nodal, and ventricular premature contractions occur.[151, 216] Direct stimulation of peripheral alpha and beta adrenergic endings in peripheral tissues appears to be one mechanism by which amphetamines act. Release of catecholamines from nerve terminals within the CNS is another mode of amphetamine action; doses of amphetamines too small to affect re-uptake of catechols have a stimulant effect in the CNS.[151, 217] A third mechanism is the inhibition by amphetamine of the re-uptake of catechols into adrenergic nerve endings, both centrally and peripherally.[151]

Some information is also available concerning the mechanism of tolerance to the amphetamines. A small per cent of amphetamine is oxidized to 4-hydroxynorephedrine. With repeated doses, this latter compound accumulates in sympathetic nerve endings, replacing norepinephrine. The 4-hydroxynorephedrine then acts as a false transmitter. Lewander ascribed tolerance to the cardiovascular, pyrogenic, and lipolytic effects of amphetamine to the accumulation of 4-hydroxyephedrine in sympathetic nerve endings. It is not yet known whether this mechanism might explain CNS tolerance to the alerting or euphoric effects of amphetamines.[151] The cortical alerting effects of the amphetamines do not depend on intact connections between the medulla or midbrain and the cortex. In this regard, the amphetamines appear to differ from the hallucinogenic indoles and phenylethylamines.[132]

Twenty-seven per cent of a single dose of amphetamine is excreted in the urine as benzoic acid, while approximately 20 per cent is excreted unchanged.[219] After a single dose, amphetamines are excreted in the urine over a period of five to seven days.[214] Acidification of the urine with ammonium chloride greatly increases the excretion of amphetamine by ionizing it, preventing tubular reabsorption. There is as yet no evidence that enzyme induction occurs with chronic amphetamine administration.[151]

Cross tolerance develops among the amphetamines, which include amphetamine

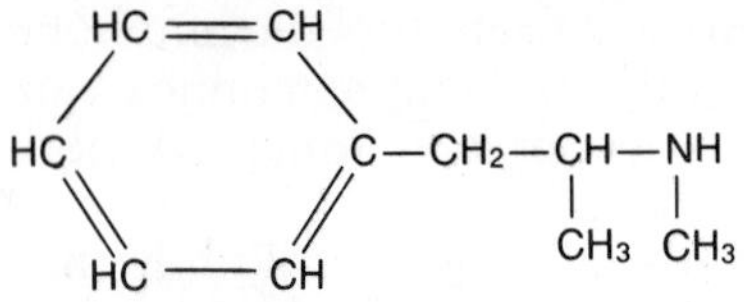

Methamphetamine

Figure 18–24.

(Benzedrine), dextroamphetamine (Dexedrine), and methamphetamine (Desoxyn, Methedrine). The *d* isomer, dextroamphetamine, is about three times more potent than the *l* isomer in causing CNS excitation. Amphetamine itself is a racemic mixture of equal amounts of the *d* and *l* isomers. Amphetamines are often used to prolong and intensify the effects of LSD and mescaline. Amphetamines may even cause flashbacks in persons who have previously taken LSD.[2] Cross tolerance does not develop between the amphetamines and the indole or phenylethylamine hallucinogens.[1] Although tolerance is seen in amphetamine users, no physical dependence occurs, and no abstinence syndrome requiring treatment has yet been reported. The increase in REM (rapid eye motion) sleep time that occurs after withdrawal from amphetamines can be reversed by restarting amphetamines; however, this increase in REM sleep time does not constitute an abstinence syndrome.[1, 2] Nor can the spell of depression that occurs after amphetamine withdrawal be considered part of an abstinence syndrome.[1] Amphetamine toxicity may be treated by sedation with short-acting barbiturates,[212] diazepam, or chlorpromazine.[212] Chlorpromazine has been found to counteract the EEG changes, convulsions, and hyperthermia of amphetamine intoxication in animals, whereas barbiturates counteract these effects only at anesthetic doses. Espelin and others reported good results with chlorpromazine therapy, 1 mg per kg, for amphetamine intoxication in children; when a mixed barbiturate-amphetamine intoxication is suspected, they recommended 0.5 mg per kilogram as an initial dose. For severe hypertension they recommended the use of alpha blockers such as phenoxybenzamine. Regitine in small incremental doses or trimethaphan camphorsulfonate administered as a drip should control acute hypertension in patients intoxicated by amphetamines. Diazoxide (Hyperstat) should also be quite effective in controlling hypertension resulting from amphetamine overdose, since it reduces arterial resistance by a direct effect on precapillary resistance vessels, has a rapid onset of action, and lasts considerably longer than regitine or trimethaphan camphorsulfate.[221] Doses of diazoxide are 300 mg in adults or 5 mg per kg in children, administered rapidly intravenously. A second dose may be necessary if the hypertension has not responded after an interval of 30 minutes. Further doses may be employed as needed at intervals varying from every four hours to once daily until the hypertensive effect of the amphetamine subsides. If alpha-methyldopa (Aldomet) is used to treat hypertension resulting from amphetamines, an initial increase in blood pressure may occur. This effect is seen with small doses of alpha-methyldopa but is inhibited by larger doses.[222] For control of severe tachycardia or ventricular arrhythmias due to amphetamine intoxication, propranolol intravenously in small increments (1.0 mg) at 10 minute intervals should suffice. Treatment in an intensive care unit is advisable.

Therapy with large amounts of intravenous fluids is also important, as patients intoxicated by amphetamines may have poor fluid intake and may have considerable fluid loss due to fever. Temperature should be monitored, and reduced if necessary.[151] If intoxication is due to ingested amphetamines, gastric lavage may be useful to recover unabsorbed drug. Precautions to prevent aspiration are necessary; and in delirious or comatose patients, intubation prior to gavage will be necessary. Since amphetamines are excreted rather slowly in the urine, and since many metabolites of the amphetamines are pharmacologically active, the administration of ammonium chloride to acidify the urine should be considered.[151] In acid urine, the amphetamines become completely ionized, and their reabsorption from the renal tubules is greatly retarded.[223]

Espelin and others noted that patients intoxicated with amphetamine-barbiturate combinations have the clinical appearance of amphetamine intoxication on admission and that symptoms of barbiturate intoxication appear later.[212] If a differential diagnosis cannot be made between intoxication with amphetamines, belladonna alkaloids, or dimethoxymethylamphetamine (DOM), chlorpromazine should be avoided; it is contraindicated in belladonna poisoning, and is generally considered contraindicated in cases of intoxication with DOM.[133]

Users of amphetamines often treat the depression that occurs as the drugs wear off by using narcotics[209] or occasionally large doses of barbiturates.[127] Psychoses resulting from amphetamine abuse may be treated with promethazine, haloperidol, or large doses of diazepam or chlordiazepoxide.[151] Psychiatric consultation should be obtained; any amphetamine abuser whose delirium or paranoid illusions last more than a week after amphetamines are discontinued is likely to have an underlying psychosis.

Amphetamines have been implicated as a cause of necrotizing angiitis histologically indistinguishable from periarteritis nodosa. This syndrome has been reported in 14 patients, one of whom used only methamphetamine. The most common combinations used by the other patients were methamphetamine and heroin, or methamphetamine and d-lysergic acid diethylamide. Four of these patients died with renal failure and hypertensive encephalopathy. Episodes of pulmonary edema frequently appeared prior to death. Autopsy showed multiple renal and splenic infarcts; microaneurysms, intimal proliferation, and medial fibrosis were seen in the arteries of many organs (kidneys, adrenals, brain, gastrointestinal tract, and muscle). An unexplained hemolytic anemia was present in four patients.[224] A similar angiitis with microaneurysm formation has recently been noted in abusers of methylphenidate (Ritalin).[225] The development of these vascular lesions appears unrelated to the intravenous injection of talc present in tablets of methylphenidate, but may be related to the amphetamine or methylphenidate itself. Both of these agents, used intravenously, cause hypertensive episodes that may play a role in the development of lesions in the systemic arteries. Except for this syndrome and except for occasional cerebrovascular accidents, there is no evidence at present that amphetamines may cause pathologic changes in major organ systems, including the central nervous system, in man.

Amphetamines and MAC of General Inhalational Anesthetics

During the past decade Johnston and his coworkers have studied the interactions between the amphetamines and the minimal alveolar concentrations (MAC) of several general inhalational anesthetics. Their work has both theoretical and practical implications. In an initial study in dogs, Johnston, Way, and Miller found that dextroamphetamine, 0.1, 0.5, and 1.0 mg per kg given as a single dose, increased the minimal alveolar concentration for halothane by 19 ± 8, 67 ± 11, and 96 ± 15 per cent, respectively, above the control values.[216] They employed the method of Eger and others for determining MAC.[226] They also found that chronic administration of dextroamphetamine, 5 mg per kg per day for seven days, decreased MAC for halothane in dogs by 21 ± 3 per cent.[216] In a subsequent study, they compared the effect of acute dextroamphetamine administration (1 mg/kg) with the effect of reserpine pretreatment for two days (1 mg/kg/day).[227] The anesthetic agents they studied were cyclopropane, which increases the rate of sympathetic discharge from the CNS, and halothane, which either reduces sympathetic CNS outflow or does not stimulate the sympathetic system. They found that MAC rose proportionately more for halothane (64%) than for cyclopropane (36%) after acute administration of dextroamphetamine. Conversely, they also found a proportionately greater decrease in MAC for cyclopropane (39%) than for halothane (20%) following reserpine pretreatment (Table 18–14). They also noted that other drugs which deplete CNS catechols such as alpha methyldopa or alpha methyl-

Table 18–14A   *Effect of Dextroamphetamine on Halothane and Cyclopropane MAC (Paired Values, Group III)*

Anesthetic	Control MAC*	MAC After 1 mg/kg Dextroamphetamine
Halothane	1.06 ± 0.06	1.74 ± 0.07
Cyclopropane	20.7 ± 1.3	28.2 ± 1.2†

*Means ± SE.
†Represents a proportionately smaller increase than was measured for the halothane group ($p < 0.05$).

Table 18–14B   *Effect on Reserpine on Halothane and Cyclopropane MAC (Paired Values, Group IV)*

Anesthetic	Control MAC*	MAC After Intramuscular Reserpine, 2 mg/kg
Halothane	0.97 ± 0.05	0.78 ± 0.07
Cyclopropane	20.0 ± 1.2	$12.2 \pm 1.8†$

*Means ± SE.
†Represents a proportionately greater decrease than was measured for the halothane group ($p<0.05$).

p-tyrosine also reduce the MAC of halothane to 0.71 to 0.75 volume per cent from a control value of 1.06 per cent.[227] They propose that all anesthetics have a baseline MAC value, the value measured after reserpine pretreatment. They note that the highest value of MAC obtainable with amphetamine pretreatment for either halothane or cyclopropane is 2.3 times the baseline MAC, or 230 per cent of the baseline MAC (Fig. 18–25). They propose that where an anesthetic lies within this range depends on the extent to which the anesthetic increases sympathetic activity or releases catechols within the CNS, as described by Carr and Moore.[227] Johnston and coworkers suggest that diethyl ether and fluroxene should behave more like cyclopropane than like halothane, since both diethyl ether and fluroxene increase sympathetic activity in the CNS. Some unpublished measurements by Johnston tended to confirm that fluroxene resembles cyclopropane in its response to pretreatment with amphetamines or reserpine.[227] Whether other agents—enflurane, methoxyflurane, isoflurane—will act as Johnston and coworkers predict remains to be proved. The interaction between amphetamine acutely administered in the drug naive subject and halothane results in the largest increase in anesthetic requirement, or MAC, thus far encountered. Neither hyperthyroidism nor high fever nor interactions with other drugs can increase MAC to the same extent.[216, 227] The possibility that phenylethylamine hallucinogens (sympathetic hallucinogens—Table 18–11) might have effects on MAC similar to those of the amphetamines appears to warrant further investigation.

In the studies of Johnston and coworkers in drug naive animals pretreated with a single dose of amphetamine and then anesthetized, increases in blood pressure and temperature occurred and cardiac arrhythmias appeared. Blood pressures rose 70 to 120 per cent above control values, and sinus tachycardia as well as atrial, nodal, and ventricular premature contractions occurred.[216] The animals were cooled externally, so the extent of the temperature increase was not documented. These effects of acute amphetamine administration subsided after six hours.[216]

In animals maintained on amphetamines, 2.5 mg/kg/day, for a week prior to anesthesia, the MAC for halothane was reduced 22 ±3 per cent below the control MAC. Increases in blood pressure, heart rate, and body temperature did not appear in these animals during anesthesia, nor did cardiac arrhythmias occur.[120, 216] Animals maintained for a week on dextroamphetamine, 2.5 mg/kg/day, became lethargic. These animals responded poorly to indirect acting vasopressors. Johnston and coworkers suggest that chronic amphetamine users may respond poorly to such indirect acting vasopressors as ephedrine and metaraminol, and that therapy of hypotension in these patients may require norepinephrine or other direct acting pressors.[216]

In the naive subject acutely intoxicated by amphetamines or in the "spree" user still high on amphetamines, increased doses of general anesthetics will be necessary. It

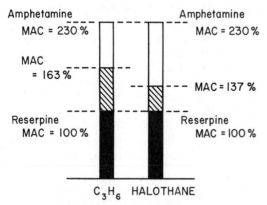

Figure 18–25. In the presence of minimal CNS catecholamines, all anesthetics have the baseline MAC value indicated by "Reserpine MAC." For both C_3H_6 and halothane, MAC with dextroamphetamine pretreatment is 230 percent greater than with reserpine. Although this range is equal for both anesthetics, the position of MAC within this range is significantly higher with cyclopropane (163 versus 137 percent). (From Johnston, R. R.: Anesth. Analg. 54:655, 1975.)

might seem wise to avoid agents that sensitize the myocardium to the effects of catecholamines such as cyclopropane, halothane, and trichloroethylene. Methoxyflurane seems satisfactory in that it does not sensitize the myocardium to catechols; however, high concentrations of this agent for prolonged periods must be avoided because of renal toxicity. Its usefulness is limited in patients requiring high concentrations for maintenance of anesthesia. Enflurane, which is negatively dromotropic, appears to be satisfactory for patients acutely intoxicated by amphetamines. A balanced anesthetic employing nitrous oxide, barbiturates, droperidol, narcotics, and muscle relaxants also seems acceptable. The mild alpha blockade of droperidol may help control hypertension. *d*-Tubocurarine appears to be the muscle relaxant of choice, in that it may reduce hypertension and may also reduce heat production. The interaction between amphetamine compounds and *d*-tubocurarine has been studied in unanesthetized dogs; the curarized animals did not become hyperthermic and survived higher doses of amphetamines than the untreated controls.[210]

In the chronic amphetamine user, reduced doses of inhalational anesthetics should be employed. Arrhythmias are unlikely, so cyclopropane or halothane may be employed. Enflurane appears satisfactory, and methoxyflurane may be used in low concentrations for limited periods of time. Nitrous oxide, narcotics, and barbiturates may be used, perhaps in reduced doses. Any muscle relaxant may be employed; however, if hypotension occurs, *d*-tubocurarine should probably be avoided. Treatment of hypotension or low cardiac output may require the use of direct acting catechols such as norepinephrine, epinephrine, or isoproterenol. Temperature should be monitored, and the patient should be warmed, when necessary.

ANESTHETIC CONSIDERATIONS IN PATIENTS USING BELLADONNA ALKALOIDS, OTHER ANTICHOLINERGICS, AND COCAINE

The belladonna alkaloids atropine and scopolamine — and cocaine, which has some resemblance to the belladonna alkaloids — have stimulating and hallucinatory effects on the central nervous system. Structurally, the belladonna alkaloids and cocaine are tropanes (Table 18–11). Because amnesia and confusion are prominent symptoms of belladonna intoxication, the belladonna alkaloids are often referred to as deliriants. Numerous other drugs and plants listed in Table 18–17 may produce a syndrome of anticholinergic intoxication resembling that of the belladonna alkaloids. Certain of these other anticholinergic drugs with hallucinogenic or deliriant effects will be discussed together with the belladonna alkaloids. Cocaine, a tropane structurally similiar to the belladonna compounds, differs sufficiently from them in its pharmacological effects as to warrant separate consideration.

Belladonna alkaloids have been used in combination with LSD to prolong the hallucinatory effects of the latter drug. Combinations of belladonna with amphetamines have become popular,[187] and the combination of cocaine and a narcotic (morphine or opium) is frequently encountered. The combination of belladonna (stramonium) and marijuana known as the "green dragon" has also become fairly popular among devotees of the drug culture.[230]

The belladonna drugs and cocaine may be used alone as stimulants or hallucinogens. Belladonna alkaloids are sold in the United States without prescription as medications for motion sickness (Triptone) or for sedation (e.g., Sominex).[231] Piperidyl glycolate and many other synthetic antispasmodics have hallucinogenic properties.[232]

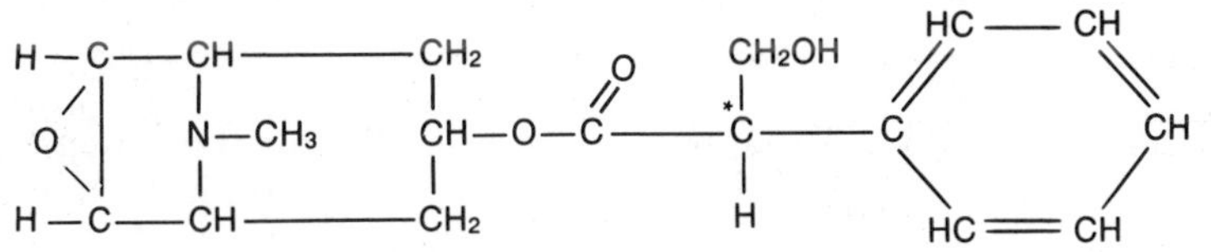

Atropine (d-l mixture)

Figure 18–26.

Many antihistamines, tricyclic antidepressants, antispasmodics, and antiparkinsonian agents also can cause delirium or hallucinations resembling the syndrome of anticholinergic intoxication (Table 18–17). Since these compounds are readily available, their potential for misuse is immense. The amnesia that accompanies the abuse of deliriants limits their popularity to some extent; if a user cannot remember the euphoria and hallucinations resulting from a particular drug, he is less likely to take the drug again.[1]

The Anticholinergic Hallucinogens

In low doses scopolamine causes drowsiness and euphoria, although doses under 1 mg may cause restlessness or hallucinations. Holzgrafe and coworkers noted that only 1.4 per cent of patients given up to 0.5 mg of scopolamine developed overt delirium.[233] With low doses of atropine, euphoria and hallucinations are seldom encountered. Higher doses of belladonna alkaloids have an excitatory effect on the CNS; restlessness, irritability, confusion, delirium, and hallucinations appear. With very high doses, coma and death occur from depression of the medullary respiratory centers. Signs of atropine intoxication include fever (particularly in children); very dry oral mucosa, mydriasis and cycloplegia; hot, flushed skin but absence of sweating; tachycardia (inconstant in young children and the aged); hypertension, nausea and vomiting; decreased intestinal motility; and urinary retention. Lilliputian hallucinations are often present. The signs and symptoms of atropine intoxication are summarized in Table 18–15, reproduced from Goodman and Gilman.[234*]

According to Goldfrank and Melinek, electrocardiographic changes observed with belladonna intoxication include generalized myocardial conduction delay similar to quinidine toxicity: specifically, a prolonged Q–T interval, S–T depression, and widening of the QRS complex to over 100 msec.[235]

---

*A mnemonic summarizing the signs of belladonna intoxication is:

  Hot as a hare
  Blind as a bat
  Dry as a bone
  Red as a beet
  Mad as a hatter.[235]

Table 18–15 *Effects of Atropine in Relation to Dosage**

Dose	Effects
0.5 mg	Slight cardiac slowing; some dryness of mouth; inhibition of sweating
1.0 mg	Definite dryness of mouth; thirst; acceleration of heart, sometimes preceded by slowing; mild dilatation of pupil
2.0 mg	Rapid heart rate; palpitation, marked xerostomia; dilated pupils; some blurring of near vision
5.0 mg	All the above symptoms marked; speech disturbed; difficulty in swallowing; restlessness and fatigue; headache; dry, hot skin; difficulty in micturition
10.0 mg and more	Above symptoms more marked; pulse rapid and weak; iris practically obliterated; vision very blurred; skin flushed, hot, dry, and scarlet; ataxia, restlessness and excitement; hallucinations and delirium; coma

*From Goodman, L. S., and Gilman, A.: The Pharmacologic Basis of Therapeutics. 4th ed. New York, Macmillan, 1970, p. 534.

The differential diagnosis between intoxication with belladonna alkaloids or hallucinogens and schizophrenia may be difficult. The absence of sweating and the presence of very dry mucous membranes indicate belladonna intoxication.[188] Absent or hypoactive bowel sounds also favor belladonna intoxication.[235]

The differential diagnosis between amphetamine and belladonna intoxication can also be difficult. In amphetamine intoxication, profuse sweating may be present, whereas cycloplegia and hot, dry skin and mucosa favor belladonna intoxication.[188] In amphetamine intoxication hyperactive bowel sounds and marked hypertension are found, whereas in belladonna intoxication an ileus is usually present and hypertension, if noted, is mild.[235]

Signs and symptoms helpful in the differential diagnosis of the various drugs that alter mood and perception, summarized by Taylor et al., are shown in Table 18–16. Urine tests for the presence of amphetamines, belladonna alkaloids, and other hallucinogens may also be helpful. The diagnosis of belladonna intoxication or anticholinergic poisoning may be confirmed by the administration of physostig-

Table 18–16 Signs and Symptoms of
Commonly Used Drugs Altering Mood
and Perception*

Agents	Effects
Hallucinogens (LSD, STP, mescaline)	Dilated pupils Reflex hyperactivity Anxiety symptoms Nausea
Anticholinergics	Tachycardia Dilated pupils Dry mouth Absence of sweating (frequently red rash around neck, face and chest) Erythema or rash on face, neck and chest Reflex hyperactivity Anxiety symptoms Fever Nausea and delirium
Amphetamines	Increased sweating Increased motor activity (variable) Tachycardia Hypertension (may be absent)
Marijuana	Tachycardia Absence of dilated pupils Dilatation of conjunctival vessels (may be absent)
Opiates	Miosis

*Modified from Taylor, R. L., et al.: J.A.M.A. 213:424, 1970.

mine, 2.0 mg in adults or 0.5 mg in children, intramuscularly, or slowly or in divided doses intravenously.[235] A favorable response with resolution of the delirium confirms the diagnosis. If the delirium and signs of intoxication persist, other intoxicants, hypoxemia, or acidosis may be present. These latter two conditions may be confirmed or ruled out by an arterial blood gas determination.[235] Since the advent of physostigmine, the mecholyl test described by Dameshek and Feinsilver appears outdated.[236] If anticholinergic poisoning is not present, physostigmine may cause cholinergic toxicity, including increased lacrimation and salivation, loss of bladder and bowel control, bradycardia, bronchospasm, and occasionally seizures.[235]

Currently the treatment for belladonna intoxication consists of physostigmine, 2.0 mg in adults and 0.5 mg in children, as outlined above as a diagnostic test for this condition. The physostigmine should be given slowly or in divided doses intravenously, or intramuscularly to minimize cholinergic side effects such as bradycardia or bronchospasm. If some improvement is seen with this initial dose, more physostigmine may be given — as much as 4.0 or 6.0 mg during the first hour.[188, 237] When signs and symptoms of belladonna intoxication recur, the physostigmine may need to be repeated several times over a 24 hour period.[235] The goal of therapy should be to alleviate the delirium and to control serious autonomic side effects such as fever and tachycardia. It is not necessary to give sufficient physostigmine to counteract the mydriasis; the pupils may remain dilated for several days following belladonna intoxication.[237] Pilocarpine eye drops may be used to alleviate photophobia, or the room lights may be dimmed.[238] Therapy with physostigmine will diminish the risk of seizures that sometimes occur with belladonna intoxication and will restore normal bladder and bowel function.[235] Physostigmine is effective in atrial or supraventricular arrhythmias resulting from anticholinergic poisoning but is not recommended for ventricular arrhythmias.[235] Therapy with lidocaine or propranolol may be necessary.

The duration of action of physostigmine is rather brief; Martin and Weiss found that nearly all of a 1.0 mg dose was eliminated within two hours.[239] Belladonna intoxication usually lasts about two days, depending on the amount and types of alkaloids ingested. Only about half of a single dose of atropine in man is excreted via the kidney in 24 hours. Hence, repeated doses of physostigmine and close observation of the patient are necessary.

Peripheral autonomic effects of belladonna intoxication may be counteracted with cholinergic drugs such as neostigmine.[240] However, neostigmine, a quaternary ammonium compound, does not cross the blood-brain barrier and therefore does not counteract the CNS effects of belladonna alkaloids. Ambenonium, edrophonium, and pyridostigmine, all quaternary ammonium compounds, likewise have little or no CNS effects.[235] Physostigmine, a tertiary amine, crosses the blood-brain barrier and may decrease cholinesterase activity, making more acetylcholine available to antagonize competitively blockade by belladonna compounds of cholinergic sites within the CNS.[241] However, the actions of belladonna compounds in the CNS are quite complex, the cholinergic receptors within the CNS have not yet been characterized, and no simple explanation of the antagonism of belladonna compounds by physostigmine in the CNS can be accepted at present. Katz suggests that physostigmine may increase afferent input to the CNS.[241] Physostigmine has been shown to counteract belladonna-induced depression of the reticular activating system in animals.[242]

Patients intoxicated by belladonna drugs may require intravenous fluids to replace losses due to fever or to diminished oral intake.[238] Gavage to remove unabsorbed drug may be helpful.[230] Sedation with diazepam or barbiturates may still be necessary in occasional cases, particularly when a mixed intoxication involving other hallucinogens (indole or phenylethylamine derivatives) is present. Sedatives had been recommended for the management of belladonna intoxication before therapy with physostigmine was developed.[187, 236] If seizures occur, therapy with phenytoin (Dilantin), 100 mg intramuscularly, has been recommended.[238] Chlorpromazine, which is a weak parasympatholytic, is generally considered contraindicated in patients who have taken large doses of belladonna alkaloids or similar compounds.[133, 188, 238, 243] Perphenazine should also be avoided because of its antimuscarinic side effects.[238] In severe cases of belladonna intoxication, mechanical ventilation and external cooling may be necessary. The use of chlorpromazine even to facilitate cooling is relatively contraindicated. In severe cases, bronchial plugging with dry, inspissated secretions can be a problem. Paralytic ileus and urinary retention may be anticipated. Postural hypotension may appear.[244] Therapy with physostigmine should rapidly control these autonomic side effects.

Some tolerance to belladonna alkaloids does appear in man, but the mild abstinence syndrome of malaise, salivation, diaphoresis, and vomiting is not clinically significant.[245]

Datura stramonium (Jimson Weed, Locoweed), Datura arborea (Trumpet Lily), and other Anticholinergic Deliriants. Many crude herbal preparations containing belladonna alkaloids are used by teenagers or devotees of the drug culture for their euphoric and deliriant effects (Table 18–17). Several of these are encountered

frequently and have received considerable attention in the medical literature. *Datura stramonium* (Jimson weed, or locoweed) contains atropine (*d*,l-hyoscyamine), and small amounts of scopolamine (hyoscine).[238] The stramonium plant grows wild in many areas of the United States. A tea may be made from its leaves,[237] or the plant may be ground to a powder and one to three teaspoonfuls of it may be washed down with soda or beer.[230] The powder contains roughly 2.5 mg of belladonna alkaloid per teaspoonful.[230] Stramonium leaves may also be smoked, alone or combined with marijuana.[230, 238]

Gowdy reviewed 212 cases of stramonium intoxication, and found that 99 developed hallucinations, 45 became disoriented, and 22 became combative. The hallucinations included color images of people, flowers, bears, etc. There were five accidental deaths in the series, including two persons who drowned while searching for red-eyed dolphins.[230] Patients delirious from stramonium have also been involved in motor vehicle accidents.[237]

Datura arborea (trumpet lily) grows in Australia and causes a syndrome similar to that of *Datura stramonium*. Its ingestion has been fatal in at least one instance.[246]

Treatment for *Datura stramonium* or *Datura arborea* intoxication is the same as that described for atropine or scopolamine poisoning. If physostigmine for parenteral use is not yet available in Australia, tetrahydroaminacrin may be employed.[246]

Many antihistamines, antiparkinsonian agents, antidepressants, antispasmodics, sedatives, and drugs used for motion sickness can cause euphoria, delirium, and the syndrome of anticholingeric intoxication (Table 18–17). Some of these drugs may be purchased without prescription, and others are frequently prescribed, making them available for abuse.

Benactyzine, which is used as a sedative, also has strong anticholinergic properties.[247] Glutethimide, which may be abused as an addicting hypnotic (see above), also has deliriant, anticholinergic properties.[247] Sominex, Compoz, Sleepeze, and Sleeptite all contain scopolamine, which has sedative as well as euphoric and deliriant properties.[247] These have been sold as nonprescription sedatives, and have been abused for their deliriant effects.

Dipheniramine, an antihistamine, has an-

Table 18–17 *Drugs and Chemicals Capable of Producing the Anticholinergic Syndrome*

Medications	Plants
Amitriptyline (Elavil, Triavil)	*Amanita muscaria* (although muscarine is present in minute amounts, major toxic effects are anticholinergic)
Anisotropine (Valpin)	
Atropine	
Belladonna	
Benactyzine (Deprol)	Bittersweet (*Solanum dulcamara*)
Chlorpheniramine (Ornade, Teldrin, etc.)	Black henbane (*Hyocyamus niger*)
Cyclopentolate (Cyclogel)	Black night shade (*Solanum nigrum*)
Desipramine (Norpramin, Pertofrane)	Deadly night shade (*Atropia belladonna*)
Dicyclomine (Bentyl)	Jerusalem cherry (*Solanum pseudocapsicum*)
Diphenhydramine (Benadryl)	
Doxepin (Sinequan)	Jimson weed (*Datura stramonium*)
Homatropine	Lantana (*Lantana camara*) (Also known as red sage, wild sage)
Hyoscine	
Hyoscyamus	Potato leaves, sprouts, tubers (*Solanum tuberosum*)
Imipramine (Tofranil, Presamine)	
Isopropamide (Darbid)	Wild tomato (*Solanum carolinense*)
Mepenzolate (Cantil)	Trumpet lily (*Datura arborea*)
Methantheline (Banthine)	
Methapyriline (Sominex, Compoz, Cope)	Many other antihistamines, antispasmodics, sleep aids, decongestants, analgesics, anti-parkinsonian agents and miscellaneous drugs, chemicals and plants may produce clinically recognizable anticholinergic findings
Nortriptyline (Aventyl)	
Pipenzolate (Piptal)	
Piperidyl isomer (Ditran, Ditropan)	
Propantheline (Probanthine)	
Protriptyline (Vivactil)	
Pyrilamine	
Scopolamine	
Stramonium (Asthmador)	
Trihexyphenidyl (Artane)	

ticholinergic side effects.[233, 247] Dimenhydrinate (Dramamine), an antihistamine used mainly in the treatment of vertigo and motion sickness, has significant anticholinergic properties.[247] It has achieved considerable popularity as a deliriant.[238] Trihexyphenidyl (Artane), used in the treatment of Parkinson's disease, has parasympathetic inhibitory effects and may produce delirium.[233]

Numerous drugs used as antispasmodics for gastrointestinal problems also have anticholinergic side effects on the CNS. Examples of this type of drug include propantheline, and piperidyl isomer (Ditran, Ditropan), which have been abused as deliriants.[1]

Therapy for delirium resulting from these drugs includes intravenous or intramuscular physostigmine, as described above for belladonna intoxication.[233, 238, 247]

The tricyclic antidepressants also have CNS anticholinergic properties and may cause many serious side effects including A–V block, ventricular fibrillation, delirium, and coma.[248] Tricyclics include amitriptyline (Elavil, Triavil), desipramine (Norpramin), doxepin (Sinequan), imipramine (Tofranil), nortriptyline (Aventyl), and protriptyline (Vivactil). In cases of intoxication, the tricyclics appear to have been taken either as suicidal overdoses or, by children, as accidental overdoses. Tricyclics apparently are not abused as pleasure-giving drugs. However, they account for up to 10 per cent of the overdoses currently seen in some centers, and anesthesiologists may need to be familiar with their toxic effects.[250] Patients presenting with tricyclic poisoning resemble those with moderate to severe belladonna intoxication. They exhibit tachycardia, normal to low blood pressure, urinary retention, and coma. However, they also have myoclonus and choreoathetosis, which may be mistaken for convulsions.[248] Sinus tachycardia, atrial fibrillation, bizarre, wide QRS complexes, A–V block, and ventricular fibrillation may occur. Treatment with physostigmine, 4 mg in adults or 0.5 mg in children, intravenously usually will restore consciousness and slow the tachycardia. Up to 26 mg of physostigmine has been given in a 24 hour period to counteract delirium and coma from tricyclic antidepressant overdose.[248]* For serious ventricular arrhythmias, lidocaine or propranolol may be necessary.[249] Transvenous pacing may be necessary if A–V block occurs.

Anesthesia for Patients Intoxicated with Belladonna or with Other Anticholinergic Deliriants

When patients intoxicated with anticholinergic agents require emergency surgery, their intoxication should first be treated with physostigmine. The patient whose delirium has resolved and whose tachycardia and arrhythmias are controlled is obviously a better risk for anesthesia than is the patient with untreated anticholinergic syndrome. Therapy with physostigmine and intravenous fluids preoperatively should counteract fever and dehydration. If treatment with physostigmine makes the patient rational and cooperative, regional anesthesia might be employed, provided that the site and nature of the surgery are consistent with its use. Additional physostigmine may be needed during operation if delirium or the autonomic signs of anticholinergic intoxication recur. Some sedation with diazepam may also be necessary.

If general anesthesia is necessary for the proposed surgery, tachycardia should be reduced with physostigmine preoperatively, and arrhythmias should be controlled with lidocaine or with small doses (0.5–1.0 mg) or propranolol intravenously. In severe intoxication, atrioventricular block may require preoperative transvenous pacing. Even in patients well prepared for anesthesia, it might seem advisable to avoid agents that sensitize the myocardium to arrhythmias (cyclopropane, halothane, trichloroethylene), because an imbalance between the sympathetic and parasympathetic systems may be present. Nodal rhythm is not uncommon in belladonna intoxication, and ventricular extrasystoles or ventricular

tachycardia may occur. Nitrous oxide, enflurane, or limited doses of methoxyflurane may be used. Diethyl ether may be used, but is hazardous because it is flammable. Diazepam or short-acting and ultra-short-acting barbiturates, which are employed as sedatives in atropine poisoning, may be used for anesthesia. Monitoring of temperature is necessary, and measures to control fever should be available. Narcotics may be employed in patients treated with physostigmine prior to surgery; muscle relaxants should probably be avoided. Physostigmine has a weak peripheral anticholinesterase blocking action and will make somewhat more acetylcholine available to compete with nondepolarizing muscle relaxants at the postjunctional membrane. Slightly increased doses of d-tubocurarine should overcome pretreatment with physostigmine, if muscle relaxation is imperative. Either d-tubocurarine or metocurine iodide may be used; gallamine or pancuronium bromide (Pavulon) can cause hypertension and tachycardia, which seem undesirable in patients intoxicated by anticholinergic drugs. Succinylcholine, 0.5 to 1.0 mg per kg, may be used for intubation in patients intoxicated with anticholinergics who have been given physostigmine to treat their intoxication. Neostigmine prolongs the duration of action of succinylcholine by inhibiting serum cholinesterase.[253] Physostigmine may have a similar effect. Hence, rather small doses of succinylcholine may be indicated. If nondepolarizing muscle relaxants are used in patients who have received physostigmine preoperatively, the increased doses of nondepolarizing drugs may still be reversible with neostigmine or other strong peripheral cholinesterase inhibitors; if not, mechanical ventilation should be utilized until the effects of the muscle relaxants wear off. Measurements of neuromuscular function with a nerve stimulator and of tidal volume and vital capacity may be helpful. The use of atropine prior to neostigmine administration for reversal of nondepolarizing relaxants would seem unnecessary. At present, in the literature there are no case reports concerning the conduct of anesthesia in patients intoxicated by anticholinergic hallucinogens.

Cocaine

Cocaine is a CNS stimulant that causes extreme euphoria and excitement and feel-

---

* Physostigmine, or eserine, apparently has analeptic effects in cases of delirium or coma resulting from drugs that do not have CNS anticholinergic properties. Physostigmine is very effective in cases of coma due to large doses of phenothiazides.[241] Physostigmine also will reverse sedation with diazepam, droperidol, or hydroxyzine.[241, 251] Physostigmine may also be used to reverse the delirium that occasionally results from benzquinamide.[252] This delirium may be an anticholinergic effect. Physostigmine should not be used for extrapyramidal reactions due to benzquinamide when consciousness is not impaired.[252]

ings of great mental and physical prowess. In chemical structure it is a tropane that resembles the belladonna alkaloids, but in its pharmacologic actions it differs from them significantly. Cocaine is usually used alone, but combinations of cocaine with LSD or mescaline or with alcohol (the "liquid lady") are seen.[187, 254] The use of cocaine together with narcotics has increased greatly since 1975.[254] A "speedball" is heroin combined with cocaine.[1, 254] Cocaine abusers may try to mitigate the dysphoria that occurs as the cocaine "high" subsides by medicating themselves with ethanol, barbiturates, diazepam, or other sedatives. After an injection of cocaine, the ecstatic effects of the drug quickly wear off and the user becomes nervous and irritable. If sufficient drug is taken, visual and auditory hallucinations with paranoid ideation appear.[79] Some chronic users acquire tactile hallucinations and may hurt themselves while scratching imaginary insects from under their skin.[256] Chronic users of cocaine — especially those on high doses — may become severely paranoid.[151, 255] Aggressive behavior may lead to traumatic injuries. The toxic delirium resembles that seen with amphetamines.

Cocaine acts as a CNS stimulant, a local anesthetic, and as a vasoconstrictor that can slow its own absorption.[151] Traditionally cocaine has been "snorted" or inhaled into the nose and has been absorbed rather quickly from the nasal mucosa, a practice that has often led to ischemic necrosis and perforation of the nasal septum in habitual users.[255] Cocaine is found in the leaves of the coca plant *Erythroxylon coca*, which grows in the Andes Mountains in South America. Over three million people in Bolivia and Peru chew coca leaves as a stimulant.[257] Coca

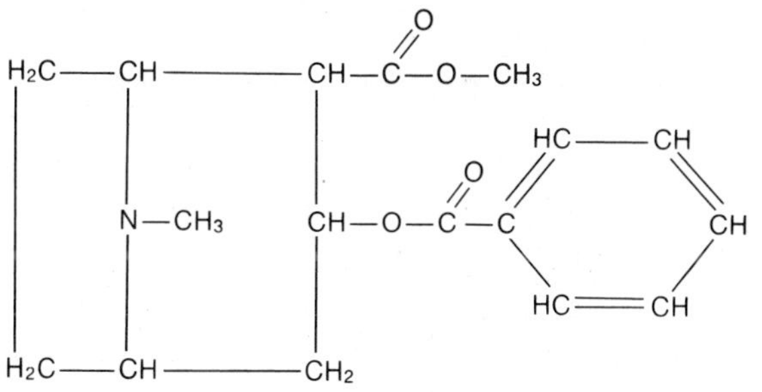

paste, a crude extract containing 40 to 85 per cent cocaine sulfate, is smoked and causes an intense, brief "high," since blood levels rise more quickly with smoking than with "snorting." With smoking, peak blood levels are close to those obtained by intravenous administration of similar doses.[258] Cocaine is also smoked as the "free base." Cocaine hydrochloride, which tends to break down when smoked, is converted to cocaine sulfate by the smoker, using a process that employs petroleum ether, before it is smoked. The conversion also eliminates mannitol, talc, ephedrine, amphetamines, and phencyclidine, substances with which cocaine is often adulterated.[258] The conversion has led to a number of serious burns among users. The free base may be smoked alone in a pipe or may be mixed with marijuana in a cigarette. There has been a recent increase in the smoking of cocaine.[258] Rather little cocaine is ingested, probably because of the widespread misconception that cocaine is inactivated by hydrolysis in the gastrointestinal tract. Van Dyke and coworkers have shown that peak plasma concentrations do not differ significantly whether the drug is ingested or administered intranasally. However, peak plasma levels occurred only 15 minutes after "snorting" cocaine, 2 mg per kg; while peak levels did not occur until 30 minutes after gelatin tablets containing the same dose of cocaine were ingested. Van Dyke and coworkers reported better "highs" after cocaine ingestion than after its intranasal application.[257] At least seven fatalities have been reported following the ingestion of large doses of cocaine in order to hide the drug from the police.[254] Cocaine has become popular as a recreational drug during the past five years — even among professional groups — perhaps because of the misconception that it is a safe drug. Since 1975 the use of intravenous cocaine has increased, and the number of fatalities attributed to cocaine abuse has also increased. The lethal dose of cocaine in man is approximately 1.2 grams, although as little as 30 mg has caused ventricular fibrillation and death.[151, 255] Wetli and Wright noted cocaine blood levels from 0.14 to 1.7 mg per ml in their study of deaths associated with cocaine abuse.[254] Death occurred at lower blood levels in intravenous cocaine users who suddenly collapsed and died, or who died after a brief period of coma. Higher blood levels were

Cocaine

Figure 18–27.

found in fatalities following oral ingestion or nasal use of cocaine. In these cases, death was preceded by convulsions or respiratory arrest, and not by sudden collapse. Wetli and Wright suggest that the rate of rise of the blood level of cocaine, not simply the peak blood level, may determine whether cocaine intoxication will be fatal.[254]

Cocaine is hydrolyzed by esterases in plasma, liver, and other organs; in man 35 to 54 per cent of a dose of cocaine is excreted as benzoylecgonine within 24 hours, while less than 9 per cent is excreted unchanged. The stimulant effects of cocaine in the CNS may result from a direct action on dopamine receptors or from release of dopamine. Thus far, no inhibition of norepinephrine uptake in the brain by cocaine has been demonstrated.[151]

Signs of sympathetic stimulation appear with administration of cocaine to unanesthetized subjects. Significant hypertension resulting from central stimulation, and tachycardia — both central and peripheral in origin — appear. The peripheral component of the tachycardia is thought to result from the ability of cocaine to interfere with the re-uptake of norepinephrine by the sympathetic nerve terminals.[259] The sympathetic receptor sites are therefore exposed to a higher concentration of sympathetic transmitter substance. The effect of cocaine on the re-uptake of the sympathetic transmitter was described as early as 1961 by Hertting et al. and by Muscholl.[261]

Symptoms of cocaine intoxication include dry throat, vertigo, and a desire to defecate or micturate as a result of smooth muscle spasm. Then confusion, diaphoresis, and vomiting occur.[255] Marked hyperpyrexia, another effect of cocaine, results from generalized vasoconstriction, from increased muscle activity, and probably from an effect on CNS centers that regulate temperature. Hyperreflexia and tonic clonic convulsions may occur.[259] Rapid and shallow breathing may be followed by Cheyne-Stokes respiration and apnea.[255] Large doses of cocaine can cause death from central depression of respiration.[259] Death may also result from cerebral hemorrhage, probably due to hypertension.[255] Cases of acute overdoses of cocaine are rarely seen in emergency rooms; Wetli and Wright note that minor reactions to cocaine appear to resolve quickly, while severe reactions are rapidly fatal.[254]

The treatment for convulsions from acute cocaine poisoning is a short-acting barbiturate given intravenously;[255, 259] if ventilation is inadequate, artificial respiration must be employed.[259] For hyperactivity, insomnia, or delirium, diazepam has been recommended.[187] Either a barbiturate or diazepam should be effective against seizure activity. In brief, the management of cocaine intoxication is the same as the management of an overdose of any local anesthetic agent. Propranolol intravenously in 1 mg increments may be used to control the tachycardia and hypertension resulting from cocaine abuse. Gay and coworkers have used propranolol successfully in at least 50 cases of acute cocainism.[255] The sympathetic effects respond to propranolol but the vomiting does not; therapy with antiemetics may be necessary. Cocaine users may have a psychological dependence on the drug; however, no report of physical dependence on cocaine or of an abstinence syndrome upon withdrawal of the drug can be found in the literature. Some tolerance, at least to the lethal effects of cocaine, seems to develop. As much as 10 grams per day may be consumed by abusers.[151, 262] According to Caldwell and Sever, the tolerance persists even during brief periods of abstinence.[151]

Anesthesia for Cocaine Users. If emergency surgery, possibly for treatment of injuries, should become necessary in a cocaine user, adequate preoperative sedation should be achieved with barbiturates or diazepam. If tachycardia and hypertension are present at the time of induction — an unlikely possibility in view of the rapid metabolism of cocaine — the anesthesiologist might do well to avoid agents such as cyclopropane and trichloroethylene, which sensitize the myocardium to catechols. Koehntop and coworkers recently found that cocaine, 2 mg per kg given intravenously during anesthesia with 1 per cent halothane and 60 per cent nitrous oxide, decreased the arrhythmogenic dose of epinephrine by up to 50 per cent in dogs.[263] It may not be necessary to avoid halothane in patients intoxicated with cocaine. Any serious arrhythmias that may occur should respond to propranolol.

Stoelting and coworkers showed that intravenous cocaine, 2 mg per kg, increased the MAC for halothane in dogs from a control level of 1.12 ± 0.03 per cent to 1.21 ± 0.06 per cent after one hour. This effect of cocaine on MAC persisted for at least three hours, but disappeared by 24 hours after cocaine administration. The effect was dose related, in that intravenous cocaine, 4 mg per kg, increased the MAC for halothane to 1.21 ± 0.06 per cent at one hour and to 1.35 ± 0.04 per cent at three hours.[262]

Somewhat smaller doses of cocaine (1.5 mg per kg) administered topically in man before nasal intubation after 25 minutes of anesthesia with 0.5 per cent halothane and 60 per cent nitrous oxide caused no apparent increase in pulse rate, mean arterial pressure, or cardiac index for nearly an hour after cocaine application.[264] Both the control group and the group given a topical cocaine anesthetic developed transient increases in pulse rate and mean arterial pressure during intubation. The maximum plasma cocaine concentration, averaging 331 μg per ml, occurred 25 minutes after intubation when the transient tachycardia and hypertension had resolved. Barash and coworkers noted that during light general anesthesia with halothane and nitrous oxide, cocaine in the dose they employed was not accompanied by clinically significant signs of stimulation.[264] No arrhythmia appeared. Effects of cocaine on MAC were not measured during this study in man. Further studies of interactions between general anesthetics and cocaine in a wider range of doses are needed, in animals, in drug naive human subjects, and in heavy cocaine abusers. Enflurane and halothane may be employed in patients intoxicated with cocaine. Increased doses of these agents may be necessary. Methoxyflurane may also be suitable, provided that the total dose of this agent can be limited to avoid renal damage. Anesthesia with nitrous oxide supplemented with barbiturates and narcotics also appears suitable. The mild alpha blockade of droperidol or the bradycardiac effect of fentanyl may be useful in patients intoxicated with cocaine. Regional anesthetics may be possible in a few well sedated patients, but general anesthesia will be necessary for surgery in most patients intoxicated by cocaine.

ANESTHETIC CONSIDERATIONS IN PATIENTS TAKING CANNABIS (MARIJUANA)

Cannabis is the genus of plants that produce hemp. Both male and female plants of the genus contain psychoactive compounds.[265] Marijuana is a general term indicating any part of the plant (chopped leaves, flowers, or stems) that can cause hallucinatory effects when ingested or smoked. The word hashish refers specifically to the resin extracted from the tops of female hemp plants. Delta[9]-3,4-trans-tetrahydrocannabinol (THC) is the most active of the 30 cannabinoids already isolated.[1, 266] A single marijuana cigarette has roughly 0.5 gm of crude marijuana or around 0.5 mg of tetrahydrocannabinol.[267] Most marijuana available in the United States contains only 1 or 2 per cent THC in its seed pods or flower tops; the leaves and stems contain considerably less. Hashish, the resin extracted from the green flowers, may contain as much as eight per cent THC.[1, 265] Therefore, hashish is between five and 10 times more potent than marijuana.[265, 266] Hashish is marketed as blocks of solid resin. Cigarettes may be laced with the resin, or

Figure 18–28.

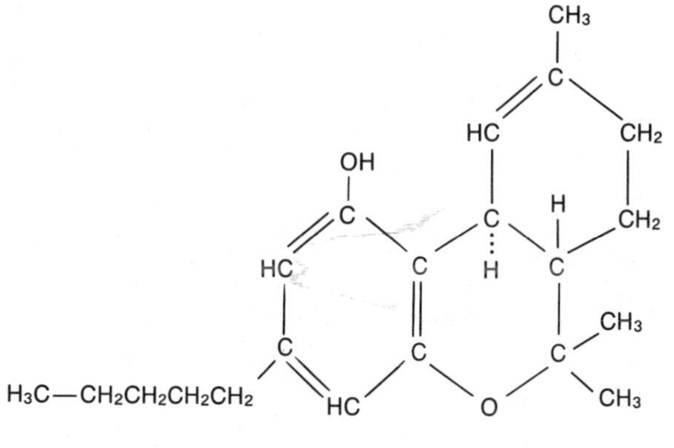

Δ^9 Tetrahydrocannabinol

bits of resin may be put on the burning end of an ordinary cigarette and the fumes inhaled.[2] The resin may also be smoked in a pipe. Although the flame destroys about half the drug, THC and marijuana are more effective when smoked than when ingested orally; however, the effects last longer, up to 12 hours, after oral ingestion.[1, 265, 266] Further extraction of cannabis plant materials or of hashish yields "hashish oil," a dark liquid containing up to 20 per cent THC. One or two drops of this liquid is as potent as the average marijuana cigarette.[268] Cannabinols are heat labile; at 70° F, 5 per cent of THC is destroyed each month.[1] The smoke is irritating, causes conjunctival injection, and smells like burning alfalfa.[1, 2]

On inhaling marijuana the user may feel a "jittery rush," followed by a mood of tranquility. He may note an increased awareness of sounds and taste; visual perceptions may be altered in shape, size, or distance from the observer. Associations between ideas may be loosened, and awareness of the passage of time may be altered. Varying degrees of anxiety, even reaching the proportions of a toxic psychosis, may appear. THC, 0.05 mg per kg, causes a "social high" or euphoria, with mild distortions in color and distance, and a slower passage of time. A floating sensation and a hunger for sweets may be experienced. With 0.1 mg per kg more perceptual distortion, memory impairment, and emotional lability occurs; and with 0.2 mg per kg, vivid hallucinations, depersonalization, and psychotic episodes will appear.[1, 2, 268] The effects are felt within minutes after smoking marijuana, are most intense at 15 to 30 minutes, and wane after two or three hours.[268]

In some users "flashbacks" similar to those seen in patients taking LSD but of lesser intensity have been reported. These "flashbacks" are extremely rare.[269] There is considerable evidence among very heavy users of tolerance to cannabis;[266, 271] however, a "reverse" tolerance may also occur, in that with repeated use the subject notes an increase in the psychic effects of marijuana.[265] There are no reports of an abstinence syndrome in man after withdrawal of cannabis. Nor are there reports of cross tolerance with major hallucinogens such as LSD, psilocybin, or the amphetamines.[1, 266]

The use of marijuana is extremely popular in the United States at present; over 43 million Americans have tried the drug, and 16 million use it monthly, according to the latest estimate.[268] No reports of death from overdose of marijuana or hashish have appeared to date; hence cannabinoids appear safer than ethyl alcohol, with respect to dose related fatalities.[270] Marijuana or hashish equivalent to 400 mg of THC per day has been consumed by persons in Morocco.[271] The tachycardia caused by cannabinols is potentially dangerous in patients with angina.[270]

The half-life of THC in plasma is 36 hours, and in tissues it is seven days.[270, 271] THC is fat soluble and is distributed into many body compartments.[271] Cannabinols are excreted in bile and reabsorbed from the intestine. A single dose of THC may require up to 30 days for complete elimination, and only 20 to 30 per cent is excreted via the kidney.[270, 271] In animals, during a four day period, THC markedly increased the activity of hepatic microsomal dechlorinase, the enzyme that cleaves the bond between carbon and chlorine in both halothane and methoxyflurane.[272]

The physiological effects of marijuana include tachycardia (greater in chronic users than in nonusers), mild tachypnea, and slight changes in blood pressure.[273, 274] The use of THC, 0.44 mg per kg, as an intravenous premedication resulted in systolic hypertension followed by hypotension (20–40 mm Hg decrease) associated with vertigo and nausea in three of 10 subjects in one study. Marked tachycardia with a shortened P-R interval and with a decrease in the height of the T wave was also observed. The tachycardia is thought to result from CNS sympathetic stimulation rather than from a peripheral vagolytic action.[270] The hunger seen with low doses of THC has been ascribed to hypoglycemia.[2] However, in one well-conducted study no alterations in pupil size or blood glucose levels were observed.[273] Marijuana also causes a dry mouth, and with moderate or higher doses, complex reaction time increases and incoordination resembling that during intoxication with alcohol occurs.[1, 2]

The intravenous use of marijuana apparently results in an acute illness characterized by chills, fever, nausea, vomiting, diarrhea, hypotension, glycosuria, leukocytosis, and a transient thrombocytopenia.[275]

Marijuana smoke often causes bronchitis with a nonproductive cough.[266] Marijuana smokers may have a decreased vital capacity and may have mild pulmonary obstructive disease. Animals exposed to marijuana smoke for over 80 days developed scattered foci of alveolitis, infiltrations of macrophages, and granulomas.[271] Marijuana smoke also appears to hinder pulmonary resistance to infection more than does tobacco smoke.[271] Although up to 20 per cent of the marijuana grown in Mexico has been contaminated with the insecticide Paraquat, and although Paraquat itself causes focal hemorrhage and fibrosis when instilled into the bronchi, no cases of lung damage due to Paraquat have yet been reported in marijuana smokers.[278, 279] Marijuana smoke also irritates the eyes; conjunctival injection is frequent in marijuana smokers.[266]

Some of the behavioral effects of marijuana may be mediated via the limbic system. Exposure to THC for six months has been shown to cause permanent brain wave changes — high amplitude spikes originating in the limbic system. Primates exposed to marijuana for three months show similar changes; and damage to synapses in the limbic system has been demonstrated by electron microscopy in these animals.[271] THC in large doses can trigger some types of epilepsy in patients with low seizure thresholds — a fact well known among devotees of the drug culture.[271] The pathophysiology of heavy doses of marijuana has not yet been thoroughly studied.[1]

Marijuana apparently prolongs barbiturate sleeping time and may potentiate the depressant effect of ethanol.[265, 270] Siemens and coworkers showed that cannabis doubled pentobarbital sleeping time in rats, while Sofia and coworkers showed that pretreatment with THC doubled the sleeping time for ketamine in mice.[276, 277] Marijuana also may enhance the effects of amphetamines.[270] The administration of barbiturates can intensify the hallucinations resulting from THC. Johnstone and coworkers found that in volunteers given pentobarbital, 100 mg per 70 kg, the administration of rather large doses of THC, 27 to 134 μg per kg, caused severe hallucinations but did not cause respiratory depression.[280] However, in volunteers whose respiration was depressed by oxymorphone, 1.0 mg per 70 kg, THC caused further respiratory depression and acted as an excellent sedative.[280] It appears that small doses of narcotics may be used with caution in patients intoxicated by marijuana.

Therapy for patients intoxicated by marijuana consists of reassurance and sedation with chlordiazepoxide or diazepam.[1] Intermediate acting barbiturates should be avoided.[280] Phenothiazides should also be avoided, since they might cause postural hypotension.[1]

The interactions between THC and two inhalational anesthetics have been studied in animals. Vietz and coworkers found that THC, 1.0 and 2.0 mg intraperitoneally, reduced the MAC of cyclopropane given two hours later by 15.4 ± 3.6 and 25.1 ± 1.4 per cent, respectively.[281] Stoelting and coworkers found that THC, 0.5 mg per kg given intravenously during anesthesia with halothane in oxygen, decreased the MAC of halothane by 32 per cent one hour after injection but that the effect disappeared after three hours. With a larger dose of THC, 2.0 mg per kg, the MAC of halothane was decreased by 42 per cent at 24 hours.[282] They also suggested that THC may inhibit cholinesterase. It is likely that THC will decrease the MAC of other inhalational anesthetics, but no studies have yet been published for other agents.

In summary, the patient acutely intoxicated with marijuana will require no belladonna premedication, since he will have a dry oropharynx and a tachycardia. Severe tachycardias may be controlled with propranolol. He may require some diazepam for sedation or for control of frightening hallucinations. Pentobarbital and other barbiturates with a medium duration of action should be avoided; barbiturates intensify the hallucinations caused by THC. If the patient is in pain, he may require small doses of narcotics; some caution is necessary, since THC increases the respiratory depression of narcotics. For induction diazepam seems preferable; however, a short acting barbiturate such as thiopental will probably not contribute to postoperative hallucinations, since short acting barbiturates redistribute rather quickly. The patient acutely intoxicated with marijuana will require less than the usual MAC dose for maintenance of anesthesia with cyclopropane or halothane, and probably with other inhalational agents as well. No agent is contraindicated in patients intoxicated with cannabis. However, methoxyflurane may be metabolized by hepatic peroxidoses to a much greater extent in marijuana users than in naive patients; it may be wise to avoid using methoxyflurane in these patients. Trichloroethylene and cyclopropane should probably be avoided in patients with marked preoperative tachycardia. Enflurane and halothane seem satisfactory for use in patients intoxicated by marijuana. These agents would counteract bronchospasm in patients whose airways have been irritated by marijuana smoke. Therapy with bronchodilators such as isoetharine aerosol (Bronkosol) or with aminophylline may be necessary in occasional cases. A balanced anesthetic consisting of nitrous oxide supplemented with muscle relaxants, diazepam, and narcotics in limited doses should be satisfactory; however, in heavy marijuana users, poor pulmonary function may limit the concentration of nitrous oxide that can be used safely. Although THC has some anticholinesterase activity, no clinical reports of problems with muscle relaxants or their reversal have yet been made in patients acutely intoxicated with cannabis. Finally, tachycardia may persist postoperatively in patients affected by cannabinols. Gregg and coworkers point out that some tachycardia may be expected during the recovery period and that the tachycardia should not be treated unnecessarily.[270]

THE CYCLOHEXYLAMINES: METHYLPHENIDATE, PHENMETRAZINE, AND PHENCYCLIDINE (PCP)

Several drugs with a phenylcyclohexylamine structure or with a structure resembling that of the phenylcyclohexylamine nucleus are used for their psychedelic effects. These drugs include methylphenidate (Ritalin), phenmetrazine (Preludin), phencyclidine (Sernylan, PCP), and analogues of phencyclidine — ethylphenylcyclohexylamine (PCE), phenylcyclohexylpyrrolidine (PHP, PCPy), and thienylcyclohexylpiperidine (TCP, TPCP) (see Table 18–11). All of these compounds may cause psychosis. Phenmetrazine rarely causes psychosis at recommended doses, but may do so at increased doses. Methylphenidate may cause psychosis, particularly when used intravenously. Phencyclidine and its analogues often produce psychosis, especially with repeated use. Prolonged psychotic reactions have occurred after only one dose of phencyclidine. Of all the drugs that alter mood or perception, phencyclidine is without a doubt the most dangerous to the user.

Methylphenidate (Ritalin). Methylphenidate is a CNS stimulant which on intravenous injection causes a "rush" resembling that experienced with the injection of heroin or cocaine.[225] Methylphenidate has been used as an analeptic in barbiturate poisoning, and currently is used in the treatment of minimal brain dysfunction in children and of narcolepsy in adults.[283] Average therapeutic doses are 20 to 30 mg per day, and not over 60 mg per day is recommended for adults. Methylphenidate abusers may inject up to 500 mg per day intravenously.[225] A powder made by grinding tablets of the drug is dissolved in water and injected. Agitation, insomnia, auditory hallucinations, delirium, and a toxic psychosis result from overdose of methylphenidate. Intravenous abuse of the drug is especially associated with the development of frank psychosis.

Methylphenidate causes sympathetic effects including hypertension, tachycardia,

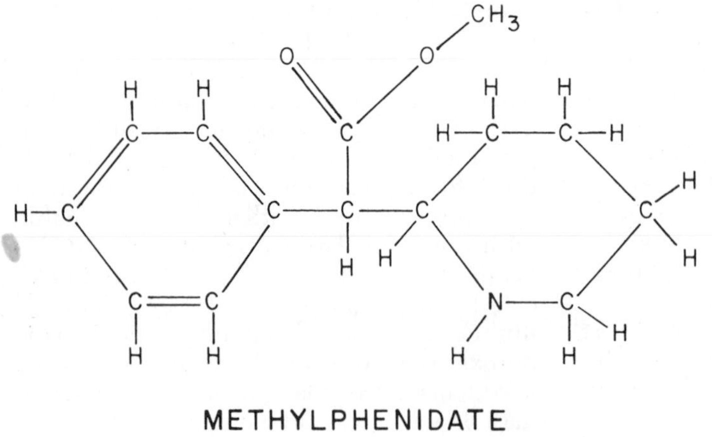

Figure 18–29.

METHYLPHENIDATE

arrhythmias, mydriasis, and fever. It also causes hyperreflexia and tremors. High doses may cause convulsions and coma. It also may cause vomiting, diaphoresis, and a dry mouth. Repeated use of intravenous methylphenidate may cause a necrotizing vasculitis with the formation of microaneurysms. Fifteen of the 16 patients with a history of methylphenidate abuse studied by Boswell had abnormalities on angiograms; five of the 15 had microaneurysms. The patients ranged in age from 26 to 53 years. Lesions appeared in smaller arteries, but in five of the patients, large arteries were also affected.[225] Citron and coworkers found similar lesions in methamphetamine abusers, as described earlier.[224] Retinal vascular damage leading to blindness was observed with methylphenidate abuse.[225, 284] Seven of the 16 methylphenidate abusers described by Boswell had dyspnea or chest pain, associated with segmental branch pulmonary artery occlusions or with occlusion of the pulmonary arterial supply to the lower lobe of one or both lungs.[225] The talc used as a filler in methylphenidate tablets may contribute to pulmonary vascular damage, but the systemic arterial lesions appear to be caused by the methylphenidate itself.[225]

Therapy for acute intoxication with methylphenidate includes sedation with barbiturates or diazepam. Arrhythmias may be controlled with propranolol; and hypertension, if severe, may be treated with phentolamine. Dilantin may be used to treat convulsions. Gastric lavage may remove unabsorbed drug. In massive overdoses of methylphenidate, external cooling may be required to control fever, and mechanical ventilation may be necessary to sustain respiration.

Phenmetrazine (Preludin). Phenmetrazine, an oxazine compound, resembles the sympathetic amines in its pharmacological effects and is used as an anorectic in the treatment of obesity. Phenmetrazine has been abused both orally and intravenously.[284] Phenmetrazine abuse, like that of the amphetamines, may evoke a strong psychological dependence, but no physical dependence leading to an abstinence syndrome upon withdrawl of the drug occurs. Therapeutic doses of 50 to 75 mg per day rarely cause psychosis; however, large amounts may cause a psychosis indistinguishable from schizophrenia. This psychosis usually

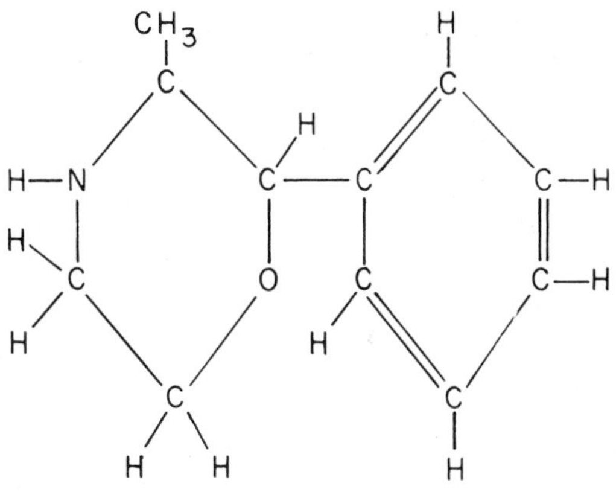

PHENMETRAZINE
Figure 18–30.

clears in a matter of days after the drug is discontinued.

The syndrome of phenmetrazine overdose resembles that described above for the amphetamines or for methylphenidate.[284] However, necrotizing angiitis and the formation of microaneurysms have not yet been described in phenmetrazine abusers. Hypertension, tachycardias, and arrhythmias occur. Insomnia, irritability, combativeness, hallucinations, panic, psychosis, hyperreflexia, convulsions, and coma are seen with overdoses. Abdominal cramps, nausea, and vomiting may also appear.[284] Treatment resembles that described for intoxication with methylphenidate or the amphetamines. Gastric lavage may be helpful. Acidification of the urine hastens excretion of the drug, as described for the amphetamines.

Phencyclidine and Analogues of Phencyclidine. Phenycyclidine (PCP) or phenylcyclohexylpiperidine and its analogues ethylphenylcyclohexylamine (PCE), phenylcyclohexylpyrrolidine (PCPy, PHP), and thienylcyclohexylpiperidine (TPCP, TCP) are all cyclohexylamines that cause violent behavior and prolonged psychosis resembling schizophrenia in abusers. Its behavioral toxicity is so severe that heavier penalties have been imposed for its manufacture or possession than for any other nonnarcotic drug.* Popular names for phen-

---

*Manufacture or possession of PCP or its analogues with intent to sell carries a federal prison term of 10 years and a $25,000 fine, or both, for a first offense. Penalties for a second offense are double those for a first offense. All sales of piperidine, its salts, and acyl derivatives must be reported to the Drug Enforcement Administration.[285]

cyclidine indicating its destructive and bizarre effects include "angel dust," "embalming fluid," "killer weed," and "super grass."[285] Phencyclidine was originally studied for possible use as an anesthetic, but its hallucinogenic and psychotic side effects made it unfit for human use. Until 1978 it was sold as a veterinary anesthetic under the name Sernylan. It is now manufactured only in clandestine laboratories and usually contains some impurities. Phencyclidine is the parent compound of ketamine, which is approved for use as a dissociative anesthetic in man.[134] The abuse of phencyclidine appears to be increasing. Showalter and Thornton note that in a 1977 study of 1000 cases of intoxication in Detroit, Michigan, phencyclidine was the most commonly abused drug.[134] Phencyclidine is available as a powder or a liquid, as well as in tablets or capsules. It is usually placed on tobacco, marijuana, or parsley and smoked. When purified, the powder is water soluble and may be mixed with any type of drink. It has been sold deceptively as lysergic acid diethylamide, mescaline, or tetrahydrocannabinol.[285]

Low doses of phencyclidine cause euphoria and a giddy feeling. Clarity of thought is decreased; sensation — particularly touch — is diminished, although vision, hearing, taste and position sense are also affected. Paresthesias involving the face and extremities occur. The kaleidoscopic visual hallucinations characteristic of the hallucinogenic indoles do not occur with phencyclidine. Distortions of body image occur, with illusory changes in size or with the sensation that the limbs are floating away. Orientation is lost, and panic and hostile actions may occur.[134, 286] Frank psychosis or an agitated delirium may occur. With higher doses a cataleptic or "dissociative" state occurs during which surgery may be performed. Persons intoxicated with PCP may become involved in accidents or may mutilate themselves severely.[286, 287]

Neurologic signs with phencyclidine intoxication vary with the dose of the drug inhaled or ingested. With low doses, slurred speech, ataxia, clonus, tremors, and increased deep tendon reflexes are present. Respiration is unaffected. With moderate or anesthetic doses, the patients appear to stare — the eyes remain open but move very little.[134, 286] The pupils may be normal or constricted, but their light reflex is diminished. Bilateral ptosis is often present, and nystagmus may be present. The most impressive neurological finding in patients intoxicated by PCP is sensory blockade resembling that due to ketamine.[134] Laryngeal and gag reflexes remain active; laryngopasm may occur. The corneal reflex may be diminished. With anesthetic doses of phencyclidine muscular rigidity occurs, and deep tendon reflexes may be decreased or absent.[134, 286] Opisthotonos may be present. The neurological signs may not be uniform, especially in lighter levels of intoxication; sensation, reflexes, or myoclonus may be present unilaterally.[286] With severe intoxication, polysynaptic reflexes are depressed, and myoclonus, convulsions, or coma is present. Respiratory depression, Cheyne-Stokes breathing, and apnea may occur. Upon awakening, the patient may have a psychosis that can last up to a year.[187] The author knows of one case in which psychosis following ingestion of a single dose of PCP has necessitated hospitalization for a year and a half.

The autonomic side effects of phencyclidine intoxication resemble those of ketamine. Elevation of blood pressure for 15 to 60 minutes occurs and is dose related; and an enhanced response to vasopressors may be present for another hour. The hypertension responds to alpha blocking agents.[134] Sinus tachycardia may occur. Tachyphylaxis to the pressor effect of PCP develops rapidly.[134] Diaphoresis, nausea, and vomiting may occur. Hyperthermia has been observed.[286]

Electroencephalographic changes reported with phencyclidine include slow waves or theta activity in the occipital, temporal, and parietal regions.[134] Hyvarinen and coworkers found that PCP in doses under 0.5 mg per kg increased spontaneous activity and responses to visual and auditory stimuli in the posterior parietal association cortex in primates. Large doses had a depressing effect.[288] Phencyclidine can interact to some extent with muscarinic receptors — an interaction that may explain some of its vagal effects.[163] Phencyclidine analgesia may be mediated by narcotic receptors, since the slope of its log concentration inhibition curve resembles that of morphine.[292] Its sympathetic effects may be mediated by dopamine receptors.

Phencyclidine is hydroxylated in the liver and is excreted principally as a 4-hydroxy piperidine derivative.[134] Acidification of the urine promotes rapid excretion of PCP.[289] Phencyclidine is reported to inhibit pseudocholinesterase; however, no report of prolonged apnea resulting from PCP has appeared in the anesthesia literature.[134] Tolerance to phencyclidine after only four days of use has been demonstrated in primates; as yet no cross tolerance between the phenylcyclohexylamines and any other drug has been proven.[290]

The diagnosis of intoxication with phencyclidine or its analogues is based on the presence of hypertension, bizarre neurological signs and behavior, and normal or increased respiration. The presence of sensory blockade and the characteristic stare suggest PCP intoxication. These features distinguish PCP intoxication from primary psychosis or from intoxication resulting from narcotics or most sedatives. However, intoxication with methaqualone is not characterized by respiratory depression and may be difficult to distinguish from PCP intoxication, particularly when the patient presents with coma. Corales and coworkers emphasize this point.[286] When a patient presents with coma, the differential diagnosis includes intoxication with phencyclidine, methaqualone, and brain injury. Radiographic examination including arteriography or computerized axial tomography (CAT-scan) may be necessary to rule out head injury. Psychosis upon awakening suggests PCP intoxication.

Therapy for patients intoxicated with phencyclidine or its analogues is as follows: For mild or moderate intoxication, the patient should be kept in a quiet environment. Restraints may be necessary. Diazepam is useful for sedation and for reducing muscle spasm.[134] Chlorpromazine should be avoided, since it has caused significant hypotension and bradycardia in patients intoxicated with PCP.[134, 286] Haloperidol, 2 to 5 mg intramuscularly, may be used to control psychotic symptoms, and may be repeated as necessary. Psychiatric consultation should be obtained for patients intoxicated with phencyclidine. If significant hypertension is present, phentolamine or diazoxide may be used to control it, as was described above for therapy of amphetamine intoxication.[134, 291] Acidification of the urine with ascorbic acid or ammonium chloride should be done to achieve more rapid excretion of PCP, which itself is slightly alkaline.[287, 289] Fever, if present, should be treated with external cooling, and adequate hydration will be necessary. In severe intoxication with PCP, gastric lavage is beneficial.[134] Respiratory depression should be treated by mechanical ventilation, and convulsions should be controlled with barbiturates, diazepam, or Dilantin.[134]

Specific descriptions of anesthetics in patients intoxicated with phencyclidine and its cogeners have not yet appeared in the literature. However, the anesthesiologist familiar with the effects of ketamine should be able to manage these patients satisfactorily. In patients mildly intoxicated with PCP, general anesthesia seems preferable to regional, since these patients are likely to exhibit violent and bizarre behavior. Induction of anesthesia can be done with barbiturates or diazepam. Maintenance with enflurane, halothane, or nitrous oxide supplemented with narcotics should prove satisfactory. For patients in a dissociated state from phencyclidine, no anesthetic will be necessary for superficial surgical procedures. For surgery in major body cavities, intubation and muscle relaxants will be required. Patients in coma from high doses of phencyclidine will require supportive measures, including mechanical ventilation, hydration, and external cooling, as described above.

ANESTHESIA FOR THE IRRADIATED PATIENT

Irradiated patients fall into two principal groups: those who have had half or whole body exposure, and those who have had exposure limited to specific, rather small regions of the body. Most of the irradiated patients having anesthesia for surgical procedures or being managed by anesthesiologists in intensive care units have had radiotherapy to specific organs or to the lymphatic drainage of limited regions of the body. However, articles concerning the use of general anesthesia for both regional and whole body radiotherapy have appeared within the last few years. The LD_{50} in man for a single whole body dose of ionizing

Table 18–18 *Irradiation Sickness in Man: Clinical Presentation Related to a Single Whole Body Radiation Dose**

A. 200–400 rads: Hematopoietic and immunologic depression
    a) prodrome of lethargy and vomiting
    b) immediate lymphocytopenia
    c) symptom free interval of 2–4 weeks
    d) granulocytopenia maximal in 4–6 weeks
    e) thrombocytopenia maximal at 4 weeks
    f) some deaths from infection or hemorrhage

B. 400–1000 rads: Gastrointestinal dysfunction
    a) prodrome of lethargy and vomiting
    b) immediate lymphocytopenia
    c) early onset of nausea, vomiting, and diarrhea
    d) dehydration, hypokalemia ⎱ possibly fatal by 2–3 weeks
    e) electrolyte imbalance ⎰
    f) anemia and thrombocytopenia – severe by 4 weeks
    g) late deaths from infection or hemorrhage

C. 3000 rads or more: Central nervous system dysfunction
    a) lethargy and coma
    b) ataxia, tremor, and convulsions
    c) erythematous radiation burns
    d) death within 48 hours

*The median lethal dose of whole body irradiation in man at six weeks following exposure is 350 rads (tissue dose). Data after Eiseman, B., and Bond, V.: Surg. Gynecol. Obstet. *146*:877, 1978.

radiation is approximately 350 rads.*[293] Patients exposed to single whole body doses of 200 to 1000 rads present problems in the medical management of marrow depression, infection, and radiation enteritis. General anesthetics have been employed during radiation therapy using up to 1000 rads given as a single whole body dose to prepare patients with leukemia for bone marrow transplants.[294] Whole body doses above 1000 rads are nearly always fatal; and after massive doses of whole body irradiation (3,000 rads (r), or more), death results within 48 hours from a CNS syndrome consisting of

*The rad is a measure of energy absorption in tissue, and applies to nonionizing as well as ionizing radiation. One rad (r) equals 100 ergs of energy absorbed in 1 gm of tissue. The roentgen (R) is a measure of ionizing energy produced when gamma rays are absorbed by air. One roentgen is the amount of gamma radiation that will produce 1 coulomb of electrostatic charge when absorbed by 0.001293 gm of air at standard temperature and pressure. For small portions of tissue the number of rads absorbed in a unit time will closely approximate the number of roentgens delivered to the tissue in a unit time. For large blocks or tissue, the absorbed dose (rads) becomes less than the air dose (roentgens) delivered to the tissue because of decreased intensity at greater distance from the radiation source. There is also an exponential attenuation of beam intensity from interaction of the gamma rays with layers of tissue near the surface of the irradiated block of tissue.

lethargy, tremors, ataxia, convulsions, and coma (Table 18–18C).[296] Some information is available concerning the effects of anesthesia on patients who are receiving high therapeutic doses of irradiation; however, very few of these patients come to surgery shortly after receiving radiation therapy. The effects of combinations of ionizing radiation, thermal burns, trauma, anesthesia, and surgery are not well understood in man.[293] A few studies of x-irradiation and thermal injury have been done in laboratory animals. The largest number of patients anesthetized after whole body irradiation were survivors of the Hiroshima and Nagasaki atomic bombs who also sustained injuries necessitating surgery. The Atomic Bomb Casualties and Control Commission tried to ascertain the effect of radiation exposure on anesthetic morbidity and mortality in this group of patients but was unable to draw any conclusions because of inadequate medical records.

The subject of anesthesia for the irradiated patient may be divided into the following topics: the effects of whole body irradiation in man; the effects of irradiation on specific organs of importance in anesthesia; the effects of irradiation on anesthetic mortality in experimental animals; the interactions between irradiation and drugs used as adjuncts during anesthesia; radioprotection or sensitization of normal and neoplastic tissue by chemical or thermal means; the anesthetic management of patients during diagnostic and therapeutic radiological procedures; and the management of combined injury from trauma and irradiation.

EFFECTS OF WHOLE BODY IRRADIATION ON THE PATIENT

Patients subjected to whole body irradiation in doses of 200 to 1000 rads display several clinical patterns of disease (Table 18-18). After a period several hours following irradiation during which the patient feels well, sudden episodes of vomiting not necessarily preceded by nausea occur. Danjoux and coworkers note that these episodes somewhat resemble those seen in patients with increased intracranial pressure.[295] Anorexia and nausea often develop, and the patient becomes lethargic and may sleep between bouts of vomiting. The pattern of vomiting alternating with sleep continues for six to eight hours, until the episodes of vomiting become less frequent and disappear, and the intervals of sleep become longer.[295] With larger doses of irradiation (600-1000 rads), this prodrome of vomiting and lethargy begins within two hours following exposure, whereas with lesser doses (200-400 rads), it may not begin for six to 12 hours. Exposure of the upper abdomen to ionizing irradiation apparently is an etiological factor in this syndrome. Danjoux and coworkers noted that 70 (83%) of 88 patients receiving high dose radiotherapy to the upper abdomen and thorax developed acute radiation sickness; yet only 39 of 101 patients receiving similar doses (mean 808 rads) to the lower half of the body including the abdomen up to the umbilicus developed the syndrome. Exclusion of the head from the field made no apparent difference in the incidence or severity of the symptoms. About a third of the patients given radiation to the upper half of the body developed chills, and low grade fevers (39°C) were noted in some patients. Five per cent of the patients developed transient diarrhea within 12 hours of irradiation. Pretreatment with antiemetics had no effect on the nausea or vomiting.[295]

The "prodrome," or first phase, of radiation sickness apparently coincides with the release of toxic products from necrosis of radiosensitive cells such as lymphocytes and intestinal epithelium.[296] These symptoms may also appear early during a course of radiotherapy for neoplasms that are especially radiosensitive, such as seminomas and lymphomas, or when large regions of tissue are irradiated for palliative treatment of widespread metastases. The dehydration and potassium loss that occur shortly after irradiation should be treated before patients are subjected to anesthesia and surgery. Hypochloremic alkalosis due to vomiting or metabolic acidosis due to diarrhea should also be corrected. The initial nausea and vomiting that occur after a single dose of radiation or early in the course of radiotherapy usually subside in one to two days.

With whole body irradiation in the dose range from 400 to 1000 rads, nausea and vomiting may continue beyond the prodromal period (see Table 18-18, B). If nausea and vomiting persist and are accompanied by severe diarrhea, the physician should suspect a widespread necrosis of intestinal mucosa. Massive replacement of electrolyte solutions, plasma, and blood may prevent death from hypovolemia. The intestinal mucosa may regenerate over four to seven days if sufficient viable epithelial cells capable of mitosis remain in the crypts of Lieberkühn.[297]

After high doses of whole body irradiation (400 to 1000 rads), mild anemia develops by the second or third week. There is an increased rate of red cell destruction, both from thrombus formation in irradiated tissues and from petechial hemorrhages. Erythropoiesis virtually stops after whole body doses of from 400 to 1000 rads, and, in patients who recover, does not resume for about a month after exposure. The hemoglobin and hematocrit should be kept sufficiently high to assure adequate tissue oxygenation. The saturation of central venous blood samples may be helpful in determining the adequacy of tissue oxygenation. Eiseman notes that transfusions of whole blood or packed cells will not be necessary unless significant hemorrhage occurs, since erythropoiesis will resume within six to eight weeks after irradiation — an interval considerably less than the half-life of the erythrocyte.[293] The physician should also be aware of Allen's failure to improve survival in sublethally irradiated animals by vigorous transfusion therapy.[298, 299]

Patients who have recieved 400 to 1000

rads of whole body irradiation and who develop radiation enteritis are poor surgical risks — as Eiseman points out — not only because of problems with fluid and electrolyte replacement but also because lethal bone marrow depression usually accompanies radiation doses sufficient to cause necrosis of the intestinal epithelium. Eiseman suggests that if these patients require surgery, they should be operated as soon after irradiation as possible, before depression of the immune system occurs.[293]

At lower whole body doses of irradiation — 200 to 400 rads — survival depends on the degree of bone marrow depression (see Table 18–18, A). As is the case with higher doses of irradiation, a prodrome of lethargy, anorexia, nausea, and vomiting appears, but it subsides within 36 hours. The patient may feel well for three to six weeks. Lymphocytopenia occurs immediately and may persist for months. An initial granulocytosis is followed by granulocytopenia. The rate of decline in the neutrophil count is dose dependent; minimal levels occur in four to six weeks after whole body doses of 200 to 300 rads. The platelet count initially increases and then declines as a function of irradiation dose. After 200 rads, the platelet count declines to minimal levels about 30 days after exposure. A hemorrhagic diathesis does occur at platelet counts below 20,000 per cubic millimeter[297] but may disappear before the platelet count actually rises.[298] Platelet transfusions or fresh whole blood may be necessary. Plasma fibrinogen is adequate or increased after sublethal irradiation. There can be an increased prothrombin time in vitro, but this increase seems related to a lack of platelets rather than to decreased enzyme synthesis or enzyme inactivation.[298]

After whole body exposure of from 200 to 800 rads, human beings have an increased susceptibility to infection. The reasons for this include 1) leukopenia; 2) decreased phagocytosis, both in leukocytes and in reticuloendothelial cells; 3) decreased production of circulating antibody; and 4) increased permeability of irradiated tissues. B- and T-cell populations are decreased and IgG and IgM production is reduced.[293] There is now considerable evidence that a decrease occurs in the numbers of alveolar macrophages in the lungs of irradiated dogs;[300, 301] one might suspect a relationship between this decrease and the high mortality from bronchopneumonia in irradiated animals[302] and in irradiated man. There are also adverse changes in the microcirculation after irradiation, as shown by Kivy-Rosenberg and Zweifach.[303] Changes in the microcirculation may play a role both in diminished resistance to infection and in altered responses to drugs.

Patients who have received over 200 rads of whole body irradiation should be managed as if they were immunologically suppressed. Prophylactic broad spectrum antibiotics should be utilized until the patient's granulocyte count is over 1500 per mm[3].[293] Careful attention to sterile technique and the use of reverse isolation may be advisable.

EFFECTS OF IRRADIATION ON SPECIFIC ORGANS OF IMPORTANCE IN ANESTHESIA

High doses of x-irradiation delivered to small volumes of tissue may cause pathological changes in specific organs that are important in anesthesia. Radiation damage in the larynx, lung, heart, adrenal glands, kidney, liver, thyroid gland, major systemic arteries, or central nervous system can cause difficulties during anesthesia. Complications of radiation enteritis may necessitate laparotomy in patients with poor wound healing and poor nutritional status.

Larynx. Irradiation of laryngeal tumors, of cervical or paratracheal nodes, or of carcinomas involving the pharynx or other tissues of the neck often leads to edema and congestion of the mucosa of the epiglottis, glottis, or cricoid cartilage, rendering the mucosa vulnerable to minor trauma such as intubation. After high voltage radiotherapy, the laryngeal mucosa becomes erythematous and edematous, and a fibrinous exudate is present over the hypopharynx and endolarynx. By two to six weeks after radiotherapy, the edema and exudates disappear, leaving only hyperemia of the laryngeal mucosa.[304] Glottic edema may persist for several months after radiotherapy.[296] The author has seen two cases of glottic edema, including massive edema of the false cords, necessitating tracheostomy after apparently atraumatic intubations. One case occurred in a patient who had received radiation for a carcinoma of the vocal cords six weeks prior to intubation. The other case occurred in a patient who had received mantle radiation to substernal and cervical nodes for Hodgkin's disease eight weeks prior to intubation. Therapy with steroids and endotracheal intubation for several days did not eliminate the need for a temporary tracheostomy. After heavy doses of irradiation (3000–6000 rads), webs of scar tissue may form in the anterior commissure, the vocal cords may not move well, and endarteritis of small arteries may lead to atrophy of one or both vocal cords.[304] Chandler noted a 12 per cent incidence of significant complications in 122 patients who had received irradiation to the larynx or neck, including 12 cases of cord paralysis or marked laryngeal edema and two cases of laryngeal necrosis necessitating permanent tracheostomy.[304] Vocal cord paralysis has also been reported after therapy of hyperthyroidism with as little as 7.3 mCi of [131]iodine.[305] Therapy with steroids prior to intubation may be helpful in patients who have had radiation to the larynx. The author has had no problems with laryngeal edema following intubation in several patients who had paralysis of one vocal cord resulting from radiation therapy for vocal cord tumors. Dexamethasone, 10 mg, several hours prior to intubation should suffice. On rare occasions, x-irradiation of laryngeal tumors can result in the later development of a fibrosarcoma of the larynx. At least 33 such cases have been reported to date.[306]

Lung. A significant number of patients irradiated for mammary carcinoma, pulmonary carcinoma, or Hodgkin's disease will develop radiation pneumonitis and subsequent pulmonary fibrosis. Seydel et al. reported a 92 per cent incidence of pulmonary fibrosis in 41 patients who received 3500 to 4500 rads (r) as treatment for Hodgkin's disease or bronchogenic carcinoma.[307] Bennett et al. reported seven deaths from radiation pneumonitis in 915 patients with bronchogenic carcinoma treated with 4000 roentgens (R) of x-irradiation. One of these deaths was from pulmonary failure shortly after surgery.[308] Collins and coworkers were consistently able to induce radiation pneumonitis and pulmonary fibrosis in animals with radiation doses between 3000 and 4000 rads.[309] Gimes reported a 13 per cent incidence of radiation pneumonitis after 2000 R of x-ray therapy for mammary carcinoma.[310] Roswit and White indicate that total doses up to 2000 r may be delivered to both lung fields without significant risk of radiation pneumonitis, provided that the radiation is delivered over a period of 12 or more days.[311] However, they do note that doses of 4000 r for Hodgkin's disease and doses of 5500 to 6000 r for carcinoma of the lung may be necessary to achieve any improvement in survival rates. With these heavy doses some radiation pneumonitis is inevitable. They have also observed that radiation pneumonitis and fibrosis in the apex of the lung is well tolerated and rarely causes symptoms, but that irradiation of the bases often results in clinical illness. Moreover, inclusion of the mediastinum or the hilum of the lung in the treatment field is most likely to cause symptomatic radiation pneumonitis, probably by interfering with the pulmonary lymphatics.[311] Radiation pneumonitis can also occur after irradiation of esophageal tumors, and has been reported in ^{131}I therapy of pulmonary metastases from thyroid carcinoma.[312]

The acute phase of radiation pneumonitis appears within a month after irradiation, whereas the later phase of chronic radiation fibrosis may not develop until 18 months following exposure. The clinical picture is variable. Although patients with acute radiation pneumonitis may be nearly asymptomatic, they usually develop cough, dyspnea, and chest pain. The cough may be dry or it may become productive of blood-tinged sputum. In severe cases, marked dyspnea and fever develop, and death may result from pulmonary insufficiency. Leukocytosis and an increased erythrocyte sedimentation rate are present. The chest x-rays show fluffy opacities that coalesce and then clear. The chest x-rays may also show a diffuse haziness with air bronchograms, or may develop a ground-glass appearance. Pleural effusions may be present.[313, 314, 315] As chronic radiation fibrosis develops, the initial opacities are replaced by fibrotic streaking and atelectasis. Approximately 70 per cent of one series of patients showed regions of moderate to severe fibrosis a year after irradiation.[307] Mediastinal shift and pleural thickening may develop; and over 5 per cent of patients who received radiation doses of 5000 rads or more will develop pleural effusions.[313]

Histologically in acute radiation pneumonitis there is pulmonary capillary congestion with necrosis of capillary endothelial cells, which may slough off the capillary basement membranes. Plasma leaks into the interstitium of the lung, and the alveoli fill with edema fluid. Alveolar lining cells become multinucleated and necrotic. An inflammatory exudate develops, and necrotic cells together with plasma proteins form hyaline membranes in the alveoli. Pulmonary lymphatics may appear dilated, and damage to pulmonary lymphatics reduces the rate at which fluid is removed from the alveoli. Gas exchange is diminished. Type II alveolar cells may proliferate, nearly filling the alveoli.[311, 314, 315] These cells may serve as scavengers, clearing the alveoli of necrotic hyalinized debris; the scavenging macrophages themselves are eliminated in the sputum. Bronchial epithelial cells also may become necrotic. The inflammatory changes of acute radiation pneumonitis may be completely reversible.[311] However, the alveolar septa may remain somewhat thickened.[314, 315] Proliferation of fibroblasts may occur rather early in radiation pneumonitis, as does proliferation of collagen in the septa.

Later, as the phase of chronic radiation fibrosis develops, collagen may proliferate within pulmonary vessels, subendothelial and perivascular fibrosis occurs, while the media becomes thickened, hyalinized, and less cellular. Peribronchial and generalized pulmonary fibrosis, partly secondary to the vascular sclerosis, occurs late in the healing process. According to Roswit and White, the longer the acute changes of radiation pneumonitis persist, the more likely it is that radiation fibrosis will develop.*

Radiation pneumonitis causes clinically significant changes in pulmonary physiology. Naimark and coworkers have shown decreases in phosphatidyl choline content and in ^{14}C palmitate incorporation, resulting in reductions in the stability of bubbles of material obtained by lung lavage in animals after irradiation of one hemithorax with 3000 r. Naimark's group found that a decrease in static compliance of the lung resulted from the alteration in pulmonary surfactant.[316] Gross was unable to duplicate these findings using radiation doses of only 1200 r, but did demonstrate that decreased compliance several months after irradiation was due to an altered alveolar surface.[301, 317]

He also found that after 3000 r, a fourfold increase in both albumin and globulin content was present in fluid lavaged from the lungs of animals irradiated four months previously (Fig. 18–31).[317] He demonstrated an increase in wet lung weight, suggesting that chronic pulmonary edema may be present four months after irradiation.[317] A trend toward increased permeability of pulmonary capillaries was detected by two months following irradiation; but by four months a significant increase ($p<0.01$) in capillary permeability to labeled albumin had appeared.[317] This increase in capillary permeability which Gross observed four months after irradiation may in part explain why patients who have survived the acute phase of radiation pneumonitis and appear to be improving may again become ill. It may even account for some of the late mortality in radiation pneumonitis. Gross speculates that by four months after exposure to ionizing radiation the capillary endothelial cells have divided to produce endothelial cells that can no longer function to prevent leakage of protein through the capillaries.[317]

Radiation pneumonitis and fibrosis also cause clinically significant changes in pulmonary function. Femirgil and Heinemann studied 15 patients who had received 4100 to 5000 R unilaterally or 2900 to 3900 R bilaterally to the thorax. The first measurable change was a diminution in lung volume, with decreases in inspiration capacity and residual volume. This was followed by hypoxemia with a median Po_2 of 78 mm Hg on room air (range, 65 to 91 mm Hg). The hypoxemia improved somewhat over the next eight months. From 60 to 120 days after irradiation the carbon monoxide diffusing capacity diminished — in two cases to as low as 4.5 and 6.5 cc per minute per mm Hg — but then returned toward normal. Lung compliance was reduced from about 1.5 L per cm H_2O to about 0.8 L per cm H_2O. The work of breathing was increased, and the maximal breathing capacity was reduced. No patient had CO_2 retention; increased respiratory rates compensated for diminished tidal volumes in this series.[318]

Bake et al. studied nine patients treated with 3000 R to supraclavicular and mammary nodes and to the chest wall after radical mastectomy. During the first series of tests, performed while chest x-rays showed opacities in the irradiated lung, there was evidence of diminished ventila-

---

*For more histologic detail, see References 309, 310, 311, and 315. For histology of experimental radiation fibrosis, see Reference 314.

Figure 18–31. Appearance of radioactivity in the lung and alveolar fluid following tail vein injection of RISA. The activity was calculated for the whole of the lavaged right lung (open circles, mean ±1 S.D.) or alveolar lavage fluid from the right lung (closed circles) and made proportional to the activity in 10 μl of blood obtained simultaneously. Significance of the difference between values in irradiated mice and corresponding control values: $+p < 0.05$; $*p < 0.01$. (From Gross, N. J.: J. Lab. Clin. Med. 95:19, 1980.)

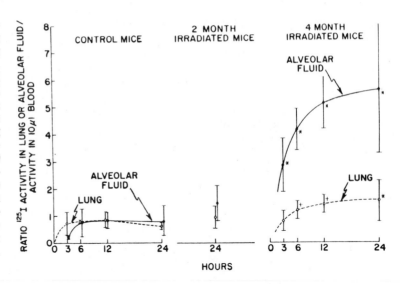

tion and perfusion on the affected side. A second study two months later, when the opacities had diminished, showed reductions in lung volume, ventilation, and perfusion on the affected side. These workers also found reductions in dynamic compliance and in diffusing capacity. They concluded that restrictive ventilatory impairment is the most common consequence of radiation pneumonitis.[319] More recent experimental work in subhuman primates confirms that restrictive impairment or loss of lung volume is the most fundamental change resulting from radiation pneumonitis. Collins and coworkers found decreases in lung compliance and diffusing capacity in baboons where upper lung zones had been treated with 3000 to 4000 r. However, these changes in function were secondary to the decrease in lung volume; the ratio D_{Lco}/V_A was normal, and the alteration in pressure/volume curves disappeared when observed lung volume rather than a predicted ideal lung volume was used. They found that radiation fibrosis essentially resulted in a "normally functioning but smaller lung." The fibrotic regions contributed little to ventilation or to gas exchange.[309] Roswit and White note that fibrosis of less than half a lung is tolerated quite well, although a fibrotic region may develop bronchiectasis, abscess, or a chronic pneumonitis.[311] If sufficient lung is involved, pulmonary hypertension and cor pulmonale may develop.

Cameron et al. studied 14 patients with bronchial compression from tumor during radiation therapy. They found initial decreases of 100 to 300 cc. in the one-second

forced expiratory volume (FEV_1), and attributed these decreases to edema in the tumors. The FEV_1 values returned to preirradiation levels after seven days — an improvement they attributed to tumor shrinkage.[320] Tewfik and coworkers studied pulmonary perfusion and ventilation scans in 14 patients with peripheral bronchogenic carcinoma and in nine patients with hilar or mediastinal lesions (six with squamous carcinomas and three with lymphoma or seminoma). The patients received 3000 to 6000 r over four to six weeks. Only five of the 14 patients with peripheral lesions showed a transient improvement in perfusion of the affected lobe four to eight weeks after treatment; decreased perfusion and ventilation eventually occurred in these patients and in the others with peripheral lesions. Patients with hilar or mediastinal lymphomas or seminomas improved both in ventilation and perfusion, while those with squamous (bronchogenic) carcinomas did not.[321] Radiation therapy occasionally results in dramatic improvement of airways obstructed by hemangioma, lymphoma, or cylindroma. Neonates with partial airway obstruction from hemangioma involving the larynx or trachea may be treated successfully with irradiation.[322] In adults with adenoid cystic carcinomas (cylindromas) inside the trachea or major bronchi, external irradiation with 6000 r doses has relieved airway obstruction in patients whose FEV_1 was as low as 28 per cent of normal. Intraluminal radiation with iridium attached to a stent made from an endotracheal tube and inserted through a tracheostomy has also relieved airway obstruction in patients with cylindroma of the trachea.[323]

Some improvement in radiation pneumonitis may occur with steroid therapy. Gimes recommends prednisolone, 50 to 100 mg daily, for six to 10 weeks.[310] Roswit and White claim that high doses of steroids can suppress the acute phase of radiation pneumonitis in about half the patients treated with them. Such therapy causes the infiltrates to clear and improves exercise tolerance. The steroids should be weaned slowly.[311] Demeter and coworkers note that the sudden withdrawal of steroids from an irradiated patient may lead to an acute radiation pneumonitis.[313] If steroids are to be used, they should be started soon after irradiation; Roswit and White claim that by the time the edges of the radiation port are visible on the chest x-ray, it is nearly too late to try to reverse radiation pneumonitis with steroids.[311] They also note that bedrest seems helpful in minimizing lung damage during acute radiation pneumonitis, while exertion or exposure to cold may cause an increase in the symptoms of acute radiation pneumonitis.[311] The treatment of radiation pneumonitis with steroids or bedrest has not yet been studied in any rigorous, double blind manner.

Heart and Pericardium. Irradiation of the thorax can cause cardiac arrhythmias, ST-T changes on the electrocardiograph, coronary artery sclerosis leading to myocardial infarction, decreased ventricular function, and pericarditis.

Preoperative irradiation for carcinoma of the lung can be associated with an increased incidence of cardiac arrhythmia. Mark et al. reported an increased incidence of tachycardia (P>110 per minute) and of atrial arrhythmias, including atrial flutter and atrial fibrillation, in 20 pneumonectomy patients treated with 6000 R over a six-week period preoperatively. In most patients the

arrhythmia or tachycardia appeared during the recovery or postoperative period. In some patients the tachycardia appeared after the irradiation but prior to surgery. The data of Mark et al. are shown in Table 18–19. The arrhythmias were treated with digitalis or quinidine. All patients responded with a slower rate or conversion to sinus rhythm.

Dick and coworkers studied the effect of gamma irradiation from ^{60}Co on the atrial septum in dogs. With doses of 4300 to 5600 R, 10 of 12 dogs developed arrhythmias from 48 to 150 days after irradiation. The arrhythmias included atrial fibrillation, atrial or junctional tachycardia, and second degree atrioventricular block. The anterior, median, and posterior internodal tracts and the SA and AV nodes showed varying degrees of damage.[325] Vaeth et al. reported on 20 patients receiving 3000 to 5000 R, which included at least 35 per cent of the myocardium in the irradiated field. Two patients showed electrocardiographic changes of pericarditis, and four patients had nonspecific ST-T changes. All patients with abnormal electrocardiograms had SGOT elevations. The clinical course of these patients was unaffected by the cardiac irradiation.[326] Approximately 15 per cent of patients irradiated for carcinoma of the breast develop transient ST-T changes on electrocardiogram.[327]

Very high doses of irradiation have caused complete heart block in man. Tzivoni and coworkers recently reported the occurrence of third degree heart block in two women who had received 10,000 to 12,000 rads to the left chest 18 and 22 years previously. Both patients had cutaneous ulcerations, edema of the left arm, fibrosis of the left lung, and rib fractures secondary to the radiation. Both patients were treated with pacemaker implants and did well.[327]

Over 15 cases of arteriosclerosis of the

Table 18–19*

	Postoperative Cardiac Complications (Number of Patients)		
	Atrial Arrhythmias	Tachycardia over 110/min.	Total
Nonirradiated	5/40 (12.5%)	11/35 (31%)	16/40
Radiated	6/20 (30%)	11/14 (79%)	17/20

*From Mark, J., et al.: J. Thorac. Cardiovasc. Surg. 51:30, 1966.

coronary arteries secondary to radiation therapy have been reported in the recent medical literature. Angina or myocardial infarction, often with a fatal outcome, has resulted from radiation-induced coronary artery disease. Most of these cases have occurred in young adults receiving 2900 to 5000 rads of mantle radiation as a treatment for Hodgkin's disease. Symptoms of coronary insufficiency may appear as early as two months following radiotherapy, but the average interval between irradiation and clinically apparent heart disease has been 47 months.[328] The anterior descending coronary artery is most frequently diseased, but lesions in the right coronary artery have also been reported.[328, 329, 330] Anterior myocardial infarction may occur; at least eight deaths from radiation-induced myocardial infarction have been reported to date.[328, 330] The coronary lesions, which are usually located proximally in the arteries, demonstrate proliferation of the intima, fragmentation of the internal elastic membrane, and irregular atrophy of the media. Fibrosis is present in both the coronary artery and the myocardium.[328, 329] A few patients have been treated successfully with coronary bypass grafts.[329, 331] The complaint of chest pain resembling angina should be taken seriously in patients who have had thoracic irradiation, even if the patient is below the usual age range for coronary artery disease.

High dose irradiation of the myocardium can cause decreased left ventricular function and congestive heart failure. Arom and coworkers measured cardiac output and left atrial and left ventricular pressures weekly in dogs whose hearts had been treated with a total of 500 rads.[332] Two weeks after irradiation the left atrial and left ventricular diastolic pressures became elevated (Fig. 18–32). Between the eighth and twelfth weeks, left ventricular dp/dt had dropped from a control mean of 2740 mm Hg/sec to a mean of only 1025 mm Hg/sec (Fig. 18–33). Resting cardiac output decreased from an initial mean of 3.9 ± 0.8 L/min to 2.1 ± 0.5 L/min by the eighth week after irradiation. Significant decreases in mean left ventricular pressure and in mean aortic blood pressure occurred after the eighth week. The animals became lethargic and tachypneic by the eleventh week, and audible rales were present. Several animals died with congestive heart failure. In surviving animals, most parameters of cardiac function returned to normal by 23 weeks after irradiation. Histologically, endothelial damage was present in myocardial capillaries. Many capillaries were occluded and some ischemic fibrosis of the myocardium was present.[332] Congestive failure as a direct result of high doses of radiation to the mediastinum has not yet been reported in man. Mild hypotension has been documented in outpatients during radiation therapy to the thorax or abdomen, but it is unlikely that irradiation of the myocardium can account for the hypotension observed.[333]

There are occasional reports of fibrinous pericarditis with tamponade and of myocardial fibrosis secondary to irradiation.[334, 335] Acute pericarditis with effusion may re-

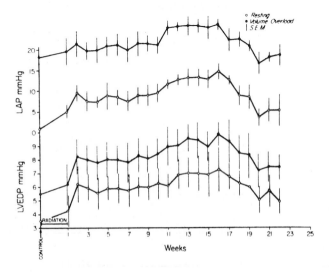

Figure 18–32. Effect of cardiac irradiation with 5000 rads on myocardial function in dogs, showing the progressive change in left atrial pressure (LAP) and left ventricular end-diastolic pressure (LVEDP). Note that the pressures had already increased during the first week after irradiation. Both LAP and LVEDP were highest, at rest and with volume overload, during the eleventh and seventeenth weeks. (SEM = standard error of the mean.) (From Arom, K. V., et al.: Ann. Thorac. Surg. 28:166, 1979.)

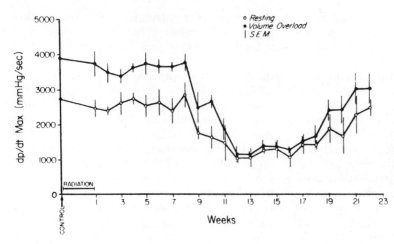

Figure 18–33. Changes in maximum rate of rise of left ventricular pressure (dp/dt Max) during the 24 weeks after cardiac irradiation. It dropped significantly after eight weeks and did not respond well to volume overload during congestive heart failure. (SEM = standard error of the mean.) (From Arom, K. V., et al.: Ann. Thorac. Surg. *28*:166, 1979.)

spond to therapy with prednisolone, 30 mg daily.[336] Large effusions may need to be tapped. Radiation may cause constrictive pericarditis; several such cases have been managed successfully by pericardectomy.[337] The presence of considerable myocardial fibrosis may indicate a poor prognosis.[338]

Adrenal. Most of our current knowledge of the effects of irradiation on adrenal function is derived from animal studies. Early work indicated a transient elevation in plasma corticosteroids after irradiation, followed by a decline in those levels. Flemming found that plasma steroids in rats rose to about 55 gamma per cent immediately after whole body irradiation and then decreased to less than normal values.[339] Some years previously, Goodall and Long had reported a large, dose-dependent reduction in the epinephrine content of the rat adrenal medulla after irradiation. After 800 R, they found that the epinephrine content de-

creased from 1300 to 300 µg per gram of tissue; after 1300 R, it declined from 1300 µg to close to zero. They suggested that some of the radioprotective effect of epinephrine may involve nothing more than the replacement of a depleted hormone.[340] More recent work does not indicate a decline in corticosteroid levels after whole body irradiation. Flemming and Hellwig did a second, well controlled study of the problem and found increases in corticosteroid levels in the adrenal glands and in the blood during the first four weeks after whole body irradiation in mice.[341] After lethal doses of irradiation (1500 R), there was an early peak in adrenal corticosteroid content that returned to normal by 90 minutes (Fig. 18–34). This peak was followed by progressive increases in adrenal and plasma corticosteroid levels during the next week, until all the animals died (Table 18–20). After sublethal doses of irradiation,

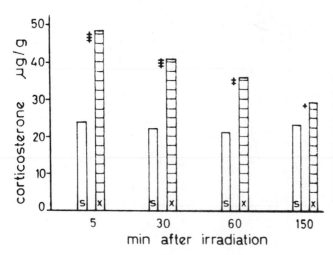

Figure 18–34. Corticosteriod increase immediately after irradiation in habituated female mice. Whole-body irradiation, with 1500 R. Corticosterone content of the adrenals. Eight animals per point. S = sham irradiation. X = irradiation. Analysis of variance: $\bar{x} \pm s\bar{x}$; $s\bar{x} \pm 2.9$. Significance: $+ = p < 0.05$; $\ddagger = p < 0.01$; $\ddagger\!\!\!= = p < 0.001$. (From Flemming, K., and Hellwig, J.: Acta Radiol. Scand. Suppl. *310*:124, 1971.)

Table 18-20 *Corticosteroid Changes Following Lethal Irradiation.*
Female Mice. Whole-Body Irradiation, 1500 R.

Day After Irradiation	No. of Mice	Corticosterone			Body Weight (g)	Adrenal Weight (mg)
		μg/g Adrenal	μg/2 Adrenals	μg/100 ml Plasma		
Unirradiated controls	8	34.4 ± 6.9	0.225 ± 0.056	22.8 ± 2.3	27.3 ± 2.5	6.5 ± 0.9
Irradiated mice						
1	8	41.9 ± 6.4	0.258 ± 0.049	27.1 ± 5.0	24.9 ± 1.6	6.0 ± 0.5
3	8	65.0 ± 3.6*	0.435 ± 0.059*	38.9 ± 7.9*	21.5 ± 1.6	6.6 ± 0.7
5	5	67.2 ± 7.8*	0.453 ± 0.081*	63.4 ± 14.3	18.9 ± 1.4*	6.7 ± 0.7
6	7	85.5 ± 5.1*	0.518 ± 0.081*	75.4 ± 6.4*	18.2 ± 0.8*	6.7 ± 0.9
7	2	99.6 ± 8.5*	0.692 ± 0.099*	89.1 ± 4.0*	18.1 ± 0.4*	7.0 ± 0.2
6 + 7**	9	101.0 ± 15.6*	0.749 ± 0.105*	—	18.3 ± 1.5*	7.6 ± 0.7

*p < 0.001.
**Animals died spontaneously; the adrenals were obtained within 30 min after death.
(From Flemming, K., and Hellwig, J.: Acta Radiol. Scand. Suppl. *310*:124, 1971.)

the early peaks in adrenal and plasma corticosteroid levels were again observed, and increases in these levels occurred on the second day and between the fifth and seventh days after irradiation. Flemming and Hellwig consider the initial peak to be an acute reaction to injury mediated via the pituitary, while they attribute the increases on the second day after exposure to radiation injury of the intestine. They suggest that the increase in plasma steroid levels may play a part in decreasing the blood lymphocyte count after irradiation. They also note that after irradiation, glucocorticoids increase more than mineralocorticoids.[341] One recent study in man has appeared concerning the late effects of irradiation on the adrenals. Sommers and Carter found fibrosis of the inner zone of the adrenal cortex in 17 patients who had had radiation to the abdomen, pelvis, or lumbar region averaging 5000 r up to 21 months before autopsy.[342] Hyaline fibrosis was present in the zona reticularis of the cortex. The vascular plexus of the region had been damaged by irradiation and the cells had apparently atrophied because of ischemia. Sommers and Carter point out that the cells of the region secrete mainly androgens, estrogens, and progesterone. Regions of the cortex that produce aldosterone or glucocorticoids appeared normal. Nor was there evidence of any damage to the adrenal medulla.[342] While Sommers and Carter suggest that no abnormalities in the production of catechols would be expected, more data are needed concerning the response of the adrenal medulla to irradiation.

Kidney. Radiation nephritis may occur when doses exceeding 2000 r are delivered to retroperitoneal nodes. In patients treated with actinomycin D, radiation nephritis has developed after irradiation with doses of only 1500 r. Hypertension related to elevated plasma renin levels may develop, and nephrectomy may be necessary.[343] Sclerosis of interlobular and arcuate arteries occurs, and glomeruli may necrose. The BUN and creatinine may become elevated, but oliguria or anuria does not usually occur unless congestive failure develops.[343, 344, 345] In rare instances disseminated intravascular coagulation may appear.[344] There is some evidence in animals that whole body irradiation with the kidneys shielded can cause nephrosclerosis, elevated renin levels, and hypertension.[346] Extrarenal factors may contribute to radiation nephritis. The anesthetic management of radiation nephritis is the same as that for any patient with hypertension and renal failure.

Liver. Radiation hepatitis may appear if the liver is subjected to over 3000 rads of ionizing radiation. Two of 117 patients reported by Kim and coworkers developed radiation hepatitis after 3000 r of abdominal irradiation for lymphoma. The patients developed abdominal distention, hepatomegaly, and tenderness to palpation over the liver. Their serum alkaline phosphatase became elevated, and liver biopsy showed marked passive congestion.[347] Mild bilirubin elevations (2.2 mg/100 ml) have been reported in radiation hepatitis from doses of 4500 r.[348] Elevations of the serum LDH and SGOT values have also been described in acute radiation hepatitis.[349] In the acute phase, angiography shows stretching of the hepatic arteries and retrograde flow in intrahepatic branches of the portal vein. As the hepatitis resolves over four to six months, there is atrophy and fibrosis of irradiated regions and compensatory hypertrophy of non-irradiated regions.[349] The cases of radiation hepatitis reported to date have resolved without treatment.

During the acute phase of radiation hepatitis, decreases occur in the activity of at least one hepatic enzyme that metabolizes drugs. In mice given 1000 rad doses of hepatic irradiation, the rate of N-demethylation of chlordiazepoxide is reduced, from three days to three weeks after irradiation.[350] In male rats given 850 to 1500 rads to the head, the lower trunk, or the whole body, the rate of oxidative demethylation of aminopyrine is also reduced. If the animals are anesthetized with sodium pentobarbital just prior to irradiation, the activity of the enzyme system is unaffected by the radiation. If the animals receive irradiation to the pituitary gland, the activity of the hepatic oxidative demethylating enzyme also decreases. Pituitary irradiation decreases the production of luteinizing hormone, which decreases the production of testosterone. The hepatic enzyme system for oxidative demethylation apparently requires the presence of testosterone for normal activity.[351] The effects of irradiation on the function of hepatic enzymes merit further study, both in experimental animals and in man. Reduced doses of diazepines, and possibly of other drugs, may be advisable during anesthesia in patients with acute radiation hepatitis.

It seems unwise to use halothane in patients during the acute phase of irradiation hepatitis. Brase and coworkers studied the morphological effects of irradiation and halothane anesthesia separately and in combination in dogs.[352] They found that by three months after irradiation with 1000 r, hepatic cells exhibited small to moderate fatty change and periportal acidophilia. There was an increase in the Kupffer cells, and some inflammatory infiltrate was present in the interlobular septa. There was some proliferation of bile ducts, but little or no hepatocellular necrosis was evident. The morphology was that of a mild toxic hepatitis. However, in dogs given only 500 rads of hepatic irradiation, and anesthetized with halothane for one hour each week during the next three months, the livers showed considerable damage. The livers appeared grossly flecked or spotted. There was widespread hepatocellular necrosis in the central and intermediate zones. Many hepatocytes had vacuolated cytoplasm, and the sinusoids were filled with a polymorphonuclear infiltrate. The morphology suggested a chronic hepatitis following a severe toxic hepatitis.[352] Although the interaction between irradiation and halothane has not been studied in man, the use of halothane up to six months after hepatic or abdominal irradiation in patients should probably be avoided.

Thyroid. Hypothyroidism frequently results from radiation therapy of head and neck cancers, from mantle radiation for Hodgkin's disease, or from the treatment of hyperthyroidism with radioactive iodine. As early as 1964 Koulumines and coworkers noted low protein bound iodine values in half of 118 patients treated with 5000 r for carcinoma of the larynx. None of the patients in their series appeared clinically hypothyroid.[353] Einhorn and Wikholm reported that three of 41 patients irradiated for carcinoma of the larynx or hypopharynx became clinically hypothyroid.[354] Schimpff and coworkers recently reported thyroid dysfunction in 112 of 169 patients who had received 4000 rads of mantle irradiation for Hodgkin's disease. Sixty-nine patients (41%) had elevated TSH levels but normal T_4 values, while 43 patients (24%) had T_4 levels below normal. Schimpff emphasizes that hypothyroidism develops gradually between one and six years after radiation therapy and recommends TSH measurements every six months for diagnosis.[355] Many patients who have had radioactive iodine (^{131}I) treatment for hyperthyroidism will become hypothyroid several years later. Hormone replacement with 1 to 3 grains of desiccated thyroid or 150 to 200 micrograms of levothyroxine daily will prevent problems during anesthesia in hypothyroid patients.

An occasional patient may become hyperthyroid after radiation therapy for lymphoma. Both Schimpff and Mahnke have reported a case of hyperthyroidism after cervical irradiation.[355, 356] Suppression with propylthiouracil, 300 mg daily, followed by total thyroidectomy may be necessary for cure.[356]

Radiation of the head, neck, or mediastinum in children for acne, tinea capitis, or hypertrophy of the adenoids, tonsils, or thymus has caused many cases of thyroid carcinoma after a latent period of over 25 years. The treatment is thyroidectomy. For more detail on this problem the reader should consult the references by Cerletty, Sener, or Wagner.[357, 358, 359]

Major Systemic Arteries. Heavy doses of irradiation occasionally cause arteriosclerosis in major systemic arteries. Ormerod reported a case of acquired coarctation of the aorta that developed 20 years after 3000 rads of mantle irradiation for Hodgkin's disease. A systemic murmur was audible over the back, and a 20 mm Hg gradient was demonstrated during aortography.[360] Dossing and coworkers reported a thickened, fibrotic aortic arch in a 21-year-old male who died from myocardial infarction 16 months after receiving 4000 rads of mantle irradiation for Hodgkin's disease. The elastic lamellae were disorganized, but no adventitial fibrosis or inflammatory exudates were present.[361] Silverberg and coworkers at Stanford reported on nine patients who had received 4400 to 12,000 rad doses of irradiation for Hodgkin's disease, carcinoma of the breast, thyroid carcinoma, or supraglottic carcinoma. These patients developed carotid artery disease 10 years earlier than a control group of patients with carotid occlusive disease due to hypertension or atherosclerosis. Eight of the nine patients developed carotid occlusions within the irradiated region, and many of their lesions were not located at the carotid bifurcation — the most common site for carotid lesions due to atherosclerotic disease. The lesions were treated surgically, and an increase in periarterial fibrous tissue was noted at operation. Silverberg and coworkers claim that radiation induced carotid artery disease is a discrete clinical entity. They also note that stenosis of the subclavian, iliac, and femoral vessels due to irradiation has been reported.[362]

Central Nervous System. Irradiation of the brain with doses of up to 2400 rads in children with leukemia or lymphoma may cause a syndrome of anorexia, irritability, lethargy, and somnolence. Parker and coworkers reported that 60 per cent of children who received cranial irradiation developed the "somnolence syndrome." Electroencephalography showed symmetrical slowing of the dominant rhythm or an increase in theta rhythm. The syndrome resolved spontaneously, and there was no difference in survival between children who became somnolent and those who did not.[363] In another series no neurological or psychological differences were found between 34 children who had craniospinal irradiation for leukemia and 27 control children who received irradiation to other parts of the body; however, four children dying with leukemia who were dropped from the series did have leukoencephalopathy at autopsy.[364]

Irradiation of the brain with doses in the range of 5000 to 7000 rads may cause cerebral vasculopathy and infarction or radiation necrosis. Brant-Zawadski and coworkers reported six cases of occlusions of the middle or posterior cerebral arteries or of the internal carotid artery within the calvarium. These occlusions appeared about four months to two years after radiotherapy of brain tumors with radiation doses exceeding 5000 r. The clinical presentation included blindness or hemiparesis, depending on the location of the infarct. Autopsy disclosed foam cells within the intima of the occluded arteries, disruption of the internal elastic membrane, hyaline changes in the subintimal region, and myointimal proliferation. There was no evidence of an inflammatory vasculitis.[365] Martins and coworkers recently described six cases of radionecrosis of the brain appearing nine months to a year after radiation therapy for intracranial tumors, particularly for pituitary tumors. Symptoms included amnesia, headache, and seizures; hemiparesis appeared in some patients, and severe dementia developed by two years after radiotherapy in most of these patients. Increases in spinal fluid protein were present, and an avascular mass was present on angiogram. To differentiate cerebral radionecrosis from tumor, brain biopsy was necessary. The gyri had a yellow appearance, and gliosis was present. Dexamethasone, 4 mg daily, caused transient improvement in brain function in most of these patients.[366]

A few cases of radiation myelopathy have been reported after large doses of radiation to the cervical or thoracic spine.[367] The onset of radiation myelopathy varies from five weeks to several years. Early symptoms include paresthesias in the trunk or limbs produced by flexion of the neck. Paresis or paralysis may occur and usually appears after the sensory symptoms.[368] However, Kristenson and coworkers recently reported four cases of radiation myelopathy resulting in flaccid paralysis and atrophy of gluteal, perineal, and leg muscles but with no detectable sensory loss. The patients were unable to walk without crutches. Kristenson postulated that doses of 5300 rads damaged the blood supply of the cord, causing necrosis of the anterior horn cells.[369] Peripheral neuropathy has also been reported after radiotherapy for carcinoma of the breast. Demyelination and fibrosis involving the brachial plexus can occur.[370] Spinal anesthesia seems acceptable in irradiated patients who are free of neurological signs or symptoms. The anesthesiologist may wish to avoid subarachnoid or epidural block if he feels that the patient may develop neurological symptoms because of progression of the neoplastic disease.

Radiation Enteritis. Up to 5 per cent of patients receiving abdominal or pelvic irradiation for carcinoma of the cervix or uterus may develop injuries requiring surgical intervention. Such injuries include ureteral obstruction, radiation cystitis or proctitis, and strictures of the small or large bowel. Mucosal ulceration, fistulae, and perforation of the small or large intestine may also occur. Irradiation of the intestine results in an obliterative angiitis of small vessels with inflammation and lymphatic obstruction, leading to ischemic strictures or necrosis and perforation. Changes in the small bowel resemble regional enteritis; changes in the colon may resemble acute diverticulitis. Anastomotic leaks, fistulae, and failure of abdominal wounds to heal occur frequently in patients who have had abdominal or pelvic irradiation.[371] Anemia and malabsorp-

tion of glucose, fats, and electrolytes may develop. Protein loss and bloody diarrhea can also occur in radiation enteritis. The diarrhea from radiation enteritis may respond to mixtures of diphenexylate and atropine contained in Lomotil, while the vomiting may respond to phenothiazines.[372] Total parenteral alimentation and transfusions are often necessary in patients requiring surgery for the complications of abdominal or pelvic irradiation.[371, 372]

A summary of radiation tolerance doses for the gastrointestinal tract is outlined in Table 18–21.

EFFECT OF IRRADIATION ON ANESTHETIC MORTALITY IN EXPERIMENTAL ANIMALS

Most of our knowledge of the effect of irradiation on the mortality and morbidity of general inhalation anesthetics is derived from animal experiments. There has been nearly no interest in the interactions between irradiation and inhalation anesthesia in the West during the past decade. A few recent studies have appeared in the Soviet or Eastern European literature and either are not available in English translation or appear of doubtful validity.

As Zauder and Orkin pointed out some years ago, all the potent inhalational anesthetic agents are associated with increased anesthetic mortality in the irradiated experimental animal.[373] The magnitude of the increase in mortality varies greatly for the different agents and depends also on the time elapsed since the radiation exposure. Differences among the effects of anesthetic agents on mortality in irradiated animals can be accounted for by variation in the design of the experiments. Other differences in the data reported on survival rates may result from infections in some of the animal colonies, varying susceptibility of animals to irradiation and anesthesia, or other factors difficult to identify or control.

Certain agents such as divinyl ether and trifluoroethyl vinyl ether (fluroxene) have been associated with such high mortality rates in irradiated animals that their use in man after whole body irradiation is contraindicated. Chloroform may be considered relatively contraindicated because of the anesthetic morbidity observed in experiments on irradiated animals. Tri-

Table 18–21   *Radiation Tolerance Doses*

Organ	Injury at 5 years	TD 5/5*
Oral mucosa	Ulcer, severe fibrosis	6000
Salivary	Xerostomia	5000
Esophagus	Ulcer, stricture	6000
Stomach	Ulcer, perforation	4500
Intestine	Ulcer, stricture	4500
Colon	Ulcer, stricture	4500
Rectum	Ulcer, stricture	5500
Liver	Liver failure, ascites	3500

*Minimal tolerance dose—the dose that, when applied to a given population of patients under standard treatment conditions, results in no more than a 5% severe complication rate within 5 years after treatment. Standard conditions refer to supervoltage therapy (1–6 MeV), fractionation of 1000 rads per week, five daily fractions. (From Donaldson, S. S., and Lenon, R. A.: Cancer *43*:2036, 1979.)

chloroethylene has not been extensively studied but is associated with increased death rates in irradiated animals anesthetized one week to one month after exposure. Cyclopropane, diethyl ether, and halothane are associated with a slight tendency toward increased mortality several weeks after exposure, but may be acceptable agents for use in irradiated humans. Nitrous oxide and ethylene, although difficult to test in small animals, increase the 30-day mortality of irradiated animals to a very small extent. Enflurane has not yet been studied. Although one might safely consider agents such as divinyl ether and fluroxene to be contraindicated in irradiated humans, it is difficult if not impossible to decide which of the agents that seem acceptable on the basis of animal experiments is optimal for use in irradiated humans.

It is necessary to review the published evidence for the effects of each inhalational anesthetic agent in irradiated animals.

Divinyl ether (Vinethene) was studied by Zauder and Orkin in mice irradiated with 350, 450, and 750 roentgens and then anesthetized with 6 per cent divinyl ether at one-, two-, four-, seven-, 21-, or 28-day inter-

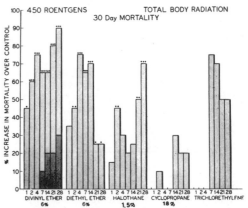

Figure 18–36. Effect of divinyl ether 6 per cent, diethyl ether 6 per cent, halothane 1.5 per cent, cyclopropane 18 per cent, and trichlorethylene 1.8 per cent on 30-day mortality in mice after 450 R of whole body irradiation. The ordinate shows percentage of increase in mortality over that of unanesthetized controls. Numbers along the abscissa indicate days between irradiation and anesthesia. (From Zauder, H. L., and Orkin, L. R.: New York State J. Med. 63:1943, 1963.)

vals after exposure.[373] After 350 roentgens, 30-day mortality in the anesthetized mice exceeded that of the unanesthetized irradiated controls by 25 to 65 per cent. The greatest increases in mortality occurred in mice anesthetized four and 28 days after exposure (p<0.001). These increases in mortality in the experimental group were significant from day two through day seven (p <0.01) (Fig. 18–35). At 450 roentgen doses, the increase in 30-day mortality in mice given Vinethene ranged from 45 to 90 per cent — obviously a statistically significant difference (Fig. 18–36). On the basis of this one study, divinyl ether would appear to be contraindicated in patients who have had large doses of whole body irradiation.

Trifluoroethyl vinyl ether (fluroxene) was tested by Young and coworkers in mice a few hours after 1100 and 800 rad doses of whole body x-irradiation.[374] All animals given fluroxene died by the fifth day after 800 rads, whereas some control animals survived until the tenth day after irradiation. The increased death rate with fluroxene was significant (p <0.05) (Fig. 18–37). At a dose of 650 rads, which resulted in a 50 per cent mortality in control mice, all animals given fluroxene died by the tenth day after irradiation and anesthesia. Young et al.

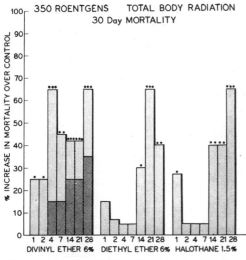

Figure 18–35. Effect of divinyl ether 6 per cent, diethyl ether 6 per cent, and halothane 1.5 per cent on 30-day mortality in mice following 350 R of external whole body irradiation. The ordinate shows percentage of increase in mortality over that of unanesthetized controls. The numbers along the abscissa indicate the number of days between irradiation and anesthesia. (From Zauder, H. L., and Orkin, L. R.: New York State J. Med. 63:1943, 1963.)

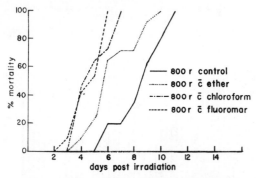

Figure 18–37. Effect of diethyl ether, chloroform, and fluroxene anesthesia on mortality rates of mice after 800 rads of whole body irradiation. (From Young, T. M., et al.: Anesthesiology 23:74, 1962.)

did not use fixed concentrations of inhalational agents in these experiments but attempted to achieve a light level of anesthesia in which the animals did not respond to tactile stimuli.[374] Pending further study, fluroxene would appear to be contraindicated in humans after large doses of ionizing radiation.

Chloroform has been tested by several authors in irradiated animals. In an early study, Burdick noted a trend toward higher 30-day mortality with this agent.[375] Young found that mice given chloroform a few hours after 650 rads all died within six days, whereas only half the unanesthetized controls were dead by the sixteenth day after exposure (Table 18–22). This result was statistically significant (p <0.05). Wilson found trends toward earlier death in rats

anesthetized after 800 rads, and noted that these animals recovered slowly from anesthesia and displayed muscle spasms.[376] Young et al. also noted this tendency for slow recovery, and stated that their rats appeared ill the day after anesthesia and showed obvious weight loss.[374] In view of these results in animals, chloroform would seem a poor choice in irradiated humans.

Trichloroethylene (Trilene) has been studied in irradiated animals only by Zauder and Orkin. In rats given 450 roentgens and anesthetized one to six days after exposure, there was no increased mortality, but when Trilene was given two to four weeks after exposure, the increase in 30-day mortality ranged from 55 to 75 per cent (Fig. 18–36). Further animal studies would appear necessary before this agent could be recommended for use in irradiated patients.[373]

Halothane has been studied extensively in irradiated rodents by Young et al. and by Zauder and Orkin. Young et al. studied it in mice at 200, 400, and 680 rad doses and at one-, three-, seven-, 14-, and 28-day intervals after exposure and found no statistically significant increase in 30-day mortality (Table 18–22). They also studied it in rats at 525 and 600 rad doses with the same results. When halothane was given a few hours after 800 rads, there was a trend toward earlier death (Fig. 18–38). Rats anesthetized with halothane after three weeks did not lose weight, whereas those anesthetized with chloroform, cyclopropane, and ether did. In these experiments, fixed concentrations of halothane were not used, but an attempt

Table 18–22 *Mortality in Mice Subjected to Anesthesia Several Hours After Irradiation**

Radiation Dose	Anesthetic Agent	Number of Days Before 100% Mortality
800 r	Chloroform	6
"	Trifluoroethyl vinyl ether	6
"	Diethyl ether	9
"	Controls (no anesthesia)	11
"	Halothane	13

Radiation Dose	Anesthetic Agent†	Mortality by 13th Postanesthetic Day
650 r	Chloroform	100%
"	Trifluoroethyl vinyl ether	100%
"	Diethyl ether	100%
"	Controls (no anesthesia)	50%

*From Young, T. M., et al.: Anesthesiology 23:74, 1962.
†Halothane was not tested after 650 r whole body radiation in mice.

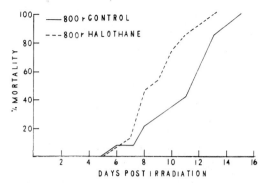

Figure 18–38. Effect of halothane anesthesia on the mortality rate of mice given 800 rads of external whole body irradiation. (From Young, T. M., et al.: Anesthesiology 23:74, 1962.)

was made to keep the animals lightly anesthetized. Young et al. concluded that halothane seems to be a satisfactory agent for use following whole body irradiation. They do suggest that anesthesia be delayed for 24 hours after exposure, if possible.[374]

Zauder and Orkin did find significant increases in 30-day mortality in mice given halothane three to four weeks after irradiation (Fig. 18–35).[373] They also found some increases in mortality when halothane was given in the first two weeks after exposure (Fig. 18–36). After 450 roentgens there was a 45 per cent increase in 30-day mortality when halothane was given two days after irradiation; when halothane was given on the twenty-first and twenty-eighth days after irradiation, the 30-day mortality was 50 to 70 per cent. Fixed concentrations of 1.5 per cent halothane for one hour were employed in this study.[373]

Bruce and Koepke also looked for an interaction between halothane and radiation in mice, using low doses per unit time.[377] They gave 881 roentgens (total dose) to mice over a 15-week period, and exposed them to 0.1 per cent halothane eight hours a day during this period. They found no synergistic effect between irradiation and halothane at these low doses.[377]

Halothane may be a safe agent to use in humans after whole body irradiation. Bruce, using subanesthetic doses, and Young et al., using light levels of halothane in irradiated animals, did not find increases in mortality with halothane anesthesia. Zauder and Orkin, employing higher doses of halothane, did find increases in mortality in ir-

radiated animals, especially three to four weeks after irradiation. The anesthesiologist must weight the advantages and disadvantages of halothane in the individual case. It would seem preferable to avoid general anesthesia in the first 24 hours after irradiation; if halothane is used in the irradiated patient, it would seem wise to keep the level of anesthesia as light as possible.

Cyclopropane has been studied in irradiated animals by at least four groups and appeared to be a fairly good agent in these animals. Burdick[375] and Young et al.[374] found no significant effect on 30-day mortality in rats anesthetized with cyclopropane after irradiation. Young et al. used doses of 525 to 600 rads and kept the levels of cyclopropane fairly light. They anesthetized the rats at three hour, three day, or three week intervals after exposure.[374] Wilson gave 615 and 730 rad doses to rats and anesthetized them with 30 per cent cyclopropane for 30 minutes. He found no significant difference in mortality by 30 days between control and anesthetized animals. In one group of rats exposed to 835 rads and a week later given 40 per cent cyclopropane for 30 minutes, there was a 100 per cent death rate during anesthesia, whereas only 65 per cent of the nonirradiated controls died. The result was significant at the 5 per cent level.[376] Yet, as Young et al. point out, the rather high mortality (25%) in a week between radiation and anesthesia raises the possibility that an uncontrolled factor such as unrecognized infection was present in this group of animals.[374] Wilson also noted some weight loss in rats given cyclopropane three weeks after 525 and 600 rads.[376] Zauder and Orkin studied cyclopropane, 18 per cent for 30 minutes, in mice after 450 roentgens of whole body irradiation. From one to seven days after exposure there was virtually no increase in 30-day mortality in anesthetized animals when compared with the controls (Fig. 18–36). At 14 days after exposure, there was a 20 per cent increase. They conclude that in the first two weeks after large doses of radiation, cyclopropane may be the safest potent agent. This conclusion has not yet been confirmed by studies in humans.[373]

Diethyl ether in irradiated animals has been studied by at least five authors. Young et al. gave light levels of ether to mice a few hours after exposure to 650 rads and found that 100 per cent of the controls died. This result was significant. However, they failed to find a significant effect of ether on 30-day mortality in rats anesthetized three hours, three days, or three weeks after 525 and 600 rads.[374] After 800 rads in mice anesthetized just after exposure, Young and coworkers found no difference in the death rate between controls and animals given light ether (Fig. 18–37). Moreover, at smaller radiation doses (525 and 600 rads) in rats given ether three hours to three weeks after exposure, they failed to observe an increase in 30-day mortality.[374]

Zauder and Orkin tested ether, 6 per cent for 30 minutes, in mice after radiation with 350 and 450 roentgens. At the lower radiation dose (350 R) there were only slight increases (5 to 15 per cent) in 30-day mortality when anesthesia was given within seven days of irradiation. Yet when ether was given 21 days after irradiation, there was a 65 per cent rise in 30-day mortality (Fig. 18–35). After 450 R in mice, when ether was given four through 14 days after irradiation, there was a 70 to 75 per cent rise in 30-day mortality — obviously an important result (Fig. 18–36). From days 21 to 28 there was only a 20 per cent increase in mortality.[373]

Zauder and Orkin demonstrated that mortality with ether in irradiated mice is dose related; a reduction in ether concentration from 7 to 6 per cent diminished the 30-day mortality ($p<0.05$), and a reduction from 7 to 5 per cent caused even less mortality ($p<0.001$).[373]

Restivo et al.[378] and Wilson[379] did not find a significant effect of ether on 30-day mortality of irradiated mice or rats. Wilson did find trends toward lower median survival times in rats given 810 to 820 rads followed by 4 to 11 per cent ether. Restivo et al. anesthetized their animals for only five minutes, a fact that may account for their failure to find increased mortality with ether.

Treatment of diethyl ether with acidified ferrous sulfate to remove peroxides resulted in a trend toward decreased mortality in mice anesthetized after 700 R. The 30-day mortality was 50 per cent in the controls, 56 per cent in mice given ferrous sulfate–treated ether, and 60 per cent in mice given untreated USP diethyl ether.[378]

There is little doubt that diethyl ether has an adverse effect on irradiated animals. Soviet authors consider ether contraindicated in patients after large doses of whole body irradiation.[380] Young et al. consider halothane preferable to diethyl ether after irradiation, whereas Zauder and Orkin consider diethyl ether to be somewhat less harmful than halothane in the second and third weeks after irradiation. If the anesthesiologist does elect to use diethyl ether in irradiated humans, he or she should try to achieve as light a level as possible. Diethyl ether should probably be avoided in the first or second weeks after exposure to radiation, the period when gastrointestinal symptoms may be present.

Nitrous oxide appears to be a good anesthetic for use in irradiated animals; a balanced technique, using nitrous oxide, narcotics, and relaxants, may well be the anesthetic of choice in irradiated humans.

Nitrous oxide is difficult to evaluate in small animals, because rats and mice are not anesthetized by 80 to 85 per cent concentrations of this agent. Hypoxic mixtures must be used to achieve anesthesia in these animals, and hypoxia after irradiation tends to delay or minimize the harmful effects of the radiation.

Burdick anesthetized mice that had been irradiated three hours earlier, using 95 per cent nitrous oxide for induction and 90 per cent for maintenance. He found a trend toward improved 30-day survival in the anesthetized mice — 70 per cent versus 56 per cent for the controls.[375]

Wilson failed to find this protective effect, using 90 per cent nitrous oxide after 620 to 745 rad doses in rats, but noted no significant differences in 30-day survival between anesthetized and control animals.[376]

Young et al.[374] and Zauder and Orkin[373] did not test nitrous oxide in irradiated animals, because control animals were not anesthetized by 85 per cent nitrous oxide.

Nitrous oxide has not been proved harmful in irradiated animals and would appear quite suitable for use in human patients after irradiation exposure. Its beneficial effects have not been demonstrated in the absence of hypoxemia.

Ethylene closely resembles nitrous oxide in its effects on irradiated animals. Burdick found no difference in survival between irradiated animals anesthetized with ethylene and unanesthetized controls.[375] Wilson found a protective effect with 85 per cent ethylene given to rats two hours after 825 rads. The median survival was prolonged by 3.1 days ($p<0.05$). Ethylene had no significant effect on 30-day mortality after irradiation and anesthesia.[379]

The effects of enflurane following irradiation have not yet been studied in animals or in humans.

INTERACTIONS OF IRRADIATION AND DRUGS USED AS ADJUNCTS DURING ANESTHESIA

Barbiturates. After exposure to higher doses of irradiation, experimental animals have a prolonged sleeping time when barbiturates are administered. Zauder and Orkin found a threefold increase in the sleeping time of rats pretreated with 450 and 750 R of x-irradiation.[373] Yam and Dubois found a similar effect for hexobarbital in irradiated rats and attributed this effect to diminished activity of the enzyme that transforms hexobarbital to hexoketobarbital.[381] This effect was demonstrated up to 44 days after x-irradiation.

When administered shortly after irradiation, barbiturates may tend to increase survival. Wilson and others gave thiopental, 30 mg per kg and 70 mg per kg, intraperitoneally to groups of rats two hours after 615 and 810 rads of whole body x-irradiation, respectively. In both groups of rats there were trends toward improved 30-day survival in the animals anesthetized with thiopental. There were 17 of 20 survivors in the 615 rad thiopental treated animals versus 14 of 20 survivors in the radiated controls, and 13 of 20 survivors in the 810 rad thiopental treated rats versus five of 20 survivors in the radiated controls.[379]

This effect was not seen in animals anesthetized with barbiturates 24 hours or more after irradiation. Wilson reports a 25 per cent 30-day mortality in rats given thiopental more than 24 hours after irradiation,[379] and Zauder and Orkin report a 42 per cent increase in mortality over unanesthetized controls in rats given thiopental two to four days after 350 r of whole body x-irradiation (p<0.01).[373] Soviet authors suggest that thiopental be avoided in patients anesthetized after exposure to large doses of radiation.[380]

Analgesics. The analgesic response to narcotics is unaltered in animals after sublethal irradiation. Doull treated rats and mice with sufficient morphine, codeine, meperidine, or methadone to double their reaction times to stimuli. He found no consistent differences between the magnitude or duration of the analgesic response of the irradiated animals and that of the nonirradiated controls.[382]

Muscle Relaxants. After irradiation, both in animals and in humans, there is evidence of a prolonged effect of succinylcholine. As early as 1959, Iwatzuki and Yokosawa tested succinylcholine, gallamine, and *d*-tubocurarine in animals. They found that the duration of action of succinylcholine was prolonged, whereas the duration of action of the nondepolarizing blockers was unaltered.[383] Belfrage and Schildt administered succinylcholine, 0.15 mg per kg, to 18 rabbits a week after 1100 R of whole body irradiation.[384] They found that a 20 per cent greater depression of muscle twitch occurred after the first dose of succinylcholine in the irradiated animals than occurred in the control animals. They also found that the duration of paralysis increased to 5.3 ± 0.9 minutes in the irradiated animals as compared with control values of 3.2 ± 0.6 minutes. Belfrage and Schildt ascribe the longer duration of the effect of succinylcholine in part to the impaired microcirculation seen after irradiation. Damage to capillaries and decreased peripheral circulation would slow the normal diffusion of succinylcholine away from the end-plates. They also note that irradiation can decrease the synthesis of pseudocholinesterase.[384] Deactivation of pseudocholinesterase by sublethal doses of x-irradiation is negligible. Nayor and Srinivasan have recently shown that massive doses of gamma radiation above 30 kilorads are required to produce a measurable decrease in pseudocholinesterase activity in vitro.[385] Although Belfrage and Schildt warn against extrapolating results obtained in experimental animals to man, they do note that at least one case of prolonged succinylcholine apnea has been reported in a human kidney transplant patient who had been irradiated previously.[386] Succinylcholine should be used cautiously during anesthesia in patients who have had recent irradiation.

Local Anesthetics. Within a few hours of exposure to whole body irradiation, there may be an increase in the systemic toxicity of local anesthetics. Young et al. gave mice xylocaine, 16 mg per kg intravenously, three hours after whole body x-irradiation with

660 rads and found an acute mortality of 52 per cent, whereas the mortality of the control animals was only 37 per cent. Using younger mice and higher xylocaine doses (25 mg per kg intravenously), they found a similar effect (56% versus 35%). The increased toxicity of xylocaine was no longer apparent three days after irradiation.[374] These effects of local anesthetics in whole animals differ from their effects on tissue cultures. Several reports have shown that 10 to 30 millimole concentrations of procaine increase cell survival during x-irradiation.[387, 388]

RADIOPROTECTION OF NORMAL AND NEOPLASTIC TISSUE BY DRUGS, ANESTHETICS, AND PHYSICAL MEANS

During irradiation, reduction of tissue oxygenation has an apparent radioprotective effect on both normal and neoplastic tissue. Drugs that cause regional vasoconstriction may have a radioprotective effect. Mechanical reduction of the blood supply to certain tissues during exposure to x-irradiation may also have a radioprotective effect. Antioxidants such as ascorbic acid are radioprotective to some degree. Furthermore, pentobarbital and chloral hydrate may have a radioprotective effect unrelated to decreased perfusion or ventilation.

Peterson and coworkers recently showed that clamping the blood supply to the intestine protects the mucosa against x-irradiation.[389] Sheldon and coworkers showed that clamping the base of cutaneous tumors in mice during x-ray therapy has a radioprotective effect on the tumors.[390] Juillard and coworkers showed that an infusion of vasopressin increases by 50 per cent the dose of radiation the canine gastrointestinal tract can tolerate.[391] Prewitt recently demonstrated a significant increase in survival of hamsters treated with phenylephrine while receiving 870 rads of gamma irradiation. Hypoxemic protection of the bone marrow evidently accounts for the radioprotection.[392] Vitamin C appears to protect against ionizing radiation by reducing the concentration of superoxides or free radicals in tissues.[393] Alkoxyglycerols have recently been used to reduce radiation injury during irradiation of cervical carcinoma.[394]

Anesthesia with pentobarbital during irradiation has a statistically significant protective effect on certain murine tumors. Sheldon and coworkers have shown that anesthesia with sodium pentobarbital, 60 mg per kg intraperitoneally, affords more radioprotection to MT-1 tumors than does occluding the tumors' blood supply (Figure 18–39).[390] The radioprotective effect of pentobarbital did not appear in several other types of murine tumors. Sheldon and coworkers also demonstrated a radioprotective effect of chloral hydrate in the MT-1 murine tumor.[395] No tumor radioprotection was found for tribromoethanol (Avertin), 200 mg per kg, or for diazepam, 15 mg per kg. Nor did the combination of fentanyl, 0.15 mg per kg, and fluanisone, 7.5 mg per kg intraperitoneally, offer any radioprotection.[395] More research should be done into the radioprotective effects of sedatives and anesthetics in both animals and humans.

ANESTHETIC MANAGEMENT OF PATIENTS HAVING THERAPEUTIC OR DIAGNOSTIC RADIOLOGICAL PROCEDURES

General anesthesia is often necessary for children having radiotherapy or certain diagnostic radiographic procedures. Anesthesia may also be necessary for adults having single, high doses of whole body irradiation.[294] General anesthesia for radiotherapy requires remote monitoring of at least one respiratory and circulatory parameter, as outlined by Feingold and his group.[396] A reliable airway is necessary. However, the repeated use of an endotracheal tube to secure an airway, particularly in children, should be avoided. Feingold and coworkers also point out that a safe, constant plane of anesthesia is desirable and that the agent must be nonexplosive. Feingold and his coworkers performed over 100 anesthetizations for biweekly radiation therapy in 12 children one to five years old using halothane, 1 per cent, or methoxyflurane, 0.5 per cent in 60 per cent nitrous oxide insufflated through a Guedel airway with a vallecular extension. Monitoring included a precordial stethoscope with an amplifier, a finger plethysmograph, and visual observation of the patient and the anesthesia machine either through an observation window or by closed circuit television. Most patients were kept in the supine position with the neck extended. No therapy session was interrupt-

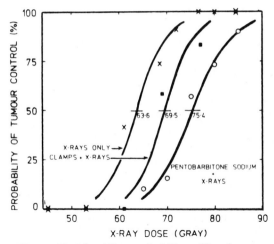

Figure 18–39. The probability of local tumor control at 80 days for 112 unanesthetized mice receiving x-rays only (x); 72 unanesthetized mice receiving x-rays while their tumors were clamped off to render them fully hypoxic (■); and 57 mice which received x-rays while anesthetized with pentobarbitone sodium (○). The TCD 50s are shown; the horizontal bars represent TCD 50 ± 1 standard error of the mean. TCD is tumor control dose. One Gray equals 100 rads. (From Sheldon, P. W., et al.: Int. J. Radiobiol. 32:571, 1977.)

ed to alter the depth of anesthesia, and no anesthetic complication occurred.[396] Although the repeated use of methoxyflurane should be avoided because of possible renal toxicity, the repeated use of halothane in children rarely has led to complications. Whitman and coworkers have described the use of general endotracheal anesthesia in older children or young adults having large single doses of whole body irradiation prior to bone marrow transplantation.[294] General anesthesia was necessary to prevent episodes of vomiting from interrupting treatment before a thousand rad dose had been delivered. Most of the anesthetics were 67 per cent nitrous oxide supplemented with fentanyl, 5 to 10 μg per kg, and pancuronium, 0.1 to 0.15 mg per kg. Barbiturates and succinylcholine were used for induction and intubation. Remote monitoring of blood pressure, electrocardiograph, tidal volume, and temperature was employed. No anesthetic complications appeared, but all patients in the series had emesis due to high doses of radiation.[294]

Amberg and Gordon have used low doses of ketamine, 2.7 to 3.6 mg per kg intramuscularly, for radiation therapy in children.[397]

When ketamine is employed, even in low doses, both circulation and respiration should be monitored adequately.[398]

Either general anesthesia or sedation is necessary for a number of diagnostic radiological procedures that are invasive and painful or that require the patient to remain motionless for a long period of time.

Bronchograms in children usually require general anesthesia with enflurane or halothane in oxygen.[399] Small doses of xylocaine intravenously or as a topical anesthetic in the trachea may depress the cough reflex.

Cerebral angiography can be done with local anesthesia and sedation in most adults. In children and in confused adults, general anesthesia is indicated.[399]

Pneumoencephalography can be quite painful; general anesthesia is usually used for both adults and children. Light levels of halothane in oxygen are recommended for this procedure; the increase in intracranial pressure due to halothane may be counteracted by hyperventilation.[399] Increases in intracranial pressure may result in herniation of the cerebellar tonsils — an event that may be fatal. Nitrous oxide should not be given to patients whose cerebral ventricles contain air. Wrapping the legs with Ace bandages decreases venous pooling when the patient is anesthetized and in an upright position. Heart sounds should be monitored, since air embolism may occur.[399]

Computerized Axial Tomography (CAT Scanning). For computerized tomography the patient must not move for prolonged periods of time. CAT scanning in infants and children is usually performed with general endotracheal anesthesia. Hyperventilation should be used if halothane is employed in patients who may have increased intracranial pressure.[399] The procedure may also be performed under sedation with rectal thiopental, 32 mg per kg.[400, 401]

Cardiac Catheterization and Aortograms. These procedures can usually be done with sedation and local anesthesia, even in infants and children.[399] Translumbar aortography may require general anesthesia. Heat loss may occur during radiographic procedures and may be minimized by wrapping the limbs and keeping the patient covered.

General anesthesia can facilitate many diagnostic or therapeutic radiologic procedures. It should cause rather little morbidity, provided the nature of the patient's disease and the requirements of the procedure are given proper consideration.

MANAGEMENT OF COMBINED TRAUMA AND IRRADIATION INJURY

Through nuclear accident or war, the medical community may have to treat numbers of patients with combinations of thermal and radiation burns and mechanical trauma. Very little information about such combined injuries is available; most irradiation accidents to date have not also included mechanical trauma; and much of the experience at Hiroshima and Nagasaki was lost because of inadequate records.

Eiseman and Bond point out that whole body irradiation with 250 to 500 rads greatly increases the mortality of thermal burns affecting 31 to 35 per cent of the body surface in experimental animals (Fig. 18–40). They suggest that active treatment may not be indicated for patients with early onset of CNS or gastrointestinal symptoms of irradiation, or with irradiation plus a 25 per cent thermal burn, or with irradiation plus trauma that might have a 50 per cent mortality. Much will depend on the availability of facilities and staff.[293] Surgical intervention, if indicated, should probably be carried out before the end of the first week to minimize the risk of bone marrow depression and infection. The anesthetic management is as described earlier, in the section concerning the effects of whole body irradiation on the patient.

SOME CONCLUSIONS

Patients who have received 200-to-800-rad doses of whole body irradiation have an increased risk during surgery and anesthesia for a period of time after their irradiation. Anesthesia should probably be avoided for 24 hours after a large dose of irradiation if the clinical situation permits.[374] By six to eight weeks after whole body irradiation, the patients are generally no longer increased risks for anesthesia and surgery.[296]

After whole body irradiation, deficits in fluids, electrolytes, and plasma volume should be corrected before patients are subjected to anesthesia and surgery. The hemoglobin should be adequate but not necessarily normal. For hemorrhagic diathesis during surgery, platelets and fresh whole blood may be needed. Broad spectrum antibiotics should be utilized.

A balanced technique using nitrous oxide, narcotics, diazepam, and nondepolarizing muscle relaxants is probably the anesthetic of choice, although light levels of cyclopropane, halothane, or enflurane seem acceptable. Barbiturates may have some protective effect during or shortly after irradiation. Judging from results in several species of experimental animals, chloroform and divinyl ether are contraindicated, and trichloroethylene and trifluorovinyl ether are probably poor choices. Soviet authors advise against the use of diethyl ether in the acute phase of nausea and vomiting after irradiation, or if gastrointestinal symptoms persist.[380] Methoxyflurane has been employed during radiotherapy but should probably be avoided in patients with the nausea and vomiting of irradiation sickness.

Succinylcholine may be used on the irradiated patient, provided that the anesthesiologist is aware of the possibility of prolonged apnea and avoids it. Narcotics and local anesthetics produce no unusual problems in patients who have had 200 to 800 rads of whole body irradiation. In the Soviet Union, local anesthesia is preferred for such patients.[380]

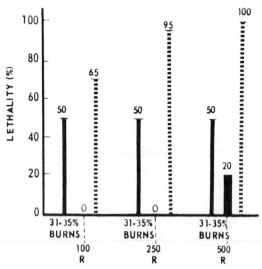

Figure 18–40. Lethality of burns to 31 to 35 per cent of the body surface area as affected by whole body irradiation between 100 and 500 rads in rats. R = Rads. (From Eiseman, B., and Bond, V.: Surg. Gynec. Obstet. *146*:877, 1978.)

Patients who have had high doses of irradiation to particular regions of the body may present problems in anesthetic management even years after irradiation. The larynx, lungs, heart, adrenal glands, kidneys, liver, thyroid gland, major systemic arteries, or the central nervous system may be damaged during regional radiotherapy. The anesthesiologist should ascertain the functional status of any irradiated organs and vary his anesthetic management appropriately. General anesthesia is necessary and can be administered safely for many diagnostic and therapeutic radiological procedures. The interactions between irradiation and general anesthesia in man warrant further study. Likewise, the possible radioprotective effects of barbiturates or other drugs used as adjuncts during anesthesia have not yet been studied in man. Finally, the effect of anesthetics in patients with combinations of thermal burns, trauma, and irradiation unfortunately is still largely a matter of conjecture.

REFERENCES

Anesthetic Management of the Narcotic Addict

1. Gay, G. R.: *In* Munson, E. S. (Ed.): Questions and Answers. Anesth. Analg. 53:838, 1973.
2. Cherubin, C. E.: The medical sequelae of narcotics addiction. Ann. Intern. Med. 67:23, 1967.
3. Isbell, H.: Clinical aspects of the various forms of non-medical use of drugs. Anesth. Analg. 50:886, 1971.
4. The National Narcotics Intelligence Consumers' Committee: The Supply of Drugs to the U.S. Illicit Market from Foreign and Domestic Sources in 1978. U. S. Govt. Printing Office GSA No. 027-004-00030-0.1980.
5. Louria, D. B.: Medical complications of pleasure-giving drugs. Arch. Intern. Med. 127:82, 1969.
6. Helpern, M.: Deaths from narcotics in New York City. New York State J. Med. 66:2391, 1966.
7. Louria, D. B.: Major medical complications of heroin addicts. Ann. Intern. Med. 67:1, 1967.
8. Baker, C. C., Peterson, S. R., and Sheldon, G. F.: Septic phlebitis: A neglected disease. Am. J. Surg. 138:97, 1979.
9. Tsueda, K., Oliver, P. B., and Richter, R. W.: Cardiovascular manifestations of tetanus. Anesthesiology 40:588, 1974.
10. Hussey, H. H., and Katz, S.: Septic pulmonary infarction. Ann. Intern. Med. 22:526, 1945.
11. Hussey, H. H., and Katz, S.: Infections resulting from narcotics addiction. Am. J. Med. 9:186, 1950.
12. Luttgens, W. F.: Endocarditis in "main line" opium addicts. Arch. Intern. Med. 83:653, 1949.
13. Olsson, R. A., and Romansky, M. J.: Staphylococcal tricuspid endocarditis. Ann. Intern. Med. 57:755, 1955.
14. Oerther, F. J., Goodman, J. L., and Lerner, A. M.: Infections in paregoric addicts. J.A.M.A. 190:683, 1964.
15. Cherubin, C. E., and Brown, J.: Systemic infections in heroin addicts. Lancet 2:298, 1968.
16. Reyes, M. P., Palutke, W. A., Wylin, R. F., and Lerner, A. M.: Pseudomonas endocarditis in the Detroit Medical Center, 1969-1972. Medicine 52:173, 1973.
17. Reyes, M. P., El-Khatib, M. R., Brown, W. J., Smith, F., and Lerner, A. M.: Synergy between carbenicillin and an aminoglycoside (gentamicin or tobramycin) against *Pseudomonas aeruginosa* isolated from patients with endocarditis, and sensitivity of isolates to normal human serum. J. Infect. Dis. 140:192, 1979.
18. Carey, J. S., and Hughes, R. K.: Cardiac valve replacement for the narcotic addict. J. Thorac. Cardiovasc. Surg. 53:663, 1967.
19. Gelfand, M. L., Hammer, H., and Hevizy, J.: Asymptomatic pulmonary atelectasis in drug addicts. Dis. Chest 53:782, 1967.
20. Egbert, L. D., and Bendixen, H. H.: Effect of morphine on breathing pattern. J.A.M.A. 188:485, 1964.
21. Wendt, V. E., Puro, H. E., Shapiro, J., Mathews, W., and Wolf, P. L.: Angiothrombotic pulmonary hypertension in addicts. J.A.M.A. 188:755, 1964.
22. Huff, B. B. (ed.): Physician's Desk Reference. 34th ed., Oradell, N. J., Medical Economics Co., 1980, p. 900.
23. Spain, D. M.: Patterns of pulmonary fibrosis as related to pulmonary function. Ann. Intern. Med. 33:1150, 1950.
24. Tinckler, L. F., and Bartham, G.: Opium addiction and surgery. Brit. J. Surg. 53:576, 1966.
25. Sapira, J. D.: The narcotics addict as a medical patient. Am. J. Med. 45:565, 1968.
26. Martin, W. R., Jasinski, D. R., Sapira, J. D., Flanary, H. G., Kelly, O. A., Thompson, A. K., and Logan, C. R.: The respiratory effects of morphine during a cycle of dependence. J. Pharmacol. Exp. Ther. 62:182, 1968.
27. Marks, V., and Chapple, P. A. L.: Hepatic dysfunction in heroin and cocaine users. Brit. J. Addict. 62:189, 1967.
28. Norris, R. F., and Potter, H. P., Jr.: Hepatic inflammation in narcotics addicts: Viral hepatitis a possible cause. Arch. Environ. Health 2:662, 1965.
29. Kaplan, K.: Chronic liver disease in narcotics addicts. Am. J. Dig. Dis. 8:402, 1963.
30. Norkrans, G., Frösner, G., Hermodsson, S., and Iwarson, S.: Multiple hepatitis attacks in drug addicts. J.A.M.A. 243:1056, 1980.
31. Eisenman, A. J., Fraser, H. F., and Brooks, J. W.: Urinary excretion and plasma levels of 17-hydroxycorticoids during a cycle of addiction to morphine. J. Pharmacol. Exp. Ther. 132:225, 1961.

32. Richter, R. W., and Rosenberg, R. N.: Transverse myelitis associated with heroin addiction. J.A.M.A. 206:1255, 1968.

33. Boak, R., Carpenter, C. M., and Miller, J. N.: Biological false positive reactions for syphilis among narcotic addicts J.A.M.A. 175:326, 1961.

34. Harris, W. D. M., and Andrei, J.: Serologic tests for syphilis among narcotics addicts. New York State J. Med. 67:2967, 1967.

35. Isbell, H.: Public Health Reports, 1947, No. 62, p. 1499.

36. Borison, H. L., Fishburn, B. R., Bhide, N. K., and McCarthy, L. E.: Morphine-induced hyperglycemia in the cat. J. Pharmacol. Exp. Ther. 138:229, 1962.

37. Goodman, L. S., and Gilman, A.: The Pharmacological Basis of Therapeutics. 3rd ed., New York., The Macmillan Co., 1965, p. 259.

38. Way, E. L., and Adler, T. K.: The pharmacologic implications of the fate of morphine and its surrogates. Pharmacol. Rev. 12:383, 1960.

39. Satoh, M., Zieglgänsberger, W., and Herz, A.: Actions of opiates upon single unit activity in the cortex of naive and tolerant rats. Brain Research 115:99, 1976.

40. Pert, C. B., and Snyder, S. H.: Opiate receptor: Demonstration in nervous tissue. Science 179:1011, 1973.

41. Lowney, L. I., Schulz, K., Lowery, P. J., and Goldstein, A.: Partial purification of an opiate receptor from mouse brain. Science 183:749, 1974.

42. Jacquet, Y. F., Klee, W. A., and Rice, K. C.: Stereospecific and nonstereospecific effects of (+) and (−) morphine: Evidence for a new class of receptors? Science 198:842, 1977.

43. Kuhar, M. J., Pert, C. B., and Snyder, S. H.: Regional distribution of opiate receptor binding in monkey and human brain. Nature 245:447, 1973.

44. Peters, R. I., and Klemm, W. R.: Electrophysiological signs of differential tolerance development to morphine in selected areas of the rabbit brain. Life Sci. 20:85, 1977.

45. Jacquet, Y. F., and Lajtha, A.: Paradoxical effects after microinjection of morphine in the periaqueductal gray matter in the rat. Science 185:1055, 1974.

46. Teitelbaum, H., Catraves, G. N., and McFarland, W. L.: Reversal of morphine tolerance after medial thalamic lesions in the rat. Science 185:449, 1974.

47. Seevers, H. M., and Woods, L. A.: The phenomenon of tolerance. Amer. J. Med. 14:546, 1953.

48. Collier, H. O. J.: A general theory of drug dependence by induction of receptors. Nature, 205, 181, 1965.

49. Wei, E., Loh, H. H., and Way, E. L.: Brain sites of precipitated abstinence in morphine dependent rats. J. Pharmacol. Exp. Ther. 185:108, 1973.

50. Cheney, D. L., and Goldstein, A.: Tolerance to opioid narcotics: Time course and reversibility of physical dependence in mice. Nature 232:477, 1977.

51. Stevens, D. R., and Klemm, W. R.: Morphine-naloxone interactions: A role for nonspecific morphine excitatory effects in withdrawal. Science 205:1379, 1979.

52. Bernheim, F., and Bernheim, M. L. D.: Action of drugs on the cholinesterase of the brain. J. Pharmacol. Exp. Ther. 57:427, 1936.

53. Wikler, A.: Sites and mechanisms of action of morphine and related drugs in the central nervous system. Pharmacol. Rev. 2:494, 1950.

54. Young, D. C., Van der Ploeg, R. A., Featherstone, R. M., and Gross, E. G.: The interrelationships among the central, peripheral and anticholinesterase effects of some morphinan derivatives. J. Pharmacol. Exp. Ther. 114:23, 1955.

55. Foldes, F. F., Erdos, E. G., Baat, N., Zwartz, J., and Zsigmond, E. K.: Inhibition of cholinesterases by narcotic analgesics — their antagonists. Arch. Int. Pharmacodyn. 120:286, 1959.

56. Domino, E. F., Vasko, M. R., and Wilson, A. E.: Mixed depressant and stimulant actions of morphine and their relationship to brain acetylcholine. Life Sciences 18:361, 1976.

57. Maynert, E. G., and Klingman, G. I.: Tolerance to morphine. I. Effects on catecholamines in the brain and adrenal glands. J. Pharmacol. Exp. Ther. 135:285, 1962.

58. Quinn, G. P., and Brodie, B. B., 1961: Quoted in Clouet, D. M.: Biochemical response to narcotic drugs in the nervous system. Int. Rev. Neurobiol. 2:99, 1968.

59. Verri, R. A., Groeff, F. G., and Corredo, A. P.: Quoted in Clouet, D. H.: Biochemical response to narcotic drugs in the nervous system. Int. Rev. Neurobiol. 2:99, 1968.

60. Iwamoto, E. T., Ho, I. K., and Way, E. L.: Elevation of brain dopamine during naloxone-precipitated withdrawal in morphine-dependent mice and rats. J. Pharmacol. Exp. Ther. 187:558, 1973.

61. Smith, C. B., Sheldon, M. I., Bednarczyk, J. H., and Villarreal, J. E.: Morphine induced increases in the incorporation of ^{14}C tyrosine into ^{14}C dopamine and ^{14}C norepinephrine in the mouse brain: Antagonism by naloxone and tolerance. J. Pharmacol. Exp. Ther. 180:547, 1972.

62. Gold, M. S., Pottash, A. C., Sweeney, D. R., and Kleber, H. D.: Opiate withdrawal using clonidine. J.A.M.A. 243, 343, 1980.

63. Gold, M. S., and Redmond, D. E., Jr.: Pharmacologic activation and inhibition of noradrenergic activity alter specific behaviors in nonhuman primates. Neurosci. Abst. 3:250, 1977.

64. Redmond, D. E., Jr., Hwang, Y. H., and Gold, M. S.: Anxiety: The locus coeruleus connection. Neurosci. Abst. 3:258, 1977.

65. Aghajanian, G. K.: Tolerance of locus coeruleus neurons to morphine and suppression of withdrawal response by clonidine. Nature 276:186, 1978.

66. Adriani, J., and Morton, R. C.: Drug dependence; important considerations from the anesthesiologist's viewpoint. Anesth. Analg. 47:472, 1968.

67. Giuffrida, J. G., Bizzarri, D. V., Saure, A. C.,

and Sharoff, R. L.: Anesthetic management of drug abusers. Anesth. Analg. 49:273, 1970.

68. Eiseman, B., Lam, R. C., and Rush, B.: Surgery in the narcotics addict. Ann. Surg. 159:748, 1964.

69. Blachly, P. H.: Management of the opiate abstinence syndrome. Am. J. Psychiat. 122:742, 1966.

70. Mark, L. C.: Hypotension during anesthesia in narcotic addicts. New York State J. Med. 66:2685, 1966.

71. Goodman, L. S., and Gilman, A.: The Pharmacological Basis of Therapeutics. 3rd ed., New York, Macmillan Co., pp. 293–294.

72. Margolis, J.: Codeine addiction with death possibly due to abrupt withdrawal. J. Amer. Geriatr. Soc. 15:951, 1967.

73. Gay, G. R., and Inaba, D. S.: Treating acute heroin and methadone toxicity. Anesth. Analg. 55:607, 1976.

74. Harris, L. S., and Pierson, A. K.: Some narcotic antagonists in the benzomorphan series. J. Pharmacol. Exp. Ther. 143:141, 1964.

75. Fraser, H. F., and Rosenberg, D. E.: Studies on the human addiction liability of 2'hydroxy-5,9-dimethyl-2(3,3-dimethylallyl)-6,7-benzomorphan (Win 20228), a weak narcotic antagonist. J. Pharmacol. Exp. Ther. 143:149, 1954.

76. Goodman, L. S., and Gilman, A.: The Pharmacologic Basis of Therapeutics. 3rd ed., New York, Macmillan Co., 1965, p. 278.

77. Jasinski, D. R., Martin, W. R., and Haertzen, C. A.: The human pharmacology and abuse potential of N-allylnormorphine (naloxone). J. Pharmacol. Exp. Ther. 157:420, 1967.

78. Kemp, W.: Abuse-liability and narcotic antagonism of pentazocine. Dis. Nerv. Syst. 29:599, 1968.

79. Stern, R.: The pregnant addict. Amer. J. Obstet. Gynecol. 94:253, 1966.

80. Perlmutter, J. F.: Drug addiction in pregnant women. Amer. J. Obstet. Gynecol. 99:569, 1967.

81. Perlmutter, J. F.: Heroin addiction and pregnancy. Obstet. Gynecol. Surv. 29:439, 1974.

82. Blinick, G., Wallach, R., and Jerez, E.: Pregnancy in narcotic addicts treated by medical withdrawal. Amer. J. Obstet. Gynecol. 105:997, 1969.

83. Stone, M., Salerno, L., Green, M., and Zelson, C.: Narcotic addiction in pregnancy. Amer. J. Obstet. Gynecol., 109:716, 1971.

84. Nathenson, G., Golden, G., and Litt, I.: Diazepam in the management of the neonatal narcotic withdrawal syndrome. Pediatrics 48:523, 1971.

85. Yarby, A.: Problem of neonatal narcotic addiction. New York State J. Med. 66:1248, 1966.

86. Blinick, G.: Menstrual function and pregnancy in narcotics addicts treated with methadone. Nature 219:180, 1968.

87. Foldes, F. F.: The human pharmacology and clinical use of nalorphine. Med. Clin. North Am. 48:421, 1964.

88. Fraser, H. F.: The human pharmacology and clinical use of nalorphine. Med. Clin. North Am. 48:421, 1964.

89. Bensinger, P. B.: Statement before the Subcommittee on Health and the Environment, U. S. House of Representatives, March, 1980.

Anesthesia for Other Drug Abusers

1. Isbell, H.: Clinical aspects of the various forms of nonmedical use of drugs. Anesth. Analg. 50:886, 1971.

2. Unwin, J. B.: Illicit drug use among Canadian youth. Canad. Med. Assoc. J. 98:402, 1968.

3. Seevers, M. H.: Adaptation to narcotics. Fed. Proc. 13:672, 1954.

4. Lee, P. K. Y., Cho, M. H., and Dobkin, A. B.: Effects of alcoholism, morphinism, and barbiturate resistance on induction and maintenance of general anesthesia. Canad. Anesth. Soc. J. 11:366, 1964.

5. Johnstone, R. E., Kulp, R. A., and Smith, T. C.: Effects of acute and chronic ethanol administration on isoflurane requirement in mice. Anesth. Analg. 54:277, 1975.

6. Smith, R. A., Winter, P. M., Smith, M., and Eger, E. I., II: Tolerance to and dependence on inhalation anesthetics. Anesthesiology 50:505, 1979.

7. Criteria Committee, National Council on Alcoholism: Criteria for the diagnosis of alcoholism. Am. J. Psychiatry 129:127, 1972.

8. Knott, D. H., and Beard, J. D.: Liver function in apparently healthy chronic alcoholic patients. Amer. J. Med. Sci. 252:261, 1966.

9. Morse, R. M., and Hurt, R. D.: Screening for alcoholism. J.A.M.A. 242:2688, 1979.

10. Randall, B.: Sudden death and hepatic fatty metamorphosis. J.A.M.A. 243:1723, 1980.

11. Dundee, J. W.: Thiopentone narcosis in the presence of hepatic dysfunction. Brit. J. Anesth. 24:81, 1962.

12. Schideman, F. E., Kelly, A. B., Lee, L. E., Lowell, V. F., and Adams, B. J.: The role of the liver in the detoxification of thiopental (Pentothal) by man. Anesthesiology 10:421, 1949. Cited in Dundee, W.: Thiopentone and Other Thiobarbiturates. Edinburgh, E. S. Livingstone, Ltd., 1956, pp 50–51.

13. Dundee, J. W., and Gray, T. C.: Resistance to d-tubocurarine in the presence of liver damage. Lancet 2:16, 1953.

14. Baraka, A., and Gabaldi, F.: Correlation between tubocurarine requirements and plasma protein pattern. Brit. J. Anesth. 40:89, 1968.

15. Ghoneim, M. M., Kramer, S. E., Bannow, R., Pandya, M. S., and Routh, J. I.: Binding of d-tubocurarine to plasma proteins in normal man and in patients with hepatic or renal disease. Anesthesiology 39:510, 1973.

16. Duvaldestin, P., Agoston, S., Kersten, J. W., and Desmonts, J. M.: Pancuronium pharmacokinetics in patients with liver cirrhosis. Brit. J. Anaesth. 50:1131, 1978.

17. McLeod, K., Watson, M. J., and Rawlins, M. D.: Pharmacokinetics of pancuronium in patients with normal and impaired renal function. Brit. J. Anesth. 48:341, 1976.

18. Somogyi, A. A., Shanks, C. A., and Triggs, E. J.: Clinical pharmacokinetics of pancuronium

bromide. Eur. J. Clin. Pharmacol. *10*:367, 1976.

19. Somogyi, A. A., Shanks, C. A., and Triggs, E. J.: Disposition kinetics of pancuronium bromide in patients with total biliary obstruction. Brit. J. Anaesth. *49*:1103, 1977.

20. Greenblatt, D. J., and Koch-Weser, J.: Clinical pharmacokinetics. N. Engl. J. Med. *293*:702, 1975.

21. Foldes, F. F.: Factors which alter the effects of muscle relaxants. Anesthesiology *20*:464, 1959.

22. McFarland, W., and Libre, E. P.: Abnormal leukocyte response in alcoholism. Ann. Intern. Med. *59*:865, 1963.

23. Sullivan, L. W., and Herbert, V.: Suppression of hematopoiesis by ethanol. J. Clin. Invest. *43*:2048, 1964.

24. Post, R. M., and Desforges, J. F.: Thrombocytopenic effect of ethanol infusion. Blood *31*:344, 1968.

25. Marks, P. A., Debellis, R. H., and Burka, E. R.: Hemolytic anemia associated with liver disease. Med. Clin. North Am. *47*:711, 1963.

26. Hall, C. A.: Erythrocyte dynamics in liver disease. Amer. J. Med. *28*:541, 1960.

27. Ratnoff, O. D.: Hemostatic mechanisms in liver disease. Med. Clin. North Am. *47*:721, 1963.

28. Evans, W.: Alcohol and the heart. Practitioner *196*:238, 1966.

29. Bashour, F. A., McConnell, T., and Miller, W. F.: Circulatory and respiratory changes in patients with Laennec's cirrhosis of the liver. Amer. Heart J. *74*:569, 1967.

30. Alexander, C. S.: Electron microscopic observations in alcoholic heart disease. Brit. Heart J. *29*:200, 1967.

31. Regan, T. J., Levinson, G. E., Oldewurtel, H. A., Frank, M. J., Weisse, A. B., and Moschos, C. B.: Ventricular function in non-cardiacs with alcoholic fatty liver: Role of ethanol in the production of cardiomyopathy. J. Clin. Invest. *48*:398, 1969.

32. Klatsky, A. L.: Alcoholism and hypertension. Hospital Physician *15*:40, 1979.

33. Keys, A., and Snell, A.: Respiratory properties of arterial blood in normal man and in patients with diseases of the liver. J. Clin. Invest. *17*:59, 1938.

34. Caldwell, P., Fritts, H., and Cournand, A.: The oxyhemoglobin dissociation curve in liver disease. J. Appl. Physiol. *20*:316, 1955.

35. Bashour, F., and Cochran, P.: Alveolar-arterial oxygen gradients in cirrhosis of the liver. Amer. Heart J. *71*:734, 1968.

36. Berthelot, P., Walker, J., Sherlock, S., and Reid, L.: Arterial changes in the lungs in cirrhosis of the liver; lung spider nevi. N. Engl. J. Med. *274*:291, 1966.

37. Kowalski, H., and Abelman, W.: The cardiac output at rest in Laennec's cirrhosis. J. Clin. Invest. *32*:1025, 1953.

38. Murray, J., Dawson, A., and Sherlock, S.: Circulatory changes in chronic liver disease. Am. J. Med. *24*:358, 1958.

39. Eisenberg, S.: Blood volume in patients with Laennec's cirrhosis of the liver, as determined by radioactive chromium-tagged red cells. Amer. J. Med. *20*:189, 1956.

40. Beard, J. D., and Knott, D. H.: Fluid and electrolyte balance during acute withdrawal in chronic alcoholic patients. J.A.M.A. *204*:133, 1968.

41. Wadstein, J., and Skude, G.: Does hypokalemia precede delirium tremens? Lancet *2*:549, 1978.

42. Lee, J. F., Giesecke, A. M., Jr., and Jenkins, M. T.: Anesthetic management of trauma: Influence of alcohol ingestion. South. Med. J. *60*:1240, 1967.

43. Barraclough, M. A., and Sharpey-Schafer, E. P.: Hypotension from absent circulatory reflexes. Lancet *1*:1121, 1963.

44. Vartia, K. O., Forsander, O. A., and Krusins, F. E.: Blood sugar values in hangover. Quart. J. Stud. Alc. *21*:597, 1960.

45. Freinkel, N., Singer, D. L., Arkey, R. A., Bleicher, S. J., Anderson, J. B., and Silbert, C. K.: Alcohol hypoglycemia. I. Carbohydrate metabolism of patients with clinical alcohol hypoglycemia and the experimental reproduction of the syndrome with pure ethanol. J. Clin. Invest. *42*:1112, 1963.

46. Forney, R. B., and Harger, R.: Toxicology of ethanol. Ann. Rev. Pharmacol. *9*:379, 1969.

47. Goodman, L. S., and Gilman, A.: The Pharmacological Basis of Therapeutics. 3rd ed., New York, Macmillan, 1965, p. 150.

48. Johnstone, R. E., Kulpus, R. A., and Smith, T. C.: Effects of acute and chronic ethanol administration on isoflurane requirement in mice. Anesth. Analg. *54*:227, 1975.

49. Dundee, J. W., Isaac, M., Pandit, S. K., and McDowell, S. A.: Clinical studies of induction agents XXXIV: Further investigations with ethanol. Brit. J. Anesth. *42*:300, 1970.

50. Keilty, S. R.: Anesthesia for the alcoholic patient. Anesth. Analg. *68*:659, 1968.

51. Morton, R. C., and Adriani, J.: Problems of drug addiction and drug abuse in surgical patients. J. La. State Med. Soc. *119*:475, 1967.

52. Morton, R. C., and Adriani, J.: Drug dependence: Important considerations from the anesthesiologist's viewpoint. Anesth. Analg. *47*:472, 1968.

53. Abreu, B. E., and Emerson, G. A.: Susceptibility to ether anesthesia of mice habituated to alcohol, morphine, and cocaine. Anesth. Analg. *18*:294, 1939.

54. Lee, J. A.: A Synopsis of Anesthesia. 4th ed., Baltimore, Williams & Wilkins Co., 1959, p. 460.

55. Sollman, T.: A Manual of Pharmacology. 8th ed., Philadelphia, W. B. Saunders Co., 1957, p. 881.

56. Han, Y. H.: Why do chronic alcoholics require more anesthesia? Reported at A. S. A. Meeting, October, 1968.

57. Dille, J. M., and Ahlquist, R. P.: The synergism of ethyl alcohol and sodium pentobarbital. J. Pharmacol. Exp. Ther. *61*:385, 1937.

58. Smith, J. W., and Loomis, T. A.: The potentiating effect of alcohol on thiopental-induced sleep. Proc. Soc. Exper. Biol. Med. *78*:827, 1952.

59. Ramsey, H., and Haag, H. B.: The synergism between the barbiturates and ethyl alcohol. J. Pharm. Exp. Ther. *88*:313, 1946.

60. Dundee, J. W.: Intravenous ethanol anesthesia: A study of dosage and blood levels. Anesth. Analg. 49:467, 1970.

61. Sandberg, F.: A quantitative study on the alcohol barbiturate synergism. Acta Physiol. Scand. 22:311, 1951.

62. Forney, R. B., Hughes, F. W., and Halpieu, H. F.: Potentiation of ethanol-induced depression in dogs by representative ataractic and analgesic drugs. Quart. J. Stud. Alc. 24:1, 1963.

63. Hubbard, T. F., and Goldbaum, L. R.: The mechanism of tolerance to thiopental in mice. J. Pharmacol. 97:488, 1949.

64. Amirdvani, M., Chalom, J., and Turndorf, H.: Murine memory and halothane, ethanol, diazepam and scopolamine. Anesthesiology 51(Suppl. 3):5, 1979.

65. Rubin, E., Gang, H., Misra, P. S., and Licker, C. S.: Inhibition of drug metabolism by acute ethanol intoxication. Postgrad. Med. 49:801, 1970.

66. Rubin, E., Gang, H., Misra, P. S., and Licker, C. S.: Inhibition of drug metabolism by acute ethanol intoxication. Postgrad. Med. 49:801, 1970.

67. Price, H. L., Deutsch, S., Cooperman, L. H., Clement, A. J., and Epstein, R. M.: Splanchnic circulation during cyclopropane anesthesia in normal man. Anesthesiology 26:312, 1965.

68. Isbell, H., Fraser, H. F., Wikler, A., Belleville, R. E., and Eisenman, A. J.: An experimental study of the etiology of "rum fits" and delirium tremens. Quart. J. Stud. Alc. 16:1, 1955.

69. Thompson, W. L., Johnson, A. D., Maddrey, W. L.: Diazepam and paraldehyde for treatment of severe delirium tremens. Ann. Intern. Med. 82:175, 1975.

70. Golbert, T. M., Sanz, C. J., Rose, H. D., and Leitschuh, T. H.: comparative evaluation of treatment of alcohol withdrawal syndrome. J.A.M.A. 201:99, 1967.

71. Muller, D. J.: A comparason of three approaches to alcohol-withdrawal states. South. Med. J. 62:495, 1969.

72. Rothfeld, V. A.: Conference, April 1967, Quoted in Kissen, B., and Gross, M. M.: Drug therapy in alcoholism. Amer. J. Psychiat. 125:69, 1968.

73. Knott, D. H., and Bear, J. H.: The study of drugs in the management of chronic alcoholism. G. P. 36:118, 1967.

74. Tavel, M. E.: A new outlook on an old syndrome: Delirium tremens. Arch. Intern. Med. 109:124, 1962.

75. Rosenbaum, M.: Cerebrospinal fluid in delirium tremens. J.A.M.A. 116:2487, 1941.

76. Isbell, H.: Addiction to barbiturates and the barbiturate abstinence syndrome. Ann. Intern. Med. 33:108, 1950.

77. Fraser, H. F., Isbell, H., Eisenman, A. J., and Pescor, F. J.: Chronic barbiturate intoxication. Arch. Intern. Med. 94:21, 1954.

78. Eddy, N. B., Halbach, H., Isbell, H., and Seevers, M. H.: Drug dependence: Its significance and characteristics. Psychopharmacology Bulletin 3(3), 1966.

79. Fraser, H. F.: Problems resulting from the use of habituating drugs in industry. Amer. J. Publ. Health 48:516, 1958.

80. Lous, P.: Barbituric acid concentration in serum from patients with severe, acute poisoning. Acta. Pharm. Toxicol. 10:261, 1954.

81. Gruber, C. M., and Keyser, G. F.: A study of the development of tolerance and cross tolerance to barbiturates in experimental animals. J. Pharmacol. Exp. Ther. 86:186, 1946.

82. Isbell, H.: Clinical characteristics of addictions. Amer. J. Med. 14:558, 1953.

83. Wikler, A.: Diagnosis and treatment of drug dependence of the barbiturate type. Amer. J. Psychiat. 125:759, 1968.

84. Wulff, M. H.: The Barbiturate Withdrawal Syndrome. Copenhagen, Munksgaard, 1960, p. 65.

85. Isbell, H.: Personal communication. Quoted in Essig, C. F.: Addiction to non-barbiturate sedatives and tranquilizers. Clin. Pharm. Ther. 5:334, 1964.

86. Gay, G. R.: Intra-arterial injection of secobarbital sodium into the brachial artery. Anesth. Analg. 50:979, 1971.

87. Dundee, J. W.: Thiopentone and other thiobarbiturates. Edinburgh, E. S. Livingstone, Ltd., 1956, pp. 121–123.

88. Giuffrida, J. G., Bizzarri, D. V., Saure, A. C., and Sharoff, R. L.: Anesthetic management of drug abusers. Anesth. Analg. 49:223, 1970.

89. Burns, J. J.: Role of biotransformation. In Papper, E. M., and Kitz, R. J. (eds.): Uptake and Distribution of Anesthetic Agents. New York, McGraw-Hill Book Co., 1963, p. 177.

90. Hitt, B. A., and Mazze, R. I.: Effects of phenobarbital and 3-methylcolanthrene on anesthetic defluorination in Fischer 344 rats. Presented at the A.S.A. Meeting, October, 1978.

91. Rice, S. A., and Mazze, R. I.: The induction of microsomal anesthetic defluorination by phenytoin. Presented at the A.S.A. Meeting, October, 1978.

92. Burstein, S., and Kaiber, E. W.: Phenobarbital-induced increase in 6-β-hydroxycortisol excretion. J. Clin. Endocrinol. 25:293, 1965.

93. Cohn, M. L., and Cohn, M.: Pentobarbital alteration of cyclic AMP metabolism. Anesthesiology 51(Suppl.3):5, 1979.

94. Setter, J. G., Maher, J. F., and Schveiner, G. E.: Barbiturate intoxication. Arch. Intern. Med. 117:224, 1966.

95. Shubin, H., and Weil, M. H.: The mechanism of shock following suicidal doses of barbiturates, narcotics, and tranquilizer drugs, with observations on the effects of treatment. Amer. J. Med. 38:853, 1965.

96. Arena, J. M.: Poisoning. 2nd ed., Springfield, Ill. Charles C Thomas, 1970, p. 312.

97. Isbell, H., and Fraser, H. F.: Addiction to analgesics and barbiturates. Pharmacol. Rev. 2:355, 1950.

98. Papper, S., Belsky, J. L., Blesfer, K. H., Saxon, L., and Smith, W. P.: Effect of meperidine and secobarbital upon renal excretion of water and solute in man. J. Lab. Clin. Med. 56:727, 1960.

99. Ellinwood, E. H., Jr., Ewing, J. A., and Hoaken, P. C. S.: Habituation to ethinamate. N. Engl. J. Med. 266:185, 1962.

100. Essig, C. F.: Addiction to non-barbiturate sedatives and tranquilizers. Clin. Pharm. Ther. 5:334, 1964.

101. Rogers, G. A.: Addiction to glutethimide (Doriden). Amer. J. Psychiat. 115:551, 1958.

102. Smith, B. E., and Pino, D. M.: Glutethimide therapy and overdosage. A review with report of a case. U. S. Armed Forces Med. J. 11:161, 1960.

103. Goodman, L. S., and Gilman, A.: The Pharmacologic Basis of Therapeutics. 3rd ed., New York, Macmillan, 1965, pp. 137–138.

104. Johnson, F. A., and Von Buren, H. C.: Abstinence syndrome following glutethimide intoxication. J.A.M.A. 180:1024, 1962.

105. Zivin, I., and Shalowitz, M.: Acute toxic reaction and prolonged glutethimide administration. N. Engl. J. Med. 266:496, 1962.

106. Reidt, W. U.: Fatal poisoning with methylprylon (Nodular), a non-barbiturate sedative. N. Engl. J. Med. 255:231, 1956.

107. Nattels, S., Bayne, L., and Ruedy, J.: Physostigmine in coma due to drug overdose. Clin. Pharm. Ther. 25:96, 1979.

108. McGuire, T. F., and Leary, F. J.: Tranquilizing drugs and stress tolerance. Amer. J. Publ. Health 48:578, 1958.

109. Hazlip, T. M., and Ewing, J. A.: Meprobamate habituation. N. Engl. J. Med. 258:1181, 1958.

110. Philips, M. D., Miya, T. S., and Yim, G. K. W.: Studies on the mechanism of meprobamate tolerance in the rat. J. Pharmacol. Exp. Ther. 135:223, 1962.

111. Goodman, L. S., and Gilman, A.: The Pharmacologic Basis of Therapeutics. 3rd ed., New York, Macmillan Co., 1965, p. 185.

112. Hollister, L. E., and Glazener, F. S.: Withdrawal reaction from meprobamate, alone and combined with promazine: A controlled study. Psychopharmacologia 1:336, 1960.

113. Bulla, J. D., Ewing, J. A., and Buffaloo, W. J.: Further controlled studies of meprobamate. Amer. Pract. Dig. Treat. 10:1961, 1959.

114. Swanson, L. A., and Olcada, T.: Death after withdrawal of meprobamate. J.A.M.A. 184:780, 1963.

115. Bensinger, P. B.: Depressants: Methaqualone. Drug Enforcement 6:22, 1979.

116. Abboud, R. J., Freedman, M. T., Rogers, R. M., and Daniels, R. P.: Methaqualone poisoning with muscular hyperactivity necessitating the use of curare. Chest 65:204, 1974.

117. Sanderson, J. H., Cowdell, R. H., and Higgins, G.: Fatal poisoning with methaqualone and diphenhydramine. Lancet 2:803, 1966.

118. Marks, P., and Sloggem, J.: Perpiheral neuropathy caused by methaqualone. Am. J. Med. Sci. 272:323, 1976.

119. Matthew, H., Proudfoot, A. T., and Brown, S. S.: Mandrax poisoning. Conservative management of 116 patients. Br. Med. J. 2:101, 1968.

120. Udall, J. A.: Clinical implications of warfarin interactions with five sedatives. Amer. J. Cardiol. 35:67, 1975.

121. Bensinger, P. B.: Depressants: Benzodiazepines. Drug Enforcement: 6:23, 1979.

122. Hollister, L. E., Matzenbacker, F. P., and Degan, R. O.: Withdrawal from chlordiazepoxide. Psychopharmacologia 2:63, 1961.

123. Blitt, C. D., and Petty, W. C.: Reversal of lorazepam delirium by physostigmine. Anesth. Analg. 54:607, 1975.

124. Liberti, J. D., O'Brien, M. L., and Turner, T.: The use of physostigmine as an antidote in accidental diazepam ingestion. Pediatrics 86:106, 1975.

125. Cahn, C. H.: Intoxication by ethchlorvynol. Canad. Med. Assoc. J. 81:733, 1959.

126. Kuenssberg, E. V.: Side effects of ethchlorvynol. Brit. Med. J. 2:1610, 1962.

127. Ellinwood, E. H., Ewing, J. A., and Hoaken, P. C. S.: Habituation to ethinimate. N. Engl. J. Med. 266:185, 1962.

128. Mendelson, J., Wexler, D., Leiderman, P. H., and Solomon, P. A.: A study of addiction to non-ethyl alcohols and other poisonous compounds. Quart. J. Stud. Alc. 18:561, 1967.

129. Beier, L. S., Pitts, W. H., and Gonick, H. C.: Metabolic acidosis occurring during paraldehyde intoxication. Ann. Intern. Med. 58:155, 1963.

130. Litt, I. F., and Cohen, M. I.: The drug using adolescent as a pediatric patient. J. Pediatr. 77:195, 1970.

131. Hall, A.: Teen-ager dies from apparent overdose; sniffed Liquid Paper. Nashville Tennessean, Fri., Jan. 11, 1980, p. 1.

132. Brawley, P., and Duffield, J. C.: The pharmacology of hallucinogens. Pharm. Rev. 24:31, 1972.

133. Domino, E. F.: The hallucinogens. In Pechter, R. W. (ed.): Medical Aspects of Drug Abuse. Hagerstown, Md., Harper & Rowe, 1975.

134. Showalter, C. W., and Thornton, W. E.: Clinical pharmacology of phencyclidine toxicity. Am. J. Psychiat. 134:1234, 1977.

135. Freedman, D. X., and Aghajanian, G. K.: Approaches to the pharmacology of LSD. Lloydia (Cincinnati) 29:309, 1967.

136. Tongue, S. R., and Leonard, B. E.: The effect of some hallucinogenic drugs upon the metabolism of 5-hydroxytryptamine in the brain. Life Sci. 8:805, 1969.

137. Snyder, S. H., and Richelson, E.: Steric models of drugs predicting psychotropic activity. In D. H. Efron (ed.): Psychotomimetic Drugs. New York, Raven Press, 1970, pp. 43–66.

138. Snyder, S. H., and Merril, C. R.: A relationship between the hallucinogenic activities of drugs and their electronic configuration. Proc. Nat. Acad. Sci. U.S.A. 54:258, 1965.

139. Kang, S., and Green, J. P.: Correlation between activity and electronic state of hallucinogenic amphetamines. Nature 226:645, 1970.

140. Abood, L. G.: Stereochemical and membrane studies with the psychotomimetic glycol esters. In D. H. Efron, (ed.): Psychotomimetic Drugs, New York, Raven Press, 1970, pp. 67–80.

141. Savage, C.: The resolution and subsequent remobilization of resistance to LSD in psychotherapy. J. Nerv. Ment. Dis. 125:434, 1957.

142. Schwarz, C. J.: The complications of LSD. J. Nerv. Ment. Dis. 146:174, 1968.

143. Griggs, E. A., and Ward, M.: LSD toxicity. A suspected cause of death. Ky. Med. Assn. J. 75:172, 1975.

144. Dolphin, A., Enjalbert, A., Tassim, J. P., Lucas, M., and Bockaert, J.: Direct interaction of LSD

with central "Beta" adrenergic receptors. Life Sci. 22:345, 1975.

145. Persson, S. A.: LSD and related drugs as dopamine antagonists: Receptor-mediated effects on the synthesis and turnover of dopamine. Life Sci. 23:523, 1978.

146. Trulson, M. E., and Jacobs, B. L.: Alterations of serotonin and LSD receptor binding following repeated administration of LSD. Life Sci. 24:2053, 1979.

147. Balestrier, A.: In Rothlin, E. (ed.): Neuropsychopharmacology. Amsterdam, Elsevier, p. 581, 1966.

148. American Academy of Clinical Toxicology Conference, San Franciso, October, 1970.

149. Freedman, D. X.: The psychopharmacology of hallucinogenic agents. Ann. Rev. Med. 20:409, 1969.

150. Horowitz, M. J.: Flashbacks; recurrent intrusive images after the use of LSD. Am. J. Psychiat. 126:565, 1969.

151. Caldwell, J., and Sever, P. S.: The biochemical pharmacology of abused drugs. I. Amphetamine, cocaine and LSD. Clin. Pharm. Ther. 16:625, 1974.

152. Hoffer, A., and Osmond, H.: The Hallucinogens. New York, Academic Press. 1967, pp. 103–104.

153. Rinkel, M., Hyde, R., Soloman, H. C., and Hoagland, H.: Clinical and physio-chemical observations in experimental psychosis. Am. J. Psychiat. 3:881, 1955.

154. Rinkel, M., Hyde, R., and Soloman, H. C.: Experimental psychiatry. IV. Hallucinogens: Tools in experimental psychiatry. Dis. Nerv. Syst. 16:229, 1955.

155. Hoffer, A., and Osmond, H.: Op. cit., p. 99.

156. Boakes, R. J., Bradley, P. B., Briggs, I., and Dray, A.: Antagonists of 5-hydroxytryptamine by LSD-25 in the central nervous system: A possible neuronal basis for the actions of LSD-25. Br. J. Pharmacol. 40:202, 1970.

157. Giarman, N. J., and Freedman, D. X.: Biochemical aspects of the actions of psychotomimetic drugs. Pharmacol. Rev. 17:1, 1965.

158. Berridge, M. J., and Prince, W. T.: The nature of the binding between LSD and a 5-HT receptor. Br. J. Pharmacol. 51:269, 1974.

159. Aghajanian, G. K., Foote, W. E., and Sheard, M. H.: Lysergic acid diethylamide: sensitive neuronal units in the midline raphe. Science 161:706, 1968.

160. Aghajanian, G. K.: LSD and CNS transmission. Ann. Rev. Pharmacol. 12:157, 1972.

161. Couch, J. R.: Responses of neurons in the raphe nuclei to serotonin, norepinephrine, and acetylcholine, and their correlation with an excitatory synaptic input. Brain Res. 19:137, 1970.

162. Bradley, P. B., and Merley, E.: Effect of tryptamine and tryptamine homologues on cerebral electrical activity and behavior in the cat. Br. J. Pharmacol. 24:669, 1965.

163. Wong, W. Y., Chiu, S., and Mishra, P. K.: Effect of D-lysergic acid diethylamide on striatal choline acetyl-transferase activity in the rat. Biochem. Pharmacol. 28:2207, 1979.

164. Aghajanian, G. K.: LSD and 2-Bromo-LSD: A comparison of effects on serotonergic neurons and on neurons in 2 serotonergic projection areas, the ventral lateral geniculate and amygdala. Neuropharmacol. 15:521, 1976.

165. Koella, W. P., and Wells, C. H.: Influence of LSD-25 on optically evoked potentials in the nonanesthetized rabbit. Amer. J. Physiol. 196:1181, 1959.

166. Schwarz, B. E., Sem-Jacobsen, C. W., and Petersen, M. C.: Effects of mescaline, LSD-25, and adrenochrome on depth electrograms in man. A.M.A. Arch. Neurol. Psychiat. 75:579, 1956.

167. Passouant, P., Passouant-Fontaine, T. H., and Cadilhac, J.: The action of LSD on the behavior and on the cortical and rhinencephalic rhythms of the chronic cat. Electroencephologr. Clin. Neurophysiol. 8:702, 1956.

168. Adey, W. R., Dennis, F. R., and Bell, F. R.: Effects of LSD-25, psilocybin, and psilocin on temporal lobe EEG patterns and learned behavior in the cat. Neurology 12:591, 1962.

169. Fox, P. C., and Dray, A.: Iontophoresis of LSD: Effects on responses of single cortical neurons to visual stimulation. Brain Res. 161:167, 1969.

170. Zahid, H., Siddik, Z. H., Barnes, R. D., Dring, L. G., Smith, P. L., and Williams, R. T.: The metabolism of lysergic acid Di ^{14}C ethylamide in the isolated perfused rat liver. Biochem. Pharmacol. 28:3081, 1979.

171. Kast, E. C., and Collins, V. J.: Lysergic acid diethylamide. Curr. Res. Anesth. Analg. 43:285, 1964.

172. Zsigmond, E.: Anesthetic considerations in patients on LSD-25. Anesthesiology 29:284, 1968.

173. Zsigmond, E. K., Foldes, F. F., and Foldes, V. M.: The inhibiting effect of psilocybin and related compounds on human cholinesterases. Fed. Proc. 20:393, 1961.

174. Winter, J. C.: Tolerance to a behavioral effect of lysergic acid diethylamide and cross tolerance to mescaline in the rat; absence of a metabolic component. J. Pharmacol. Exp. Ther. 178:625, 1971.

175. Hock, P. H.: In Cholden, L. (ed.): Lysergic Acid Diethyl Amide and Mescaline in Experimental Psychiatry. New York. Grune & Stratton, 1956, p. 8.

176. Hoffer, A., and Osmond, H.: Op. cit., p. 206.

177. Schwarz, C. J.: Paradoxical response to chlorpromazine after LSD. Psychosomatics 8:210, 1967.

178. Malitz, S., Wilkins, B., and Escover, R. A.: A comparison of drug-induced hallucinations with those seen in spontaneously occurring psychoses. In West, L. J. (ed.): Hallucinations. New York, Grune & Stratton, 1962.

179. Isbell, H., and Logan, C. R.: Studies on the diethylamide of lysergic acid (LSD-25). A.M.A. Arch. Neurol. Psychiat. 77:350, 1957.

180. Freedman, D. X., and Giarman, N. J.: LSD-25 and the status and level of brain serotonin. Ann. N.Y. Acad. Sci. 96:98, 1962.

181. Hoffer, A., and Osmond, H.: Op. cit. p. 210.

182. Bensinger, P. B.: Hallucinogens: Psilocybin and psilocyn. Drug Enforcement 6:29, 1979.

183. Hoffer, A., and Osmond, H.: Op. cit., pp. 486–495.

184. McCawley, E. L., Bennett, R. E., and Dana, G. W.: Convulsions from psilocybe mushroom poi-

soning. Proc. West. Pharmacol. Soc. 5:27, 1962.

185. Freedman, D. S., Gottlieb, R., and Lovell, R. A.: Psychotomimetic drugs and brain 5-hydroxytryptamine metabolism. Biochem. Pharmacol. 19:1181, 1970.

186. Zigsmond, E. K., Foldes, F. F., and Foldes, V. M.: The inhibiting effect of psilocybin and related compounds on human cholinesterases. Fed. Proc. 20:393, 1961.

187. Solursh, L. P., and Clement, W. R.: Use of diazepam in hallucinogenic drug crisis. J.A.M.A. 205:645, 1968.

188. Taylor, R. L., Maufer, J. I., and Tinklenberg, J. R.: Management of "bad trips" in an evolving drug scene. J.A.M.A. 213:422, 1970.

189. Hoffer, A., and Osmond, H.: Op. cit. p. 458.

190. Szara, S.: Dimethyltryptamia: Its metabolism in man; the relating of its psychotic effects to the serotonia metabolism. Experientia 12:441, 1956.

191. Aghajanian, G. K., Foote, W. E., and Sheard, M. H.: Action of psychotogenic drugs on single midbrain raphe neurons. J. Pharmacol. Exp. Ther. 171:178, 1970.

192. Silva, M. T. A., Carlini, E. A., and Clausson, U.: Lack of cross-tolerance in rats among Δ⁹cannabis extract, mescaline, and LSD-25. Psychopharmacologia 13:332, 1968.

193. Isbell, H., and Jasinski, D. R.: A comparison of LSD-25 with Δ⁹THC and attempted cross-tolerance between LSD and THS. Psychopharmacologia 14:115, 1969.

194. Rosenberg, D. E., Isbell, H., Miner, E. J., and Logan, C. R.: The effect of N,N-dimethyltryptamine in human subjects tolerant to lysergic acid diethylamide. Psychopharmacologia 5:217, 1964.

195. Snyder, S. H., Faillace, L. A., and Weingartner, H.: DOM (STP), a new hallucinogenic drug, and DOET: Effects in normal subjects. Amer. J. Psychiat. 125:357, 1968.

196. Snyder, S. H., Faillace, L. A., and Hollister, L.: 2,5-Dimethoxy-4-methyl-amphetamine (STP): A new hallucinogenic drug. Science 158:669, 1967.

197. Rosenberg, D. E., Isbell, H., Miner, E. J., and Logan, C. R.: The effect of N,N-dimethyltryptamine in human subjects tolerant to lysergic acid diethylamide. Psychopharmacologia 5:217, 1964.

198. Shulgin, A. T.: Psychotomimetic agents related to mescaline. Experientia 20:366, 1964.

199. Shulgin, A. T.: 3-methoxy-4,5-methylenedioxyamphetamine, a new psychotomimetic agent. Nature 201:1120, 1964.

200. Alles, G. A.: In Abramson, H. A. (ed.): Neuropharmacology. New York, Josiah Macey, Jr. Foundation, 1959.

201. Fairchild, M. D., Alles, G. A., Jenden, D. J., and Mickey, M. R.: The effects of mescaline, amphetamine and four ring-substituted amphetamine derivatives on spontaneous brain electrical activity in the cat. Int. J. Neuropharmacol. 6:151, 1967.

202. Kapida, G., and Fayez, M. B. E.: Peyote constituents: Chemistry, biogenesis, and biological effects. J. Pharm. Sci. 59:1699, 1970.

203. Goodman, L. S., and Gilman, A.: Op. cit., p. 205.

204. Smithies, J. R., Koella, W. P., and Levy, C. K.: The effect of mescaline on optic evoked potentials in the unanesthetized rabbit. J. Pharmacol. Exp. Ther. 129:462, 1960.

205. Balestrier, A.: In Rothlin, E. (ed.): Neuropsychopharmacology. Amsterdam, Elsevier, pp. 581–582, 1968.

206. Stevenson, I., and Richards, T. W.: Prolonged reactions to mescaline. A report of two cases. Psychopharmacologia 7:24, 1960.

207. Schapp, T. R., Kreuter, W. F., and Guzak, S. V.: Neuromyal blocking action of mescaline. Amer. J. Physiol. 200:1226, 1961.

208. Peretz, D. I., Smythies, J. R., and Gibson, W. C.: A new hallucinogen: 3,4,5-trimethoxyphenyl-B-aminopropane. J. Ment. Sci. 101:317, 1955.

209. Kramer, J. C., Fishman, V. S., and Littlefield, D. C.: Amphetamine abuse. J.A.M.A. 201:89, 1967.

210. Zalis, F. G., Kaplan, G., Lundberg, G. O., and Knutson, R. A.: Acute lethality of amphetamine in dogs and its antagonism by curare. Proc. Soc. Exp. Biol. Med. 118:557, 1955.

211. Connell, P. H.: Clinical manifestations and treatment of amphetamine type of dependency. J.A.M.A. 196:718, 1966.

212. Espelin, D. E., and Done, A. K.: Amphetamine poisoning: Effectiveness of chlorpromazine. N. Engl. J. Med. 278:1361, 1968.

213. Geerlings, P. J.: Social and psychiatric factors in amphetamine users. Psychiatr. Neurol. Neurochir. 75:219, 1972.

214. Goodman, L. S., and Gilman, A.: Op. cit., p. 298.

215. Ong, B. H.: Hazards to health: Dextroamphetamine poisoning. N. Engl. J. Med. 266:134, 1962.

216. Johnson, R. R., Way, W. L., and Miller, R. D.: Alteration of anesthetic requirement by amphetamine. Anesthesiology 36:357, 1972.

217. Glowinski, J.: Effects of amphetamine on various aspects of catecholamine metabolism in the central nervous system of the rat. In Costa, E., and Garattini, S. (eds.): Amphetamine and Related Compounds. New York, Raven Press, 1970, p. 301.

218. Lewander, T. A.: A mechanism for the development of tolerance to amphetamine in rats. Psychopharmacologia 21:17, 1971.

219. Caldwell, J., Dring, L. G., and Williams, R. T.: Metabolism of [¹⁴C] methamphetamine in man, the guinea pig, and the rat. Biochem. J. 129:11, 1972.

220. Lasagna, L., and McCann, W. P.: Effect of tranquilizing drugs on amphetamine toxicity in aggregated mice. Science 125:1241, 1957.

221. Goodman, L. S., and Gilman, A.: Op. cit., p. 723.

222. Goodman, L. S., and Gilman, A.: Op. cit., p. 573.

223. Änggård, E., Gunne, L.-M., Jönsson, L.-E., and Niklasson, F.: Pharmacokinetic and clinical studies on amphetamine dependent subjects. Eur. J. Clin. Pharmacol. 3:3, 1970.

224. Citron, H. P., Halpern, M., McCann, M., Lundberg, G. D., McCormick, R., Pincus, I. J., Tat-

ter, D., and Haverback, B. J.: Necrotizing angiitis associated with drug abuse. N. Engl. J. Med. 283:1003, 1970.

225. Boswell, W. D., Jr.: Angiitis from IV methylphenidate. Medical World News, Jan. 9, 1978, p. 62.

226. Eger, E. I., Saidman, L. J., and Brandstater, B.: Minimum alveolar concentration: A standard of anesthetic potency. Anesthesiology 26:756, 1965.

227. Johnston, R. R., White, P. F., and Eger, E. I.: Comparative effects of dextroamphetamine and reserpine on halothane and cyclopropane anesthetic requirements. Anesth. Analg. Curr. Res. 54:655, 1975.

228. Johnston, R. R., Way, W. L., and Miller, R. D.: Amphetamine users require double dose of anesthetic. Academy News Bulletin, 1970, p. 2.

229. Carr, L. A., and Moore, K. E.: Norepinephrine release from brain by d-amphetamine in vivo. Science, 164:322, 1969.

230. Gowdy, J. M.: Stramonium intoxication. J.A.M.A. 221:585, 1972.

231. Smith, D. E.: The trip there and back. Emerg. Med. 1:26, 1969.

232. Waser, P.: Personal communication, 1970.

233. Holzgrafe, R. E., Vondrell, J. J., and Mintz, S. M.: Reversal of postoperative reactions to scopolamine with physostigmine. Anesth. Analg. Curr. Res. 52:921, 1973.

234. Goodman, L. S., and Gilman, A.: Op. cit., p. 531.

235. Goldfrank, L., and Melinek, M.: Locoweed and other anticholinergics. Hospital Physician 15 (8):18, 1979.

236. Dameshek, W., and Feinsilver, O.: Human autonomic pharmacology. XIV. J.A.M.A. 109:561, 1937.

237. Orr, R.: Reversal of Datura stramonium delirium with physostigmine. Report of three cases. Anesth. Analg. Curr. Res.: 54:158, 1975.

238. DeYoung, G., and Cross, E. G.: Stramonium psychedelic. Canad. Anesth. Soc. J. 16:429, 1969.

239. Martin, H. E., and Weiss, S.: Persistence of action of physostigmine, and the atropine physostigmine antagonism in animals and in man. Pharm. Expl. Ther. 27:181, 1926.

240. Meiring, P. D.: Poisoning by Datura stramonium. South Afr. Med. J. 40:311, 1966.

241. Katz, R., quoted in Bernards, W.: Case number 74: Reversal of phenothiazine-induced coma with physostigmine. Anesth. Analg. Curr. Res. 52:938, 1973.

242. Exley, K. A., Flemming, M. C., and Espelin, A. D.: Effects of drugs which depress the peripheral nervous system on the reticular activating system of the cat. Brit. J. Pharm. Chemother. 13:485, 1958.

243. Gershon, S., Nembauer, H., and Sunderland, D. M.: Interactions between some anticholinergic agents and phenothiazide. Clin. Pharmacol. Ther. 6:749, 1965.

244. Goodman, L. S., and Gilman, A.: Op. cit., pp. 528–532.

245. Gosselin, R. E., Gabourel, J. O., and Willis, J. H.: The fate of atropine in man. Clin. Pharmac. Ther. 14:597, 1960.

246. Mendelson, G.: Letter to the Editor. Anesth. Analg., Curr. Res. 55:260, 1976.

247. Duvoisin, R. C., and Katz, R.: Reversal of central anticholinergic syndrome in man by physostigmine. J.A.M.A. 206:1963, 1968.

248. Burks, J. S., Walker, J. E., Rumack, B., and Ott, J. E.: Tricyclic antidepressant poisoning. J.A.M.A. 230:1405, 1974.

249. Fowler, N. O., McCall, D., Chou, T.-C., Holmes, J. C., and Hanenson, I. B.: Electrocardiographic changes and cardiac arrhythmias in patients receiving psychotropic drugs. Amer. J. Cardiol. 37:223, 1976.

250. Newton, R. W.: Physostigmine salicylate in the treatment of tricyclic antidepressant overdosage. J.A.M.A. 231:941, 1975.

251. Rosenberg, H.: Physostigmine reversal of sedative drugs. J.A.M.A. 229:1168, 1974.

252. Chapin, J. W., and Wingard, D. W.: Physostigmine reversal of benzquinimide-induced delirium. Anesthesiology 46:364, 1977.

253. Stovner, J.: Clinical use of relaxants in Europe. In Katz, R. L. (ed.): Muscle Relaxants. New York, American Elsevier Co. 1975, p. 250.

254. Wetli, C. V., and Wright, R. K.: Death caused by recreational cocaine use. J.A.M.A. 241:2519, 1979.

255. Gay, George R., Inaba, D. S., Rappolt, R. T., Gushue, G. F., and Perkner, J. J.: Cocaine in current perspective. Anesth. Analg. Curr. Res. 55:582, 1976.

256. Bensinger, P. B.: Op. cit., p. 25.

257. Van Dyke, C., Jatlow, P., Ungerer, J., Barash, P. G., and Byck, R.: Oral cocaine; plasma concentrations and central effects. Science 200:211, 1978.

258. Allport, S.: Epidemic of cocaine smoking seen. Medical Tribune, Jan. 16, 1980, p. 12.

259. Ritchie, J. M., Cohen, P. J., and Dripps, R. D.: Cocaine procaine, and other synthetic local anesthetics. In Goodman, L. S., and Gilman, A. (eds.): Op. cit., p. 376.

260. Hertting, G., Axelrod, J., and Whitby, L. G.: Effect of drugs on the uptake and metabolism of H³ norepinephrine. J. Pharm. Exp. Ther. 134:146, 1961.

261. Muscholl, E.: Effect of cocaine and related drugs on the uptake of noradrenalin by heart and spleen. Brit. J. Pharm. Chemother. 16:352, 1961.

262. Stoelting, R. K., Creassor, C. W., and Martz, R. C.: Effect of cocaine administration on halothane MAC in dogs. Anes. Analg. Curr. Res. 54:422, 1975.

263. Koehntop, D. E., Liao, J.-C., and Van Bergan, F. H.: Effects of pharmacologic alterations of adrenergic mechanisms by cocaine, tropolone, aminophyllin, and ketamine on epinephrine-induced arrhythmias during halothane-nitrous oxide anesthesia. Anesthesiology 46:83, 1977.

264. Barash, P. G., Kupriva, C. J., Langou, R., VanDyke, C., Jatlow, P., Stahl, A., and Byck, R.: Is cocaine a sympathetic stimulant during general anesthesia? J.A.M.A. 243:1437, 1980.

265. Pillard, R. C.: Marihuana. N. Engl. J. Med. 283:294, 1970.

266. Lieberman, C. M., and Lieberman, B. W.: Marihuana — a medical review. N. Engl. J. Med. 284:88, 1971.

267. Mikuriya, T. H.: Historical aspects of Cannabis sativa in western medicine. Committee on

Problems of Drug Dependence, NRC-NAS, Palo Alto, Calif., Feb., 1969.

268. Bensinger, P. B.: Cannabis. Drug Enforcement 6:34, 1979.

269. Keeler, M. H., Reifler, C. B., and Liptzin, M. B.: Spontaneous recurrence of marihuana effect. Amer. J. Psychiat. *125*:384, 1968.

270. Gregg, J. M., Campbell, R. L., Levin, K. J., Ghis, J., and Elliott, R. A.: Cardiovascular effects of cannabis during oral surgery. Anesth. Analg. *55*:203, 1976.

271. Nahas, G. G.: Current status of marijuana research. J.A.M.A. *242*:2775, 1979.

272. Berman, M. L., and Bochautin, J. F.: Effect of delta 9 tetrahydrocannabinol (marihuana) on liver microsomal dechlorinase activity: a preliminary report. Anesth. Analg. Curr. Res. *51*:929, 1972.

273. Weil, A. T., Zinberg, N. E., and Nelson, J. M.: Clinical and psychological effects of marihuana in man. Science 62:1234, 1968.

274. Goodman, L. S., and Gilman, A.: Op. cit. pp. 300–301.

275. King, A. B., Pechet, G. S., and Pechet, L.: Intravenous injection of crude marihuana. J.A.M.A. *214*:1711, 1970.

276. Siemons, A. J., Kalant, H., and Khanna, J. M.: Effect of cannabis on pentobarbital-induced sleeping time and pentobarbital metabolism in the rat. Biochem. Pharmacol. *23*:447, 1974.

277. Sofia, R. D., and Knoblock, L. C.: The effect of delta-9-tetrahydrocannabinol pretreatment on ketamine, thiopental, or CT-1341-induced loss of righting reflex in mice. Arch. Int. Pharmacodyn. Ther. *207*:270, 1974.

278. Zavala, D. C., and Rhodes, M. L.: An effect of paraquat on the lungs of rabbits. Chest 74:418, 1978.

279. Fawshter, R. D., and Wilson, A. F.: Paraquat and marihuana. Chest 74:357, 1978.

280. Johnstone, R. C., Lief, P. L., Kulp, R. A., and Smith, T. C.: Combination of delta-9-tetrahydrocannabinol with oxymorphone or pentobarbital. Anesthesiology *42*:674, 1975.

281. Vietz, T. S., Way, W. L., Miller, R. D., and Eger, E. I. II: Effects of delta-9-tetrahydrocannabinol on cyclopropane MAC in the rat. Anesthesiology 38:525, 1973.

282. Stoelting, R. K., Martz, R. C., Gartner, J., Creasser, C., Brown, D. J., and Forney, R. B.: Effects of delta-9-tetrahydrocannabinol on halothane MAC in dogs. Anesthesiology 38:521, 1973.

283. Koppanyi, T., and Richards, R. K.: Treatment for barbiturate poisoning — with or without analeptics. Anesth. Analg. Curr. Res. 37:182, 1958.

284. Bensinger, P. B.: Op. cit., pp. 26–27, 1979.

285. Bensinger, P. B.: Op. cit., pp. 29–31, 1979.

286. Corales, R. L., Maull, K. I., and Becker, D. P.: Phencyclidine abuse mimicking head injury. J.A.M.A. *243*:2323, 1980.

287. Grove, V. E., Jr.: Painless self-injury after ingestion of "angel dust." J.A.M.A. *242*:655, 1979.

288. Hyvarinen, J., Lassko, M., Roine, R., and Leimonen, L.: Effects of phencyclidine, LSD, and amphetamine on neuronal activity in the posterior parietal association cortex of the monkey. Neuropharmacol. *18*:237, 1979.

289. Cohen, S.: PCP (angel dust): New trends in treatment. Drug Abuse Alcoholism Newsletter 7, 1978.

290. Balster, R. L., Johanson, C. E., and Harris, R. T.: Phencyclidine self-administration in the rhesus monkey. Pharmacol. Biochem. Behav. *1*:167, 1973.

291. Eastman, J. W., and Cohen, S. W.: Hypertensive crisis and death associated with phencyclidine poisoning. J.A.M.A. *235*:1708, 1976.

292. Finck, A. D., and Ngai, S. H.: A possible mechanism of ketamine-induced analgesia. Anesthesiology *51*:S-34, 1979.

Anesthesia for the Irradiated Patient

293. Eiseman, B., and Bond, V.: Surgical care of nuclear casualties. Surg. Gynec. Obstet. *146*:877, 1978.

294. Whitman, J. G., Owen, J. R., Spiers, A. S. D., Morgan, M., Guolden, A. W. G., Goldman, J. M., and Gordon-Smith, E. C.: General anesthesia for high-dose total body irradiation. Lancet *1*:128, 1978.

295. Danjoux, C. E., Rider, W. D., and Fitzpatrick, P. J.: The acute radiation syndrome. Clin. Radiol. *30*:581, 1979.

296. Little, J. R., and Radford, E. P., Jr.: Effects of ionizing radiation and their importance in anesthesiology. Anesthesiology 25:479, 1963.

297. Cronkite, E. P.: Radiation injury. In Harrison, T. R., et al. (eds.): Principles of Internal Medicine. 4th ed., New York, McGraw-Hill, 1962, p. 852.

298. Allen, J. G.: Radiation injury. In Harkins, H. N., Moyer, C. A., Rhoads, J. E., and Allen, J. G. (eds.): Surgery, Principles and Practice, 2nd ed. Philadelphia, J. B. Lippincott Co., 1961, pp. 319, 323–324.

299. Allen, J. G., Basinger, C. E., Landy, J. J., Sanderson, M. H., and Emerson, D. E.: Blood transfusion in irradiation hemorrhage. Science, *115*:523, 1952.

300. Moyer, R. F., and Riley, R. F.: Effect of whole body and particle x-irradiation on the extractable cellular components of the lung, with special consideration to the alveolar macrophage. Radiation Res. *39*:716, 1969.

301. Gross, N. J.: Early physiologic and biochemical effects of thoracic x-irradiation on the pulmonary surfactant system. J. Lab. Clin. Med. *91*:537, 1978.

302. Brooks, J. W., Evans, E. I., Ham, W. T., Jr., and Reid, J. D.: Influence of external body radiation on mortality for thermal burns. Ann. Surg. *136*:533, 1952.

303. Kivy-Rosenberg, E., and Zweifach, B. W.: Microcirculatory effect of serotonin on hemostasis following whole body x-irradiation. Amer. J. Physiol. *211*:730, 1966.

304. Chandler, J. R.: Radiation fibrosis and necrosis of the larynx. Ann. Otol. 88:509, 1979.

305. Snyder, S.: Vocal cord paralysis after radioiodine therapy. J. Nuclear Med. *19*:975, 1978.

306. Donaldson, I.: Fibrosarcoma in a previously irradiated larynx. J. Laryngol. Otol. *92*:425, 1978.

307. Seydel, H. G., and Mann, J.: Pulmonary fibrosis following radiotherapy for bronchogenic carci-

noma and Hodgkin's disease. Maryland Med. J. *18*:61, 1964.

308. Bennett, D. E., Million, R. R., and Ackerman, L. V.: Bilateral radiation pneumonitis, a complication of the radiotherapy of bronchogenic carcinoma. Cancer *23*:1001, 1969.

309. Collins, J. F., Johanson, W. G., Jr., and McCullough, B.: Effects of compensatory lung growth in irradiation-induced regional pulmonary fibrosis in the baboon. Am. Rev. Resp. Dis. *117*:1079, 1978.

310. Gimes, B.: Radiation pneumonitis as a complication of radiotherapy of mammary carcinoma. Fortsch. Roent. *108*:638, 1968.

311. Roswit, B., and White, D. C.: Severe radiation injuries of the lung. Am. J. Roentgenol. *129*:127, 1977.

312. Rall, J. F., Alper, J. D., Lewallen, C. C., Sonnenberg, M., Berman, M., and Rawson, R. W.: Radiation pneumonitis and fibrosis, a complication of radioiodine treatment of pulmonary metastases for cancer of the thyroid. J. Clin. Endocrinol. *17*:1263, 1957.

313. Demeter, S. L., Ahmad, M., and Tomashefski, J.: Drug-induced pulmonary disease. Part III. Agents used to treat neoplasms or alter the immune system including a brief review of radiation therapy. Cleve. Clin. Quart. *46*:113, 1980.

314. deVillers, A. J., and Gross, P.: Radiation pneumonitis. Arch. Environ. Health *15*:560, 1967.

315. Robin, E.: Restrictive pulmonary diseases and disorders of pulmonary diffusion. *In* Harrison, T. R. (ed.): Principles of Internal Medicine, 4th ed., 1962, p. 1528.

316. Naimark, A., Newman, D., and Bowden, D. H.: Effect of radiation on lecithin metabolism, surface activity, and compliance of rat lung. Canad. J. Physiol. Pharmacol. *48*:685, 1970.

317. Gross, N. J.: Experimental radiation pneumonitis IV. Leakage of circulatory proteins onto the alveolar surface. J. Lab. Clin. Med. *95*:19, 1980.

318. Femirgil, C., and Heineman, H. O.: Effects of irradiation of the chest on pulmonary function in man. J. Appl. Physiol. *16*:331, 1961.

319. Bake, B., Bjure, J., Johansson, J., Rosengren, B., and Stiksa, J.: Regional lung function in patients with local pulmonary radiation reaction studied by isotope techniques. Scand. J. Resp. Dis. *50*:235, 1969.

320. Cameron, S. J., Grant, I. W. B., Lutz, W., and Pearson, J. G.: The early effect of irradiation on ventilatary function in bronchial carcinoma. Clin. Radiol. *20*:12, 1969.

321. Tewfik, H. H., Abdel-Dayen, H. M., Tewfik, F. A., and Latourette, H. B.: Changes in patterns of pulmonary perfusion and ventilation after radiation therapy of intrathoracic malignancies. J. Iowa Med. Soc. *68*:54, 1978.

322. Glicksman, A. S.: Malignant radiation of benign conditions, Ann. Intern. Med. *89*:130, 1978.

323. Price, J. C., Percarpio, B., Murphy, P. W., and Henderson, R. L.: Recurrent adenoid cystic carcinoma of the trachea: Intraluminal radiotherapy. Otolaryngol. Head and Neck Surg. *87*:614, 1979.

324. Mark, J., Call, E. P., and Von Essen, C. F.: Preoperative irradiation in patients undergoing pneumonectomy for carcinoma of the lung. J. Thorac. Cardiovasc. Surg. *51*:30, 1966.

325. Dick, H. L. H., Saylor, C. B., Reeves, M. M., and Davies, M. J.: Chronic cardiac arrhythmias produced by focused cobalt-60 gamma irradiation of the canine atria. Radiat. Res. *78*, 390, 1979.

326. Vaeth, J. M., Feigenbaum, L. Z., and Merrill, M. D.: Effects of intense radiation on the human heart. Radiology *76*:755, 1961.

327. Tzivoni, D., Ratkowski, E., Biran, S., Brook, J. G., and Stern, S.: Complete heart block following therapeutic irradiation of the left side of the chest. Chest *71*:231, 1977.

328. Rasmussen, S., Døssig, M., Walbom-Jørgensen, S.: Coronary heart disease — a possible risk of megavoltage therapy. Acta. Med. Scand. *203*:237,1978.

329. Alibelli, M. J., Marco, J., Fournial, G., Subatie, J. P., and Dardenne, P.: Severe coronary insufficiency in a young woman after mediastinal radiotherapy. Arch. Mal. Coeur. *71*:1311, 1978.

330. Rogers, D. L.: Precocious myocardial infarct after radiation treatment for Hodgkin's disease. Chest *70*:675, 1976.

331. Iqbal, S. M., Hanson, E. L., and Gensini, G. G.: Bypass graft for coronary arterial stenosis following radiation therapy. Chest *71*:664, 1977.

332. Arom, K. V., Bishop, V. S., Grover, F. L., and Trinkle, J. K.: Effect of therapeutic-dose irradiation on left ventricular function in conscious dogs. Ann. Thorac. Surg. *28*:166, 1979.

333. Larsson, L., Lindahl, J., and Unsgaard, B.: Fall in blood pressure during radiation therapy. Acta Radiol. Ther. Phys. Biol. *15*:241, 1976.

334. Teng, C. Y., Nemickes, R., Tobin, J. R., Jr., Szanto, P. B., and Gunnar, R. M.: Pericardial effusion following radiation to the chest. Dis. Chest *52*:549, 1967.

335. Fajardo, L. F., Stewart, R., and Cohen, K. E.: Morphology of radiation-induced heart disease. Arch. Pathol. *86*:512, 1968.

336. Biran, S., Corticosteroids in radiation-induced pericarditis. Chest *74*:97, 1978.

337. Schneider, J. S., and Edwards, J. E.: Irradiation-induced pericarditis. Chest *75*:560, 1979.

338. Scott, D. L., and Thomas, R. D.: Late onset constrictive pericarditis after thoracic radiotherapy. Brit. Med. J. *1*:(6019):341, 1978.

339. Flemming, K.: Radiation effects and the adrenal cortex. Internat. J. Rad. Biol. *14*:91, 1968.

340. Goodall, M. C., and Long, M.: Effect of whole body x-irradiation on the adrenal medulla and the hormones adrenalin and noradrenalin. Amer. J. Physiol. *197*:1265, 1959.

341. Flemming, K., and Hellwig, J.: Radiation effects and adrenal cortex. VII. Corticosteroid changes in mice following whole body irradiation. Acta Radiol. Scand. Suppl. *310*:124, 1971.

342. Sommers, S. C., and Carter, M. E.: Adrenocortical postirradiation fibrosis. Arch. Pathol. *99*:421, 1975.

343. Dhaliwal, R. S., Adelman, R. D., Turner, E., Russo, J. C., and Ruebner, B.: Radiation nephritis with hypertension and hyperreninemia following chemotherapy. Cure by nephrectomy. J. Pediat. *96*:68, 1980.

344. Cogan, M. G., and Arieff, A. I.: Radiation nephritis and intravascular coagulation. Clin. Nephrol. *10*:74, 1978.

345. Luxton, R. W.: Radiation nephritis. Quart. J. Med. *22*:215, 1953.

346. Lurie, A. G., and Casarett, G. W.: Influence of adrenalectomy on radiation hypertension and nephrosclerosis. Radiat. Res. 61:80, 1975.

347. Kim, J. H., Panahon, A. M., Friedman, M., and Webster, J. H.: Acute transient radiation hepatitis following whole abdominal irradiation. Clin. Radiol. 27:449, 1976.

348. Lansing, A. M., Davis, W. M., and Brizel, H. E.: Radiation hepatitis. Arch. Surg. 96:878, 1968.

349. Nebesar, R. A., Tefft, M., Vawter, G. F., and Filler, R. M.: Angiography in radiation hepatitis. Br. J. Radiol. 47:588, 1974.

350. Sukol, G. H., Greenblatt, D. J., Littman, P., Franke, K., and Koch-Weser, J.: Chlordiazepoxide metabolism in mice following hepatic irradiation. Pharmacology 13:248, 1975.

351. McTaggert, J., and Wills, E. D.: The effects of whole- and partial-body irradiation on circulating anterior pituitary hormones and testosterone, and the relationship of these hormones to drug-metabolizing enzymes in the liver. Radiat. Res. 72:122, 1977.

352. Brase, A., Emminger, E., and Bockslaff, H.: The influence of halothane on liver parenchyma after previous irradiation. Strahlentherapie 149:296, 1975.

353. Koulumies, M., Voultilaine, A., and Koulumies, R.: Effect of x-ray irradiation in laryngeal cancer on the function of the thyroid gland. Ann. Med. Intern. Fenn. 53:89, 1964.

354. Einhorn, J., and Wikholm, G.: Hypothyroidism after external irradiation to the thyroid region. Radiology 88:326, 1967.

355. Schimpff, S. C., Diggs, C. H., Wiswell, J. G., Salvatore, P. C., and Wiernik, P. H.: Radiation-related thyroid dysfunction: Implications for the treatment of Hodgkin's disease. Ann. Intern. Med. 92:91, 1980.

356. Mahnke, D. F.: Hyperthyroidism associated with radiation for lymphoma. Rocky Mt. Med. J. 76:187, 1979.

357. Cerletty, J. M., Guansing, A. R., Engbring, N. H., Hagen, T. C., Kim, H., Shetty, K. R., Rosenfeld, P. S., and Wilson, S.: Radiation-related thyroid carcinoma. Arch. Surg. 113:1072, 1978.

358. Sener, S. F., Scanlon, E. F., Garces, R. M., Khandetsar, J. D., and Murphy, E. D.: Preoperative physical assessment of thyroid glands in previously irradiated patients. Am. J. Surg. 138:666, 1979.

359. Wagner, D. H., Recant, W. M., and Evans, R. H.: A review of 150 thyroidectomies following prior irradiation to the head, neck, and upper part of the chest. Surg. Gynecol. Obstet. 147:903, 1978.

360. Ormerod, L. P.: Acquired coarctation of the aorta: a long-term complication of irradiation. Br. Med. J. 2(6042): 977, 1976.

361. Dossing, M., Rasmussen, S., Fischer-Hansen, B., and Walbom-Jorgensen, S.: Radiation-induced lesions of the aorta. Br. Med. J. 1(6066):973, 1977.

362. Silverberg, G. D., Britt, R. H., and Goffinet, D. R.: Radiation-induced carotid artery disease. Cancer. 41:130, 1978.

363. Parker, D., Malpas, J. S., Scandland, R., Sheaff, P. C., Freeman, J. E., and Paxton, A.: Outlook following "somnolence syndrome" after pro-

phylactic cranial irradiation. Br. Med. J. 1:(6112):544, 1978.

364. Soni, S. S., Marten, G. W., Pitner, S. E., Duenas, D. A., and Powazek, M.: Effects of central nervous system irradiation on neuropsychologic functioning of children with acute lymphocytic leukemia. N. Engl. J. Med. 293:113, 1975.

365. Brant-Zawadski, M., Anderson, M., DeArmond, S., Conley, F. K., and Jahnke, R.: Radiation-induced large intracranial vessel vasculopathy. Am. J. Roentgenol. 134:51, 1980.

366. Martins, A. N., Johnston, J. S., Henry, J. M., Stoffel, T. J., and DiChiro, G.: Delayed radiation necrosis of the brain. J. Neurosurg. 47:336, 1977.

367. Kristenson, K.: Delayed radiation lesions of the human spinal cord. Acta Neuropath. 9:34, 1967.

368. Howell, D. A.: Radiation myelopathy. Devel. Med. and Child Neurol. 21:655, 1979.

369. Kristensen, O., Melgård, B., and Schiødt, A. V.: Radiation myelopathy of the lumbo-sacral spinal cord. Acta. Neurol. Scand. 56:217, 1977.

370. Stoll, B. A., and Andrews, J. T.: Radiation-induced peripheral neuropathy. Brit. Med. J. 1:834, 1966.

371. Dirksen, P. K., Matolo, N. M., and Trelford, J. D.: Complications following operation in the previously irradiated abdominopelvic cavity. Am. Surg. 43:234, 1977.

372. Donaldson, S. S., and Lenon, R. A.: Alterations of nutritional status: Impact of chemotherapy and radiation therapy. Cancer 43:2036, 1979.

373. Zauder, H. L., and Orkin, L. R.: Effect of radiation on response to anesthetic agents. New York State J. Med. 63:1943, 1963.

374. Young, M. T., Parsons, S. A. A., Mezistrono, J., and Morris, L. E.: Effects of anesthesia in irradiated animals. Anesthesiology 23:74, 1962.

375. Burdick, K. H.: Effect of anesthetic agents in rats after whole body irradiation. Anesth. Analg. 32:319, 1953.

376. Wilson, J. E.: Pharmacological actions of anesthetics in irradiated animals. Anesthesiology 16:503, 1955.

377. Bruce, D. L., and Koepke, J. A.: Interaction of halothane and irradiation in mice: Possible implications. Anesth. Analg. 48:687, 1969.

378. Restivo, S. R., and Meffird, R. T.: Effects of postirradiation surgical stress, anesthesia, and spleen transplantation on survival of mice. Radiation Res. 6:153, 1957.

379. Wilson, J. E.: Pharmacological action of anesthetic agents in irradiated animals. Anesthesiology 16:503, 1955.

380. Khrmor, K. K.: Anesthetization in radiation sickness. Vestnik, Khirurgh, 77:65, 73, 1956. Reprinted in Anesthesiology 19:792, 1958.

381. Yam, K. M., and Dubois, K. P.: Effects of x-irradiation of the hexobarbital-metabolizing enzyme system of rat liver. Radiation Res. 31:315, 1967.

382. Doull, J.: Pharmacologic responses in irradiated animals. Radiation Res. 31:315, 1967.

383. Iwatzuki and Yokosawa: Tokoku J. Exper. Med. 71:79, 1959; quoted in Belfrage, P., and Schildt, B.: Op. cit.

384. Belfrage, P., and Schildt, B.: Increased sensitivity

to the muscle-relaxing effect of succinylcholine in irradiated rabbits. Acta Anesth. Scand. *11*:65, 1967.

385. Nayor, G. N. A., and Srinivasan, S.: The effects of gamma irradiation in solutions of acetylcholinesterase. Radiation. Res. *64*:657, 1975.

386. Vourc'h G., Winckler, C., Germain, A., Miraille, A., Pelatti, J., and Cakmar, D.: Problèmes anesthésiques posés par les griffes du rein. Acta de l'Institut d'Anesth. *10*:91, 1961.

387. Yau, T. M.: Procaine-mediated modification of membranes and of the response to x-irradiation and hyperthermia in mammalian cells. Radiation Res. *80*:523, 1979.

388. Yau, T. M., and Kim, S. C.: Radioprotection of mammalian cells by procaine. Br. J. Radiol. *51*:551, 1978.

389. Peterson, C. E., Eddy, H. A., and Patterson, W. B.: Hypoxic protection of canine jejunum from radiation injury. Surg. Forum *28*:426, 1977.

390. Sheldon, P. W., Hill, S. A., and Moulder, J. E.: Radioprotection by pentobarbitone sodium of a murine tumor in vivo. Int. J. Radiat. Biol. *32*:571, 1977.

391. Juillard, G. J. F., Peter, H. H., Weisenburger, T. H., Tesler, A. S., Langdon, E. A., Barenfus, M., Lagasse, L., Watring, W. E., and Smith, M. L.: Radioprotection of the digestive tract by intravenous infusion of vasopressin. Gynec. Oncol. *3*:233, 1975.

392. Prewitt, R. L., and Musacchia, X. J.: Mechanism of radio-protection by catecholamines in the hamster. Int. J. Radiat. Biol. *27*:181, 1975.

393. Gregory, N. L.: Mechanism of radioprotection by vitamin C. (letter). Br. J. Radiol. *51*:473, 1978.

394. Brohult, A., Brohult, J., Brohult, S., and Joelsson, I.: Effect of alkoxyglycerols on the frequency of injuries following radiation therapy for carcinoma of the uterine cervix. Acta Obstet. Gynecol. Scand. *56*:441, 1977.

395. Sheldon, P. W., and Chu, A. M.: The effect of anesthetics on the radiosensitivity of a murine tumor. Radiation Res. *79*:568, 1979.

396. Feingold, A., Lowe, H., Holiday, D. A., and Griem, M. L.: Inhalation anesthesia and remote monitoring during radiotherapy for children. Anesth. Analg. *49*:656, 1970.

397. Amberg, H. L., and Gordon, G.: Low dose intramuscular ketamine for pediatric radiotherapy. Anesth. Analg. Curr. Res. *55*:92, 1976.

398. Feingold, A.: Use of monitor for ketamine in radiotherapy (letter). Anesth. Analg. Curr. Res. *55*:895, 1976.

399. Korten, K.: Anesthesia for diagnostic procedures. Am. Fam. Phys. *15*(3):103, 1977.

400. Ferrer-Brechner, T., and Winter, J.: Anesthetic considerations for cerebral computer tomography. Anesth. Analg. Curr. Res. *56*:344, 1977.

401. Kallar, S., Vasinanukorn, M., Rah, K. H., and Boyan, C. P.: The use of rectal thiopental in children for computerized axial tomography. Anesthesiol. Rev. *7*(8):30, 1980.

Index

Page numbers in *italic* type refer to illustrations.
Page numbers followed by (t) refer to tables.

Abdomen, in Weber-Christian disease, 72
Abdominal muscle deficiency syndrome, in infants,
        description of, 147
    treatment of, 148
Abdominal pain, in type 1 hyperlipoproteinemia, 58
Abdominal wall defects, in infants, 146–150
    anesthetic management of, 148–150
        postoperative care in, 149
        preoperative evaluation in, 148–149
        ventilation control in, 149
    embryonic development of, 147
    treatment of, 148
Abetalipoproteinemia, 66
    anesthesia in, 67
Abortion, tubal, 92
Abscess, liver, amebic, 420–421
    pyogenic, 420
Acanthocytosis, in abetalipoproteinemia, 66
Achalasia, 401–402
Acid aspiration syndrome, in incompetent cervix
    patient, 94
Acid-base balance, kidney and, 465
    vomiting and, 430–431
Acidosis, in gastrointestinal disorders, 430
    in parenteral hyperalimentation, 459
Acromegaly, 181
Acrosclerosis, 569
ACTH. See *Adrenocorticotrophic hormone.*
ACTH syndrome, oat cell carcinoma of the lung and,
    192
Actinomycosis, of large intestine, 416
Acute glomerulonephritis, 470–472
    anesthetic considerations in, 471–472
    renal function tests in, 471
Acute gouty arthritis, factors disposing to, 50
    treatment of, 50–51
Addiction, narcotics, theories of, 677–681, *680*
Addison's disease, 187–191, 189(t), 190(t). See also
    Adrenocortical hypofunction.
Adenocarcinoma, of small intestine, 409
Adenoma, adrenal, vs. adrenal hyperplasia, 194
    gastric, 407
    villous, diarrhea in, 391
        of large intestine, 417
Adenosine diphosphate (ADP), in thrombocytopenic
    purpura, 349
Adenosine 3', 5'-phosphate, in fatty acid metabolism,
    55
Adenosine triphosphate, 3
Adenyl cyclase, in fatty acid metabolism, 55
ADH. See *Antidiuretic hormone.*
ADP. See *Adenosine diphosphate.*
Adrenal adenoma, vs. adrenal hyperplasia, 194

Adrenal cortex, ACTH influence on, 187
    diseases of, 187–198
        anesthesia in, 195
            agents and methods of, 195
            premedication for, 195
        pathophysiology of, 187
Adrenal dysfunction, in connective tissue disease,
        509
    in narcotics addiction, 677
    steroids and, 406, 509
Adrenal genital syndrome, hirsutism from, 194
Adrenal gland, adenoma of, pre- and postoperative
        management of, 193–194
    carcinoma of, pre- and postoperative management
        of, 193–194
    disorders of, in geriatric patients, 110–111
    metastatic carcinoma from, chemotherapy for, 192
    sex hormone secreting tumors of, 194–195
    tumor of, metapyrone in, 193
        removal of, 192
Adrenal hyperplasia, metapyrone in, 193
    vs. adrenal adenoma, 194
    vs. Conn's syndrome, 194
Adrenal medulla, pheochromocytoma of, 198–204
    pathophysiology of, 198–199
Adrenalectomy, bilateral, for hypercortisolism, 192
    in hypokalemic periodic paralysis, 556
    total, substitution therapy for, 196
Adrenocortical hyperfunction, 191–195
    anesthesia in, operative problems of, 195–196
    causes of, 191
    diabetes in, operative management of, 196
    hypertension in, operative management of, 196
    hypokalemia in, operative management of, 196
    management of, 192–195
    osteoporosis in, operative management of, 196
    postoperative problems in, 196
    pre- and postoperative management of, 192–195
    symptoms of, 191
    tests for, 191–192
Adrenocortical hypofunction, 187–191, 189(t), 190(t)
    causes of, 188
    from pituitary hypofunction, 188
    from steroids, 188
    hormone therapy of, 189
    management of, 188–190, 189(t), 190(t)
    operative and postoperative problems, 196–197
    plasma cortisol test for, 188
    pre- and postoperative management of, 190–191,
        190(t)
    tests for, 188–190
Adrenocortical insufficiency, in diabetes inspidus,
    182

Adrenocortical insufficiency (*Continued*)
  in diabetes mellitus, 207
Adrenocorticotrophic hormone (ACTH), adrenal
    cortex target of, 187
Adrenogenital syndrome, 188
Agammaglobulinemia, 513
Age, body fluid composition and, 99
Aging. See *Geriatric patient(s)*.
Aglossia adactylia, 581
Agranulocytosis, 339–340
  drugs causing, 339–340
  treatment of, 340
AHF. See *Antihemophilic factor*.
δ-ALA synthetase, biosynthesis of, 24–25
  induction of, 25
Albinism, oculocutaneous, in Chediak-Higashi
    syndrome, 71
Albright's syndrome, 582
Alcohol abstinence syndrome, 699–701
  death during, 701
  hypokalemia in, 700
  management of, 700
  symptoms of, 700
  treatment of, 700–701
Alcohol abuse, anesthetic considerations in, 439
Alcoholic patient, abstinence syndrome in, 699–701
  anesthesia for, 691–692, 692, 696–699
    alcohol interaction with, 698, 698(t)
    general, 699
    induction of, 696–699
    maintenance of, 696–699
    regional, 699
  beriberi in, 694
  blood volume in, 695
  circulation in, 695
  gastric acidity in, 696
  heart disease in, 694–695
  hemorrhage in, 694
  hydration in, 696
  hypertension in, 695
  hypoglycemia in, 696
  liver disease in, 693–694, 693(t)
  liver function tests in, 693(t)
  medical profile of, 693–696, 693(t), 695(t)
  myocardiopathy in, 694–695
  neurological disease in, 696
  paralytic ileus in, 696
  polyneuritis in, 696
  pulmonary dysfunction in, 695, 695(t)
Aldosterone, anesthesia and, 465
  function of, 187
  plasma, in primary aldosteronism, 194
Aldosteronism, primary, 194
    operative problems of, 197–198
    postoperative problems of, 198
Alkaline phosphatase, elevation of, in osteomalacia,
    159
  in Paget's disease, 159
Alkalosis, extracellular, in gastrointestinal disorders,
    432
  metabolic, in gastrointestinal disorders, 430, 432
Alleles, 1
Allergic alveolitis, anesthetic considerations in,
    258–259
  extrinsic, 257–259
    pathogenesis of, 258
  pulmonary function in, 258
  roentgenography of, 258
  symptoms of, 258
  treatment of, 258

Allopurinol, in therapy of gouty arthritis, 52
Alpha-amino acids, general structure of, 31
Alpha₁-antitrypsin deficiency, 262
  anesthetic considerations in, 262
Alveolar disorders, infiltrative, 232–236
Alveolar hypersensitivity, 257–259. See also *Allergic
    alveolitis, extrinsic*.
Amebiasis, intestinal, 437
  of large intestine, 416
Amebomas, in amebiasis, 416
Ames Eyetone Reflectometer, 207, 214
Amino acid(s), for protein sparing, 397
  metabolism of, 32
    inborn errors of, 31–40
  sources of, 31
Aminoacidurias, 32
Aminorex fumarate, pulmonary hypertension with,
    230
Amphetamine(s), action of, 713
  inhalational anesthetics and, 727–729, 728, 727(t),
    728(t)
  intoxication with, anesthetic considerations in,
    724–729, 724, 726, 728, 725(t), 727(t), 728(t)
    necrotizing angiitis and, 727
    signs and symptoms of, 725, 725(t)
    treatment of, 726
    vs. belladonna intoxication, 730
  tolerance to, 725
Amyloidosis, aortic stenosis and, 297
  in rheumatoid arthritis, 512
  mitral stenosis and, 304
  renal disease in, 474
Amylopectinosis, 21
Amyotrophic lateral sclerosis, 489–491
  anesthetic considerations in, 492
  carcinoma with, 491
  clinical course of, 489–499
  epidemiology of, 489
  laboratory findings in, 490–491
Anaphylactic shock, antibiotics and, 593
Anatomy, infant, 119–120
Andersen's disease, 21, 540
Anemia(s), aplastic, 318–319
    causes of, 318
    symptoms of, 318
  blood loss, 316–317
    hypovolemia in, 317
  Cooley's, 331–332
  Heinz body, 320
  hemolytic, 319–336, *322, 323, 329*, 319(t), 325(t)
    autoimmune, 332–334
      "warm type," 333
    congenital, 320–321
    drug-induced, 334
    microangiopathic, 335
    nonspherocytic, 320
  hepatic failure, 318
  in cirrhotic liver disease, 439
  in lymphocytic leukemia, 342
  in rheumatoid arthritis, 512, 516
  Mediterranean, 331–332
  megaloblastic, 314–316
    hepatic dysfunction in, 316
    in gastrectomy, 392–393
    surgery in, 316
    transfusion in, 316
  pernicious, 314–315
    causes of, 314
    clinical findings in, 314
    laboratory findings in, 314

Anemia(s) (*Continued*)
  renal failure and, 317–318
  sickle cell, 325, 327–331, *329*
    aplastic crises in, 328
    blood oxygen tension in, 330
    crises in, 328
      physiopathologic development of, *329*
    epidemiology of, 327
    hematologic crises in, 328
    hemolytic crises in, 328
    molecular character of, 327
    organ system involvement in, 328
    painful crises in, 328
    preoperative preparation in, 328–330
      exchange transfusion for, 328
      respiratory function in, 329
    serum cholinesterase activity in, 329
    surgery in, blood oxygen tension during, 330
      postoperative precautions for, 330
    symptoms of, 327–328
    treatment of, 330–331
    two forms of, 327–328
  sideroblastic, 319
  spur cell, 334–335
  target cell, 331–332
Anesthetists, health of, 371
Angiodysplasia, 392, 418
Angiokeratoma corporis diffusum, 575–576
Ankylosing spondylitis, 512–513
  anesthesia in, 516
  aortic insufficiency and, 301
Anorexia nervosa, 455
Antibiotic(s), anaphylactic shock with, 593
  anesthesia and, adverse effects of, 593–595, *594, 595*
  anesthetic drugs and, 590–595, *594, 595*, 591(t)
    neuromuscular blockade with, 591–593, 591(t)
    respiratory depression with, 591–593
  cardiac arrest with, 594
  convulsions with, 593
  hemolysis with, in glucose-6-phosphate
    dehydrogenase deficiency, 595
  myocardial depression with, 593
  nephrotoxicity of, 475
  ototoxicity of, 594
Anticholinergic deliriants, intoxication with, 732–734, 733(t)
  anesthesia in, 729–737
Anticholinergic drugs, for vomiting control, 428
Anticonvulsants, in epileptic phenylketonuric
  patients, 40
Antidiuretic hormone (ADH), in Guillain-Barré
  disease, 491
  renal function and, 464, 465
Antiemetics, in gastrointestinal disorders, 428
Antihemophilic factor (AHF), concentrates of, 359(t)
  deficiency of. See *Hemophilia.*
  genetic pattern of, 359(t)
  half-life of, 359(t)
  normal range of, 359(t)
  storage stability of, 359(t)
  surgical requirements for, 359(t)
"Anti-insulin" hormones, 3
Aorta, trauma to, 658–660
Aortic insufficiency, 300–301, 302(t)
  anesthesia and monitoring in, 308–309
  diseases causing, 302(t)
  Frank-Starling mechanism in, 300
Aortic rupture, 658–660
  anesthetic considerations in, 659–660

Aortic rupture (*Continued*)
  clinical findings in, 659
  "pseudocoarctation" syndrome in, 658
  thoracotomy in, 659
Aortic stenosis, 297, 298(t)
  anesthesia and monitoring in, 308–309
  causes of, 298(t)
Aortocaval compression, uteroplacental perfusion
  and, 85
Aortogram, anesthesia for, in children, 763
Apert's syndrome, 580
Apnea, in the newborn, 121
Apolipoproteins, structure and function of, 56(t)
Apparent volume of distribution (AVD), in infants,
  123–124, 124(t)
Arachnodactyly, in Marfan's syndrome, 68
Arcus cornea, in familial hypercholesterolemia, 60
Arnold-Chiari malformation, 501–502
Arrhythmias, in geriatric patients, 113
Arteriosclerosis, in geriatric patients, 102
Arthritis, acute gouty, 50–51
  anti-inflammatory drugs in, 51
  arthrocentesis in, 51
  in Behçet's disease, 569
  rheumatoid, 510–512, *511*
  renal disease in, 473–474
Asbestosis, 248–249
  neoplastic change and, 249
  pathogenesis of, 249
  roentgenograph of, 249
  symptoms of, 249
Ascending cholangitis, 424–425
Ascites, 400, 439
L-asparaginase, pulmonary disease from, 253
Aspergillosis, 262–263
  anesthetic considerations in, 263
  clinical features of, 263
Aspiration pneumonitis, in endotracheal intubation,
  429–430
    treatment of, 429–430
Asthma, physical findings in, 225(t)
Asymmetric septal hypertrophy. See *Idiopathic
  hypertrophic subaortic stenosis.*
Ataxia, in abetalipoproteinemia, 66
Atelectasis, in narcotics addicts, 674–675
  in newborns, 121–122
  physical findings in, 225(t)
  radiography of, 226
Atherosclerosis, in diabetes mellitus, 204
Atlanto-axial instability, in dwarfism, 579
ATP. See *Adenosine triphosphate.*
Atropine, in laryngeal papillomas, 132
  in newborn, 126
  intoxication with, 730, 730(t)
Autonomic dysreflexia, anesthetic considerations in,
  651
  in spinal cord injuries, 650–651
Azathioprine, pulmonary disease from 253

Bacteremia, 597
Bacteremic shock, 604–607
Bacterial endocarditis, aortic insufficiency and, 301
  subacute, renal disease in, 474
Bagassosis, 257
Barbiturate(s), addiction to, acute, 701–702
  anesthetic management of, 703–704
  chronic, 702
  overdose in, 704

Barbiturate(s) (*Continued*)
  vs. narcotics addiction, 685
  withdrawal from 702, 703, 703(t)
  in renal disease, 468
  irradiation and, 761
  porphyric activity of, 29
Barbiturate abstinence syndrome, 702–703, 703(t)
Baritosis, 251
Barrett's syndrome, 404
Basal ganglia degeneration, 485–489
  clinicopathological correlations of, 486
  neuroanatomy of, 485–486
  neurophysiology of, 485–486
  primary symptoms of, 486
Basal skull fractures, 647
Batten-Curschmann's disease, 533–537
Becker dystrophy, 532
Beckwith-Wiedemann syndrome, omphalocele and, 148
Behavioral and environmental disorders, 672–777
Behcet's disease, 568–569
  anesthetic management of, 569
Belladonna alkaloids, in renal disease, 468
  intoxication with, anesthetic considerations in, 729–737
    treatment for, 731–732
    vs. amphetamine intoxication, 730
    vs. hallucinogenic intoxication, 730
    vs. schizophrenia, 730
Benign chronic bullous dermatosis of childhood, 565
Benign familial pemphigus, 565
Benzene, anemia from, 334
Benzodiazepine compounds, addiction to, 708–709, 708
  in renal disease, 468
Beri-beri, 459
  in alcoholic patients, 694
Besnier's fever, 525–527, 526, 527
Bezoars, 405
Bile, 430
Biliary disease, in infants, 141–143
  anesthetic management in, 140–141
    anesthetic choice for, 143
    blood loss in, 143
    clinical characteristics of, 142–143
  therapy for, 142
Biostator, 214, 215
Bladder, perforation of, in geriatric patient, 109
Bland-White-Garland syndrome, in coronary artery disease, 282
Bleeding, gastrointestinal, 391–392
  in ruptured tubal pregnancy, 92
Bleomycin, pulmonary disease from, 252
Blind loop syndrome, 393
Blindness, in cranial (temporal) arteritis, 521, 522
  in diabetes mellitus, 204
Bloch-Sulzberger syndrome, 576
Blood, bank, vs. normal blood, 368(t)
  rat, gas inhalation effects on, 371(t)
  replacement of, in newborns, 128
  transfused, bacterial contamination of, 366
    reactions to, 364–372, 368(t), 371(t)
    temperature in, 369
Blood cells, generation of, 315
Blood coagulation, test for, 364(t)
Blood glucose, concentration of, in operating room, 9
  factors influencing, 4(t)
  monitoring of, in hyperinsulinism, 214, 215
Blood platelet function, blood coagulation and, 360–364

Blood pressure, in geriatric patients, 102
Blood urea nitrogen (BUN), in renal disease, 467
Blood vessel function, blood coagulation and, 360–364
Boeck's fever, 525–527, 526, 527
Boerhaave's syndrome, 385, 402, 403
Bone disorders, 562–587
Bourneville's disease, 504
Bowel, disorders of, anesthetic considerations in, 436–437
Bradykinin, in carcinoid tumors, 437, 438
Brain, effect of phenylketonuria on, 37
  in geriatric patients, 107
  in Wilson's disease, 42
Brancher deficiency, 540
Brazilian pemphigus, 565
Bronchial asthma, physical findings in, 225(t)
Bronchitis, chronic, cor pulmonale from, 286–287
    pathophysiology of, 286–287
  industrial, in coal miners, 251
  physical findings in, 225(t)
Bronchopulmonry dysplasia, in infants, treatment plan for, 139–140
Bronchopulmonary lavage, for pulmonary alveolar proteinosis, 234–235
  in cystic fibrosis, 261
Bronchoscopy, in major airways trauma, 655
Bullous disease of the lung, 263–264
  pulmonary function in, 264
  roentgenography of, 264
BUN. See *Blood urea nitrogen.*
Burkitt's lymphoma, 346
Burns, malnutrition state in, 454–455
  pharmacokinetics of drugs in, 455
Byssinosis, 263

Cachexia of malignancy, 455–456
Calcitonin, in calcium metabolism, 156
  in thyroid cancer, 174
Calcium, in blood transfusion, 368
  in hemorrhagic shock, 639
  level of, in malignant hyperthermia, 547
    in thyroid cancer, 175
  metabolism of, disorders of, 155–164
    excessive absorption in, 157
    physiology of, 155–156
  therapy with, in osteoporosis, 164
Calculi, renal, in cystinuria, 33
Calorie-to-nitrogen ratio, 434
Cancer, hypercalcemia in, 159
  thyroid, 174–175
Cannabinols, action of, 713
Capillary vessels, abnormalities of, 349–352
Caplan's syndrome, 242, 243, 250
Carbohydrates, functions of, 2
  metabolism of, inborn errors of, 2–17
    fatty acids and, 54
Carbon tetrachloride, nephrotoxicity of, 475
Carcinoid syndrome, 409
Carcinoid tumors, anesthetic considerations in, 437–438
  of small intestine, 409–410
  preoperative management in, 438
Carcinoma, in amyotrophic lateral sclerosis, 491
  in dermatomyositis, 523
  in Eaton-Lambert syndrome, 553
  in myasthenic syndrome, 553
  in ulcerative colitis, 415

Carcinoma (*Continued*)
  of extrahepatic bile duct, 425–426
  of liver, 421
  of lung, in geriatric patients, 106
Cardiac arrest, antibiotics and, 594
Cardiac catheterization, anesthesia for, in children, 763
Cardiac disease(s), 268–312
  in abetalipoproteinemia, 66
  in alcoholic patients, 694–695
  in Down's syndrome, 71
  in Duchenne dystrophy, 531, 532
  in dwarfism, 580
  in geriatric patients, 101–105
  in malignant hyperthermia, 545
  in Marfan's syndrome, 68
  in myotonic muscular dystrophy, 534
  in pregnancy, 83–84
  in sarcoidosis, 526, *526*
  in Weber-Christian disease, 72
  irradiation and, 750–752, *751*, *752*, 750(t)
Cardiac pacemakers, in geriatric patients, 103–105
Cardiac tamponade, 290–291, 294, *291*, 292–293(t), 656–657
  anesthesia and monitoring in, 294–296, *294*
  assessment of severity of, 295
  causes of, 292–293(t)
  central venous pressure monitoring in, 294, *294*
  circulatory therapy in, 295
  pathophysiology of, 291, *291*
  symptoms of, 291
Cardiac trauma, 655–658
Cardiac valve(s), disruption of, 657–658
  lesions of, 296–309, 298–299(t), 302–303(t), 305(t), 307(t)
Cardiomyopathy(ies), 269–279, *276*, *279*, 270–271(t), 272–274(t), 277(t)
  classification of, 269
  congestive, 269–277, *276*, 270(t), 272(t)
    anesthesia and monitoring in, 276–277
    inflammatory, 269, 275, 270–271(t)
      causes of 270–271(t), 275
      circulatory problems with, 270–271(t)
      mechanisms of, 270–271(t)
      symptoms of, 269
    non-inflammatory, 275–276
      alcoholic, 275
      causes of, 272–274(t)
      circulatory problems with, 272–274(t)
      mechanisms of, 272–274(t)
    stroke volume in, 276, *276*, 277
  obstructive, 277–278, 277(t)
    anesthesia and monitoring in, 278, *279*
    causes of, 277(t)
    circulatory problems in, 277(t)
    mechanisms of, 277(t)
  restrictive, 278–279, 280(t)
    vs. constrictive pericarditis, 290
    vs. endocardial fibroelastosis, 279
    with pheochromocytoma, 198
Cardiovascular system, disease of, in geriatric patients, 101–105
  in pregnancy, 83–84
  in diabetic patient, 206
  in Ehlers-Danlos syndrome, 69
  in hemochromatosis, 74
  in hyperthyroidism, 176–177, 178
  in Marfan's syndrome, 68
  in newborns, 122–123, *123*, 123(t), 126
  in pregnancy, 81–82, 83

Carnitine deficiency, 541
Carnitine palmityl transferase deficiency, 541–542
Catecholamines, in pheochromocytoma, 199
CDH. See *Congenital diaphragmatic hernia.*
Cell membrane, phospholipid structure of, 65
Cell metabolism, in septic shock, 600
Central core disease, 544
  vs. McArdle's disease, 544
Central nervous system, effect of hypoglycemia on, 8
  in narcotics addicts, 677
  role of ceruloplasmin in, 41
Central nervous system depressants, abuse of, anesthesia in, 690, 691–696, *692*
  miscellaneous, anesthesia for, 704–709
  prothrombin times and, 707–708
  warfarin anticoagulants and, 707–708
Ceruloplasmin, copper content of, 41
Cervical spondylosis, anesthesia in, 514–515, *515*
Cervix, incompetent, 93–94
  anesthesia in, 93–94
Chagas' disease, 417
  achalasia in, 402
  cardiomyopathy and, 275
Charcot-Marie-Tooth disease, 492
Chediak-Higashi syndrome, 71–72
  anesthesia in, 72
Chemopallidectomy, in Parkinson's syndrome, 488–489
Chest, trauma to, 655–660
Chest pain, in pulmonary disease, 222
Chlorambucil, pulmonary disease from, 252
Chlordiazepoxide addiction, anesthesia in, 708, *708*
Chlorthalidone, for hypoparathyroidism, 161
Choanal atresia, in infants, anesthesia in, 129
  laser correction of, 129
Cholangioma, 421
Cholangitis, ascending, 424–425
  sclerosing, primary, 425
  suppurative, 425
Choledochal cyst, 423
Cholelithiasis, in gallstone ileus, 424
Cholestasis, drug-induced, 423
Cholesterol, 54
  sources of, 59
Cholinesterase, functions of, 66
  serum, in sickle cell anemia, 329
Chorea, adult, 487
  chronic progressive, 487
Christmas disease, 357–358
Christmas factor, concentrates of, 359(t)
  deficiency of, genetic pattern of, 359(t)
  half-life of, 359(t)
  normal range of, 359(t)
  storage stability of, 359(t)
  surgical requirements of, 359(t)
Chromophobe adenoma, 179, 181
  differential diagnosis of, 183–184
  in Cushing's syndrome, 192
Chronic myeloid leukemia (CML), 341–342
  treatment of, 342
Chronic obstructive pulmonary disease, in geriatric patients, 106
Chronic tophaceous gout, 49
Chylomicrons, properties and composition of, 56(t)
Cirrhosis, hepatic, renal disease in, 474
  in hemochromatosis, 73
CLE. See *Congenital lobar emphysema.*
Clot retraction, measurement of, 363
Clotting, dynamics of, 348, *348*

Clotting factor(s), deficiency of, laboratory characteristics of, 354(t)
CML. See *Chronic myeloid leukemia.*
Coagulation, abnormalities of, 352–360, *353,* 354(t), 359(t)
  anesthetic gas and vapor effects on, 371–372
  mechanism of, *349*
Coal-workers' pneumoconiosis (CWP), 243, 249–252
  anesthetic considerations in, 251–252
  pathogenesis of, 250
  pulmonary function in, 250
Cocaine, abuse of, 734–737, *735*
  intoxication with, anesthetic consideration in, 729–737
  symptoms of, 736
Cogan's syndrome, aortic insufficiency and, 301
Cohn's fraction, for hemophilia, 355
Cold agglutination disease, 333
Colitis, granulomatous, 415
  ischemic, of large intestine, 416–417
  pseudomembranous, 415–416
  ulcerative, 414–415
Collagen diseases, 516–523, *517, 519, 523*
  of the lung, 241–244
Collagen synthesis, disorders of, 69–70
Coma, hepatic, 400
Computerized tomography (CT), for adrenal gland tumors, 193
  for pituitary tumors, 184
  in children, 763
Congenital cystic adenomatoid malformation, vs. congenital diaphragmatic hernia, 144
Congenital diaphragmatic hernia (CDH), 143–146
  anesthetic management in, 145–146
    precautions in, 145–146
  clinical characteristics of, 144
  embryonic development of, 143–144
  postoperative care in, 146
  respiratory distress in, 145
  vs. congenital cystic adenomatoid malformation, 144
Congenital fibrinogen deficiency, 358
Congenital lobar emphysema (CLE), 140–141
  anesthetic management of, 140–141
    review of systems in, 140–141
    technique in, 141
  clinical characteristics of, 140
Congenital lung cysts, in infants, 141
Connective tissue diseases, 508–529
  adrenal competency in, diagnostic tests for, 510
  anesthetic considerations in, 508–509
  anesthetic management of, 509–510, 510(t)
  of the lung, 241–244
  postoperative adrenocortical failure in, 509
Conn's syndrome, 194
  vs. adrenal hyperplasia, 194
Constipation, 390–391
Convulsions, antibiotics and, 593
  prevention of, 88
Copper, body requirement of, 40–41
  deficiency of, 41
  excess of, 41
Coproporphyria, hereditary, 29
Cor pulmonale, 224, 286–290, 289(t)
  acute, 286
  anesthesia and monitoring in, 287–290, 289(t)
  bronchitis and, 286–287
  chronic, 286
  definition of, 286
  in cystic fibrosis, 261

Cor pulmonale *(Continued)*
  in pulmonary alveolar microlithiasis, 234
  types of, 286
  ulcers and, 407
Cori's disease, 20
Coronary artery disease, 279, 281–284, *281,* 282(t)
  anatomical considerations in, 281–282
  anesthesia and monitoring in, 283–284
  Bland-White-Garland syndrome in, 282
  causes of, uncommon, 282(t)
  disease modification of, 281
  familial hypercholesterolemia and, 60
    anesthetic management in, 63–64
  gout and, 49
  in geriatric patient, 113
  physical findings in, 279
  physiology of, 281–283, *281,* 282(t)
Corticosteroid therapy, in adrenocortical hypofunction, 197
  in hypercalcemia, 159
Cortisol, function of, 187
  secretion of, with surgery, 195
  synthetic analogues of, 189, 189(t)
    potencies and half-lives of, 189(t)
Cortisone, withdrawal of, 509
Cough, in pulmonary disease, 222
Coxiella burnetti, metabolic response to, 589
Coxsackie-B virus, cardiomyopathy from, 275
C-peptide test, in islet cell tumors of the pancreas, 213
Cranial (temporal) arteritis, 521–522
  anesthetic management of, 522
CREST syndrome, 569
Creutzfeldt-Jacob disease, 489
Cricoarytenoid arthritis, 513–514, *514*
Crohn's disease, 410–411, 415
Crouzon's syndrome, 580
Cryoprecipitate fractions, for hemophilia, 356, 355(t)
CT. See *Computerized tomography.*
Culdocentesis, in suspected ectopic pregnancy, 92
Curare, in infants, 124, 124(t)
  in renal disease, 469
  lincomycin and, respiratory paralysis with, 591–592
Curling's ulcers, 406
Cushing response, after head trauma, 646–647
Cushing's disease, 191
Cushing's syndrome, 191–195. See also *Adrenocortical hyperfunction; Hypercortisolism.*
Cushing's ulcer, 406
CWP. See *Coal workers' pneumoconiosis.*
Cyclic neutropenia, 340
Cyclohexylamines, abuse of, 740–743, *740, 741*
Cyclophosphamide, pulmonary disease from, 252
Cyclopropane, circulatory effects of, 463
Cyst(s), choledochal, 423
  pancreatic, 419–420
Cystic fibrosis, 259–262
  anesthetic considerations in, 261–262, 438
  biliary disease in, 260
  diagnosis of, 260
  gastrointestinal problems in, 260
  genitourinary problems in, 260
  in adults, 420
  pathogenesis of, 259
  pulmonary function in, 260
  symptoms of, 259–260
  treatment of, 260–261
Cystine, 32
Cystinuria, anesthetic considerations in, 34–35
  cause of, 32

Cystinuria (*Continued*)
  cystine calculi in, 33
  renal disorders associated with, 33

Dantrolene, for malignant hyperthermia, 549, 550
  pharmacology of, 550
Datura arborea, intoxication with, 732
Datura stramonium, intoxication with, 732
Debrancher deficiency, 539–540
Decoppering therapy, in Wilson's disease, 43
Dego's disease, 574–575
Dehydration, in gastrointestinal disorders, 431–432
  in protein-calorie deficiencies, 456
Déjérine-Sottas disease, 492
Deliriants, action of, 713
Delta⁹-3,4-trans-tetrahydrocannabinol (THC), 737,
  738–740, *737*
Demyelinating diseases, 495–496
Deoxyribonucleic acid (DNA), 1
Dermatomyositis, 522–523, *523*
  anesthetic management of, 523
  carcinoma in, 523
  clinical features of, 522
Dermatosis, bullous, of childhood, 565
Dexamethasone suppression study, for adrenocortical
  hyperfunction, 191
Dextrostix, 207
Diabetes insipidus, 181–183
  after hypophysectomy, 184
  after pituitary gland surgery, 186
  drug treatment of, 182
  surgical management of, 182
  tests for, 182
Diabetes mellitus, 204–212
  after pituitary gland surgery, 186
  complications of, 204–205
  definition of, 204
  diagnosis of, 205
  early, late hypoglycemia in, 8
  emergency surgery in, 208
  hemochromatosis and, 73
  hyperglycemia in, drug production of, 206
  hypertension in, propranolol for, 206
  in adrenocortical hypofunction, 190–191
  in geriatric patients, 111
  ketoacidosis in, correction of, 208–209
  pathophysiology of, 204
  pre- and postoperative management in, 206–209
  renal involvement in, 473
  renin deficiency in, 188
  surgery in, 209–213
    anesthetic agents and methods in, 211–212
    hypertension during, 207–208
    insulin after, 210
    insulin during, 206–208, 208(t)
    ketosis following, 207
    management during, 209–210, 212–213
    oral drug cessation in, 210
    premedication and preparation in, 211
    problems during, 210–211
Dialysis, 478–479
  renal transplantation and, 478–481
Diaphragm, trauma to, 660–661
Diarrhea, 391
  causes of, 391
  in carcinoid syndrome, 409
Diazepam, addiction to, anesthesia in, 708–709, *708*
  in hemorrhagic shock, 642

Diazepam (*Continued*)
  in laryngeal papillomas, 132
DIC. See *Disseminated intravascular coagulation.*
Diethyl ether, circulatory effects of, 463
  in diabetes mellitus, 211–212
  in hyperinsulinism, 215
  in infections, 596
  neomycin and, respiratory depression with, 591
Diethyltryptamine, 718–719, *719*
Diffuse esophageal spasm, 402
Diffuse systemic sclerosis, 241–242
DiGeorge syndrome, 161
Digitalis, hypercalcemia and, 166, 167
  in renal disease, 470
  in septic shock therapy, 623, *613*
  toxicity within, in hypercalcemic therapy, 159
DiGuglielmo's disease, 343
Dihydropteridine reductase deficiency, 37(t)
2,5-Dimethoxy-4-ethylamphetamine (DOET), 721,
  721
2,5-Dimethoxy-4-methylamphetamine (STP; DOM),
  721–722, *720*
Dimethyltryptamine, 718–719, *718*
2,3-Diphosphoglycerate (2,3-DPG), 338–339
  abnormal shifts of, 338–339
  production of, 339
Disseminated Intravascular Coagulation (DIC),
  361–363
  causes of, 361–362
  microangiopathic hemolytic anemia and, 335
  therapy in, 363–364, 364(t)
Diuresis, for cystinuric patient, 34
Diverticulum(a), 401
  epiphrenic, 401
  of small intestine, 411–412
  pharyngoesophageal, 401
  supradiaphragmatic, 401
  thoracic, 401
  traction, 401
  Zenker's, 401
  vomiting in, 428
DNA. See *Deoxyribonucleic acid.*
DOET. See *2,5-Dimethoxy-4-ethylamphetamine.*
DOM. See *2,5,-Dimethoxy-4-methylamphetamine.*
Dopamine, in septic shock therapy, 622
Down's syndrome, 70–71, 500–501
  anesthesia in, 71
  immunologic deficiency in, 71
  soft tissues in, 71
2,3-DPG. See *2,3-Diphosphoglycerate.*
Droperidol, circulatory effects of, 464
Drowning, near-, 662–663
Drug(s), antibiotic, pulmonary disease from, 253–254
  antineoplastic, pulmonary disease from, 252–253
  intoxication with, differential diagnosis in, 730–731,
    731(t)
  liver and, 422–423, 424(t)
  psychedelic, abuse of, 711–743, 743(t)
    action of, 712–714
  pulmonary disease from, 252–255
  vasoactive, pulmonary disease from, 254
Drug abuse, dependence produced by, 690, 690(t)
  narcotic, 673–689. See also *Narcotics addict.*
  non-narcotic, 689–710. See also specific drug name.
  abstinence syndromes in, 691
Dubin-Johnson syndrome, 422
Duchenne dystrophy, 531–532
  anesthetic experience in, 532
  cardiac abnormalities in, 531
  cardiac dysfunction in, 532

Duchenne dystrophy (*Continued*)
    female, 531
    Gowers' sign in, 531
    postoperative complications in, 532
    respiratory dysfunction in, 532
    serum enzymes in, 531
Duodenum, disorders of, 405–409
Dwarfism, 578–580
    abnormalities in, 579
    airway management difficulties in, 579
    anesthetic management in, 580
    classification of, 578
Dysfibrinogenemia, 358
Dysostoses, craniofacial, 580–581
        anesthetic management of, 581
    mandibulofacial, 580–581
Dysphagia, in scleroderma, 519
Dysplasia, fibrous, 582–583
Dyspnea, 222
    in choanal atresia, 129
Dystrophic epidermolysis bullosa, dominant, 563
    recessive, 563
Dystrophy, Duchenne, 531–532
    muscular, 530–537

Eaton-Lambert syndrome, 553–554
ECG. See *Electrocardiogram.*
Echinococcosis, of liver, 421
Eclampsia, 87
Ectopic pregnancy, 92–93
Edema, in gastrointestinal malabsorption, 394
    laryngeal, in preeclampsia, 89
    of preeclampsia, 88
Ehlers-Danlos syndrome, 69–70
    anesthesia in, 69–70
    connective tissue failure in, 69
Eisenmenger syndrome, 285
Elderly patient(s). See *Geriatric patient(s).*
Electrocardiogram (ECG), in renal disease, 467
Electrolytes, serum, in renal disease, 456
Elliptocytosis, hereditary, 320
Embden-Meyerhof pathway, 2
Embolism, pulmonary, 227–230
Emphysema, alpha$_1$-antitrypsin deficiency and, 262
    chronic, ulcers in, 407
    in coal miners, 251
    in Marfan's syndrome, 68
    physical findings in, 225(t)
    radiography of, 226
Empty sella syndrome, 184
Encephalopathy, hepatic, 439
Endocardial fibroelastosis, vs. cardiomyopathy, 279
Endocarditis, bacterial, in narcotics addicts, 673–674
Endocrine system, diseases of, anesthesia in, 155–220
    disorders of, in geriatric patients, 110–112
Endoscopy, in major airways trauma, 655
Endotracheal intubation, aspiration pneumonitis
        following, 429–430
    in ectopic pregnancy, 93
    in gastrointestinal disorders, 429–430
        aspiration pneumonitis following, 429–430
        technique for, 429
    in newborn, 127
End-tidal CO_2 determination, in newborns, 127
Energy, metabolism of, 433
Enflurane, in aortic rupture, 659
    in diabetes mellitus, 212
    in infections, 596

Enteritis, actinic, of small intestine, 412
    radiation, of small intestine, 412
    regional, clinical manifestations of, 411
        indications for surgery of, 411
        of small intestine, 410–411
        treatment of, 411
    tuberculous, of small intestine, 411
    typhoid, of small intestine, 411
Enteropathy, protein-losing, 393–394
Environmental disorders, behavioral and, 672–777
Eosinophilic granuloma, 244
Eosinophilic infiltration, of stomach, 407
Eosinophilic lung disease, 235–236
    anesthetic considerations in, 236
    causes of, 236
    chronic, 235–236
Epidermolysis, categories of, 562
Epidermolysis bullosa, 562–564
    acquired, 563
    anesthetic management of, 563–564
        airway care in, 563–564
        friction prevention in, 563
        intubation in, 564
    associated disease states of, 564
    junctional, 563
    nonscarrring, 562–563
    scarring, 563
Epidermolysis bullosa simplex, 562
Epilepsy, in phenylketonuria, 39–40
Epinephrine, anesthesia with, in scleroderma, 520
    in carbohydrate homeostasis, 3
    in septic shock therapy, 624
Erythema multiforme, 566–567
    anesthetic management of, 566–567
Erythema multiforme minor, 566
Erythema nodosum, 572–573
    anesthetic management of, 573
Erythroblastosis fetalis, increased glucose
        concentration and, 8
Erythrocytes, in septic shock, 601
Erythroleukemia, 343
Erythropoietic porphyria, 320
Erythropoietin, 337–339, *338*
    action of, 337
    production of, 337
Escherichia coli, endotoxin effects of, 601, 602
    platelet effects in, 598
Esophageal moniliasis, 403
Esophageal obstruction, 387
Esophageal perforation, 402–403
Esophageal ring, lower, 405
Esophageal webs, 405
Esophagitis, corrosive, 403
    reflux, 403–404
        operative repair for, 404
Esophagus, disorders of, 401–405
        anesthetic considerations in, 436
        systemic disease and, 405
    moniliasis of, 403
    perforation of, 402–403
    spasm of, 402
Essential fructosuria, 11
Estrogen, concentration of, in postmenopausal
        women, 111
    for panhypopituitarism, 185
Ethanol, induction of gout and, 46
Ethchlorvynol addiction, 709, *709*
Ethinamate addiction, 709, *709*
Ethyl alcohol, abuse of, anesthesia in, 691–692, *692*
Ethylene, in infections, 596

Ethylene glycol, nephrotoxicity of, 475
Eventration, 144
Excretory system disorders, in geriatric patients, 108–109
Exophthalmos, 172–173
Exsanguination, 637–644, 637
  anesthetic management in, 641–644
    procedure for, 643–644
    rapid-sequence induction for, 643–644
  fluid volume replacement in, 637–641
    acellular fluid for, 639–641
    acid-base status in, 639
    blood filtration in, 639
    blood for, 638–639
    blood temperature in, 639
    blood type for, 638–639
    citrate intoxication in, 639
    "clear fluid" for, 638, 639–641
    "colloid" solutions for, 639–640
    "crystalloid" solutions for, 639–640
    human plasma for, 640
    human serum albumin solution for, 640–641
    non-protein colloid solutions for, 641
    plasma protein fraction for, 640
    Ringer's lactate solution for, 640
    saline for, 640
  pathophysiologic events in, 637–638, 637
  position for treatment of, 641
  treatment of, diuretics for, 641
    fluid volume replacement for, 637–641
    lower-body compression for, 641
    position for, 641
    vasodilators for, 641
    vasopressors for, 641
Extrahepatic bile duct, carcinoma of, 425–426
Extrahepatic biliary system, disorders of, 423–426
Extremity replantation, 661–662
Eye, disease of, in sarcoidosis, 526
  effect of familial hypercholesterolemia on, 60

Fabry's disease, 575–576
  coronary artery disease and, 281, 283
Factor I, concentrates of, 359(t)
  deficiency of, 358
    genetic pattern of, 359(t)
    laboratory characteristics of, 354(t)
  half-life of, 359(t)
  normal range of, 359(t)
  storage stability of, 359(t)
  surgical requirements of, 359(t)
Factor II, concentrates of, 359(t)
  deficiency of, genetic pattern of, 359(t)
    laboratory characteristics of, 354(t)
  half-life of, 359(t)
  normal range of, 359(t)
  storage stability of, 359(t)
  surgical requirements of, 359(t)
Factor V, concentrates of, 359(t)
  deficiency of, genetic pattern of, 359(t)
    laboratory characteristics of, 354(t)
  half-life of, 359(t)
  normal range of, 359(t)
  storage stability of, 359(t)
  surgical requirements of, 359(t)
Factor VII, concentrates of, 359(t)
  deficiency of, 358, 360
    genetic pattern of, 359(t)
    laboratory characteristics of, 354(t)
Factor VII (Continued)
  half-life of, 359(t)
  normal range of, 359(t)
  storage stability of, 359(t)
  surgical requirements of, 359(t)
Factor VIII, concentrates of, 359(t)
  deficiency of, genetic pattern of, 359(t)
    laboratory characteristics of, 354(t)
  half-life of, 359(t)
  normal range of, 359(t)
  storage stability of, 359(t)
  surgical requirements of, 359(t)
  See also Hemophilia.
Factor IX, concentrates of, 359(t)
  deficiency of, genetic pattern of, 359(t)
    laboratory characteristics of, 354(t)
  half-life of, 359(t)
  normal range of, 359(t)
  storage stability of, 359(t)
  surgical requirements of, 359(t)
  See also Christmas disease.
Factor X, concentrates of, 359(t)
  deficiency of, 358
    genetic pattern of, 359(t)
  half-life of, 359(t)
  normal range of, 359(t)
  storage stability of, 359(t)
  surgical requirements of, 359(t)
Factor XI, concentrates of, 359(t)
  deficiency of, genetic pattern of, 359(t)
  half-life of, 359(t)
  normal range of, 359(t)
  storage stability of, 359(t)
  surgical requirements of, 359(t)
Factor XII, concentrates of, 359(t)
  deficiency of, genetic pattern of, 359(t)
    laboratory characteristics of, 354(t)
  half-life of, 359(t)
  normal range of, 359(t)
  storage stability of, 359(t)
  surgical requirements of, 359(t)
Factor XIII, concentrates of, 359(t)
  deficiency of, 360
  half-life of, 359(t)
  normal range of, 359(t)
  storage stability of, 359(t)
  surgical requirements of, 359(t)
Fallopian tube, pregnancy in, 92
Familial combined hyperlipoproteinemia, 63–64
  anesthesia in, 63
Familial dysautonomia, 502
Familial endocrine adenomatosis type II, pheochromocytoma in, 198
Familial hypercholesterolemia, 60–62
  anesthesia in, 61
Familial hyperlipoproteinemia, cholinesterase levels in, 66
Familial hypertriglyceridemia, 63
Familial hypolipoproteinemias, 66–67
Familial lipoprotein lipase deficiency, 58–60
Familial periodic paralysis, 554–557
Familial type 3 hyperlipoproteinemia, 62–63
Familial type 4 hyperlipoproteinemia, 63
Familial type 5 hyperlipoproteinemia, 63
Farmer's lung, 257
Fasting hypoglycemia, 5
Fat emulsions, complications of, 435
  for nutrition, 397
  for parenteral nutrition, 435
Fat malabsorption, in abetalipoproteinemia, 66

Fatty acids, carbohydrate metabolism and, 54
  metabolism of, 55
Feces, heme precursor and/or converted porphyrin
  in, 27(t)
Felty's syndrome, 336
Fentanyl, acid-base effect of, 431
Fetus, effects of maternal hypotension on, 84
Fever, in septic shock, 598
FFA. See Free fatty acids.
Fibrin stabilizing factor, 359(t)
  concentrates of, 359(t)
  deficiency of, 360
    genetic pattern of, 359(t)
  half-life of, 359(t)
  storage stability of, 359(t)
  surgical requirements of, 359(t)
Fibrinogen, concentrates of, 359(t)
  deficiency of, 358
    congenital, 358
    genetic pattern of, 359(t)
    laboratory characteristics of, 354(t)
  half-life of, 359(t)
  normal range of, 359(t)
  storage stability of, 359(t)
  surgical requirements of, 359(t)
Fibrinolysis, of pulmonary embolism, 228
  primary, in hypovolemic shock, 363
Fibrothorax, physical findings in, 225(t)
Fibrotic lung diseases, 245–259
Fibrous dysplasia, 582–583
Fistulas, 386–387
  biliary, 387
  colonic, 386
  duodenal, 386
  gastric, 386
  gastroileal, 387
  gastrojejunocolic, 386
  pancreatic, 386
  planned, 387
  small bowel, 386
  urinary enteric, 387
Fluid balance, in gastrointestinal disorders, 431, 432
Fluid metabolism, in the newborn, 125
Fluid therapy, intraoperative, in newborns, 127–128
Fluoride, nephrotoxicity of, 475
Folate deficiency, 315–316
  causes of, 315
Folic acid deficiency, in renal failure anemia, 317
Forbes' disease, 539–540
Foreign bodies, of stomach and duodenum, 405
Fractures, basal skull, 647
Frank-Starling function curve, definition of, 288
Frank-Starling mechanism, in aortic insufficiency,
  300
Free fatty acids (FFA), plasma, elevation of, 665
Friedreich's ataxia, 492
Fructose, metabolism of, 11
  inborn errors of, 10–14
  structure of, 10
Fructose intolerance, hereditary, 11
  anesthesia in, 12–13, 14
Fructose-1,6-diphosphatase deficiency, hereditary, 13
Fructosuria, essential, 11
Furosemide, for hypercalcemia, 159

Gaisböck's disease, 347
Galactokinase deficiency galactosemia, 16
Galactose, conversion to glucose of, 14–15

Galactose (Continued)
  metabolism of, inborn errors of, 14–17
  structure of, 10
Galactosemia, galactokinase deficiency, 16
  transferase deficiency, 2, 15, 16
  α-Galactosidase A deficiency, 575–576
Gallbladder, disorders of, 423–426
  in geriatric patients, 110
Gallstone ileus, 423–424
Ganglionic blockers, in renal disease, 469–470
Gangliosidoses, 499–500
Gardner's syndrome, 417
Gas anesthesia, effects of, on human blood, 369–372
  on rat blood, 371(t)
Gastrectomy, for Zollinger-Ellison syndrome, 406
Gastric adenomas, 407
Gastric bypass surgery, for obesity, 454
Gastric dilatation, acute, 390
Gastric volvulus, 408
Gastritis, atrophic, macrocytic anemia from, 436
  corrosive, 405
  granulomatous, 407
  necrotizing, 407
  phlegmonous, 407
  suppurative, 407
Gastrointestinal bleeding, 391–392
Gastrointestinal disorders, 384–449, 389, 433, 395(t),
  398(t), 424(t)
  acid-base status in, anesthetic effects on, 431
    vomiting and, 430–431
  anesthetic considerations in, 426–440
    endotracheal intubation in, 429–430
      aspiration pneumonitis following, 429–430
      technique for, 429
    fluid replacement in, 431–432, 433(t)
    pathophysiologic status of patient in, 426–427
  dehydration in, 431–432
  electrolyte abnormalities with, 432
  extracellular alkalosis in, 432
  fluid abnormalities with, 432
  fluid balance in, 431
  fluid replacement in, requirements of, 432
  in geriatric patients, 109–110
  malnutrition in, 432–433
  metabolic alkalosis in, 432
  parenteral nutrition in, 432–435
    indications for, 433–434
  potassium deficit in, 432, 433(t)
  vomiting in, causes of, 428–429
    complications of, 427
    pharmacologic pretreatment of, 428
Gastrointestinal obstruction, 387–390
Gastrointestinal system, in pregnant patient, 83, 84
Gastroschisis, in infant, anesthetic management of,
  150
  description of, 147
  treatment for, 148
Gastrostomy, in Pierre Robin syndrome, 129
Gaucher's disease, 335–336, 499
Gene mutation, 1
Generalized glycogenosis, 19
Geriatric patient, adrenal gland disorders in, 110–111
  airway management in, 100
  airways of, 105–107
  anesthesia for, body fluid composition and, 99
    body mass and, 99
    general, 115
    hypotensive, 115
    management of, 113–116
      during recovery period, 116
      monitoring in, 114

Geriatric patient (*Continued*)
    pharmacology of, 112–113
      preanesthetic medication in, 114
    progeria and, 99
    regional, 116
    temperature regulation and, 99
    cardiovascular disease in, 101–105
      anesthesia in, 103
    endocrine system disorders in, 110–112
    evaluation of physical characteristics of, 99–101
    excretory system disorders in, 108–109
      anesthesia in, 109
    gastrointestinal system disorders in, 109–110
    hypertension in, 113
    nervous system disorders in, 107–109
      anesthesia in, 108
    nutritional deficiencies in, 110
    organic dementia in, 107
    osteoarthritis in, 100
    ovarian disorders in, 111
    pacemakers for, 103–105
      anesthesia in, 104
    pancreatic disorders in, 111–112
    parathyroid gland disorders in, 111
    physiologic and behavioral responses in, 107
    pituitary gland in, 110
    posture in, 100
    preanesthetic medication for, 114
    pulmonary system of, 105–107
      anesthesia and, 106–107
    surgical and anesthetic risk in, 98
    surgical complications of, 98–99
    testicular disorders in, 111
    thyroid gland disorders in, 111
    total hip replacement in, 101
      anesthesia for, 101
    transurethral resection of prostate in, 109
      anesthesia in, 109
GH. See *Growth hormone.*
Gilbert's syndrome, 422
Glanzmann's disease, 361
Glomerular filtration rate (GFR), anesthesia and, 464, 466(t)
Glomerulonephritis, acute, 470–472
    anesthetic considerations in, 471–472
    renal function tests in, 471–472
  in geriatric patient, 108
  membranous, 471
Glucagon, deficiency of, 6
  in carbohydrate metabolism, 3
Glucocorticoids, hepatic gluconeogenesis and, 6
Glucocorticoid deficiency, effects of, 6
Gluconeogenesis, 3
Glucose, cell transport of, anesthetics and, 5
  requirements of, 2
  structure of, *10*
Glucose metabolism, anesthetic action on, 5
Glucose-insulin-potassium therapy, for septic shock, 623–624
Glucose-6-phosphate dehydrogenase deficiency, 320–321
"Glue sniffing," 710
Glutethimide addiction, anesthesia in, 705, *705*
Glycogenolysis, 3
Glycogen, metabolism of, *538*
  inborn errors of, 17–23
  synthesis of, 17
Glycogen storage diseases, 537–541, *538*
  classification of, 537–541
  type 1, 18
  type 2, 19

Glycogen storage diseases (*Continued*)
  type 3, 20
  type 4, 21
  type 5, 21
  type 6, 23
  type 7, 23
  type 8, 23
Glycogenosis, Cori type I, 537–539
    anesthetic experience with, 538–539
    diagnosis of, 537
    therapy of, 537
  Cori type II, 539
  Cori type III, 539–540
  Cori type IV, 540
  Cori type V, 540
  Cori type VI, 540
  generalized, 19, 539
  type VII, 540–541
  type VIII, 541
  type IX, 541
  type X, 541
Glycosuria, in renal disease, 467
Goiter, nodular, in hyperthyroidism, 170
  toxic, 172
  simple, 175
Goldenhar's syndrome, 581
Goodpasture's syndrome, 255–257
  laboratory findings in, 256
  pathology of, 256
  pulmonary function in, 256
  roentgenography of, 256
  symptoms of, 256
  therapy of, 256
Gorlin formula, 296
Gout, alcohol induction of, 46
  coronary artery disease and, 49
  drugs inducing, 46
  mitral stenosis and, 304
  pathology of, 45
  progression of, 50
  renal disease in, 49, 474
Gouty arthritis, anesthesia in, 53–54
  treatment of, 50–54
Gouty nephropathy, 49
Gowers' sign, in Duchenne dystrophy, 531
Granuloma, cotton fiber, in narcotics addicts, 675
  drug-induced, in liver, 423
Granulomatous colitis, 415
Granulomatous diseases, 524–527, *526*, *527*
Graves' disease, 167
  causes of, 170
  exophthalmos in, 172–173
Growth hormone (GH), in acromegaly, 181
Guillain-Barré disease, 491–492

Hageman factor, 359(t)
  concentrates of, 359(t)
  deficiency of, genetic pattern of, 359(t)
  half-life of, 359(t)
  laboratory characteristics of, 354(t)
  storage stability of, 359(t)
  surgical requirements of, 359(t)
Hailey-Hailey disease, 565
Hairy cell leukemia, 343
Hallervorden-Spatz disease, 489
Hallucinogens, 714–719, *718*, *719*, 717(t)
  action of, 712–713
  anesthesia with, 719–720
  anticholinergic, 730–734, 733(t)

Hallucinogens (*Continued*)
  comparative strengths of, 717(t)
  physiologic and anesthetic considerations in,
    714–717, 717(t)
  sympathetic, 720–724
    intoxication with anesthetic management in,
      722–723
Halothane, cellular effects of, 369, 370
  circulatory effects of, 464
  in aortic rupture, 659
  in diabetes mellitus, 212
  in hemorrhagic shock, 642
  in infections, 596
  in narcotics addicts, 683
  in sarcoidosis, 526–527
  MAC for, in infants, 124
  resistance to infection and, 590
Hamman-Rich syndrome. See *Pulmonary fibrosis,
  idiopathic.*
Hand-Schüller-Christian disease, 244
Hanhart syndrome, 581
Hashimoto's thyroiditis, hyperthyroidism and, 170,
    173
  thyroid antibodies in, 169
  vs. subacute thyroiditis, 173
Hb M syndrome, abnormality in, 324–325
Head trauma, 644–647
Heart, trauma to, 655–658
Heat loss, in infant, during anesthesia, 125
Heavy γ-chain disease, 346
Heinz body anemia, 320
Hemangiomas, of small intestine, 410
Hematemesis, 391
Hematochezia, 392
Hematocrit, in newborn, preoperative, 126, 128
    intraoperative, 128
Hematologic diseases, 313–383
Hematopoietic system, anesthetic agents and,
    369–371
Heme, biosynthesis of, 23–25
Heme precursor and/or converted porphyrin, in urine
    and feces, 27(t)
Hemifacial microsomia, 581
Hemochromatosis, 73–74, 336
  anesthesia in, 73
Hemoglobin(s), abnormal, production of, 324
    saturation curves in, *323*
  amino acid abnormalities of, 325(t), 326(t)
  oxygen dissociation curve and, *323*
  respiratory role of, 322–332, *323*
  sickle, molecular abnormality of, 324
  structure of, 322, *322*
  synthesis of, 322
Hemoglobin SC disease, 332
Hemoglobinopathies, 321–332, *322, 323, 329,* 325(t),
    326(t)
  amino acid abnormalities of, 325(t), 326(t)
  hereditary, molecular changes in, 324–325
Hemoglobinuria, march, 335
  paroxysmal cold, 333
Hemolysis, antibiotic-caused, in glucose-6-phosphate
    dehydrogenase deficiency, 595
Hemolytic streptococcus, in gastritis, 407
Hemophilia, 352–357, *353,* 354(t), 355(t)
  anesthetic considerations in, 356–357
  dental procedures in, 357
  Factor VIII preparations for, 355–356, 355(t)
  genetics of, *353*
  laboratory characteristics of, 354(t)

Hemophilia (*Continued*)
  pain alleviation in, 357
  preoperative preparation in, 356
  replacement therapy for, 355–356
Hemophilia B Layden, 357
Hemophilus influenza, in cystic fibrosis, 260
Hemorrhage, intraventricular, in premature infants,
    139
Hemorrhagic shock. See *Exsanguination.*
Hemostasis, disorders of, 347–360, *348, 349, 353,*
    350(t), 354(t), 355(t), 359(t)
Henoch-Schönlein purpura, renal disease in, 474
Heparin, for disseminated intravascular coagulation,
    363
  for pulmonary embolism, 229
Hepatic coma, 400
Hepatic disease, in alcoholic patient, 693–694, 693(t)
  in narcotics addicts, 676–677
Hepatic encephalopathy, 439
Hepatic fibrosis, 439
Hepatic phosphorylasekinase activity, deficient, 541
Hepatic porphyria(s), biosynthesis of porphyrins or
    porphyrin precursors in, 26, 27(t)
  clinical manifestations of, 26
  description of, 26
  hereditary, 23–31
    anesthesia in, 28(t), 30–31
Hepatitis, drug-induced, 423
  in narcotics addicts, 676–677
Hepatoma, 421
Hepatomegaly, in hereditary fructose intolerance, 12
Hepatophosphorylase deficiency, 540
Hepatorenal glycogenosis, 537–539
Hepatorenal syndrome, 400
Hepatosplenomegaly, in type 1,
    hyperlipoproteinemia, 59
  in Wilson's disease, 42
Hereditary anhidrotic ectodermal dysplasia, 575
Hereditary coproporphyria, pathology of, 29
Hereditary elliptocytosis, 320
Hereditary fructose intolerance, 11
  anesthesia in, 12
Hereditary hemorrhagic telangiectasia, 231, 352, 410
Hereditary hepatic porphyrias, 23–31
Hereditary spherocytosis, 319–320
Hernia, diaphragmatic, 660–661
  paraesophageal, 402
Hers' disease, 23, 540
Heterozygosity, 1
Hirsutism, from adrenal tumor, 194
Histiocytosis X, 244–245
  anesthetic considerations in, 245
  roentgenography of, 244
HLA-B8 antigen, in diabetes mellitus, 204
Homozygosity, 2
Hoover's sign, 223
Hormone therapy, replacement, in
    panhypopituitarism, 185
Hunter's syndrome, 497
Huntington's chorea, 487
Hurler's syndrome, 497
  in coronary artery disease, 282
Hydatid disease of liver, 421
Hydrocortisone therapy, in panhypopituitarism, 185
17-Hydroxycorticoid urinary excretion, test for, in
    adrenocortical hypofunction, 188–189
  in adrenocortical hyperfunction, 191
21-Hydroxylase deficiency syndrome, 188
Hydroxyproline, 31

Hyperalimentation, 434, 435
  CO_2 increase with, 435
  intravenous, metabolic complications of, 398(t)
  parenteral, 457–459, 458(t)
    complications of, 457, 459, 458(t)
  See also *Parenteral nutrition.*
Hypercalcemia, 156–160, 158(t)
  cancer and, 157, 159
  clinical features of, 157
  differential diagnosis of, 158(t)
  digitalis and, 166, 167
  in multiple myeloma, 344
  in sarcoidosis, 239
  thiazide diuretics and, 157
  treatment of, 159–160
    corticosteroids for, 159
    digitalis toxicity in, 159
    furosemide for, 159
    mithramycin for, 159–160
    potassium infusion for, 159
    rehydration in, 159
Hyperceruloplasminemia, 41
Hyperchylomicronemia, 58
Hypercortisolism, management of, 192–195
  pre- and postoperative management of, 192–195
Hypercupriuria, in Wilson's disease, 43
Hyperglycemia, and neonatal intracerebral
      hemorrhage, 8
  drug production of, 206
  halothane and, 10
  in parenteral hyperalimentation, 457
Hyperinsulinemia, insulinomas and, 6
Hyperinsulinism, anesthesia for, 214–215
  in islet cell tumors of the pancreas, 213–215
Hyperkalemia, in adrenocortical hypofunction, 189,
      190
  in blood transfusion, 368
  in parenteral hyperalimentation, 457
Hyperkalemic periodic paralysis, 556–557
  anesthetic considerations in, 557
  myotonia in, 556
  pathogenesis of, 556
  therapy for, 556
Hyperlipidemia, 57
  ileal bypass for, 414
Hyperlipoproteinemia(s), 57
  familial, 58–68
Hyperlordosis, anesthesia in, 67
Hyperparathyroidism, 160–161, 406
  anesthesia in, 165–167
    agents and methods for, 165–166
    operative problems with, 166
      circulatory, 166
      neuromuscular, 166
      respiratory, 166
    postoperative problems with, 166–167
  causes of, 157
  management of, 160–161
    operative, 160
    postoperative, 160–161
  normocalcemic, 159
  osteitis fibrosa cystica and, preoperative treatment
      of, 160
  parathyroid hormone level in, 157
  surgery for, hypoparathyroidism after, 166–167
Hyperphenylalaninemias, 37(t)
Hyperpyrexia, hypoglycemia and, 10
Hypersensitivity, to organic dust, 257–259
Hypersplenism, in cirrhotic liver disease, 439

Hypertension, chronic, in hepatic porphyrias, 26
  hyperuricemia and, 49
  in adrenocortical hyperfunction, operative
      management of, 196
  in alcoholic patients, 695
  in diabetes mellitus, propranolol for, 206
  in geriatric patient, 113
  in hypercortisolism, 193
  in pheochromocytoma surgery, 202
  in preeclampsia, 88
  in primary aldosteronism, 194
  intracranial, in leukemia, 341
  portal, 399–400
  pulmonary, 224
    in narcotics addicts, 675
    primary, 230–231
  whole body irradiation and, 753
Hyperthermia, in epileptic phenylketonuric patients,
      40
  in hereditary anhidrotic ectodermal dysplasia, 575
  in hyperthyroidism, 177
  in osteogenesis imperfecta, 578
  in pituitary gland surgery, 186
  malignant, 545–550, *546*
Hyperthyroidism, anesthesia in, 175–178
    agents and techniques for, 176
    operative problems during, 176–177
    premedication for, 175–176
  antithyroid drugs for, 175
  causes of, 170
  irradiation and, 754
  neonatal, 171
    management of, 172
  occult, crisis of, 172
  operation for, circulatory problems in, 176–177
    hyperthermia during, 177
    hypoxia during, 177
    substitution therapy in, 178–179
  postoperative problems of, 177–178
  preoperative medication for, 170–171
  radioactive iodine uptake test in, 169
  surgical preparation in, 170–171
  T3 excess in, 168
  T4 level in, 167
  thyrotoxic crisis in, postoperative, 177–178
  treatment of, 175
Hypertriglyceridemia, 58
Hyperuricemia, acute gouty arthritis and, 50
  drugs inducing, 48
  etiology of, 45
  hypertension and, 49
  in type 1 glycogen storage disease, 18
Hyperventilation, in the newborn, 121
Hypnosis, in hemophilia, for dental extractions, 357
Hypobetalipoproteinemia, 66
Hypocalcemia, 161–164
  after parathyroidectomy, 160–161
  cardiac effects of, 163–164
  differential diagnosis of, 162(t)
  in parenteral hyperalimentation, 457
  parathyroid hormone levels in, 163, 162(t)
  phosphorus levels in, 161, 163, 162(t)
  symptoms of, after parathyroidectomy, 160
  vitamin D therapy of, 163
Hypocalcemic tetany, postoperative, in
      hyperthyroidism, 178
Hypoceruloplasminemia, 41
  in Wilson's disease, 41, 42
Hypocupremia, in Wilson's disease, 42

Hypoglycemia, anesthesia in, 4, 9–10
  causes of, 5, 6(t)
  central nervous system and, 8
  clinical manifestations of, 8
  definitive therapy for, 9
  extrapancreatic neoplasms and, 7
  factitious, 7
  fasting, 5
  glucose metabolism and, 5–10
  hyperpyrexia and, 10
  in adrenocortical hypofunction, 190
  in alcoholic patients, 696
  in epileptic phenylketonuric patients, 40
  in hereditary fructose-1,6-diphosphatase deficiency,
    13
  in type 3 glycogen storage disease, 20
  ketotic, 6
  neonatal, 6
  reactive, diagnosis of, 8
Hypokalemia, in hypercortisolism, 193
  in parenteral hyperalimentation, 457
  in primary aldosteronism, 194
  in Zollinger-Ellison syndrome, 406
  operative management of, in adrenocortical
    hyperfunction, 196
Hypokalemic periodic paralysis, 554–556
  adrenalectomy in, 556
  anesthetic considerations in, 555
  drug action in, 554
  monitoring of, 555–556
  pathogenesis of, 554
  therapy of, 554
Hypolipoproteinemias, familial, 66–67
    anesthesia in, 63, 67
Hyponatremia, in adrenocortical hypofunction, 189,
    190
  in pancreatic disorders, 438
Hypoparathyroidism, calcium therapy for, 161
  surgical, vitamin D therapy for, 161
  vitamin D therapy for, 163
Hypophosphatemia, in parenteral hyperalimentation,
    457
Hypophysectomy, management of, 184–185
  transsphenoidal, indications for, 185
Hypopituitarism, 179–181
  diagnosis of, 180
  insulin tolerance test for, 180–181
  metapyrone test for, 180
Hypoproteinemia, after intestinal bypass surgery, 454
  enteropathic, 394
  in protein-calorie deficiencies, 457
Hypoprothrombinemia, anesthesia in, 67
Hypotension, in adrenocortical hypofunction, 191,
    197
  in gastrointestinal disorders, 428
  in narcotics addicts, 682, 683–684
  in pheochromocytoma surgery, 202–203
  uteroplacental perfusion and, 84
Hypothalamic pituitary thyroid axis, 169
Hypothermia, in hyperthyroidism, 178
Hypothyroidism, 173–175
  anesthesia in, 178–179
    agents and methods for, 178
    operative problems of, 178–179
    premedication for, 178
  diagnosis of, 174
  irradiation and, 754
  myxedema coma with, 173–174

Hypothyroidism (Continued)
  neonatal, 171
    management of, 171
  postoperative, 172
  preoperative preparation in, 173
  T4 level in, 167
  treatment for, 175
  TSH level in, 168
Hypovolemia, in blood loss anemia, 317
  in ectopic pregnancy, 92
Hypovolemic shock, fibrinolysis in, 363
Hypoxia, in hyperthyroidism, 177

I cell disease, 498
Idiopathic hypertrophic subaortic stenosis (IHSS),
    269, 277–278, 279
Idiopathic pulmonary fibrosis, 245–247
Idiopathic pulmonary hemosiderosis (IPH), 256–257
  anesthetic considerations in, 257
  diagnosis of, 257
Idiopathic thrombocytopenic purpura (ITP), 350,
    350(t)
Idiopathic unconjugated hyperbilirubinemia, 422
IHSS. See Idiopathic hypertrophic subaortic
    stenosis.
Ileojejunostomy, malnutrition after, 453–454
Ileostomy, 387
Ileus, paralytic, 390
    fluid loss in, 431
Inborn errors, of carbohydrate metabolism, 2–17
  of fructose metabolism, 10–14
  of galactose metabolism, 14–17
  of metabolism, 1–68
Incompetent cervix, 93–94
Incontinentia pigmenti, 576
Indocin, for cancer-associated hypercalcemia, 159
Indomethacin, for gouty arthritis, 51
Infants, diseases of, 119–154
  See also Newborns.
Infarction, rarity of, in pulmonary embolism, 228
Infection(s), anemia from, 334
  anesthesia and, leukocyte function in, 590–591
  anesthetic blocks for, 596
  anesthetic choice in, 595–597
  antibiotics for, anesthetic drugs and, 590–595, 594,
    595, 591(t)
  bacterial, in narcotics addicts, 673
  iatrogenic, 588
  metabolic response to, 589
  protein catabolism in, 589
  resistance to, anesthesia and, 589–591
    cyclopropane and, 590
    diethyl ether and, 589
    enflurane and, 590
    halothane and, 590
    ketamine and, 590
    methoxyflurane and, 590
    morphine and, 590
    nitrous oxide and, 590
    pentobarbital and, 589
    thiopental-Innovar-nitrous oxide and, 590
  septic shock with, 597–628
  temperature monitoring in, 596
  whole body irradiation and, 746
Infectious diseases, 588–634, 594, 595, 599, 603, 606,
    610, 612, 614, 616, 617, 608(t), 609(t), 614(t)

Infiltrates, alveolar, in pulmonary disease, 225
  interstitial, in pulmonary disease, 225–226
Infiltrative alveolar disorders, 232–236
Inhalation agents, pharmacology of, in newborns, 124
Inspissated bile syndrome, in newborns, 142
Insulin, deficiency of, in hemochromatosis, 73
  in carbohydrate metabolism, 3
  surgical requirement for, in diabetes mellitus,
    207–208, 208(t)
Insulin tolerance test, for hypopituitarism, 180–181
Insulinoma(s), 213–215
  anesthetic considerations in, 438–439
  diagnosis of, 213–214
  hyperinsulinemia and, 7
  surgery for, 214
Intermittent acute porphyria, biochemical lesion of,
    28
  clinical pattern of, 28
  heme precursors and/or converted porphyrin in,
    27(t)
Interstitial lung disease, physical findings in, 225(t)
Intestinal bypass, problems following, 453–455
Intestine(s), disorders of, in geriatric patients, 110
  large, 414–418
  small, adenocarcinoma of, 409
    benign neoplasms of, 410
    carcinoid of, 409–410
    disorders of, 409–414
    neoplasms of, 409–410
    sarcoma of, 409
    vascular lesions of, 410
Intra-abdominal bleeding, in ectopic pregnancy, 92
Intracranial pressure, acute control of, 647
Intrathoracic airway trauma, 654–655
Intravenous agents, pharmacology of, in newborns,
    124
Intubation, in Pierre Robin syndrome, 130
IPH. See Idiopathic pulmonary hemosiderosis.
Iron absorption, in hemachromatosis, 73
Irradiated patient, anesthesia for, 743–765
Irradiation, adrenal function and, 752–753, 752, 753(t)
  anesthesia and, analgesics with, 761
    barbiturates with, 761
    drug adjuncts with, 761–762
    in experimental animals, 756–761, 757, 758, 759,
      758(t)
    management of, 762–764, 763
    muscle relaxants with, 761
  central nervous system disease and, 755–756
  chloroform and, in experimental animals, 758, 758,
    758(t)
  cyclopropane and, in experimental animals, 759
  diethyl ether and, in experimental animals,
    759–760
  divinyl ether and, in experimental animals, 757,
    757
  enteritis and, 756
  ethylene and, in experimental animals, 760
  for hypercortisolism, 192
  halothane and, in experimental animals, 758–759,
    759
  injury from, trauma and, 764, 764
  kidney function and, 753
  local anesthetics and, 761–762
  myelopathy and, 755–756
  nitrous oxide and, in experimental animals, 760
  of gastrointestinal tract, tolerance doses in, 756
  of heart and pericardium, 750–752, 751, 752, 750(t)

Irradiation (Continued)
  of larynx, 747
  of liver, 753–754
  of lung, 747–750, 749
    pulmonary fibrosis in, 747, 748, 749
    pulmonary function in, 748, 749
    radiation pneumonitis in, 747–749, 750
  of thyroid, 754–755
  organ specific, 746–756
  sickness following, 744, 744(t)
    prodome of, 745
  systemic artery disease and, 755
  tissue protection during, 762
  trichloroethylene and, in experimental animals, 758
  trifluoroethyl vinyl ether and, in experimental
    animals, 757
  whole body, anesthesia and, 764–765
    effects of, 745–746, 744(t)
    high dose, 744(t), 745
    low dose, 744(t), 746
Ischemic colitis, 416–417
Islet cell tumors of the pancreas, 213–215
Isoflurane, in diabetes mellitus, 212
Isopropyl alcohol addiction, 709–710
Isoproterenol, in septic shock therapy, 622–623

Jaundice, 400–401
  in cirrhotic liver disease, 439
  in gallstone ileus, 424
  in newborns, 142
Jimson weed. See Datura stramonium.
Jodbasedow effect, in nodular thyroid disease, 172
Joints, in geriatric patients, 100
Junctional epidermolysis bullosa, 563

Kallikrein(s), 599
  in carcinoid tumors, 410
Kallman's syndrome, 180
Kanamycin, myocardial depression with, 593
Kasabach-Merritt syndrome, 362
Kayser-Fleischer rings, 42
Ketamine, in head trauma, 645
  in hemorrhagic shock, 642, 644
  in infants, 124
Ketoacidosis, diabetic, management of, 206, 208–209
17-Ketosteroid urinary excretion, level of, in
    hirsutism, 194
Ketotic hypoglycemia, 6
Kidney(s), age related changes in, 108
  diseases of, 463–484, 466(t)
  function of, in newborn, 125
Kininogens, 599
Kinins, plasma, in infections, 599, 599
Klippel-Feil syndrome, 501
Krebs cycle, 2
Kveim test, in sarcoidosis, 239
Kwashiorkor, 456
Kyphoscoliosis, in dwarfism, 580

Laennec's cirrhosis, lung disease in, 695
Landouzy-Dejerine muscular dystrophy, 532
Laparoscopy, in ectopic pregnancy patient, 93

Laryngeal edema, in preeclampsia, 89
Laryngeal papillomas, in infants, 130–133
    anesthesia in, induction in, 132
        intubation for, 132
        monitoring of, 132
        premedication for, 132
        technique of, 132–133
    hospitalization for, 133
    intravenous steroids in, 132
    laser removal of, 131
Laryngotracheoesophageal cleft, anesthetic
    management in, 136
Larynx, fracture of, 654
    papillomas of. See Laryngeal papillomas.
Laser(s), CO₂, 131
    intratracheal fires from, prevention of, 131
    precautions during use of, 131
    removal of laryngeal papillomas by, 131
Lead toxicity, anemia from, 334
Leiomyosarcoma, of small intestine, 409
    of stomach, 408
Lethal midline granuloma, 524
    anesthetic management of, 524–525
Letterer-Siwe disease, 244
Leukemia, 340–343
    acute, granulocytopenia in, 341
        presentation of, 341
        pseudomonas septicemia in, 597
        therapeutic agents for, 341
    epidemiology of, 340–341
    hairy cell, 343
    lymphocytic, 342
    mast cell, 573
    monocytic, 342–343
        laboratory findings in, 342
    myelocytic, acute, sideroblastic anemia and, 319
    myeloid, chronic, 341–342
    pathology of, 341
    renal disease in, 474
Leukemic reticuloendotheliosis. See Leukemia, hairy
    cell.
Leukocyte(s), diseases of, 339–347
Leukopenia, anesthetic gases and, 370
    drug-induced, 340
    nitrous oxide and, 369–370
Limit dextrinosis, 20, 539–540
Lincomycin, anesthesia and, respiratory paralysis
        with, 591–592
    cardiac arrest with, 594
Lipase, in fatty acid metabolism, 55
Lipid(s), constitution of, 54
    infusions of, 435
        complications of, 435
    metabolism of, anesthetic drugs and, 64
        inborn errors of, 54–58
Lipid storage myopathies, 541–542
    type I, 541
    type II, 541–542
Lipoprotein(s), properties and composition of, 56(t)
Lipoprotein lipase, 57
Lithium carbonate, for hyperthyroidism, 170
Liver, abscess of, amebic, 420–421
        pyogenic, 420
    carcinoma of, 421
        types of, 421
    diseases of, 399–400
        after intestinal bypass surgery, 454
        anesthetic drug effects in, 440
        drug use in, 423
        gastric disease and, 407

Liver (Continued)
    disorders of, 420–423, 439–440
        in geriatric patients, 110
    drugs and, 422–423, 424(t)
    echinococcosis of, 421
    hydatid disease of, 421
    in abetalipoproteinemia, 66
    in hemochromatosis, 73
    in Wilson's disease, 42
    regeneration of, 422
    resection of, 421–422
Lobectomy, in cystic fibrosis, 261
Locoweed. See Datura stramonium.
Loeffler's syndrome, 235
LSD. See Lysergic acid diethylamide.
Luft's disease, 542
Lung, bullous disease of, 263–264
    collagen diseases of, 241–244
        anesthetic considerations in, 243–244
    of geriatric patients, 105
    of pregnant patient, 82–83, 84
    trauma to, 654–655
Lye solution, esophagitis from, 403
Lyell's disease, 567–568
Lymphoma, Burkitt's, 346
    of small intestine, 409
    of stomach, 408
Lymphoplasmacytic cells, in Waldenström's
    macroglobulinemia, 346
Lyon hypothesis, in female Duchenne dystrophy, 531
Lysergic acid diethylamide, action of, 712–713, 713
    anesthesia with, 717, 719–720
    anxiety from, treatment for, 717
    autonomic effects of, 714
    electrophysiological effects of, 716
    physiologic and anesthetic considerations in,
        714–717
    psychic effects of, 715, 716
    tolerance to, 714–715
Lysine, 32
Lysosomal acid maltase deficiency, 539

Macroglobulinemia, renal disease in, 474
Malabsorption, 392–394
    biliary cause of, 393
    blind loop syndrome, 393
    gastrectomy causing, 392–393
    gastric disorders causing, 392–393
    hepatic cause of, 393
    pancreatic causes of, 393
    protein-losing enteropathic, 393–394
    small intestine causes of, 393
    with diverticula of small intestine, 412
Malignant atrophic papulosis, 574–575
Malignant hyperthermia, 545–550, 546
    anesthetic considerations in, 546
    cardiac dysfunction in, 545
    clinical features of, 545–546
    dantrolene for, 549, 550
    diagnosis of, 547, 548
        biopsy for, 547
        laboratory tests for, 547
    elective anesthesia in, 549–550
    intraoperative management of, 548
    morphological studies of, 547
    pathogenesis of, 546–547, 546
    therapeutic regimen for, 548
Mallory-Weiss syndrome, 385, 405

Malnutrition, in gastrointestinal disorders, 432–433
  in obesity, 453–454
  protein-calorie, 454–457
    anesthetic management in, 456–457
    burn-caused, 454–455
Malt-worker's lung, 258
Marasmus, 456
March hemoglobinuria, 335
Marchiafava-Micheli syndrome, 333
Marfan's syndrome, 68–69
  anesthesia in, 69
  renal disease in, 474
Marijuana, behavioral effects of, 739
  inhalation anesthetics and, 739
  intoxication with, therapy for, 739
  physiological effects of, 738
  use of, anesthetic considerations with, 737–740, 737
Maroteaux-Lamy syndrome, 498
Mass casualties, 663–664
  anesthetic technique in, 664
    drugs for, 664
    personnel for, 664
  fluid resuscitation in, 664
  triage of, 663–664
Mass motor reflexes, in spinal cord trauma, 651–652
Mast cell leukemia, 573
Mastocytosis, 573–574
  anesthetic management of, 574
  pathophysiology of, 573
Maxillofacial trauma, 652–654
McArdle's disease, 22, 540
  vs. central core disease, 544
MDA. See 3,4-Methylenedioxphenylethyl amine.
MEA. See Multiple endocrine adenomatosis syndrome.
Meckel syndrome, 581
Mediastinitis, in esophageal disorders, 436
Megaconical myopathy, 543
Megakaryocytic myelosis, 345
Melena, 391
Melnick-Needles syndrome, 581
Melphalan, pulmonary diseases from, 252
Mendelson's syndrome, 385
Menkes' disease, 41
Menopause, endocrine changes associated with, 111
Meperidine, addiction to, 677
  in infants, 124
Meprobamate addiction, anesthesia in, 706, 706
Mescaline, 719
  ingestion of, anesthesia with, 723–724, 723
Messenger RNA, 1
Metabolic bone disease, 164–165
Metabolism, inborn errors of, 1–68
  regulation of, 3
Metal(s), heavy, nephrotoxicity of, 475
Metapyrone, in adrenal hyperplasia, 193
  in adrenal tumors, 193
  in ectopic ACTH syndrome, 193
Metapyrone test, for hypopituitarism, 180
  in hypercortisolism, 193
Metaraminol, for septic shock therapy, 624
Methadone, for narcotic withdrawal, 685
  narcotic equivalents of, 682, 682(t)
Methaqualone addiction, anesthesia in, 707, 707
Methemoglobinemia, antimalarial-caused, 595
Methimazole, for hyperthyroidism, 170, 175
Methohexital, in hemorrhagic shock, 643
Methotrexate, pulmonary disease from, 253
Methoxyflurane, coagulation changes with, 372
  contraindications to, in gouty arthritis patients, 54

Methoxyflurane (Continued)
  in infections, 596
  nephrotoxicity of, 475
3-Methoxy-4,5-methylene-dioxyamphetamine (MMDA), 722, 722
Methyl alcohol addiction, 709–710
3,4-Methylenedioxyphenylethyl amine (MDA), 722
Methylphenidate, abuse of, 740–741, 740
Methyprylon addiction, anesthesia in, 705–706, 705
Methysergide, pulmonary disease from, 254
Metocurine, in infants, 124, 124(t)
Microangiopathy, in diabetes mellitus, 204
Milk-alkali syndrome, 157
Mineralocorticoid(s) therapy, in panhypopituitarism, 185
Mitochondrial myopathies, 542–543
Mitral regurgitation, 306, 307(t)
  anesthesia and monitoring in, 308–309
Mitral stenosis, 304, 305(t)
  anesthesia and monitoring in, 308–309
  diseases causing, 305(t)
MMDA. See 3-Methoxy-4,5-methylene-dioxyamphetamine.
Mongolism, 500–501
  anesthetic considerations in, 500–501
Morphea, 518, 569
Morphine, analgesic response to, 679
  CNS tolerance to, 679
  experimental addiction to, 675–676, 675, 676
  in infants, 124
  opiate receptors for, 678–679
  tolerance to, 678
Morquio's syndrome, 497
Moschcowitz's disease, 351
Motor neuron degeneration, 489–491
Movement disorders, 485–489
Mucopolysaccharidoses, 496–499
  anesthetic considerations in, 498
  premedication in, 498–499
  preoperative preparation in, 498–499
Mucoviscidosis, of pancreas, 438
Multiple endocrine adenomatosis syndrome (MEA),
  adrenocortical hyperplasia in, 191
  type I, insulinoma in, 214
  type II, 174–175, 181
  type III, pheochromocytoma in, 198
  with pheochromocytoma, 200
Multiple myeloma, 343–345
  amyloidosis in, 344
  hyperviscosity syndrome in, 344
  plasma protein abnormalities in, 343–344
  radiography of, 344
  renal insufficiency in, 344
  symptoms of, 344
Multiple sclerosis, 495–496
  anesthetic considerations in, 496
  clinical course of, 495–496
  pathology of, 495
Multisystem disease, pulmonary disease in, 236–245
Muscle diseases, 530–561, 538, 546
  anesthesia for, general principles of, 530
Muscle phosphofructokinase deficiency, 540–541
Muscle relaxants, antibiotics and, 596
  in renal disease, 469
Muscular dystrophy, 530–537
  Becker type, 532
  distal form of, 533
  Erb's type, 533
  fascioscapulohumeral, 532
  Leyden-Mobius type, 533

Muscular dystrophy (*Continued*)
  limb girdle, 533
  myotonic, 533–537
  ocular, 533
Mushroom-worker's lung, 257
Myasthenia(s), 550–554
Myasthenia gravis, 550–553
  anesthetic considerations in, 551–552
    anticholinesterase in, 552
  cholinergic crisis of, 551
  classification of, 550
  crisis of, 551
  esophageal disturbances in, 405
  extubation in, 553
  intubation in, 552
  pathogenesis of, 551
  pediatric types of, 550–551
  postoperative care in, 552
  pregnancy in, 553
  premedication in, 552
  therapy of, 551
Myasthenic syndrome, 553–554
  carcinoma in, 553
Mycobacteriosis, in silicosis, 248
Mycoplasma pneumoniae, in erythema multiforme, 566, 567
Myelofibrosis, 345
Myeloid metaplasia, 345
Myelomatosis, renal disease in, 474
Myeloproliferative diseases, 340–347
Myocardial contusion, 655–656
Myocardial depression, antibiotic-caused, 593
Myocardial rupture, 656–657
Myocardiopathy, alcoholic, 694–695
Myocarditis. See *Cardiomyopathy, congestive, inflammatory.*
Myocardium, diseases of. See *Cardiomyopathy.*
Myopathy, lipid storage, 541–542
  mitochondrial, 542–543
  myotubular, 544–545
  nemaline, 543–544
  sarcoplasmic, 543–545
Myophosphorylase deficiency, 540
Myositis ossificans, 542
Myotonia atrophica, 533–537
Myotonia congenita, 537
Myotonic muscular dystrophy, 533–537
  anesthetic management of, 535–537
  cardiorespiratory abnormalities in, 534–535
  clinical features of, 534–535
  CNS manifestations in, 535
  muscle pathology of, 533–534
  muscle relaxation in, 536
  postoperative complications in, 536
  pregnancy with, 537
  procainamide for, 535
  respiratory dysfunction in, 536
  somnolence in, 535
  swallowing difficulty in, 535
  therapy of, 535
Myotubular myopathy, 544–545
Myxedema, in geriatric patients, 111
Myxedema coma, 173–174
  symptoms of, 173

Narcotics, addiction and tolerance to, abstinence syndrome in, 679–680, *680*, 684–685, 685(t)

Narcotics (*Continued*)
  addiction and tolerance to, acetylcholine release in, 680–681
    acetylcholinesterase inhibition in, 680–681
    analgesic response in, 679
    catechol metabolism in, 681
    opiate receptors in, 678–679
    single neuron effects in, 678
    theories of, 677–681, *680*
  in hemorrhagic shock, 642
  in renal disease, 468
  opiate receptors for, 678–679
Narcotics abstinence syndrome, 679–680, 684–684, 685(t)
  catechol release in, 681
Narcotics addicts, acute narcotism in, 688–689
  adrenal cortical function in, 677
  anemia in, 677
  anesthetic management of, 673–689
    anesthetic choice in, 682–683
    general, 683
    halothane use in, 683
    maintenance of, 683–684
    methadone for, 682
    premedication in, 681, 682
    regional, 682–683
  atelectasis in, 674–675
  bacterial endocarditis in, 673–674
    anesthesia in, 683
  bacterial infection in, 673
  central nervous system effects in, 677
  false positive serology in, 677
  hematocrit in, 677
  hemoglobin in, 677, 684
  hepatitis in, 676–677
  hyperglycemia in, 677
  hypotension in, 682, 683–684
  infants of, withdrawal in, 687–688, 687(t)
  liver disease in, 676–677
  medical profile of, 673–677, *675*, *676*
  methadone for, 685
  overdose in, treatment of, 688–689
  pneumonia in, 674
  postoperative management of, 684–686, 685(t)
    synthetic analgesics for, 686
  pregnancy and, 686–688, 687(t)
  pulmonary disease in, 674–676, *675*, *676*
  pulmonary hypertension in, 675
  respiratory function in, 675–676, *675*, *676*
  synthetic analgesics for, 686
  tetanus in, 673
  transverse myelitis in, 677
  withdrawal in, 681, 682, 684–686, 685(t)
    clonidine hydrochloride for, 686
Nausea, 385
Near-drowning, 662–663
  associated conditions and, 663
  biochemical disturbances and, 663
  hemolysis and, 663
  hypothermia in, 663
Necrotizing angiitis, 521
Nelson's syndrome, 192
Nemaline myopathy, 543–544
Neomycin, anesthesia and, respiratory depression with, 591
Neonatal hyperinsulinemia, 7
Neonatal hypoglycemia, 6
Neonatal respiratory distress syndrome (RDS), 136–140

Neonatal respiratory distress
syndrome (RDS) (Continued)
  anesthetic management in, 138–140
    fluid therapy in, 139
    general anesthesia for, 139
    intubation in, 139
    monitoring in, 138–139
    respiratory support in, 138
    ventilation in, 139
  bronchopulmonary dysplasia in, 137
  clinical characteristics of, 137
  ductus arteriosus in, 138
  necrotizing enterocolitis in, 138
  postoperative management of, 139
  therapy of, 137
Neoplasm, benign, of esophagus, 404
  of stomach, 407–408
Nephrotic syndrome, 473
  in geriatric patients, 108
Nephrotoxins, 474–476
Neuroectodermal disorders, 502–504
Neuroendocrine system, feedback mechanisms of,
  179, 180
Neurofibromatosis, 503, 571–572
  anesthetic management of, 572
  pheochromocytoma in, 198
Neuroleptanalgesia, in renal disease, 469
Neurological disorders, 485–507
Neuromuscular blockade, treatment for, 592–593
  with antibiotics and anesthesia, 591–593, 591(t)
Neuromuscular blocking agents, acid-base effect of,
  431
  in elderly, 115
Neuromyositis, 522–523, 523
Neuropathy, in diabetes mellitus, 204
Neutropenia, cyclic, 340
Newborns, anatomy of, 119–120
  anesthetic considerations in, 119–129
  anesthetic management of, 126–129
    drug effects in, 86–87
    emergence in, 128–129
    inhalation drugs in, 124
    intraoperative, 126–128
    intravenous, 124
    preanesthetic evaluation in, 126
    relaxants in, 124, 124(t)
  apnea in, 121
  apparent volume of distribution in, 123–124, 124(t)
  atelectasis in, 121–122
  cardiovascular physiology of, 122–123, 123, 123(t)
  cardiovascular system in, 122–123, 123, 123(t), 126
  choanal atresia in, 129
  fluid metabolism in, 125
  heat loss in, 125
  hyperventilation in, 121
  inhalation agents in, 124
  intravenous agents in, 124
  kidney function in, 125
  medical history in, 126
  narcotics withdrawal in, 687–688, 687(t)
  neostigmine in, 124, 124(t)
  oxygen therapy in, 124–126
  pharmacology in, 123–125, 124(t)
  physiology of, 120–123, 121(t), 123(t)
  premature, oxygen therapy in, 124–125
  relaxants in, 124, 124(t)
  respiration in, 119, 120–122
    vs. adult respiration, 121
  temperature regulation in, 125

Niemann-Pick disease, 499
Nitrofurantoin, pulmonary disease from, 253
Nitrous oxide, in acute leukemia, 341
  in bowel obstruction, 437
  in infections, 596
  in reduced renal function, 469
  lincomycin and, respiratory paralysis with, 591–592
  megaloblastic bone marrow depression with,
    369–370
  vitamin B_{12} interaction with, 314–315
Nonphosphorylated lipids, 54
Norepinephrine, fatty acid metabolism and, 54–55
  for septic shock therapy, 624
  in carbohydrate homeostasis, 3
Normokalemic periodic paralysis, 557
Nutmeg, intoxication with, 722
Nutrition, amino acid, for protein sparing, 397
  baseline, 394
  parenteral, complications of, 396, 398(t)
    in gastrointestinal disorders, 432–435
    indications for, 396
  supportive, 394
  surgical, 394–397, 395(t)
    baseline needs for, 394
    elemental diets for, 394–395, 395(t)
    fat emulsions for, 397
    gastrostomy for, 394
    jejunostomy for, 394
    method for, 394
    nasogastric tube for, 394
    parenteral, 395–397
      access routes for, 396
Nutritional disorders, 450–462

Obesity, bypass operation for, 412–414
    complications of, 413
    gastric, 413–414
    methods of, 413
    results of, 413·
  morbid, 450–454
    circulatory function in, 451
    classification of, 451
    functional alterations in, 450–451
    intra-abdominal surgery for, 453
    other nutritional disorders and, 450–462, 458(t)
    preoperative examination of, 453
    pulmonary function in, 451
    respiratory problems in, 451, 453
    surgical problems in, 452–454
Obstipation, 390
Obstruction, bowel, anesthetic considerations in,
    436–437
  closed loop, 388–389
  colonic, 390
  esophageal, 387
  gastrointestinal, 387–390
    pre-induction management in, 428
    vomiting potential of, 428
  intestinal, fluid loss in, 431
  pyloric, 387–388
  small intestine, 388–390, 389
  strangulated, 389
Oculoauriculovertebral dysplasia, 581
17-OHS. See 17-Hydroxycorticosteroid urinary
    excretion.
Omphalocele, in infants, anesthetic management of,
    149

Omphalocele (*Continued*)
  in infants, complications with, 148
    description of, 147
    surgical treatment of, 148
O-negative blood, in hemorrhagic shock, 639
  in mass casualties, 664
"Opium lung," 675
Oppenheim's disease, 488
Oral-facial-digital syndrome, 581
Orthostatic hypotension syndrome of Shy-Drager, 502
Osler-Weber-Rendu syndrome, 410, 437
Osteitis deformans, 581–582
Osteitis fibrosa cystica, bone resorption in, 164
  hyperparathyroidism and, preoperative treatment
    of, 160
Osteodysplasty, 581
Osteogenesis imperfecta, 577–578
  anesthetic management in, 578
Osteogenesis imperfecta congenita, 578
Osteogenesis imperfecta tarda, 578
Osteomalacia, 164–165, 576–577
  alkaline phosphatase excess in, 159
  differential diagnosis of, 165
  steroid-induced, 165
  treatment of, 165
Osteopetrosis, 576–577
Osteoporosis, 164–165, 576–577
  detection of, 164
  differential diagnosis of, 164
  in geriatric patient, 100
  operative management of, in adrenocortical
    hyperfunction, 196
  treatment of, 164
Ototoxicity, amikacin and, 594
  kanamycin and, 594
  streptomycin and, 594
Oxygen therapy, in infants, 124–125
  in premature newborns, 124–125

Pacemakers, electrocautery hazard of, 104
  in geriatric patients, 103–105
  interference with during surgery, 104
Paget's disease, 581–582
  alkaline phosphatase excess in, 159
  aortic stenosis and, 297
  treatment of, 165
Pancreas, deficiency of, causes of, 393
  disorders of, 418–420
    anesthetic considerations in, 438
    in geriatric patients, 110, 111–112
  exocrine disease of, gastric disease and, 407
Pancreatic cysts, 419–420
  true, 419
    vs. pancreatic pseudocysts, 419
Pancreatic juice, 430
Pancreatitis, acute, 418–419
  complications of, 419
  manifestations of, 419
  chronic, 419
  in type 1 hyperlipoproteinemia, 59
Pancuronium, in infants, 124, 124(t)
  in renal disease, 469
Panhypopituitarism, hormone therapy in, 185
  management of, 184–185
Panniculitis, nodular nonsuppurative, 72–73
Papulosis, atrophic, malignant, 574–575
Paraesophageal hernia, 402

Paraldehyde addiction, 709, *709*
Paralysis, periodic, 554–557
  hyperkalemic, 556–557
  hypokalemic, 554–556
  normokalemic, 557
  thyrotoxic, 555
Paralytic ileus, 390
Paramyotonia congenita, 537
Paraplegic syndrome, 494
Parathyroid gland(s), diseases of, anesthesia for,
    155–167
  in geriatric patients, 111
Parathyroid hormone (PTH), assays for, 156
  forms of, 156
  in calcium metabolism, 155–156
  levels of, in hypocalcemia, 163, 162(t)
Parathyroidectomy, for hyperparathyroidism, 160
Parenteral hyperalimentation, 457–459, 458(t)
  complications of, 457, 459, 458(t)
    etiologies of, 458(t)
  total, in infections, 589
Parenteral nutrition, 457–459, 458(t)
  complications of, 434–435, 457, 458(t), 459
  fat emulsions for, 435
    complications of, 435
  indications for, 433–434
  metabolic implications of, 435
  requirements for, 434
  solutions for, 434
Parkinson's syndrome, 486, 488–489
  chemopallidectomy in, 488–489
  metabolic pathology of, 488
Pasteurella tularemia, metabolic response to, 589
PCP. See *Phencyclidine.*
Pectus excavatum, in Marfan's syndrome, 68
PEEP. See *Positive end-expiratory pressure.*
Pemphigoid, 564–566
  anesthetic management of, 565–566
  bullous, 565
  cicatricial, 565
Pemphigus, 564–566
  anesthetic management of, 565–566
  associated disease states of, 565
  familial, benign, 565
Pemphigus erythematosus, 565
Pemphigus foliaceus, 565
Pemphigus vegetans, 564–565
Pemphigus vulgaris, 564
Penicillin, adverse reactions with, 593
Perforations, esophageal, 436
Periarteritis, 521
Periarteritis nodosa, coronary artery disease and, 281,
    283
  renal disease in, 474
Pericardial rupture, 658
Pericardiectomy, special problems with, 295–296
Pericarditis, constrictive, 290, 292(t), 294–296
  anesthesia and monitoring in, 294–296, *294*
  cardiac tamponade and, 290–296, *291, 294,*
    292–293(t)
  causes of, 292(t)
  circulatory therapy in, 295
  vs. restrictive cardiomyopathy, 290
Pericardium, normal function of, 290
Peritonitis, 397
Peutz-Jeghers syndrome, 410, 437
PFC. See *Pulmonary fetal circulation.*
pH, preoperative, in newborn, 126
Phenacetin, as cause of DiGuglielmo's disease, 343

Phencyclidine, intoxication with, 741–743
    anesthesia in, 743
    diagnosis of, 743
    effects of, 742
    therapy for, 743
Phenmetrazine, abuse of, 741, *741*
Phenothiazine, in renal disease, 468
Phenotypic expression, 2
Phenylalanine, 31, 35, *36*
    analgesic properties of, 40
Phenylalanine hydroxylase, 35
Phenylhydrazine, anemia from, 334
Phenylketonuria, 2, 35–40
    anesthesia in, 38–40
    epilepsy in, 39–40
    incidence of, 37
    mental retardation in, 39
    pathology of, 37
    presenting symptoms of, 38
    preventive therapy in, 38
    surgery in, anesthesia for, 39
Pheochromocytoma, 198–204
    anesthesia for, agents and methods of, 201
        monitoring during, 201
        operative problems of, 201–204
        premedication in, 200–201
    cardiac arrhythmia in surgery for, 203
    hypertension in, 199, 200
    hypotension in, 202–203
    laboratory evaluation of, 198–199
    methyltyrosine in, 200
    postoperative problems of, 203
    pre- and postoperative management of, 199–200
    pregnancy precipitation of, 200
    removal of, anesthesia for, 200–204
    surgery for, special preparations for, 203–204
    symptoms of, 198
Philadelphia chromosome, in chronic myeloid
    leukemia, 342
Phlebotomus fever, metabolic response to, 589
Phosphate, for hypercalcemia, 160
Phosphohexoisomerase deficiency, 541
Phospholipase, anesthetics and, 65
Phospholipids, 54, 65
Phosphorus, in hypocalcemia, 161, 163, 162(t)
Pickwickian syndrome, 450, 451
Pierre Robin syndrome, 129–130, 581
    anesthetic management in, 130
Pituitary gland, anterior, diseases of, 179–181
        hyperfunction of, 181
        hypofunction of, 179–181
    diseases of, 179–186
        anesthesia for, 185–186
            preoperative considerations of, 185–186
            postoperative considerations of, 186
    in geriatric patient, 110
    pathophysiology of, 179
    posterior, disorders of, 181–184
    tumor of, 181
        adrenocortical hyperfunction and, 191
        prolactin-secreting, 181
Plasma, fresh-frozen, for hemophilia, 355, 355(t)
    lyophilized, for hemophilia, 355
Plasma cortisol, in adrenocortical hyperfunction,
    191
    in adrenocortical hypofunction, 188
Plasma insulin/blood glucose concentration, in
    carbohydrate metabolism, 4–5
Plasma lipoproteins, in fatty acid metabolism, 55

Plasma thromboplastin component, deficiency of,
    laboratory characteristics of, 354(t)
    See also *Christmas disease.*
Plasmin inhibitor, in primary pulmonary
    hypertension, 230–231
Platelet function, abnormalities of, 349–352
Pleoconical myopathy, 543
Pleural effusion, physical findings in, 225(t)
    radiography of, 226
Pleurisy, in systemic lupus erythematosus, 517
Pleuritic pain, 222
Plummer-Vinson syndrome, 405
PMF. See *Progressive massive fibrosis.*
Pneumatosis cystoides intestinalis, 412
Pneumoconioses, 247–252
    coal-workers', 249–252
    graphite, 251
    other, 251
Pneumocystis carinii, pulmonary alveolar proteinosis
    with, 233
Pneumoencephalogram, in empty sella syndrome,
    184
Pneumomediastinum, 658
Pneumonia, in geriatric patients, 106
    in narcotics addicts, 674
Pneumothorax, physical findings in, 255(t)
    radiography of, 226
Poiseuille's law, 285
Poisonous compounds, abuse of, 710
Polyarteritis nodosa, 521
    anesthetic management of, 522
    clinical features of, 521
Polyarthralgia, in hemochromatosis, 73
Polyarthritis, after intestinal bypass surgery, 454
Polycystic ovarian disease, hirsutism from, 194
Polycythemia, 346–347
    primary, 346–347
    pseudo-, 347
    secondary, 347
Polymyositis, 522–523, *523*
Polyneuropathies, chronic, 492
Pompe's disease, 19, 277, 539
    aortic stenosis and, 297
Porphyria(s), anesthetic drugs for, 28(t)
    care of skin in, 30
    drug-induced, 29, 29(t)
    heme precursor and/or converted porphyrin in,
        27(t)
    hepatic, hereditary, 23–31
    intermittent acute, 28
    undetected, anesthesia and, 31
    variegate, pathology of, 28
Porphyrin(s), 23
Portal hypertension, 399–400
    etiology of, 399
    surgical therapy for, 399–400
        fresh blood transfusion in, 400
Positive end-expiratory pressure (PEEP), in
    pulmonary hypertension, 289
Potassium, deficits of, in gastrointestinal disorders,
    432, 433(t)
    infusion of, for hypercalcemia, 159
Preeclampsia, 87–88
    anesthetic considerations in, 89–90
    blood volume in, 89
    pathophysiologic alterations of, 88
    therapy of, 88–89
Pregnancy, disorders of, 87–94
    ectopic, 92–93

Pregnancy (*Continued*)
  in myasthenia gravis, 553
  in myotonic muscular dystrophy, 537
  pheochromocytoma precipitation by, 200
  physiologic alterations of, anesthesia and, 83–84
    clinical application of, 83–84
  thyrotoxicosis during, management of, 170–171
  toxemia of, 87–90
  tubal, anesthesia for, 92–93
    hemorrhagic shock in, 92
Pregnant patient, 81–87
  anesthesia for, 81–87
  blood volume in, 81
  cardiac output of, 82
  cardiovascular changes in, 81–82
  cardiovascular disease in, 83–84
  gastrointestinal system of, 83, 84
  narcotics addiction and, 686–688, 687(t)
  respiratory system in, 82–83, 84
  uteroplacental perfusion in, 84–86
  vena caval occlusion in, 85
Preludin. See *Phenmetrazine*.
Premature newborns, oxygen therapy in, 124–125
Primary sclerosing cholangitis, 425
Proaccelerin, concentrates of, 359(t)
  deficiency of, genetic pattern of, 359(t)
  half-life of, 359(t)
  normal range of, 359(t)
  storage stability of, 359(t)
  surgical requirements of, 359(t)
Probenecid, in treatment of gouty arthritis, 51
Procainamide, in malignant hyperthermia, 550
  in myotonic muscular dystrophy, 535
Procarbazine, pulmonary disease from, 253
Proconvertin, concentrates of, 359(t)
  deficiency of, genetic pattern of, 359(t)
  half-life of, 359(t)
  normal range of, 359(t)
  storage stability of, 359(t)
  surgical requirements of, 359(t)
Progeria, 99
Progressive massive fibrosis (PMF), 250
Progressive systemic sclerosis, 518–519, *519*
Prolactin-secreting tumors, 181
Proline, 31
Propoxyphene, addiction to, 689
Propranolol, for hyperthyroidism, 170
Propylthiouracil, for hyperthyroidism, 170, 175
Prostate, transurethral resection of, in geriatric
    patient, 109
Prostatism, in geriatric patients, 108
Proteins, 31
Proteinuria, in preeclampsia, 88
  in renal disease, 467
Prothrombin, concentrates of, 359(t)
  deficiency of, genetic pattern of, 359(t)
    laboratory characteristics of, 354(t)
  half-life of, 359(t)
  normal range of, 359(t)
  storage stability of, 359(t)
  surgical requirements of, 359(t)
"Prune belly." See *Abdominal muscle deficiency
    syndrome*.
Pseudogout, acute arthritis in, 52
Pseudohemophilia A, laboratory characteristics of,
    354(t)
Pseudohemophilia B, laboratory characteristics of,
    354(t)
Pseudohypoparathyroidism, 163

Pseudomembranous colitis, 415–416
Pseudomonas, endocarditis with, in narcotics addicts,
    674
  in cystic fibrosis, 260
Pseudomonas aeruginosa, endotoxins of, 598
Pseudopolycythemia, 347
Psilocybin, 714, 718, *718*
Psoriasis, 571
Psoriatic erythroderma, 571
PTA, concentrates of, 359(t)
  deficiency of genetic pattern of, 359(t)
  half-life of, 359(t)
  normal range of, 359(t)
  storage stability of, 359(t)
  surgical requirements of, 359(t)
PTH. See *Parathyroid hormone*.
Pulmonary alveolar microlithiasis, 233–234
  roentgenography of, 234
Pulmonary alveolar proteinosis, 232–233, 234–235
  anesthetic considerations in, 234–235
  bronchopulmonary lavage for, 234–235
  laboratory investigation of, 233
  pathological changes in, 232–233
  roentgenography of, 233
  symptoms of, 233
  treatment of, 233
Pulmonary arteriovenous fistula, 231–232
  anesthetic considerations in, 232
  laboratory examination in, 232
  roentgenography of, 232
  symptoms of, 232
Pulmonary disease, antibiotic-induced, 253–254
    anesthetic considerations in, 254–255
  antineoplastic-drug-induced, 252–253
    anesthetic considerations in, 254–255
  L-asparaginase-induced, 253
  azathioprine-induced, 253
  bleomycin-induced, 252
  bullous, 263–264. See also *Lung*.
  busulfan-induced, 252
  chlorambucil-induced, 252
  cyclophosphamide-induced, 252
  drug-induced, 252–255
  gastric disorder and, 407
  general considerations of, 222–227
  history of, 222
    chest pain in, 222
    cough in, 222
    dyspnea in, 222
    sputum in, 222
  in alcoholic patients, 695, 695(t)
  in dermatomyositis, 522–523
  in geriatric patients, 105–107
  in multisystem diseases, 236–245
  in narcotics addicts, 675–676, *675, 676*
  in polyarteritis nodosa, 521
  in sarcoidosis, 525–526
  intraoperative monitoring of, 227
  melphalan-induced, 252
  methotrexate-induced, 253
  methysergide-induced, 254
  nitrofurantoin-induced, 253
  obstructive, 259–263
  P-A chest films for, 224–225
  physical examination in, 222–224
    breath sounds in, 223–224, 223(t), 225(t)
    chest inspection in, 223
    general observation in, 222–223
    vocal fremitus in, 223

Pulmonary disease (*Continued*)
  physical findings in, outline of, 225(t)
  preoperative preparation in, 227
  procarbazine-induced, 253
  radiation-induced, 254
    anesthetic considerations in, 254–255
  radiography for, 224–226
    alveolar infiltrates on, 225
    atelectasis on, 226
    chest film in, 224–225
    emphysema on, 226
    interstitial infiltrates on, 225–226
    pleural effusion on, 226
    pneumothorax on, 226
    pulmonary embolus on, 226
    specialized tests for, 227
    sulfonamide-induced, 253
    vascular, 227–232
    vasoactive-drug-induced, 254
  anesthetic considerations in, 254–255
Pulmonary edema, physical findings in, 225(t)
Pulmonary embolectomy, for pulmonary embolism, 229
Pulmonary embolism, 227–230
  anesthetic considerations in, 229–230
  conditions causing, 228
  diagnosis of, 228, 229
  in blood transfusion, 369
  laboratory tests for, 229
  physiologic effects of, 228
  radiography of, 226
  resolution of, 228
  risk factors of, 228
  surgery for, 229
    anesthesia in, 229–230
  treatment of, 229
Pulmonary fetal circulation (PFC), therapy of, 146
Pulmonary fibrosis, idiopathic, 245–247
  anesthetic considerations in, 246–247
  histology of, 245
  pathogenesis of, 245
  roentgenography of, 246
  symptoms of, 246
  treatment of, 246
  physical findings in, 225(t)
Pulmonary function, in allergic alveolitis, 258
  in bullous disease of the lung, 264
  in cystic fibrosis, 260
  in Goodpasture's syndrome, 256
  in myotonic muscular dystrophy, 534–535
  in obesity, 451
  in sarcoidosis, 525–526, 527
  in scleroderma, 519
  in silicosis, 248
Pulmonary function testing, 226–227
  in histiocytosis X, 245
  in sarcoidosis, 239
  in systemic sclerosis, 242
  obstructive pattern of, 226
  restrictive pattern of, 226–227
Pulmonary hemosiderosis, idiopathic, 256–257
Pulmonary hypertension, 224, 284–286, 284(t)
  anesthesia and monitoring in, 287–290, 289(t)
  cor pulmonale and, 284–290, 284(t), 289(t)
  pathologic causes of, 284, 284(t)
  primary, 230–231
    anesthetic considerations in, 231
    clinical features of, 230
    diagnosis of, 230–231

Pulmonary hypertension (*Continued*)
  primary, pathologic findings in, 230
    roentgenography of, 230
    treatment of, 231
  secondary, in pulmonary alveolar microlithiasis, 234
  symptoms of, 285
Pulmonary sequestration. See *Congenital lung cysts.*
Pulmonic stenosis, 297, 300, 299(t)
  diseases causing, 299(t)
Pulmonary vascular pharmacopeia, 289(t)
Pulmonary vascular resistance, 224–225
Pulmonic insufficiency, 301, 303(t), 304
  anesthesia and monitoring in, 308–309
  diseases causing, 303(t)
Pulmonic stenosis, anesthesia and monitoring in, 308–309
  causes of, 299(t)
  compensatory mechanisms in, 300
Purine, biosynthesis of, 45, *46*
Purpura, allergic, 351
  anesthetic considerations in, 351–352
  idiopathic thrombocytopenic, 350, 350(t)
  infectious, 351
  nonthrombocytopenic, 351
  post-transfusion, 351
  thrombocytopenic, 349–351, 350(t)
    idiopathic, 350, 350(t)
    neonatal, 351
    secondary, 350–351
    thrombotic, 351
Pyelonephritis, 472
  differential diagnosis of, 472
Pyloric obstruction, 387–388
Pyridoxine, deficiency of, 459

Rad(s), definition of, 744
Radiation, ionizing, LD_{50} of, 743
  pulmonary disease from, 254
  See also *Irradiation.*
Radioactive iodine, for hyperthyroidism, 175
Radioactive iodine uptake (RAIU), for thyroid function test, 168–169
Radiologic contrast material, nephrotoxicity of, 475
Radiological procedures, anesthesia for, 762–764, 763
RAIU. See *Radioactive iodine uptake.*
Raynaud's phenomenon, in scleroderma, 519, 520
  in systemic lupus erythematosus, 241
RDS. See *Neonatal respiratory distress syndrome.*
Reactive hypoglycemia, diagnosis of, 8
Rectal bleeding, 391–392
Red cell, production of, 338
Reflex apnea, in tracheal esophageal fistula, 135
Reiter's syndrome, 513
Relaxants, pharmacology of, in newborns, 124, 124(t)
Renal blood flow (RBF), depression of, 463–464
  age related changes in, 108
Renal calculi, in ileostomy, 387
Renal colic, cystinuria and, 33
Renal disease(s), 463–484, 466(t)
  antihypertensives in, 470
  in diabetes mellitus, 473
  in geriatric patients, 108–109
  in gout, 49, 474
  in periarteritis nodosa, 474
  in systemic lupus erythematosus, 474

Renal disease(s) (*Continued*)
  neuromuscular blockade resolution and, 593
  toxin-caused, 474–476
Renal dysfunction, in Wilson's disease, 42
Renal failure, acute, 476–478
    emergency surgery in, 478
    nonoliguric, 477
    prerenal causes of, 477–478
    urinary output in, 477–478
  in diabetes mellitus, 204
  in liver disease, 439
Renal function, after transplantation, 481
  depression of, 463
  evaluation of, in diabetic patient, 206
  impaired, diagnosis of, 465, 467
    in paraplegic syndrome, 494
    in rheumatoid arthritis, 512
    in scleroderma, 519
    in systemic lupus erythematosus, 517
  normal, anesthetic effects on, 463–465, 466(t)
    antidiuretic hormone and, 464
    circulatory effects on, 463–464, 466(t)
    endocrine system effects on, 464–465, 466(t)
    sympathetic nervous system effects on, 464,
      466(t)
  reduced, anesthetic agents in, 468–470
    antihypertensives in, 470
    digitalis in, 470
    drug alterations in, 457–470
    ganglionic blockers in, 469–470
    inhalation agents in, 468–469
    intravenous agents in, 469
    muscle relaxants in, 469
    premedicant agents in, 468
    vasopressors in, 470
  studies of, interpretation of, 465, 467
Renal osteodystrophy, 165
Renal papillary necrosis, 472
Renal transplantation, 479–481
  donor for, anesthetic management of, 479
    preoperative treatment of, 479
  recipient of, anesthetic management of, 480–481
Rendu-Osler-Weber's disease, 231, 232
Renin, plasma, in primary aldosteronism, 194
  secretion of, failure of, 188
    in anesthesia, 465
Renin-angiotensin system, during anesthesia, 465
Replantation, extremity, 661–662
Respiration, in newborns, 119, 120–122
  vs. adult, 121
  in pregnant patient, 83
Respiratory dysfunction, in Duchenne dystrophy, 532
  in myotonic muscular dystrophy, 534–535
Respiratory obstruction, in tracheal esophageal
  fistula, 135
Respiratory paralysis, treatment for, 592
Respiratory system, embryonic development of, 133,
    136–137
  in paraplegic syndrome, 494
  in pregnant patient, 82–83, 84
  obstruction of, in hyperthyroidism, 177
  problems of, in hyperthyroidism, 178
Retina, in abetalipoproteinemia, 66
Retinopathy, in diabetes mellitus, 204
Retrolental fibroplasia, in newborn, 124
Rheumatoid arthritis, 510–512, *511*
  amyloidosis in, 512
  anemia in, 512, 516
  anesthetic management of, 513–516, *514, 515*

Rheumatoid arthritis (*Continued*)
  clinical picture of, 511–512
  etiology of, 510
  of cervical spine, 515
  pathology of, 511, *511*
  pulmonary manifestations of, 511–512
  renal disease in, 473–474
  renal function in, 512
  salicylates in, 512
  subcutaneous nodules in, 512
  treatment of, 512
Rheumatoid disease, of lungs and pleura, 242–243
    anesthetic considerations in, 243–244
    arteritis in, 243
Rheumatoid factor, in sarcoidosis, 239
  in systemic sclerosis, 241
"Rheumatoid lung," 511
Rheumatoid pneumoconiosis, 250
Riboflavin, deficiency of, 459
Ribonucleic acid, 1
Rickets, 460
Right ventricular hypertrophy (RVH), 224
Riley-Day syndrome, 502
Ritalin. See *Methylphenidate.*
Ritter's disease, 568
RLF. See *Retrolental fibroplasia.*
RNA. See *Ribonucleic acid.*
Rocaltrol, for hypoparathyroidism, 161
Roentgen (R), definition of, 744
RVH. See *Right ventricular hypertrophy.*

Salicylates, platelet function and, 512
Salmonella, endotoxins of, 598
Salpingitis, and ectopic pregnancy, 92
Sanderhoff's disease, 499
Sanfilippo's syndrome, 497
Sarcoidosis, 238–240, 525–527, *526, 527*
  anesthetic considerations in, 239–240
    cardiac system and, 240
    renal function and, 240
  anesthetic management of, 526–527, *527*
  aortic stenosis and, 297
  calcium absorption in, 157
  cardiac, 526, *526*
  clinical features of, 239, 525–526
  diagnosis of, 526
  laboratory investigation of, 239
  mitral stenosis and, 304
  pathology of, 525
  pulmonary function changes in, 239
  renal disease in, 474
  roentgenography of, 238
Sarcoma, of small intestine, 409
  of stomach, 408
Schaumann's fever, 525–527, *526, 527*
Scheie's syndrome, 498
Schistosomiasis, of large intestine, 417
Schmidt's syndrome, 188
Schönlein-Henoch syndrome, 351
Scleredema, 520
  anesthetic management of, 520–521
Scleredema adultorum of Buschke, 520
Sclerodactyly, in scleroderma, 519
Scleroderma, 241–242, 518–519, *519*, 569–570
  anesthetic management of, 520–521, 570
  cardiac function in, 519
  clinical features of, 518–519

Scleroderma (*Continued*)
  diffuse, 569
  esophageal disturbances in, 405
  localized, 569
  regional anesthesia in, 520
Sclerosteosis, 577
Scoliosis, in dwarfism, 580
  in Marfan's syndrome, 68
Scopolamine, intoxication with, 730, 730(t)
Scurvy, 460
Sella turcica, abnormal, 183–184
  in adrenocortical hyperfunction, 192
Senile muscle atrophy, 101
Sepsis, causes of, 597
  examination for, in newborn, 126, 127
  gram-negative, 604–607
    blood lactate levels in, 605
    coagulation changes in, 605
    electrolyte pattern of, 604
    glucose tolerance curve in, 605
    in infants, 607
    jaundice in, 607
    laboratory findings in, 605–606
    physical findings in, 605–606
    vs. gram-positive, 608–609, 609(t)
  gram-positive, 607
    vs. gram-negative, 608–609, 609(t)
  hemodynamic changes in, 607–615, *610, 612, 613,
    614,* 609(t), 614(t)
  hyperalimentation and, 435
  pathogens in, 597, 597(t)
  rickettsial, 607
  tetanus, 607
  viral, 607
Septal rupture, 657
Septic shock, anesthesia in, 597–628, 626–629
    barbiturates in, 628
    diazepam for, 628
    diethyl ether for, 628
    ethylene for, 628
    fentanyl-oxygen for, 628
    general, 627–629
    ketamine for, 628
    nitrous oxide for, 628
    preoperative considerations in, 626–627
    scopolamine for, 628
  anesthetic block in, epidural, 627
    spinal, 627
  arteriovenous shunting in, 611, 615–616, *616, 617*
  AV O_2 difference vs. peripheral resistance in, *616*
  capillary blood flow and cardiac index in, *617*
  cardiac function in, 609–610, *610*
  cardiac index in, *616*
    oxygen consumption vs., *616*
  cirrhosis with, 611
  clinical findings in, 608(t)
  heart failure in, 611–612, *612*
    glucose-insulin-potassium therapy in, 612–613,
      614, 614(t)
    inotropic therapy for, 612, *613*
  hemodynamic changes in, 607–615, *610, 612, 613,
    614,* 609(t), 614(t)
  intravascular coagulation in, 603
  lactic acidosis in, 616–617, *617*
  multiple sclerosis with, 611
  myocardial depressant factor in, 617–618
  pathophysiology of, 598–604, *599, 603*
    capillary morphology in, 602
    cell metabolism effects of, 600

Septic shock (*Continued*)
  pathophysiology of, clotting system in, 603–604
    controversial areas in, 615–618, *616, 617*
    erythrocyte effects in, 601
    fever in, 598
    microcirculation effects in, 601–602
    plasma effects in, 598–599
    platelet and leukocyte effects in, 598
    regional blood flow effects in, 602
    reticuloendothelial system effects of, 600–601
    serum complement effects in, 599
    sympathetic system effects in, 601
    venous return in, 602–603, *603*
  respiratory function in, vs. hemorrhagic shock, 606,
    606
  reticuloendothelial system in, 600–601
  steroids for, actions of, 621
  systemic resistance measure in, 619
  therapy for, 618–624
    acidosis and, 620
    anti-inflammatory drugs in, 625–626
    aprotinin in, 625
    chlorpromazine in, 625
    dextran in, 625
    digitalis in, *613,* 623
    dopamine in, 622
    experimental drugs and adjuncts to, 624–626
    glucose-insulin-potassium solution for, 623–624
    inotropic, 621–624
    isoproterenol in, 622–623
    monitoring of, 618–619
    nitrol paste in, 625
    respiratory failure and, 619
    steroids in, 620–621
    α_2-surface binding globulin in, 626
    vasodilation, 624–625
    vasopressor drugs for, 624
    volume deficits and, 619–620
  tissue hypoxia in, 616–617, *617*
  types of, 604–607
  vs. hemorrhagic shock, 606, *606*
  vs. myocardial infarction, 607
Serotonin, abnormalities of, in mongolism, 500
  in carcinoid syndrome, 409
  in carcinoid tumors, 410, 437, 438
  release of, in pulmonary embolism, 228
Shivering, postoperative, in myotonic muscular
  dystrophy, 536
Shock, bacteremic, 604–607
  hemorrhagic, in tubal pregnancy, 92
    sodium thiopental in, 642–643
  hypovolemic, fibrinolysis in, 363
  septic, 597–628, 626–629
Shwartzman reaction, generalized, 361–362
Shy-Drager syndrome, 502
  Sia test, in Waldenström's macroglobulinemia,
    346
SIADH. See *Syndrome of inappropriate ADH
  secretion.*
Sickle cell anemia, 325, 327–331, *329*
  coronary artery disease and, 281, 283
  renal disease in, 474
Sickle cell trait, 327
Silicoproteinosis, 248
Silicosiderosis, 251
Silicosis, 247–248
  connective tissue disorders in, 248
  diagnosis of, 248
  in coal miners, 251

Silicosis (*Continued*)
  pathogenesis of, 247–252
  pulmonary function in, 248
  roentgenography of, 248
  symptoms of, 248
  therapy of, 248
Sipple's syndrome, pheochromocytoma in, 198
Sjögren's syndrome, 513, *513*, 516, 570
Skeletal muscle, biochemical action in, 546, *546*
  in geriatric patients, 100
Skeleton, in Down's syndrome, 71
  in Marfan's syndrome, 68
Skin, in geriatric patients, 100
  in hemochromatosis, 73
  in phenylketonuric patients, 40
Skin and bone disorders, 562–587
Skull, trauma to, 647
SLE. See *Systemic lupus erythematosus.*
Small bowel, resection of, gastric disease and, 407
Small intestine, obstruction of, 388–390, *389*
    causes of, 388
    pathology of, 388, *389*
    surgical management of, 389–390
Solvent abuse, 710, 710(t)
Sorbitol, functions of, 10
Spherocytosis, hereditary, 319–320
Spinal cord trauma, 494–495, 647–652
Spinal stenosis, in dwarfism, 579
Spinocerebellar degeneration, 492–493
Splenectomy, in hereditary spherocytosis, 320
Splenomegaly, in type 3 glycogen storage disease, 21
Spondylosis, cervical, anesthesia, in, 514–515, *515*
Sputum, in pulmonary disease, 222
Stannosis, 251
Staphylococcal scalded-skin syndrome, 568
Staphylococcus aureus, in psoriasis, 571
  in staphylococcal scalded-skin syndrome, 568
  infection with, in narcotics addicts, 673, 674
Starvation, metabolism during, 433
Status marmoratus, 489
Steinert's disease, 533–537
Stenosis, valvular, grading of, 296
Steroids, adrenocortical, after pituitary gland surgery,
      186
    for myxedema coma, 174
  adrenocortical hyperfunction with, 191
  adrenocortical hypofunction with, 188
  in adrenocortical hypofunction, 190, 190(t)
  intravenous, in laryngeal papillomas, 132
Stevens-Johnson syndrome, 565
Stomach, disorders of, 436
  in geriatric patients, 110
  neoplasms of, 407–408
Stomach and duodenum, disorders of, 405–409
STP. See *2,5,-dimethoxy-4-methylamphetamine.*
Streptomycin, myocardial depression with, 593, *594*
Stress ulcers, 406–407
Stricture, reflux, 404
Stuart factor, concentrates of, 359(t)
  deficiency of, 358
    genetic pattern of, 359(t)
  half-life of, 359(t)
  normal range of, 359(t)
  storage stability of, 359(t)
  surgical requirements of, 359(t)
Sturge-Weber disease, 502, 503
Succinylcholine, in hallucinogenic intoxication, 717,
    720

Succinylcholine (*Continued*)
  in infants, 124, 124(t)
  in renal disease, 469
  spinal cord trauma and, 652
Sudden death, from hydatid disease, 421
  in primary pulmonary hypertension, 231
Suicide rate, in anesthetists, 371
Sulfonamide(s), nephrotoxicity of, 475
  pulmonary disease from, 253
Sulfones, anemia from, 334
Superior caval syndrome, from goiters, 175
Supine hypotensive syndrome, 85
Surgical nutrition, 394–397, 395(t)
Surgical traction, in gastrointestinal disorders, 428
Sydenham's chorea, 486–487
Sympathetic nervous system, in metabolic process, 3
  in septic shock, 601
Syndrome of inappropriate ADH secretion, 183
Syphilis, gastric lesions in, 407
Syringomyelia, 493–494
Systemic lupus erythematosus (SLE), 240–241
  anesthetic considerations in, 243–244
  anesthetic management of, 518
  aortic insufficiency and, 301
  clinical course of, 518
  clinical features of, 517–518, *517*
  lung and pleura involvement in, 241
  pleurisy in, 517
  pulmonary function tests in, 241
  renal disease in, 474
  renal function in, 517
Systemic sclerosis, diffuse, 241–242
  anesthetic considerations in, 243–244
  organ involvement in 242
  pulmonary function tests in, 242
  pulmonary pathology in, 241–242
  treatment of, 242

T3. See *Triiodothyronine.*
T3-RIA test, for thyroid function, 168
T4. See *Tetraiodothyronine.*
T4-RIA test, thyroid function by, 167–168
Tamponade, atrial rupture and, 656
  cardiac, 656–657
    anesthetic considerations in, 656–657
Tangier disease, 66
Tauri, 540–541
Tay-Sachs disease, 499
TBG. See *Thyroid binding globulin.*
TEF. See *Tracheal esophageal fistula.*
Temperature, in newborn, 125, 126–127
  in protein-calorie deficiencies, 456–457
Temporomandibular joint, gouty arthritic
    involvement of, 54
Tendons, xanthomas of, in familial
    hypercholesterolemia, 60
Teratogenicity, anesthetic drugs and, 86–87
Testes, disorders of, in geriatric patients, 111
Testosterone therapy, in, panhypopituitarism, 185
Tetanus, 607
  in narcotics addicts, 673
Tetracycline, myocardial depression with, 593, *594,*
    595
  neuromuscular blockage with, 592
Tetracycline steatosis, 423

Tetraiodothyronine (T4), 167, *168*, 169
  deiodination of, 167, *168*
Tetralogy of Fallot, omphalocele and, 148
Thalassemia, biochemistry of, 331
  clinical types of, 331
  hemoglobin abnormality of, 324
  treatment for, 331–332
THC. See *Delta⁹-3,4-trans-tetrahydrocannabinol.*
Thermal injury, malnutrition state in, 454–455
  pharmacokinetics of drugs in, 455
Thiopental, acid-base effect of, 431
  circulatory effects of, 464
  in diabetes mellitus, 212
  in renal disease, 469
Thoracic dystrophy, in dwarfism, 579
Thrombasthenia, 361
Thrombocytopenia, in cirrhotic liver disease, 439
  in hemolytic reactions, 367
  laboratory characteristics of, 354(t)
Thrombocytopenic purpura, 349–351, 350(t)
  clinical development of, 349
Thrombocytosis, 361
Thrombopathia, 361
Thrombophoresis, in megakaryocytic myelosis, 345
Thromboplastin generation test, in hemophilia, 353
Thymectomy, in myasthenia gravis, 551
Thyroglobulin, serum levels of, in papillary cancer,
    169–170
Thyroid binding globulin, 167
Thyroid function test(s), 167–170
  corrected T4, 168
  radioactive iodine uptake, 168–169
  serum T4 by radioimmunoassay, 167–168
  serum thyroid stimulating hormone, 168
  serum triiodothyronine, 168
  thyroid scan, 169
Thyroid gland, disease(s) of, 167–179
    general surgical problems in, 175
  in geriatric patients, 111
  nodular, 174–175
  hormones of, 167
  pathophysiology of, 167
  tests of, resin triiodothyronine uptake, 168
Thyroid stimulating immunoglobulin (TSI), in
    Graves' disease, 170
Thyroid storm, in occult hyperthyroidism, 172
  postoperative, in hyperthyroidism, 177–178
Thyroidectomy, hypothyroidism after, 172
  subtotal, for hyperthyroidism, 175
Thyroiditis, subacute, vs. Hashimoto's thyroiditis, 173
Thyrotoxic crisis, postoperative, in hyperthyroidism,
    177–178
Thyrotoxic periodic paralysis, 555
Thyrotoxicosis, in pregnancy, management of,
    170–171
Thyrotropin releasing factor, test for, 169
Thyrotropin stimulating hormone (TSH), 167
L-thyroxine, for hypothyroidism, 173, 175
  for myxedema coma, 173–174
TMA. See *3,4,5-Trimethoxyamphetamine.*
Torsion dystonia, 488
Torticollis, 487–488
  surgery for, 487–488
Total parenteral hyperalimentation, in infections, 589
Total parenteral nutrition (TPN), 395–397
Toxemia of pregnancy, 87–90
Toxic epidermal necrolysis, 567–568
  associated diseases of, 567

Toxic megacolon, ulcerative colitis and, 415
TPN. See *Total parenteral nutrition.*
TR3U test, for thyroid gland function, 168
Tracheal esophageal fistula (TEF), in infants,
    133–136
  anatomic variants of, 133–134
  anesthetic management of, 135–136
    monitoring in, 135
    postoperative, 136
    premedication in, 135
    preoperative history in, 135
  diagnosis of, 134
  surgical management of, 134–135
    respiratory obstruction after, 135
  symptoms of, 134
Transaminase deficiency, 37(t)
Transcutaneous O_2 and CO_2 determinations, in
    newborns, 127
Transfer RNA, 1
Transferase deficiency galactosemia, 2, 15
Transfusion, blood, calcium in, 368
    citrate administration effects in, 367–368
    detritus in, 369
    hyperkalemia in, 368
    of 2,3-diphosphoglycerate depleted blood, 368
    pulmonary emboli in, 369
    temperature in, 369
Transfusion reactions, 364–372, 368(t), 371(t)
  allergic, 365
  diagnosis of, 364
  febrile, 365
  hemolytic, 366–367
    simulated, 367
  pyrogen, 365–366
Transsphenoidal hypophysectomy, diabetes mellitus
    and, 207
  for hypercortisolism, 192
Transverse myelitis, in narcotics addicts, 677
Trauma, acute, 635–671, 636, 637
  basic care of, 635–637, 636
  aortic, 658–660
    head and, 660
  basal skull, 647
  cardiac, blunt, 655–658
    penetrating, 658
  chest, 655–660
  diaphragm, 660–661
  head, 644–647
    airway control in, 644
    and accompanying trauma, 644–646
    anesthetic agent and technique in, 645
    hypertension following, 646–647
    intracranial pressure monitoring in, 645–646, 647
    positioning in, 645
    pulmonary edema after, 646
    ventilation in, 644–645
  intrathoracic airway, 654–655
  larynx, 654
  major airways, 654–655
  maxillofacial, 652–654
    airway problems in, 652–653
    eye injuries in, 653–654
    intraoperative problems in, 653
    intubation techniques for, 652–653
  spinal cord, 494–495, 647–652
    chronic injuries in, 650–652
      autonomic dysreflexia in, 650–651
      complications in, 652

Trauma (*Continued*)
  spinal cord, chronic injuries in, mass motor
        reflexes in, 651–652
      succinylcholine and, 652
    high acute injuries in, 648–650
      airway control for, 648–649
      autonomic dysfunction in, 649
      intubation for, 648–649
      motor dysfunction in, 649–650
      pulmonary edema in, 649
    low acute injuries in, 648
Treacher Collins syndrome, 581
Tricuspid insufficiency, 306, 308, 307(t)
  anesthesia and monitoring in, 308–309
Tricuspid stenosis, 304, 306, 305(t)
  anesthesia and monitoring in, 308–309
  diseases causing, 305(t)
Tricyclic antidepressants, intoxication with, 733–734
Triglycerides, 54, 55
Triiodothyronine (T3), 167, *168, 169*
  for hypothyroidism, 175
  for myxedema coma, 174
3,4,5-Trimethoxyamphetamine, ingestion of,
    anesthesia with, 724, *724*
Trisomy 21, 70–71
Trumpet lily. See *Datura arborea.*
Trypanosomiasis, cardiomyopathy from, 275
TSH. See *Thyrotropin stimulating hormone.*
TSH level test, for thyroid function, 168
Tubal pregnancy, 92
Tuberculosis, anesthetic equipment for, 265
  in coal worker's pneumoconiosis, 250
  isolation precautions for, 264–265
  of large intestine, 416
  of stomach, 407
Tuberous sclerosis, 502, 504
Tumor(s), carcinoid, anesthetic considerations in,
        437–438
    preoperative management in, 438
  intramural, of stomach, 407–408
  parathyroid, in geriatric patients, 111
Type 1 glycogen storage disease, anesthesia for
    patient with, 19
Type 1 hyperlipoproteinemia, 58–60
Type 2 glycogen storage disease, 19
  anesthesia for infants with, 20
Type 2 hyperlipoproteinemia, 60–62
Type 3 glycogen storage disease, anesthesia for
    patients with, 20
Type 4 glycogen storage disease, anesthesia for
    infants with, 21
Type 5 glycogen storage disease, anesthesia in, 22
Tyrosine, conversion of phenylalanine to, 35, *36*
  synthesis of, 31
Tyrosinemia, 37(t)

Ulcer(s), anesthetic considerations with, 436
  decubitus, in paraplegic syndrome, 495
  stress, 406–407
Ulceration, gastric and duodenal, other diseases and,
    406–407
Ulcerative colitis, 414–415
  carcinoma with, 415
  clinical features of, 414
  complications of, 414
  surgical intervention for, 414

Ulcerative colitis (*Continued*)
  toxic megacolon and, 425
  treatment of, 414
University Group Diabetes Project, 205
Uric acid, 45
  biosynthesis of, 45, *46*
  hyperexcretion of, 47–48
Urinalysis, for renal function diagnosis, 465, 467
Urinary osmolality, in renal function, 465, 467
Urine, heme precursor and/or converted porphyrin
    in, 27(t)
Urine VMA, test of, for pheochromocytoma, 199
Uteroplacental perfusion, effect of aortocaval
        compression on, 85
  hypotension and 84
  in incompetent cervix patient, 94
Uveoparotid fever, 525–527, *526, 527*

Vagotomy, intraoperative testing with, 408–409
Valvular lesions, 296–309, 298–299(t), 302–303(t),
    305(t), 307(t)
  anesthesia and monitoring in, 308–309
  rheumatic, 296
Variegate porphyria, pathology of, 28
Vascular disease, pulmonary, 227–232
Vascular ectasias, 418
Vascular reactivity, in preeclampsia, 89
Vasculitis, allergic, in hereditary hemorrhagic
    telangiectasia, 352
Vasopressors, in renal disease, 470
  in treatment of maternal hypotension, 85–86
VATER association, 133
VDRL, false positive, in narcotics addicts, 677
Vena caval interruption, for pulmonary embolism,
    229
Vena caval occlusion, in pregnant patients, 85
Venous return, in septic shock, 602–603, 603(t)
Venous thrombosis, 227, 228
  diagnosis of, 228
Vitamin B, deficiency of, in blind loop syndrome, 393
  in gastrectomy, 392
  in ileum resection, 393
Vitamin B$_1$, deficiency of, 459
Vitamin B$_6$, deficiency of, 459
Vitamin B$_{12}$ deficiency of, 314–315, 459
  nitrous oxide interaction with, 314–315
Vitamin C, deficiency of, 460
Vitamin D, deficiency of, 460
  in calcium metabolism, 156
  in hypercortisolism, 193
  intoxication by, 157
    in hypoparathyroidism therapy, 161
  therapy with, after parathyroidectomy, 160–161
    for steroid-induced osteomalacia, 165
Vitamin deficiencies, 459–460
Vitamin K$_1$, preoperative, in newborn, 126
Volvulus, cecal, 418
  gastric, 408
  of large intestine, 417–418
    symptoms of, 418
    treatment of, 418
Vomiting, 385–386
  acid-base changes in, 430–431
  anesthetic precautions against, 427–428
  antihistamines for, 428
  causes of, in gastrointestinal disorders, 428–429

Vomiting (*Continued*)
   etiologies of, 385
   fluid therapy for, 385–386
   in gastrointestinal disorders, 427–431
   mechanism of, 427
   pharmacologic pretreatment of, 428
   physiologic alterations in, 385
   prolonged, in gastrointestinal disorders, 430
von Gierke's disease, 18, 537–539
von Hippel-Lindau disease, 502, 503
   pheochromocytoma in, 198
von Recklinghausen's disease, 502, 503, 571–572
von Willebrand's disease, 355, 360–361
   laboratory characteristics of, 354(t)

Waldenström's macroglobulinemia, 345–346
Weber-Christian disease, 72–73
   anesthesia for, 72
Wegener's granulomatosis, 236–238, 524
   anesthetic considerations in, 237–238
   anesthetic management of, 524–525
   biopsy in, 237
   cardiovascular disease in, 237, 238
   clinical features of, 237
   laboratory findings in, 237
   renal disease in, 237, 238
   treatment of, 237

Werdnig-Hoffmann disease, 489, 491
   anesthetic considerations in, 493
Werner-Morrison syndrome, 406
White cell diseases, 339–347
Wilson's disease, 40–45, 439
   anemia of, 44
   anesthesia in, 43–45
   clinical diagnosis of, 42
   clinical manifestations of, 41
   cornea in, 42
   organs affected by, 42
   pathology of, 41
   treatment of, 43
Wilson-Mikity syndrome, 137, 138
   anesthetic management for, 140

Xanthoma, in familial type 3 hyperlipoproteinemia, 62
Xanthomatosis, primary, in coronary artery disease, 282(t)

Zollinger-Ellison syndrome, 406
   clinical features of, 406
   gastrectomy for, 406
   hypokalemia in, 406